Textbook of Neurointensive Care: Volume 1

Elizabeth Mahanna Gabrielli
Kristine H. O'Phelan
Monisha A. Kumar • Joshua Levine
Peter Le Roux • Andrea Gabrielli
A. Joseph Layon
Editors

Textbook of Neurointensive Care: Volume 1

Neuroanatomy, Diagnostic Assessment, Disease Management

Third Edition

Springer

Editors

Elizabeth Mahanna Gabrielli
University of Miami Health System
Miami, FL, USA

Monisha A. Kumar
Hospital of the University of Pennsylvania
Philadelphia, PA, USA

Peter Le Roux
Bassett Healthcare Network
Cooperstown, NY, USA

A. Joseph Layon
College of Medicine
University of Central Florida
Orlando, FL, USA

Kristine H. O'Phelan
Miller School of Medicine
University of Miami
Miami, FL, USA

Joshua Levine
Hospital of the University of Pennsylvania
Philadelphia, PA, USA

Andrea Gabrielli
Miller School of Medicine
University of Miami
Miami, FL, USA

ISBN 978-3-031-62222-9 ISBN 978-3-031-62220-5 (eBook)
https://doi.org/10.1007/978-3-031-62220-5

Layon, A Joseph, Gabrielli, Andrea, Friedman, William A. (Eds), Textbook of Neurointensive Care 2e, ISBN 978-1-4471-5225-5, 2014, $189.00, 988 pp, Hardcover, Total Sales 411, Total Usage 197,293.

This Springer imprint is published by the registered company Springer Nature Switzerland AG
The registered company address is: Gewerbestrasse 11, 6330 Cham, Switzerland

To the memory of my sister, who was always my biggest fan and supporter. To my parents for giving me the foundation to dream big.

To my husband and my children for helping me grow in ways I didn't know were possible and continuously showing me the fun side of life.

To my patients and their families from whom I continuously learn and for whom I strive to be better.

Elizabeth Mahanna Gabrielli, MD

To the memory of my Chairman, Ralph Sacco, for his unwavering support, patience, and mentorship.

Kristy O'Phalen, MD

To my parents, Prasanna and Savitri, who never doubted my successes even when I did.

To my husband, Josh, my bashert, who inspires me to be the best person I can be.

To my children, Lake and Phoenix, my moon and stars: you have the power to change the world with your thoughts and actions. Dream big!

Monisha Kumar, MD

To my family, teachers, students, colleagues, and patients. You have taught me, shaped me, and inspired me. For that, I am eternally grateful.

Joshua Mark Levine

To the ICU staff who take care of all our patients

Peter Le Roux, MD

To my wife Elizabeth and my children Rachelle, Vera, and Marcus, for bringing me endless joy and energy.

To the memory of my parents, Pietro and Giuliana. They would have been proud to see the results of this effort.

To my brother Marco, living the best lifestyle I know.

To our patients: our inspiration for learning and providing compassionate care.

Andrea Gabrielli, MD

To my family, teachers, students, colleagues, and patients. You have taught me, shaped me, and inspired me. For that, I am eternally grateful.

For my wife and comrade of 43 years, Susana

For my children Maria, Nicolas, and Daniel, of whom I am so proud and love

For my grandchildren Marianna, Sloane, and Harlow, each brilliant in her own right

For those who struggle for justice, even at the cost to themselves

For my comrades-in-arms, always

This book is dedicated.

AJ Layon, MD

Foreword

Something over two decades ago, Andrea Gabrielli, William Friedman, and I thought it would be a challenge, as well as a service to our colleagues, to write a textbook on neurocritical care medicine. So, with some trepidation, we did. In 2004, the first edition was released by Saunders. We worked on a second edition in 2014 and we are now releasing our third edition, in early 2024, both published by Springer.

We have attempted to hone our work so that it will be of maximal use to clinicians and clinicians in training, a task—we hope—that has been accomplished.

Yet 20 years on, more than the science has changed. As my colleague and comrade-in-arms, Stanley Cohen (@StanleyCohenLaw), has commented, our generation is now beginning to pass into the twilight. It is time for our younger colleagues—our students and former fellows, our junior faculty partners—to pick up the banner that we, now, are no longer able to carry forward. This is as true in the realm of neurocritical care as it is in other arenas.

Thus, this will be the last edition with which Doctor Andrea Gabrielli and I are involved. Going forward, this textbook will be written and edited by the superb team of Elizabeth Mahanna Gabrielli, MD (exm1044@med.miami.edu), Kristine H. O'Phelan, MD (KOPhelan@med.miami.edu), Monisha Kumar, MD (monisha.kumar@pennmedicine.upenn.edu), Joshua Levine, MD (jolevine@pennmedicine.upenn.edu), and Peter D. Leroux, MD (lerouxpeterd@gmail.com). We wish them well.

In some manner, Doctor Gabrielli and I have had a good run. We cared for very sick fellow humans, taught students, carried out investigations, published papers, and enjoyed friends, food, and wine. We did battle with some administrative colleagues who seemed to place quality and safety of care, as well as patient satisfaction, in secondary positions of importance. These were not, and are not, enemies, merely colleagues with a different view of things. Overall, at times we prevailed, and at others we did not, but it was always our hope that our efforts made our world—within medicine and without—slightly better.

Our hope, indeed.

Yet in some ways, our failures are evident to all who have eyes to see. In our United States, some 50 million of us are uninsured or underinsured; indeed, why do we continue to talk about insurance as if it were a good? Something between 500,000 and 600,000 of us declare bankruptcy yearly primarily due to medical expenses. This is, of course, unheard of in the wealthy world except in our country. And, how many of us die because we cannot access medical care in a timely manner?

Again, this is the last time I will edit this textbook. If my words upset, well, take them as the not-so-random thoughts of a man who has spent a lifetime actively in the arena of medical politics and politics in general.

So, my colleagues, take up the banner of neurocritical care, advance our knowledge and ability to care for our fellow humans. Do not lose sight, I ask of you, of the imperative statement: Healthcare is a right, not a privilege.

And be willing to do battle for that which you deeply believe. For one day you, too, will be writing the last preface of your career and, looking over the landscape, will ask yourself, over and over, $10 \times 10 \times 10$ times: As I prepare to leave, have I made our world just a bit better? Have I kept faith with all who preceded me?

An answer to that query is needed.

Gainesville, FL, USA
31 August 2023

A. Joseph Layon

Preface

Something over two decades ago, Andrea Gabrielli, William Friedman, and I thought it would be a challenge, as well as a service to our colleagues, to write a textbook on neurocritical care medicine. So, with some trepidation, we did. In 2004, the first edition was released by Saunders. We worked on a second edition in 2014 and we are now releasing our third edition, in mid-to-late 2024, both published by Springer.

This extensively updated edition provides a comprehensive review of intensive care for neurologically injured patients from the emergency room through the operating room and post-surgical period, including the ICU. It consists of two comprehensive volumes.

The first volume presents a comprehensive view that incorporates best practice/evidence-based medicine and performance improvement while championing the three characteristics needed in our neuro-ICUs: patient and family centered high-quality care, education, and discovery.

Volume 1 concentrates on neuroanatomy, diagnostic assessment, and disease management, examining the neurological problems most frequently seen in intensive care, and describes the various types of neurosurgical interventions and critical features in the management of such patients. General issues are discussed across the textbook, such as cardiac care, fluids and electrolytes, nutrition, and monitoring as well as more specific conditions and complications including elevated intracranial pressure, seizures, and altered mental states.

"Listening" to an injured brain is not easy. It requires knowledge, dedication, and an understanding of the critically ill patient and their family.

Textbook of Neurointensive Care Volume 1: Neuroanatomy, Diagnostic Assessment, Disease Management provides the reader with a detailed resource for studying this most complex area of medicine. We think it will be helpful—indeed, essential—reading for all trainees and professionals in critical care, neurosurgery, anesthesiology, and neurology.

All of the editors trust you will find this textbook useful and enjoyable.

Gainesville, FL, USA — A. Joseph Layon
28 April 2024

Contents

Part I

Neuroanatomy, Physiology and Neurological Examination

The Functional Organization of the Nervous System

1

William A. Friedman, Or Cohen-Inbar, Jackson Narett, William Lombardi, Jessica Johns, and Jose Javier Provencio

Contents

W. A. Friedman (✉)
Department of Neurological Surgery, University of Florida College of Medicine, Gainesville, FL, USA
e-mail: friedman@neurosurgery.ufl.edu

O. Cohen-Inbar
Department of Neurological Surgery, University of Pittsburg Medical Center and School of Medicine, Cumberland, MD, USA

J. Narett
School of Medicine, University of Virginia, Charlottesville, VA, USA
e-mail: jan3dw@virginia.edu

W. Lombardi · J. Johns
Department of Neurology, University of Virginia, Charlottesville, VA, USA
e-mail: wl5r@virginia.edu; jmj7uu@virginia.edu

J. J. Provencio
Department of Neurology, University of Virginia School of Medicine, Charlottesville, VA, USA
e-mail: jp3b@virginia.edu

Abstract

The nervous system is organized in such a way that a careful history and physical examination will almost always allow the clinician to localize the site of disease. This requires basic knowledge of the neurological exam and the anatomy that underlies that exam. In this chapter, we will review the examination of mental status, cranial nerves, and motor, reflex, and sensory systems. We will then illustrate the application of those exams in multiple example cases.

E. Mahanna Gabrielli et al. (eds.), *Textbook of Neurointensive Care: Volume 1*, https://doi.org/10.1007/978-3-031-62220-5_1

Introduction

> If the nervous communication be cut off between the brain and other parts, the experiences of those other parts are non-existent for the mind. The eye is blind, the ear deaf, the hand insensible and motionless. And conversely, if the brain be injured, consciousness is abolished or altered, even although every other organ in the body be ready to play its normal part.
> —William James, 1890[1]

This quote illustrates the centrality of the nervous system to our ability to interact with and experience the world. Central and peripheral nervous system diseases are different from most other medical problems in one fascinating and important way: The precise site of the neurological disorder can almost always be determined from a careful history and neurological examination. Once the site of disease is elucidated, a differential diagnosis, drawing from the basic categories of neurological illness, can be constructed. Patient history is particularly valuable in ordering the differential diagnosis from the most to least probable. When this intellectual process is finished, appropriate diagnostic tests can be ordered and a precise diagnosis may be established.

Neurological Examination

A neurological examination is generally divided into the following parts: mental status, cranial nerves, motor examination (including cerebellar function), reflexes, and sensory examination. As in other parts of the physical exam, adhering to a strict order helps the physician avoid errors of omission.

Mental Status

Examination of the mental status focuses on the level of consciousness, orientation, memory, emotional state, and higher cortical functions (including language). Orientation to the person, place, and time is typically tested. Patients are frequently described as "oriented times three." Typically, recent memory is tested by asking the patient to remember three objects and then testing them 2 and 5 min later for recall. Long-term memory may be tested by asking for their address, phone number, the names of presidents, capitals, etc.

Consciousness is a hallmark property of animals from fish to humans. It can be defined as a state of wakeful awareness but is much harder to categorize based on a particular set of qualities. To be conscious, one must have arousal and content; that is to say, a conscious person is both awake (or wake-able) and is able to organize external or internal sensory information. In patients with brain injury, good neurological outcomes are often defined by the recovery of consciousness. Disorders of consciousness (DoC) are an important aspect of many injuries in the neurointensive care unit.

The anatomical features of consciousness can be separated into wakefulness (arousal) and awareness (content of consciousness). The reticular activating system (RAS, also called the ascending arousal pathway) of the brain stem is a diffuse integrated system that rhythmically signals the subcortical and cortical structures of the brain to maintain attentiveness. Disorders of the RAS lead to DoC (specifically wakefulness), the depth of which tracks the amount of input by the RAS and its proximity to deep brain structures that are impaired. Scattered cortical and/or subcortical damage can also lead to impaired wakefulness and awareness, but this is less well understood.

Recent data have suggested a network for cortical processing, termed the "default mode network (DMN)" or the "medial frontoparietal network (M-FPN)," which is impaired in patients in coma who later do not recover consciousness but is preserved in patients who do [1]. Although still debated, the network that is composed of the areas of the medial temporal lobe, including the hippocampus, dorsomedial prefrontal cortex, angular gyrus, and posterior cingulate cortex, appear to be the most likely network in which damage is associated with impaired awareness.

The content of consciousness is more widely distributed in the cortical and subcortical structures of the brain. Impairment of consciousness solely based on lack of content requires large-scale damage to multiple cortical and subcortical areas. What is more common is a "fractional" loss of the content of consciousness due to the focal damage to brain structures, such as the hippocampus, leading to loss of short-term memory, which, in turn, limits the content of consciousness.

Altered states of consciousness are described by a variety of terms, including, in order of severity, "clouded," "lethargic," "obtunded," "stuporous," and "comatose." A "clouded" patient refers to an individual with a mildly depressed level of awareness and slowing of mentation. A "lethargic" patient will lie quietly or sleep in the absence of stimulation but can interact fairly well when prompted. An "obtunded" patient will sleep in the absence of stimulation, can be aroused with some difficulty, and has generally depressed intellectual function. A "stuporous" patient requires vigorous stimulation to provoke any arousal and is incapable of meaningful verbal exchange. A "comatose" patient fits the following precise definition: "incapable of following commands, does not speak, and does not open eyes to pain." Dementia, unlike the

[1] James, William. *The Principles of Psychology* (Vol. 1) 1890. Henry Holt and Co. New York City

previous descriptors, refers only to a loss of intellectual function and does not imply any alteration of consciousness.

Unfortunately, the terms described previously are rather imprecise. To eliminate interobserver variability in describing decreased levels of consciousness, the Glasgow Coma Scale (GCS) was developed. It relies upon three simple tests: best eye opening response, best verbal response, and best motor response (Fig. 1.1). The worst score is 3, and the best score is 15. The earlier cited definition of coma corresponds to a GCS score of ≤8.

The differential diagnosis of coma is broad. It includes toxic/metabolic disorders like electrolyte imbalance, endocrine dysfunction, toxin ingestion, infection, nutritional deficiency, organ failure, and epilepsy. A wide variety of structural disorders can also cause coma, including hemorrhage, ischemic stroke, brain abscess, brain tumor, and trauma. When this impairment is long-lasting or permanent, it is called prolonged disorders of consciousness (PDoC), a spectrum of disorders best characterized in patients with traumatic brain injury. From the most to least severe, PDoC include coma, a persistent vegetative state, minimally conscious states, and neurological impairments that affect consciousness. It is common for patients to progress from one state to another after brain injury. Coma can be defined as the inability to interact with the environment both internally and externally. It is usually a transient condition where severely brain-damaged individuals show no ability to communicate and have limited ability to regulate their bodily functions. Patients in a persistent vegetative state show no ability to communicate but can regain control of their bodily functions such as breathing and sleeping. Patients in minimally conscious states show many of the same findings as do those in persistent vegetative states, except that the former patients have transient, non-sustained episodes of attentiveness. Finally, the catchall phrase of neurological impairment that affects consciousness describes other neurological impairments that affect awareness or content to a lesser degree than a minimally conscious state.

Eye opening

- Spontaneous ⇒ 4
- To speech ⇒ 3
- To pain ⇒ 2
- None ⇒ 1

Best verbal response

- Oriented ⇒ 5
- Confused speech ⇒ 4
- Inappropriate ⇒ 3
- Incomprehensible ⇒ 2
- None ⇒ 1

Best motor response

- Obeys commands ⇒ 6
- Localizes pain ⇒ 5
- Withdraws ⇒ 4
- Abnormal flexion ⇒ 3
- Extension ⇒ 2
- None ⇒ 1

Fig. 1.1 The Glasgow Coma Scale (modified with permission of Elsevier from Teasdale and Jennett [2])

The Pupil

Close attention to pupil size and reactivity can provide valuable information to many diagnoses of concern. Conversely, it is equally important to be able to recognize common pupil abnormalities that do not warrant further investigation. Pupillary size is determined by the net outcome balancing parasympathetic innervation of the strong pupillary sphincter (via the oculomotor nerve (the third cranial nerve; CN-III) and sympathetic innervation of the much weaker pupillary dilator muscle, together with local iris-related factors that affect the "stiffness" of the iris stroma.

Anisocoria (uneven pupils) is never caused by visual loss. Pupillary size equality is not affected even if one eye is normal and the other is blind. Anisocoria is an efferent problem arising from abnormalities in ocular sympathetic or parasympathetic innervation/tone. *Ptosis* of the upper eyelid is an important accompanying clinical sign. The oculomotor nerve CN-III and the sympathetic nervous system (SNS) are involved in lid position balance as well. CN-III innervates the powerful levator muscle, and SNS contributes a few millimeters of lid lift through the Müller muscle [3].

The first and most important step in examining the pupils of a patient with anisocoria is to determine whether the larger or the smaller pupil is abnormal. In a patient with parasympathetic system problem on one side, that pupil will be larger. In this setting, the difference in pupillary size is most apparent under bright light because that pupil does not constrict well. In a patient with a sympathetic nervous system outflow deficiency, the difference in pupillary size is greatest in the dark, implicating the smaller pupil.

When the larger pupil is abnormal, the most important concerns are oculomotor CN-III palsy, Adie's pupil, or pharmacologic mydriasis. CN-III palsy will typically manifest with more than isolated pupillary dilation. One should look for disturbances in oculomotor functions as well. The Adie "tonic" pupil manifests as unilateral mydriasis with the pupillary response to near focus being far better than the response to light. Also termed "light-near dissociation," this is seen in "blind" eyes and bilaterally in patients with neurosyphilis or dorsal midbrain syndrome.

When the smaller pupil is abnormal, an oculosympathetic cause (aka Horner's syndrome) must be considered. Relative miosis and a slight ptosis (1–2 mm) may result from interruption of the SNS pathway anywhere along the path from the hypothalamus to the ciliospinal center of Budge–Waller (C8–T1), across the lung apex to the superior cervical ganglion, or from the superior cervical ganglion by means of the carotid plexus SNS nerves to the pupillary dilator. Postganglionic interruption (at or distal to the superior cervical ganglion) is most commonly benign or idiopathic, whereas preganglionic (central) oculosympathetic paresis is associated with malignancy in about 50% of cases [3–7].

The Cranial Nerves (Fig. 1.2)

The Olfactory Nerve

The olfactory nerve mediates the sense of smell. This can be tested by asking the patient to identify vials containing common substances (coffee, orange extract, etc.) by smell alone while alternately occluding each nostril. The olfactory nerve is the most frequently injured by head trauma. It can also be affected by neoplasms growing near the olfactory groove area intracranially, including meningiomas and esthesioneuroblastomas.

The Optic Nerve

The optic nerve connects the retina to the optic chiasm and, hence, to the posterior visual pathways (Fig. 1.3). Unlike other cranial nerves, it can be directly viewed via fundoscopic examination. Increased intracranial pressure (ICP) will often be manifested as papilledema of the optic nerve head. Long-standing pressure or inflammation of the optic nerve will cause fundoscopically visible optic pallor (optic atrophy). The most valuable localizing test of visual pathway function involves "visual fields." Visual fields are tested in the clinic by having the patient occlude one eye. The examiner then directs the patient to look straight ahead and tests

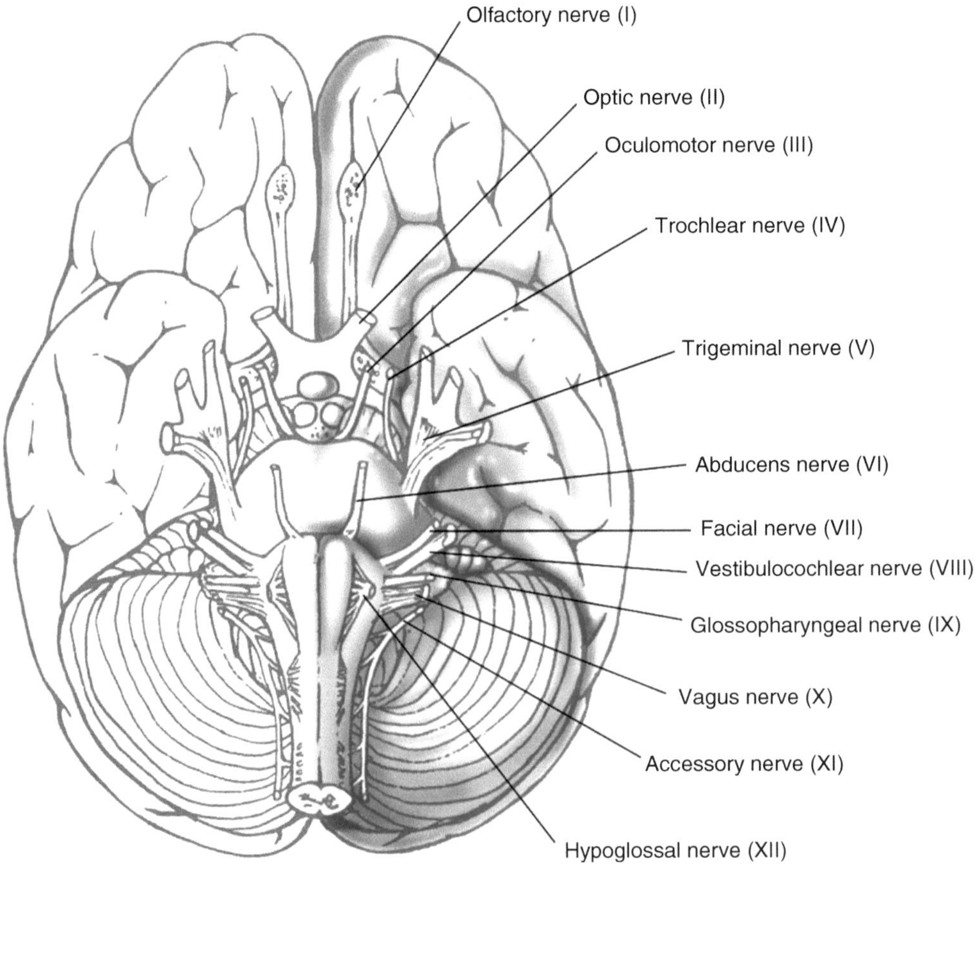

Fig. 1.2 An anterior inferior view of the brain shows the 12 paired cranial nerves (with permission from David Peace, illustrator. Reproduced with permission from Friedman et al. [8])

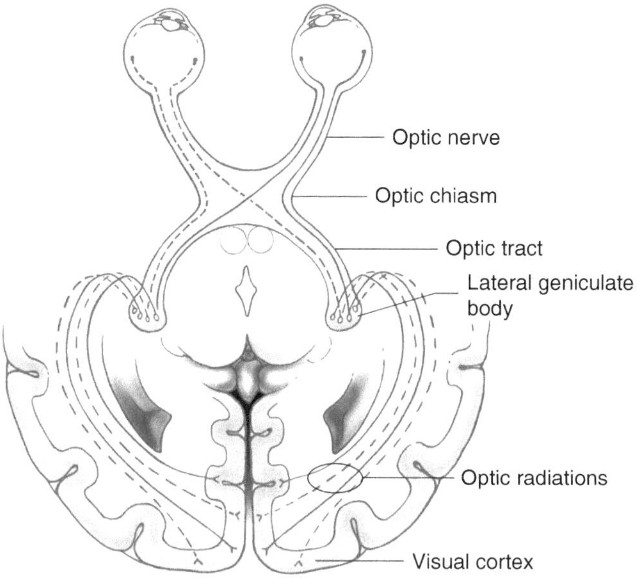

Fig. 1.3 The optic nerves meet at the optic chiasm. The optic tracts run from the chiasm to the lateral geniculate nuclei of the thalamus. The optic radiations run from these nuclei to the primary visual cortex in the occipital lobe. The nasal retinal fibers cross in the chiasm, so a lesion there tends to produce the characteristic "bitemporal visual field cut." Lesions of the tract, radiations, or the occipital lobe tend to cause complete loss of vision on the opposite side (a homonymous hemianopia) (with permission from David Peace, illustrator. Reproduced with permission from Friedman et al. [8])

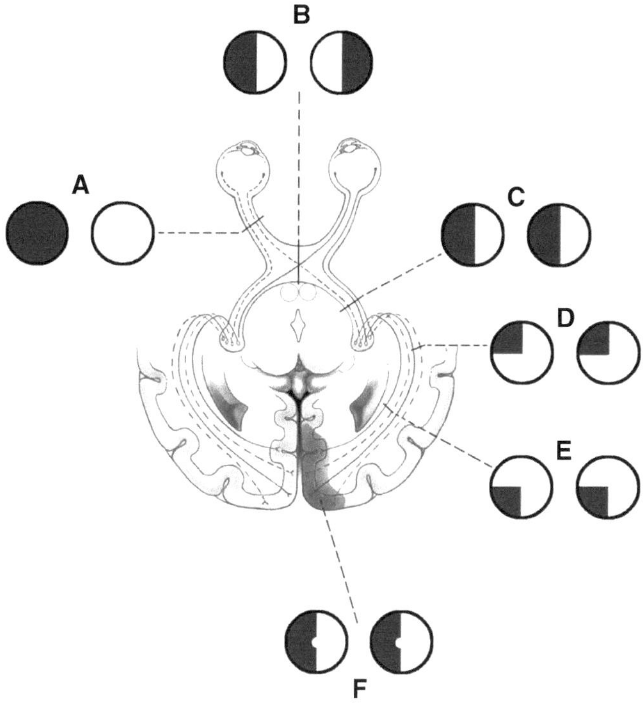

Fig. 1.4 Lesions in various parts of the visual pathways lead to highly characteristic and localizing visual field defects: (**a**) optic nerve, (**b**) optic chiasm, (**c**) optic tract, (**d**) temporal optic radiations, (**e**) parietal optic radiations, and (**f**) primary visual cortex (with permission from David Peace, illustrator. Reproduced with permission from Friedman et al. [8])

their ability to count fingers in the four quadrants of that eye's visual field. Formal visual fields can be performed by an ophthalmologist if this is abnormal. A variety of visual field abnormalities are described, which very accurately localize the site of the lesion within the nervous system (Fig. 1.4): unilateral visual loss, junctional scotoma, bitemporal hemianopia, and homonymous hemianopia.

The Oculomotor Nerve

The oculomotor nerve innervates the levator palpebrae, the medial rectus, the superior rectus, the inferior oblique, the inferior rectus, the pupilloconstrictor muscle, and the muscle that controls accommodation of the lens within the eye (Fig. 1.5). Lesions of the third nerve result in movement of the globe into a "down-and-out" position, ptosis, and pupillary dilatation. Temporal lobe herniation can cause a unilateral third nerve injury, with, usually, contralateral hemiplegia. Direct compression of the third nerve by an aneurysm or tumor can produce these findings, as can diabetes or stroke.

The Trochlear Nerve

The trochlear nerve innervates the superior oblique muscle (Fig. 1.6). Lesions of this nerve result in vertical diplopia, with the affected eye elevated and externally rotated. The patient will attempt to correct this condition by tilting their head away from the affected side (to internally rotate the eye). The trochlear nerve is rarely affected in isolation but is frequently affected in combination with the III and VI nerves by lesions of the cavernous sinus area.

The Trigeminal Nerve

The trigeminal nerve provides sensation to the face (Fig. 1.7). It has three divisions: the ophthalmic division innervates the forehead and eye; the maxillary division innervates the upper jaw and side of the nose; and the mandibular division innervates the lower jaw, teeth, and tongue. The trigeminal nerve also innervates the muscles of mastication. Injuries to this nerve will result in ipsilateral loss of facial sensation and atrophy and weakness of the masseter muscle. This most frequently results from tumors (acoustic schwannoma, trigeminal schwannoma, nasopharyngeal carcinoma, etc.). The trigeminal nerve is also involved in a severe, lancinating pain disorder, called trigeminal neuralgia, which is frequently treated with surgery.

The Abducens Nerve

The abducens nerve innervates the lateral rectus muscle, which moves the globe laterally (Fig. 1.8). Lesions of the nerve will cause inward deviation of the eye. Because of its long subarachnoid course, this nerve is commonly affected by increased intracranial pressure, which can cause a unilateral or bilateral sixth nerve palsy (a so-called false localizing sign).

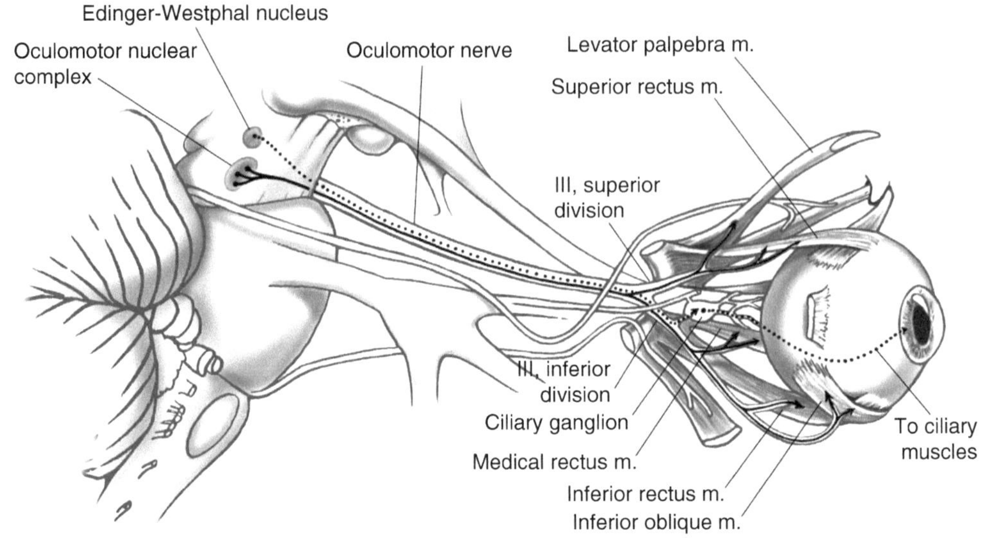

Fig. 1.5 The oculomotor nerve exits the brain stem between the mesencephalon and pons and travels to the cavernous sinus and on to the orbit. The motor nucleus innervates multiple extraocular muscles. The Edinger–Westphal nucleus provides parasympathetic innervation to the pupil and the lens of the eye (with permission from David Peace, illustrator. Reproduced with permission from Friedman et al. [8])

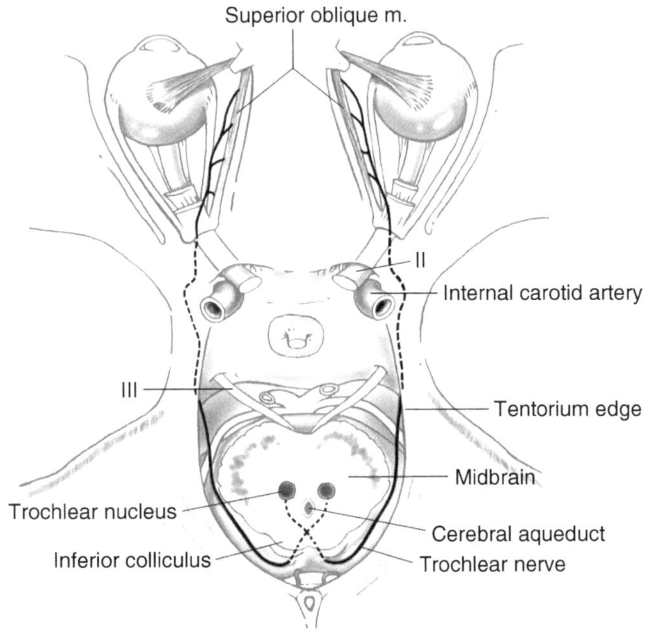

Fig. 1.6 The fourth cranial nerve is the only one that decussates (crosses the midline). It exits just below the collicular plate and travels along the tentorium to the cavernous sinus. It enters the orbit and innervates one extraocular muscle—the superior oblique (with permission from David Peace, illustrator. Reproduced with permission from Friedman et al. [8])

The Facial Nerve

The facial nerve innervates the muscles of facial expression (Fig. 1.9). It is also responsible for salivary gland activity, lacrimation, and taste over the anterior two-thirds of the tongue. Peripheral lesions of the nerve (such as trauma or Bell's palsy) cause weakness of the upper and lower face. Lesions of the upper motor neuron pathways from the motor cortex innervating the facial nerve nucleus in the brain stem cause weakness of only the contralateral lower face. The upper face receives bilateral cortical innervation and remains normal. This type of facial paralysis is called a "central seventh."

The Vestibulocochlear Nerve

The vestibulocochlear nerve innervates the cochlea (the organ of hearing) and the vestibular complex (the organ of balance). Lesions of this nerve are seen after basilar skull fractures and with tumors of the cerebellopontine angle (usually acoustic schwannomas). Hearing is usually tested at the bedside by determining whether a patient can hear fingers rubbing together outside the external ear canal (a high-frequency sound) and whether a patient can hear the pads of the thumb and a finger tapping together (a low-frequency sound). Formal audiometry is performed if these are abnormal.

The Glossopharyngeal Nerve

The glossopharyngeal nerve innervates the stylopharyngeus muscle, which is involved in swallowing (Fig. 1.10). This nerve supplies taste sensation to the posterior tongue. Lesions of the ninth nerve rarely occur in isolation, and sectioning of the nerve usually does not result in any significant deficit.

The Vagus Nerve

The vagus nerve innervates most of the muscles responsible for swallowing and supplies sensory input to the pharynx as well (Fig. 1.11). Lesions of the nerve result in asymmetry of palatal movement. The vagus also supplies parasympathetic input to the heart and gastrointestinal (GI) tract. The ninth, tenth, and eleventh nerves exit through the jugular foramen, where they can be jointly affected by tumors (especially jugular foramen schwannomas and meningiomas).

The Spinal Accessory Nerve

The spinal accessory nerve innervates the trapezius and sternocleidomastoid muscles (Fig. 1.12). These muscles are tested by shoulder shrug and head turning. Trauma is the

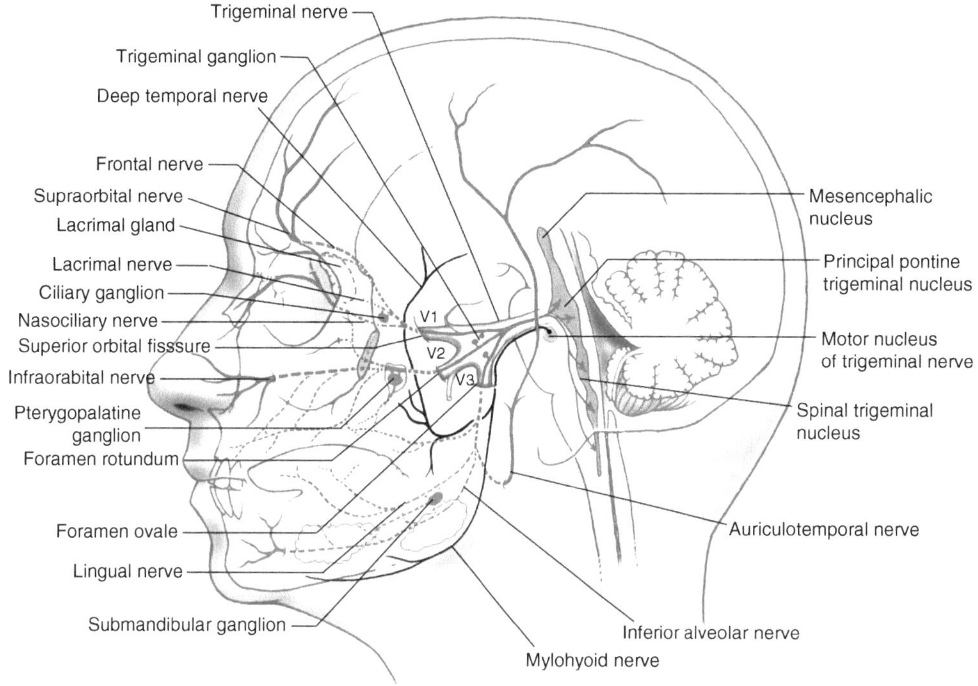

Fig. 1.7 The trigeminal nerve exits the brain stem at the pontine level. The trigeminal (Gasserian) ganglion is just lateral to the cavernous sinus. Three branches enter the cavernous sinus and innervate the face: the ophthalmic branch (V1), the maxillary branch (V2), and the mandibular branch (V3). The trigeminal nerve also mediates motor function (the muscles of mastication and the tensor tympani) (with permission from David Peace, illustrator. Reproduced with permission from Friedman et al. [8])

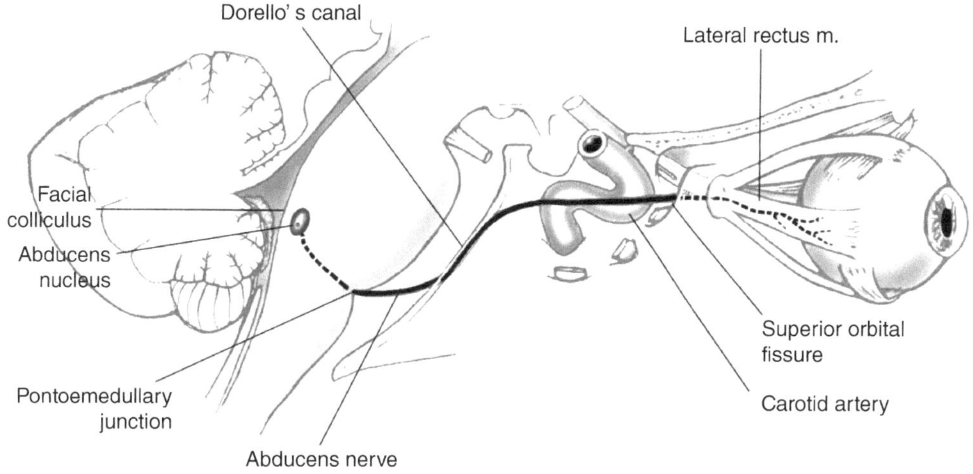

Fig. 1.8 The sixth nerve nucleus is on the floor of the fourth ventricle. The nerve exits the *midline* at the junction of the pons and medulla. It travels along the clivus and through the Dorello canal to reach the cavernous sinus. This nerve innervates one extraocular muscle—the lateral rectus (with permission from David Peace, illustrator. Reproduced with permission from Friedman et al. [8])

most frequent cause of an isolated XI nerve injury; not infrequently, injury occurs due to iatrogenic causes such as surgery in the posterior cervical triangle.

The Hypoglossal Nerve

The hypoglossal nerve innervates the muscles of the tongue. Dysfunction leads to protrusion of the tongue toward the affected side and atrophy of the affected side. This nerve may be affected by tumor, trauma, or stroke.

The Motor Function

The motor system consists of neural structures that create voluntary and some involuntary movements and involves the motor cortex of the brain, the corticospinal (and other descending) tracts, the motor pathways within the spinal cord, the motor neurons within the brain stem and spinal cord, the nerve roots, the peripheral nerves, the neuromuscular junction, and the muscles. In addition, normal motor function is heavily dependent on the complex circuitry within the basal ganglia and the cerebellum.

Disease at any of these sites will lead to alterations in the motor examination and, in many cases, will clearly localize to a specific part of the nervous system (Fig. 1.13).

Diseases of the motor cortex and descending motor pathways are called "upper motor neuron" disorders and are characterized by weakness of the opposite side of the body, lack of atrophy, spasticity, and increased reflexes (Fig. 1.14). Diseases of the motor neurons in the brain stem and spinal

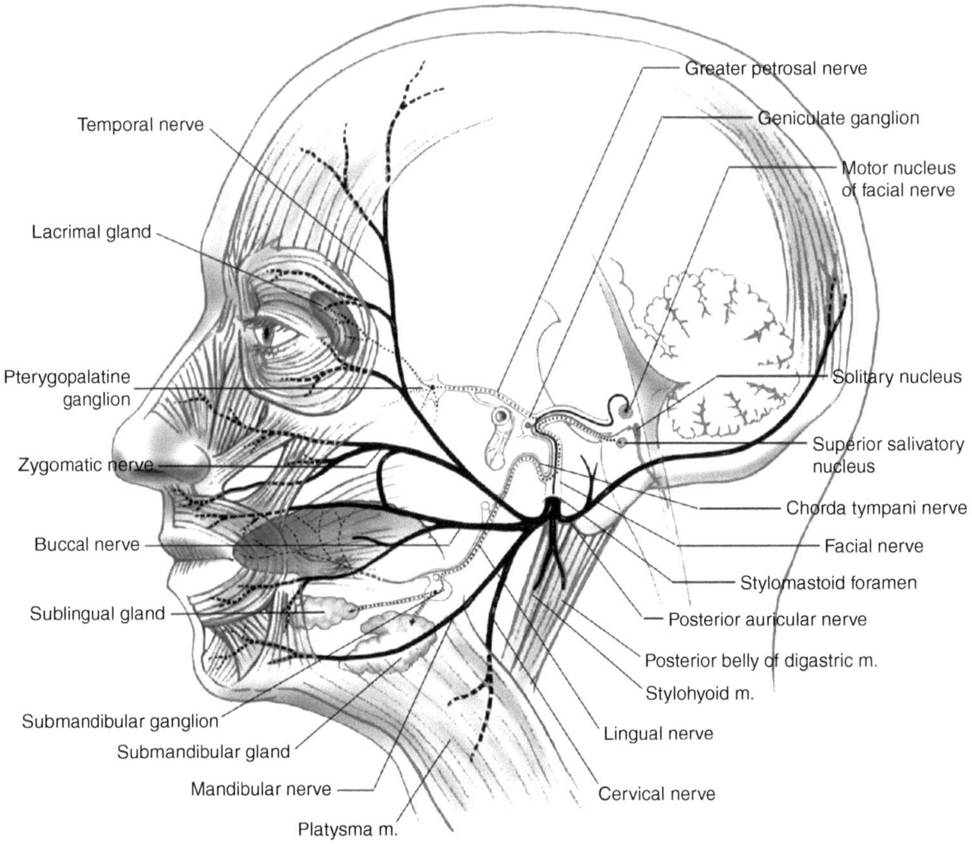

Fig. 1.9 The seventh nerve exits lateral to the sixth, in the pontomedullary groove. It innervates the muscles of facial expression through multiple branches after exiting the stylomastoid foramen. This nerve also provides parasympathetic innervation to the geniculate and sphenopalatine ganglia and, hence, to the lacrimal and salivary glands. The chorda tympani branch provides taste sensation to the anterior two-thirds of the tongue (with permission from David Peace, illustrator. Reproduced with permission from Friedman et al. [8])

cord, as well as the peripheral and cranial nerves, are called "lower motor neuron" disorders (Fig. 1.15). They are characterized by weakness, atrophy, decreased tone, and decreased reflexes. Diseases of the neuromuscular junction (such as myasthenia gravis) result in fluctuating weakness affecting cranial and limb muscles, normal tone and reflexes, and no atrophy. Table 1.1 compares upper and lower motor neuron injuries. Diseases affecting the muscle (like polymyositis) result in atrophy, weakness, and decreased reflexes and tone. Diseases affecting the basal ganglia and its related pathways (like Parkinson's disease) are called "extrapyramidal" disorders. They are frequently associated with normal strength, increased tone, unchanged reflexes, and tremor. Diseases of the cerebellar pathways can result in decreased tone and reflexes, normal strength, limb incoordination, and gait ataxia.

Examination of the motor systems should include evaluation for atrophy, changes in tone, strength, and coordination. Strength is usually tabulated on a 0–5 scale: 0 is total paralysis; 1 is a visible flicker of movement only; 2 is movement weaker than antigravity; 3 is full movement against gravity; 4 is full movement overcome by resistance; and 5 is normal strength.

Coordination is tested by having the patient touch their fingertip to their nose and by observing their gait. Lateral cerebellar lesions tend to affect extremity coordination. Vermian lesions tend to cause ataxic gait. In Parkinson's disease and other extrapyramidal disorders, gait tends to be stooped and shuffling. A hemiparesis will typically cause a spastic gait. Waddling gait is associated with muscular dystrophy affecting the hips. Table 1.2 reviews the motor landmarks for a neurological physical examination.

Reflexes

A reflex examination centers on determination of the deep tendon reflex responses at the elbows, knees, and ankles. This reflex arc requires integrity of the sensory neurons, motor neurons, and muscle. The rating is 0–4, with 0 signifying absence, 2+ being normal, and 4+ being very hyperactive. Hyperactive reflexes may be seen with upper motor neuron disease. Hypoactive reflexes may be seen with diseases of the peripheral nerve (i.e., polyneuritis), sensory root (i.e., tabes dorsalis), anterior horn cell (i.e., polio), proximal nerve root (i.e., lumbar disc herniation), peripheral motor nerve (i.e., trauma), and muscle (i.e., myopathy).

Various superficial (cutaneous) reflexes are "released" in upper motor neuron disease. The most commonly tested are the Babinski (Fig. 1.16), a dorsiflexion of the toes to plantar stimulation, and the Hoffman, twitching of the distal thumb in response to "flicking" the distal fingers (Fig. 1.17a, b).

Nucleus ambiguus

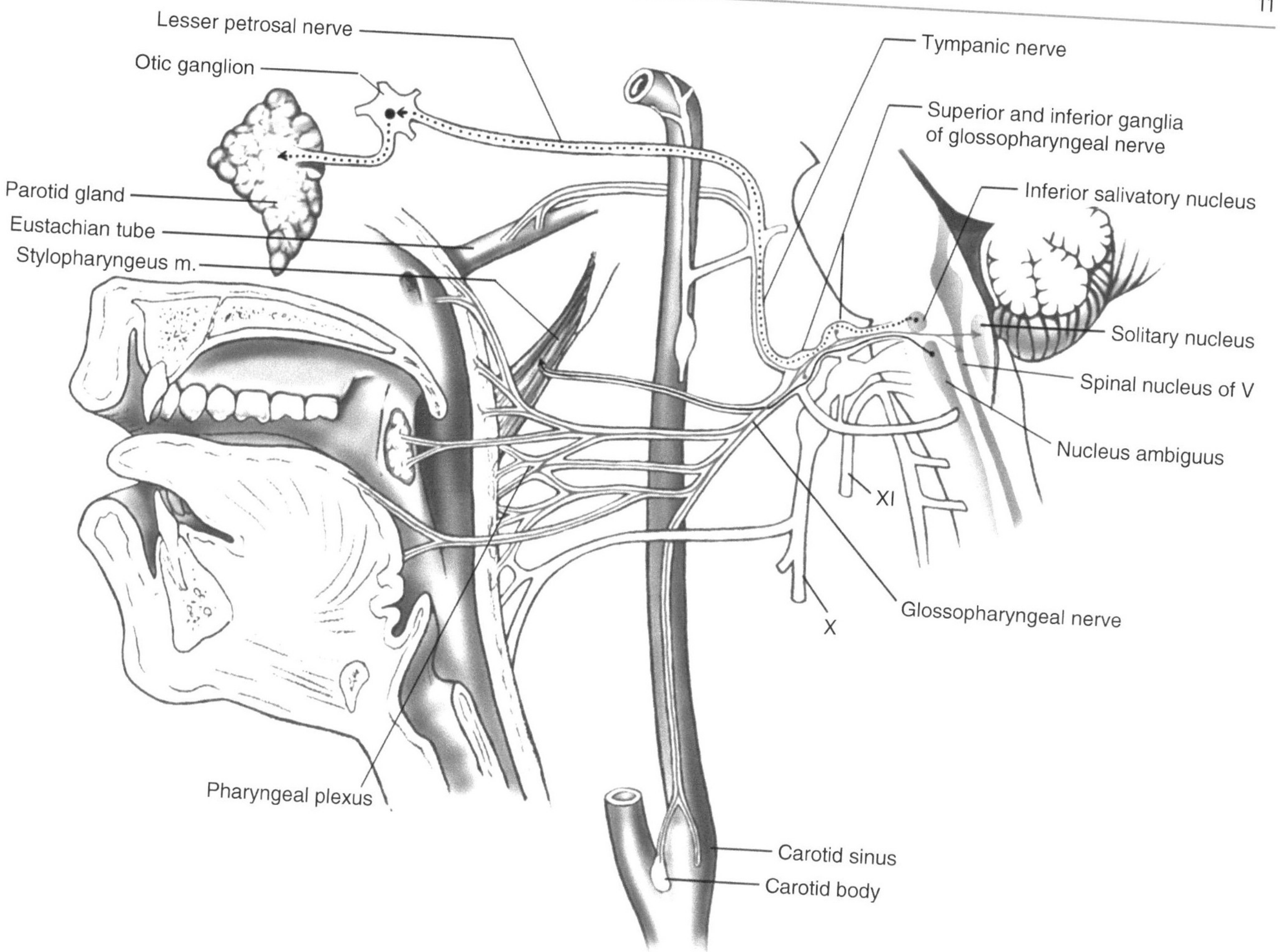

Fig. 1.10 The glossopharyngeal nerve provides motor innervation to the stylopharyngeus muscle and parasympathetic innervation to the parotid gland and carotid body (with permission from David Peace, illustrator. Reproduced with permission from Friedman et al. [8])

Sensation

Pain and temperature sensation are mediated via the spinothalamic tracts, which cross in the spinal cord and ascend to the opposite side of the brain stem and cortex (Figs. 1.18 and 1.19). Touch and proprioception are mediated by the dorsal columns of the spinal cord. These pathways remain ipsilateral until they reach the sensory decussation in the lower brain stem. Consequently, lesions of the hemispinal cord will result in loss of pain and temperature on the opposite side of the body and loss of touch and proprioception on the ipsilateral side of the body.

A sensory exam should include tests of pain fibers (pin), light touch (fingers), proprioception (checking that the patient can tell whether their toes or fingers are being moved up or down), and vibration (tuning fork). Various patterns of sensory loss can localize to specific areas of the nervous system and/or to certain well-known disease processes (Figs. 1.20 and 1.21). For example, loss of all sensory modalities in the distribution of one peripheral or cranial nerve clearly localizes to that nerve. Loss of all modalities below a given spinal level localizes to the spinal cord. Loss of sensation on one side of the face and the opposite side of the body localizes to the brain stem. Loss of sensation of one side of the body and face localizes to the opposite cerebrum. Loss of dorsal column modalities only usually indicates a metabolic disease such as B_{12} deficiency. Table 1.2 reviews the sensory landmarks for a neurological physical examination.

Special Senses

The ability of humans to interact with their environment depends a great deal on the special senses. Somatic sensory function will be addressed separately; here, we will focus on vision, hearing, smell, and taste. Together, these four senses make up most of the non-tactile sensory environment. Large areas of the cerebral cortex are dedicated to the processing of

herniation var-
of patients have
outcome, 10%
e. Factors asso-
ge and anisoco-
e are bilaterally
–7, 10–14].
refers to the her-
orly through the
low lateral hemi-
fracture-induced
ma. The clinical
egia, and coma.
ough the tentorial
ve arterial territo-
n 24–48 hours (if

in rapidly expand-
the lateral middle
ial uncus and hip-
tentorium cerebri,
, and directly com-
occluded (as with
ness is NOT a reli-
arly and consistent
ed by the compres-
brain stem and not
opic organization of
that its vasomotor
eas its somatomotor
central artery of the
h as in uncal hernia-
ng ophthalmoplegia.
in diabetes mellitus),
h pupil sparing.
pocampal herniation
the lateral aspect of
its normal pentago-
ging may show brain
ession of the contra-
paradoxical ipsilat-
enomenon) [15], or
ease of ipsilateral
parasellar and inter-
or hippocampus is
erniation is also seg-
worsening progno-
3–7, 10–14].
a refers to a condi-
hemispherical pres-
dial aspect of the
cerebri. It is usually
bral artery (ACA)

Fig. 1.13 This coronal

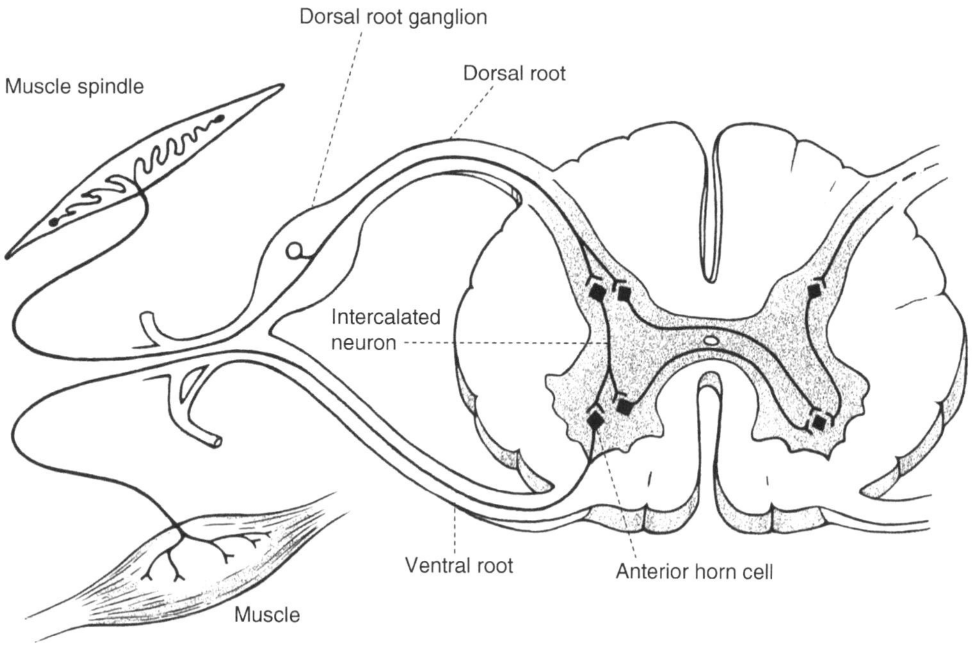

Fig. 1.15 The corticospinal (and other) axons synapse with the motor neurons of the ventral spinal gray matter. The lower motor neuron axons exit through the ventral root and travel through the spinal roots and peripheral nerves to reach the neuromuscular junction. This diagram also illustrates the basic spinal reflex arc, whereby a stretch of the muscle spindle leads to synaptic connections with the motor neurons leading to the muscle involved in the reflex (with permission from David Peace, illustrator. Reproduced with permission from Friedman et al. [8])

Table 1.1 Upper and lower motor neuron (UMN and LMN, respectively) injury comparison [4]

Parameters	UMN[a] injury	LMN[b] injury
Possible etiologies	Stroke, spinal cord injury	Herniated disc, nerve entrapment, polio
Muscle tone	Initially flaccid than spastic (with clasp-knife resistance)	Flaccid
Tendon reflexes	Hyperactive, clonus	Absent
Pathological reflexes (Babinski, Hoffman)	Present (after days to weeks)	Absent
Muscle manifestations	Spasms and extremely mild atrophy due to disuse may occur	Fibrillations, fasciculations, atrophy within days to weeks

[a] Upper motor neuron
[b] Lower motor neuron

Table 1.2 Motor and sensory landmarks for a physical neurological examination [3, 4]

Level	Muscle	Action to test	Reflex	Sensory dermatome
C2				Occipital protuberance
C3				Supraclavicular fossa
C4	Diaphragm	Tidal volume, vital capacity		Top of the acromioclavicular joint
C5	Biceps, deltoid	Flex elbow, abduct arm	Biceps	Lateral antecubital fossa
C6	Wrist extensors	Cock up wrist	Supinator	Dorsal thumb, proximal phalanx
C7	Triceps	Extend elbow	Triceps	Middle finger, dorsal surface, proximal phalanx
C8	FDP[a]	Grasp		Dorsal little finger, proximal phalanx
T1	Hand intrinsics	Abduct little finger		Medial side of the antecubital fossa
T2–9	Intercostals	Use sensory level, abdominal reflexes, Beevor's sign[b] [9]		T2—Apex of the axilla, T4—Nipple line
T9–10	Upper abdomen			T10—Umbilicus
T11–12	Lower abdomen			T12—Mid-inguinal ligament
L2	Iliopsoas	Hip flexion	Cremasteric	Mid-anterior thigh
L3	Quadriceps	Knee stretch	Knee jerk	Medial femoral condyle
L4	Tibialis anterior	Ankle dorsiflexion	Medial hamstrings	Medial malleolus
L5	Extensor hallucis longus	Dorsiflex big toe		Dorsum foot at the third metatarsal phalangeal joint
S1	Gastrocnemius	Plantar flexion	Achilles	Lateral heel
S2	Flexor digitorum, flexor halluces			Popliteal fossa in the midline
S3	Bladder, bowel, anal sphincter			Ischial tuberosity
S4–5				Perianal region

[a] Beevor's sign refers to a medical sign in which the navel moves toward the head upon flexing the neck, indicating selective weakness of the lower abdominal muscles. Causes include spinal cord injury, amyotrophic lateral sclerosis (ALS), and facioscapulohumeral muscular dystrophy (FSHD) [9]
[b] Flexor digitorum profundus

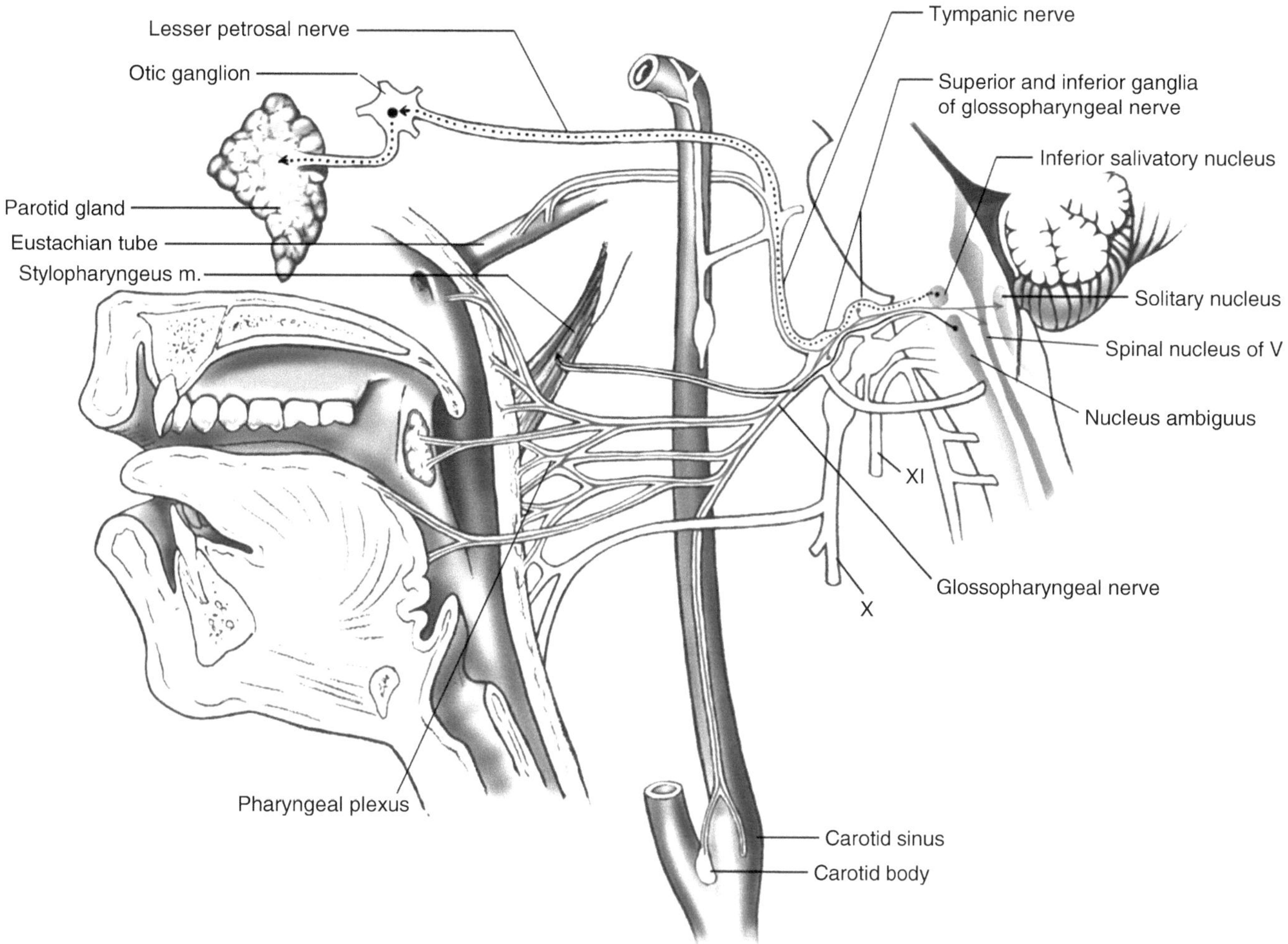

Fig. 1.10 The glossopharyngeal nerve provides motor innervation to the stylopharyngeus muscle and parasympathetic innervation to the parotid gland and carotid body (with permission from David Peace, illustrator. Reproduced with permission from Friedman et al. [8])

Sensation

Pain and temperature sensation are mediated via the spinothalamic tracts, which cross in the spinal cord and ascend to the opposite side of the brain stem and cortex (Figs. 1.18 and 1.19). Touch and proprioception are mediated by the dorsal columns of the spinal cord. These pathways remain ipsilateral until they reach the sensory decussation in the lower brain stem. Consequently, lesions of the hemispinal cord will result in loss of pain and temperature on the opposite side of the body and loss of touch and proprioception on the ipsilateral side of the body.

A sensory exam should include tests of pain fibers (pin), light touch (fingers), proprioception (checking that the patient can tell whether their toes or fingers are being moved up or down), and vibration (tuning fork). Various patterns of sensory loss can localize to specific areas of the nervous system and/or to certain well-known disease processes (Figs. 1.20 and 1.21). For example, loss of all sensory modalities in the distribution of one peripheral or cranial nerve clearly localizes to that nerve. Loss of all modalities below a given spinal level localizes to the spinal cord. Loss of sensation on one side of the face and the opposite side of the body localizes to the brain stem. Loss of sensation of one side of the body and face localizes to the opposite cerebrum. Loss of dorsal column modalities only usually indicates a metabolic disease such as B_{12} deficiency. Table 1.2 reviews the sensory landmarks for a neurological physical examination.

Special Senses

The ability of humans to interact with their environment depends a great deal on the special senses. Somatic sensory function will be addressed separately; here, we will focus on vision, hearing, smell, and taste. Together, these four senses make up most of the non-tactile sensory environment. Large areas of the cerebral cortex are dedicated to the processing of

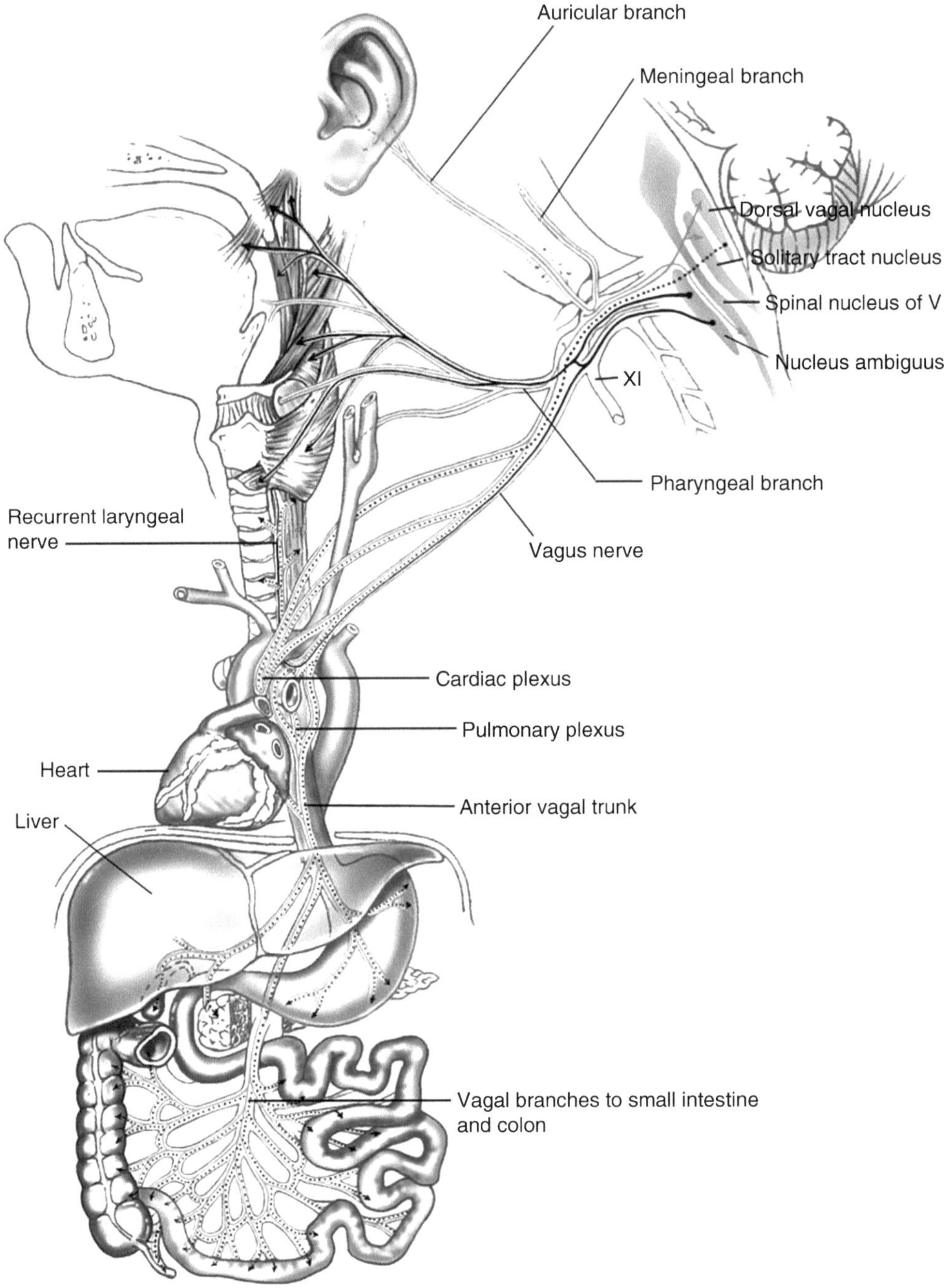

Fig. 1.11 The vagus nerve provides motor innervation to the pharyngeal muscles and parasympathetic innervation to the heart and gut (with permission from David Peace, illustrator. Reproduced with permission from Friedman et al. [8])

sensory data. In addition, the localization of their nuclei in the brain stem makes them important landmarks for localization of abnormalities. We will look at each one in turn.

Vision

The visual system in humans is a robust binocular system that allows depth perception in the primary fields and almost 180 degrees of vision with the head stationary (more than 240 degrees with the head turning). It coordinates the retinal function, pupillary opening, and extraocular muscle movements to see, react, and accommodate to different stimuli and light states. This system can be thought of as two coordinated systems: one that develops images (the retino-cortical tract) and a motor system that coordinates the binocular, conjugate gaze. The retino-cortical tract sends signals from the retina to the optic nerve (cranial nerve 2), to the lateral geniculate nucleus of the thalamus, through the optic radiations, to the medial occipital cortex. Since the optic path traverses the entire base of the cerebrum and passes through three vascular territories, it is extremely useful for localization of some cerebral injuries.

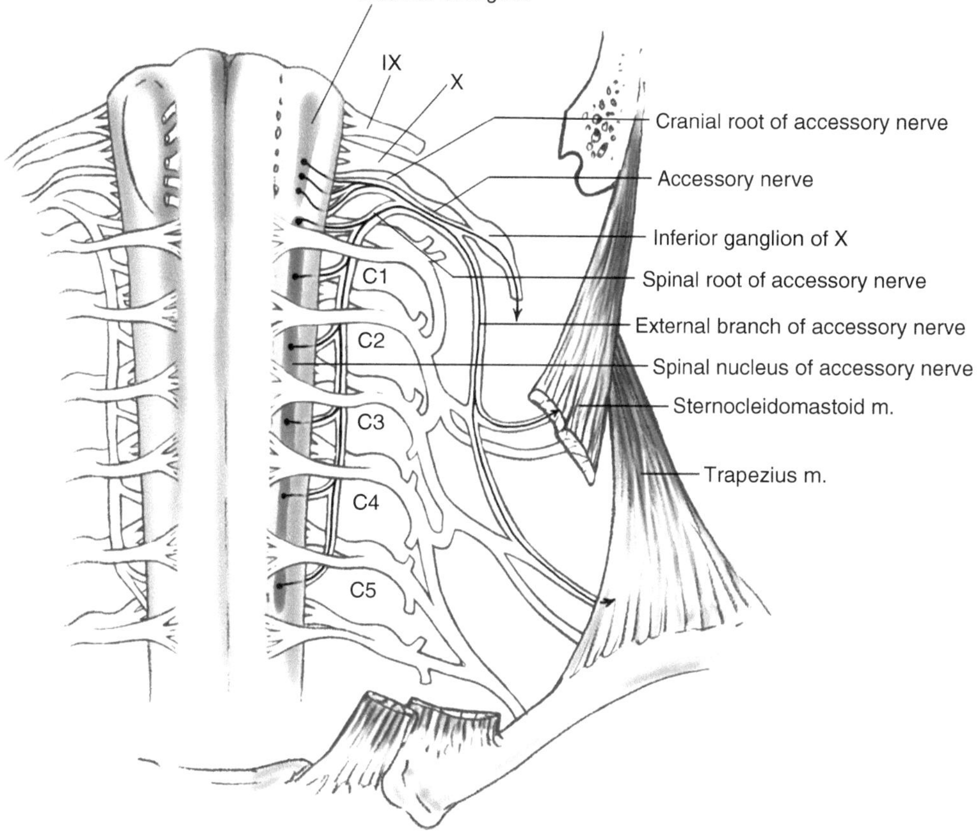

Fig. 1.12 The spinal accessory nerve has branches from the brain stem (nucleus ambiguous) and the upper cervical spinal cord. It provides motor innervation to the trapezius and sternocleidomastoid muscles (with permission from David Peace, illustrator. Reproduced with permission from Friedman et al. [8])

The motor coordination system is more complex as it involves the third, fourth, and sixth cranial nerves and includes the autonomic functions of the eye. Signals from the optic nerve diverge at the level of the geniculate to pass to the superior colliculus and coordinate the function of the cranial nerves so that they fluidly move in all directions and allow conjugate gaze. Localization of the third nerve nucleus in the rostral midbrain and the sixth nerve nucleus in the caudal pons makes interrogating this system important for localizing brain stem injuries.

Hearing

The tympanic membrane oscillates with molecular movement within a range that we define as the audible hearing range. The anatomical pathway for hearing starts with movement of the tympanic membrane through three oscillating bones, which stimulate fluid perturbation through the auditory cochlea, thus stimulating the eighth nerve. The eighth nerve ends in the eighth nerve nucleus which sends fibers to the cochlear nucleus to the superior olivary nucleus the lateral lemniscus to the inferior colliculus and finally to the medial geniculate nucleus of the thalamus. Information from the thalamus is passed to the primary auditory cortex in the temporal lobe and to the secondary sites. Importantly, the superior olivary nuclei are bilaterally innervated by the cochlear nuclei, and, therefore, a unilateral lesion causing hearing loss in the central nervous system (CNS) is not likely.

Taste and Smell

Taste and smell are integrally associated with each other. The receptors for smell are in the nose and interact directly with the olfactory bulb (a brain tract that is also designated the first cranial nerve), and taste passes from the receptors on the taste buds through the facial (fifth cranial nerve) and glossopharyngeal (ninth cranial nerve) nerves to the thalamus on to the parietal and insular cortices. The cortical areas for the two senses are closely integrated.

Herniation Syndromes

The term "brain herniation" refers to the abnormal shift of the brain tissue through a rigid opening in the skull or across a meningeal folding, causing compression of other structures of the CNS and producing symptoms. Herniation syndromes require, by definition, a change in consciousness (either deteriorating or a comatose state). The shift of brain struc-

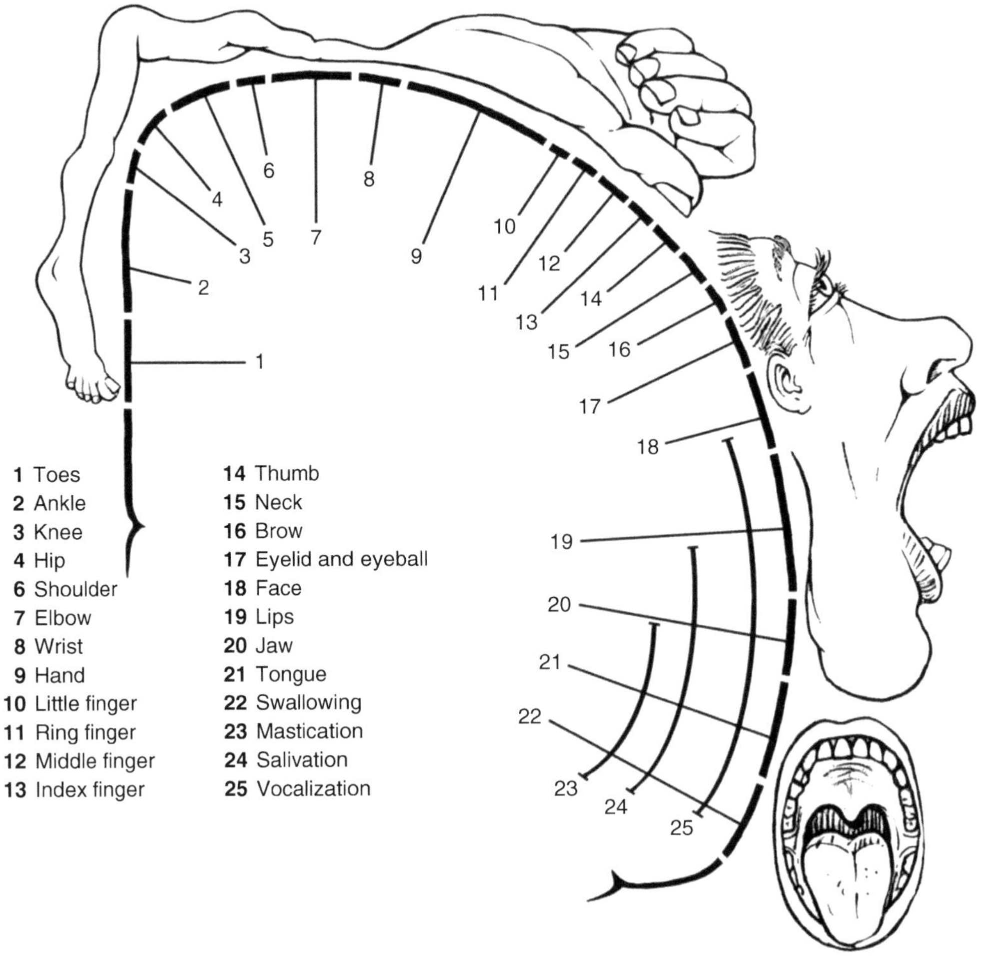

Fig. 1.13 This coronal section through the primary motor strip of the brain illustrates the "motor homunculus." The parts of the body that are innervated by different motor strip areas are shown (with permission from David Peace, illustrator. Reproduced with permission from Friedman et al. [8])

tures as seen on imaging (the radiological correlate) may not always be accompanied by clinical manifestations and may actually represent an epiphenomenon occurring late in the process (like cerebellar tonsillar descent found incidentally in an asymptomatic patient indicative of radiographic Chiari I malformation). Table 1.3 provides a concise overview of the neuroanatomical correlates of the herniation syndromes discussed. An important note is that predicting the location of the lesion based on the herniation syndrome type is unreliable. Etiologies for cerebral herniation range from vascular (stroke, intracerebral hemorrhage, subarachnoid hemorrhage), inflammatory (cerebral abscess, subdural empyema, herpes simplex encephalitis), neoplastic, or traumatic (epidural or subdural hematomas). There are many possible herniation syndromes, divided herein into five clinical entities.

Central (aka transtentorial) herniation refers to a central downward displacement of the brain stem. In milder cases, it results in traction of the abducens nerve (CN-VI) as it courses over the clivus of the occipital bone. Larger supratentorial lesions or lesions in the posterior fossa may cause pressure to convey further through the foramen magnum, resulting in *cerebellar tonsillar herniation*, associated with compression of the medulla oblongata and resulting in respiratory arrest, blood pressure instability, and death.

Central herniation may be either chronic (due to the presence of tumors, especially in the frontal, parietal, or occipital lobes) or acute in the setting of rapidly increasing space-occupying lesions such as a hemorrhage. Central herniation results in the sequential failure of the diencephalon, midbrain, pons, and medulla oblongata. The diencephalon (the thalamus and related structures) is gradually forced through the tentorial incisura. The pituitary stalk may be sheared, resulting in diabetes insipidus. The posterior cerebral arteries (PCAs) may be trapped along the open edge of the incisura and may occlude, producing bilateral occipital infarcts with resultant cortical blindness. The brain stem suffers from ischemia as a result of compression and shearing of the perforating arteries arising from the basilar artery. This results in hemorrhages within the brain stem parenchyma (so-called Duret hemorrhages). Imaging shows a downward displacement (seen more in the pineal region). The perimesencephalic cisterns are compressed. The "classic" signs of increased intracranial pressure (ICP) are hypertension, bradycardia, and an altered respiratory pattern. These are usu-

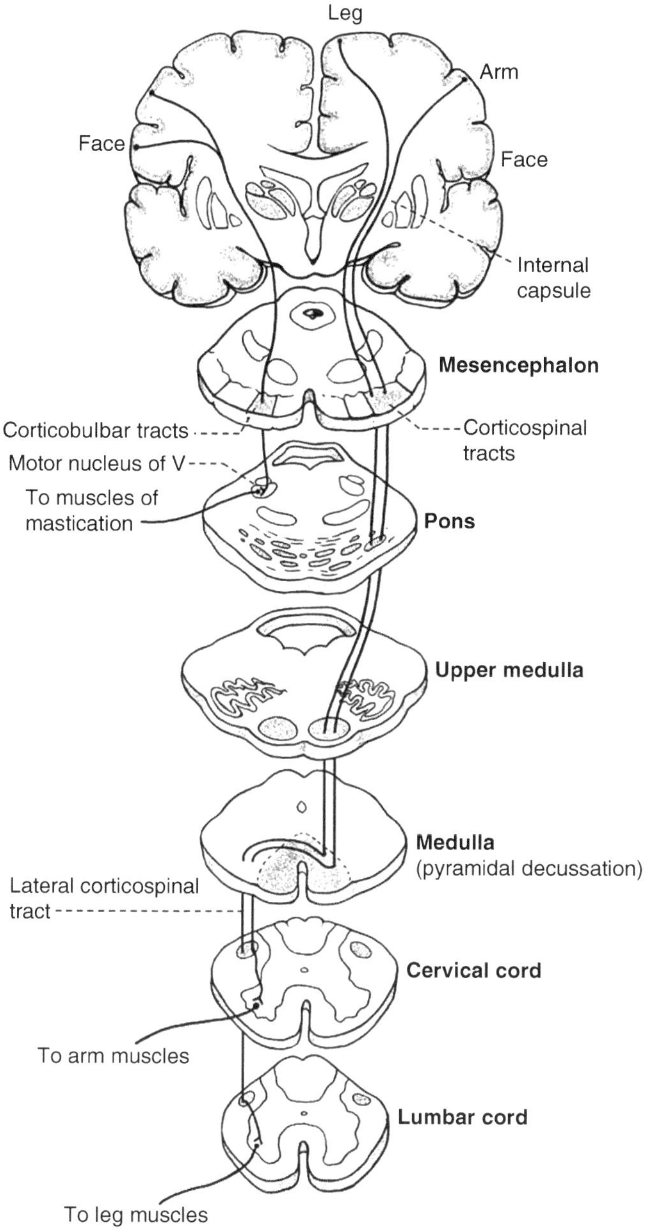

Fig. 1.14 The upper motor neuron fibers descend through the internal capsule into the ventral mesencephalon to the pyramids of the medulla. There, the pathways decussate and form the corticospinal tracts in the posterolateral spinal cord (with permission from David Peace, illustrator. Reproduced with permission from Friedman et al. [8])

ally seen with a posterior fossa lesion and may be absent in slowly developing supratentorial masses.

Central herniation typically progresses through several stages, named according to the compromised structure at that stage (summarized in Table 1.4). These stages are successive steps, which, if halted sooner, carry a better prognosis. The diencephalic stage warns of impending (irreversible) midbrain damage but is frequently reversible if the cause is promptly treated. The midbrain–upper pons stage occurs when midbrain signs fully develop, at which point prognosis is extremely poor. The outcome after central herniation varies but is generally dismal. As few as 9% of patients have good recovery, 18% have a good functional outcome, 10% are severely disabled, and 60% of patients die. Factors associated with a better outcome include young age and anisocoria. Factors associated with a poor outcome are bilaterally fixed pupils, indicating midbrain damage [3–7, 10–14].

Uncal (aka mesial temporal) herniation refers to the herniation of the medial temporal lobe inferiorly through the tentorial notch. This is typically caused by low lateral hemispheral (temporal lobe) pressure such as a fracture-induced middle meningeal artery epidural hematoma. The clinical triad includes a "blown" pupil, hemiplegia, and coma. Compression of the PCAs as they pass through the tentorial notch may cause infarctions in the respective arterial territories as well. This typically manifests within 24–48 hours (if the patient survives the acute phase).

This type of herniation usually occurs in rapidly expanding traumatic hematomas, frequently in the lateral middle fossa or temporal lobe, pushing the medial uncus and hippocampal gyrus over the edge of the tentorium cerebri, entrapping the oculomotor nerve (CN-III), and directly compressing the midbrain. The PCAs may be occluded (as with central herniation). Impaired consciousness is NOT a reliable early sign in uncal herniation. An early and consistent sign is a unilaterally dilating pupil, caused by the compression of the CN-III nerve (after leaving the brain stem and not due to CNS compression). The somatotopic organization of the nerve fibers within CN-III is such that its vasomotor fibers are located at its periphery, whereas its somatomotor fibers are located at its center, around the central artery of the nerve. Thus, external compression (such as in uncal herniation) causes a blown pupil prior to causing ophthalmoplegia. A vascular event (most commonly seen in diabetes mellitus), conversely, causes ophthalmoplegia with pupil sparing.

On imaging, impending uncal or hippocampal herniation may be indicated by encroachment on the lateral aspect of the suprasellar cistern with flattening of its normal pentagonal shape. Once herniation occurs, imaging may show brain stem displacement and flattening, compression of the contralateral cerebral peduncle (at times with paradoxical ipsilateral motor signs, aka Kernohan's phenomenon) [15], or midbrain rotation with a slight increase of ipsilateral subarachnoid space. Obliteration of the parasellar and interpeduncular cisterns occurs as the uncus or hippocampus is forced through the hiatus. This type of herniation is also segregated into stages with a progressively worsening prognosis, as summarized, again, in Table 1.3 [3–7, 10–14].

Cingulate (aka subflacine) herniation refers to a condition typically caused by a higher lateral hemispherical pressure, causing the cingulate gyrus (medial aspect of the hemispheres) to herniate under the falx cerebri. It is usually asymptomatic unless the anterior cerebral artery (ACA)

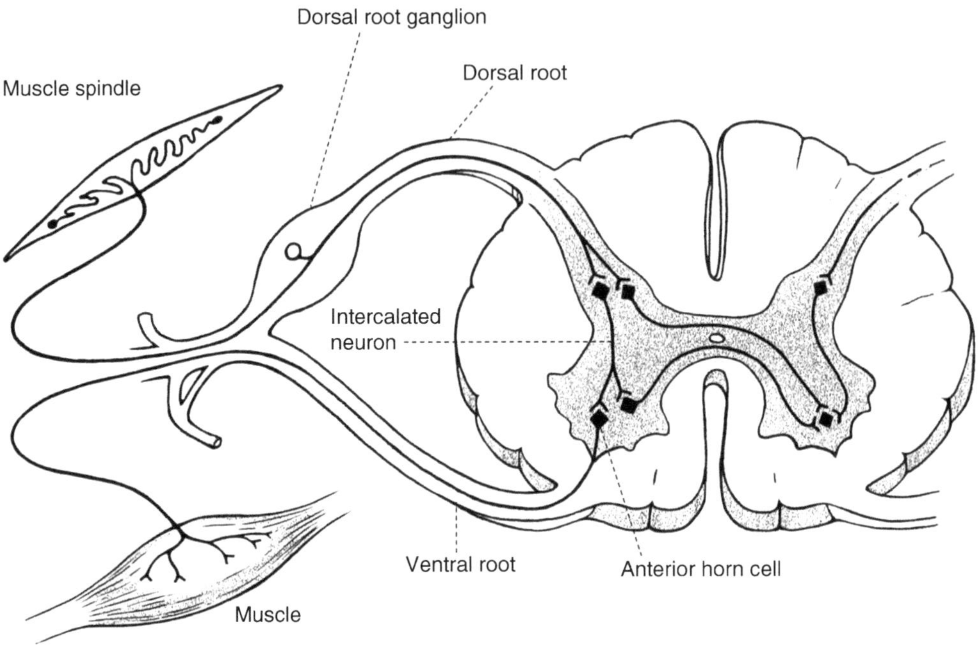

Fig. 1.15 The corticospinal (and other) axons synapse with the motor neurons of the ventral spinal gray matter. The lower motor neuron axons exit through the ventral root and travel through the spinal roots and peripheral nerves to reach the neuromuscular junction. This diagram also illustrates the basic spinal reflex arc, whereby a stretch of the muscle spindle leads to synaptic connections with the motor neurons leading to the muscle involved in the reflex (with permission from David Peace, illustrator. Reproduced with permission from Friedman et al. [8])

Table 1.1 Upper and lower motor neuron (UMN and LMN, respectively) injury comparison [4]

Parameters	UMN[a] injury	LMN[b] injury
Possible etiologies	Stroke, spinal cord injury	Herniated disc, nerve entrapment, polio
Muscle tone	Initially flaccid than spastic (with clasp-knife resistance)	Flaccid
Tendon reflexes	Hyperactive, clonus	Absent
Pathological reflexes (Babinski, Hoffman)	Present (after days to weeks)	Absent
Muscle manifestations	Spasms and extremely mild atrophy due to disuse may occur	Fibrillations, fasciculations, atrophy within days to weeks

[a] Upper motor neuron
[b] Lower motor neuron

Table 1.2 Motor and sensory landmarks for a physical neurological examination [3, 4]

Level	Muscle	Action to test	Reflex	Sensory dermatome
C2				Occipital protuberance
C3				Supraclavicular fossa
C4	Diaphragm	Tidal volume, vital capacity		Top of the acromioclavicular joint
C5	Biceps, deltoid	Flex elbow, abduct arm	Biceps	Lateral antecubital fossa
C6	Wrist extensors	Cock up wrist	Supinator	Dorsal thumb, proximal phalanx
C7	Triceps	Extend elbow	Triceps	Middle finger, dorsal surface, proximal phalanx
C8	FDP[a]	Grasp		Dorsal little finger, proximal phalanx
T1	Hand intrinsics	Abduct little finger		Medial side of the antecubital fossa
T2–9	Intercostals	Use sensory level, abdominal reflexes, Beevor's sign[b] [9]		T2—Apex of the axilla, T4—Nipple line
T9–10	Upper abdomen			T10—Umbilicus
T11–12	Lower abdomen			T12—Mid-inguinal ligament
L2	Iliopsoas	Hip flexion	Cremasteric	Mid-anterior thigh
L3	Quadriceps	Knee stretch	Knee jerk	Medial femoral condyle
L4	Tibialis anterior	Ankle dorsiflexion	Medial hamstrings	Medial malleolus
L5	Extensor hallucis longus	Dorsiflex big toe		Dorsum foot at the third metatarsal phalangeal joint
S1	Gastrocnemius	Plantar flexion	Achilles	Lateral heel
S2	Flexor digitorum, flexor halluces			Popliteal fossa in the midline
S3	Bladder, bowel, anal sphincter			Ischial tuberosity
S4–5				Perianal region

[a] Beevor's sign refers to a medical sign in which the navel moves toward the head upon flexing the neck, indicating selective weakness of the lower abdominal muscles. Causes include spinal cord injury, amyotrophic lateral sclerosis (ALS), and facioscapulohumeral muscular dystrophy (FSHD) [9]
[b] Flexor digitorum profundus

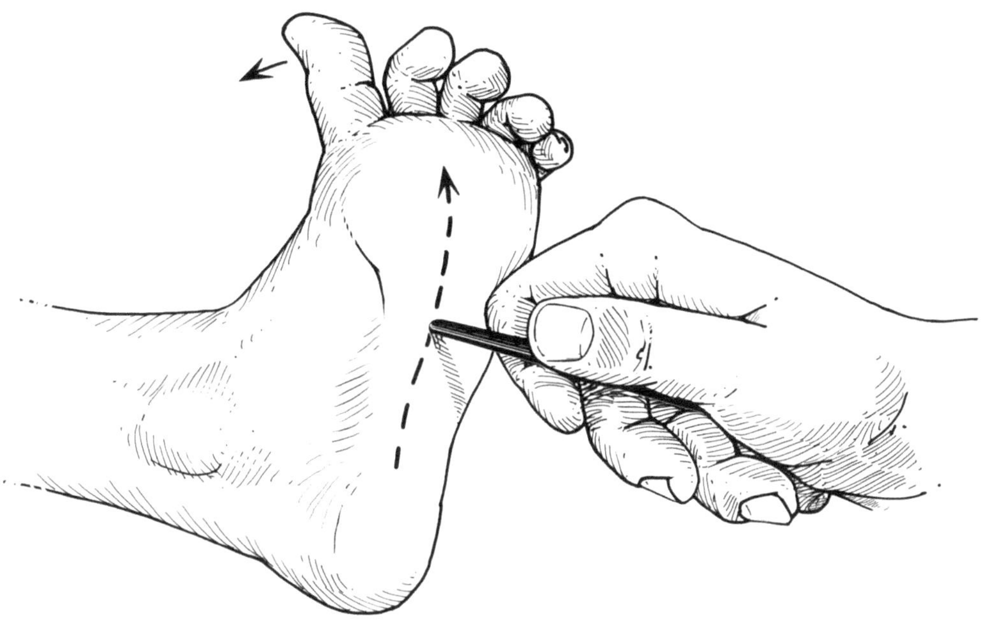

Fig. 1.16 The Babinski sign (with permission from David Peace, illustrator. Reproduced with permission from Friedman et al. [8])

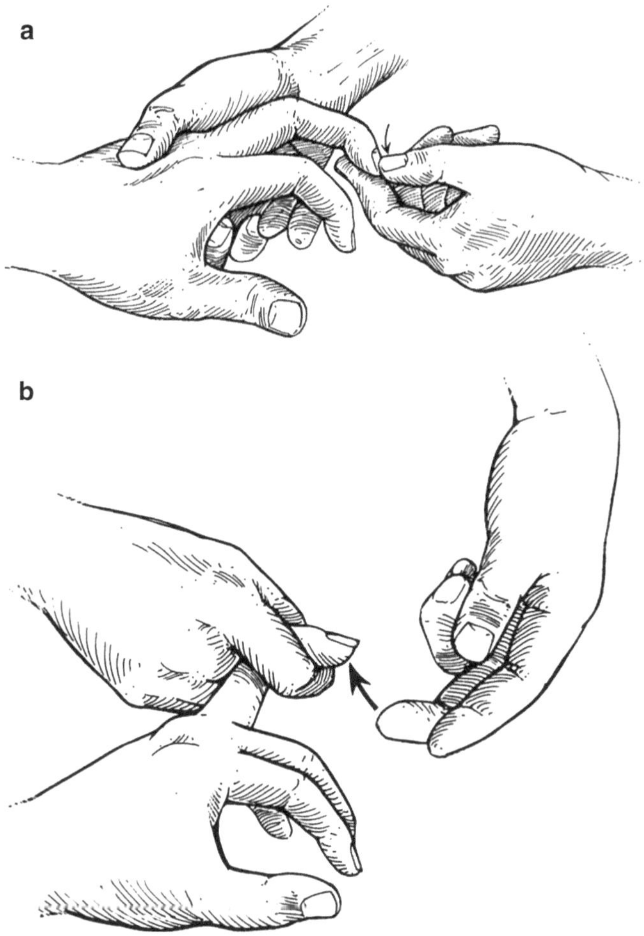

Fig. 1.17 The Hoffman (**a**) and Trömner(**b**) reflexes cause flexion of the distal thumb if upper motor neuron disease is present (with permission from David Peace, illustrator. Reproduced with permission from Friedman et al. [8])

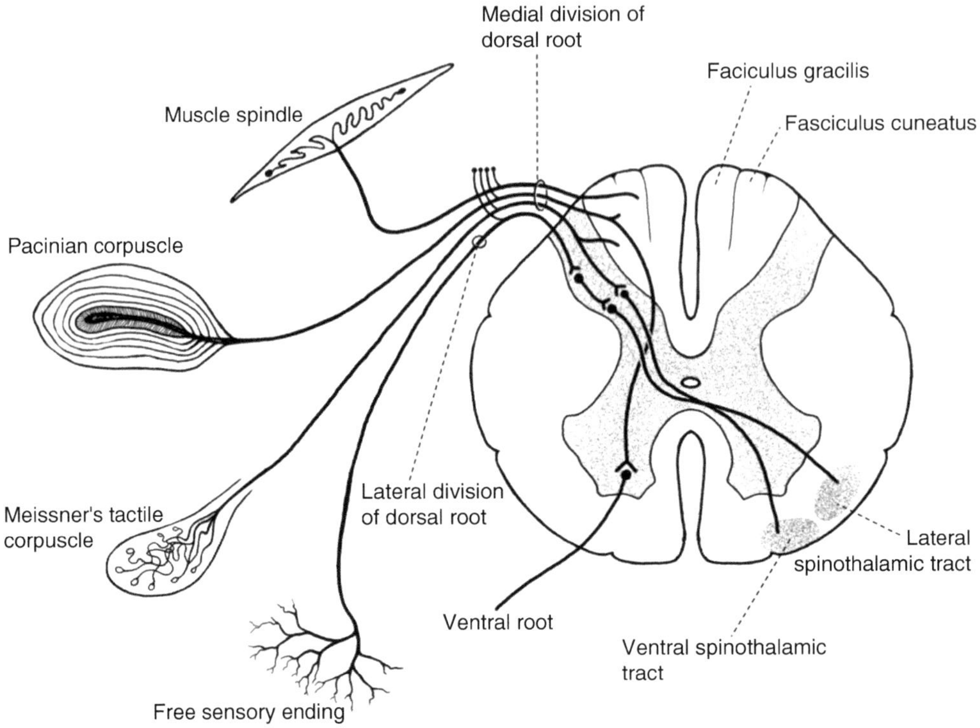

Fig. 1.18 All sensory neurons reside in the dorsal root or brain stem ganglia. Sensory fibers enter the spinal cord through the dorsal root. Those mediating proprioception, vibration, and fine touch enter the dorsal columns and ascend ipsilaterally. Those mediating pain and temperature sensation cross the midline and ascend to the spinothalamic tracts (with permission from David Peace, illustrator. Reproduced with permission from Friedman et al. [8])

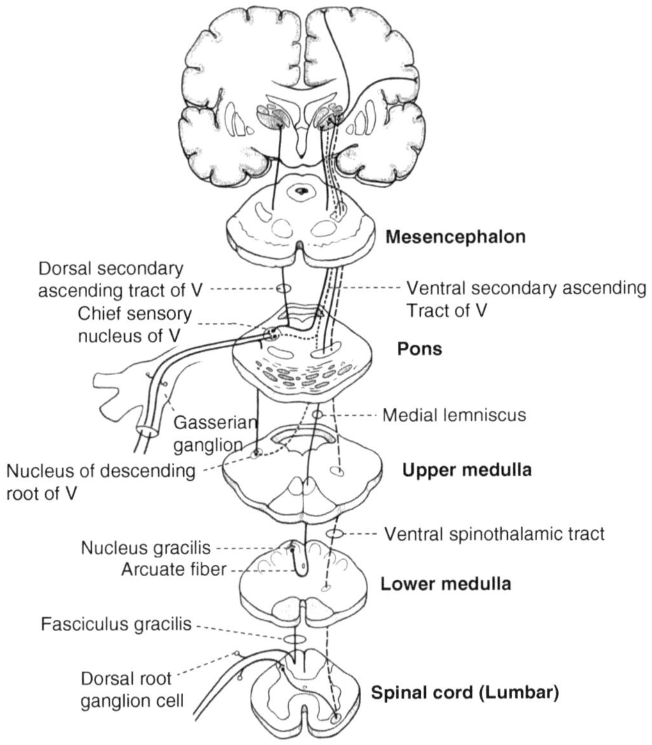

Fig. 1.19 The spinothalamic tracts ascend to the sensory thalamic nuclei and on to the sensory cortex. The dorsal column fibers synapse in the dorsal column nuclei of the medulla, decussate, and ascend to the thalamus and then to the cortex (with permission from David Peace, illustrator. Reproduced with permission from Friedman et al. [8])

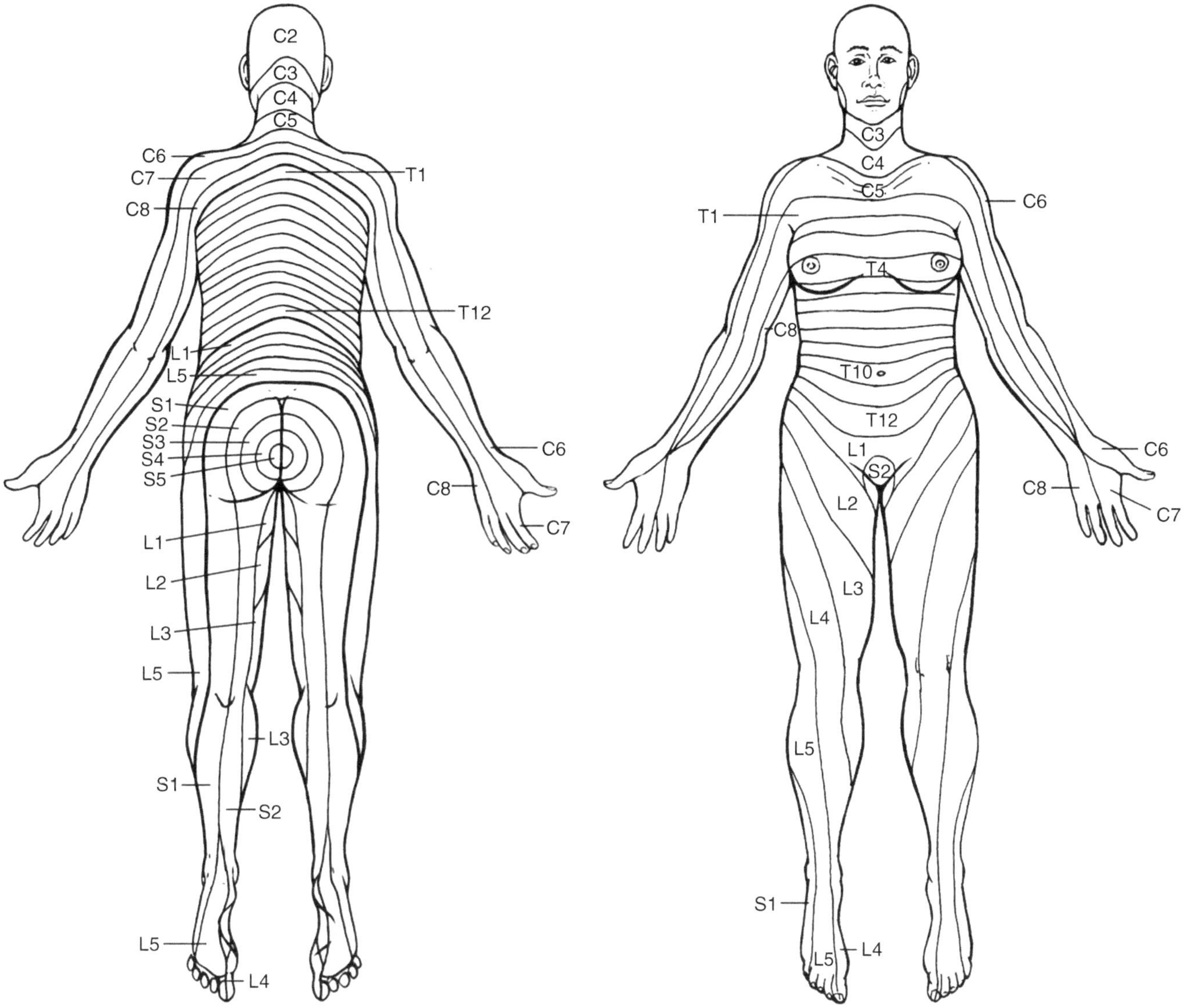

Fig. 1.20 Each spinal sensory root, from C2 to coccygeal 5, innervates a specific skin area, called a "dermatome" (with permission from David Peace, illustrator. Reproduced with permission from Friedman et al. [8])

trunk is compressed under the falx as well, causing bifrontal infarctions. This herniation type usually warns of an impending transtentorial herniation.

Upward cerebellar herniation is a rare, iatrogenic entity, caused when a ventricular external drain is allowed to overdrain, causing a shift of the cerebellum and brain stem structures through the tentorial incisura. The cerebellar vermis ascends above the tentorium, compressing the midbrain and possibly occludes both superior cerebellar arteries (SCAs), resulting in cerebellar infarction. The cerebellar vermis may also compress the sylvian aqueduct at the tentorial incisura level, resulting in secondary obstructive hydrocephalus.

External (aka transcalvarial) herniation refers to the brain tissue extending through an opening in the dura matter and skull (into the nasal cavity in trauma or pediatrics or externally). This type is not always accompanied by loss of consciousness and may at times manifest with rhinorrhea or noticeable scalp asymmetry. There is danger of vascular strangulation with compromised blood supply or draining veins from the herniated segment compressed against the free bone or dural edge of the herniated tissue, resulting in secondary arterial or venous infarcts (ischemic or hemorrhagic) [3–7, 10–14].

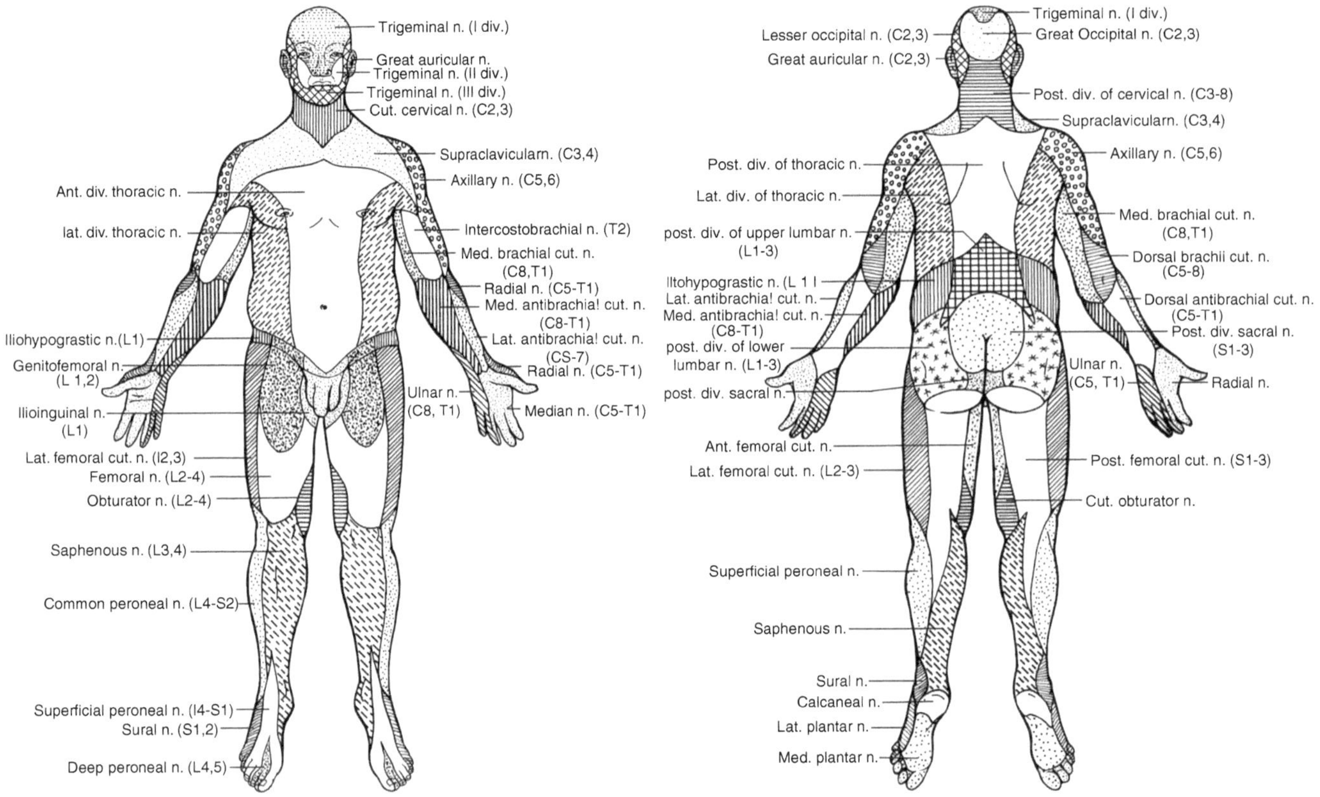

Fig. 1.21 Spinal nerves combine to form multiple peripheral nerves. Each peripheral nerve also has a known sensory skin representation. Careful attention to the sensory exam can localize the nervous system lesion to a peripheral nerve, a spinal nerve, the spinal cord, the brain stem, or the cerebrum (with permission from David Peace, illustrator. Reproduced with permission from Friedman et al. [8])

Table 1.3 Herniation syndromes: an overview of neuroanatomical clinical correlations [3, 4]

Herniation	Anatomical structures involved	Clinical correlates
Subfalcine (cingulate)	Cingulate gyrus	Leg weakness
	Pericallosal arteries (from the ACA)	
Transtentorial (uncal)	CN-III palsy	Ipsilateral ptosis and mydriasis
	Cerebral peduncle	Contralateral/ipsilateral hemiparesis
	PCA	Cortical blindness
	Brain stem reticular formation	Decreased consciousness
Posterior (tectal)	Superior colliculi	Bilateral ptosis
	Brain stem compression	Vertical gaze paralysis
Central (axial)	Basilar artery perforators	Depressed consciousness, impaired eye movements (medial longitudinal fasciculus (MLF))
		Respiratory irregularity, apnea
		Hypertension, bradycardia
Tonsillar	Medulla oblongata	Apnea, respiratory depression

Table 1.4 Central and uncal herniations: stages and clinical correlates [3, 4]

	Consciousness	Respiration	Pupils	Oculomotor	Motor
Central herniation	Diencephalic	Sighs, yawns, later Cheyne–stokes	Small (1–3 mm)	Positive doll's eyes and conjugate ipsilateral response to cold water caloric test	Early bilateral Babinski sign may later become motionless and then decorticate posturing
	Upper pons	Cheyne–stokes	Mid-position (3–5 mm)	Doll's eyes; caloric test impaired. MLF lesions may cause internuclear ophthalmoplegia	Initially decorticate, then bilateral decerebrate posturing
	Lower pons–upper medullary	Regular shallow, rapid (20–40/min)			Flaccid, bilateral Babinski
	Medullary (terminal)	Slow, irregular rate and depth	Widely dilated		
Uncal herniation	Early CN-III	Normal	Unilateral dilated, 85% ipsilateral to the lesion	Doll's eye is normal or dysconjugate	Contralateral Babinski
	Late CN-III	Sustained hyperventilation	Blown	After blown pupil, external ophthalmoplegia may occur	Contralateral or ipsilateral weakness (Kernohan's), bilateral decerebration
	Midbrain/upper pons	Sustained hyperpnea	Blown and fixed	Absent movement	Rigidity, bilateral decerebration

Clinical Anatomical Correlation in Neurological Disease

In this section of the chapter, we will briefly review the neurological functions that commonly localize to the major anatomical divisions of the nervous system.

The Cerebral Cortex

It is possible that, more than any other parts of the CNS, the cerebral cortex and hemispheres have captured the imagination of clinicians and researchers alike. The discussion on the biology that forms one's soul and personality is fascinating, since the essence of human behavior is processed and formed in the cerebral hemispheres. This short overview of higher-order cerebral functions is quickly followed by a brief review of dominant and nondominant hemispherical syndromes as well as a table-formatted review of regional cerebral and hemispherical brain syndromes (Table 1.5).

The Dominant Hemisphere

Language processing and related functions is a hallmark function of the dominant lobe. Auditory information reaches the primary auditory cortex located on the banks of the sylvian fissure in the temporal lobe. Initial processing occurs in Wernicke's area (primary sensory speech area, aka Brodmann's area 22) [16, 17] in the posterior two-thirds of the dominant superior temporal gyrus. Articulation of sounds depends on the combined activity of the face area of the primary motor cortex (located in the inferior precentral gyrus). The motor planning of speech occurs in the nearby motor association cortices termed "Broca's area" (Brodmann 44–45) [16, 17], (Fig. 1.22)located in the pars operculum and pars triangularis of the inferior frontal gyrus. The ability to hear and repeat a word requires proper transfer of information across the sylvian fissure (between Broca's and Wernicke's centers) (Fig. 1.23). This is conveyed via the arcuate fasciculus (part of the superior longitudinal fasciculus subcortical white matter pathway) that connects these two speech centers. Other cortical centers involved in language functions include the premotor, prefrontal, and supplementary motor cortices, all acting in concert with Broca's area. The supramarginal and angular gyri act in concert with Wernicke's area and are important for reading functions. The nondominant hemisphere, connected to the dominant one via the corpus callosum, participates in language processing as well. Its contribution is important for the recognition and production of the affective elements of speech. The subcortical structures involved in language processing and functions to different degrees are the thalamus and basal ganglia [3–7].

Aphasia speech defect classification is based on three parts of the physical examination: speech fluency, comprehension, and repetition. *Broca's (motor) aphasia* (most commonly caused by an infarct in the left middle cerebral artery (MCA)s superior division) manifests with decreased fluency of spontaneous speech (phrase length of less than five words, and the noun number is more than function words). Prosody (normal melodious intonation of speech) is characteristically absent in motor aphasia. Repetition is impaired due to the disconnection from Wernicke's. Comprehension is relatively intact (which tends to aggravate the patient's anxiety of the deficit). "Big Broca's aphasia" is the clinical manifestation caused by large lesions, initially presenting as global aphasia

Table 1.5 Regional cerebral and hemispherical brain syndromes

Location or name			Clinical correlation
Frontal lobe			
Unilateral large lesions			Apathy, abulia
Frontal eye field			Lesions cause impaired contralateral eye movement (looking "toward" the lesion)
			Seizures cause stimulation of the contralateral center (looking "away" from the lesion)
Foster Kennedy syndrome			Olfactory groove Ipsilateral anosmia, central scotoma, contralateral papilledema
Prefrontal lobe			Executive functions
Parietal lobe			
Cortical sensory syndrome			Lesion of the postcentral gyrus, mainly in the hand region
			Loss of position sense, inability to localize tactile stimuli
			Astereognosis (inability to judge size and shape by touch)
			Agraphesthesia (inability to detect numbers written on hand)
			Sensory extinction
			Contralateral homonymous hemianopia
			Contralateral neglect
Dominant	Aphasia	Wernicke's	Sensory aphasia, commonly caused by an infarct in the left MCA inferior division or a lesion in the auditory association cortex
		Broca's	Apraxia of motor sequencing Commonly caused by an infarct in the left MCA superior division
		Global	Lesion/stroke involving large portions of the language centers Fluency, comprehension, and repetition are all disturbed
		Conduction	Disruption of connections (arcuate fasciculus, typically infarct) between cortical centers Clinically similar to Wernick's aphasia with impaired repetition and the patient is *aware* of the deficit
		Pure word blindness	Alexia without agraphia. Patients can write but are unable to read A rare lesion in the parieto-occipital lobe, which interrupts connections between the left angular gyrus and both occipital lobes
		Transcortical motor	Impaired fluency, normal comprehension, spared repetition, commonly caused by an infarct in the ACA–MCA watershed zone
		Transcortical sensory	Normal fluency, no comprehension, spared repetition Commonly caused by an infarct in the MCA–PCA watershed zone
	Gerstmann's syndrome		Agraphia without alexia, right–left confusion, digit agnosia, acalculia
	Bilateral astereognosis		
Nondominant			Topographic memory loss, anosognosia, dressing apraxia
Occipital lobe			
Homonymous hemianopia			
Pineal region			
Parinaud's syndrome			Convergence and supranuclear upward gaze palsy, normal response to vertical doll's eyes, lid retraction (aka "setting sun sign")
Sylvian aqueduct syndrome			When Parinaud's is combined with downward gaze palsy

and later settle into Broca's aphasia. "Little Broca's aphasia" refers to the clinical presentation of smaller lesions confined to the frontal operculum, presenting as Broca's aphasia with a partial recovery thereafter. *Wernicke's (sensory) aphasia* (most commonly caused by an infarct in the left MCA's inferior division) manifests with marked impaired comprehension. The patient does not follow any commands. Spontaneous speech has normal fluency, normal prosody, and normal grammatical structure, but impaired lexical function results in speech that is empty and meaningless. Paraphasic errors (inappropriate substitutions of a word) and neologism (invented words) may occur. Naming is similarly impaired, as does repetition (due to disconnection from Broca's). In contrast to Broca's, patients are unaware of their deficit (anosognosia).

Impaired reading or writing abilities (*alexia* or *agraphia*, respectively) are caused by deficits in central language processing and not by simple motor or sensory deficits. These may occur in isolation or together. When these present with aphasia, the clinical manifesting abnormalities tend to parallel those of the aphasic syndrome for spoken language. The syndrome of *alexia without agraphia* (when the patient can write but not read) is caused by a lesion in the dominant occipital cortex extending to the posterior corpus callosum

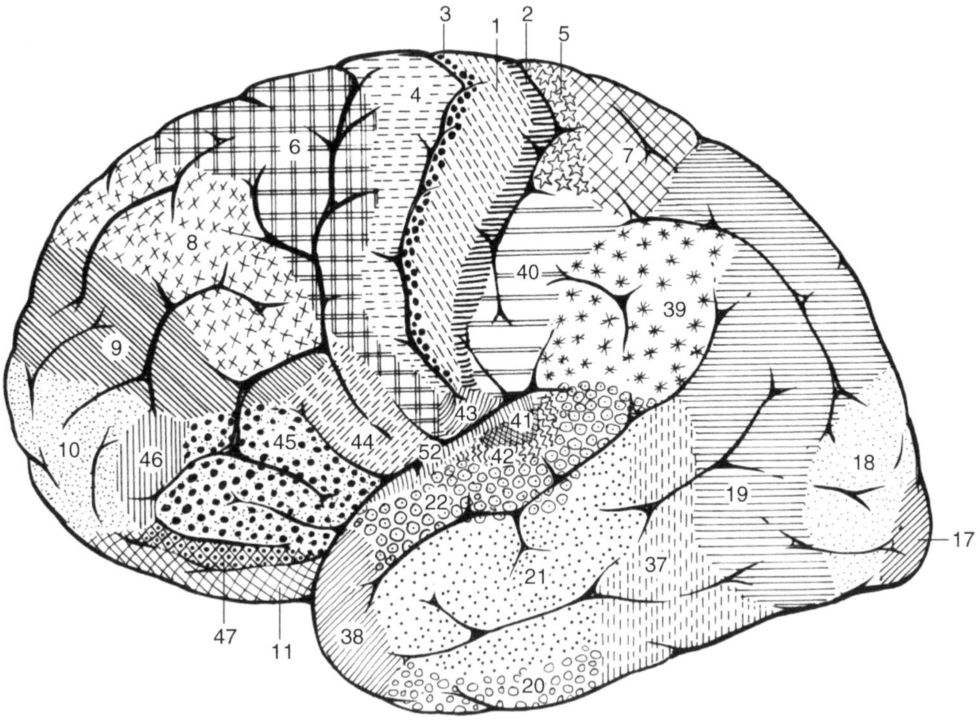

Fig. 1.22 Brodmann functional areas of the brain into approximately 52 areas

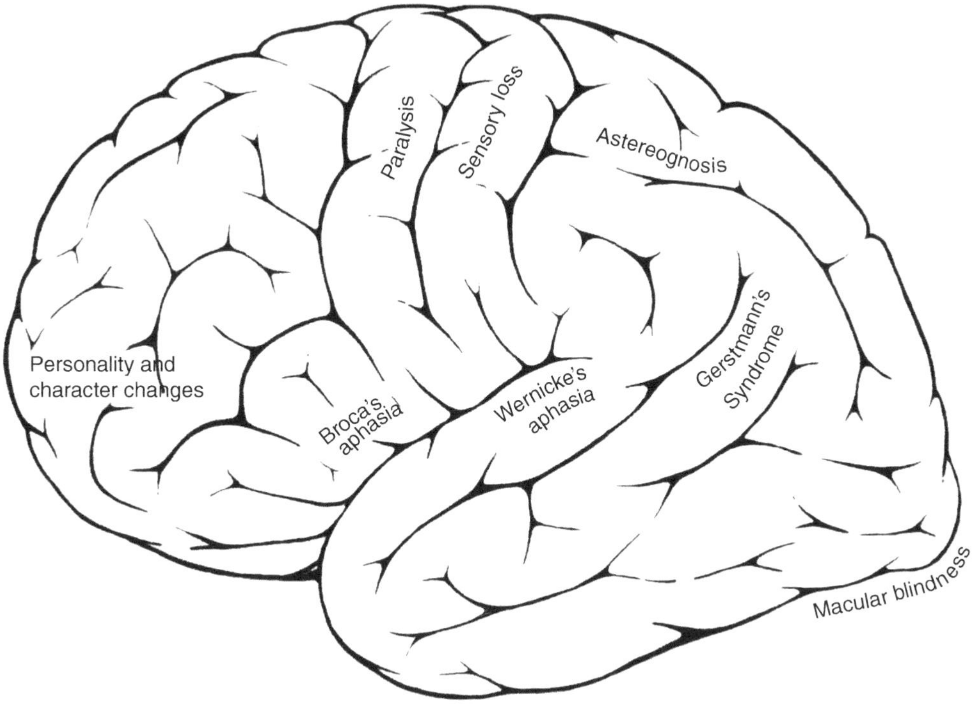

Fig. 1.23 Functional areas of the cortex of the brain

(often due to a PCA infarct, typically presenting with right hemianopia).

Gerstmann's syndrome refers to the presence of four seemingly unrelated signs, with each having very little localizing power by itself, but when presenting together in combination (in the absence of global confusion), it strongly localizes to the dominant inferior parietal lobule. These signs are agraphia, acalculia (for basic mathematics), left–right disorientation, and finger agnosia.

Apraxia refers to the loss of a previously learned motor skill. A good example is an adult patient presenting with an infant-like walk, characterized by asymmetric steps and leg movements (termed "motor apraxia"). This can be seen in conditions such as normal pressure hydrocephalus (NPH), secondary to white matter hemispherical changes mainly in the depth of the frontal lobes. "Ideomotor apraxia" is the term that refers to the inability to carry out an action in response to a verbal command (the patient initiates motor actions on their own, speaks, and understands but is unable to follow commands). *Verbal apraxia* (aka *aphemia*) refers to apraxia of the speech and articulatory apparatus, without language disturbances, with a normal written language (unlike Broca's). Commonly caused by small lesions in the dominant frontal operculum, speech is referred to as *foreign accent syndrome*.

In *cortical deafness*, patients are aware of an existing sound but are unable to interpret verbal or nonverbal stimuli. It is commonly caused by bilateral lesions of the primary auditory cortex (Heschl's gyrus in the temporal lobe). *Pure word deafness* (aka verbal auditory agnosia) is a subset of cortical deafness, in which patients can identify nonverbal sounds but cannot understand any spoken words. This is commonly caused by an infarct in the auditory area of the dominant hemisphere, extending to the subcortical white matter [3–7].

The Nondominant Hemisphere

Attention has several components. Global attention manifests in functions such as vigilance and concentration. Selective directed attention manifests in focusing attention on a particular domain. Attention like alertness depends on activating systems such as the pontomesencephalic reticular formation, different diencephalic structures, limbic structures, etc. Nondominant (typically right) hemispherical lesions may lead to prominent and long-lasting deficits in attention on the contralateral side. Under normal conditions, the nondominant (typically right) hemisphere strongly attends to the left side and less to the right side, whereas the dominant (typically left) hemisphere mainly attends to the right side.

Visuospatial analysis is performed by a distributed network and depends on the bilateral regions of the frontal and parietal association cortices. Visual information is processed by two streams: one ventral question dealing with the "what?" and the second dorsal stream dealing with the "where?" question. The "what" question's processing occurs in the ventral occipital, temporal, and prefrontal cortices. The "where" question's processing takes place in the dorsal occipital, parietal, and prefrontal cortices. The parietal association cortex (located at the junction of the parietal–temporal–occipital lobes) is especially important for visuospatial analysis. It is part of the dorsal stream and analyzes the location and movement of visual objects in space. Spatial analysis encompasses both the surrounding environment and the relative position of one's body in space using visual, proprioceptive, vestibular, and auditory information.

Hemineglect syndrome appears in patients presenting with profound neglect for the contralateral half of the external world and of their body. Patients are often unaware of the deficit, at times not even recognizing the left side of the body as theirs. Lesions causing hemineglect symptoms are located in the right parietal or frontal cortex and may involve the cingulate gyrus, thalamus, basal ganglia, or midbrain reticular formation.

As discussed previously, the nondominant hemisphere participates in language processing as well, important for the recognition and production of the affective elements of speech. Thus, in right hemispherical lesions, no obvious language disturbance can be observed but difficulty judging the intended expression by a particular tone or difficulty producing and attaching an emotional expression to a sentence is seen. Please refer to Table 1.5 for a short and organized summary of regional cerebral and hemispherical brain syndromes [3–7].

The Frontal Lobes

The frontal lobes of the brain subserve many important neurological functions. First, the frontal association areas are responsible for personality and level of energy. Frontal lobe lesions can result in apathy, inactivity, depression, changes in personality, inappropriate actions, etc. Severe bilateral frontal lobe injury leads to a condition called akinetic mutism. Alternatively, some frontal lesions lead to a sense of euphoria accompanied by inappropriate jocularity (Witzelsucht).

The frontal eye fields (Brodmann's area 8) direct both eyes to the opposite side of the body. Damage to this area of the brain will frequently result in head and eye turning toward the side of injury. This is seen after trauma and stroke.

The posterior portion of the frontal lobes contains the primary motor cortex (Brodmann's area 4). This strip is organized in a somatotopic pattern, with the face most inferior, then the hand, and then the arm. The hips and shoulders are near the top of the strip. Leg function is localized to the mesial hemisphere. Injury to this area will result in paralysis of an "upper motor neuron" variety.

The inferior posterior surface of the dominant (usually left) frontal lobe is called Broca's area (Brodmann's area 45).

The Temporal Lobes

The temporal lobes, especially the mesial limbic structures (including the hippocampus), are an important part of the neurological circuits involved in memory. Disease of the temporal lobes, especially when bilateral, can lead to profound recent memory loss.

The dominant temporal lobe (usually left) is involved in language function. The posterior superior temporal gyrus is called Wernicke's area (Brodmann's area 22). Lesions of this area cause Wernicke's aphasia, which is characterized by an inability to understand spoken or written speech. Speech output is fluent but is nonsensical.

Lesions of both temporal tips can cause a condition called the Kluver–Bucy syndrome, which is characterized by oral automatisms and hypersexuality. This condition is rare and is most commonly seen with head trauma.

The Parietal Lobes

The anterior parietal lobes contain the primary somatosensory cortex (Brodmann's areas 3,1,2). Like the motor strip, this area is organized somatotopically. Lesions of the primary sensory cortex cause loss of all sensory modalities in the corresponding opposite body parts. Posterior to the primary sensory cortex, in the superior parietal lobules, are the sensory association areas. Lesions of these areas cause "agnosias," wherein objects cannot be recognized by a sensory input even though the primary sensory modalities are intact. Parietal lesions can cause "neglect" of the opposite hemibody, wherein the patient tends to ignore stimuli to that side. Severe neglect can lead to autotopagnosia or the inability to recognize one's own body. Anosognosia refers to ignorance of the existence of disease and has been specifically applied to denial of hemiplegia. A more subtle test for parietal lobe dysfunction involves simultaneous stimulation of bilateral body parts. With parietal lesions, the sensation over the opposite body will frequently not be perceived.

The left inferior parietal lobe integrates many sensory modalities. Lesions in this area can cause Gerstmann's syndrome, which is characterized by finger agnosia, acalculia, left–right confusion (allochiria), and agraphia. Lesions in the angular gyrus area of the inferior parietal lobe are particularly likely to cause anomia, the inability to remember the names of objects.

The right parietal lobe is implicated in higher sensory processing as well. Lesions in this area can cause "dressing apraxia," wherein a patient cannot figure out how to properly put on clothing because of their inability to integrate sensory information.

The Occipital Lobes

The occipital lobes contain the primary visual cortex. Lesions of the occipital lobe tend to cause loss of vision in the opposite visual fields of both eyes (homonymous hemianopia). The macular (central) fields may be spared.

More anterior occipital areas contain the visual association cortex. Lesions here will cause a variety of "visual agnosias." The inability to recognize faces is called "prosopagnosia."

The Brain Stem

The brain stem is usually divided into three parts: the mesencephalon, the pons, and the medulla. The brain stem connects the cerebral hemispheres and deep structures to the spinal cord, so it contains the long motor and sensory tracts, which connect these structures as well as the cranial nerve nuclei. Because so many important structures are crowded into such a small area, even small injuries to the brain stem cause highly localizable deficits. Large brain stem insults frequently lead to coma or death. The vascular territories of the brain stem are described in Table 1.6.

Table 1.6 Vascular territories of the brain stem [3, 4, 6, 7, 18]

Anatomical site		Vascular supply
Medulla	Medial	Paramedian branches of the ASA caudally
		Paramedian branches of the VA rostrally
	Lateral	Penetrating branches of the VA and PICA
Pons	Medial	Paramedian branches of the BA
	Lateral	Circumferential branches of the BA
		AICA in the caudal pons
		Inner ear is supplied by the labyrinthine artery, arising from the AICA
	Rostral	Pontine artery, a short circumferential artery
	Superior dorsolateral	SCA
Midbrain	Paramedian branches from the BA and proximal PCA enter the interpeduncular fossa to supply to the medial midbrain and thalamus	
	Medial	The artery of Percheron

VA vertebral artery, *PICA* posterior inferior cerebral artery, *BA* basilar artery, *AICA* anterior inferior cerebral artery

Ventral mesencephalic lesions tend to cause an ipsilateral third nerve palsy and contralateral hemiplegia. This symptom complex, called Weber's syndrome, can be seen with stroke and tumors. Dorsal mesencephalic lesions are often associated with Parinaud's syndrome that is characterized by decreased pupillary light reflex, preserved pupillary constriction to accommodation, paralysis of upward gaze, retraction–convergence nystagmus, and other anomalies. Parinaud's syndrome is most often seen with pineal region tumors but can also be seen with severe hydrocephalus.

Ventral pontine lesions cause an ipsilateral sixth nerve palsy and contralateral weakness (Millard–Gubler syndrome). This is most often seen with stroke. More dorsolateral lesions are associated with hearing loss, vertigo, facial weakness, and ataxia.

Ventral medullary lesions cause an ipsilateral twelfth nerve palsy and contralateral hemiplegia (Hughlings Jackson syndrome). Dorsal lateral lesions cause Wallenberg's syndrome, usually associated with vertebral artery occlusion and characterized by dysphonia, Horner's syndrome, dysphagia, ataxia, ipsilateral facial numbness, and contralateral body numbness.

Table 1.7 Clinical vascular syndromes of the brain stem [3–7, 10–14, 18]

Syndrome	Anatomical location	Clinical manifestation
Anton	Bilateral PCA/top of the basilar bilateral occipital lobe stroke	Visual deficit without recognition of blindness (visual agnosia)
Claude	Dorsal midbrain syndrome Ipsilateral CN-III palsy with contralateral ataxia	
Dejerine	Medial medullary syndrome BA, VA, ASA	Contralateral spastic weakness sparing face, loss of vibration/position sense, ipsilateral tongue weakness
Dejerine–Roussy	PCA thalamic perforators	Hemisensory loss, hemibody pain
Foville	Inferior medial pontine syndrome BA perforators	Contralateral weakness, facial weakness, lateral gaze deficit
Locked-in	BA	Paralysis of all movements, except vertical gaze and eyelid opening Sensation and conscious preserved
Marie-Foix	AICA occlusion	Ipsilateral ataxia, nausea, vertigo, decreased hearing, contralateral hemiparesis
Millard–Gubler	Aka base of pons syndrome BA perforators	Contralateral weakness, diplopia, strabismus, ipsilateral facial weakness
Raymond	BA perforators	Lateral gaze deficit (CN-VI), weakness
Top of the basilar	Sudden-onset altered mental status, ophthalmoplegia, papillary/visual field deficits Embolic or stent deployment complication	
Wallenberg	VA occlusion/dissection, PICA occlusion	Facial pain and sensory loss, ataxia, nystagmus, Vertigo, nausea, vomiting, dysphagia, hoarseness, Dysarthria, ipsilateral Horner's syndrome, contralateral loss of pain and temperature, hiccups
Weber	Ventral midbrain infarct PCA midbrain perforators	Contralateral weakness, lateral gaze deficit and ipsilateral pupillary dilatation, contralateral corticobulbar dysfunction
Benedict	A combination of Claude's and Weber's syndromes (large infarct containing ventral and dorsal-central midbrain)	

VA vertebral artery, *BA* basilar artery, *PICA* posterior inferior cerebral artery

Many other brain stem syndromes have been described (Table 1.7); a comprehensive review is beyond the scope of this chapter.

The Spinal Cord

The spinal cord may be injured by trauma, tumors, degenerative disease, vascular lesions, infection, and metabolic disorders. A complete spinal cord injury results in loss of all motor and sensory functions below the level of the lesion. If the thoracic cord is involved, then this results in paraplegia. If the cervical cord is involved, then quadriplegia is seen. In the acute phase of an injury, all reflexes are lost; this is termed a "spinal shock." Because sympathetic outflow to the body is interrupted, hypotension and bradycardia are often seen (a "neurogenic shock"). Gradually, reflexes return and, because of the upper motor neuron nature of the injury, become hyperactive.

A variety of partial spinal cord injury syndromes are commonly described (Table 1.8). Brown-Sequard syndrome refers to a "hemispinal cord" injury which can be caused by trauma or neoplasm. This is characterized by loss of ipsilateral motor function as well as proprioception and vibratory sensation below the lesion. Contralateral pain and temperature sensation are lost.

Anterior spinal artery syndrome is usually associated with trauma but can be caused by vascular disease of the aorta. It can be seen after prolonged clamp times during aortic aneurysm or coarctation repair. It is characterized by bilateral paralysis and loss of pain and temperature sensation, with preservation of dorsal column function (touch and proprioception).

Dorsal column syndrome refers to isolated injury of the dorsal columns, most commonly associated with metabolic disease. This results in loss of touch and proprioception below the lesion, with preservation of other functions.

The motor neurons of the spinal cord can be selectively injured in certain diseases, including poliomyelitis, and some forms of amyotrophic lateral sclerosis. This results in weakness and atrophy of the associated muscles, without sensory loss.

The Peripheral Nerves

The peripheral nerves contain motor and sensory axons. The cell bodies of origin of the sensory axons are found in the

Table 1.8 Clinical syndromes in spinal cord injury [3–5, 10, 19–21]

Lesion	Description		Scheme
Transverse cord lesion	All sensory and motor pathways are interrupted		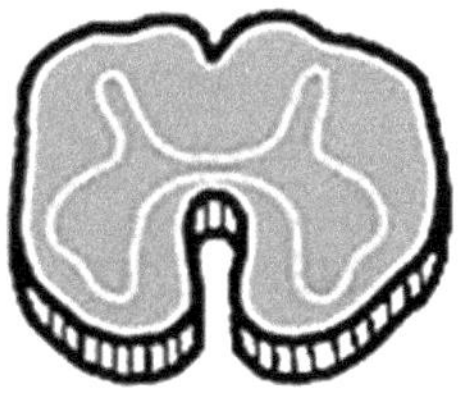
Central cord syndrome	A lesion occurring almost exclusively in the cervical region that produces sacral sensory sparing and greater weakness in the upper limbs than in the lower limbs		
	Small lesions	Damage to spinothalamic fibers, crossing the anterior commissure, causes bilateral regions of suspended sensory loss to pain and temperature (termed sensory dissociation). When in cervical region, classical cape distribution.	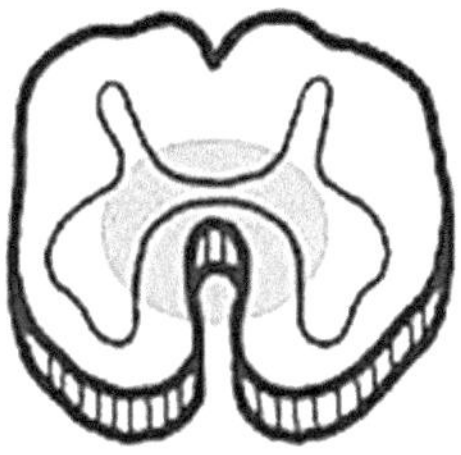
	Larger lesions	Anterior horn cells are also damaged, producing LMN. The corticospinal tract is also affected causing UMN signs. Dorsal columns and ALS may be involved.	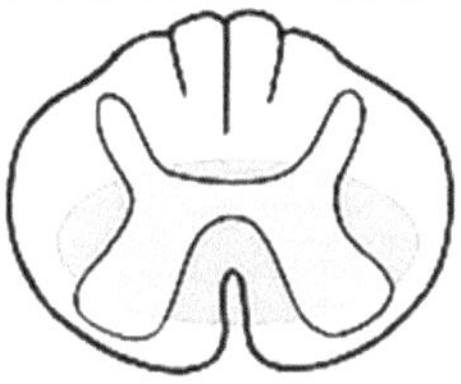
Posterior cord	Dorsal (Posterior) Columns are affected (due to trauma, compression, Multiple sclerosis, B12 deficiency, Tabes dorsalis).		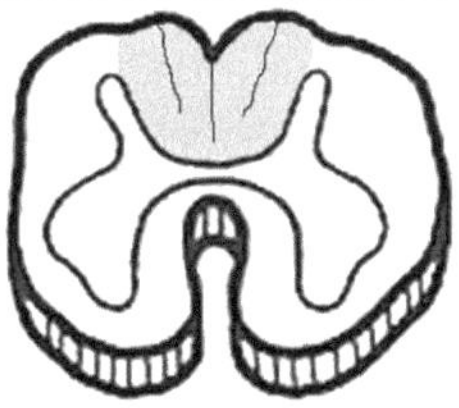
Anterior cord	A lesion that produces variable loss of motor function and of sensitivity to pain and temperature while preserving proprioception (sensory dissociation). Damage to anterior horn may cause LMN weakness.		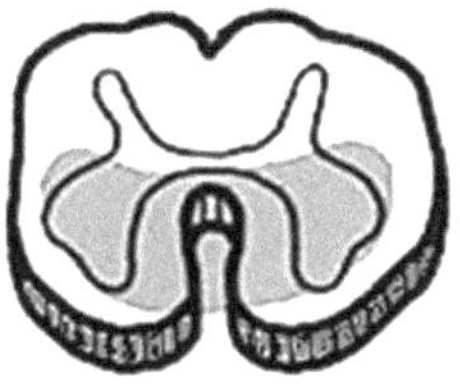
Brown-Sequard syndrome	Hemicord lesion, producing an ipsilateral motor weakness, ipsilateral proprioceptive loss and contralateral loss of sensitivity to pain and temperature (because of the different levels of decussation of the dorsal columns versus the ALS).		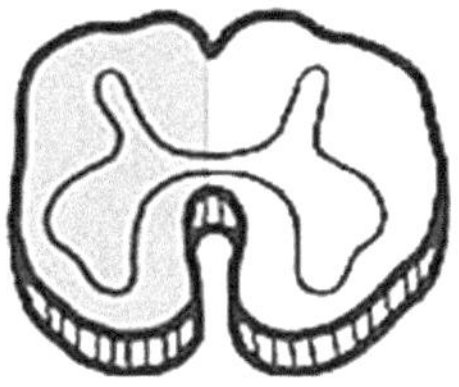

LMN lower motor neuron, *UMN* upper motor neuron

dorsal root ganglia, and those of the motor axons are found in the ventral horn of the spinal cord. The sensory axons subserve the many peripheral sensory organs, which convey pain, temperature, touch, special sensory function, etc. The motor axons conduct impulses from the lower motor neurons to the muscles.

Hundreds of disorders can affect the peripheral nerves. Peripheral nerve disease typically leads to weakness and atrophy of the involved muscles. Disease of a specific nerve will lead to sensory loss in the known distribution of that nerve. Generalized peripheral neuropathy tends to cause loss of sensation in a "stocking-glove" distribution, although there are many exceptions.

The reader is referred to several excellent texts for a detailed discussion of peripheral neuropathy [22–27].

The Neuromuscular Junction

The synapse between the motor axon and the muscle is called the neuromuscular junction. It is probably the best-studied and understood synapse in the body. Diseases of the neuromuscular junction (like myasthenia gravis) tend to cause fluctuating weakness, with no signs of atrophy, involvement of the cranial and peripheral muscles, and respond to anticholinesterase inhibitors.

The Muscle

Diseases of the muscle are called "myopathies." A myopathy can be congenital, metabolic, inflammatory, infectious, or can present as a remote effect of carcinoma. Myopathies are characterized by weakness, most frequently affecting the proximal more than the distal musculature. Often, atrophy is present, and reflexes are reduced. Muscle pain may be present, and muscle enzymes may be elevated.

Conclusions

An understanding of the functional anatomy of the nervous system is important for diagnosing patients with neurological injury. Although brain imaging and physiological assessment of neuronal function are improving rapidly, evaluating the connectivity and responsiveness of multiple parts of the nervous system by examination allows the observer to make an intellectual map of the areas of the brain, spinal cord, or peripheral nervous system that are dysfunctional. By searching for points where separate systems anatomically colocalize, one can predict where in the nervous system a lesion is located, i.e., "localization of lesions." This allows for differential diagnosis development, fine-tuning of imaging, and prediction of the disease course.

References

1. Edlow BL, Claassen J, Schiff ND, Greer DM. Recovery from disorders of consciousness: mechanisms, prognosis and emerging therapies. Nat Rev Neurol. 2021;17(3):135–56.
2. Teasdale G, Jennett B. Assessment of coma and impaired consciousness. A practical scale. Lancet. 1974;2:81–4.
3. Cohen-Inbar O. Focused neurosurgery textbook. 1st ed. Jaypee Brothers; 2016.
4. Cohen-Inbar O. Focused neuroanatomy for medical students. 1st ed. Nova Science; 2015.
5. Winn HR. Youmans and Winn neurological surgery. 8th ed. Elsevier; 2022.
6. Mancall EK, Brock DG. Gray's clinical neuroanatomy: the anatomic basis for clinical neuroscience. 1st ed. Elsevier; 2011.
7. Standring S. Gray's anatomy, the anatomical basis of clinical practice. 39th ed. Elsevier; 2008.
8. Friedman WA, Foote KD, Peace D. Neurologic disease: an overview. In: Layon AJ, Gabrielli AG, Friedman WA, editors. Textbook of neurointensive care. Philadelphia: W.B. Saunders; 2004.
9. Pearce JM. Beevor's sign. Eur Neurol. 2005;53(4):208–9.
10. Greenberg MS. Handbook of neurosurgery. 7th ed. Thieme; 2010.
11. Ramina R, Pires de Aguiar PH, Tatagiba M. Samii's Essentials in Neurosurgery. 2nd ed. Springer-Verlag; 2014.
12. Yasargil MG. Microneurosurgery in 4 volumes. Thieme Stratton Inc.; 1988.
13. Rhoton AL. The Rhoton collection. Neurosurgery. 2000;47(3) Rhoton.inerurodb.org.
14. Carpenter MB. Core text of neuroanatomy. 3rd ed. The Williams & Wilkins Company; 1985.
15. Zafonte RD, Lee CY. Kernohan-Woltman notch phenomenon: an unusual cause of ipsilateral motor deficit. Arch Phys Med Rehabil. 1997;78(5):543–5.
16. Brodmann K. Vergleichende Lokalisationslehre der Grosshirnrinde (in German). Leipzig: Johann Ambrosius Barth; 1909.
17. Garey LJ. Brodmann's localization in the cerebral cortex. New York: Springer; 2006.
18. Neuroangio. www.neuroangio.org.
19. Brown AG. Organization in the spinal cord. The anatomy and physiology of identified neurons: Springer-Verlag; 1981.
20. Davies AM, Lumsden A. Ontogeny of the somatosensory system: origins and early development of primary sensory neurons. Ann Rev Neurosci. 1990;13:61–73.
21. Eccles, J.C. and Schade, J.P. Organization of the Spinal Cord. Progress in Brain Research Volume 11. , 1964.
22. Aronson AE, et al. Clinical examination in neurology. 4th ed. Philadelphia: W.B. Saunders; 1977. p. 1–235.
23. Heilman KM, Watson RT, Greer M. Differential diagnosis of neurologic signs and symptoms. London: Appleton; 1977. p. 1–231.
24. Newman NJ. Practical neuro-ophthalmology. In: Tindall GT, Cooper PR, Barrow DL, editors. The practice of neurosurgery. Baltimore: Williams and Wilkins; 1996. p. 159–85.
25. Rengachary SS. Cranial nerve examination. In: Wilkins RH, Rengachary SS, editors. Neurosurgery. New York: McGraw-Hill; 1985. p. 50–70.
26. Ropper AH, Samuels M. Adams and Victor's principles of neurology. 9th ed. New York: McGraw-Hill; 2001. p. 1–1572.
27. Winn HR. Youman's neurological surgery, vol. I. Philadelphia: W.B. Saunders; 2011.

A Multidisciplinary Approach to Neurocritical Care

2

Sayona John

Contents

Abstract

This chapter provides a brief introduction into the history, need, development, and staffing of neurological intensive care units (ICUs). It describes the different models of ICUs that currently exist and their pros and cons. It also describes staffing models for physicians and advance practice providers (APPs). A special note has been made of the workflows in an ICU and the quality metrics of importance.

S. John (✉)
Department of Neurological Sciences, Rush University Medical Center, Chicago, IL, USA
e-mail: sayona_john@rush.edu

History and Evolution of Intensive Care Medicine

Intensive care or critical care medicine is the science and art of detecting and managing patients with life-threatening illnesses while preventing further deterioration, to achieve the best possible outcomes. It is a multidisciplinary and interprofessional specialty dedicated to the comprehensive management of patients having, or at risk of developing, acute, life-threatening organ dysfunction. The primary goal is to prevent further physiological deterioration while the underlying disease is treated and resolved [1].

The intensive care unit (ICU) is a specialized hospital unit dedicated to the care of patients requiring life support and those at an extremely high risk of organ failure and death.

Intensive care medicine as a specialty emerged in the 1950s with its beginnings in Copenhagen during the polio-

E. Mahanna Gabrielli et al. (eds.), *Textbook of Neurointensive Care: Volume 1*, https://doi.org/10.1007/978-3-031-62220-5_2

myelitis epidemic, where patients with respiratory failure were artificially ventilated [2]. The first known neurological ICU was established at the University of Colorado by Michael P. Earnest in 1969 [3]. The medical subspecialty of neurocritical care is devoted to the comprehensive multisystem care of critically ill neurology and neurological surgery patients. Like other intensivists, the neurointensivist assumes either primary or shared responsibility for the care of patients in the ICU, coordinating their neurological, surgical, and medical management..

The ICU is commonly located in proximity to other acute areas in the hospital such as the emergency room and the operating rooms, as most situations in the ICU are critically time-dependent. This also permits optimization of the timing of admissions to the ICU and safe, effective discharge of patients to a less intensive area of the hospital for the continued monitoring of resolving organ dysfunction [4].

The concept of levels of care was defined by a National Institutes of Health (NIH) consensus conference of critical care medicine at the Bethesda Conference in 1960 [5]. Based on the differences in staffing, available technology, and professional organizational structure of ICUs, the Bethesda Conference proposed the division of intensive care facilities into four groups: intensive care, high care, medium care, and low care. The two main criteria used in this classification were the availability of technological resources (type and intensity of use of specific monitoring and therapeutic interventions) and the availability of human resources (training and coverage by medical leadership and nurse-to-patient ratio).

The field of critical care medicine has embraced a standard, whereby care is provided by an interprofessional team that includes many disciplines [6]. This standard includes the collaboration of intensivists with specialty-trained nurses, advance practice providers (APPs), respiratory therapists, clinical pharmacists, clinical nutritionists, and physical, occupational, and speech therapists to provide optimal care to critically ill patients. Adherence to this standard has resulted in lower morbidity and mortality rates among ICU patients [7].

The limiting factor in the practice of intensive care at the ICU level is resource limitations or capacity strain. This occurs when the demand rises relative to supply, including more patients, shortage of supplies, or clinician shortage. A given number of practitioners in an ICU can take care of patients with varying complexities if other variables such as occupancy rate and length of stay are considered. The care of critically ill patients by intensivists and critical care nurses can improve patient-related outcomes as well as achieve a more efficient use of available resources. Improved outcomes include reduction in the rates of infections, decreased complications, reduced length of stay, and decreased mortality.

The concept of life support now extends to include other acute, potentially reversible disorders. Care now includes prevention of secondary complications of critical illnesses such as pressure ulcers, deep vein thrombosis, and stress ulcers. In the USA, a separate subspecialty of intensive care medicine has been created with specific training requirements and accreditation as an extension of internal medicine, anesthesiology, general surgery, pediatrics, and neurology training.

Need for Specialized Units

Several studies have now shown that it is important that patients in the ICU are cared for by physicians specialized in critical care medicine. Units with intensivists present lower mortality, better resource allocation with lower costs, and also shorter length of stay than do units without permanent doctors or specialists [8].

A recent meta-analysis of 12 studies encompassing 24,520 patients has presented original data comparing models of care for critically ill neurological patients and has revealed clear reduction in mortality and improved neurological outcomes for patients cared for in a specialized critical care unit [9].

Neurocritical Care as a Subspecialty

In the 1970s, stroke units began to appear, which were dedicated to the care of stroke patients, and are some of the direct precursors to modern neurocritical care units. Advances in anesthesiology for neurosurgery also generated a need for specialized postoperative care units. In the 1980s, evidence-based research in clinical neurology and neurosurgery began to take root, leading to improved diagnosis and therapy and prompting the inception of the first specialized neurocritical care units. This led to the need for physicians with expertise not only in the neurological and neurosurgical aspects of these patients but also in the principles of hemodynamic monitoring, mechanical ventilation, and management of multiple organ dysfunctions.

Despite the existence of specialized neurointensive care units, the presence of specialists in the area was not considered obligatory for the care of these patients. In the last decade, steps have been taken toward the recognition of this expertise. Neurocritical care as a subspecialty was accepted in the USA by the United Council of Neurologic Subspecialties (UCNS) in 2006 [10]. Medical training standards were established, and a period of 2 years was determined as the period needed for training of which 1 year must comprise continuous clinical work in an ICU [10]. Effective September 26, 2021, the Accreditation Council for Graduate

Medical Education (ACGME) has approved accreditation of programs in the subspecialty of neurocritical care and will be a multidisciplinary certificate cosponsored by the American Board of Psychiatry and Neurology (Administrative Board), the American Board of Anesthesiology, the American Board of Emergency Medicine, and the American Board of Neurological Surgery. The first certification exam was conducted in October of 2021.

The Neurocritical Care Society was founded in the USA in 2002 with the mission of promoting better quality of care for critically ill neurological and neurosurgical patients along with collaboration, research, training, and education..

Based on a proposed classification of ICUs, level I units are receiving centers for patients with complex neurological emergencies who require advanced interventions; these centers provide the most comprehensive neurocritical care. These units should be equipped to provide definitive and expert care to a wide variety of neurocritical care disorders using an interdisciplinary approach. Level I units offer a full complement of advanced monitoring and surgical and medical treatments, have the capability to provide physician fellowship and advanced practice professional training, and, as such, are often associated with an academic program. Level II units can stabilize acutely ill patients and safely manage stable neurocritical disease processes while having established relationships with level I neurocritical care units. Level III units can provide emergent evaluation and stabilization of patients presenting with neurological emergencies and facilitate transfer of these patients to level I and level II units when appropriate. Clearly delineated protocols and processes are necessary to identify patients for rapid referral and safe transfer once stable for advanced subspecialty care. Although a variety of systems to stratify stroke and trauma centers exist, and geographical and economic factors may shape the services offered, the system of stratification proposed here recognizes that high-quality neurocritical care services may be delivered in units without advanced research or academic or surgical programs, thus allowing for flexibility in developing a program to meet the needs of the patients of any region [11] (Table 2.1).

Table 2.1 ICU levels of care [12]

	Level 1	Level 2	Level 3
Therapeutic capacity	Physiologic stabilization and short-term support of mild organ dysfunction	Basic support of failing organ function	Complex, comprehensive support and management of organ dysfunction
Personnel	Physicians with some experience in critical care available at least during the day	Physicians with ICU training or comparable experience present during day and available at night	Physicians with formal ICU training on call 24/7; immediate in-hospital availability of medical staff with ICU experience
	Experienced nurses provide 24/7 care	Nurses have extra training or comparable experience in critical care and provide 24/7 care	Nursing staff with specialist ICU training provide 24/7 care
	Other personnel available	Variable inclusion of allied health personnel–respiratory therapists, physiotherapists, dieticians, pharmacists, etc–as part of ICU care team	Allied health personnel–respiratory therapists, physiotherapists, pharmacists, dieticians, etc–as regular members of ICU team
	Nurse-patient ratio higher than on ward; preferably 1:4 or 1:3 (1 nurse for 4 patients)	Nurse-patient ratio appropriate to patient needs but usually no less than 1:3	Nurse-patient ratio appropriate to patient needs and no less than 1:2
	Daily rounds; ad hoc structure	Formal daily ICU rounds with physicians and nurses	Formal multidisciplinary ICU rounds daily and as needed based on patient complexity and acuity
	Variable engagement in critical care continuing professional education	Engagement in continuing professional education	Regular engagement in continuing medical/nursing education
	Variable access to other medical specialties in hospital	Ready access to respirologists, nephrologists, cardiologists, infectious disease specialists, general surgeons	Rapid access to and variable engagement of full complement of medical and surgical consultant specialists
Monitoring capacity	Noninvasive or minimally invasive monitoring–transcutaneous oxygen saturation, cardiac monitoring, urine output	Invasive monitoring of blood pressure and central venous pressures as dictated by patient status	Advanced hemodynamic monitoring (cardiac catheterization, ultrasonography, etc); advanced monitoring of pulmonary, cerebral, and other physiology as directed by clinical needs
		Blood gas analyzer immediately available	Blood gas analyzer and star lab associated with ICU

(continued)

Table (continued)

	Level 1	Level 2	Level 3
Unit design and organ support	Dedicated geographic area	Dedicated geographic area with central monitoring station	Dedicated geographic area with individual patient care areas and central monitoring station
	Capacity for oxygen therapy and noninvasive respiratory support	Basic mechanical ventilatory support, pharmacologic support of cardiovascular function, intermittent renal replacement therapy, parenteral nutrition	Advanced ventilator and hemodynamic support, continuous renal replacement therapy, capacity for tracheostomy and other basic surgical procedures
			Capacity for isolation of patients needing contact or airborne precautions
Integration within the hospital	Defined geographic area only	Ad hoc interactions with other acute care areas such as emergency department	Outreach team(s), integration, with step-down or high-dependency unit; close collaboration, with emergency department
Research and education	Ad hoc activity	Organized educational activities for staff	Formal educational programs for staff
	Basic quality improvement program	Formal quality improvement program	Formal quality improvement program
		Ad hoc engagement in clinical research	Active involvement in clinical research
			Training of residents and fellows as available
Responsiveness to regional and societal needs	Ad hoc only, but available and responsive in event of disaster	Serves as resource for critically ill patients within hospital	Referral resource for community and district hospitals and for other ICUs
	Formal policy outlining criteria for patient transfer to higher level ICU		Disaster preparedness plan and capacity

Intensive Care Unit Organization

There are three common models of ICU organization:

- *An Open Unit*: Any physician with privileges to admit patients to the hospital can admit and care for patients in the ICU. Medical decisions are made by the admitting physician, often with the input of consultants, which may include intensivists. The perceived benefit of this model is continuity of care.
- *A Closed Unit*: All patients entering the ICU are admitted to the care of an intensivist for the duration of their ICU stay. The patient's primary physician may or may not remain closely involved in the care of the patient while in the ICU. This model is gaining acceptance in the United States based on research findings and response to the Leapfrog standard [13] and has shown lower mortality, fewer complications, and shorter ICU and hospital length of stay.
- *A Semi-Closed Unit*: In this model, the intensivist may participate in some or all of the patient's care while in the ICU, in conjunction with the patient's attending physician. The intensivist's role may be limited to triage functions and emergency response but more often includes hemodynamic, respiratory, fluid, and nutritional management. This model is common in surgical practices where the attending surgeon addresses the operative aspects of a patient's care, with the rest of the management directed by the intensivist[14].

Pronovost, et al. conducted a systematic review examining physician staffing patterns and clinical outcomes [8]. The model of care in each of 17 studies was classified as either low intensity (no intensivist or elective consultation) or high intensity (mandatory critical care consultation or a closed ICU). The high-intensity model was associated with lower ICU and hospital mortality. There is also evidence that hospital investment in physician intensivist services is recouped with better patient flow and lower utilization of pharmacy, laboratory, and radiology services. Having an intensivist round on postoperative patients shortens the length of stay, reduces complications, and lowers total hospital cost.

ICU Staffing

Physicians

The Leapfrog Organization ICU physician staffing (IPS) standards [13] were established after reviewing the published literature and have since been reviewed and revised incorporating current data and input from hospital and physician communities. Hospitals fulfilling the IPS standard operate ICUs that are managed or comanaged by:

1. Intensivists who are present during daytime hours and provide clinical care exclusively in the ICU.
2. Intensivists who, when not present on site or via telemedicine, return pages at least 95% of the time within 5 min and arrange for a physician, a physician assistant (PA), a nurse practitioner (NP), or an FCCS-certified nurse to reach ICU patients within 5 min [13] (FCCS is the course on Fundamental Critical Care Support of the Society of Critical Care Medicine.)

The number of physicians needed to adequately staff an ICU depends on the number of beds, the severity of illness, the number of hours spent in-house and on-call, the intensity of the services provided, the availability of consultants, nursing, and patient and family expectations. A clinical full-time equivalent (FTE) represents the amount of work done by one individual working only on patient care tasks in the intensive unit with in-house coverage for the ICU 24 h of the day, 7 days a week for 365 days; 4.2 FTEs would be needed to cover the workload. This workload might be met by five FTE physicians [14].

Nurses

The knowledge and expertise of the bedside nurse is a critical component in the delivery of high-quality neurocritical care. Nurses are generally the first provider to identify deterioration in patients and activate immediate responses. Nursing expertise in the management of neurocritical care patients requires additional orientation, ongoing education, and competency assessment. While specialty certification in neurocritical care is currently unavailable, nursing staff are generally specialty certified in critical care, neuroscience, stroke, neurovascular etc. Specialty certification in nursing allows nurses to demonstrate specialty knowledge in their area of practice and may be associated with improved patient outcomes [15].

Advance Practice Providers

The term "advance practice providers (APPs)" encompasses the roles that include nurse practitioners (NPs), clinical nurse specialists (CNSs), and physician assistants (PAs). NPs working in an ICU generally complete a 2-year master's degree after a 4-year registered nursing degree and undergo training in acute care (adult gerontology acute care NPs). NPs have to pass a national examination to obtain a license. Each state has established NP practice regulations, which vary from independent practice to restricted practice under the supervision of a physician. PAs must complete an accredited training program, usually 2 years in duration, and pass a national examination to obtain a license. PAs practice medicine under a physician's supervision [14]. Additional training in neurocritical care is necessary for all APPs prior to practice in a neurocritical care ICU.

The need for APPs in recent years has been primarily driven by cutbacks in federal funding for residency training, by the Accreditation Council for Graduate Medical Education standards placing limits on the duty hours for medical trainees, and by increasing patient care needs [14].

A few studies have shown that introduction of collaborative care by APPs and an intensivist is beneficial to patient outcomes, financial outcomes, length of stay, and patient satisfaction. In one study, patients managed by acute care nurse practitioners had a significantly shorter overall length of stay, a shorter mean length of stay in the ICU, lower rates of urinary tract infection and skin breakdown, and a shorter time to discontinuation of the Foley catheter and mobilization with total cost savings [16]. In addition, APPs can be trained and credentialed in procedures necessary in an ICU, which are within the scope of their practice and include line placements (triple lumen, hemodialysis catheters, and arterial) as well as lumbar puncture. APPs can also be engaged in quality and safety measures for the ICU.

Pharmacists

Pharmacy service is an essential component of ICU care. The Joint Commission and the Society of Critical Care Medicine recommend the integration of a dedicated pharmacist in the ICU [17, 18]. Medication errors are common, particularly during transition of care, leading to mortality and morbidity. Pharmacist interventions are an effective strategy to reduce these errors and improve the length of stay. Involvement of pharmacy service in an ICU also leads to reduction in medication costs and adverse drug interactions [17–19].

Additional Disciplines

Respiratory therapists skilled in the management of neurocritically ill patients require additional competency and training. Neurocritically ill patients may have clinical concerns, such as increased intracranial pressure, which may warrant a different approach to endotracheal intubation and mechanical ventilation. Patients in a neurocritical care unit, who are on the ventilator, may require a different level of ventilatory support as often the indication for ventilatory support is not primary pulmonary failure. Specific weaning parameters and ventilator settings are necessary for this patient population, especially in the setting of intracranial pressure crisis, status epilepticus, and coma. Effective communication with the respiratory therapist in defining the implications of ventilatory support and weaning is integral to safe patient care.

Physical, occupational, and speech language therapists are essential service providers in an ICU and should have expertise in the management of neurocritical care patients. Additionally, clinical nutritionists should also be available for the evaluation and management of these patients.

Workflow in an ICU

Optimal patient care in an ICU involves a complex interplay between multiple medical services utilizing a wide range of medicines, treatments, and procedures. Communication and information transfer within the team and between teams are key. A workflow describes a sequence of specific tasks performed by a single person or a team and is generally based on a set of procedural rules and aims at realization of an objective. A process is a specific notion that has a well-defined input, output, and purpose. Analyzing the workflow may help redesign work allocation strategies and improve productivity. Various scoring systems have been used to analyze nursing activities and workload. In contrast, few studies have been conducted to analyze physicians activities and workload [20].

Quality Metrics in an ICU

Quality of healthcare and intensive care unit care has become a national and international policy issue. Practice patterns and quality of medical care vary widely, and health-care providers are interested in having objective information about their performance. Publicly reported measures of quality of care are readily available for patients to review..

Health-care quality is defined as “the degree to which health services for individuals and populations increase the likelihood of desired health outcomes and are consistent with current professional knowledge.” The Institute of Medicine (IOM)s definition suggests a broad approach to measuring health-care quality, desired outcomes, and related processes of care. Outcomes are relative improvement in health and in experience/satisfaction that are achieved by the use of processes of care that are supported by scientific evidence and consumer preference [21].

Global quality measures include readmission to the ICU, ICU length of stay greater than 7 days, and ICU mortality rates. Complication measures include ventilator-associated pneumonia, infections related to the central venous catheter and indwelling urinary catheter, gastrointestinal bleeding, prolonged mechanical ventilation, transfusion-related complications, postoperative myocardial infarctions or cardiac death, deep vein thrombosis and pulmonary embolism, decubitus ulcers, and medication errors per ICU days. Quality measure also include patient and family satisfaction.

To improve quality of care, performance must be measured. By improving ICU quality measures, it may be possible to improve outcomes, such as reducing mortality, morbidity, and ICU length of stay. Controversy exists regarding whether performance measures should be interventions (process or structural) or outcomes. Process measures are easier to measure than are outcome measures and can be used to provide immediate feedback to providers regarding their performance and also provide validity of performance. However, outcome measures are the most important as they are ultimately what patients care about most. It is more important to select measures in which evidence regarding the association between the intervention and outcome is strong. Quality of care cannot improve in the absence of an intervention that improves patient outcomes [22].

The neurocritical care patient often requires multiple subspecialists, including neurosurgeons, neurointerventionalists, and stroke neurologists in addition to the neurointensivists. Interpersonal (including interprofessional) communication and collaboration are the key features of intensive care and the likely “critical zones” for medical errors [23]. Coordinating care amongst multiple specialties in order to avoid errors and duplication is a core skill of the intensivist. Four key teamwork processes have been consistently shown to predict outcomes in intensive care and include team communication, team leadership, team coordination, and team decision-making [24]. Standardized processes of care, including protocols, guidelines, checklists, and order sets, along with a predefined process of communication, can help prevent errors and reduce complications.

Pronovost, et al. focused on developing and implementing measures of ICU quality of care aimed at improving quality, noticing that many patients were not receiving the right therapy, which resulted in significant and preventable morbidity, mortality, and increased costs [25] (Table 2.2). Their results included suggestions on how to design and implement measures of quality using primary data collection. Suggested mechanisms to reduce errors included implementation of protocols, checklists, and scheduled multiple physician rounds. Protocols have been promoted as enhancing the efficiency, safety, and efficacy of care, as enabling more rigorous clinical research, and as facilitating education. Although protocols are easily applied to simple processes, their usefulness is debatable when more complex issues are involved [26]. An alternative to the protocol is the checklist. Vincent created the “Fast Hug” checklist, which highlights seven key aspects in the general care of all critically ill patients listing feeding, analgesia, sedation, thromboembolic prevention, head of the bed elevation, stress ulcer prophylaxis, and glucose control [27]. Checklists such as this may help improve quality of care in ICUs.

Table 2.2 Quality measures, definitions, and design specifications

Quality measure	Definition	Specifications
Outcome measures		
ICU mortality rate	Percentage of ICU discharges who die in the ICU (no risk adjustment; to be used for comparison over time within an ICU)	Numerator: Total number of ICU deaths
		Denominator: Total number of ICU discharges (including deaths and transfers)
Percentage of ICU patients, with ICU LOS >7 days	Percentage of ICU discharges with ICU LOS >7 days	Numerator: All ICU patients with ICU LOS >7 days
		Denominator: Total number of ICU discharges (including deaths and transfers)
Average ICU LOS	Average ICU LOS	Numerator: Sum of ICU length of stay for all discharges
		Denominator: Total number of ICU discharges (including deaths and transfers)
Average days on mechanical ventilation	Average days on mechanical ventilation	Numerator: Total number of ventilator days
		Denominator: Total number of intubated/trached patients, who were mechanically ventilated
Suboptimal management of pain	Percentage of 4-h intervals with a pain score > 3	Numerator: Number of 4-h intervals in which the pain score was >3
		Denominator: Total number of 4-h intervals
Patient/family satisfaction	To be developed	To be developed
Access measures		
Rate of delayed admissions	Rate of delay admissions to the ICU	Numerator: Number of admissions that are delayed for ≥4 h to the ICU (exclude transfers from outside hospitals)
		Denominator: Total number of ICU admissions (exclude transfers from outside hospitals)
Rate of delayed discharges	Rate of delay discharges from the ICU	Numerator: Number of discharges that are delayed for ≥4 from the ICU
		Denominator: Total number of ICU discharges
Canceled OR cases	Number of canceled OR cases due to lack of ICU beds	Numerator: Number of canceled OR cases owing to lack of ICU beds
		Denominator: None (if total number of OR cases are available, than these data can be presented as a rate)
Emergency department by-pass hours	Emergency department by-pass hours per month owing to lack of ICU beds	Numerator: Total by-pass hours per month that are caused by a lack of ICU beds
		Denominator: None
Complication measures		
Rate of unplanned ICU readmissions	Rate of unplanned ICU readmission	Numerator: Number of patients who had an unplanned ICU readmission within 48 h of ICU discharge
		Denominator: Total number of ICU discharges
Rate of catheter-related bloodstream infections	Rate of catheter-related bloodstream infections per 1000 catheter days	Numerator: Number of patients with catheter-related bloodstream; infections as defined by the CDC
		Denominator: Total number of catheter days in the ICU
Rate of resistant infections	Rate of new-onset resistant infections per ICU patient day	Numerator: Number of patients who developed resistant infections in the ICU (defined as MRSA or VRE infections)
		Denominator: Total ICU patient days
Process measures		
Appropriate sedation	The percentage of ventilator days on which: (1) sedation was held for at least 12 h or until the patient could follow commands or (2) if the patient followed commands without the need to hold sedation	Numerator: Number of ventilator days on which (1) sedation was held for ≥12 h or until the patient followed commands or (2) the patient followed commands without sedation held
		Denominator: Total ventilator days
Prevention of ventilator-associated pneumonia	The percentage of ventilator days on which the head of bed is elevated ≥30°	Numerator: Number of ventilator days on which the head of the bed was elevated ≥30°
		Denominator: Total number of ventilator days
Appropriate PUD prophylaxis	The percentage of ventilator days on which the patient received PUD prophylaxis	Numerator: Number of ventilator days on which the patient received PUD prophylaxis
		Denominator: Total ventilator days

(continued)

Table 2.2 (continued)

Quality measure	Definition	Specifications
Appropriate DVT prophylaxis	The percentage of ventilator days on which the patient received DVT prophylaxis	Numerator: Number of ventilator days on which the patient received DVT prophylaxis
		Denominator: Total ventilator days
Appropriate use of blood transfusions	The percentage of packed red blood cell transfusions for which the hemoglobin level before transfusion was <8 g/dL	Numerator: Number of packed red blood cell transfusions for which the hemoglobin level immediately before transfusion was <8 g/dL (include transfusions during episodes of massive bleeding (≥4 U/ h) and assume that these transfusions all had hemoglobin levels <8)
		Denominator: Total number of transfusions
Effective assessment of pain	Percentage of 4-h intervals for which each patient had a pain score documented with the visual analogue scale	Numerator: Number of 4-h intervals for each patient had their pain score measured with the visual analogue scale
		Denominator: Total number of 4-h intervals

Reprinted with permission of Elsevier from Pronovost et al. [23]

Abbreviations: *LOS* length of stay, *OR* operating room, *PUD* peptic ulcer disease, *DVT* deep vein thrombosis, *CDC* centers for disease control and prevention, *MRSA* methicillin-resistant *Staphylococcus aureus*, *VRE* vancomycin-resistant enterococcus

Teleneurointensive Care Unit (Teleneuro-ICU)

Telehealth is the delivery of health-care services by health-care professionals, where distance is a critical factor, through using information and communication technologies (ICTs) for the exchange of valid and correct information [28]. Teleneuro-ICUs provide the ability to conduct remote assessment of critically ill patients with neurological issues utilizing audiovisual (AV) technology [29]. When the physician performing the evaluation is a neurointensivist, the term "teleneurointensivist" is applicable. Given the shortages in physicians specialized in neurocritical care, telemedicine has provided a platform to expand provider reach in an efficient and cost-effective manner [30].

The basic requirement for Teleneuro-ICU evaluations is to have a reliable, high-quality AV conference call camera and interface. Several commercially available robotic platforms now exist, permitting network reliability and security as well as 24/7 on-call tech support to regain access immediately in case connectivity issues arise. Regulations associated with the Health Insurance Portability and Accountability Act (HIPAA) require any patient-related communication to be secured with encrypted information to protect the patient's confidentiality. Additional data that enhance evaluation include access to information, including neuroimaging via a picture archiving and communications system (PACS), laboratory data, electronic record data review of vital signs, and electroencephalography (EEG) data [29]. The ideal Teleneuro-ICU system is one that includes a high-quality, real-time, encrypted, audiovisual teleconferencing system; neuroimaging integration; mobility for site independence; decision and technical support features; electronic medical record integration; and billing and documentation that can be implemented across the World Wide Web [31].

To perform Teleneuro-ICU consultations effectively, a bedside nurse or physician is often necessary due to limitation of technology in performing parts of the neurological examination, particularly the cranial nerve exam. These personnel need to be trained in administration of the neurological exam, including the Glasgow Coma Scale (GCS) or the National Institutes of Health Stroke Scale (NIHSS). It is also critical to establishing protocols on when to activate Teleneuro-ICU evaluations for proper utilization and efficiency [29].

Benefits of Teleneuro-ICUs include increasing access to expert neurological consultations, improved access to specialists and emergency management of neurological injuries, faster transfers for emergent cases, and improved patient outcomes [32].

Limitations include costs associated with implementation and maintenance, lack of service providers, clinical limitations compared to bedside clinical examination, and availability of adequately trained support staff and equipment [32].

Impact of COVID-19 on Healthcare

International hospitals and health-care facilities faced catastrophic financial challenges related to the COVID-19 pandemic [33]. During the first wave of the COVID-19 pandemic, use of health-care services dropped precipitously, with most healthcare not directly related to treating patients with COVID-19 shut down [34]. Shutting down non-COVID-19-related care also drove down the demand for health-care workers not directly involved in COVID-19 care [35]. Additionally, large numbers of health-care workers left healthcare as a result of stress and burnout that occurred due to the pandemic, seeking work in other sectors or leaving the labor market altogether [34]. Although health employment in many facilities has nearly returned to pre-pandemic levels, the effects of the pandemic linger [36]. Nurses have experienced many untoward effects on their physical, psychological, and social health [37]. The health-care industry reported a loss of 30% of the nursing workforce, leading to the era of "the great resignation" [38]. The pandemic has also significantly undermined health insurance coverage in the United States [39]. All these factors have led to telemedicine emerging as an indispensable resource to improve the surveillance of patients, curb the spread of disease, facilitate timely identification and management of ill people, and guarantee continuity of care for patients.

Conclusions

Neurocritical care like other critical care specialty is driven by a multidisciplinary approach. Providers with expertise in neurocritical care are the foundation of this specialty. The goal of a multidisciplinary approach is to leverage the expertise of each of these specialists in providing high-quality care, leading to improved outcomes for patients.

References

1. Marshall JC, Bosco L, Adhikari NK, et al. What is an intensive care unit? A report of the task force of the world Federation of Societies of intensive and critical care medicine. J Crit Care. 2017;37:270–6.
2. Lassen HC. A preliminary report on the 1952 epidemic of poliomyelitis in Copenhagen with special reference to the treatment of acute respiratory insufficiency. Lancet (London, England). 1953;1:37–41.
3. Bleck TP. Historical aspects of critical care and the nervous system. Crit Care Clin. 2009;25(153–64):ix.
4. Moreno R, Miranda DR, Matos R, Fevereiro T. Mortality after discharge from intensive care: the impact of organ system failure and nursing workload use at discharge. Intensive Care Med. 2001;27:999–1004.
5. Lockward HJ, Giddings L, Thoms EJ. Progressive patient care. A preliminary report. JAMA J Am Med Assoc. 1960;172:132–7.
6. Weled BJ, Adzhigirey LA, Hodgman TM, et al. Critical care delivery: the importance of process of care and ICU structure to improved outcomes: an update from the American College of Critical Care Medicine Task Force on models of critical care. Crit Care Med. 2015;43:1520–5.
7. Curtis JR, Cook DJ, Wall RJ, et al. Intensive care unit quality improvement: a "how-to" guide for the interdisciplinary team. Crit Care Med. 2006;34:211–8.
8. Pronovost PJ, Angus DC, Dorman T, Robinson KA, Dremsizov TT, Young TL. Physician staffing patterns and clinical outcomes in critically ill patients: a systematic review. JAMA. 2002;288:2151–62.
9. Kramer AH, Zygun DA. Do neurocritical care units save lives? Measuring the impact of specialized ICUs. Neurocrit Care. 2011;14:329–33.
10. Mayer SA, Coplin WM, Chang C, et al. Core curriculum and competencies for advanced training in neurological intensive care: united Council for Neurologic Subspecialties guidelines. Neurocrit Care. 2006;5:159–65.
11. Moheet AM, Livesay SL, Abdelhak T, et al. Standards for neurologic critical care units: a statement for healthcare professionals from the Neurocritical care society. Neurocrit Care. 2018;29:145–60.
12. Marshall JC, Bosco L, Adhikari NK, Connolly B, Diaz JV, Dorman T, Fowler RA, Meyfroidt G, Nakagawa S, Pelosi P, Vincent JL, Vollman K, Zimmerman J. What is an intensive care unit? A report of the task force of the world Federation of Societies of intensive and critical care medicine. J Crit Care. 2017;37:270–6.
13. The Leapfrog Group. http://www.leapfroggroup.org. Accessed 12 Dec 2021.
14. Irwin RS. Irwine and Rippe's intensive care medicine. 6th ed. Philadelphia: Lippincott Williams & Wilkins; 2007.
15. Fleischman RK, Meyer L, Watson C. Best practices in creating a culture of certification. AACN Adv Crit Care. 2011;22:33–49.
16. Russell D, VorderBruegge M, Burns SM. Effect of an outcomes-managed approach to care of neuroscience patients by acute care nurse practitioners. Am J Crit Care. 2002;11:353–62.
17. Weant KA, Armitstead JA, Ladha AM, Sasaki-Adams D, Hadar EJ, Ewend MG. Cost effectiveness of a clinical pharmacist on a neurosurgical team. Neurosurgery. 2009;65:946–50; discussion 50–1.
18. Oliveira D, Gildasio S Jr, Castro-Alves LJ, Kendall MC, McCarthy R. Effectiveness of pharmacist intervention to reduce medication errors and health-care resources utilization after transitions of care: a meta-analysis of randomized controlled trials. J Patient Saf. 2021;17:375–80.
19. MacLaren R, Bond CA, Martin SJ, Fike D. Clinical and economic outcomes of involving pharmacists in the direct care of critically ill patients with infections. Crit Care Med. 2008;36:3184–9.
20. Flaatten HMR, Putensen C, Rhodes A. Organization and management of intensive care. Berlin: Medical Scientific Publishing GmbH; 2010.
21. Palmer RH. Process-based measures of quality: the need for detailed clinical data in large health care databases. Ann Intern Med. 1997;127:733–8.
22. Berenholtz SM, Dorman T, Ngo K, Pronovost PJ. Qualitative review of intensive care unit quality indicators. J Crit Care. 2002;17:1–12.
23. Malhotra S, Jordan D, Shortliffe E, Patel VL. Workflow modeling in critical care: piecing together your own puzzle. J Biomed Inform. 2007;40:81–92.
24. Reader TW, Flin R, Mearns K, Cuthbertson BH. Developing a team performance framework for the intensive care unit. Crit Care Med. 2009;37:1787–93.
25. Pronovost PJ, Berenholtz SM, Ngo K, et al. Developing and pilot testing quality indicators in the intensive care unit. J Crit Care. 2003;18:145–55.
26. Brattebø G, Hofoss D, Flaatten H, Muri AK, Gjerde S, Plsek PE. Effect of a scoring system and protocol for sedation on duration of patients' need for ventilator support in a surgical intensive care unit. BMJ. 2002;324:1386–9.
27. Vincent JL. Give your patient a fast hug (at least) once a day. Crit Care Med. 2005;33:1225–9.
28. Monaghesh E, Hajizadeh A. The role of telehealth during COVID-19 outbreak: a systematic review based on current evidence. BMC Public Health. 2020;20(1):1193.
29. William D, Freeman MD, Rincon F, Vatz KA. Teleneurointensive Care Unit (TeleneuroICU): Expanding the reach of subspecialty neuroicu care. teleneurology in practice, a comprehensive clinical guide. New York, NY: Springer New York. p. 59–74.
30. Angus DC, Kelley MA, Schmitz RJ, White A, Popovich J Jr. Committee on manpower for pulmonary and critical care societies (COMPACCS). Caring for the critically ill patient. Current and projected workforce requirements for care of the critically ill and patients with pulmonary disease: can we meet the requirements of an aging population? JAMA. 2000;284(21):2762–70.

31. Switzer JA, Levine SR, Hess DC. Telestroke 10 years later–'telestroke 2.0'. Cerebrovasc Dis. 2009;28:323–30.
32. Klein KE, Rasmussen PA, Winners SL, Frontera JA. Teleneurocritical care and telestroke. Crit Care Clin. 2015 Apr;31(2):197–224. https://doi.org/10.1016/j.ccc.2014.12.002.
33. Kaye AD, et al. Economic impact of COVID-19 pandemic on healthcare facilities and systems: international perspectives. Best Pract Res Clin Anaesthesiol. 2021;35(3):293–306.
34. Wilensky GR. The COVID-19 pandemic and the US health care workforce. JAMA Health Forum. 2022;3(1):e220001.
35. Cutler D. How COVID-19 changes the economics of health care. *JAMA health*. Forum. 2021;2(9):e213309. https://doi.org/10.1001/jamahealthforum.2021.3309.
36. Zhang X, Tai D, Pforsich H, Lin VW. United States registered nurse workforce report card and shortage forecast: a revisit. Am J Med Qual 2018;33(3):229–236. doi:https://doi.org/10.1177/1062860617738328.
37. Lopez V, et al. Does the COVID-19 pandemic further impact nursing shortages? Issues Ment Health Nurs. 2022;43(3):293–5.
38. Kurtzman ET, et al. Nursing workforce challenges in the postpandemic world. J Nurs Regul. 2022;13(2):49.
39. Blumenthal D, et al. Covid-19—implications for the health care system. N Engl J Med. 2020;383(15):1483–8.

Fundamentals of Neuroradiological Imaging

3

Otto Rapalino

Contents

O. Rapalino (✉)
Neuroradiology Division, Department of Radiology, Massachusetts General Hospital, Boston, MA, USA
e-mail: orapalino@mgh.harvard.edu

E. Mahanna Gabrielli et al. (eds.), *Textbook of Neurointensive Care: Volume 1*, https://doi.org/10.1007/978-3-031-62220-5_3

Abstract

Radiological imaging techniques have a central role in the management of critically ill neurological patients. This chapter describes the basic physical concepts, potential clinical applications, strengths, and weaknesses of neuroradiological imaging. It provides examples of the rational use of the most frequently used imaging modalities, including plain radiographs, computed tomography (CT), magnetic resonance imaging (MRI), ultrasound, positron emission tomography (PET), and digital subtraction angiography (DSA). This chapter aims to equip healthcare personnel with a basic understanding of the neuroimaging techniques that are essential for making accurate clinical decisions in the neurointensive care unit (neuro-ICU) environment. These techniques have undergone significant advancements and can now be performed at the bedside, which decreases the need to move patients out of the neuro-ICU. It is important to use these techniques rationally by considering both their strengths and weaknesses, which will optimize their use in the neurointensive care setting.

Introduction

In the neurointensive care unit (neuro-ICU), where critical patients require fast and accurate diagnostic and therapeutic decisions, neuroradiological imaging plays a crucial role. These imaging techniques allow the neuro-ICU team to visualize pathological changes, which are used for diagnostic, therapeutic, and prognostic purposes. Some of the most frequent clinical indications for these imaging modalities include ischemic stroke, hemorrhage, traumatic brain injury, and central nervous system (CNS) infections [1] (Table 3.1). Additionally, this chapter summarizes the status of advanced imaging techniques, such as photon-counting computed tomography (PCCT), computed tomography (CT) perfusion (CTP) and magnetic resonance imaging (MRI)-based perfusion, diffusion imaging, and functional MRI (fMRI).

Table 3.1 Accuracy of different imaging modalities for the common pathologies seen in the neuro-ICU

Pathology	CT	MRI	PET
Infarcts	Low to moderate (depending on lesional size)	High	Low
Hemorrhage	High for acute hemorrhage	High	Low
Intracranial neoplastic disease	Low to moderate (depending on lesional size)	High	Low
Nonconvulsive status	Low	High (particularly with perfusion imaging)	High
Encephalitis	Low to moderate	High	Low
Hydrocephalus	High	High	Low

Plain Radiographs

Basic Concepts

Radiographs, or X-rays, generate medical images using ionizing radiation. An X-ray tube produces photons called X-rays by accelerating electrons and colliding them with a metallic target, usually tungsten, in a vacuum-sealed tube. These X-rays are then directed through the desired anatomical target onto a detector film on the other side. As these X-rays pass through different tissues, they are attenuated to varying degrees based on the density and composition of the tissues. The detector captures the two-dimensional (2D) pattern of differential X-ray attenuation within the target anatomy.

Strengths and Weaknesses

The main strengths of plain radiographs are its wide availability, fast acquisition times, and portability owing to its convenience of use in the neuro-ICU. Although plain radiographs are frequently used in the neurointensive care setting to image the chest, abdomen, and extremities, this modality has a limited role in imaging the central nervous system due to its poor visualization of intracranial contents. Plain radiographs are often reserved for evaluating ventricular shunts and foreign bodies (e.g., clearance of orbits before MRI). Other weaknesses include the requirement of ionizing radiation and the overlap of anatomical structures intrinsic to 2D imaging using a single beam of X-rays. Despite these limitations, plain radiographs are one of the most used imaging techniques in the neuro-ICU.

Clinical Applications

Plain radiographs are typically used for imaging the chest and abdominal cavities in neuro-ICU patients. Neuroimaging applications of plain radiographs include evaluating ventricular shunt systems [2] (to detect focal disconnection or programmable valve settings) or foreign bodies (e.g., metallic fragments near the orbits). Plain radiographs that are used for evaluating craniofacial and spinal trauma are increasingly being replaced by computed tomography due to the latter's higher accuracy in detecting fractures and in identifying other post-traumatic abnormalities.

Rational Use

The judicious use of plain radiographs for chest and abdominal imaging in the neuro-ICU is a well-established protocol. Plain radiographs still provide the best possible in-plane resolution for applications such as the noninvasive visualization of ventriculoperitoneal (VP) shunt valve parameters. Their convenience makes portable plain radiographs easier to obtain for some applications, such as the assessment of VP shunt tubes and foreign bodies. However, computed tomography is likely more accurate for these indications. Computed tomography has a well-established superior accuracy for evaluating craniofacial and spinal trauma and should be an imaging modality of choice.

Computed Tomography

Basic Concepts

Similar to plain radiographs, computed tomography (CT) imaging depends on the distinct attenuation of X-ray beams that pass through the body's various tissues. CT scanners have X-ray tubes that rotate and emit fan-shaped beams of X-rays, which detectors on the opposite side receive. Different tissues have distinct attenuation coefficients measured in Hounsfield units, which result in varying amounts of X-rays hitting the detectors. The detectors then convert the detected X-rays into electrical signals that a computer with specialized reconstruction algorithms processes to create cross-sectional images. The use of contrast-containing iodine enables the visualization of blood vessels and areas of higher vascular permeability due to the greater attenuation of iodine present in the contrast material at typical energy levels of the X-ray beams.

Strengths and Weaknesses

Computed tomography imaging is a quick and efficient technique that can produce a non-contrast head CT acquisition in under 60 s. This is especially useful for patients who cannot tolerate longer acquisition times, such as children or uncooperative patients. Head CT is particularly good at evaluating high- and low-attenuation densities, such as osseous, metal, fat, or air pathologies. However, its specificity decreases in the intermediate range of attenuation values. The in-plane spatial resolution of CT imaging is generally excellent, but differentiating between tissues with similar attenuation values can be challenging. It is worth noting that the use of ionizing radiation is a potential drawback, particularly for patients who require repeated imaging or multiple CT modalities, including CT perfusion.

Clinical Applications

In clinical practice, there are various CT techniques that allow for the visualization of intracranial contents with or without contrast, assessment of vascular anatomy and pathology, intracranial perfusion, and tissue characterization. CT is commonly used as the first neuroimaging step, especially for adult patients in the emergency room and outpatient setting. For pathologies such as acute ischemic stroke, trauma, or intracranial hemorrhage, computed tomography is the preferred imaging method. Additionally, CT is ideal for evaluating pathologies that affect osseous structures and the overlying soft tissues.

Rational Use

Computed tomography is indicated in the evaluation of intracranial hemorrhage, acute ischemic stroke, intracranial traumatic injury, and craniocervical fractures. CT angiography (CTA) will provide a more accurate visualization of the intracranial and cervical arteries compared to MR angiography (MRA). CT techniques are much faster compared to MR and nuclear medicine techniques and are particularly helpful in patients who cannot tolerate long scanning times. MRI should be considered in patients with pathologies such as acute cerebral ischemia, encephalitis, and other nonhemorrhagic cerebral pathologies [3] that are stable enough to travel to the MRI suite and tolerate the length of a brain MRI examination.

Conventional Computed Tomography

The attenuation values on CT images (Hounsfield units) are used for tissue characterization, and the typical ranges and relevant tissue identities are the following: air <−1000; fat between −120 and − 30; cerebrospinal fluid (CSF) 0–10; white matter 25; muscle/soft tissues 20–40; gray matter 35; hemorrhage 60–100; calcifications 60–>1000; and iodinated CT contrast 100–600.

Computed tomography is often used to diagnose acute ischemic stroke, intracranial hemorrhage, intracranial masses, hydrocephalus, or brain herniation. Non-contrast CT imaging is superior to magnetic resonance imaging in visualizing osseous structures and calcified lesions. However, MRI is superior to CT for visualizing most intracranial pathologies.

Intracranial hemorrhage will appear hyperdense on CT images during the acute to early subacute stages, but it will become isodense and eventually hypodense during the subacute and chronic stages, respectively (Fig. 3.1) (Table 3.2).

Hyperacute cerebral ischemia is often difficult to detect on CT images, but the sensitivity of CT is higher after 6–12 h and in the later stages of ischemic lesions (Table 3.3). Subacute infarcts can sometimes be more difficult to visualize due to the development of "fogging."

Non-contrast CT images have limited sensitivity for detecting intracranial masses, and the use of contrast increases the sensitivity of the CT technique. However, even with contrast, CT imaging has lower sensitivity for detecting intracranial neoplastic disease compared to MRI. Additional CT signs, such as the hyperdense vessel sign, increase the sensitivity of CT imaging to detect acute cerebral ischemia.

CT imaging is helpful for the assessment of the ventricular system and cortical sulci. The development of hydrocephalus or cerebral edema can be diagnosed using CT images in the intensive care unit (ICU).

Table 3.2 Appearance of intracranial hemorrhage on different imaging techniques

Stage	CT	T1-weighted MRI	T2-weighted MRI
Hyperacute	Hyperdense	Hypointense or isointense	Isointense to hyperintense
Acute	Hyperdense	Hypointense to isointense	Hypointense
Early subacute	Isodense to hyperdense	Hyperintense	Hypointense
Late subacute	Isodense to hyperdense	Hyperintense	Hyperintense
Chronic	Hypodense	Centrally T1 isointense to hypointense, peripherally hypointense	Centrally hyperintense, peripherally hypointense

Table 3.3 Appearance of cerebral infarcts on different imaging modalities

Stage	CT	DWI	ADC
Hyperacute	Isointense to hypodense	Hyperintense	Hypointense
Acute	Hypodense	Hyperintense	Hypointense
Early subacute (1–7 days)	Hypodense with variable mass effect	Hyperintense	Hypointense
Late subacute (7–21 days)	Hypodense with or without local mass effect	Hyperintense	Isointense to hyperintense
Chronic	Hypodense with volume loss	Hyperintense to isointense	Isointense

DWI diffusion-weighted imaging, *ADC* apparent diffusion coefficient

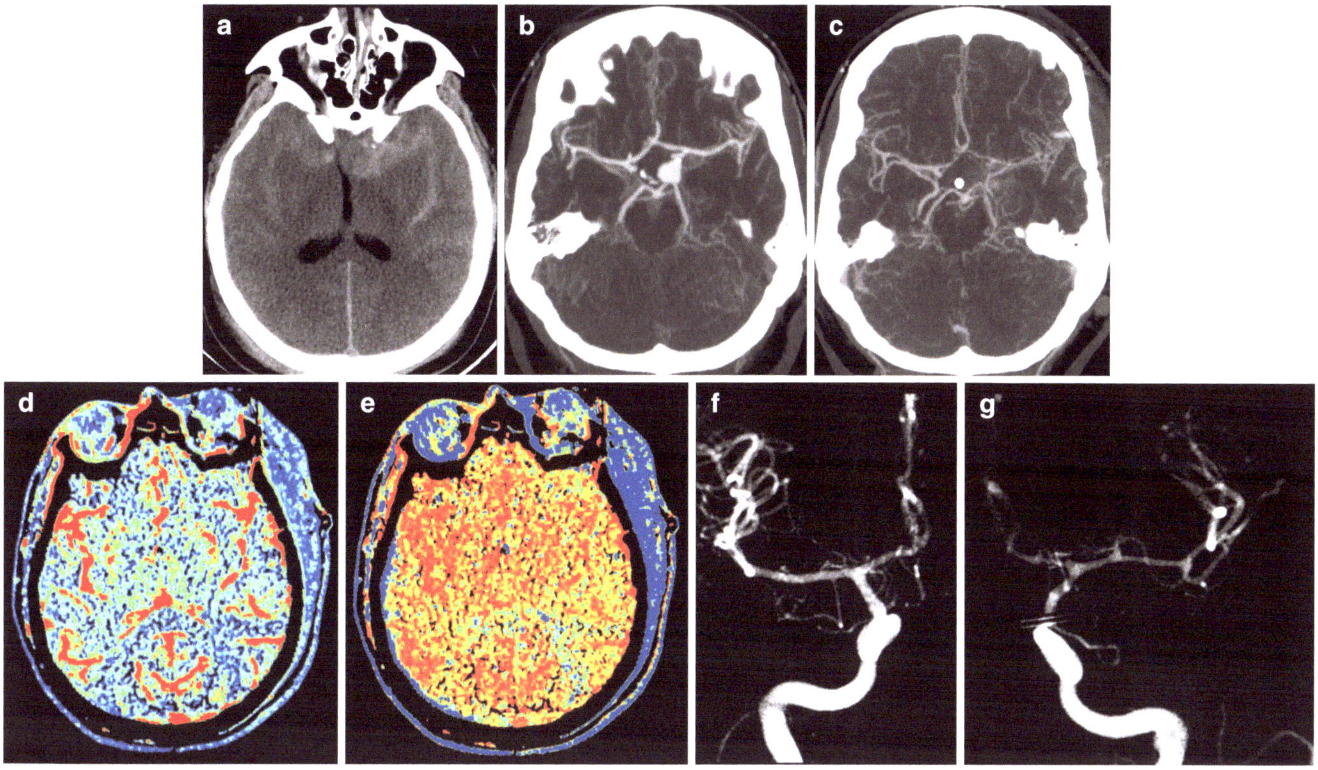

Fig. 3.1 Subarachnoid hemorrhage secondary to a ruptured left posterior communicating artery aneurysm complicated with vasospasm. Non-contrast head CT (**a**) shows extensive areas of acute subarachnoid hemorrhage in the left supraclinoid region and bilateral MCA cisterns (left greater than right). Head CT angiograms before (**b**) and after (**c**) the surgical clipping of the aneurysm show the interval development of extensive segments of luminal narrowing in the left M1, bilateral A1, and left P2 segments compatible with vasospasm. Similar vascular changes can be seen in DSA (**f**, **g**). CT perfusion maps show minimally decreased CBF (**d**) but a more significant increase of MTT values (**e**) in the left MCA territory. *MCA* middle cerebral artery, *DSA* digital subtraction angiography

Computed Tomography Angiography

CT angiography (CTA) is a commonly used imaging modality when evaluating the cerebral and cervical vasculature. This technique involves administering an iodine-based contrast agent through an intravenous (IV) route, followed by fast high-resolution CT scanning timed either at a specific interval or with aortic arch opacification. This allows visualization of the vascular lumen in the arteries or veins depending on the timing after contrast administration. CT angiography plays a critical role in the imaging assessment of patients with suspected acute ischemic stroke for identifying large vessel occlusion, sites of arterial stenosis, or dissection. Additionally, it is used to evaluate acute intracranial hemorrhage for determining the presence of an aneurysm, vascular malformation, vasospasm, or focal extravasation within the hematoma (spot sign) (Fig. 3.1) [4]. This technique is also vital for the planning and postprocedural follow-up of endovascular or surgical vascular interventions in critically ill neuro-ICU patients. Although CT angiography is more accurate than is non-contrast MRA for detecting vascular abnormalities, it is not as precise as conventional angiography.

Computed Tomography Perfusion (CTP)

CT perfusion of the brain is an advanced technique that allows the noninvasive evaluation of different perfusion parameters in the brain parenchyma [5, 6]. It involves obtaining a series of CT images before, during, and after administering an intravenous iodine-based contrast agent to analyze attenuation changes in the cerebral vessels and parenchyma. Semiquantitative maps of cerebral blood flow (CBF), cerebral blood volume (CBV), mean transit time (MTT), and time to peak (TTP) are generated to provide information about the hemodynamics and perfusion of the brain parenchyma. CT perfusion is particularly useful for managing acute ischemic stroke as it helps identify the ischemic core (CBF <30%) and ischemic penumbra (Tmax >6 s). It is also helpful for assessing vasospasm after subarachnoid hemorrhage, brain tumors, cerebral perfusion in patients with high-grade arterial stenosis, or moyamoya after a revascularization procedure (Fig. 3.1). CT scanners can also use xenon to obtain perfusion images [7].

Dual-Energy Computed Tomography (DECT) and Spectral Computed Tomography

Dual-energy CT (DECT) and spectral CT are state-of-the-art computed tomography techniques that utilize two X-ray energy levels to create images and enable the identification of materials based on their energy-dependent attenuation properties. Dual-energy CT scanners use two X-ray tubes with different energy levels or rapidly alternate between energies using a single tube. On the other hand, spectral CT scanners use detectors that can distinguish and sort incoming X-rays into different energy levels. The data gathered through these modalities can be processed after scanning to produce material-specific images and quantitative maps, such as virtual non-contrast images and iodine maps, respectively. Dual-energy and spectral CT have numerous clinical uses in neuroimaging, such as distinguishing between hemorrhage and contrast staining following endovascular procedures and enhancing the quality of intravascular angiographic opacification.

Portable Computed Tomography (PCT)

Portable CT scanners are smaller and mobile versions of conventional fixed CT scanners, with similar physical principles, and have been created to be movable and available at the patient's bedside, particularly helpful in the neuro-ICU for patients that are unstable or critically ill, thus avoiding their transportation outside of the monitored ICU environment [8, 9]. Portable CT scanners help evaluate major acute neurological events, including large acute intracranial hemorrhage, large territorial infarcts, progressive mass effect, or brain herniation. These portable CT scanners also allow the follow-up imaging of intracranial pathologies at the bedside.

Photon-Counting Computed Tomography

Photon-counting computed tomography (PCCT) is a relatively new advanced CT imaging modality that allows the detection of and digitally quantifies individual X-ray photons [10]. Due to these capabilities, PCCT enables the acquisition of CT images with higher resolution and contrast-to-noise ratios. It also allows better material differentiation (e.g., distinguishing between iodine and calcium) and lower radiation exposures.

Magnetic Resonance Imaging

Basic Concepts

Magnetic resonance imaging is a revolutionary medical imaging modality based on the differential excitation of cerebral tissues by magnetic fields and uses the signal generated after these excitations to create images [11].

Strengths and Weaknesses

MRI is the most accurate technique for diagnosing acute cerebral ischemia, intracranial hemorrhage, intracranial neoplastic disease, and many other intracranial pathologies. It has a more limited sensitivity for diagnosing some osseous pathologies (e.g., skull fractures). The use of magnetic fields can be a contraindication in patients with passive and active metallic implants. Acquisition times are typically longer compared to those of CT imaging.

Clinical Applications [11]

Magnetic resonance techniques can be used for structural imaging (brain MRI), visualization of vascular structures (MR angiography), cerebral perfusion, functional activity (fMRI), and assessment of cerebral metabolism (MR spectroscopy) [11].

MRI has a high sensitivity (>85%) for detecting acute cerebral ischemia. However, false-negative MRI scans occasionally occur. The rate of these diffusion-negative infarcts varies from 5% to 15%, and these diffusion-negative infarcts are often located in the brain stem.

MRI has a high sensitivity for detecting all stages of intracranial hemorrhage, often with a higher sensitivity than CT.

MRI is the gold standard for diagnosing many pathologies seen in the neuro-ICU, including acute infarcts, white matter disorders, and neoplastic processes.

Portable MRI scanners that can be helpful for limited structural imaging [12–16] are now commercially available.

Rational Use

Magnetic resonance imaging is the radiological modality of choice for many clinical indications [11, 17]. If the patient is clinically stable, then MRI will be the most accurate imaging modality for detecting ischemic changes, hemorrhage, metabolic changes, CNS infection, and CNS inflammation. Patients requiring fast imaging will benefit from using CT imaging instead, as most of the MRI sequences are significantly longer compared to the typical acquisition time of a CT scan (Fig. 3.2) (Table 3.4).

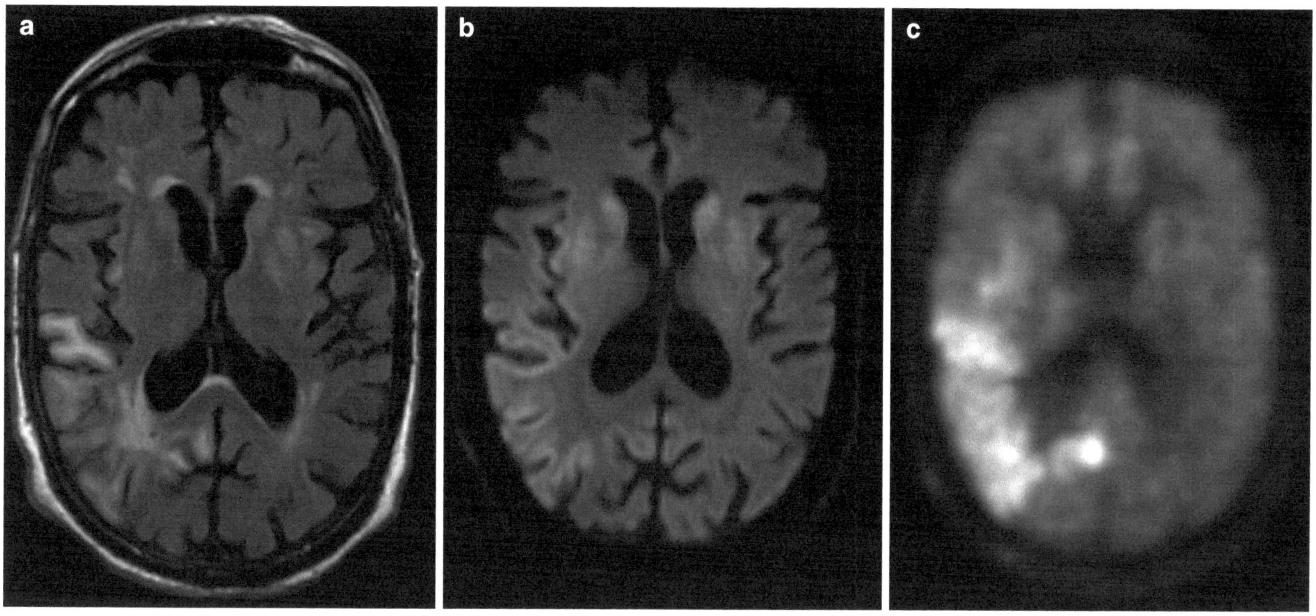

Fig. 3.2 Focal encephalitis with nonconvulsive partial status. Axial FLAIR image (**a**) shows focal FLAIR hyperintense signal abnormalities in the right temporoparietal parenchyma associated with subtle cortical restricted diffusivity on the diffusion-weighted image (**b**) and focal hyperperfusion on the ASL image (**c**). *FLAIR* fluid attenuated inversion recovery, *ASL* arterial spin labeling

Table 3.4 Main MRI sequences used in clinical practice

Sequence	Clinical value
T1	Accurate anatomical definition, detection of fat-containing lesions, proteinaceous material, mineralization, and subacute hemorrhage. Enhancement after injection of gadolinium
T2	Visualization of fluid-containing structures or abnormalities
FLAIR	Suppression of the CSF signal allows improved visualization of white matter or sulcal abnormalities
T2* (e.g., GRE, SWI)	Detection of hemorrhage or mineralization. SWI is the most sensitive imaging modality for detection of hemorrhage
Diffusion-weighted imaging and diffusion tensor imaging (DWI and DTI, respectively)	Restricted diffusion with low ADC values seen in hyperacute to early subacute infarcts, pyogenic infections with purulent material, and hypercellular lesions (e.g., lymphoma, medulloblastoma)
Perfusion: Arterial spin labeling (ASL), dynamic susceptibility contrast (DSC), and dynamic contrast enhanced (DCE) techniques	Penumbral stroke imaging, detection of vasospasm, and evaluation of intracranial masses. ASL relies on the CBF maps, DSC perfusion allows the creation of multiple DSC perfusion-derived maps, and DCE describes vascular permeability
Contrast-enhanced post-contrast T1-weighted images	Enhancement reflects increased vascular permeability with leakage of contrast. This can be helpful in the evaluation of many different neurological disorders, including infectious, inflammatory, and neoplastic pathologies
Magnetic resonance angiography	Visualization of arteries and/or veins using endogenous (non-suppressed incoming intraluminal protons) and exogenous contrast material (gadolinium-containing compounds)
Functional MRI	Changes in local tissue perfusion during neuronal activity result in increased washout of deoxyhemoglobin, resulting in increased signal on echo planar images (EPI) images (blood oxygen-level-dependent effect). These changes can occur secondary to specific tasks (task-based) or during rest (resting state fMRI)
Magnetic resonance spectroscopy	Noninvasive assessment of specific metabolites based on their signal characteristics (including N-Acetylaspartate (NAA), choline, lactate, etc.)

ADC apparent diffusion coefficient, *FLAIR* fluid attenuated inversion recovery, *GRE* gradient echo sequence, *SWI* susceptibility-weighted imaging
*T2-weighted MRI

Nuclear Medicine

Basic Concepts

Several nuclear medicine techniques are used in the neuro-ICU, including single-photon emission computed tomography (SPECT) and positron emission tomography (PET). SPECT is a radiological technique that uses the gamma radiation directly produced by a radiopharmaceutical to create medical images and is often used to diagnose brain death and epilepsy cases [18, 19] (Fig. 3.3). PET imaging (18) is another nuclear imaging technique based on positron-emitting radioisotopes, and it can be used to detect nonconvulsive status and characterize focal intracranial pathologies [20, 21] (Table 3.5).

Strengths and Weaknesses

Nuclear medicine techniques allow the visualization of pathological conditions using specific molecular probes that can be incorporated into their metabolic pathways. The visualization of metabolic changes with these imaging techniques provides alternative information compared to conventional structural imaging techniques and can be more sensitive or specific for some conditions. The relatively lower spatial and temporal resolution of these imaging modalities and the use of ionizing radiation constitute these techniques' main limitations and weaknesses.

Clinical Applications

Nuclear medicine techniques in the neuro-ICU, particularly PET, have multiple clinical applications, including the evaluation of epileptic syndromes and status epilepticus, autoimmune encephalopathies, large vessel vasculitis, and the determination of brain death [18, 20, 22, 23].

Rational Use

SPECT and PET techniques have specific clinical indications highlighted in the previous paragraphs. These imaging techniques take longer to acquire, and patients should

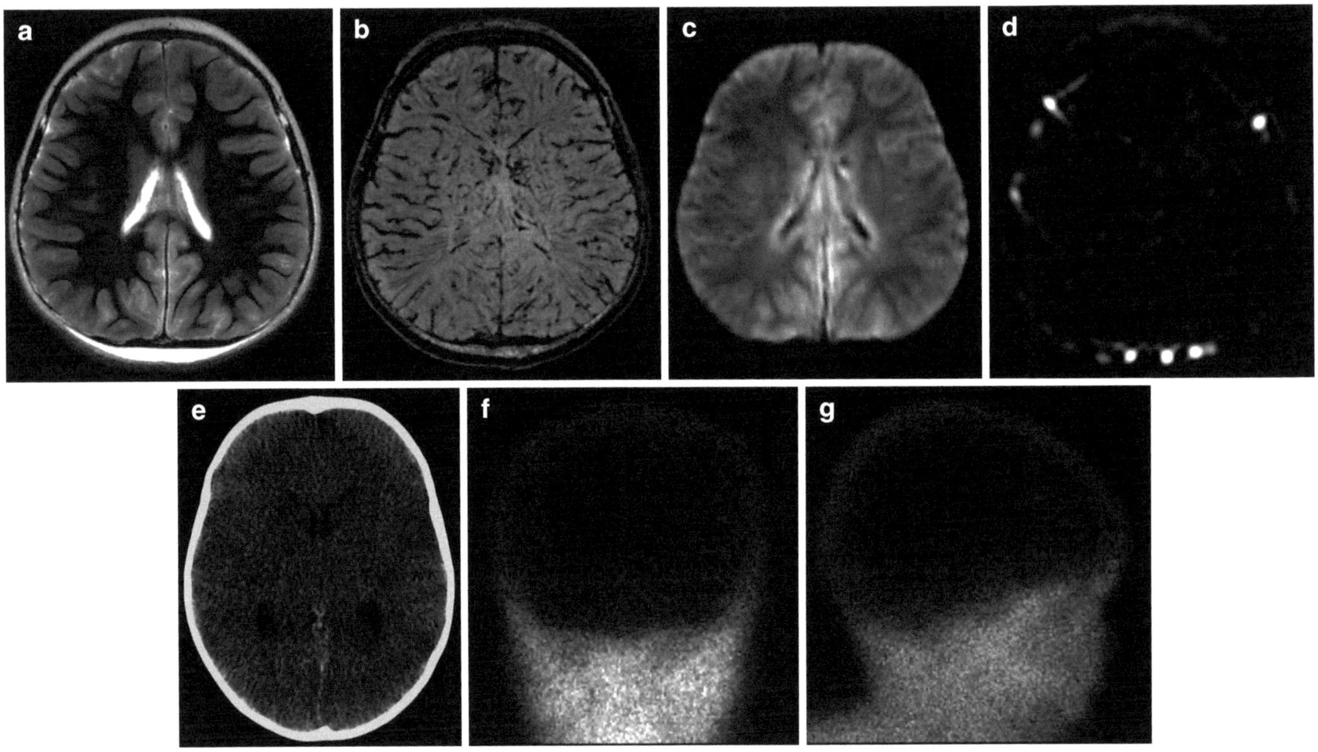

Fig. 3.3 Brain death examples. Axial T2 image (**a**) shows diffuse cerebral edema with bilateral partial effacement of the lateral ventricles. Prominent engorged/thrombosed vessels are seen throughout the brain parenchyma on the susceptibility-weighted image (**b**) in a pattern typically described with brain death [28]. Axial diffusion image (**c**) shows extensive bilateral areas of restricted diffusivity in the brain parenchyma. ASL demonstrates no flow within the brain parenchyma but preserved extracranial flow within the distal ECA branches (**d**). A noncontrast CT from the same patient shows extensive areas of hypoattenuation, loss of gray–white matter differentiation, and edema (**e**). A ^{99}mTc exametazime scan from a different patient shows absent cerebral uptake compatible with brain death (**f**, **g**). *ASL* arterial spin labeling, *ECA* external carotid artery

Table 3.5 Nuclear medicine techniques in the neuro-ICU [18]

Pathology	SPECT	PET
Brain death and cerebral perfusion	[^{99}mTc(V)-HMPAO]; ^{99}mTc ethyl cysteinate dimer (ECD)	[^{18}F]-FDG
Parkinsonism	[^{123}I]-ioflupane, [^{99}mTc(I)]-TRODAT-1	[^{18}F]-FDG
Dementia	Experimental (DRM10 and [123I]-I-ABC577)	[^{18}F]-FDG; amyloid tracers such as [^{18}F]-flutemetamol, [^{18}F]-florbetapir, and [^{18}F]-florbetaben; tau tracers such as [^{18}F]-flortaucipir
Epileptic syndromes [19]	[^{99}mTc(V)-HMPAO]; ^{99}mTc ethyl cysteinate dimer (ECD)	[^{18}F]-FDG

HMPAO hexamethylpropyleneamine oxime, *[^{18}F]-FDG* [^{18}F]-fluorodeoxyglucose

be stable enough to travel outside of the neuro-ICU and tolerate these imaging modalities' relatively longer acquisition times.

Ultrasound

Basic Concepts

Ultrasound imaging utilizes high-frequency sound waves to visualize relatively superficial soft tissues in real time based on the differences in sound attenuation [3]. Ultrasound techniques include 2D and three-dimensional (3D) conventional ultrasound, color Doppler, and catheter-based ultrasound, among others [3].

Strengths and Weaknesses

Ultrasound imaging has multiple advantages over other modalities. These include the lack of ionizing radiation, wide availability (even capable of connecting to smartphones or tablets), portability, lower costs, easy acquisition with basic technical training, real-time imaging, and easy inclusion of Doppler vascular imaging. Unfortunately, ultrasound has limited penetration into soft tissues, and ultrasonic waves cannot penetrate spaces with high acoustic impedance (e.g., air, bone). Due to this limitation, the cranial vault markedly affects the direct application of these techniques for neuroimaging. Ultrasound techniques are also operator-dependent, and their accuracy will depend on the skill of the sonographer and interpreting healthcare professional.

Clinical Applications

Ultrasound is often used in the ICU [24] as a portable imaging modality to evaluate the cervical (e.g., carotid Doppler) and intracranial (e.g., transcranial Doppler) arteries [24–26]. It is also used for brain imaging in newborns while the fontanelles are open [27] and real-time imaging of the exposed brain parenchyma during surgery or bedside procedures through burr holes. Ultrasound probes are also used for imaging-guided procedures due to their high spatial resolution and real-time visualization of the target anatomy. In addition to diagnostic applications, ultrasound is increasingly used for therapeutic purposes owing to its thermal and mechanical properties [25].

Rational Use

Ultrasound is frequently used in the neuro-ICU as a bedside imaging technique for evaluation of the intracranial circulation in the setting of vasospasm, for ultrasound-guided interventions, or for brain imaging in newborns through open fontanelles [27]. Ultrasound imaging has many limitations and pitfalls, and, in many cases, the findings will need confirmation with CT or MRI techniques [25].

Digital Subtraction Angiography (DSA)

Basic Concepts

Digital subtraction angiography is a fluoroscopic vascular imaging technique involving the initial acquisition of a mask image of the anatomy of interest before contrast injection, followed by the serial acquisition of images during the injection of a radiopaque contrast material. The post-contrast images can be subtracted from the initial mask image to create subtracted images without overlapping radiopaque structures and clearly showing the vascular structures.

Strengths and Weaknesses

The main drawbacks of DSA are related to the invasive nature of its acquisition, its potential technical complications, and the use of ionizing radiation.

Clinical Indications

DSA is considered the gold standard for vascular imaging and is often used to diagnose vasospasm, CTA-negative subarachnoid hemorrhage, or before endovascular interventions. Despite the technological advances of CT and MRI techniques, conventional digital subtraction angiography (DSA) is still widely used for the fine-detail evaluation of the arterial and venous circulations. Its main advantages are its high spatial resolution, allowing the visualization of small distal branches that can be helpful for the assessment of diagnostically challenging disorders such as primary CNS vasculitis or vasospasm. Conventional angiography is often used as a roadmap before the endovascular treatment of hyperacute ischemic stroke and many CNS vascular pathologies.

Rational Use

Diagnostic DSA is indicated in cases in which the noninvasive angiographic techniques do not provide enough spatial and/or temporal resolution to answer the clinical question or characterize in detail a vascular finding (e.g., vasospasm, CNS vasculitis, mycotic aneurysm) (Table 3.6).

Table 3.6 Comparison of the angiographic techniques commonly used in the neuro-ICU

Pathology	CTA	MRI/MRA	DSA
Atherosclerotic disease	High	High, particularly with contrast	Highest (gold standard)
Vasculitis	High	Moderate to high, wall enhancement aids in the diagnosis	Highest
Aneurysm	High	Moderate to high	Highest (gold standard)
AVM	High	High	Highest
Vasospasm	High (higher with CT perfusion)	Moderate to high (higher with perfusion imaging)	Highest (gold standard)

AVM arteriovenous malformation

Conclusions

Imaging techniques are crucial components of the diagnostic and prognostic techniques in the neuro-ICU. Basic knowledge of their strengths and weaknesses and their rational use will allow the neuro-ICU team to maximize their value and avoid unnecessary imaging studies.

References

1. Williamson C, Morgan L, Klein JP. Imaging in Neurocritical care practice. Semin Respir Crit Care Med. 2017;38(6):840–52.
2. Smith G, Pace J, Scoco A, Singh G, Kandregula K, Manjila S, et al. Shunt devices for Neurointensivists: complications and management. Neurocrit Care. 2017;27(2):265–75.
3. Akhtar H, Chaudhry SH, Bortolussi-Courval E, Hanula R, Akhtar A, Nauche B, et al. Diagnostic yield of CT head in delirium and altered mental status-a systematic review and meta-analysis. J Am Geriatr Soc. 2023;71(3):946–58.
4. Kamalian S, Lev MH. Stroke Imaging. Radiol Clin North Am. 2019;57(4):717–32.
5. Fang H, He G, Cheng Y, Liang F, Zhu Y. Advances in cerebral perfusion imaging techniques in acute ischemic stroke. J Clin Ultrasound. 2022;50(8):1202–11.
6. Heit JJ, Sussman ES, Wintermark M. Perfusion computed tomography in acute ischemic stroke. Radiol Clin North Am. 2019;57(6):1109–16.
7. Rostami E, Engquist H, Enblad P. Imaging of cerebral blood flow in patients with severe traumatic brain injury in the neurointensive care. Front Neurol. 2014;5:114.
8. John S, Stock S, Cerejo R, Uchino K, Winners S, Russman A, et al. Brain imaging using Mobile CT: current status and future prospects. J Neuroimaging. 2016;26(1):5–15.
9. Carlson AP, Yonas H. Portable head computed tomography scanner--technology and applications: experience with 3421 scans. J Neuroimaging. 2012;22(4):408–15.
10. Abel F, Schubert T, Winklhofer S. Advanced neuroimaging with photon-counting detector CT. Investig Radiol. 2023;58(7):472–81.
11. Patra A, Janu A, Sahu A. MR imaging in Neurocritical care. Indian J Crit Care Med. 2019;23(Suppl 2):S104–S14.
12. Krupinski EA, Harris D, Arlinghaus LR, Schlemper J, Sofka M. Image quality assessment of advanced reconstruction algorithm for point-of-care MRI scanner. J Med Imaging (Bellingham). 2023;10(Suppl 1):S11913.
13. Iglesias JE, Schleicher R, Laguna S, Billot B, Schaefer P, McKaig B, et al. Quantitative brain morphometry of portable low-field-strength MRI using super-resolution machine learning. Radiology. 2023;306(3):e220522.
14. Yuen MM, Prabhat AM, Mazurek MH, Chavva IR, Crawford A, Cahn BA, et al. Portable, low-field magnetic resonance imaging enables highly accessible and dynamic bedside evaluation of ischemic stroke. Sci Adv. 2022;8(16):eabm3952.
15. Mazurek MH, Cahn BA, Yuen MM, Prabhat AM, Chavva IR, Shah JT, et al. Portable, bedside, low-field magnetic resonance imaging for evaluation of intracerebral hemorrhage. Nat Commun. 2021;12(1):5119.

16. Cooley CZ, McDaniel PC, Stockmann JP, Srinivas SA, Cauley SF, Sliwiak M, et al. A portable scanner for magnetic resonance imaging of the brain. Nat Biomed Eng. 2021;5(3):229–39.
17. Algethamy HM, Alzawahmah M, Young GB, Mirsattari SM. Added value of MRI over CT of the brain in intensive care unit patients. Can J Neurol Sci. 2015;42(5):324–32.
18. Crisan G, Moldovean-Cioroianu NS, Timaru DG, Andries G, Cainap C, Chis V. Radiopharmaceuticals for PET and SPECT imaging: a literature review over the last decade. Int J Mol Sci. 2022;23(9):5023.
19. Kim S, Mountz JM. SPECT imaging of epilepsy: an overview and comparison with F-18 FDG PET. Int J Mol Imaging. 2011;2011:813028.
20. Kampe KK, Rotermund R, Tienken M, Thomalla G, Regier M, Klutmann S, et al. Diagnostic value of positron emission tomography combined with computed tomography for evaluating critically ill neurological patients. Front Neurol. 2017;8:33.
21. van Leer B, van Rijsewijk ND, Nijsten MWN, Slart R, Pillay J, Glaudemans A. Practice of (18)F-FDG-PET/CT in ICU patients: a systematic review. Semin Nucl Med. 2023;53(6):809–19.
22. Vander Borght T, Laloux P, Maes A, Salmon E, Goethals I, Goldman S, et al. Guidelines for brain radionuclide imaging. Perfusion single photon computed tomography (SPECT) using Tc-99m radiopharmaceuticals and brain metabolism positron emission tomography (PET) using F-18 fluorodeoxyglucose. The Belgian Society for Nuclear Medicine. Acta Neurol Belg. 2001;101(4):196–209.
23. Drake M, Bernard A, Hessel E. Brain death. Surg Clin North Am. 2017;97(6):1255–73.
24. Zhu H, Geng X, Rajah GB, Fu P, Du H. Brain ultrasound for diagnosis and prognosis in the neurological intensive care unit: a mini review for current development. Neurol Res. 2019;41(8):691–6.
25. Klibanov AL, Hossack JA. Ultrasound in radiology: from anatomic, functional, molecular imaging to drug delivery and image-guided therapy. Investig Radiol. 2015;50(9):657–70.
26. Millet A, Evain JN, Desrumaux A, Francony G, Bouzat P, Mortamet G. Clinical applications of transcranial Doppler in non-trauma critically ill children: a scoping review. Childs Nerv Syst. 2021;37(9):2759–68.
27. Ko TS, Catennacio E, Shin SS, Stern J, Massey SL, Kilbaugh TJ, et al. Advanced Neuromonitoring modalities on the horizon: detection and Management of Acute Brain Injury in children. Neurocrit Care. 2023;38(3):791–811.
28. Sohn CH, Lee HP, Park JB, Chang HW, Kim E, Kim E, et al. Imaging findings of brain death on 3-tesla MRI. Korean J Radiol. 2012;13(5):541–9.

Clinical Neuroimaging in the Intensive Care Unit

4

Hera A. Kamdar and Brian L. Edlow

Contents

H. A. Kamdar
Department of Neurology, The Ohio State University, Columbus, Ohio, United States

B. L. Edlow (✉)
Department of Neurology, Harvard Medical School, Massachusetts General Hospital, Center for Neurotechnology and Neurorecovery (CNTR), Laboratory for NeuroImaging of Coma and Consciousness (NICC), Athinoula A. Martinos Center for Biomedical Imaging, Boston, MA, USA
e-mail: bedlow@mgh.harvard.edu

Abstract

Neurological emergencies involve a vast range of neurological diseases from acute ischemia to intracerebral hemorrhage, infection, herniation, or edema that require immediate assessment and management to prevent irreversible injury. Many of these disease processes require close monitoring in the intensive care unit. Neuroimaging is not only a critical tool in diagnosis, but also is paramount

E. Mahanna Gabrielli et al. (eds.), *Textbook of Neurointensive Care: Volume 1*, https://doi.org/10.1007/978-3-031-62220-5_4

in informing prognosis and guiding management. This chapter focuses on highlighting hallmark radiologic features of high-yield neurological disease states on different neuroimaging modalities to optimize clinical care.

Introduction

Neuroimaging is a key component in the diagnosis and management of neurological diseases. Standard imaging modalities used within the intensive care unit include: computed tomography (CT) of the head, CT of head and neck vasculature (i.e., CT arteriography and CT venography), and CT perfusion; magnetic resonance imaging (MRI) of the brain, MRI of head and neck vasculature (i.e., MRI arteriogram and MRI venogram), MRI spectroscopy and perfusion, and functional MRI; and positron emission tomography (PET) scan. This chapter will highlight the critical role of these neuroimaging modalities as a salient resource for clinical practice.

Chapter Goals

- To identify the imaging modality of choice for the diagnosis and management of high-yield neurological diseases.
- To identify key sequences within these imaging modalities needed for the diagnosis and management of high-yield neurological diseases.
- To identify the key radiologic features or hallmarks of high-yield neurological diseases.
- To learn the differential diagnosis for common findings on neuroimaging.
- To learn how imaging assists in management and prognostication of certain neurological diseases.

Take Home Message

Neuroimaging plays a critical role in not only the diagnosis of neurological disease, but also as paramount in informing prognosis and guiding management. Learning hallmark radiologic features of high-yield neurological disease processes on neuroimaging is vital for optimizing patient care.

Neurovascular Diseases

Acute Ischemic Stroke

Acute ischemic stroke (AIS) is defined as time-sensitive irreversible cerebral injury secondary to insufficient blood supply to the brain. It has been estimated that a patient loses approximately 1.9 million neurons every minute that treatment is not given, and thus, AIS is deemed a neurological emergency [1]. This has led to the need for immediately available neuroimaging techniques to promptly diagnose AIS, quantify the burden of ischemia, and ultimately guide treatment decisions in a time-efficient manner. Imaging modalities used in AIS include: noncontrast CT head (CTH), CT angiography (CTA) of the head and neck, CT perfusion (CTP), and MRI [2–4].

Noncontrast CT Head

Noncontrast CTH is the universal primary imaging modality of choice for AIS [2–4]. It is not only used for rapid assessment of the structures within the bony skull such as the brain parenchyma and ventricular system but is also used to identify and quantify the degree of acute large territory infarct and rule out other acute intracranial processes, such as hemorrhage, space occupying lesion (e.g., brain tumor), or cerebral edema. These findings inform decision-making about administration of thrombolytic therapy or mechanical thrombectomy in patients with clinical concern for AIS [2–4]. When reviewing a noncontrast CTH, a three-step approach can be utilized to guide management of AIS:

Step 1: Evaluate for other acute intracranial processes such as intracranial hemorrhage or space occupying lesions (e.g., brain tumors). Intracranial hemorrhage can be intracerebral, intraventricular, subarachnoid, subdural, or epidural. These are hyperdense on CTH. Primary brain tumors are typically single solitary lesions with surrounding vasogenic edema and have a heterogeneous core with surrounding hypodensity on CTH. Secondary or metastatic brain tumors are typically smaller multiple lesions along the gray-white junction and have variable degrees of surrounding edema. Presence of either of these typically precludes thrombolytic therapy. Endovascular thrombectomy can be considered on a case-by-case basis, carefully weighing the benefits of thrombectomy versus the risks of hemorrhagic reperfusion injury.

Step 2: Evaluate for signs of ischemia and grade the extent. The hallmark radiologic signs of early ischemia include loss of signal due to cytotoxic edema resulting in the tissue becoming darker or hypodense on CTH. This results in loss of gray-white differentiation superficially around the cortex, as well as within the deep gray structures like the lentiform nucleus. This area of hypodensity (aka "infarct core") typically depicts irreversible damage to the brain and can be seen as early as 1 h after stroke onset [2–4]. The extent of ischemia can be assessed with the widely used Alberta Stroke Program Early CT Score (ASPECTS). ASPECTS is a 10-point scale that quantifies the MCA-supplied regions in the brain: three subcortical structures (caudate, internal capsule, and lentiform nucleus) and seven cortical structures (six cortical MCA regions and the insular ribbon). Each region is given a point, and one point is subtracted from the total 10 for any evidence of early ischemic change within that region. Thus, a normal CTH would receive an ASPECTS of 10, while a score of 0 indicates ischemia of MCA structures. Previous literature correlated a score of 7 or less with poor functional outcome, assuming this radiographic change indicated a decreased amount of salvageable brain tissue [5, 6]. This led to a standard practice of ASPECT of 6 or higher as a requirement for pursuing mechanical thrombectomy. However, new clinical trial data has revealed potential benefit of mechanical thrombectomy, even in those with lower range ASPECT of 3–5, or apparently higher ischemic burden on CTH [7, 8]. Ultimately, this score is important for selecting patients for acute interventions and stratifying risks versus benefits of therapy, as it helps to determine if there is salvageable brain tissue within the area of risk.

Step 3: Evaluation for hyperdense artery sign. A hyperdense sign within the intracranial vasculature may represent an acute thrombus. This sign has a specificity of approximately 95% to detect intra-arterial thrombus but has low sensitivity and may be confounded by false positives [9]. Although highly indicative of a proximal large vessel occlusion, particularly of the MCA, this method of detection is not preferred over the standard vessel imaging like CTA. It is important to note that patients with hyperdense artery signs on CTH are associated with more severe clinical deficits and less rapid clinical recovery, underscoring this sign's importance in prognosis [10].

CT Angiogram

A noncontrast CTH is typically followed by further contrasted imaging to evaluate the intracranial vasculature. CTA utilizes contrast to visualize the cerebral vessels, and in the case of AIS, to identify a thrombus blocking a proximal blood vessel or severe stenosis warranting mechanical thrombectomy or carotid intervention, respectively; both of which are time-sensitive interventions (Fig. 4.1) [11].

CT Perfusion

In the setting of a proximal large vessel occlusion, a contrasted CTH can be further processed with advanced software to provide real-time measurement of cerebral blood flow that can help differentiate between salvageable brain parenchyma (i.e., penumbra) to permanently infarcted brain tissue (i.e., core). In recent clinical trials, the infarcted brain, or core, has been quantified as the volume of parenchyma with relative cerebral blood flow of less than 30% compared to the contralateral hemisphere; and the penumbra equates to the volume of parenchyma with time to peak of more than 6 seconds (T max >6), which is at high risk of infarction if not intervened upon (Fig. 4.2) [12, 13]. Radiological algorithms based on these two volumes, along with clinical presentation and baseline disability, have now become the standard in assessing candidacy for mechanical thrombectomy.

MRI

MRI of the brain can also be used to diagnose and guide management of AIS. However, given the broad availability, rapid access, and cost efficiency of CT, the latter is more widely used. Comprehensive stroke MR sequences should ideally include T1-weighted (T1), T2-weighted (T2), T2 fluid-attenuated inversion recovery (FLAIR), gradient-recalled echo (GRE) or susceptibility-weighted imaging (SWI), diffusion-weighted imaging (DWI), and perfusion-weighted imaging. The ideal sequences to evaluate and quantify the age of an ischemic stroke include DWI and T2 FLAIR (Fig. 4.3). The DWI sequence can detect cytotoxic edema within 30 min of ischemia onset and has a sensitivity of approximately 90% [4, 14]. Acute ischemia appears as

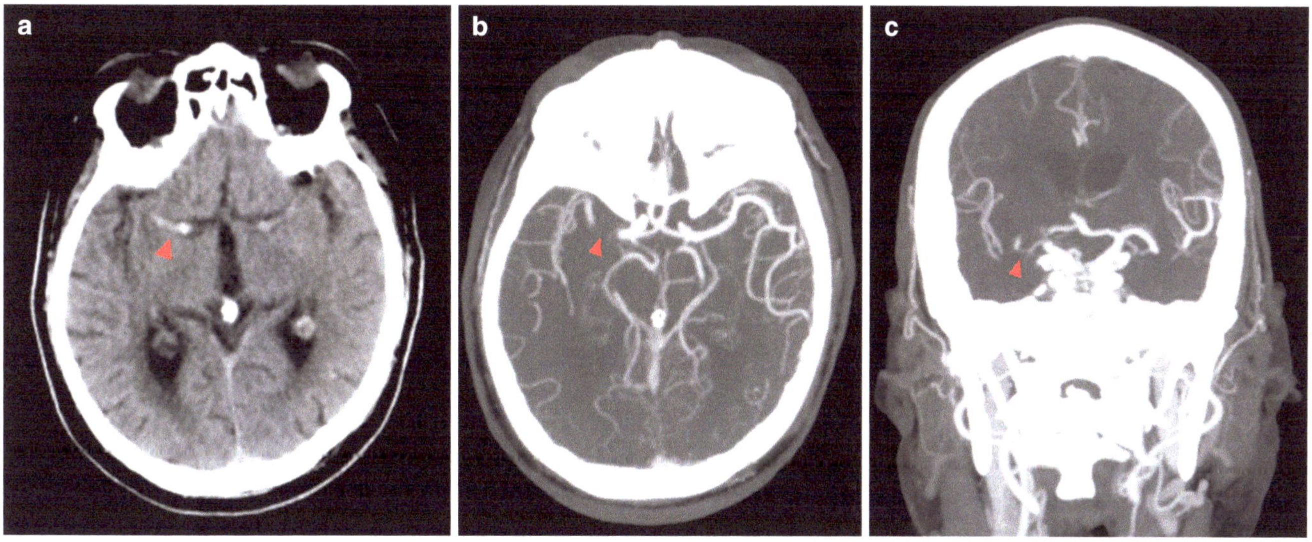

Fig. 4.1 Acute ischemic stroke. (**a**) Noncontrast CT head, axial view, with hyperdense right M1 MCA. (**b**) Contrasted CT angiogram head and neck, axial view, with right M1 MCA occlusion with paucity of cortical branches. (**c**) Contrasted CT angiogram head and neck, coronal view, with right M1 MCA occlusion with paucity of cortical branches

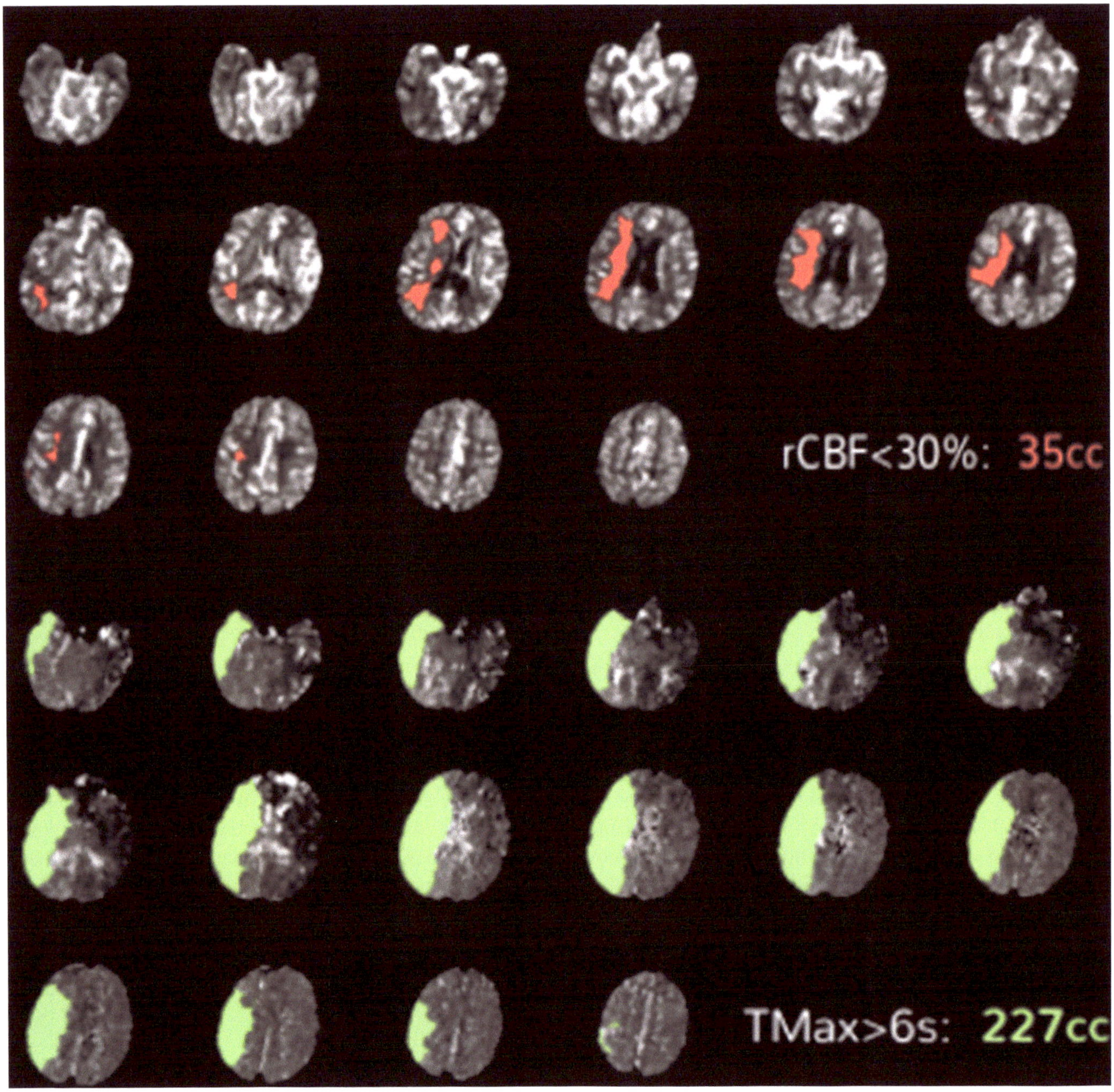

Fig. 4.2 Acute ischemic stroke. Contrasted CT perfusion with RAPID sequence processing showing core infarct (rCBF < 30%) of 35 cc with volume at total risk (Tmax > 6 s) of 227 cc within the right cerebral hemisphere, suggestive of large penumbra (mismatch volume = 192 cc)

high signal (i.e., hyperintensity) on DWI with corresponding low signal on the apparent diffusion coefficient (ADC) map within this hyperacute phase. The T2 FLAIR sequence appears hyperintense approximately 3–8 h after ischemia onset [15]. Thus, a mismatch between hyperintense DWI with a normal T2 FLAIR sequence is useful in determining candidacy for acute interventions with thrombolytics or mechanical thrombectomy. This modality is more widely used as an option in centers where MRI is available in the acute setting and is being used in studies to determine a patient's eligibility for intervention beyond the current standard of time. Additionally, the gradient-recalled echo (GRE) or susceptibility-weighted imaging (SWI) sequences may be helpful in the peri-thrombolytic management of acute stroke. These sequences can identify the location and extent of thrombus, along with the ischemic penumbra. They are also sensitive in the detection of microbleeds, which do not necessarily contraindicate thrombolytic therapy, but may stratify risk of intraparenchymal hemorrhage after thrombolysis based on the extent of microbleeds [16].

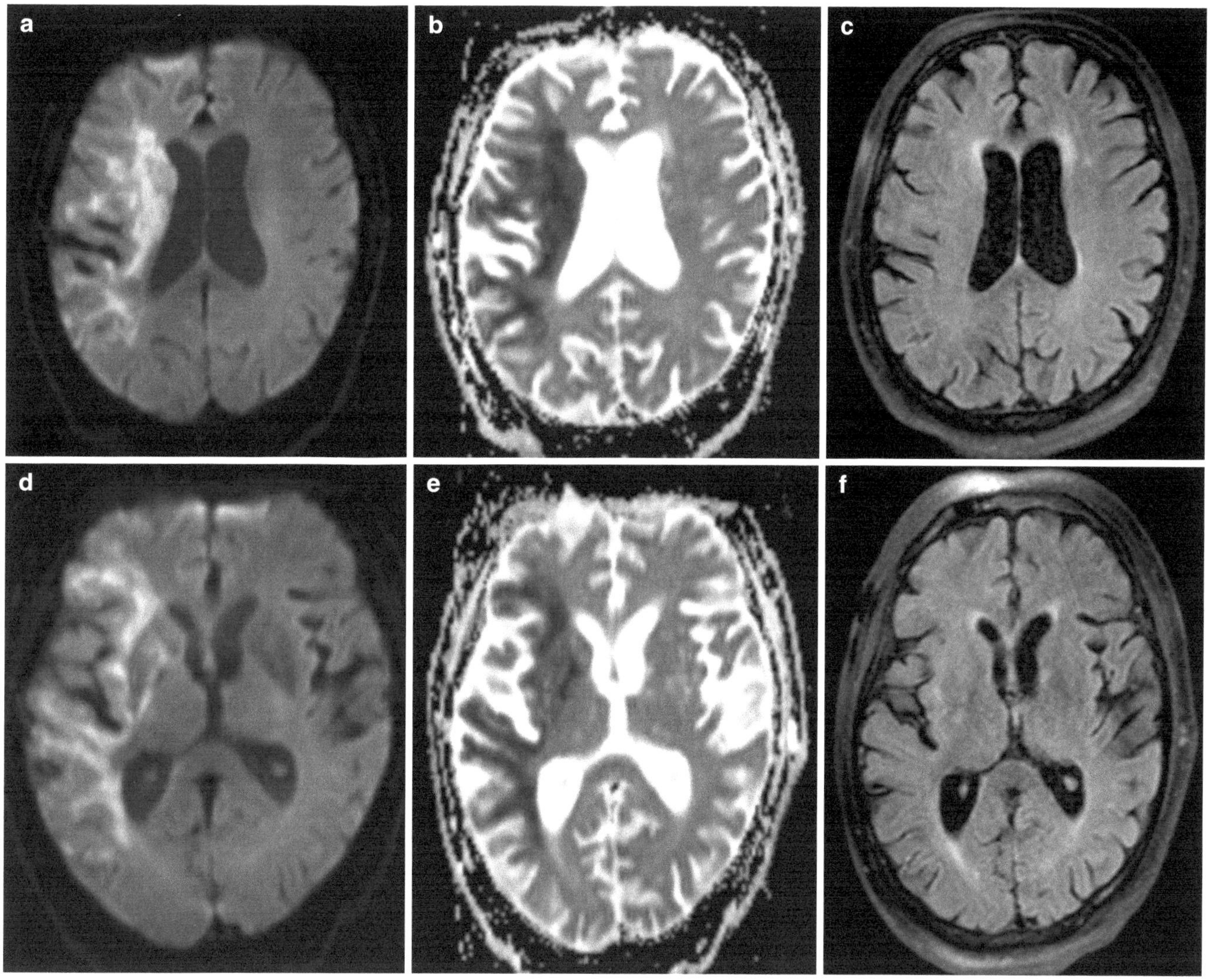

Fig. 4.3 Acute ischemic stroke. There is a large area of reduced diffusivity in the right MCA territory associated with mild T2/FLAIR hyperintensity, consistent with early acute infarct. There are also scattered and confluent foci of T2/FLAIR hyperintensity in the white matter that are nonspecific, but likely reflect sequelae of mild to moderate chronic small vessel disease. (**a** and **d**) MRI DWI sequence that appears hyperintense in setting of acute ischemia. (**b** and **e**) MRI ADC sequence that appears hypointense in correlation to DWI in setting of acute ischemia. (**c** and **f**) MRI T2/FLAIR sequence with mild correlating hyperintensity, consistent with early acute infarct

Intracerebral Hemorrhage

The different types of intracranial hemorrhage based on location include: intraparenchymal (IPH), intraventricular, subarachnoid, subdural, and epidural. This section will focus primarily on IPH. Atraumatic, spontaneous IPH is the second most common type of stroke, accounting for approximately 20% of strokes [17]. The imaging modality of choice for acute assessment and management for IPH is a noncontrast CTH. Other imaging modalities also used, particularly for determination of etiology include MRI, MRA, and CTA.

Noncontrast CTH

A noncontrast CTH is the imaging modality of choice for acute diagnosis and management of IPH. Immediate diagnosis is imperative to ensure measures are taken to stabilize the patient and determine if acute medical or surgical interventions are needed.

Hemorrhage on a noncontrast CTH appears hyperdense (Fig. 4.4). The first radiologic feature that should be assessed is IPH location (i.e., lobar or deep). IPH location helps in differentiating between common etiologies including traumatic, hypertensive, or secondary to cerebral amyloid angiopathy (CAA). Hypertensive bleeds are mostly found in the deep structures of the brain including the basal ganglia, thalamus, pons, and cerebellum, while IPH secondary to CAA is mostly restricted to the lobar region of the brain including cerebral cortex, gray-white junction, and subcortical white matter [18, 19].

The second feature that should be assessed is IPH volume, a significant independent predictor of mortality and is determined by the widely used ABC/2 score, where A is the value

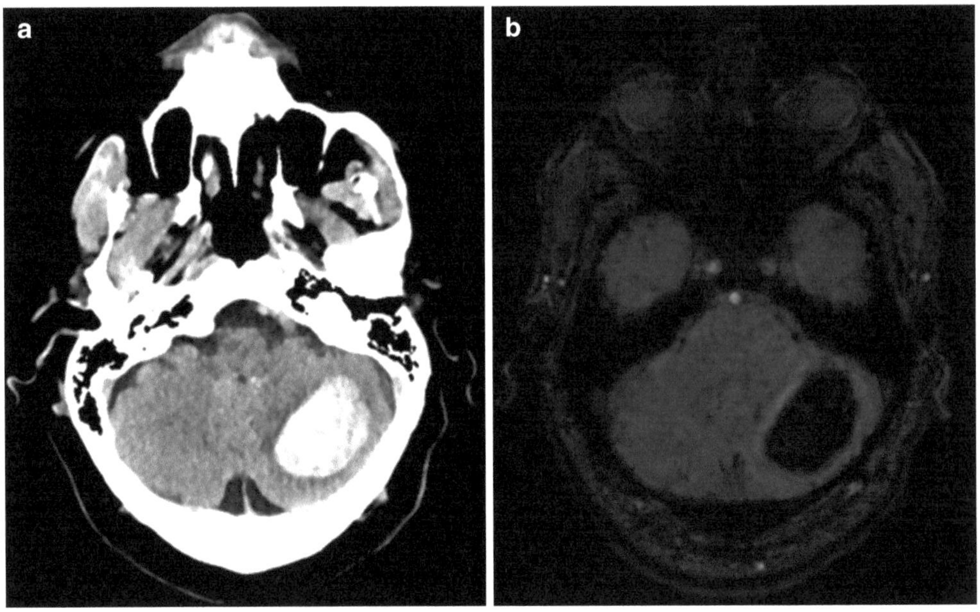

Fig. 4.4 Intracerebral hemorrhage. (**a**) Noncontrast CT head with left cerebellar 4 cm hyperdensity consistent with acute parenchymal hematoma (estimated volume 13 mL) with mild local mass effect. (**b**) MRI SWI sequence with corresponding left cerebellar hypointensity consistent with parenchymal hematoma

of the largest hematoma diameter, B is the value of the diameter perpendicular to A, and C is the number of CT slices with ≥75% of hemorrhage multiplied by the slice thickness [20, 21]. IPH volume is utilized within the clinicoradiologic scoring tool, the IPH score, and is associated with 30-day mortality rates among patients with IPH. Along with the IPH volume, key radiographic features that contribute to overall mortality include presence of IVH and infratentorial location of IPH. Along with these 3 radiographic findings, Glasgow Coma Scale (GCS) score and age are also used. Age over 80, presence of IVH, infratentorial location of IPH, and IPH volume > 30 mL all are scored with a single point, whereas GCS is given one or two points depending on severity of neurological deficits. A lower IPH score is associated with a low mortality rate, while a score of >5 correlates with a 100% mortality rate [22]. It is important to note that this score is not intended to predict 30-day mortality; clinicians should use this score with caution as to avoid self-fulfilling prophecies [23].

Other important features to appreciate on CTH include perihematomal edema, midline shift, hydrocephalus, and herniation. Midline shift can be evaluated by identifying three anatomical landmarks: the septum pellucidum, the third ventricle, and the pineal gland [24, 25]. If any of these 3 midline structures are out of alignment, then there is evidence of midline shift, which can be measured by the perpendicular distance between the shifted midline structure and the midline. Radiological features of hydrocephalus include enlargement of ventricles (particularly the inferior temporal horns of the lateral ventricles, superior horns of the lateral ventricles, and the third ventricle) and transependymal flow of cerebrospinal fluid, which appears as hypodensity on CTH around the margins of the enlarged ventricles [24].

Multiple radiographic signs are associated with hematoma expansion and poor functional outcome, including black hole sign, swirl sign, blend sign, and island sign [26–30]. The black hole sign is defined as a region of hypoattenuation encapsulated within the hyperdense hematoma with a clearly defined border [27]. The swirl sign is defined as heterogeneous collection of hyperdense and lower attenuating material representing older clotted blood and new fresh blood and is indicative of acute extravasation of blood into a hematoma [28, 29]. Similarly, the blend sign is defined as two components of a hyperattenuating region adjacent to a relatively hypoattenuating region [30]. The island sign is defined as three or greater smaller hemorrhages in addition to main hemorrhage [31].

CT Angiogram

Once a noncontrast CTH has identified a hemorrhage, a contrast-based CTA is performed to evaluate for intracranial vascular abnormalities. As previously stated, CTA utilizes contrast to visualize the cerebral vessels, and in the case of IPH, can assist in determining whether there is an underlying vascular malformation. CTA has a sensitivity of 95% and specificity of 99% to detect intracranial vascular malformations after an IPH [32]. CTA also can assist with predicting hematoma expansion. The presence of a spot sign, which is defined as a greater than 1 millimeter focus of enhancement within the hematoma representing contrast extravasation, is indicative of active bleeding [33].

MRI

As with AIS, comprehensive MR sequences for IPH should ideally include T1, T2, T2 FLAIR, GRE or SWI, contrast-enhanced, diffusion-weighted, and perfusion-weighted images [34]. MRI detects IPH with great accuracy, particularly acute large bleeds on the GRE sequence. The GRE sequence has comparable sensitivity to the noncontrast CTH and may be detected within 23 min of symptom onset (Fig. 4.4) [35–38]. However, the GRE sequence is limited in its ability to differentiate acuity with small hemorrhages or microbleeds, and it may not be readily available in the acute setting [39, 40]. Thus, noncontrast CTH remains the modality of choice for evaluating acute IPH [34].

The appearance of an IPH on MRI differs based on sequence and age of the bleed, as blood products are degraded from oxyhemoglobin to deoxyhemoglobin, methemoglobin, and ultimately hemosiderin. In the hyperacute stage (< 6 h), oxyhemoglobin predominates and appears isointense on T1, but hyperintense on T2/GRE. In the acute stage (7–72 h) deoxyhemoglobin predominates and appears isointense on T1, but hypointense on T2/GRE. In the early subacute stage (3–7 days), methemoglobin predominates and appears hyperintense on T1, and hypointense on T2/GRE. In the late subacute stage (1–4 weeks), methemoglobin again predominates but appears hyperintense on both T1 and T2/GRE. Finally, in the chronic stage (months to years), hemosiderin predominates and appears hypointense on both on T1and T2/GRE [34, 41, 42].

MRI can be useful in detecting underlying causes of secondary hemorrhages, such as tumors, cerebral venous thrombosis, or vascular malformations [34]. It is also helpful in differentiating primary IPH from hemorrhagic transformation of an ischemic stroke, which is typically irregular in shape, smaller in size compared to the total area of infarction and follows a vascular territory [43].

Subarachnoid Hemorrhage

Subarachnoid hemorrhage (SAH) is defined as bleeding within the subarachnoid space and can be caused by a myriad of etiologies, of which, spontaneous SAH secondary to aneurysmal rupture is of particular importance given its significant morbidity and mortality. Thus, imaging modalities focus on diagnosing the bleed, determining severity, and evaluating for aneurysm.

Aneurysmal Subarachnoid Hemorrhage

Noncontrast CTH

Noncontrast CTH is the most common imaging modality used to diagnose acute SAH (Fig. 4.5). It is most sensitive within the first 6–12 h, with a sensitivity of approximately 99% to 93%, respectively, but decreases overtime to approximately 60% at 7 days [44–47]. Although CTH is primarily

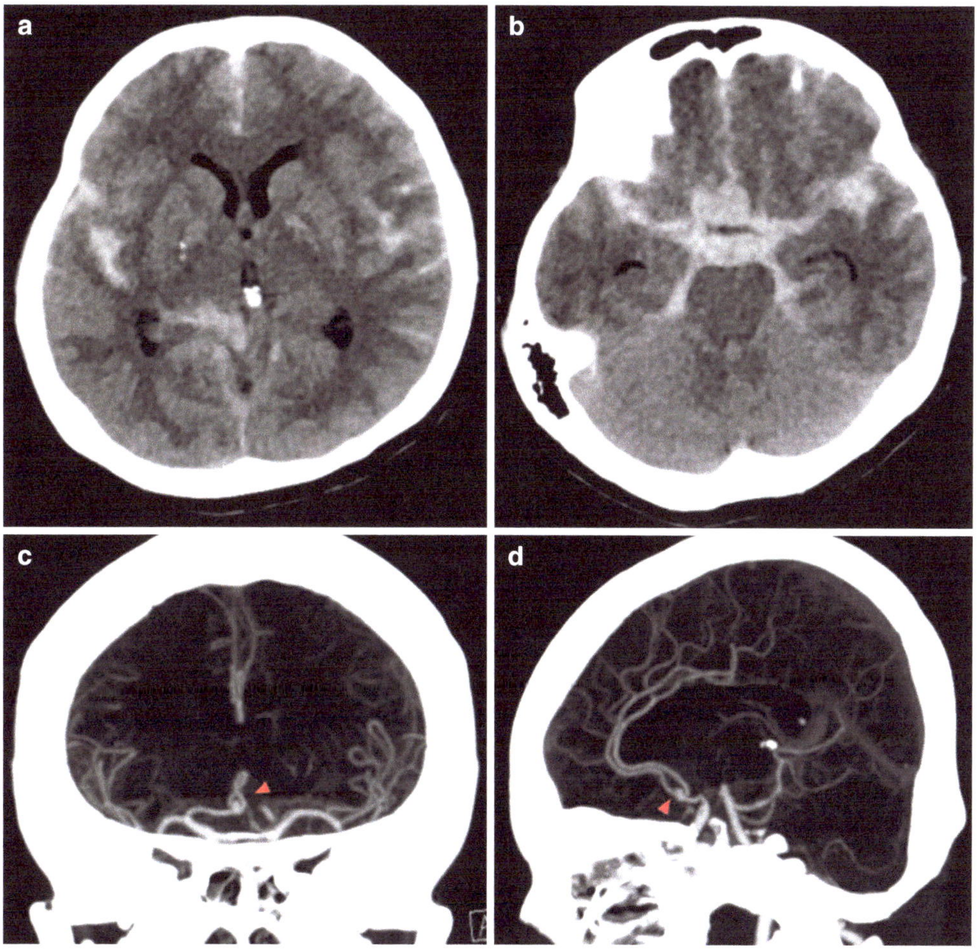

Fig. 4.5 Subarachnoid hemorrhage. (**a** and **b**) Noncontrast CT head with extensive subarachnoid hemorrhage within the basal cisterns, sylvian fissures, interhemispheric fissure, bilateral cerebral sulci, and prepontine cisterns. (**c** and **d**) Contrasted CT angiography in coronal and sagittal views, respectively, showing a superiorly oriented 2 mm anterior communicating artery aneurysm (arrow)

Table 4.1 Modified Fisher scale

Grade	Definition
1	Thin SAH (< 1 mm) No IVH
2	Thin SAH (< 1 mm) IVH present
3	Thick SAH (> 1 mm) No IVH
4	Thick SAH (> 1 mm) IVH present

SAH Subarachnoid hemorrhage, *IVH* Intraventricular hemorrhage

used for the acute detection of SAH, the pattern or location of the hemorrhage on CTH may suggest a specific site of aneurysmal rupture. For example, the presence of subarachnoid blood within the sylvian fissure is more commonly seen with middle cerebral artery aneurysms, while interhemispheric fissure blood is seen with anterior communicating artery or anterior cerebral artery aneurysms. Common locations of subarachnoid blood, regardless of aneurysm location, include the interpeduncular and basal cisterns [47].

Radiological grading scores have been developed to predict surgical risk and mortality. The most common radiographic grading score used is the modified Fisher scale [44, 48], an adaptation of the original Fisher scale [44]. Other scales include the Hijdra scale [49]. The modified Fisher scale (Table 4.1) is graded from 1 to 4, with 4 being the most severe grading. It considers the presence of SAH, whether it is localized or diffuse, thick or thin, and if there is presence of IVH.

As mentioned with IPH, other important features to evaluate on CTH include midline shift, hydrocephalus, and/or evidence of herniation, all of which impact acute management.

MRI

After the first 6–12 h, sensitivity of noncontrast CTH decreases. Thus, for subacute or chronic SAH, MRI sequences including GRE, SWI, and T2 FLAIR are superior to noncontrast CTH and should be obtained if noncontrast CTH is negative [46].

CT Angiogram

If there is evidence of SAH on CTH, then a CTA should be performed to evaluate the intracranial vasculature for potential abnormalities, particularly aneurysms (Fig. 4.5). A CTA or MRA has a reported sensitivity of 76–98% and a specificity of 85–100% in identifying aneurysms; however, digital subtraction angiography (DSA) remains the gold standard diagnostic test [50], particularly in the detection of aneurysms <5 mm in diameter [51, 52]. In patients with characteristic noncontrast CTH findings of aneurysmal SAH (i.e., non-perimesencephalic), with imaging and initial DSA negative for aneurysm, repeat DSA detects an aneurysm at a rate of 7–14%, and thus should be completed within days to weeks after initial imaging [53].

Delayed Cerebral Ischemia

Delayed cerebral ischemia is a phenomenon in aneurysmal SAH patients where patients experience either reversible or irreversible neurological changes that are associated with worse functional outcomes. DCI is defined as the occurrence of focal neurological impairment, or a decrease of at least 2 points on the Glasgow Coma Scale, that lasts for at least 1 h, is not apparent immediately after aneurysm occlusion, and cannot be attributed to other causes. It is suspected when a patient has clinical decompensation after presenting with aneurysmal SAH. The etiology of DCI is multifactorial although arterial narrowing or cerebral vasospasm has predominantly investigated etiology. The most common modality of non-invasive monitoring for DCI is transcranial Doppler (TCD), but the sensitivity and specificity of this diagnostic study are operator dependent [54]. Additional modalities include CTA and MRA, but the gold standard remains DSA [55].

Nonaneurysmal SAH

Nonaneurysmal SAH tends to have different characteristics on noncontrast CTH, particularly with respect to location: foci of SAH are often observed within cerebral sulci rather than the basal cisterns [56]. Nonaneurysmal causes of SAH include trauma, reversible cerebral vasoconstriction syndrome (RCVS), cerebral venous sinus thrombosis (CVST), posterior reversible encephalopathy syndrome (PRES), cerebral amyloid angiopathy (CAA), Moya Moya syndrome, and infectious or autoimmune vasculitis [56].

Reversible Cerebral Vasoconstrictive Syndrome (RCVS)

RCVS is characterized by segmental cerebral vessel narrowing and dilatation that typically resolves within 1–3 months [57]. Patients typically present with a thunderclap headache and may experience focal neurological deficits [57]. Precipitating factors and conditions associated with RCVS include: postpartum cerebral angiopathy (e.g., eclampsia), drugs of abuse (e.g., cannabis, cocaine, ecstasy, amphetamines, LSD), anti-migraine medications (e.g., sumatriptan, ergotamine tartrate), antidepressants (e.g., SSRIs), nasal decongestants (e.g., pseudoephedrine, ephedrine), immunosuppressants (e.g., tacrolimus, cyclophosphamide, interferon alpha), binge drinking alcohol, and/or nicotine patches [57, 58].

Noncontrast CTH

As RCVS typically presents as a sudden onset thunderclap headache with or without neurological deficits, a noncontrast CTH is performed first to rule out hemorrhage, edema, or space occupying lesion. Of note, initial brain imaging can be negative, but a majority of patients may develop a combination of one or more of the following radiologic findings; convexity SAH, IPH, AIS, or PRES. In a cohort study of 139 patients, approximately 55% had normal admitting CTH and MRI; however, 81% ultimately developed clinicoradiologic sequelae including AIS (39%), convexity SAH (34%), IPH (20%), and cerebral edema (38%) [59]. AIS is typically located within the "watershed" zones [58].

MRI Brain

As previously mentioned, initial brain imaging including MRI brain is typically normal, particularly during the first week of symptom onset, with up to 70% of patients presenting with normal MRIs despite the presence of diffuse cerebral vasoconstriction. Thus, a second scan 1–2 weeks later may be required to demonstrate radiologic abnormalities typical of RCVS.

CT Angiogram, MR Angiogram

As its name indicates, arterial imaging shows multiple areas of vasoconstriction (i.e., multifocal areas of stenosis and dilatation) within the intracranial cerebral vasculature. This is seen in the acute stage and usually reverses within days to weeks [58]. Multifocal vasoconstriction produces a classic "sausage on a string" appearance (Fig. 4.6). High-resolution vessel wall imaging, in areas of stenosis, shows loss of normal arterial contrast enhancement that classically resolves over time, differentiating it from vasculitic processes [60].

It is also important to utilize vascular imaging to evaluate for concomitant vascular lesions, as up to 20% of patients may have simultaneous cervical artery dissection, unruptured aneurysms, cavernous malformations, and/or fibromuscular dysplasia [61, 62].

Cerebral Venous Sinus Thromboses (CVST)

CVST can be provoked or unprovoked and presents with a wide spectrum of clinical symptoms from headache to focal neurological deficits, seizure, and altered level of consciousness depending on extent, location, and presence of intracranial hypertension. As with any thromboses, CVST can occur in a hypercoagulable state (e.g., malignancy, inherited coagulopathy, estrogenic oral contraceptives, pregnancy), in the setting of cerebral infection (e.g., meningitis, brain abscess, or tracking sinusitis), brain trauma, or the post-operative state [63, 64]. CVST can ultimately lead to sinus occlusion, venous congestion, and relative decrease in cerebral perfusion pressure, with development of hemorrhage and infarction [63].

Noncontrast CTH

Given new onset neurological symptoms at presentation, noncontrast CTH is the most common initial imaging test performed on the undifferentiated patient [65]. The most common radiological finding, present in up to 40% of patients, is hemorrhage [66]. Additional direct signs of CVST on noncontrast CTH include the "dense triangle sign," and "cord or string sign." [65] The dense triangle sign may be present in patients with superior sagittal sinus thrombosis (SSS) and is characterized by hyperdensity or opacification within the SSS appearing as a bright triangle in the inferior pole of the axial view of a noncontrast CTH, as clot is more dense than free flowing blood [65, 67, 68]. The cord or string sign may be present when there is cortical vein thrombosis and appears as an elongated hyperdense clot in the distribu-

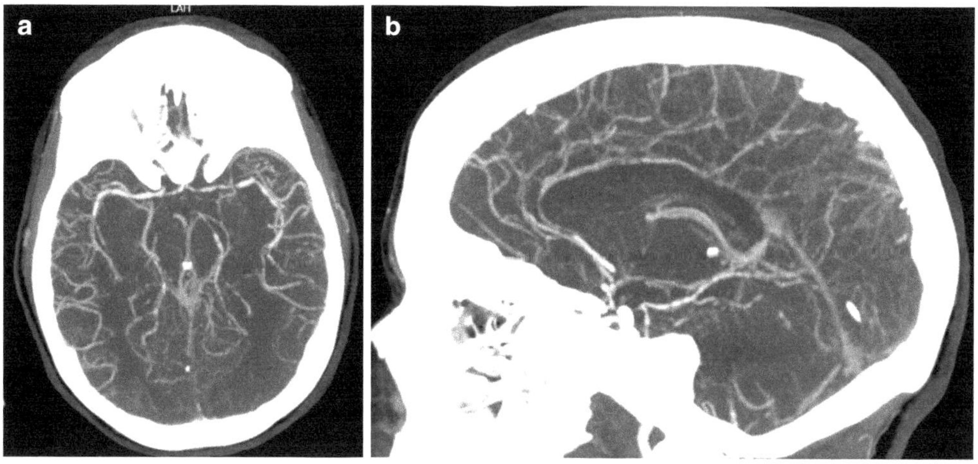

Fig. 4.6 Reversible cerebral vasoconstrictive syndrome (RCVS). Contrasted CT angiography in axial (**a**) and sagittal (**b**) views, respectively, showing segmental arterial vasoconstriction followed by abnormal dilatation, appearing with the classic "string and beads" pattern

tion of a cortical vein [63, 65, 67, 68]. Additionally, the "sigmoid notch sign" on CTH has 91% sensitivity and 86% specificity in differentiating between a transverse sinus clot and an atretic sinus, by observing the bony sigmoid notch on a CTH. A "negative" sign demarcates a normal notch size, indicating that the reason for vessel signal dropout is an acute clot. A "positive" sign demarcates a smaller bony notch that is suggestive of an atretic sinus [69].

MRI

Similar to noncontrast CTH, MRI will show hemorrhage and acute clot burden. Utilizing the T2-weighted sequences, particularly GRE/SWI are highly sensitive and specific and show changes related to the age of the hemorrhage, as detailed in the IPH section [63, 64, 70].

CT and MR Venography

CT or MR venography are the modalities of choice to diagnose CVST [63, 64]. They have comparable sensitivity and sensitivity, and thus either can be chosen based on availability, comorbidities related to contrast exposure, and cost [71]. Features on vessel imaging are flow voids or non-visualization of the vessel in the region of clot, also known as a flow defect (Fig. 4.7) [63, 64]. Of note, patients with hyperdensity within the posterior portion of the SSS on CTH presenting as a dense triangle sign will have a corresponding "empty delta sign" where the thrombus within the SSS will appear hypodense within its core, with a rim of enhancement around the clot [63–65].

Posterior Reversible Encephalopathy Syndrome (PRES)

PRES is characterized by a spectrum of neurological symptoms ranging from headache and vision loss to confusion, altered level of consciousness, and seizures secondary to vasogenic edema particularly within the posterior region of the cerebrum [72]. Risk factors for PRES include acute severe hypertension, renal failure, organ transplantation, collagen vascular or autoimmune diseases, immunosuppressants (e.g., cyclosporine, tacrolimus, cisplatin, IVIg), or eclampsia in pregnancy [72].

Noncontrast CTH

Noncontrast CTH is less sensitive than MRI in detecting initial findings and can be normal in up to 22% of people [73]. Given that these patients typically present with acute undifferentiated neurological symptoms, an initial noncontrast CTH is the first imaging modality performed. In patients with abnormalities on initial CTH, the lesions present with the characteristic pattern of vasogenic edema (i.e., focal or multifocal hypodensities), as described below [72].

MRI

MRI brain is the imaging modality of choice for prompt diagnosis and management of PRES. Key sequences to review include the T2-weighted, T2 FLAIR, DWI, and GRE/SWI sequences. The T2-weighted and T2 FLAIR sequences show characteristic hyperintensities in three discrete patterns: (1) the most commonly described dominant "parietal-occipital pattern"; (2) the "superior frontal sulcus pattern," where there are hyperintensities on the posterior surface of the superior frontal sulcus; and (3) the "holohemispheric watershed pattern" where there are linear hyperintensities within the frontal, parietal, and occipital lobes at watershed zones [72–74]. Furthermore, the MRI can distinguish vasogenic edema, present in PRES, from cytotoxic edema, most commonly seen with ischemic strokes, by DWI. On DWI, both forms of edema appear hyperintense, but the vasogenic edema of PRES on ADC will be isointense or hyperintense (i.e., "T2 shine through"), rather than hypointense in the setting of acute ischemia and cytotoxic edema [72].

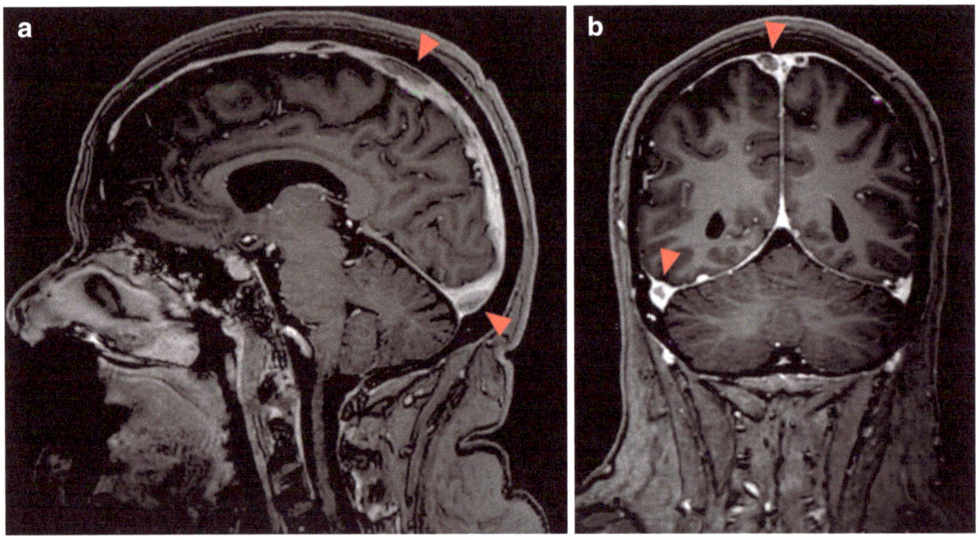

Fig. 4.7 Extensive cerebral venous sinus thrombosis involving the middle third and posterior third of the superior sagittal sinus, bilateral transverse sinus, and sigmoid sinus. (**a**) Contrasted MRV, sagittal view, with flow void in SSS and transverse sinus. (**b**) Contrasted MRV, coronal view, with flow void in SSS, and transverse sinus

Spinal Cord Infarction

Spinal cord infarction is an uncommon cause of acute myelopathy or extremity weakness, ranging from mild weakness to paraplegia [75]. Of note, acute onset back pain has been reported in up to 70% of patients [76]. Etiologies within the adult population include thoracoabdominal aneurysms, dissections, or thromboembolic disease, as well as aortic surgery, spinal arteriovenous malformations, coagulopathies, and sickle cell disease, among others [75]. Unfortunately, imaging to diagnose acute spinal cord infarcts continues to remain a challenge due to the small size of the cord, along with other technical difficulties [75].

MRI

MRI is the imaging modality of choice for the diagnosis of spinal cord ischemia. In the acute stage, there will be hyperintensity on DWI, T2, and STIR sequences, while the T1 sequence will remain isointense, but may be associated with slight enlargement of the cord [75]. There is no enhancement on contrasted sequences. These changes may present in different patterns and anatomic regions based on the spinal artery involved. For example, if there is involvement of the anterior spinal artery, there will be ischemia in the anterior horns of gray matter and adjacent white matter; while if there is involvement of the posterior spinal artery, there will be involvement of the posterior columns and/or the adjacent white matter [75].

Non-Neurovascular Diseases

Brain Tumors

Brain tumors are divided into primary, originating from the central nervous system (CNS), and metastatic tumors originating from other sources within the body. Metastatic disease is substantially more common than primary and is most commonly derived from melanoma, renal, breast, and colorectal cancer [77]. Adult primary brain tumors are classified by the World Health Organization, based on their histological variation, and more recently, their genetic profile. Imaging can be used to assist in the diagnosis, surveillance, and response to treatment of disease.

Noncontrast CT Head

The imaging modality of choice to detect, characterize, and diagnose primary or metastatic brain tumors is an MRI [78]. However, as earlier described, a noncontrast CTH is the most common initial imaging modality of choice in a patient with new acute neurological symptoms. The role of CTH is primarily in the emergent setting, to detect hemorrhage, edema, midline shift, hydrocephalus, or evidence of herniation.

MRI Brain

An MRI brain with gadolinium contrast is the imaging modality of choice for the detection, diagnosis, and surveillance of brain tumors (Fig. 4.8). A broad array of MRI sequences, including pre- and post-gadolinium contrast T1 sequence, T2/T2 FLAIR, GRE, SWI, DWI/ADC, DTI, perfusion, MR spectroscopy, and functional MRI, have shown utility in describing hallmark features of specific brain tumors and are further elucidated in Table 4.2 [78].

Of these sequences, the post-contrast T1 sequence plays a fundamental role in diagnosis and treatment response. A widely used post-contrast T1 sequence is Magnetization Prepared Rapid Gradient Echo Imaging (MPRAGE), which has been applied in clinical trials and in the Response Assessment in Neuro-Oncology (RANO) criteria [79].

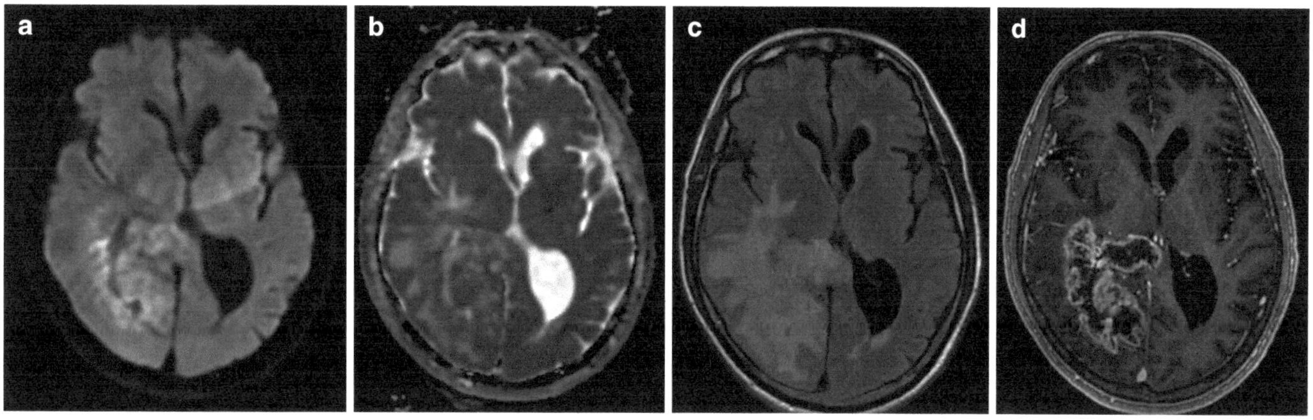

Fig. 4.8 Glioblastoma multiforme. (**a** and **b**) MRI DWI and ADC sequences, respectively, with DWI and ADC hyperintensity in the right posterior temporal and occipital lobes. (**c**) MRI T2/FAIR sequence with large area of diffuse hyperintensity in the right posterior temporal and occipital lobes without disruption of the gray-white junction, consistent with vasogenic edema. (**d**) MRI post-contrast T1 sequence with a large and irregular, rim-enhancing right posterior temporal and occipital lobe mass with extension across the midline through the splenium, suspicious for glioblastoma multiform

Table 4.2 MRI sequence role in brain tumor imaging [78]

MRI sequence	Role in brain tumor imaging
Pre- and post-contrast T1	Determine location of tumor, whether it is intra-axial or extra-axial, and enhancement characteristics
T2/T2 FLAIR	Identify extent of adjacent vasogenic edema
SWI	Evaluate the presence of blood or calcification within or surrounding the tumor bed
DWI/ADC	Differentiate stroke from solid tumor with the presence of DWI without ADC correlation
Diffusion tensor imaging (DTI) tractography	Assist in surgical planning, as tractography identifies white matter tracts which is important in determining critical sites to avoid during surgical resection
Perfusion	Determine vascular supply
MR spectroscopy	Determine the metabolic characteristics of tumors through the identification of neuronal markers (N-acetylaspartate), cellular metabolism markers (creatine), and markers of cell membrane turnover (choline)
Functional MRI (fMRI)	Assist in surgical planning, as fMRI identifies critical sites to avoid during surgical resection

Additional post-contrast T1 sequences including SPACES and VIBE may be beneficial for characterizing lesions with low gadolinium concentration [79].

Positron Emission Tomography (PET) Scan

PET scan utilizes a glucose derived radioactive substance known as fluorodeoxyglucose (FDG), which is known to collect in high-grade tumor cells, assisting in the diagnosis and surveillance of malignancy. FDG PET can also help differentiate tumor from other post treatment related changes that can be difficult to interpret on MRI [78]. An abnormal increase in FDG uptake within cells is indicative of abnormal cellular growth and can be deduced to be cancer in an appropriate clinical setting.

CNS Infection

The spectrum of CNS infection includes meningitis, encephalitis, and brain abscess, all of which require prompt diagnosis and management. Although imaging and CSF analysis are the primarily modalities of diagnosis, these may be negative early within the course, and if clinical suspicion is high enough, early empiric therapy is recommended. Standard imaging modalities include CTH and MRI [80].

Noncontrast CT Head

A noncontrast CTH is initially utilized to assess for mass effect from an intracranial space occupying lesion or edema. This CTH helps to determine the safety of a lumbar puncture, given the possible complication of brain herniation [81]. It is recommended to obtain a noncontrast CTH prior to an LP when there are focal neurological deficits, decreased level of consciousness, evidence of papilledema, seizures, or those who are immunocompromised or have a history of prior intracranial pathology [82]. While a noncontrast CTH is largely unrevealing in patients with early meningitis or encephalitis, a brain abscess appears as a hypointense area of edema concerning for a space occupying lesion, while a contrasted CTH will reveal a ring-enhancing lesion [83].

MRI

MRI with gadolinium is vital to the diagnosis of CNS infection, in particular brain abscess. On MRI, an abscess will have internal diffusion restriction (hyperintensity on DWI with hypointensity on ADC), surrounding vasogenic edema on T2 FLAIR, and a smooth rim of enhancement on T1 post-contrast (Fig. 4.9) [80, 83]. If multiple ring-enhancing lesions are observed in the setting of a suspected brain abscess, then consider septic emboli and pursue vessel imaging to evaluate for mycotic aneurysms. Of note, although CTA or MRA may be used, DSA is the gold standard modality for diagnosis [84]. It is important to consider the entire differential diagnosis for ring-enhancing lesions, which includes infection (abscess, toxoplasmosis, neurocysticercosis, septic emboli), malignancy (lymphoma), and inflammatory disease (tumefactive multiple sclerosis with open ring). The differential diagnosis can be narrowed by clinical presentation, features on brain imaging, as well as pathology after biopsy. Other common radiologic features of CNS infection are elaborated in Table 4.3.

CSF Shunt or Device Infection

A CSF shunt infection is a known complication of permanent CSF diversion procedures and may result in shunt failure. Shunt failure presents with symptoms consistent with raised intracranial pressure. Evaluation of such patients is done with a CTH or brain MRI, along with radiographic shunt series. Neuroimaging may reveal hydrocephalus and signs of ventriculitis [80].

Ventriculitis

When the inflammation from a cerebral infection involves the ependymal lining of the ventricles, it is termed ventriculitis. Noncontrast CTH may show hydrocephalus, periventricular hypodensity (representative of transependymal edema), and hyperdense layering of inflammatory cells in the ventricles. Contrasted CTH may show an enhancement of the ependymal lining of the ventricles as well [85]. MRI

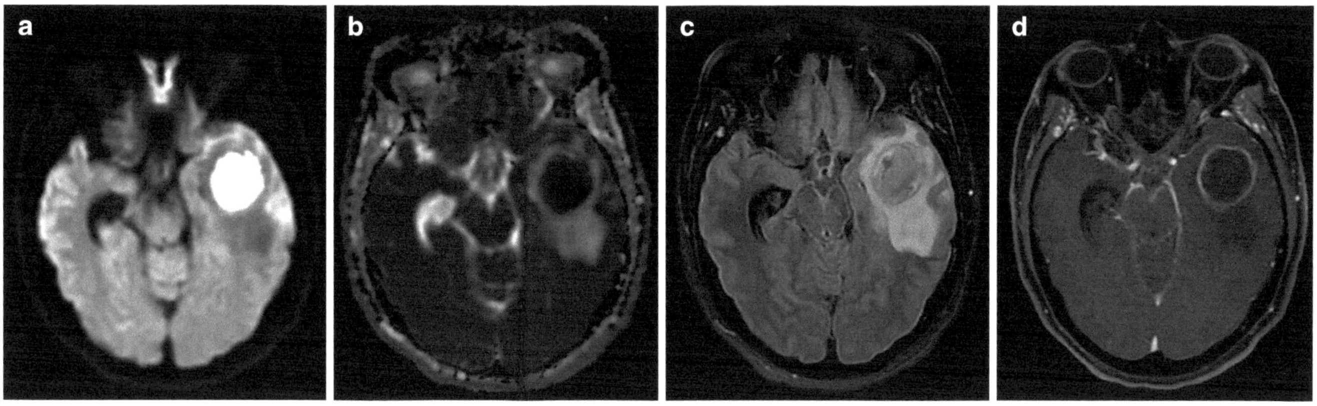

Fig. 4.9 Cerebral abscess. (**a** and **b**) MRI DWI and ADC sequences, respectively, with diffusion restriction of a circular mass within the left temporal lobe. (**c**) MRI T2/FLAIR sequence with large area of hyperintensity in the left temporal lobe without disruption of the gray-white junction consistent with vasogenic edema, and local mass effect with evidence of left uncal herniation. (**d**) MRI post-contrast T1 sequence with a large, circular, rim-enhancing left temporal lesion consistent with cerebral abscess

Table 4.3 Common radiographic features of CNS infections [80, 83]

CNS infection	Common radiologic features
Bacterial meningitis	• CT head: Normal, cerebral sulcal effacement, hydrocephalus • MRI T2 FLAIR: T2 hyperintensity in cerebral sulci • MRI T1 post-contrast: Leptomeningeal enhancement
Listeria meningitis	• MRI T1 post-contrast: Leptomeningeal enhancement, particularly in the brainstem (rhomboencephalitis)
Fungal meningitis	• CT head: Normal, cerebral sulcal effacement, hydrocephalus • MRI T2 FLAIR: T2 hyperintensity in cerebral sulci • MRI T1 post-contrast: Thick, nodular leptomeningeal enhancement
Cryptococcal meningitis	• CT head: Normal, cerebral sulcal effacement, hydrocephalus, mass lesions • MRI T2 FLAIR: T2 hyperintensity in cerebral sulci, T2+ cystic lesions, described as gelatinous pseudocysts that give a "soap bubble" or "punched-out" appearance • MRI T1 post-contrast: Range of contrast enhancing cystic lesions
Tubercular meningitis	• CT head: Normal, cerebral sulcal effacement, hydrocephalus, mass lesions • MRI T2 FLAIR: T2 hyperintensity in cerebral sulci • MRI T1 post-contrast: Thick leptomeningeal enhancement, particular in the basal cisterns; ring-enhancing abscess or tuberculomas
HSV encephalitis	• CT head: Normal, cerebral sulcal effacement particularly within the medial temporal lobes, hemorrhage • MRI T2 FLAIR: T2 hyperintensity in the orbital frontal lobes, and medial temporal lobes (Fig. 4.10) • MRI DWI/SWI: Restricted diffusion and microhemorrhages may be seen in the same region of abnormal T2 signal • MRI T1 post-contrast: Heterogeneous enhancement in the same region of abnormal T2 signal
CMV encephalitis	• CT head: Normal, hydrocephalus • MRI T2 FLAIR: Periventricular T2 hyperintesity, and ventriculomegaly • MRI T1 post-contrast: Periventricular enhancement
VZV encephalitis	• CT head: Normal, cortical and subcortical areas of hypodensity consistent with infarction • MRI DWI/ADC: Cortical and subcortical areas of diffusion restriction consistent with infarction; classically involving the gray-white junction • MRI T2 FLAIR: T2 hyperintensity correlating with areas of infarction • MRI SWI: Possible microhemorrhages correlating with areas of infarction
Toxoplasmosis	• CT head: Mass lesions • MRI T2 FLAIR: T2 hyperintensity correlating with areas of ring-enhancing lesions • MRI T1 post-contrast: Ring-enhancing lesions; classically in deep regions of the cerebrum.
PML	• CT head: Normal • MRI T2 FLAIR: T2 hyperintensities in the juxtacortical white matter • MRI T1 post contrast: Non-enhancing lesions
CJD	• CT head: Normal, cerebral sulcal effacement • MRI DWI/ADC: Superficial cortical ("cortical ribboning") and deep gray (pulvinar, caudate, and putamen) diffusion restriction • MRI T2 FLAIR: T2 hyperintensities correlating to areas of diffusion restriction • MRI T1 post-contrast: Non-enhancing lesions
Neurocysticercosis	• CT head: Hyperdense round lesions with cystic and calcified components, classically at the gray-white junction or intra/periventricular; ventricular cysts may show obstructive hydrocephalus • MRI T2 FLAIR: T2 hyperintensity correlating with areas of ring-enhancing lesions • MRI T1 post-contrast: Ring-enhancing lesions

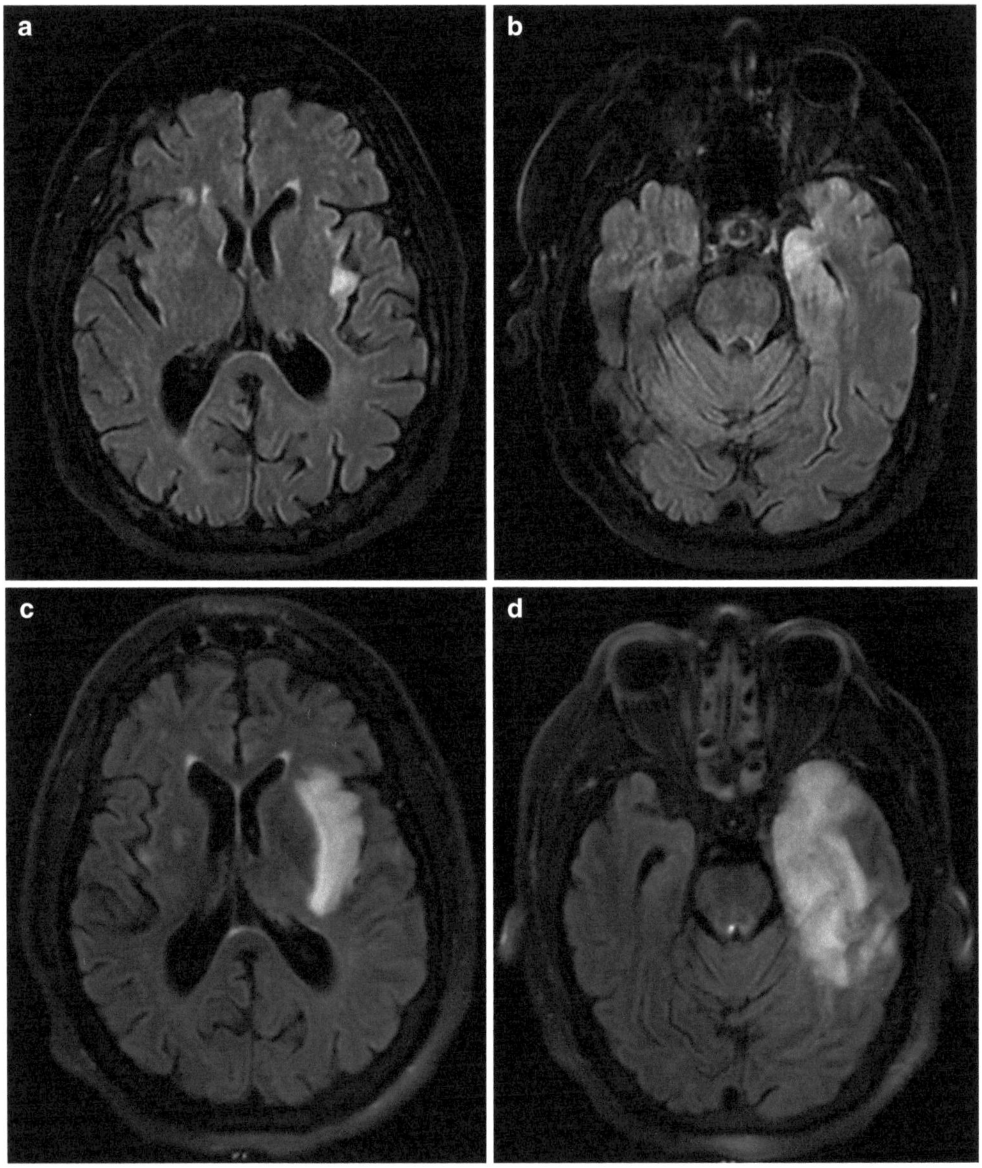

Fig. 4.10 Progressive course of HSV encephalitis. (**a** and **b**) MRI T2/FLAIR sequences showing hyperintensity within the insular region (**a**) and mesial temporal lobe (**b**), classic for patients with HSV encephalitis. (**c** and **d**) MRI T2/FLAIR sequences 1 month later showing increased hyperintensity within the same insular region (**c**), and mesial temporal lobe (**d**)

can be helpful in determining the presence and extent of ventriculitis with certain sequences. The T2 sequence may show periventricular hyperintensity, representative of the transependymal edema. Furthermore, the periventricular region may show restricted diffusion on DWI and ADC. The post-contrast T1 sequence may particularly be useful, showing contrast enhancement along and within the ventricles [85].

Traumatic Brain Injury

Traumatic brain injury (TBI) is a major cause of morbidity and mortality across the world. However, with the rapid advancement of neuroimaging and neuromonitoring techniques, there is now great potential to improve the accuracy of diagnosis and prognosis, as well as to guide development of new therapeutic interventions. Clinical classification of TBI severity is based on the admission Glasgow Coma Scale (GCS) score, with mild defined as a GCS of 13 to 15, moderate as a GCS of 9 to 12, and severe as a GCS of 8 or less [86].

Noncontrast CT Head

As with all acute neurological symptoms, the preferred acute neuroimaging technique is a CTH given its ease of accessibility and the rapidity at which it can be completed. A noncontrast CTH is able to detect emergent sequelae of TBI, such as large skull fractures or mass-occupying hemorrhages that warrant immediate neurosurgical intervention (Fig. 4.11) [87]. Furthermore, there are two CTH classification systems that utilize radiographic changes to classify and prognosticate TBI. First, there is the Marshall CT Classification Scale (Table 4.4) [88], which defines categories of diffuse injury

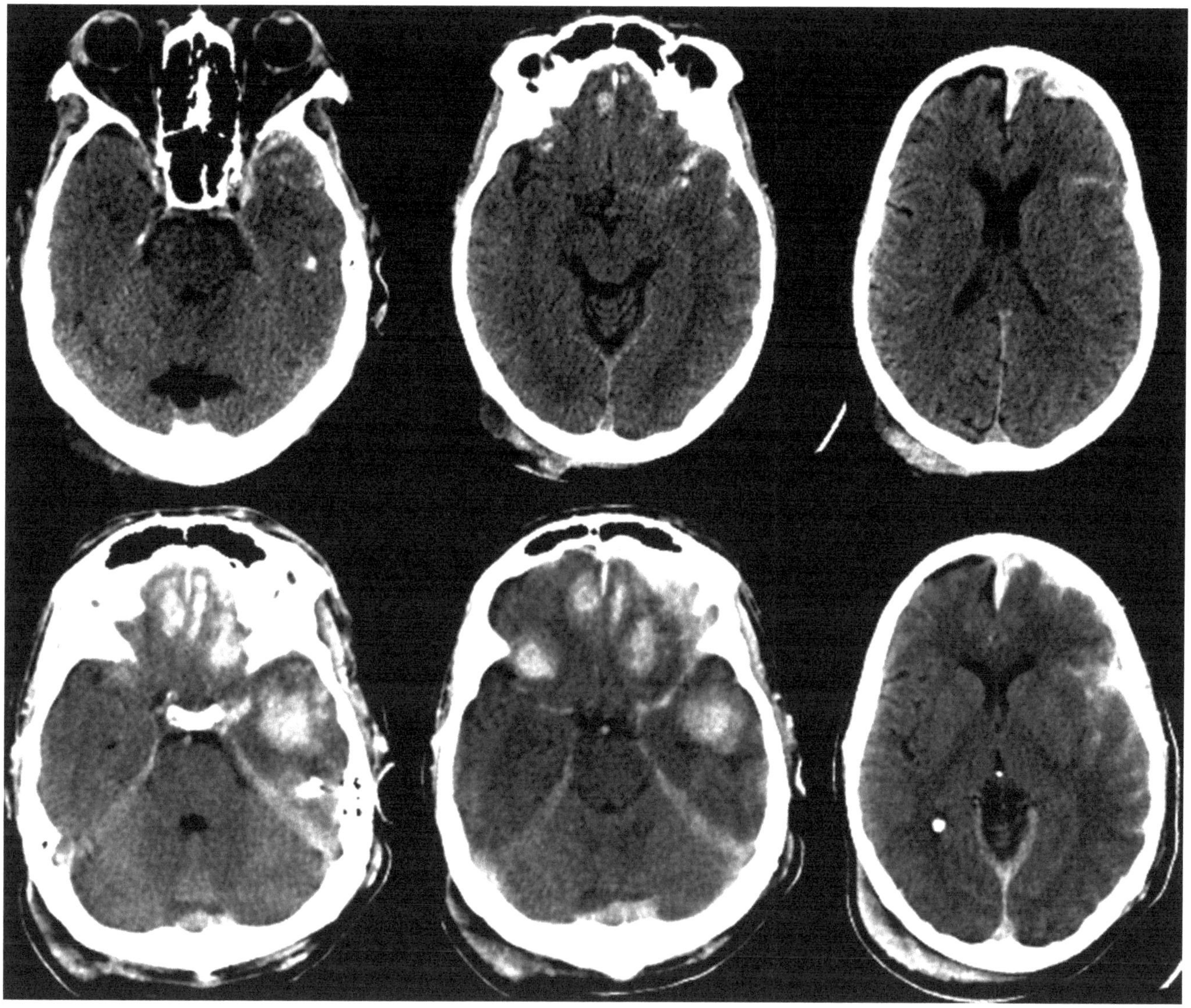

Fig. 4.11 Traumatic Brain Injury (TBI). Noncontrast CT head with bilateral frontal and temporal contusions, and diffuse left > right traumatic subarachnoid hemorrhage at time of presentation to the emergency room (Row 1), with interval progression and "blooming" of contusions with progressive subarachnoid hemorrhage on repeat 6-h scan (Row 2)

Table 4.4 Marshall CT classification scale for traumatic brain injury [88]

Scale	Definition
1	Diffuse injury I: No visible intracranial pathology
2	Diffuse injury II: Cisterns appear present; 0–5 mm of midline shift and/or lesion present; no high- or mixed-density lesion >25 mL
3	Diffuse injury III: Cisterns appear compressed or are absent; 0–5 mm of midline shift; no high- or mixed-density lesion >25 mL
4	Diffuse injury IV: >5 mm of midline shift; no high- or mixed-density lesion >25 mL
5	Any lesion surgically evacuated
6	Presence of high- or mixed-density lesion >25 mL, not surgically evacuated

and mass lesions with their associated 6-month mortality. Second, there is the Rotterdam CT Score [89] (Table 4.5) which scores the presence or absence of basal cisterns, midline shift, mass lesion, and intraventricular or subarachnoid blood to prognosticate outcomes.

MRI

A conventional MRI is routinely obtained in patients with TBI once they have acutely stabilized. MRI provides better detection of traumatic axonal injury (TAI) than noncontrast CTH [90–93] and is a more useful prognostication tool as well [90, 94, 95]. The T2 FLAIR sequence helps to evaluate white matter changes and assists in characterizing the extent of TAI. The DWI sequence, as seen with ischemic stroke, may show restricted diffusion by DWI hyperintensity with ADC hypointensity. However, unlike acute ischemic stroke, which takes minutes for diffusion restriction to appear, TAI-related diffusion restriction may be delayed and persist up to 18 days post initial injury [96]. Furthermore, diffusion restriction related to TAI is often reversible, and thus diffusion restriction should not be interpreted as infarction in patients with TBI [97, 98]. Studies of the GRE and SWI sequences within the TBI population have demonstrated that up to 80% of TAI lesions are associated with traumatic microbleeds (TMBs) [95, 99]. Historically TMBs have been associated with duration of post-traumatic unconsciousness and degree of neurological recovery [100, 101]. However, despite this potential correlation with severity and outcomes, there is inconsistent data about utilizing TMBs to predict long-term outcomes [45, 93, 99, 102, 103].

Other MRI sequences currently under investigation to enhance the characterization of TBI, define the degree of TAI, and provide new insights into pathophysiology, diagnosis, and prognostication include diffusion tensor imaging (DTI), diffusion tensor tractography, high angular resolution diffusion imaging (HARDI) tractography, resting state functional MRI (rs-fMRI), stimulus- and task-based fMRI, arterial-spin labeled (ASL) perfusion MRI, and magnetic resonance spectroscopy (MRS). Additional imaging techniques that are not part of the standard protocols at this time include PET scan, which may be considered to measure changes in brain metabolism.

Table 4.5 Rotterdam CT score [89]

Radiographic feature	Score
Basal cisterns	
Normal	0
Compressed	1
Absent	2
Midline shift	
None; < 5 mm	0
> 5 mm	1
Epidural mass lesion	
Present	0
Absent	1
Intraventricular or subarachnoid hemorrhage	
Present	0
Absent	1
Sum score: Calculate all variables and add 1 point to the total	+1

Hypoxic Ischemic Encephalopathy

Hypoxic Ischemic Encephalopathy (HIE) is a severe complication of global hypoperfusion of the brain, which may result in death or long-term disability. The most common etiology in the adult population is cardiac arrest or cerebrovascular disease. Neuroimaging not only plays an important role in the diagnosis of HIE, but also is essential in guiding clinical practice, which focuses largely on supportive care. Furthermore, imaging plays a critical role in determining the extent and severity of injury, which may help predict long-term outcomes.

Noncontrast CT Head

The noncontrast CTH is the initial screening test for patients with concern for acute neurological injury. However, it has a limited role in determining the extent of brain injury and is relatively insensitive in detecting early injury [104]. Diffuse cerebral edema may be seen as loss of cortical gray-white matter differentiation, effacement of the CSF-containing spaces, and loss of delineation of bilateral basal ganglia structures (Fig. 4.12) [105]. The reversal of normal gray-white matter junction characteristics has been termed the "reversal sign" and is often apparent within the first 24 h of acute injury. This sign indicates severe injury with a poor

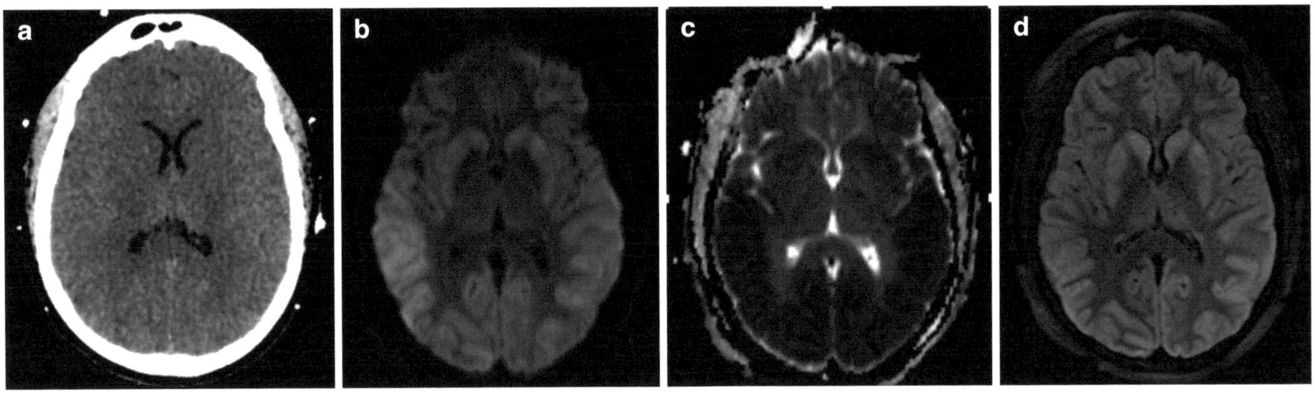

Fig. 4.12 Hypoxic ischemic encephalopathy (HIE). (**a**) Noncontrast CT head with complete loss of gray-white differentiation in the cerebrum consistent with diffuse cerebral edema in severe HIE. (**b** and **c**) MRI brain DWI and ADC sequences, respectively, with gyral diffusion restriction involving the posterior frontal, perirolandic, and occipital cortices. (**d**) MRI brain T2/FLAIR with associated hyperintensity in the same region of diffusion restriction

prognosis [106–108]. The "white cerebellum sign" has been described in conjunction with the reversal sign, where the cerebellum is relatively spared and thus appears hyperdense in comparison to the affected cerebral hemispheres [108]. In severe cases, a "pseudosubarachnoid hemorrhage sign" may also be seen, described as hyperdensity of the basal cisterns and sulci compared to the surrounding hypodense brain parenchyma, mimicking the presence of subarachnoid blood within this space [108].

MRI Brain

A negative CTH should prompt further evaluation with MRI, the neuroimaging modality of choice, not only to assist in the diagnosis of HIE, but also to determine the extent of injury. The neuroanatomic distribution of changes on MRI depends on the duration of injury, time from initial insult, and severity of disease. The pattern of disease in mild to moderate HIE presents as injury to the watershed zones, whereas severe HIE presents as injury to the parieto-occipital cortex, basal ganglia, thalami, hippocampus, and cerebellum (Fig. 4.12) [104, 109–111]. These regions have increased signal intensity on DWI with corresponding low signal on ADC due to cytotoxic edema, within the first 24 h of injury. It is important to note that these changes may normalize after 1 week [109, 112]; time to MRI acquisition impacts MRI characteristics and may complicate the use of MRI to prognosticate outcomes in these patients. T2 FLAIR imaging may show hyperintensity in these regions as early as 24 h, and up to 2 weeks of injury, with decreased intensity as time advances [109]. During the late subacute to chronic phase, signs of cortical laminar necrosis, seen as gyriform hyperintensity on T1-weighted imaging, may be seen. Ultimately, cortical atrophy and progressive white matter changes will be seen [109]. Of note, contrast enhancement typically is seen within 1–2 weeks up to 1–2 months, with resolution approximately after 6 months [109, 113].

MR Spectroscopy

Along with the DWI sequence on conventional MRI, MR spectroscopy has been described as a sensitive neuroimaging modality for the detection of HIE in the acute phase [104]. In cases of HIE, MR spectroscopy will demonstrate lactate elevation within the areas previously described to be at most risk, including the deep gray nuclei, parieto-occipital cortex, and watershed zones. There will typically be an acute rise in lactate initially after injury, followed by a second peak after 24–48 h, which may be an indicator of poor prognosis [104, 114].

Spinal Cord Compression

Spinal cord compression is a neurological emergency requiring prompt diagnosis to ensure timely management and minimize permanent neurological injury. The differential diagnosis of spinal cord compression can be classified by mechanism (traumatic or nontraumatic) or based on the site of origin (bony compartment, epidural space, or intradural space) [115] (Table 4.6). Neuroimaging plays a critical role in the diagnosis of compression and elucidating the integrity of the spinal cord along with the surrounding soft and bony tissue.

CT Spine

CT spine is the first-line imaging modality for acute spinal trauma, as it is able to definitively detect bony injury and elucidate significant soft tissue injury such as severe ligament hypertrophy, epidural collections, and/or disc herniations [115, 116].

MRI Spine

MRI is the imaging modality of choice to assess the soft tissue compartments, including the vertebral ligaments, intervertebral discs, and spinal cord. It can further differentiate the extradural and intradural compartments and is thus the imaging modality of choice for evaluation of nontraumatic myelopathy. Typical sequences used to distinguish between intrinsic versus extrinsic spinal cord lesions include unenhanced and post-gadolinium enhanced T1, unenhanced T2, and the T2-weighted fat-suppressed sequence in both axial and sagittal views. Importantly, the T2-weighted fat-suppressed sequence, also known as the STIR sequence, delineates fat as a dark signal and fluid as a bright signal, which makes edema more prominent and easier to detect. Additionally, any acute compression will result in an ill-defined area of abnormal T2 signal hyperintensity above and below the site of compression to the spinal cord, along with displacement of the surrounding CSF [115] (Fig. 4.13).

CT Myelography

CT myelography is contrasted fluoroscopic imaging of the spinal cord, which can be used to assess the nerve roots and meningeal lining [117]. It has largely been replaced by noninvasive MRI but is still used in situations where MRI is unable to be obtained. Furthermore, CT myelography remains the preferred imaging modality for certain indica-

Table 4.6 Differential diagnosis of spinal cord compression with key radiologic features [115]

Bony structures	Epidural space	Intradural space
Vertebral fractures	Disc herniation	
Osseous spine tumors (e.g., metastatic or primary)	Tumors	Tumor
Degenerative disease (e.g., RA, OA)	Epidural hematoma	Hematoma
	Epidural abscess	

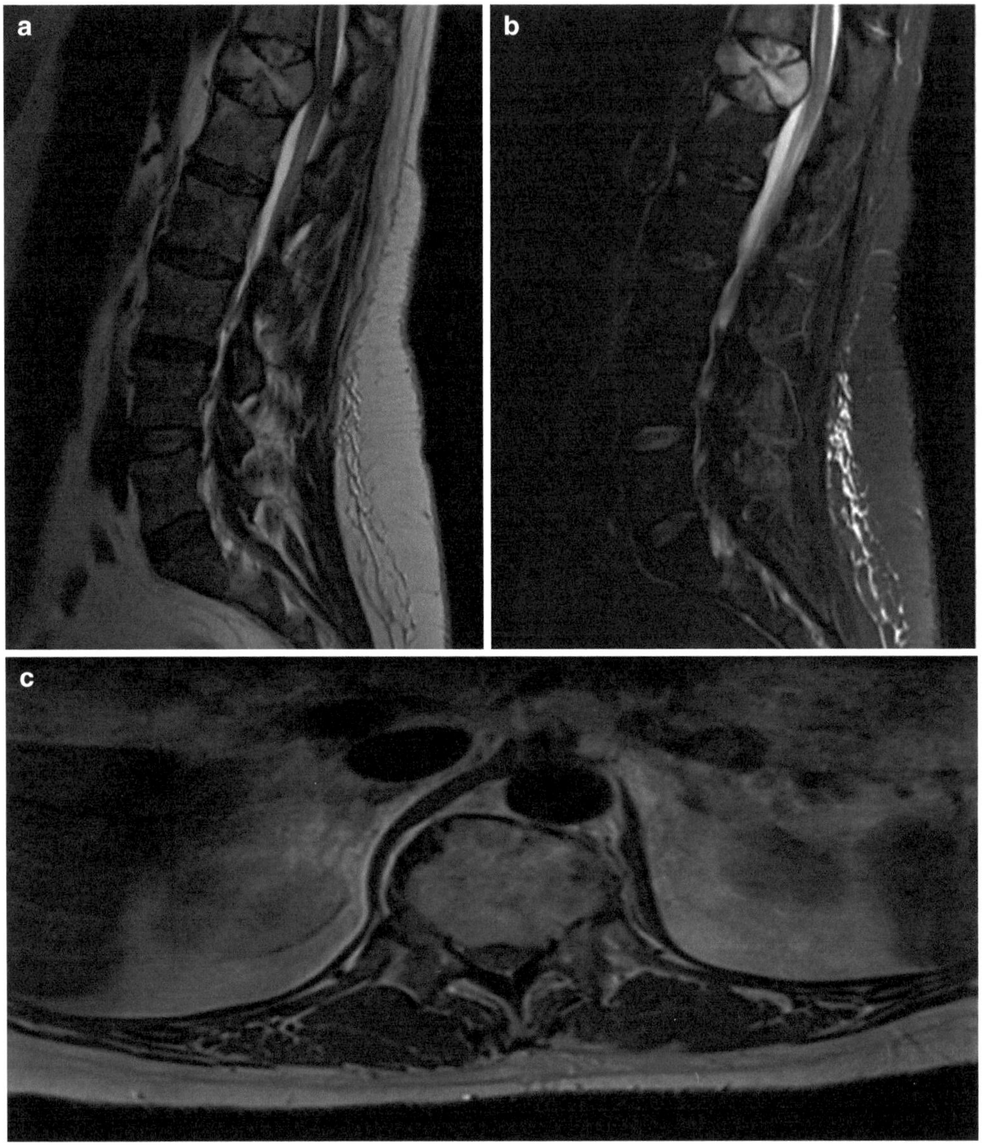

Fig. 4.13 Spinal cord compression. (**a**) MRI T2/FLAIR sequence, sagittal view, with severe compression deformity at T12 vertebral body with retropulsion resulting in moderate to severe spinal canal stenosis with complete effacement of the CSF spaces and flattening of the cord. There is also faint associated T2 hyperintense signal within the cord. (**b**) MRI STIR sequence, sagittal view, with abnormal hyperintense signal and enhancement throughout this vertebral body and corresponding spinal cord. (**c**) MRI T2/FLAIR sequence, axial view, with effacement of the left T11–T12 neural foramen

tions, including arachnoid disease (e.g., spinal arachnoid cyst, arachnoid web, arachnoiditis), superficial spinal siderosis, suspected CSF leak, or in some cases of suspected nerve root avulsion [117].

Conclusion

Neuroimaging is a rapidly evolving and improving tool that plays a critical role in not only the diagnosis of acute neurological disease, but also is paramount in informing prognosis and guiding management. Thus, learning hallmark radiologic features of high-yield neurological disease processes on neuroimaging is vital for optimizing patient care.

References

1. Saver JL. Time is brain--quantified. Stroke. 2006;37(1):263–6. https://doi.org/10.1161/01.STR.0000196957.55928.ab.
2. Ciccone A, Sterzi R, Munari L, paper sat. MRI versus CT in acute stroke. Lancet. 2007;369(9570):1342–3. https://doi.org/10.1016/S0140-6736(07)60624-2.
3. El-Koussy M, Schroth G, Brekenfeld C, Arnold M. Imaging of acute ischemic stroke. Eur Neurol. 2014;72(5-6):309–16. https://doi.org/10.1159/000362719.
4. Jadhav AP, Desai SM, Liebeskind DS, Wechsler LR. Neuroimaging of acute stroke. Neurol Clin. 2020;38(1):185–99. https://doi.org/10.1016/j.ncl.2019.09.004.
5. Pexman JH, Barber PA, Hill MD, et al. Use of the Alberta stroke program early CT score (ASPECTS) for assessing CT scans in patients with acute stroke. AJNR Am J Neuroradiol. 2001;22(8):1534–42.

6. Kuang H, Qiu W, Najm M, et al. Validation of an automated ASPECTS method on non-contrast computed tomography scans of acute ischemic stroke patients. Int J Stroke. 2020;15(5):528–34. https://doi.org/10.1177/1747493019895702.
7. Huo X, Ma G, Tong X, et al. Trial of endovascular therapy for acute ischemic stroke with large infarct. N Engl J Med. 2023;388(14):1272–83. https://doi.org/10.1056/NEJMoa2213379.
8. Sarraj A, Hassan AE, Abraham MG, et al. Trial of Endovascular Thrombectomy for Large Ischemic Strokes. N Engl J Med. 2023;388(14):1259–71. https://doi.org/10.1056/NEJMoa2214403.
9. Mair G, Boyd EV, Chappell FM, et al. Sensitivity and specificity of the hyperdense artery sign for arterial obstruction in acute ischemic stroke. Stroke. 2015;46(1):102–7. https://doi.org/10.1161/STROKEAHA.114.007036.
10. Li Q, Davis S, Mitchell P, Dowling R, Yan B. Proximal hyperdense middle cerebral artery sign predicts poor response to thrombolysis. PLoS One. 2014;9(5):e96123. https://doi.org/10.1371/journal.pone.0096123.
11. Demchuk AM, Menon BK, Goyal M. Comparing vessel imaging: noncontrast computed tomography/computed tomographic angiography should be the new minimum standard in acute disabling stroke. Stroke. 2016;47(1):273–81. https://doi.org/10.1161/STROKEAHA.115.009171.
12. Campbell BC, Mitchell PJ, Kleinig TJ, et al. Endovascular therapy for ischemic stroke with perfusion-imaging selection. N Engl J Med. 2015;372(11):1009–18. https://doi.org/10.1056/NEJMoa1414792.
13. Olivot JM, Mlynash M, Thijs VN, et al. Optimal Tmax threshold for predicting penumbral tissue in acute stroke. Stroke. 2009;40(2):469–75.
14. Edlow BL, Hurwitz S, Edlow JA. Diagnosis of DWI-negative acute ischemic stroke: A meta-analysis. Neurology. 2017;89(3):256–62. https://doi.org/10.1212/WNL.0000000000004120.
15. Leiva-Salinas C, Wintermark M. Imaging of acute ischemic stroke. Neuroimaging Clin N Am. 2010;20(4):455–68. https://doi.org/10.1016/j.nic.2010.07.002.
16. Li L, Liu MS, Li GQ, et al. Susceptibility-weighted imaging in thrombolytic therapy of acute ischemic stroke. Chin Med J (Engl). 2017;130(20):2489–97. https://doi.org/10.4103/0366-6999.216401.
17. Virani SS, Alonso A, Benjamin EJ, et al. Heart disease and stroke statistics-2020 update: a report from the american heart association. Circulation. 2020;141(9):e139–596. https://doi.org/10.1161/CIR.0000000000000757.
18. Greenberg SM, Charidimou A. Diagnosis of cerebral amyloid Angiopathy: evolution of the Boston criteria. Stroke. 2018;49(2):491–7. https://doi.org/10.1161/STROKEAHA.117.016990.
19. Freeman WD, Aguilar MI. Intracranial hemorrhage: diagnosis and management. Neurol Clin. 2012;30(1):211–40., ix. https://doi.org/10.1016/j.ncl.2011.09.002.
20. Khan M, Baird GL, Elias R, et al. Comparison of intracerebral hemorrhage volume calculation methods and their impact on scoring tools. J Neuroimaging. 2017;27(1):144–8. https://doi.org/10.1111/jon.12370.
21. Aytuluk HG, Basaran S, Dogan NO, Demir N. Comparison of conventional intensive care scoring systems and prognostic scores specific for intracerebral hemorrhage in predicting one-year mortality. Neurocrit Care. 2021;34(1):92–101. https://doi.org/10.1007/s12028-020-00987-3.
22. Hemphill JC, Bonovich DC, Besmertis L, Manley GT, Johnston SC. The ICH score: a simple, reliable grading scale for intracerebral hemorrhage. Stroke. 2001;32(4):891–7. https://doi.org/10.1161/01.str.32.4.891.
23. McCracken DJ, Lovasik BP, McCracken CE, et al. The Intracerebral Hemorrhage Score: A Self-Fulfilling Prophecy? Neurosurgery. 2019;84(3):741–8. https://doi.org/10.1093/neuros/nyy193.
24. Brant WE, Helms CA. Fundamentalse of diagnostic radiology. 3rd ed; 2007.
25. Ropper AH. Lateral displacement of the brain and level of consciousness in patients with an acute hemispheral mass. N Engl J Med. 1986;314(15):953–8. https://doi.org/10.1056/NEJM198604103141504.
26. Morotti A, Arba F, Boulouis G, Charidimou A. Noncontrast CT markers of intracerebral hemorrhage expansion and poor outcome: A meta-analysis. Neurology. 2020;95(14):632–43. https://doi.org/10.1212/WNL.0000000000010660.
27. Li Q, Zhang G, Xiong X, et al. Black hole sign: novel imaging marker that predicts hematoma growth in patients with intracerebral hemorrhage. Stroke. 2016;47(7):1777–81. https://doi.org/10.1161/STROKEAHA.116.013186.
28. Al-Nakshabandi NA. The swirl sign. Radiology. 2001;218(2):433. https://doi.org/10.1148/radiology.218.2.r01fe09433.
29. Ng D, Churilov L, Mitchell P, Dowling R, Yan B. The CT swirl sign is associated with hematoma expansion in intracerebral hemorrhage. AJNR Am J Neuroradiol. 2018;39(2):232–7. https://doi.org/10.3174/ajnr.A5465.
30. Li Q, Yang WS, Wang XC, et al. Blend sign predicts poor outcome in patients with intracerebral hemorrhage. PLoS One. 2017;12(8):e0183082. https://doi.org/10.1371/journal.pone.0183082.
31. Sporns PB, Kemmling A, Schwake M, et al. Triage of 5 Noncontrast Computed Tomography Markers and Spot Sign for Outcome Prediction After Intracerebral Hemorrhage. Stroke. 2018;49(10):2317–22. https://doi.org/10.1161/STROKEAHA.118.021625.
32. Josephson CB, White PM, Krishan A, Al-Shahi SR. Computed tomography angiography or magnetic resonance angiography for detection of intracranial vascular malformations in patients with intracerebral haemorrhage. Cochrane Database Syst Rev. 2014;9:CD009372. https://doi.org/10.1002/14651858.CD009372.pub2.
33. Wada R, Aviv RI, Fox AJ, et al. CT angiography "spot sign" predicts hematoma expansion in acute intracerebral hemorrhage. Stroke. 2007;38(4):1257–62. https://doi.org/10.1161/01.STR.0000259633.59404.f3.
34. Macellari F, Paciaroni M, Agnelli G, Caso V. Neuroimaging in intracerebral hemorrhage. Stroke. 2014;45(3):903–8. https://doi.org/10.1161/STROKEAHA.113.003701.
35. Patel MR, Edelman RR, Warach S. Detection of hyperacute primary intraparenchymal hemorrhage by magnetic resonance imaging. Stroke. 1996;27(12):2321–4. https://doi.org/10.1161/01.str.27.12.2321.
36. Schellinger PD, Jansen O, Fiebach JB, Hacke W, Sartor K. A standardized MRI stroke protocol: comparison with CT in hyperacute intracerebral hemorrhage. Stroke. 1999;30(4):765–8. https://doi.org/10.1161/01.str.30.4.765.
37. Linfante I, Llinas RH, Caplan LR, Warach S. MRI features of intracerebral hemorrhage within 2 hours from symptom onset. Stroke. 1999;30(11):2263–7. https://doi.org/10.1161/01.str.30.11.2263.
38. Fiebach JB, Schellinger PD, Gass A, et al. Stroke magnetic resonance imaging is accurate in hyperacute intracerebral hemorrhage: a multicenter study on the validity of stroke imaging. Stroke. 2004;35(2):502–6. https://doi.org/10.1161/01.STR.0000114203.75678.88.
39. Chalela JA, Kidwell CS, Nentwich LM, et al. Magnetic resonance imaging and computed tomography in emergency assessment of patients with suspected acute stroke: a prospective compari-

son. Lancet. 2007;369(9558):293–8. https://doi.org/10.1016/S0140-6736(07)60151-2.
40. Kidwell CS, Chalela JA, Saver JL, et al. Comparison of MRI and CT for detection of acute intracerebral hemorrhage. JAMA. 2004;292(15):1823–30. https://doi.org/10.1001/jama.292.15.1823.
41. Bradley WG. MR appearance of hemorrhage in the brain. Radiology. 1993;189(1):15–26. https://doi.org/10.1148/radiology.189.1.8372185.
42. Wintermark M, Fiebach J. Imaging of brain parenchyma in stroke. Handb Clin Neurol. 2009;94:1011–9. https://doi.org/10.1016/S0072-9752(08)94049-5.
43. Kidwell CS, Saver JL, Villablanca JP, et al. Magnetic resonance imaging detection of microbleeds before thrombolysis: an emerging application. Stroke. 2002;33(1):95–8. https://doi.org/10.1161/hs0102.101792.
44. Fisher CM, Kistler JP, Davis JM. Relation of cerebral vasospasm to subarachnoid hemorrhage visualized by computerized tomographic scanning. Neurosurgery. 1980;6(1):1–9.
45. Perry JJ, Stiell IG, Sivilotti ML, et al. Sensitivity of computed tomography performed within six hours of onset of headache for diagnosis of subarachnoid haemorrhage: prospective cohort study. BMJ. 2011;343:d4277. https://doi.org/10.1136/bmj.d4277.
46. da Rocha AJ, da Silva CJ, Gama HP, et al. Comparison of magnetic resonance imaging sequences with computed tomography to detect low-grade subarachnoid hemorrhage: role of fluid-attenuated inversion recovery sequence. J Comput Assist Tomogr. 2006;30(2):295–303. https://doi.org/10.1097/00004728-200603000-00025.
47. Dubosh NM, Bellolio MF, Rabinstein AA, Edlow JA. Sensitivity of early brain computed tomography to exclude aneurysmal subarachnoid hemorrhage: a systematic review and meta-analysis. Stroke. 2016;47(3):750–5. https://doi.org/10.1161/STROKEAHA.115.011386.
48. Frontera JA, Claassen J, Schmidt JM, et al. Prediction of symptomatic vasospasm after subarachnoid hemorrhage: the modified fisher scale. Neurosurgery. 2006;59(1):21–7; discussion 21–7. https://doi.org/10.1227/01.NEU.0000218821.34014.1B.
49. Hijdra A, Brouwers PJ, Vermeulen M, van Gijn J. Grading the amount of blood on computed tomograms after subarachnoid hemorrhage. Stroke. 1990;21(8):1156–61. https://doi.org/10.1161/01.str.21.8.1156.
50. Marcolini E, Hine J. Approach to the diagnosis and Management of Subarachnoid Hemorrhage. West J Emerg Med. 2019;20(2):203–11. https://doi.org/10.5811/westjem.2019.1.37352.
51. Wardlaw JM, White PM. The detection and management of unruptured intracranial aneurysms. Brain. 2000;123(Pt 2):205–21. https://doi.org/10.1093/brain/123.2.205.
52. Howard BM, Hu R, Barrow JW, Barrow DL. Comprehensive review of imaging of intracranial aneurysms and angiographically negative subarachnoid hemorrhage. Neurosurg Focus. 2019;47(6):E20. https://doi.org/10.3171/2019.9.FOCUS19653.
53. Bakker NA, Groen RJ, Foumani M, et al. Repeat digital subtraction angiography after a negative baseline assessment in nonperimesencephalic subarachnoid hemorrhage: a pooled data meta-analysis. J Neurosurg. 2014;120(1):99–103. https://doi.org/10.3171/2013.9.JNS131337.
54. Naqvi J, Yap KH, Ahmad G, Ghosh J. Transcranial Doppler ultrasound: a review of the physical principles and major applications in critical care. Int J Vasc Med. 2013;2013:629378. https://doi.org/10.1155/2013/629378.
55. Sharma S, Lubrica RJ, Song M, Vandse R, Boling W, Pillai P. The role of transcranial Doppler in cerebral vasospasm: a literature review. Acta Neurochir Suppl. 2020;127:201–5. https://doi.org/10.1007/978-3-030-04615-6_32.
56. Marder CP, Narla V, Fink JR, Tozer Fink KR. Subarachnoid hemorrhage: beyond aneurysms. AJR Am J Roentgenol. 2014;202(1):25–37. https://doi.org/10.2214/AJR.12.9749.
57. Ducros A, Boukobza M, Porcher R, Sarov M, Valade D, Bousser MG. The clinical and radiological spectrum of reversible cerebral vasoconstriction syndrome. A prospective series of 67 patients. Brain. 2007;130(Pt 12):3091–101. https://doi.org/10.1093/brain/awm256.
58. Calabrese LH, Dodick DW, Schwedt TJ, Singhal AB. Narrative review: reversible cerebral vasoconstriction syndromes. Ann Intern Med. 2007;146(1):34–44. https://doi.org/10.7326/0003-4819-146-1-200701020-00007.
59. Singhal AB, Hajj-Ali RA, Topcuoglu MA, et al. Reversible cerebral vasoconstriction syndromes: analysis of 139 cases. Arch Neurol. 2011;68(8):1005–12. https://doi.org/10.1001/archneurol.2011.68.
60. Mandell DM, Matouk CC, Farb RI, et al. Vessel wall MRI to differentiate between reversible cerebral vasoconstriction syndrome and central nervous system vasculitis: preliminary results. Stroke. 2012;43(3):860–2. https://doi.org/10.1161/STROKEAHA.111.626184.
61. Topcuoglu MA, Kursun O, Singhal AB. Coexisting vascular lesions in reversible cerebral vasoconstriction syndrome. Cephalalgia. 2017;37(1):29–35. https://doi.org/10.1177/0333102416637826.
62. Mawet J, Boukobza M, Franc J, et al. Reversible cerebral vasoconstriction syndrome and cervical artery dissection in 20 patients. Neurology. 2013;81(9):821–4. https://doi.org/10.1212/WNL.0b013e3182a2cbe2.
63. Gokey R, Das JM. Venous sinus thrombosis. StatPearls [Internet]: Treasure Island (FL):. StatPearls Publishing; 2021.
64. Sader N, de Lotbinière-Bassett M, Tso MK, Hamilton M. Management of Venous Sinus Thrombosis. Neurosurg Clin N Am. 2018;29(4):585–94. https://doi.org/10.1016/j.nec.2018.06.011.
65. Alvis-Miranda HR, Milena Castellar-Leones S, Alcala-Cerra G, Rafael M-SL. Cerebral sinus venous thrombosis. J Neurosci Rural Pract. 2013;4(4):427–38. https://doi.org/10.4103/0976-3147.120236.
66. Fischer C, Goldstein J, Edlow J. Cerebral venous sinus thrombosis in the emergency department: retrospective analysis of 17 cases and review of the literature. J Emerg Med. 2010;38(2):140–7. https://doi.org/10.1016/j.jemermed.2009.08.061.
67. Guenther G, Arauz A. Cerebral venous thrombosis: a diagnostic and treatment update. Neurologia. 2011;26(8):488–98. https://doi.org/10.1016/j.nrl.2010.09.013.
68. Poon CS, Chang JK, Swarnkar A, Johnson MH, Wasenko J. Radiologic diagnosis of cerebral venous thrombosis: pictorial review. AJR Am J Roentgenol. 2007;189(6 Suppl):S64–75. https://doi.org/10.2214/AJR.07.7015.
69. Chik Y, Gottesman RF, Zeiler SR, Rosenberg J, Llinas RH. Differentiation of transverse sinus thrombosis from congenitally atretic cerebral transverse sinus with CT. Stroke. 2012;43(7):1968–70. https://doi.org/10.1161/STROKEAHA.112.656124.
70. Bidar F, Faeghi F, Ghorbani A. Assessment of cerebral venous sinus thrombosis using T2 (*)-weighted gradient echo magnetic resonance imaging sequences. Iran J Neurol. 2016;15(2):96–9.
71. Leach JL, Fortuna RB, Jones BV, Gaskill-Shipley MF. Imaging of cerebral venous thrombosis: current techniques, spectrum of findings, and diagnostic pitfalls. Radiographics. 2006;26(Suppl 1):S19–41.; ; discussion S42–3. https://doi.org/10.1148/rg.26si055174.
72. Shankar J, Banfield J. Posterior reversible encephalopathy syndrome: a review. Can Assoc Radiol J. 2017;68(2):147–53. https://doi.org/10.1016/j.carj.2016.08.005.

73. Bartynski WS, Boardman JF. Distinct imaging patterns and lesion distribution in posterior reversible encephalopathy syndrome. AJNR Am J Neuroradiol. 2007;28(7):1320–7. https://doi.org/10.3174/ajnr.A0549.
74. Tetsuka S, Ogawa T. Posterior reversible encephalopathy syndrome: a review with emphasis on neuroimaging characteristics. J Neurol Sci. 2019;404:72–9. https://doi.org/10.1016/j.jns.2019.07.018.
75. Vargas MI, Gariani J, Sztajzel R, et al. Spinal cord ischemia: practical imaging tips, pearls, and pitfalls. AJNR Am J Neuroradiol. 2015;36(5):825–30. https://doi.org/10.3174/ajnr.A4118.
76. Novy J, Carruzzo A, Maeder P, Bogousslavsky J. Spinal cord ischemia: clinical and imaging patterns, pathogenesis, and outcomes in 27 patients. Arch Neurol. 2006;63(8):1113–20. https://doi.org/10.1001/archneur.63.8.1113.
77. Barnholtz-Sloan JS, Sloan AE, Davis FG, Vigneau FD, Lai P, Sawaya RE. Incidence proportions of brain metastases in patients diagnosed (1973 to 2001) in the metropolitan Detroit cancer surveillance system. J Clin Oncol. 2004;22(14):2865–72. https://doi.org/10.1200/JCO.2004.12.149.
78. Mabray MC, Barajas RF, Cha S. Modern brain tumor imaging. Brain Tumor Res Treat. 2015;3(1):8–23. https://doi.org/10.14791/btrt.2015.3.1.8.
79. Danieli L, Riccitelli GC, Distefano D, et al. Brain tumor-enhancement visualization and morphometric assessment: a comparison of MPRAGE, SPACE, and VIBE MRI techniques. AJNR Am J Neuroradiol. 2019;40(7):1140–8. https://doi.org/10.3174/ajnr.A6096.
80. Dorsett M, Liang SY. Diagnosis and treatment of central nervous system infections in the emergency department. Emerg Med Clin North Am. 2016;34(4):917–42. https://doi.org/10.1016/j.emc.2016.06.013.
81. van Crevel H, Hijdra A, de Gans J. Lumbar puncture and the risk of herniation: when should we first perform CT? J Neurol. 2002;249(2):129–37. https://doi.org/10.1007/pl00007855.
82. Tunkel AR, Hartman BJ, Kaplan SL, et al. Practice guidelines for the management of bacterial meningitis. Clin Infect Dis. 2004;39(9):1267–84. https://doi.org/10.1086/425368.
83. Rath TJ, Hughes M, Arabi M, Shah GV. Imaging of cerebritis, encephalitis, and brain abscess. Neuroimaging Clin N Am. 2012;22(4):585–607. https://doi.org/10.1016/j.nic.2012.04.002.
84. Hui FK, Bain M, Obuchowski NA, et al. Mycotic aneurysm detection rates with cerebral angiography in patients with infective endocarditis. J Neurointerv Surg. 2015;7(6):449–52. https://doi.org/10.1136/neurintsurg-2014-011124.
85. Fukui MB, Williams RL, Mudigonda S. CT and MR imaging features of pyogenic ventriculitis. AJNR Am J Neuroradiol. 2001;22(8):1510–6.
86. Maas AI, Stocchetti N, Bullock R. Moderate and severe traumatic brain injury in adults. Lancet Neurol. 2008;7(8):728–41. https://doi.org/10.1016/S1474-4422(08)70164-9.
87. Douglas DB, Ro T, Toffoli T, et al. Neuroimaging of traumatic brain injury. Med Sci (Basel). 2018;7(1):2. https://doi.org/10.3390/medsci7010002.
88. Marshall LF, Marshall SB, Klauber MR, et al. The diagnosis of head injury requires a classification based on computed axial tomography. J Neurotrauma. 1992;9(Suppl 1):S287–92.
89. Maas AI, Hukkelhoven CW, Marshall LF, Steyerberg EW. Prediction of outcome in traumatic brain injury with computed tomographic characteristics: a comparison between the computed tomographic classification and combinations of computed tomographic predictors. Neurosurgery. 2005;57(6):1173–82.; ; discussion 1173–82. https://doi.org/10.1227/01.neu.0000186013.63046.6b.
90. Firsching R, Woischneck D, Diedrich M, et al. Early magnetic resonance imaging of brainstem lesions after severe head injury. J Neurosurg. 1998;89(5):707–12. https://doi.org/10.3171/jns.1998.89.5.0707.
91. Paterakis K, Karantanas AH, Komnos A, Volikas Z. Outcome of patients with diffuse axonal injury: the significance and prognostic value of MRI in the acute phase. J Trauma. 2000;49(6):1071–5. https://doi.org/10.1097/00005373-200012000-00016.
92. Gentry LR, Godersky JC, Thompson B, Dunn VD. Prospective comparative study of intermediate-field MR and CT in the evaluation of closed head trauma. AJR Am J Roentgenol. 1988;150(3):673–82. https://doi.org/10.2214/ajr.150.3.673.
93. Lee H, Wintermark M, Gean AD, Ghajar J, Manley GT, Mukherjee P. Focal lesions in acute mild traumatic brain injury and neurocognitive outcome: CT versus 3T MRI. J Neurotrauma. 2008;25(9):1049–56. https://doi.org/10.1089/neu.2008.0566.
94. Skandsen T, Kvistad KA, Solheim O, Lydersen S, Strand IH, Vik A. Prognostic value of magnetic resonance imaging in moderate and severe head injury: a prospective study of early MRI findings and one-year outcome. J Neurotrauma. 2011;28(5):691–9. https://doi.org/10.1089/neu.2010.1590.
95. Lagares A, Ramos A, Pérez-Nuñez A, et al. The role of MR imaging in assessing prognosis after severe and moderate head injury. Acta Neurochir. 2009;151(4):341–56. https://doi.org/10.1007/s00701-009-0194-8.
96. Liu AY, Maldjian JA, Bagley LJ, Sinson GP, Grossman RI. Traumatic brain injury: diffusion-weighted MR imaging findings. AJNR Am J Neuroradiol. 1999;20(9):1636–41.
97. Edlow BL, Giacino JT, Hirschberg RE, Gerrard J, Wu O, Hochberg LR. Unexpected recovery of function after severe traumatic brain injury: the limits of early neuroimaging-based outcome prediction. Neurocrit Care. 2013;19(3):364–75. https://doi.org/10.1007/s12028-013-9870-x.
98. Muccio CF, De Simone M, Esposito G, De Blasio E, Vittori C, Cerase A. Reversible post-traumatic bilateral extensive restricted diffusion of the brain. A case study and review of the literature. Brain Inj. 2009;23(5):466–72. https://doi.org/10.1080/02699050902841912.
99. Scheid R, Preul C, Gruber O, Wiggins C, von Cramon DY. Diffuse axonal injury associated with chronic traumatic brain injury: evidence from T2*-weighted gradient-echo imaging at 3 T. AJNR Am J Neuroradiol. 2003;24(6):1049–56.
100. Tong KA, Ashwal S, Holshouser BA, et al. Diffuse axonal injury in children: clinical correlation with hemorrhagic lesions. Ann Neurol. 2004;56(1):36–50. https://doi.org/10.1002/ana.20123.
101. Yanagawa Y, Tsushima Y, Tokumaru A, et al. A quantitative analysis of head injury using T2*-weighted gradient-echo imaging. J Trauma. 2000;49(2):272–7. https://doi.org/10.1097/00005373-200008000-00013.
102. Scheid R, Walther K, Guthke T, Preul C, von Cramon DY. Cognitive sequelae of diffuse axonal injury. Arch Neurol. 2006;63(3):418–24. https://doi.org/10.1001/archneur.63.3.418.
103. Izzy S, Mazwi NL, Martinez S, et al. Revisiting grade 3 diffuse axonal injury: not all brainstem microbleeds are Prognostically equal. Neurocrit Care. 2017;27(2):199–207. https://doi.org/10.1007/s12028-017-0399-2.
104. Huang BY, Castillo M. Hypoxic-ischemic brain injury: imaging findings from birth to adulthood. Radiographics. 2008;28(2):417–39; quiz 617. https://doi.org/10.1148/rg.282075066.
105. Kjos BO, Brant-Zawadzki M, Young RG. Early CT findings of global central nervous system hypoperfusion. AJR Am J Roentgenol. 1983;141(6):1227–32. https://doi.org/10.2214/ajr.141.6.1227.
106. Vergote G, Vandeperre H, De Man R. The reversal sign. Neuroradiology. 1992;34(3):215–6. https://doi.org/10.1007/BF00596339.

107. Bird CR, Drayer BP, Gilles FH. Pathophysiology of "reverse" edema in global cerebral ischemia. AJNR Am J Neuroradiol. 1989;10(1):95–8.
108. Chua W, Lim BK, Lim TC. Clinics in diagnostic imaging (153). Severe shypoxic ischaemic brain injury. Singapore Med J. 2014;55(7):393–6; quiz 397. https://doi.org/10.11622/smedj.2014093.
109. Maurya VK, Ravikumar R, Bhatia M, Rai R. Hypoxic-ischemic brain injury in an adult: magnetic resonance imaging findings. Med J Armed Forces India. 2016;72(1):75–7. https://doi.org/10.1016/j.mjafi.2015.06.016.
110. Norton L, Hutchison RM, Young GB, Lee DH, Sharpe MD, Mirsattari SM. Disruptions of functional connectivity in the default mode network of comatose patients. Neurology. 2012;78(3):175–81. https://doi.org/10.1212/WNL.0b013e31823fcd61.
111. Snider SB, Bodien YG, Frau-Pascual A, Bianciardi M, Foulkes AS, Edlow BL. Ascending arousal network connectivity during recovery from traumatic coma. Neuroimage Clin. 2020;28:102503. https://doi.org/10.1016/j.nicl.2020.102503.
112. Els T, Kassubek J, Kubalek R, Klisch J. Diffusion-weighted MRI during early global cerebral hypoxia: a predictor for clinical outcome? Acta Neurol Scand. 2004;110(6):361–7. https://doi.org/10.1111/j.1600-0404.2004.00342.x.
113. Siskas N, Lefkopoulos A, Ioannidis I, Charitandi A, Dimitriadis AS. Cortical laminar necrosis in brain infarcts: serial MRI. Neuroradiology. 2003;45(5):283–8. https://doi.org/10.1007/s00234-002-0887-7.
114. Penrice J, Cady EB, Lorek A, et al. Proton magnetic resonance spectroscopy of the brain in normal preterm and term infants, and early changes after perinatal hypoxia-ischemia. Pediatr Res. 1996;40(1):6–14. https://doi.org/10.1203/00006450-199607000-00002.
115. Distefano D, Cianfoni A. Imaging of spinal cord compression. Imaging in Medicine. 2014;6(1):89.
116. Seidenwurm DJ, Wippold FJ, Cornelius RS, et al. ACR appropriateness criteria(®) myelopathy. J Am Coll Radiol. 2012;9(5):315–24. https://doi.org/10.1016/j.jacr.2012.01.010.
117. Patel DM, Weinberg BD, Hoch MJ. CT Myelography: clinical indications and imaging findings. Radiographics. 2020;40(2):470–84. https://doi.org/10.1148/rg.2020190135.

Part II

Signs, Symptoms and Management

Diagnosis and Treatment of Altered Mental Status

5

Christopher P. Robinson

Contents

C. P. Robinson (✉)
Departments of Neurology and Neurosurgery, University of Florida College of Medicine, Gainesville, FL, USA
e-mail: crobinson2@ufl.edu

E. Mahanna Gabrielli et al. (eds.), *Textbook of Neurointensive Care: Volume 1*, https://doi.org/10.1007/978-3-031-62220-5_5

Abstract

Altered mental status is commonly encountered in the neurological intensive care unit, and the differential diagnosis is broad. The general and neurological examinations can give many clues both to the neurological and non-neurological causes. Neuroimaging, neurophysiological tests, and laboratory studies are often helpful in identifying the etiology, which can run the entire gamut of disease processes including vascular, neoplastic, metabolic, or infectious. In cases of brain death, it is essential to understand the diagnostic criteria as well as adjunctive studies.

Chapter Objectives

- Identify the presentations and clinical descriptions of altered mental status.
- Recognize neurological exam findings in patients with altered mental status.
- Understand and evaluate patients with altered mental status in the ICU.
- Apply a standardized work up including laboratory and imaging modalities to assess altered mental status in the ICU.
- Analyze the various neurological diagnoses presenting as altered mental status.

Introduction

Altered mental status is a commonly encountered phenomenon in the Neurological Intensive Care Unit (NICU), but the reported range can be quite broad (13–70%) [1]. It may occur secondary to a variety of neurological and non-neurological etiologies. The differential diagnosis of altered mental status in the NICU is dauntingly large. It is important to narrow the differential by employing an understanding of the mechanisms underpinning arousal, by acquiring a careful history and physical examination, and by running carefully through the list of potential medical and neurological causes of an alteration of mental status.

Presentations and Descriptions of Acute Alterations in Consciousness

The clinical descriptors of the acutely altered states of consciousness [2] are helpful to determine severity of illness and for communication between healthcare providers. Classification of such altered states relies on both the patient's level of arousal and environmental perceptivity (content). They may or may not help in discerning a specific diagnosis or neurologic localization, but can be helpful in understanding the overall clinical picture. Below, we will review common classifications of altered consciousness used by ICU practitioners and discuss their clinical features. It is important to use the terms with consistency.

Clouding of consciousness refers to a patient that is inattentive without frank confusion and without disorientation. These individuals are usually not anosognosic—they are aware of their deficit—which differs from other forms of altered mentation. This term is commonly used to describe individuals who use certain medications or have mild metabolic disturbances [3].

A confusional state is similar to clouding of consciousness but has the additional feature of added confusion and/or disorientation. These individuals can be hypervigilant and can be combative. This state may result from medication use but more commonly is associated with infections or is encountered in individuals with very little cognitive reserve. When seen in those with poor cognitive reserve, these individuals usually have baseline physical, medical, or environmental stressors that contribute to the confusional state [3].

Lethargy refers to individuals who spontaneously sleep most of the day. Defined as a mild reduction in alertness, these individuals will wake with only mild stimulation but may also be confused. They may easily drift back to sleep if left unstimulated. During a bedside interview, they may require repeated stimuli to maintain appropriate attention and wakefulness. Often, these patients will be incomprehensible to a bedside examiner's ear, but they may occasionally provide useful historical and examination clues, especially if continuously stimulated. Lethargy is commonly associated with metabolic disturbances as well as other toxic etiologies [3].

Obtundation or "mental blunting" is a state of mild or moderate reduction in alertness and decreased interest in the environment. Obtunded patients may be difficult to arouse and may require deep pain to assess appropriate responses. Obtunded patients are slowed in their responsiveness and may stop interacting with their environment if not constantly stimulated. This state can be caused by a multitude of etiologies including metabolic disturbances, intoxications, brain lesions (with mild to moderate mass effect), CNS infections, and seizures [3].

Stupor or "to be stunned" is a moderate or severe reduction in arousal with severely decreased interest in the environment. These individuals may react to deep pain with eye opening, but do not interact with their environment. They may only grimace or withdraw from noxious stimuli. A stuporous patient may otherwise not perform purposeful actions.

Coma describes a state of general unconsciousness in which patients have no response to their environment. Coma patients do not respond to deep pain, have no eye opening, and commonly have impaired brainstem reflexes. Coma occurs due to severe impairment of the ascending reticular activating system (ARAS), bilateral thalami, or bilateral cortex from either metabolic or structural lesions. Common causes of coma include anoxic brain injury, traumatic brain injury, brainstem lesions, severe stroke or hemorrhage (usually with significant mass effect), and severe intoxications [3].

Neurocircuitry Underpinning the Level of Arousal

The level of arousal and the circuits that modulate consciousness have not been fully elucidated. It is believed that the reticular activating system plays a very important role in mediating wakefulness. [4] The reticular formation (throughout the brainstem), particularly in the periventricular region, gives rise to the ARAS. This system is thought to play a key role in activating the thalamocortical unit and in attentional processes. Once ascending to the level of the thalamus, the ARAS has a bilateral representation [5]. A depressed level of arousal can be induced by bilateral disruption of this system in the brainstem, thalamus, or cortex. At the level of the brainstem, discrete lesions will commonly include or compromise a significant portion of the reticular formation or even the ARAS. Supratentorial lesions manifesting in depressed arousal and coma must involve bilateral thalamo-cortical structures [6]. Initially, Plum and Posner theorized that supratentorial mass lesions resulting in a depressed level of arousal were secondary to downward forces impinging upon the brainstem reticular formation [2]. However, this notion has now been expanded to include lateral forces that can (in the case of mass effect) also contribute to arousal issues [5–7]. These arousal systems have a fair amount of redundancy, and it is this redundancy that may account for the relatively short-lived attentional problems in many patients, regardless of the etiology [7].

CNS insults other than focal lesions can also disturb the level of arousal. Toxic or metabolic derangements that disturb the ARAS and/or the cortex more diffusely may result in alterations in consciousness. It is not uncommon for toxic substances associated with systemic disease such as urea or ammonia to impair the function of the cerebral cortex more diffusely and therefore impair the terminal connections of the ARAS. This diffuse dysfunction of the cerebral cortex and ARAS may result in a depressed level of arousal and can be manifested by diffuse slowing on the electroencephalogram (EEG) [8].

Physical Examination and Evaluation in the ICU Setting

General

The importance of a complete general physical examination in the ICU setting cannot be overemphasized. Much information can be gained from observing the level of arousal prior to stimulation, as well as by observing the individual's reaction to verbal and tactile stimulation [2]. It is important to observe if an individual appears to be responding to internal-based stimuli, exhibition of abnormal movements, or manifestation of a normal or abnormal breathing pattern. Such observations can aid in narrowing the differential diagnosis for altered mental status. Examining specific systems can also reveal signs that may be directly or indirectly related to the cause of the altered mental status. Some of the issues uncovered may necessitate treatment, but the patient themselves cannot relay symptoms as a result of their state of diminished cognition. Examining specific organ systems can be helpful in both determining organ specific conditions that could cause or contribute to an altered mental status or contribute to the manifestations of the process underlying the altered state [9].

Cardiac and Carotid Examination

Auscultation of the chest can reveal evidence of a murmur, distant heart sounds, or a pericardial rub, all of which may be clues to underlying hypoxemia or hemodynamic dysfunction. It is important to keep in mind that aortic stenosis may present with syncope and a systolic ejection murmur radiating to the carotid artery region. The sound heard with aortic stenosis that radiates to the carotid artery region can be distinguished from that of carotid stenosis simply by auscultating over the ipsilateral eye (utilizing the bell of the stethoscope) [10]. If a sound is heard over the eye, it could be a referred sound emanating through the ophthalmic artery (the first branch off of the internal carotid artery) or secondary to reversal of flow from a completely occluded contralateral carotid artery [11]. In aortic stenosis, the pulse may also be appreciated as late and as weak (a pulsus parvus et tardus). A pericardial rub may be a clue to underlying pericarditis or a cardiac tamponade, both of which may contribute to, or be associated with, an altered mental status (presumably due to a decreased cardiac outflow and hypoperfusion). Listening for carotid bruits proximally and/or distally may clue the examiner in to potential stroke and arterial dissection risk [12].

Acute low output heart failure and acute myocardial infarction can also result in altered mental status [13], through mechanisms of hypoxemia and decreased cerebral perfusion pressure. In the ICU, a thorough cardiac examination should always be performed to evaluate for a S3/S4 heart sound, a Kussmaul's sign or hepatojugular reflux—all of which may offer clues to an underlying etiology that may contribute to an altered mental status.

In addition to classical use of the stethoscope, advances in the use of point of care ultrasound (POCUS) in the ICU setting has allowed clinicians to rapidly assess and diagnose acute conditions leading to decreased perfusion. Use of such techniques can aid physicians in the diagnosis of such disorders as pulmonary embolism, myocardial infarction, tamponade, left ventricular thrombus, biventricular failure, and carotid occlusion [14].

Pulmonary Examination and Respiratory Patterns

The pulmonary examination focuses on both the auscultation of the chest and bedside observation of overall breathing patterns. Abnormal breath sounds can be indicative of pulmonary pathology such as pneumonia, pneumothorax, acute obstruction, and foreign bodies—all of which may result in hypoxemia and altered mental status.

Abnormal respiratory patterns may offer clues to the underlying etiology of a mental status change [15]. Occasionally, an abnormal respiratory pattern can be indicative of brainstem damage [16]. A summary of centrally mediated abnormal breathing patterns has been provided in Table 5.1.

Persistent hyperventilation can be seen in many conditions such as intoxication with acidifying compounds (e.g., aspirin), hepatic coma, metabolic acidosis, and fever. In cases of central nervous system (CNS) lesions, there may be *central neurogenic hyperventilation*. This condition is often precipitated by processes affecting the function of the midbrain and the pons or as a direct result of increased intracranial pressure (ICP). Neurogenic hyperventilation may also be associated with primary CNS lymphoma [17].

Apneustic breathing has been described as a sudden, prolonged, gasping inspiration followed by a pause and then followed by an inadequate expiration. This breathing pattern should raise concern as it is commonly a clue that there is damage in the pneumotaxic centers located in the pons and medulla [18]. Other findings on physical examination that may be associated with apneustic breathing include absent or impaired brainstem reflexes. Occasionally, apneustic breathing can result from an acute intoxication.

Kussmaul respirations have been described as slow, deep, labored, almost gasping respirations. They have been associated with severe metabolic acidosis and have been classically described in diabetics in ketoacidosis. Kussmaul respirations represent the later stages of acidosis. Earlier in acidosis, respirations are shallow and rapid as the brain attempts to compensate by hyperventilating and reducing the blood pH to near normal. Therefore, when the breathing pattern truly becomes slow and laborious, it is an ominous sign.

Cheyne-Stokes respirations have been classically described as a crescendo-decrescendo breathing pattern. Periodically, they alternate every 30–120 s, and the breathing pattern slowly shifts back and forth from that of rapid and deep to slow and shallow and eventually to a period of apnea. The slower and shallower breathing results in ineffective ventilation, due to the increase in alveolar dead space. Cheyne-Stokes can be the respiratory pattern indicating imminent death; however, it may be encountered in reversible conditions. Cheyne-Stokes has been described in metabolic encephalopathy, heart failure, intoxication, and carbon monoxide poisoning. It is also encountered in conditions that damage the pontine/medullary respiratory centers [2].

Biot's respirations are similar to Cheyne-Stokes breathing with the important exception that the tidal volume usually does not fluctuate, and there are regular periods of apnea. This type of breathing may be indicative of a CNS lesion and usually localizes to the medullary region [19]. Biot's respirations have also been described in narcotic overdose [20].

Ataxic breathing has been described as a completely disordered breathing pattern intermixed with irregular periods of apnea. This breathing pattern may progress to agonal respirations, apnea, and death. Like Biot's respirations, the localization is usually medullary [21].

Table 5.1 Summary of abnormal breathing patterns

Respiratory pattern	Description	Localization	Etiologies
Persistent hyperventilation	Hyperpnea	Cortex, midbrain, pons	Acidosis, hepatic coma, fever, CNS lymphoma, elevated ICP
Apneustic breathing	Sudden, prolonged, gasping inspiration followed by a pause and then followed by an inadequate expiration	Pons, medulla	Lower brainstem lesion, acute intoxication
Kussmaul respirations	Slow, deep, labored, almost gasping respirations	Metabolic	Acidosis, particularly diabetic ketoacidosis
Cheyne-Stokes respirations	Crescendo-decrescendo breathing pattern with irregular periods of apnea	Rarely pons and/or medulla, metabolic, hemodynamic failure	Metabolic encephalopathy, acute heart failure, intoxication, and carbon monoxide poisoning. Can rarely be caused by pontine/medullary lesions
Biot's respirations	Periods of alternating hyperpnea and hyperventilation with regular periods of apnea and constant tidal volumes	Medulla	Medullary lesions, narcotic overdose
Ataxic breathing	Completely disordered breathing pattern intermixed with irregular periods of apnea progressing to agonal respirations and eventually apnea	Medulla	Medullary lesions

Abdominal Examination

The abdominal examination, when considering altered mental status, should focus on a search for stigmata of liver disease. These stigmata can include spider angiomata, ascites, hepatomegaly, or caput medusa. The abdomen should be auscultated and palpated to evaluate for signs of intussusception, small bowel obstruction, bowel ischemia, bowel perforation, or appendicitis. The clinician should look for scars revealing prior surgeries, as these may offer important clues to etiology and especially prior history of organ transplantation [12].

Skin/Nail Examination

The skin and nails should be examined as they may reveal evidence of systemic disease that could contribute to altered mental status. The skin and nail examination may include evidence of yellowing (e.g., jaundice), petechiae, microangiopathic hemolytic anemia, and splinter hemorrhages (a sign of systemic embolization). Clinicians should also evaluate for stigmata of intravenous drug use such as track marks or skin abscesses from intramuscular injection [12].

Neurological Examination

Glasgow Coma Scale (GCS)

The GCS, although simplistic and criticized for its lack of specificity, is the most commonly used scale to assess level of consciousness in clinical medicine. It is composed of the summation of three scores: one each for motor, verbal, and eye opening. Table 5.2 shows these responses and the corresponding scores for each. The sum of these three scores gives the GCS which lies with the range of 3–15 points, 3 being the worst and 15 being normal. This scale has less meaning than the levels of consciousness described previously, but is commonly used to communicate with other practitioners, and should therefore be thoroughly understood.

Modified with permission of Elsevier from Teasdale and Jennett [22].

Table 5.2 Glasgow Coma Scale responses and scores

Score	Eye response	Verbal response	Motor response
1	No eye opening	No sounds	No response to pain
2	Opens eyes to pain	Incomprehensible noises	Decerebrate posturing (extension) in response to pain
3	Opens eyes to voice	Uses inappropriate words	Decorticate posturing (flexion) in response to pain
4	Opens eyes spontaneously	Confused or disoriented	Withdrawal to pain
5		Carries out normal conversation	Localizes to pain
6			Able to follow commands appropriately

Full Outline of Unresponsiveness (FOUR) Score

The FOUR score was developed specifically due to the lack of specificity seen with the GCS score. In addition to classical eye and motor testing, the FOUR score adds in elements of brainstem and respiratory function to specifically test brainstem response and provide objective evidence of brainstem injury severity. The score itself includes the modalities of eye response, motor response, brainstem reflexes, and respiratory pattern as shown below in Table 5.3 [23]. The sum of the scores ranges from 0 to 16 points and more specifically predicts in-hospital mortality and odds of poor outcome [23]. As is related to the neurological examination in altered mental status, the FOUR score, unlike the GCS score, can specifically identify patients whom are locked-in and have progressive herniation syndromes. Its use in the neurological ICU should be routine and standard due to its superiority over the GCS.

Higher Cortical Function

Often, a detailed higher cortical function examination is difficult to perform when altered mental status in the ICU is encountered. This should not stop an examiner from attempting this examination each day, especially as there may be

Table 5.3 Full Outline of Responsiveness (FOUR) Score

Eyelid response
4 = Eyelids open, tracking or blinking to command
3 = Eyelids open but do not track examiner
2 = Eyelids closed, open to loud voice
1 = Eyelids closed, open to pain
0 = Eyelids remain closed with pain
Motor response
4 = Patient can give thumbs up or make peace sign
3 = Localization to pain
2 = Flexion or decorticate response to pain
1 = Extension or decerebrate response to pain
0 = No response to pain or myoclonic status epilepticus
Brainstem response
4 = Both pupil and corneal reflexes present
3 = One, unilateral pupil fixed and dilated
2 = Either a pupil or corneal reflex are absent
1 = Both pupil and corneal reflexes absent
0 = Absence of pupillary, corneal, and gag reflexes
Respiratory patterns
4 = Regular breathing pattern, not intubated
3 = Cheyne-Stokes pattern, not intubated
2 = Irregular pattern, not intubated
1 = Intubated breathing above ventilator rate
0 = Intubated breathing at the ventilator rate

Modified from Wijdicks et al. [3]

fluctuations in the level of consciousness. Also, importantly in some conditions, there may be cognitive fluctuations at certain hours, so careful monitoring of the cortical examination and changes in mental status throughout the day and night can be critical.

Arousal should be tested on every patient in the neurological ICU and documented daily to assess progression or improvement of disease. Typically, level of arousal is obtained by using either the GCS or FOUR scores and can provide anatomical localization on examination. Both eye and motor responses provide specific cortical and diencephalic localization, whereas cranial nerves and respiratory patters provide brainstem localization.

Attention, on the other hand, requires intact arousal and may be difficult in the ICU. Typically, attention is tested by asking the patient to spell a word backward (e.g., WORLD), performing a digit span [24] or counting backward by sevens (which can also be used to test acalculia) [25]. Such testing should be performed in normal or sub-normal levels arousal and can provide specific focal localization to areas including the frontal lobes, temporal lobes, and angular gyrus.

Other aspects of the higher cortical function examination that may be of particular value include noting abnormalities in language and in hemispatial/hemibody attention. These tests are likely to be disrupted in large hemispheric lesions; these lesions would typically depress consciousness, and they may show lateralization of the dysfunction to one or another brain hemisphere [26, 27].

Language is usually represented in the left hemisphere, and in many cases it is perisylvian in location [28]. Some general principles that may be helpful include examining fluency (e.g., getting words or letters out of the mouth), which may reflect more anterior lesions, and problems the patient has with comprehension, as this may reflect relatively more posterior lesions or dysfunction. Also, the more dorsal the lesion, the more likely the patient is to have spared repetition (e.g., transcortical aphasia), but if the lesion is causing dysfunction of the perisylvian cortex, especially caudally, they may be less likely to be able to repeat a phrase.

In the patient with right hemispheric damage, there may be hemispatial or hemibody neglect, especially if the lesion compromises the junction of the parietal, temporal, and occipital lobes. Hemispatial neglect is a syndrome where the individual manifests decreased spatial attention to people, objects, or any other stimuli in the environment, but this syndrome must be in the left of their plane of orientation. This is due to damage of the systems primarily in the right parietal lobe that may be responsible for spatial attention (e.g., although frontal and thalamic lesions may also result in these deficits) [26]. Lesions of the left parietal lobe rarely cause neglect, as the right parietal lobe services human attention to both hemispaces, while the left side gives only weak attention to the right hemispace [29].

Cranial Nerves

The cranial nerve examination is critical in a patient with altered mental status, especially in the ICU setting. The ARAS originates in the pons and medulla and is condensed into a relatively small space running along with the corticobulbar tract, the cranial nerve nuclei, and the fascicles that interconnect these nuclei [5]. By these simple anatomical connections, a CNS lesion that is relatively localized within the brainstem can result in a disruption of a significant proportion of these ARAS fibers which may in turn result in an alteration of the level of consciousness. CNS lesions in the brainstem can result in deficits of cranial nerve function and level of arousal. It should be noted that many patients with altered mental status cannot fully participate in cranial nerve testing.

Pupillary Reflex

The afferent (cranial nerve II) and efferent (cranial nerve III) pupillary responses can be examined by shining a bright light into one eye and observing the response (i.e., the direct response) and then by examining the contralateral eye for a response (e.g., a consensual response) [12]. The pupil should constrict briskly and equally in both eyes. It is not uncommon for a patient in the ICU to be on multiple medications including sedatives and paralytics that may slow, dampen, or abolish a pupillary reaction. Medications therefore must be considered as a factor when examining the eyes and recording abnormal responses [30].

The neuroanatomy of the pupillary response is important. The light response begins with the photosensitive retinal ganglion cells which project via the optic nerve to the optic chiasm. At this point, 53% of these fibers decussate, and 47% stay ipsilateral. The optic tract, a continuation of the chiasm, terminates in the pretectal nucleus ipsilaterally, and this termination is located in the dorsal midbrain. The pretectal nuclei project bilaterally to the Edinger–Westphal nuclei, which are the parasympathetic subnuclei of the oculomotor nerve. The fibers decussate to synapse in the contralateral Edinger–Westphal nucleus and then travel through the posterior commissure [31]. The Edinger–Westphal nucleus has cholinergic neurons that project to the ipsilateral ciliary ganglion, which in turn projects to the pupillary constrictor muscles in an ipsilateral fashion. Understanding the neuroanatomy of this pathway can help to localize a neurological deficit. If, for example, the pupillary reaction is brisk and equal to direct and consensual response bilaterally, the entire systems—including the optic pathways, the dorsal midbrain, the posterior commissure, the third nerve nuclear complex, the third nerve, and the pupillary constrictor muscles—are likely intact.

A frequently encountered examination finding in the NICU is that of asymmetric pupils. Determination of which pupil is abnormal, the larger or smaller, is imperative. If a pupil is abnormally large because it fails to constrict, the likely pathology is due to cranial nerve III parasympathetic dysfunction from either ischemia or compression. If the smaller pupil is abnormal, this usually reflects intrinsic or extrinsic sympathetic dysfunction such as in diencephalic herniation and Horner's syndrome, respectively. A frequently encountered and concerning examination finding is a unilaterally fixed and dilated pupil. This situation may be encountered when there is compromise to a unilateral third nerve. A "blown pupil" that is dilated and poorly reactive to light, especially when more severe than the oculomotor deficits encountered, indicates an extrinsic compression of the nerve. Such manifestation results due to the peripheral orientation of parasympathetic fibers in the third nerve. Emergent pathologies when faced with such an exam finding include uncal or transtentorial herniation or aneurysmal compression commonly from the posterior communicating artery (PCOM) [32]. Because this is an emergent situation, it is important to obtain CNS imaging as quickly as possible. A CT scan of the brain is usually adequate to rule out herniation, and a CT angiogram is required to evaluate properly for an aneurysm.

In contrast, if the smaller pupil is abnormal, this usually indicates a failure of the sympathetic system in dilating the pupil. Several conditions can account for this issue, but the one of particular concern is a Horner's syndrome. The Horner's syndrome is characterized by the triad of miosis, anhidrosis, and ptosis. This can be caused by a lesion anywhere along the central or peripheral pathways containing axons related to the oculosympathetic system. If caused by a brainstem lesion, Horner's syndrome is commonly accompanied by alteration in mental status and a contralateral loss of pain and temperature, as descending sympathetics travel in close proximity to the spinothalamic tract. In certain instances, an ipsilateral ataxia and vertigo can also be seen as in cases of a lateral medullary syndrome. A Horner's syndrome can also be caused by lesions of the stellate ganglion as in the case of a pancoast tumor, or within the cavernous sinus, and/or as a result of a carotid dissection. Pharmacological testing can confirm a Horner's syndrome [33, 34]. One to two drops of 0.5% apraclonidine in each eye will result in a reversal of anisocoria in the case of a Horner's syndrome. This reversal is due to the weak alpha-1 agonist properties, which cause a significant mydriasis in the Horner's eye because of denervation hypersensitivity, and the strong alpha-2 properties that result in miosis in the unaffected eye [31, 35].

Corneal Reflex

The corneal reflex is a monosynaptic connection composed of two cranial nerves and connections within the pons. The afferent limb is the nasociliary branch of cranial nerve V1. When the cornea is touched with a sterile cotton swab, this signal travels into the brainstem at the level of the pons, descends to the caudal pons, and terminates in the bilateral facial nerve motor nuclei. The motor nucleus of VII projects ipsilaterally to the muscles of facial expression resulting in contraction of the orbicularis oculi bilaterally when either cornea is touched. If only one side of the face blinks when either cornea is touched, this indicates either a central or peripheral lesion on the side of decreased orbicularis oculi contraction. If both sides of the face manifest a decreased blink when one cornea is touched, but both contract normally when the other is touched, it is likely that there is either damage to the peripheral trigeminal nerve or to the fascicle that contains the fibers descending to the bilateral motor nuclei of VII. The corneal reflex specifically should be used in the evaluation of altered mental status to localize pathology to the pontomedullary junction.

Vestibulo-Ocular Reflex and Cold Caloric Testing

The brainstem connections in the lower pons and upper medulla can be tested by using the vestibulo-ocular reflex (VOR). The vestibulo-ocular reflex involves connections between medial vestibular nucleus, the medial longitudinal fasciculus (MLF), and the lateral gaze centers (III,IV,VI). VORs can be tested by performing a rapid head movement test, effectively turning the patient's head from side to side and observing for contralateral eye movement as well as nystagmus. This examination maneuver has been famously called a "doll's eyes" maneuver because the eye movements resemble that of an old-fashioned doll that would move with head turning. In this circuit [36, 37], the vestibular systems project to the vestibular nuclei, which in turn stimulate the abducens nucleus on the side opposite to the direction of head rotation and in turn inhibit the abducens nucleus on the side in which the head is turning. The abducens nucleus then projects via the abducens nerve to the ipsilateral lateral rectus and also, via the MLF, to the contralateral medial rectus sub-nucleus of the oculomotor complex. These eventually stimulate the medial rectus on the ipsilateral side. The connections result in both eyes moving in the direction opposite of head rotation. A diagram of these important eye movements is shown in Fig. 5.1. If the patient is awake, the vestibulo-ocular reflex is usually suppressed due to cortical projections overriding the internuclear mechanisms. If the patient is comatose and these systems remain intact, the eyes should move conjugately in the direction opposite to the head rotation [38]. Prior to performing this test, particularly in cases of trauma, it should be confirmed that the cervical spine is stable.

An alternative method, by which these systems can be tested, especially when the cervical spine is unstable, is to employ caloric testing [39, 40]. This can be performed with either warm or cold water, but cold water is usually utilized as it provides a more potent stimulus. After ensuring that the tympanic membrane is intact, the ear canal is irrigated with cold

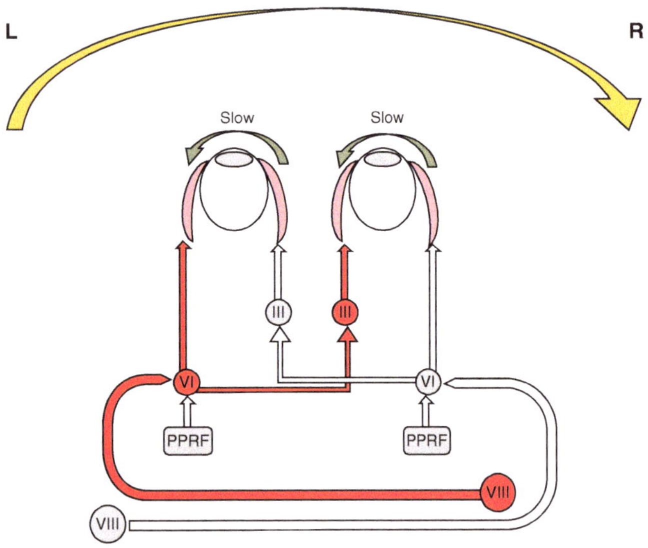

Fig. 5.1 Diagram of important eye movements in an examination maneuver that has been famously called a "doll's eyes" maneuver

water. The typical response when using cold water is for both eyes to slowly move in the direction toward irrigation. Similar to the neural networks described with VORs, the cold-water stimulus inhibits the ipsilateral medial vestibular nucleus, disinhibiting the contralateral nucleus allowing for contralateral evoked haze. In a conscious patient, or in one with intact cerebral hemispheres, a fast corrective eye movement back toward primary position should manifest. The repetitive slow eye movements toward the irrigated ear and the fast movements away result in a phenomenon referred to as nystagmus. Since nystagmus is named for the fast phase, cold-water calorics result in nystagmus beating in the opposite direction of the irrigated ear. This can be easily remembered by the mnemonic "COWS." This stands for cold-opposite, warm-same.

An internuclear ophthalmoplegia, which is a disruption of the medial longitudinal fasciculus, can also be identified by a careful eye exam when the adducting eye does not move fully medially, and the abducting eye either does not move past midline or has slowed saccades such that the eyes are dysconjugate [37]. This maneuver can also aid in localizing the lesion to the dorsal pons/midbrain. In a comatose patient, the vestibulo-ocular reflex can be utilized to evaluate for this phenomenon.

Cough and Gag Reflex

Obtaining the gag reflex is accomplished by pressing a sterile tongue blade or cotton swab against the oropharynx region and by observing for symmetric palatal elevation without uvula deviation. The afferent limb of this reflex is largely mediated by cranial nerve nine, which terminates in the nucleus solitaries and the efferent limb, which is largely cranial nerve X originating in the nucleus ambiguus. This reflex indicates cranial nerve ten dysfunction, especially if the palate elevates asymmetrically and/or if the uvula deviates away from the side of weaker palate elevation. A weak gag reflex without asymmetric palate elevation or uvula deviation can indicate a cranial nerve nine lesion, but it can also be seen in perfectly normal individuals since up to one-third of healthy people have an absent gag reflex [41].

Funduscopic Examination

The funduscopic examination is an often-overlooked portion of the physical examination in a patient with altered mental status, yet it can provide some important clues to the diagnosis or clues to associated conditions. Commonly in the ICU setting, the pupils can be quite small, making the fundus difficult to visualize. A better examination can be achieved by applying mydriatic eye drops, either using a sympathomimetic like phenylephrine or an anticholinergic such as tropicamide. It is extremely important, especially in patients with alteration of consciousness, to document in the chart what kind of dilation you have performed, what time the dilation was performed, and to ensure that you dilate both eyes equally. Failure to do so could result in the inappropriate assumption that the patient could have a compressive third nerve palsy, and this could lead to unnecessary imaging studies and/or possibly even interventions, both of which could pose potential harm to the patient.

Evaluation of both the optic disk and the retinal vasculature can provide clues as to the underlying etiology of altered mental status. If the margins of the optic disk are indistinct, optic disk edema could be present. If optic disk edema is present, it could be the result of increased intracranial pressure, in which case the edema observed is called papilledema. True optic disk edema that is not caused by increased intracranial pressure includes: optic neuritis associated with demyelinating disease, certain infectious etiologies, or some vascular causes. Papilledema, caused by increased intracranial pressure, can be a result of multiple etiologies including brain neoplasm, infections such as meningitis or abscess, cerebral sinus thrombosis, idiopathic intracranial hypertension, or any other intracranial space occupying lesion. Optic disk edema uncommonly results from an acute process other than increased intracranial pressure such as a subarachnoid hemorrhage. The retinal vessels should also be inspected for attenuation, embolus, or evidence of cuffing, which can indicate CNS vasculitis. Hollenhorst plaques are bright, yellow, refractile plaques made of cholesterol in the retinal arterioles [42]. These indicate embolic disease, possibly from the internal carotid artery, which would corroborate carotid disease in cases of anterior circulation ischemic events.

Motor Examination

The motor examination should include descriptions of bulk, tone, and strength, as well as observations of any abnormal hypo- or hyperkinetic movements. In a patient manifesting with altered mental status, this examination may prove to be a challenge. Patients may not follow commands, or alternatively they may be intubated, sedated, or paralyzed. When it is not possible to grade strength formally, tone and asymmetry of spontaneous movements can be observed, as well as potentially abnormal postures (such as external rotation of a weak lower extremity). Typically, with a peripheral nervous system lesion, tone is decreased, and with a central nervous system lesion, tone is increased. An exception to this is in cases of spinal pathology, when in the acute setting, the patient may have a flaccid paralysis, the so-called spinal shock syndrome [43].

Another portion of the motor examination is observation of the response to a painful stimulus as is performed with the GCS. Such an example is when the trapezius is squeezed with enough force to result in pain, and the pain elicits a movement. A response to pain that would indicate at least partial preservation of neurological function would be for the patient to reach toward the source of the noxious stimulus, which would be a localizing and an appropriate response [39].

If there is a significant disruption of the motor systems above the level of the midbrain, the inhibition of the rubrospinal tract by the corticospinal systems is released, and the patient will usually exhibit decorticate posturing, which is elbow flexion, forearm supination, and wrist and finger flexion. If there is significant damage to the motor systems below the red nucleus, the rubrospinal tract is also affected, and therefore the tract that provides the dominant tone is the vestibulospinal tract, and this response results in decerebrate posturing, which is extension at the elbow, pronation of the forearm, and extension of the wrist [3].

Basal Ganglia Examination

Hyperkinetic movements (e.g., tremor, chorea) or hypokinetic movements (e.g., parkinsonism) should clue the clinician to the possibility of basal ganglia dysfunction. An MRI study and possibly follow-up laboratory analysis may be necessary. Clinicians should be aware of the chorea syndrome that may appear during diabetic ketoacidosis and also the chorea and other movement disorders that may appear as a result of liver, thyroid, or metabolic dysfunction. Finally, abrupt withdrawal of dopamine or dopamine agonists (i.e., carbidopa/levodopa) can result in the neuroleptic malignant syndrome and should be avoided. The use of neuroleptic medications can exacerbate or unmask basal ganglia features and should be avoided if possible in ICU patients.

Deep Tendon Reflex Examination

Abnormal reflexes are an important adjunct to the motor examination, particularly when accompanied by weakness. The reflexes may help to determine if the weakness is central or peripheral in origin. If a central nervous system lesion is present, the inhibition on the alpha motor neuron in the anterior horn cells of the spinal cord will be released, and there would be hyperexcitability of the myotatic stretch reflex. When the tendon is tapped with a reflex hammer, the primary afferent fibers directly synapse on the motor neuron that supplies the attached muscles. Given that the descending inhibition on these neurons is released, the resulting contraction of the muscles is exaggerated. If a peripheral lesion is present, the reflex may be decreased, although the afferent limb of the stretch reflex is intact. If the motor neuron is damaged, the muscle cannot contract with full force, resulting in hyporeflexia [44].

The Babinski response is also a useful part of the motor examination. In testing the Babinski response, the lateral aspect of the plantar surface of the foot is scratched hard enough to produce a noxious stimulus. If the first movement of the great toe is upward, this is a Babinski sign. Experimental data in mice and humans indicate that this response results from damage to the medullary reticulospinal tract; however, in clinical practice, it is used to identify individuals simply with potential CNS damage [39, 45, 46].

Cerebellar Examination

The cerebellar examination is often difficult to test in an ICU setting and especially with altered mental status. When present, cerebellar findings may be clues to posterior fossa lesions that may progress to include compromise of the ARAS in the brainstem and eventually cause depressed consciousness. Cerebellar findings include appendicular ataxia, dysmetria, rebound, dysdiadochokinesia, rhythm problems, and, in select cases, associated tremor. In the more mobile patient truncal titubation, wide-based gait, and eye movement abnormalities may be present with more midline and anterior cerebellar lesions [12, 39, 44].

Sensory Examination

The sensory examination can be tricky in the ICU and even trickier in the setting of AMS. It is extremely subjective. A crude way of testing sensation in this setting is to provide a painful stimulus to each extremity, and if the patient responds to this pain, it is inferred that, grossly, the anterolateral system known as the spinothalamic tract may be intact. Testing for neuropathy, radiculopathy, plexopathy, or other issues may require a more intact mental status.

Laboratory Workup

Complete Blood Count (CBC)

The CBC can be helpful in cases of altered mental status for several reasons. A leukocytosis can indicate an infectious or neoplastic process, either of which can cause confusion, particularly in patients with decreased functional cognitive reserve. This does not exclude a CNS structural process as the cause, but it can be useful in pointing a clinician in a different direction. A low hemoglobin and hematocrit, indicating anemia, either may be completely unrelated to the altered mental status or can be symptoms of a systemic process causing the altered mental status such as a microangiopathic hemolytic anemia or can worsen cognition in patient with decreased cognition at baseline such as encountered in dementing illnesses [47, 48]. Thrombocytosis can either indicate a neoplastic process or could be reactive and support an infectious/inflammatory diagnosis. Thrombocytopenia can be seen in multiple conditions but particularly in microangiopathic hemolytic anemias [49] and disseminated intravascular coagulopathy, both of which can cause altered mental status.

Chemistries

Patients manifesting an acute confusional state/delirium or coma should at a minimum have a complete metabolic panel performed. Often, hyponatremia, diabetic ketoacidosis, acute uremia, and hepatic encephalopathy can be quickly uncovered. Also, certain treatable issues such as hypercapnia due to pulmonary insufficiency may result in an impairment of consciousness that requires ICU monitoring. Early treatment aids in prevention of complications and potentially death. Further workup is usually warranted to find the underlying etiology causing any metabolic disturbance.

Elevated ammonia levels can be encountered in the setting of severe liver damage and also as a result of medications such as valproate, which can also be associated with encephalopathy [50]. Often, if you treat the underlying etiology of the hyperammonemia, the encephalopathy can resolve. Treatment with lactulose, which is the mainstay of treatment, can increase the gastrointestinal excretion of ammonia and may speed the reversal of alterations in mental status, but the evidence here is lacking [51].

Neuroimaging

The history and examination should guide the clinician to a localization and, subsequently, an appropriately limited differential diagnosis. Based on this, imaging of the central nervous system may be warranted. Several modalities are available, each having advantages and disadvantages. The most pertinent imaging studies in most cases include computed tomography (CT) and magnetic resonance imaging (MRI) of the brain. The advantage of CT is that it is fast, readily available, and less susceptible to movement artifact, while with MRI, the images are usually better quality, more sensitive in detecting pathology, and will usually give more information about a specific etiology. Selecting which study to utilize should vary depending on the clinical scenario encountered.

CT

CT of the brain is a fast and extremely efficient way to evaluate for structural abnormalities in a patient with an AMS. Especially in cases of an acute stroke, cerebral edema, intracerebral hemorrhage, subdural hematoma, or epidural hematoma, the brain CT is very useful to quickly ascertain an underlying cause for an AMS. CT has an excellent spatial resolution [52, 53] but lacks the contrast resolution of MRI, which often makes it an inferior modality if searching for lesions within the CNS.

MRI

MRI of the brain can be particularly useful for the evaluation and further characterization of lesions that may cause AMS (stroke, hemorrhage, venous issues, and intracranial hypotension). The evaluation of posterior fossa lesions causing alterations in mental status is particularly useful as some of these etiologies may not be adequately imaged on CT. MRI is particularly important to fully characterize lesions, their appearance, involvement of adjacent structures (or lack thereof), and patterns of appearance on the various sequences, all of which aid in making a diagnosis. The excellent contrast resolution is quite useful in MRI given that many lesions within the CNS are often of similar density, resulting in similar contrast, and thus may be missed by CT scan. In acute stroke, the diffusion-weighted MRI is quite useful. In this condition, the brain CT may be normal early, and the diffusion-weighted MRI will show an acute brainstem infarct that may require close observation in the ICU setting or potentially warrant a surgical or endovascular intervention. Acute thalamic infarcts interrupting the reticular activating system may result in an alteration in mental status, which may not be seen on CT imaging; these also sometimes respond to dopamine or dopamine agonist therapy and manifest with fluctuating levels of consciousness.

The clinician should never hesitate to use a brain CT, MRI, or potentially both tests to uncover the etiology of any case of AMS, especially when the history and examination do not point clearly to the etiology.

Neuro-diagnostics

Lumbar Puncture

The lumbar puncture is particularly important in the altered mental status workup, especially if an infectious or autoimmune etiology is suspected, if the patient is immunocompromised, or if a diagnosis remains elusive after an initial workup. Sampling of the CSF allows for evaluation of the

Table 5.4 Commonly found values in some infectious CSF processes in lumbar punctures

Component	Viral	Bacterial	Tuberculosis	Fungal
WBC	<300	>1000	50–500	50–500
Cell-type predominance	Mostly lymphocytes	Mostly neutrophils	Mostly lymphocytes and monocytes	Mostly lymphocytes
Glucose	>40	<40	<40	<40
Protein	Often normal or mildly elevated	Elevated (sometimes markedly so)	Elevated	Elevated

chemical composition, quantification of the number of erythrocytes and leukocytes, culture of the fluid, polymerase chain reaction for DNA of infectious organisms, evaluation of abnormal cells, and detection of the presence of abnormal proteins such as specific antibodies. The spinal needle can also be attached to a manometer so that the CSF pressure can be measured. A normal CSF constitution is less than five leukocytes without any polymorphonuclear cells, no erythrocytes, 15–50 mg/dL of protein, and a glucose concentration that is about 2/3 that of the serum glucose; it is important to get a peripheral blood stick at the exact time of the LP [54]. A description of the commonly found values in some infectious CSF processes is depicted in Table 5.4.

EEG

The electroencephalogram (EEG) is commonly performed in the critical care setting, especially in patients with nonconvulsive status epilepticus, where clinical presentation may prove hard to decipher. Continuous EEG monitoring in the ICU allows the physician to monitor the progress of antiepileptic treatment and to decide whether or not the patient will require more aggressive management. EEG is commonly abnormal in the setting of an alteration of consciousness and can offer clues as to elusive diagnoses [55]. EEG is particularly useful in situations in the ICU when the patient is delirious or having an AMS, and the history is unable to be obtained. It is common that patients with delirium from a metabolic disturbance, hypoglycemia, diabetic coma, or excess use of sedatives will have a slowing of the posterior dominant rhythm which is normally in the alpha frequency. In patients with hepatic encephalopathy or uremic states, the EEG may show triphasic waves [56]. When there has been a benzodiazepine overdose, excessive beta activity may be seen. In the setting of CNS infections, such as herpes encephalitis, the EEG may show focal abnormalities as well as periodic lateralized discharges [57]. In the setting of severe anoxic brain injury where the patient is unresponsive and lacks brainstem reflexes, the EEG may reveal diffuse slowing or even a flat line. In the setting of a rapidly progressive dementia (e.g., Creutzfeldt-Jacob disease), the EEG may show periodic sharp wave complexes [58].

A flat line seen on EEG with no electrical potential of more than 2 mV during 30 min of recording is concerning for brain death [59]. Thus, EEG may aid in further treatment of underlying infection, seizures, metabolic disturbances, and brain death.

Diseases and Disease-Specific Treatments

Delirium

Delirium is an extremely common phenomenon in ICU patients and is reported as high as 82% [60, 61]. Development of delirium can be associated with a worse prognosis [60], and delay in treating delirium has been associated with increased mortality, increased nosocomial infections, a longer length of stay [62], and an increased rate of mechanical ventilation [63]. Delirium is defined as an acute fluctuating change in consciousness and cognition that develops over a brief period of time [64]. A hallmark of delirium is waxing and waning alteration of consciousness along with profound inattentiveness. Interestingly, patients with delirium usually have a sense of heightened awareness to their surroundings.

Causes of delirium may include infection, metabolic disturbances, medications, alcohol withdrawal, and postoperative states, especially in the elderly population. This could be due to a lack of cognitive functional reserve leading to a state of confusion. If treatment of the underlying cause of delirium is found early, it may be resolved more expeditiously.

There is no specific treatment for delirium but rather an approach to minimize physical, medical, and emotional stresses should be undertaken in addition to treating the underlying cause(s).

Intoxications

Sedatives

Sedative hypnotic medications as well as ethanol cause depressed level of arousal by modulation of the $GABA_A$ (gamma-amino butyric acid) chloride channel. Benzodiazepines increase the frequency of channel opening by increasing the channel affinity for GABA [65]. Barbiturates increase the duration of channel opening when stimulated by GABA [66]. This mechanism explains why barbiturates are inherently more dangerous than benzodiazepines in overdose due to the fact that the chloride channel could potentially remain open nearly constantly with a barbiturate, but it still closes periodically with a benzodiazepine overdose. With the channel being open for a greater percentage of the time, the chloride will continue to influx and hyperpolarize the neuron, making it more resistant to depolarization, thus slowing signal propagation within the CNS. Flumazenil is an antagonist at the benzodiazepine binding site on the $GABA_A$ receptor. It reverses the action of benzodiazepines.

Cocaine and Other Sympathomimetics

Intoxication with cocaine leads to increased sympathetic stimulation by blocking reuptake of monoamines into the presynaptic nerve terminal [67]. This produces an excessive "fight or flight" response and a hyperdynamic state with patients usually having hypertension, tachypnea, tachycardia, diaphoresis, mydriasis, hyperthermia, and occasionally paranoia [68]. Individuals suffering from sympathomimetic intoxication may appear to be altered in the sense that they are hypervigilant, but will not often have frank confusion. However, excessive alpha stimulation, especially in the setting of beta blockade, can cause vasospasm, which can produce ischemia throughout the body, but if it occurs in the brain, it can cause stroke. If the stroke affects the ARAS as mentioned in the stroke section earlier, depressed level of consciousness can occur.

LSD

Lysergic acid diethylamide (LSD) is a hallucinogen that can cause inattentiveness, lethargy, hallucinations, and illusions. Patients will usually only present with "bad trips" that are prolonged and composed of worrisome hallucinations or illusions and profound anxiety as well as gastrointestinal upset. It is commonly ingested by saturated pieces of paper. LSD has no specific antidote, but rather supportive care such as benzodiazepines and a calm, soothing environment are mainstays of treatment until the intoxication wears off [68].

GHB

Gamma-hydroxybutyric acid (GHB) is a commonly abused drug that acts on GABA receptors [69, 70] and likely a novel GHB receptor in the central nervous system to produce a syndrome of CNS depression. This drug has the effect of producing a very short-lived coma in overdoses but can also produce confusion, ataxia, nystagmus, and occasionally seizures if taken in smaller amounts [68]. Along with CNS depression effects, it can cause respiratory suppression and patients may require intubation. The drug can also have a withdrawal syndrome that can be quite similar to alcohol in that it features tremors, anxiety, tachycardia, visual and auditory hallucinations, and can even cause a Wernicke-Korsakoff syndrome [71]. One of the most worrisome effects of GHB is the sudden awakening phenomenon that can lead to self-extubation and aspiration [72].

Narcotics

Opioids are synthetic and semisynthetic derivatives of the poppy plant. They have long been used for therapeutic and recreational effects. In fact, heroin was once marketed by Bayer pharmaceuticals for its antitussive properties [10]. These compounds typically cause depressed consciousness, the degree of which is dependent on the dose, the route of administration, and the tolerance of the individual. In addition to depressed consciousness, decreased respiratory drive, miosis, and a host of idiosyncratic reactions can result from opioids [68]. By definition, the effects of an opioid can be reversed by naloxone, and this can be used as an antidote as it is a pure (mu) antagonist and will reverse the mental status changes and respiratory depression if given in an appropriate dose. Some opioids have a very long half-life which may outlast the effects of naloxone, so observation for repeated worsening of the initial symptoms should be considered.

Ischemic Disease

Stroke

Ischemic stroke is discussed elsewhere in this book. It is quite rare for ischemic stroke to present with an isolated alteration of consciousness due to the unilaterality of the blood supply to many regions of the brain and the preservation of the contralateral ARAS in the majority of cases. In a study by Benbadis, only 4% of patients had altered mental status due to a unilateral stroke, and the neurological exam is helpful in detecting those patients who need neuroimaging, with a 97% negative predictive value [73]. In particular, strokes that cause depression of consciousness and altered mental status tend to be caused by thrombosis or by embolus of the basilar artery. This artery has penetrating branches that supply both sides of the brainstem in the area where the ARAS is confined to a small region. The majority of brainstem strokes are caused by small vessel lacunar strokes which are unilateral and do not usually cause altered mental status. However, in many cases of strokes caused by the basilar artery, the brainstem may be damaged bilaterally, and consciousness and mentation can be affected. In many of these cases, there is acute onset of cranial nerve deficits, and these are often associated with contralateral motor deficits. If extensive bilateral damage to the brainstem occurs, the patient will often manifest with significant bilateral weakness, cranial nerve palsies, dysarthria, dizziness, depressed consciousness, and in arguably the worst-case scenario, a locked-in syndrome [74]. The paramedian thalamic arteries normally arise from the P1 to supply the mesial thalamus ipsilaterally through which the ARAS travels. Occasionally, a common trunk, called the artery of Percheron [75], arises from one PCA to supply both mesial thalami. In such a situation, a stroke of this artery can result in coma due to bilateral disruption of the ARAS [76]. Another cause of depressed consciousness is a posterior cerebral artery stroke or a large hemispheric stroke. Both of these clinical conditions can result in these findings, due to shifting of the intracranial contents and compromise of the contralateral ARAS [2].

Hemorrhagic Disease

Intraparenchymal Hemorrhage

Intraparenchymal hemorrhage can result from many causes but is usually associated with uncontrolled hypertension, amyloid angiopathy, underlying neoplasm, or alternatively vascular lesions. The location of these hemorrhages can often be a clue to the underlying etiology [77]. Hypertensive bleeds are usually located in the basal ganglia, pons, cerebellum, and thalamus. Those caused by amyloid angiopathy are commonly lobar in location. The location of the bleed will determine the resulting deficits. The sudden expansion of the intracranial contents and the resulting increased intracranial pressure can cause profound mass effect and compromise the ARAS bilaterally, especially when blood products are located within or near the more internal structures where the bilateral ARAS is confined to a relatively small space. This phenomenon may explain why patients with intraparenchymal bleeds have focal neurological deficits and also manifest with a state of stupor. Patients with increased intracranial bleeds will often present with nausea and vomiting from the increased intracranial pressure.

Subarachnoid Hemorrhage

Subarachnoid hemorrhage (SAH) is a potentially life-threatening condition usually caused by either trauma or a ruptured aneurysm. Patients with SAH often present with the "worst headache of their life," nuchal rigidity, cranial neuropathies, motor deficit, and altered mental status. The mortality rate of aneurysmal SAH is 7% in those patients who are admitted to neurointensive care units. Therefore, it is paramount that this diagnosis does not get missed. Careful monitoring in the ICU can help prevent cerebral vasospasm and aneurysmal rupture. Complications of vasospasm include hydrocephalus and hyponatremia. Subarachnoid hemorrhage in the ICU setting can also result in seizures due to cortical irritability from the collection of blood: iron on the cortex is irritating and can cause seizures. This may result in more complications not only from a medical standpoint but also from the need of an antiepileptic medication. Antiepileptic medications can in some cases result in more complications.

Cerebral angiography remains the gold standard for diagnosis of cerebral vasospasm. Transcranial Dopplers can also be performed to diagnose vasospasm, and these are becoming a more popular method of assessing vasospasm. The treatment of SAH consist of coiling or clipping. Afterward, if delayed cerebral ischemia (DCI) occurs, the triad of hypervolemia, hypertension, and hemodilution is often used. Early treatment of subarachnoid hemorrhage can prevent further future complications. Around 70% of patients who receive the treatment can reverse neurological complications from SAH [78].

Neoplasm

As described previously, mass lesions of any etiology can cause increased pressure on other parts of the ARAS and, if significant enough, can cause depressed level of consciousness. Any neoplasm that either compromises the brainstem or has a significant mass effect such that both cerebral hemispheres are affected can cause an alteration of consciousness. In addition to this phenomenon, cerebral neoplasms, especially when cortically based, can cause cortical irritation and result in seizures. If a patient with a cerebral neoplasm presents with an altered mental status, the main considerations are increasing cerebral edema, decreased mental status, and seizures. As discussed earlier, neuroimaging and EEG are both useful in correctly diagnosing this potential etiology.

Posterior Reversible Encephalopathy Syndrome (PRES)

PRES can potentially be life threatening if not diagnosed and recognized early. Often, if this condition goes unrecognized and causes seizures, the patient may slip into status epilepticus. Treatment of HTN is crucial especially early as it can reverse fatal complications [79]. Clinical symptoms of PRES include headache, seizures, alteration in mental status, and visual changes. Imaging, particularly MRI in PRES, shows a parietal and occipital-predominant leukoencephalopathy. It is rare to have DWI positivity, but when present, this may indicate that the damage is irreversible. Etiologies include uncontrolled HTN, eclampsia, preeclampsia, collagen vascular diseases, infections, and shock [80, 81].

Demyelinating Disease

Rarely can demyelinating disease cause an alteration of consciousness as rarely does it cause bilateral dysfunction of the ARAS. Typically, demyelinating disease will affect discrete areas of the CNS and cause focal deficits that do not influence consciousness, such as weakness, sensory loss, ataxia, central vision loss, and diplopia. Two examples of demyelinating disease that can cause alterations of consciousness are acute demyelinating encephalomyelitis (ADEM) and tumefactive multiple sclerosis (MS).

ADEM is an acute, usually monophasic demyelinating illness that is typically considered to be postinfectious or postvaccination and/or autoimmune in etiology. It is much more common in children, and typically children have a worse prognosis. Almost universally, these patients present with fever, altered mental status, headache, and focal or multifocal exam findings. Due to the presentation, it is prudent to include encephalitis and meningitis in the differential diagnosis. Imaging will often show large "fluffy" areas of increased T2 signal in various areas of the deep cerebral white matter, but unlike MS, these lesions are usually not well circumscribed or ovoid, not periventricular in location, and can often involve areas of gray matter such as the basal ganglia [82]. Treatment for ADEM is supportive, and many individuals use pulse steroids although the data for this are limited in adults. There is a particularly severe variant of ADEM called hemorrhagic leukoencephalopathy in which there is a particularly aggressive amount of edema as well as hemorrhage. This disorder can have a mortality rate as high as 70%, but evidence points toward less residual deficits with aggressive therapies with corticosteroids [82, 83], intravenous immunoglobulins (IVIG), and plasma exchange [84].

Tumefactive MS is a disorder in which a patient either with undiagnosed MS or with longstanding disease develops a lesion that is particularly large, with significant cerebral edema to the point that there could be a potential herniation syndrome [85]. There is breakdown of the blood–brain barrier, and the lesion enhances with contrast material, so many times this can be indistinguishable from a brain tumor or cerebral abscess [86]. If there are no other radiographic lesions that will help make a diagnosis of MS, a brain biopsy might be necessary to confirm this. There have been reports of mitoxantrone, rituximab, and alemtuzumab having beneficial results as well as autologous stem cell transplantation, but it is usually a fatal disease and often challenging to diagnose and treat [87].

Infections

Meningitis

Meningitis commonly presents with photophobia, altered mental status, headache, neck pain, seizures, and fevers. This condition can be caused by bacteria and viruses but can also be caused by fungi. Meningitis results from pathology of the meninges, if the brain parenchyma is affected it is evidenced by seizures, cortical dysfunction, or memory disturbances. Meningitis can be diagnosed by CSF analysis showing a pleocytosis. Bacterial causes tend to show a neutrophil-predominant CSF leukocytosis, whereas viral and tuberculous meningitis have a lymphocyte-predominant pleocytosis [88, 89].

Bacterial and fungal meningitis, if left untreated, can lead to fatal outcomes. The common causes of bacterial meningitis include *Streptococcus pneumoniae*, *Neisseria meningitidis*, and (in individuals over the age of 50) *Listeria monocytogenes*. Commonly, because of the broad spectrum of action and the good CNS coverage, a third- or fourth-generation cephalosporin such as ceftriaxone or cefepime is usually used [90]. Due to the rise of multidrug resistant *S. pneumoniae*, vancomycin is also commonly used. In elderly patients, ampicillin is usually added as a third drug to cover for *L. monocytogenes*. *Mycobacterium tuberculosis* can cause a monocyte and lymphocyte-predominant basilar meningitis that can present like other bacterial meningitis but can also have cranial nerve palsies. This condition is particularly prevalent in individuals with the human immunodeficiency virus (HIV) and in patients from areas where *M. tuberculosis* is endemic. Recent trauma can also introduce atypical organisms into the CSF and result in meningitis. These organisms commonly include Staphylococci species and gram-negative organisms such as *Pseudomonas aeruginosa* [91].

Fungal meningitis is usually seen in patients with immunodeficiencies or immunosuppressed states. The common cause of fungal meningitis is *Cryptococcus neoformans*. Viral meningitis typically has similar but milder symptoms and is usually self-limiting [92]. The causes of viral meningitis are multiple and include many enteroviruses and arboviruses. Other causes of viral meningitis include organisms such as cytomegalovirus, Epstein–Barr virus, and varicella zoster virus.

Encephalitis

Encephalitis can present similarly to meningitis but has additional features of parenchymal involvement including seizures, alterations in consciousness, memory loss, and headache. Nearly all cases of encephalitis are caused by viruses. The most frequent and treatable cause of encephalitis that always must be considered is *Herpes simplex*. This virus causes an encephalitis that is fatal in 70% of untreated patients [93]. HSV encephalitis can be treated using acyclovir, but most patients with this disorder will have some sequelae and will not regain full function—although most regain meaningful function [94]. The CSF analysis will show a lymphocytic pleocytosis in cases of encephalitis. In encephalitis caused by HSV, there is often hemorrhagic necrosis, particularly of the temporal lobes, so the CSF can show many erythrocytes as well. MRI of brain may be obtained to evaluate for such hemorrhagic necrosis of the temporal lobes. EEG may show diffuse slowing or periodic lateralized epileptiform discharges.

Cerebral Abscess

Cerebral abscesses typically present with headaches and focal neurological deficits. They do not typically manifest with the common findings of CNS infection such as stiff neck, headache, nausea, vomiting, fever, lethargy, photophobia, or optic disk edema [95, 96]. Many times, cerebral abscesses are discovered in the workup of a patient with a fever of unknown origin or in a stroke workup. The mass effect from the abscess compromises the nearby brain tissue, and therefore symptoms vary based on location. Cerebral abscesses can be a result of either direct spread from the sinuses [97] and also from occasionally dental infections or as a result of hematogenous spread. Hematogenous spread will usually result in multiple abscesses at the gray-white junction, whereas local spread usually results in a single abscess [8]. Hematogenous spread usually takes place in the setting of a compromised immune system. Diagnosis is made using neuroimaging with CT and/or MRI. The abscess is usually hypointense and, if contrast is administered, a rim of peripheral enhancement can be seen. LP is rarely helpful and occasionally can potentiate a herniation syndrome if mass effect is significant. Treatment is with empiric antibiotics and likely neurosurgical drainage of the lesion may be necessary [8].

Intracranial Hypotension

Intracranial hypotension can be either spontaneous or associated with trauma (including fenestration of the dural sac by lumbar puncture) [98]. It is caused by an insufficient hydrostatic pressure to keep the cerebrum, brainstem, and other CNS tissue suspended above the bony calvarium. When this occurs, the base of the brain and brainstem sag down and often rest on the skull base, occasionally causing damage to these structures. These patients almost all universally have headaches, but they can also present with lethargy/stupor, cranial neuropathies, or even as a discrete brainstem syndrome [99]. A frontotemporal dementia-like picture can also be seen in this condition [100]. Due to the compression of the brainstem against the skull base, the ARAS can be compromised, leading to an alteration of mental status. Up to 2/3 of patients have spontaneous intracranial hypotension and have a diagnostic or a physical exam indicative of a connective tissue disorder, leading to the presumption that these disorders have something to do with the pathogenesis [101]. Diagnosis is made by the clinical picture of postural headache worsened by standing or sitting up. The MRI can show diffuse enhancement of the pachymeninges, "slumping" of the midbrain and sometimes subdural hygromas. In the case of an LP-associated event, treatment with a blood patch is usually attempted first, and if unsuccessful, a surgical repair can be performed.

Epileptiform Activity

Convulsive Status Epilepticus

Convulsive status epilepticus is defined as seizure activity without a recovery of consciousness that lasts longer than 5 min [102]. Convulsive status epilepticus is a life-threatening condition that needs to be identified and treated early to prevent continued neuronal damage to the brain and to other organ systems. This is especially true since the chances that a seizure will resolve spontaneously decrease as the length of time that the seizure lasts increases [103]. Mortality rates are around 20% according to studies [104]. Aggressive treatment with benzodiazepines and antiepileptic treatment should be initiated. The Veterans Affairs Status Epilepticus Cooperative Study showed us that lorazepam should be considered first-line therapy for patients in status epilepticus [105]. For refractory status, general anesthesia is usually needed in order to suppress epileptic activity. Burst suppression may be needed to break refractory status and to prevent severe neuronal damage from occurring. Different etiologies of status epilepticus include drug toxicity, stroke, alcohol intoxication, chronic epilepsy with subtherapeutic antiepileptic levels, metabolic abnormalities such as hyponatremia or hypocalcemia, CNS infections such as toxoplasmosis, or any space occupying lesions. Patients who end up in status epilepticus due to stroke, anoxic brain injury, and the elderly population have a high incidence of mortality [106].

Nonconvulsive Status Epilepticus (NCSE)

NCSE is a commonly missed diagnosis and is often hard to identify clinically. Morbidity and mortality are difficult to assess in this condition, but an article by Shneker and Fountain indicated that NCSE secondary to a medical condition can have a mortality of 18% [107], which approaches that of convulsive status epilepticus. They also describe that NCSE can occur without an underlying medical condition and when this occurs it has a much lower mortality rate. EEG is the only way to diagnose this condition, so this test is especially useful in patients with AMS and a known history of seizures who are not having generalized convulsions. Although nonconvulsive status does not seem to be as fatal as convulsive status, it is still important to identify and treat earlier rather than later to prevent neuronal. It should be considered in the setting of AMS when the patient does not have metabolic/toxic/infectious or structural abnormality.

Immune-Mediated Encephalopathies

Recently, immune-mediated encephalopathies have emerged in the literature due to the advent of new assays, increasing recognition, and the concern over missing possible treatable conditions. These encephalopathies can be either idiopathic, autoimmune, or paraneoplastic in nature. As investigation into these entities progresses, the pathogenesis will be elicited and fewer will be classified as idiopathic [108]. Many of these disorders (but not all) are associated with tumors. They all have an immune-mediated pathogenesis and may respond to immune-active therapy as antibody-associated encephalopathies [109].

These disorders have an extremely varied presentation but nearly always have a rapidly progressive encephalopathy with superimposed delirium as a feature. Other manifestations include seizures, movement disorders, psychiatric symptoms (mania, hallucinations, paranoia), and fluctuating symptoms. Many of these disorders have recently had autoantibodies discovered, particularly to neuronal membrane channel proteins. These antibodies can be detected with serological testing. Many of the encephalopathies that affect the limbic system will have MRI T2 signal abnormalities in the mesial temporal lobes. Some of the more common antibodies associated with immune-mediated encephalopathy include voltage-gated potassium channel [110], NMDA receptor [111], amino-3-hydroxy-5-methyl-4-isoxazolepropionic acid (AMPA) receptor [112], and gamma-aminobutyric acid (GABA) B receptor [113]. These antibodies do not necessarily predict clinical course, clinical manifestations, or even whether or not a patient will develop symptoms. The responsiveness to immunosuppressive therapies seems to be greater in patients with subacute onset, fluctuating course, tremor, short delay to treatment, seropositivity for a known antibody, and CSF abnormalities [114].

Another disorder that seems to have immune-mediated pathogenesis is steroid responsive encephalopathy associated with autoimmune thyroiditis (SREAT) [115]. The most common manifestations of this disorder include altered mental status, seizures, stroke-like signs, EEG abnormalities, and increased CSF protein [116]. This disorder is often but not always associated with thyroid function abnormalities and antithyroid peroxidase antibodies.

Acknowledgments I would like to thank Dr. Michael Okun for his previous contributions to the manuscript.

References

1. Dubin WR, Field HL, Gastfriend DR. Postcardiotomy delirium: a critical review. J Thorac Cardiovasc Surg. 1979;77(4):586–94.
2. Plum F, Posner JB. The diagnosis of stupor and coma. Contemp Neurol Ser. 1972;10:1–286.
3. Tindall SC. Level of consciousness. In: Walker HK, Hall WD, Hurst JW, et al., editors. Clinical methods: the history, physical, and laboratory examinations. 3rd ed. Boston: Butterworths; 1990.
4. Edlow BL, Takahashi E, Wu O, Benner T, Dai G, Bu L, et al. Neuroanatomic connectivity of the human ascending arousal system critical to consciousness and its disorders. J Neuropathol Exp Neurol. 2012;71(6):531–46.
5. Reinoso-Suárez F, de Andrés I, Garzón M. Functional anatomy of the sleep-wakefulness cycle: wakefulness. Adv Anat Embryol Cell Biol. 2011;208:1–128.
6. Fisher CM. Brain herniation: a revision of classical concepts. Can J Neurol Sci. 1995;22(2):83–91.
7. Young GB. Coma. Ann N Y Acad Sci. 2009;1157(1):32–47.
8. Kaplan PW. The EEG, in metabolic encephalopathy and coma. J Clin Neurophysiol. 2004;21(5):307–18.
9. Fisher CM. The neurological examination of the comatose patient. Acta Neurol Scand. 1969;45(Suppl 36):1–56.
10. Lilly LS. Pathophysiology of heart disease. Philadelphia: Wolters Kluwer/Lippincott Williams & Wilkins; 2007.
11. Pessin M, Panis W, Prager R, Millan V, Scott R. Auscultation of cervical and ocular bruits in extracranial carotid occlusive disease: a clinical and angiographic study. Stroke. 1983;14(2):246–9.
12. Bickley LS, Bates B, Szilagyi PG. Bates' pocket guide to physical examination and history taking. 6th ed. Philadelphia: Wolters Kluwer Health/Lippincott Williams & Wilkins; 2009.
13. Rich MW. Epidemiology, clinical features, and prognosis of acute myocardial infarction in the elderly. Am J Geriatr Cardiol. 2006;15(1):7–11. quiz 12
14. Hussain A, Via G, Melniker L, Goffi A, Tavazzi G, Neri L, et al. Multi-organ point-of-care ultrasound for COVID-19 (PoCUS4COVID): international expert consensus. Crit Care. 2020;24(1):702.
15. Garcia AJ, Zanella S, Koch H, Doi A, Ramirez JM. Chapter 3 – networks within networks: the neuronal control of breathing. Prog Brain Res. 2011;188:31–50.
16. Wasserman AM, Sahibzada N, Hernandez YM, Gillis RA. Specific subnuclei of the nucleus tractus solitarius play a role in determining the duration of inspiration in the rat. Brain Res. 2000;880(1–2):118–30.
17. Pauzner R, Mouallem M, Sadeh M, Tadmor R, Farfel Z. High incidence of primary cerebral lymphoma in tumor-induced central neurogenic hyperventilation. Arch Neurol. 1989;46(5):510–2.
18. Mador MJ, Tobin MJ, Apneustic breathing. A characteristic feature of brainstem compression in achondroplasia? Chest. 1990;97(4):877–83.
19. Wijdicks EF. Biot's breathing. J Neurol Neurosurg Psychiatry. 2007;78(5):512–3.
20. Farney RJ, Walker JM, Boyle KM, Cloward TV, Shilling KC. Adaptive servoventilation (ASV) in patients with sleep disordered breathing associated with chronic opioid medications for non-malignant pain. J Clin Sleep Med. 2008;4(4):311–9.
21. Levitzky MG, Cairo JM, Hall SM. Introduction to respiratory care. Philadelphia: Saunders; 1990.
22. Teasdale G, Jennett B. Assessment of coma and impaired consciousness. A practical scale Lancet. 1974;2:81–4.
23. Wijdicks EF, Bamlet WR, Maramattom BV, Manno EM, McClelland RL. Validation of a new coma scale: The FOUR score. Ann Neurol. 2005;58(4):585–93.
24. Rosenthal EN, Riccio CA, Gsanger KM, Jarratt KP. Digit span components as predictors of attention problems and executive functioning in children. Arch Clin Neuropsychol. 2006;21(2): 131–9.
25. Pennington LA. The serial sevens test as a psychometric instrument. Am J Orthopsychiatry. 1947;17(3):488–99.
26. Heilman KM, Valenstein E. Mechanisms underlying hemispatial neglect. Ann Neurol. 1979;5(2):166–70.
27. Heilman KM, Watson RT. Mechanisms underlying the unilateral neglect syndrome. Adv Neurol. 1977;18:93–106.
28. Knecht S, Drager B, Deppe M, et al. Handedness and hemispheric language dominance in healthy humans. Brain. 2000;123(Pt 12):2512–8.
29. Huntley A. Documenting level of consciousness. Nursing. 2008;38(8):63–4.

30. Sigg EB, Sigg TD. The modification of the pupillary light reflex by chlorpromazine, diazepam, and pentobarbital. Brain Res. 1973;50(1):77–86.
31. Miller NR, Walsh FB, Hoyt WF. Walsh and Hoyt's clinical neuro-ophthalmology. 6th ed. Philadelphia: Lippincott Williams & Wilkins; 2005.
32. Yanovitch T, Buckley E. Diagnosis and management of third nerve palsy. Curr Opin Ophthalmol. 2007;18(5):373–8.
33. Brown SM. The utility of 0.5% apraclonidine in the diagnosis of horner syndrome. Arch Ophthalmol. 2005;123(4):578:author reply 578.
34. Freedman KA, Brown SM. Topical apraclonidine in the diagnosis of suspected Horner syndrome. J Neuroophthalmol. 2005;25(2):83–5.
35. Thompson HS. Diagnosing Horner's syndrome. Trans Sect Ophthalmol Am Acad Ophthalmol Otolaryngol. 1977;83(5):840–2.
36. Angelaki DE. Eyes on target: what neurons must do for the vestibuloocular reflex during linear motion. J Neurophysiol. 2004;92(1):20–35.
37. Leigh RJ, Zee DS. The neurology of eye movements. 3rd ed. New York: Oxford University Press; 1999.
38. Roberts TA, Jenkyn LR, Reeves AG. On the notion of doll's eyes. Arch Neurol. 1984;41(12):1242–3.
39. Biller J, Gruener G, Brazis PW, DeMyer W. Technique of the neurologic examination: a programmed text. 6th ed. New York: McGraw-Hill Medical Publishing Division; 2011.
40. Gonçalves DU, Felipe L, Lima TMA. Interpretação e utilidade da prova calórica. Rev Bras Otorrinolaringol. 2008;74:440–6.
41. Davies AE, Kidd D, Stone SP, MacMahon J. Pharyngeal sensation and gag reflex in healthy subjects. Lancet. 1995;345(8948):487–8.
42. Walker HK. The origins of the history and physical. In: Walker HK, Hall WD, Hurst JW, et al., editors. Clinical methods: the history, physical, and laboratory examinations. 3rd ed. Boston: Butterworths; 1990.
43. Sherrington CS. The integrative action of the nervous system. New York: C. Scribner's Sons; 1906.
44. Brazis PW, Masdeu JC, Biller J. Localization in clinical neurology. 6th ed. Philadelphia: Wolters Kluwer Health/Lippincott Williams & Wilkins; 2011.
45. Floeter MK, Fields HL. Evidence that inhibition of a nociceptive flexion reflex by stimulation in the rostroventromedial medulla in rats occurs at a premotoneuronal level. Brain Res. 1991;538(2):340–2.
46. Sandrini G, Serrao M, Rossi P, Romaniello A, Cruccu G, Willer JC. The lower limb flexion reflex in humans. Prog Neurobiol. 2005;77(6):353–95.
47. Shah RC, Wilson RS, Tang Y, Dong X, Murray A, Bennett DA. Relation of hemoglobin to level of cognitive function in older persons. Neuroepidemiology. 2009;32(1):40–6.
48. Shah RC, Buchman AS, Wilson RS, Leurgans SE, Bennett DA. Hemoglobin level in older persons and incident Alzheimer disease: prospective cohort analysis. Neurology. 2011;77:219–26.
49. Moschcowitz E. An acute febrile pleiochromic anemia with hyaline thrombosis of the terminal arterioles and capillaries; an undescribed disease. Am J Med. 1952;13(5):567–9.
50. Zaret BS, Beckner RR, Marini AM, Wagle W, Passarelli C. Sodium valproate-induced hyperammonemia without clinical hepatic dysfunction. Neurology. 1982;32(2):206–8.
51. Cook ND. The neuron-level phenomena underlying cognition and consciousness: synaptic activity and the action potential. Neuroscience. 2008;153(3):556–70.
52. Hounsfield GN. Computerized transverse axial scanning (tomography). 1. Description of system. Br J Radiol. 1973;46(552):1016–22.
53. Ambrose J. Computerized transverse axial scanning of the brain. Proc R Soc Med. 1973;66(8):833–4.
54. Roos KL. Lumbar puncture. Semin Neurol. 2003;23(1):105–14.
55. Husain AM. Electroencephalographic assessment of coma. J Clin Neurophysiol. 2006;23(3):208–20.
56. Bickford RG, Butt HR. Hepatic coma: the electroencephalographic pattern. J Clin Invest. 1955;34(6):790–9.
57. Chien LT, Boehm RM, Robinson H, Liu C, Frenkel LD. Characteristic early electroencephalographic changes in herpes simplex encephalitis. Arch Neurol. 1977;34(6):361–4.
58. Levy SR, Chiappa KH, Burke CJ, Young RR. Early evolution and incidence of electroencephalographic abnormalities in Creutzfeldt-Jakob disease. J Clin Neurophysiol. 1986;3(1):1–21.
59. International Federation of Societies for Electroencephalography and Clinical Neurophysiology. Recommendations for the practice of clinical neurophysiology. Amsterdam/New York: Elsevier; 1983.
60. Dubois MJ, Bergeron N, Dumont M, Dial S, Skrobik Y. Delirium in an intensive care unit: a study of risk factors. Intensive Care Med. 2001;27(8):1297–304.
61. Ely EW, Shintani A, Truman B, et al. Delirium as a predictor of mortality in mechanically ventilated patients in the intensive care unit. JAMA. 2004;291(14):1753–62.
62. Ely EW, Gautam S, Margolin R, et al. The impact of delirium in the intensive care unit on hospital length of stay. Intensive Care Med. 2001;27(12):1892–900.
63. Heymann A, Radtke F, Schiemann A, et al. Delayed treatment of delirium increases mortality rate in intensive care unit patients. J Int Med Res. 2010;38(5):1584–95.
64. American Psychiatric Association. Diagnostic criteria from DSM-IV-TR. Washington DC: American Psychiatric Association; 2000.
65. Campo-Soria C, Chang Y, Weiss DS. Mechanism of action of benzodiazepines on GABAA receptors. Br J Pharmacol. 2006;148(7):984–90.
66. Study RE, Barker JL. Diazepam and (−)-pentobarbital: fluctuation analysis reveals different mechanisms for potentiation of gamma-aminobutyric acid responses in cultured central neurons. Proc Natl Acad Sci USA. 1981;78(11):7180–4.
67. Benowitz NL. Clinical pharmacology and toxicology of cocaine. Pharmacol Toxicol. 1993;72(1):3–12.
68. Meehan TJ, Bryant SM, Aks SE. Drugs of abuse: the highs and lows of altered mental states in the emergency department. Emerg Med Clin North Am. 2010;28(3):663–82.
69. Williams SR, Turner JP, Crunelli V. Gamma-hydroxybutyrate promotes oscillatory activity of rat and cat thalamocortical neurons by a tonic GABAB, receptor-mediated hyperpolarization. Neuroscience. 1995;66(1):133–41.
70. Mathivet P, Bernasconi R, De Barry J, Marescaux C, Bittiger H. Binding characteristics of gamma-hydroxybutyric acid as a weak but selective GABAB receptor agonist. Eur J Pharmacol. 1997;321(1):67–75.
71. Friedman J, Westlake R, Furman M. "Grievous bodily harm:" gamma hydroxybutyrate abuse leading to a Wernicke-Korsakoff syndrome. Neurology. 1996;46(2):469–71.
72. Okun MS, Boothby LA, Bartfield RB, Doering PL. GHB: an important pharmacologic and clinical update. J Pharm Pharm Sci. 2001;4(2):167–75.
73. Benbadis SR, Sila CA, Cristea RL. Mental status changes and stroke. J Gen Intern Med. 1994;9(9):485–7.
74. Kubik CS, Adams R. Occlusion of the basilar artery; a clinical and pathological study. Brain. 1946;69(2):73–121.
75. Percheron G. The anatomy of the arterial supply of the human thalamus and its use for the interpretation of the thalamic vascular pathology. Z Neurol. 1973;205(1):1–13.

76. Reilly M, Connolly S, Stack J, Martin EA, Hutchinson M. Bilateral paramedian thalamic infarction: a distinct but poorly recognized stroke syndrome. Q J Med. 1992;82(297):63–70.
77. McCormick WF, Rosenfield DB. Massive brain hemorrhage: a review of 144 cases and an examination of their causes. Stroke. 1973;4(6):946–54.
78. Kassell NF, Sasaki T, Colohan AR, Nazar G. Cerebral vasospasm following aneurysmal subarachnoid hemorrhage. Stroke. 1985;16(4):562–72.
79. Byrom FB. The pathogenesis of hypertensive encephalopathy and its relation to the malignant phase of hypertension; experimental evidence from the hypertensive rat. Lancet. 1954;267(6831):201–11.
80. Bartynski WS. Posterior reversible encephalopathy syndrome, part 1: fundamental imaging and clinical features. AJNR Am J Neuroradiol. 2008;29(6):1036–42.
81. Bartynski WS, Boardman JF, Zeigler ZR, Shadduck RK, Lister J. Posterior reversible encephalopathy syndrome in infection, sepsis, and shock. AJNR Am J Neuroradiol. 2006;27(10):2179–90.
82. Okun MS, Millar B, Watson R. Early diagnostic magnetic resonance imaging in acute disseminated encephalomyelitis. South Med J. 2000;93(8):793–6.
83. Nishimura A, Fuchigami T, Izumi H, Okubo O, Takahashi S, Harada K. A case of early-onset acute disseminated encephalomyelitis. No To Hattatsu. 1997;29(5):396–400.
84. Stricker RB, Miller RG, Kiprov DD. Role of plasmapheresis in acute disseminated (postinfectious) encephalomyelitis. J Clin Apher. 1992;7(4):173–9.
85. Tan HM, Chan LL, Chuah KL, Goh NS, Tang KK. Monophasic, solitary tumefactive demyelinating lesion: neuroimaging features and neuropathological diagnosis. Br J Radiol. 2004;77(914):153–6.
86. De Stefano N, Caramanos Z, Preul MC, Francis G, Antel JP, Arnold DL. In vivo differentiation of astrocytic brain tumors and isolated demyelinating lesions of the type seen in multiple sclerosis using 1H magnetic resonance spectroscopic imaging. Ann Neurol. 1998;44(2):273–8.
87. Launay M, Lebrun C, Giordana E, Chanalet S, Thomas P. Clinical, radiographic, prognostic and therapeutic aspects of demyelinating disease with tumefactive demyelinating lesions. Rev Neurol (Paris). 2011;167(1):14–22.
88. Zunt JR, Marra CM. Cerebrospinal fluid testing for the diagnosis of central nervous system infection. Neurol Clin. 1999;17(4):675–89.
89. Arevalo CE, Barnes PF, Duda M, Leedom JM. Cerebrospinal fluid cell counts and chemistries in bacterial meningitis. South Med J. 1989;82(9):1122–7.
90. Chaudhuri A, Martin PM, Kennedy PGE, et al. EFNS guideline on the management of community-acquired bacterial meningitis: report of an EFNS Task Force on acute bacterial meningitis in older children and adults. Eur J Neurol. 2008;15(7):649–59.
91. Tunkel AR, Hartman BJ, Kaplan SL, et al. Practice guidelines for the management of bacterial meningitis. Clin Infect Dis. 2004;39(9):1267–84.
92. Attia J, Hatala R, Cook DJ, Wong JG. Does this adult patient have acute meningitis? JAMA. 1999;282(2):175–81.
93. Whitley RJ. Herpes simplex encephalitis: adolescents and adults. Antivir Res. 2006;71(2–3):141–8.
94. Whitley RJ, Gnann JW. Viral encephalitis: familiar infections and emerging pathogens. Lancet. 2002;359(9305):507–13.
95. Xiao F, Tseng MY, Teng LJ, Tseng HM, Tsai JC. Brain abscess: clinical experience and analysis of prognostic factors. Surg Neurol. 2005;63(5):442–9; discussion 449–50.
96. Carpenter J, Stapleton S, Holliman R. Retrospective analysis of 49 cases of brain abscess and review of the literature. Eur J Clin Microbiol Infect Dis. 2007;26(1):1–11.
97. Nunez DA, Browning GG. Risks of developing an otogenic intracranial abscess. J Laryngol Otol. 1990;104(6):468–72.
98. Schievink WI, Louy C. Precipitating factors of spontaneous spinal CSF leaks and intracranial hypotension. Neurology. 2007;69(7):700–2.
99. Fedi M, Cantello R, Shuey NH, et al. Spontaneous intracranial hypotension presenting as a reversible dorsal midbrain syndrome. J Neuroophthalmol. 2008;28(4):289–92.
100. Wicklund MR, Mokri B, Drubach DA, Boeve BF, Parisi JE, Josephs KA. Frontotemporal brain sagging syndrome. Neurology. 2011;76(16):1377–82.
101. Schievink WI, Gordon OK, Tourje J. Connective tissue disorders with spontaneous spinal cerebrospinal fluid leaks and intracranial hypotension: a prospective study. Neurosurgery. 2004;54(1):65–70; discussion 70–1.
102. Lowenstein DH. Status epilepticus: an overview of the clinical problem. Epilepsia. 1999;40(Suppl 1):3–8; discussion S21–2.
103. Garcia Penas JJ, Molins A, Salas PJ. Status epilepticus: evidence and controversy. Neurologist. 2007;13(6 Suppl 1):62–73.
104. DeLorenzo RJ, Hauser WA, Towne AR, et al. A prospective, population-based epidemiologic study of status epilepticus in Richmond. Virginia Neurology. 1996;46(4):1029–35.
105. Treiman DM, Meyers PD, Walton NY, et al. A comparison of four treatments for generalized convulsive status epilepticus. Veterans Affairs Status Epilepticus Cooperative Study Group. N Engl J Med. 1998;339(12):792–8.
106. Litt B, Wityk RJ, Hertz SH, et al. Nonconvulsive status epilepticus in the critically ill elderly. Epilepsia. 1998;39(11):1194–202.
107. Shneker BF, Fountain NB. Assessment of acute morbidity and mortality in nonconvulsive status epilepticus. Neurology. 2003;61(8):1066–73.
108. Pruitt AA. Immune-mediated encephalopathies with an emphasis on paraneoplastic encephalopathies. Semin Neurol. 2011;31(02):158:168.
109. Tuzun E, Dalmau J. Limbic encephalitis and variants: classification, diagnosis and treatment. Neurologist. 2007;13(5):261–71.
110. Thieben MJ, Lennon VA, Boeve BF, Aksamit AJ, Keegan M, Vernino S. Potentially reversible autoimmune limbic encephalitis with neuronal potassium channel antibody. Neurology. 2004;62(7):1177–82.
111. Dalmau J, Gleichman AJ, Hughes EG, et al. Anti-NMDA-receptor encephalitis: case series and analysis of the effects of antibodies. Lancet Neurol. 2008;7(12):1091–8.
112. Lai M, Hughes EG, Peng X, et al. AMPA receptor antibodies in limbic encephalitis alter synaptic receptor location. Ann Neurol. 2009;65(4):424–34.
113. Lancaster E, Lai M, Peng X, et al. Antibodies to the GABA(B) receptor in limbic encephalitis with seizures: case series and characterisation of the antigen. Lancet Neurol. 2010;9(1):67–76.
114. EiP F, McKeon A, Lennon VA, et al. Autoimmune dementia: clinical course and predictors of immunotherapy response. Mayo Clin Proc. 2010;85(10):881–97.
115. Brain L. Hashimoto's disease and encephalopathy. Lancet Neurol. 1966;2(7462):512–4.
116. Chong JY, Rowland LP, Utiger RD. Hashimoto encephalopathy: syndrome or myth? Arch Neurol. 2003;60(2):164–71.

Seizures in the Intensive Care Unit

6

Manuel Melo Bicchi, Kelsey Ladd,
and Ayham Alkhachroum

Contents

M. M. Bicchi · A. Alkhachroum (✉)
Department of Neurology, University of Miami, Miller School of Medicine, Miami, FL, USA

Department of Neurology, Jackson Memorial Hospital, Miami, FL, USA
e-mail: mmbic@miami.edu; axa2610@med.miami.edu

K. Ladd
Department of Pharmacy, Jackson Memorial Hospital, Miami, FL, USA
e-mail: kelsey.ladd@jhsmiami.org

E. Mahanna Gabrielli et al. (eds.), *Textbook of Neurointensive Care: Volume 1*, https://doi.org/10.1007/978-3-031-62220-5_6

Abstract

Early recognition and treatment of seizures in critically ill patients remains an essential factor for a favorable outcome. In this chapter, we review common electroencephalographic patterns and pharmacological and non-pharmacological treatments of seizures and status epilepticus (SE) in the intensive care unit (ICU). Most seizures are nonconvulsive in nature. In critically ill patients with altered mental status, nonconvulsive seizures (NCSs) should be suspected early and screened with an electroencephalogram (EEG). Adequate EEG interpretation should be performed by a trained electroencephalographer to guide treatment decisions.

Introduction

Seizures in the intensive care unit (ICU) have been increasingly recognized with the increased use of continuous electroencephalogram (EEG). Although still underutilized, EEG is becoming an essential screening tool in critically ill patients [1]. Seizures in the ICU population commonly evolve into status epilepticus (SE), often associated with severe central nervous system (CNS) and systemic complications if left untreated [2]. Although clinicians may promptly recognize overt convulsive seizures, subclinical seizures and nonconvulsive status epilepticus (NCSE) remain a diagnostic challenge in the ICU. Critically ill patients with traumatic brain injury (TBI), ischemic or hemorrhagic strokes, metabolic abnormalities, and brain tumors are among the most commonly seen etiologies of NCSE in the ICU [3].

Epidemiological studies have shown that SE affects approximately 16–40 cases per 100,000 people annually, with the bimodal distribution highest in children (<1 year) and in the elderly (>70 years) [4, 5]. If SE persists after the first- (i.e., benzodiazepines) and second- (i.e., antiseizure medications) or third-line agents (i.e., anesthetics), then SE is considered refractory status epilepticus (RSE) and super-refractory status epilepticus (SRSE), respectively [6, 7]. Approximately 15–45% of SE cases will progress to RSE, with 13–42% of the latter progressing to SRSE [8, 9]. The most common causes of SE include low levels of antiseizure medications (ASMs) in patients with a prior history of epilepsy (35%), remote symptomatic seizures such as stroke and trauma (25%), acute cerebrovascular injury (22%), metabolic disorders (15%), alcohol-related seizures (13%), and anoxic brain injury (5%), among others [3, 10].

Seizures may occur in up to 50% of patients with altered mental status admitted to the ICU [11]. A 30-min EEG (routine or intermittent) can detect seizures in approximately 11% of patients [12], whereas prolonged EEG can detect up to 93% of seizures over the first 48 hours in this patient population, thus highlighting the importance of continuous EEG monitoring [13, 14]. In many cases, obtaining EEG in a timely manner is crucial for rapid determination of treatment escalation in patients with nonconvulsive seizures (NCSs) or for de-escalation of treatment. Multiple challenges may lead to the delay of connecting patients to EEG, including the availability of an EEG technologist, of continuous EEG, and of trained electroencephalographers to provide a prompt reading, among others. Other options such as rapid response EEG should be considered. Rapid response EEG is an Food and Drug Administration (FDA)-approved point-of-care EEG system intended to be used in the emergency room and critical care settings, which can be easily applied by any provider in under 5 min [15].

In this chapter, we discuss the pathophysiology and etiologies of seizures in the ICU, EEG monitoring, commonly seen patterns on EEG, challenging patterns on EEG, and the treatment of seizures and status epilepticus.

The Pathophysiology of Status Epilepticus

Despite many advancements in the treatment of SE, its pathophysiology is still poorly understood. Studies have demonstrated a cascade of maladaptive changes occurring from a single seizure progressing to SE. During the initial seconds of a prolonged seizure, there is an increase in neurotransmitter release and protein phosphorylation. These molecular changes set the stage for internalization of inhibitory γ-aminobutyric acid type A ($GABA_A$) receptors and an increase of excitatory *N*-methyl-D-aspartate (NMDA) receptors [16, 17]. Animal models of status epilepticus have shown that $GABA_A$ internalization is believed to contribute to the pharmacoresistance to benzodiazepines, which becomes more prominent as the seizure duration increases [18]. Furthermore, other models of convulsive seizures have demonstrated hypoxia, hypotension, and hyperthermia with neuronal injury in the neocortex, thalami, and hippocampi [19].

Definition and Classification of Seizures and Status Epilepticus

A seizure is defined as a transient occurrence of signs and symptoms due to abnormal excessive or synchronous neuronal activity in the brain [20]. Status epilepticus is a neurological emergency that leads to an increased risk of morbidity and mortality. The International League Against Epilepsy defines status epilepticus as a condition resulting from either the failure of mechanisms responsible for seizure termination or the initiation of mechanisms, which leads to abnormally prolonged seizures (T1). If left untreated, seizures can have long-term consequences, including neuronal injury or death (T2) [21]. This definition encompasses both a conceptual and operational definition with the introduction of T1 and T2 concepts. "T1" refers to the point in time of the seizure at which it is regarded as a "prolonged seizure." "T2" refers to the point in time of an ongoing seizure activity at which there is risk of irreversible neuronal damage. For example, generalized tonic-clonic (GTC) seizures will likely continue if they last for more than 5 min (T1), with irreversible damage after 30 min (T2). Similarly, focal seizures with loss of awareness will likely continue if they last for more than 10 min (T1), with neuronal damage after 60 min (T2) [21]. These are approximate times and will vary depending on the anatomical location, age, and etiology of seizures.

The classification of SE has been evolving since the 1970s. Trinka et al. classified status epilepticus into four axes: semiology, etiology, EEG correlation, and age [21]. Although all axes play an important role in the classification, the most widely used by neurologists is semiology. This axis is broadly classified into motor activity and impairment of consciousness. Motor activity includes convulsive, myoclonic, focal motor, tonic, and hyperkinetic SE. Impaired consciousness alludes to NCSE with and without coma such as absence, aphasic, visual, psychiatric/emotional, etc. [22].

When to Suspect Seizures

Any patient with altered mental status is at risk of developing seizures, particularly if there is history of acute brain injury. Seizures may occur in 10–70% of patients with altered mental status in the ICU, with the majority (92%) of these being nonconvulsive [11, 14]. NCSE lacks obvious motor manifestations but can be associated with other subtle signs such as pupillary hippus (spasmodic or rhythmic variations in pupillary size regardless of light intensity), gaze deviation, nystagmus, subtle muscle twitching (e.g., eyelids, mouth, fingers, etc.), and autonomic instability. Several studies have revealed that 14–20% of patients with successful treatment of convulsive seizures will continue to have ongoing nonconvulsive seizures on EEG [23, 24]. These results suggest that continuous video or multiple intermittent EEGs should be obtained after cessation of convulsive seizures, especially if there is no return to the individual's cognitive baseline.

Table 6.1 Focal motor seizure mimics

Movement disorders (tremor, chorea, dystonia, choreoathetosis, hemiballismus)
Psychogenic non epileptic spells
Spasticity
Decorticate and decerebrate posturing (sometimes seen in basilar artery strokes)
Spinal reflexes (triple flexion) seen in both upper and lower extremities
Roving eye movements of coma (secondary to toxic, metabolic, or bilateral hemispheric lesions)

In critically ill patients, physical examination may not be revealing or at times may be limited due to sedation or neuromuscular blockers and the diagnosis may be missed or misinterpreted as metabolic encephalopathy, post-ictal state, or mutism or hallucinations due to a psychiatric condition [25]. Additionally, various movement disorders and psychiatric and metabolic states can mimic seizures (Table 6.1). At times, the EEG recording may be contaminated by patient movement, agitation, electrical artifact, and, frequently, myogenic artifacts. For the latter, physicians may consider using a short trial of a neuromuscular blocking agent, providing skeletal muscle relaxation to lessen the myogenic artifact in patients who are already sedated and mechanically ventilated to better evaluate the underlying EEG activity.

Interictal and Ictal EEG Patterns

Commonly seen electrographic findings include a spectrum of slow frequencies such as theta (5–7 Hz) and delta (<4 Hz), indicating mild/moderate and severe encephalopathy, respectively. These slow frequencies can be part of a focal (e.g., stroke, subdural hematoma, tumor, etc.) or a diffuse encephalopathic process (i.e., toxic metabolic encephalopathy). Widespread alpha frequencies (8–12 Hz) on EEG can be seen in patients with "alpha coma" after a cardiac arrest and are typically associated with a poor outcome [26]. Interictal findings include epileptiform discharges such as sharp and/or spike and slow wave and can be identified in an array of combinations of generalized, lateralized, multifocal, or sporadic discharges [27] (Fig. 6.1). A key publication by Treiman et al. identified a continuum of predictable electrographic changes during the natural history of generalized convulsive

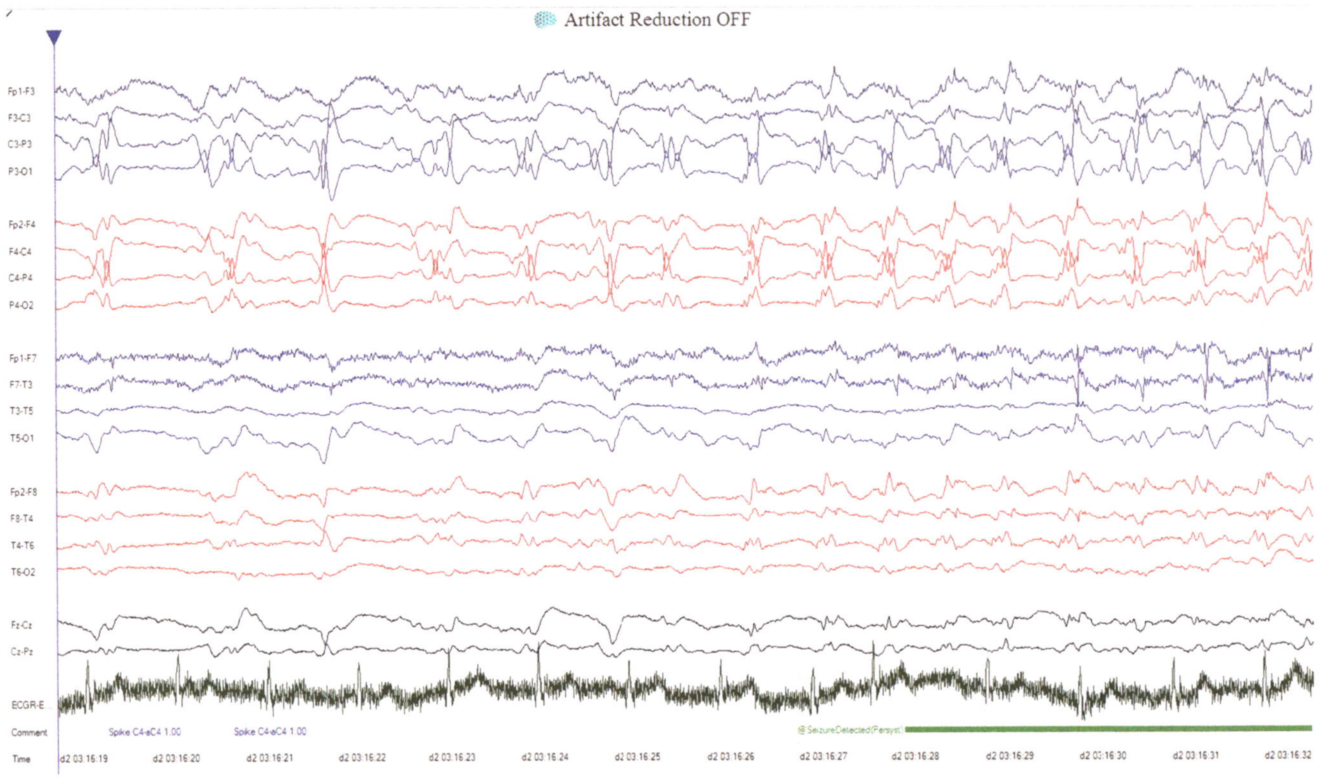

Fig. 6.1 84-year-old male admitted to the intensive care unit after a traumatic brain injury. Bipolar montage EEG shows in the initial half on the recording 0.5–1 Hz bifrontally predominant GPDs with a polyspike component. Note the increased frequency during the second half of the epoch to approximately 2 Hz. The spatiotemporal evolution indicates ictal activity

SE [28]. These include (1) discrete seizures, (2) merging seizures with waxing and waning amplitude and frequency of EEG activity, (3) continuous ictal activity, (4) continuous ictal activity punctuated by low-voltage "flat periods," and (5) periodic discharges on a "flat" background. Continuous video EEG provides timely and robust data regarding cerebral function with important therapeutic implications. This information is generally used for seizure detection, spell characterization in patients with altered mental status, managing or starting ASMs, other neuroimaging studies (e.g., vascular studies in patients with loss of beta frequencies and suspected vasospasm [29]), and managing metabolic coma (e.g., a triphasic wave pattern) and may aid in prognostication after a cardiac arrest [30, 31].

Electrographic seizures correspond to abnormal periodic and/or rhythmic neuronal electrical activity with evolution or progression in the electrical field, frequency, and/or amplitude lasting for at least 10 s [32] (Fig. 6.2). Focal seizures with a clear electrographic onset, progression, and termination are relatively easy to identify by a trained electroencephalographer. However, similar electrographic patterns (e.g., triphasic waves, periodic discharges, rhythmic slowing [lateralized or generalized theta/delta activity]) can be identified in various pathological conditions, leading to complex interpretation of the EEG. NCSE poses a greater challenge since there are no widely accepted evidence-based EEG criteria [33]. Experts in the field have proposed working diagnostic criteria also known as the Salzburg criteria for NCSE, which include generalized periodic discharges (GPDs) >2.5 Hz or ≤ 2.5 Hz, or generalized rhythmic delta activity (GRDA), or lateralized rhythmic delta activity (LRDA) >0.5 Hz associated with any of the following: subtle clinical phenomena, spatiotemporal evolution on EEG, or clinical and EEG improvement after ASM or benzodiazepine trial [34, 35]. Figure 6.3 demonstrates an example of NCSE.

The identification of electrographic interictal patterns for seizure risk stratification or "seizure forecasting" has proven beneficial in recognizing those patients at risk of NCSE or NCS. The 2HELPS2B score assigns a score (1–7) to five electrographic variables and one clinical variable: frequency > 2 Hz for LRDA, lateralized periodic discharges (LPDs), GPDs, and bilateral independent periodic discharges (BIPDs) (1 point); "plus" features such as superimposed rhythmic fast or sharp activity associated with LRDA, BIPDs, and LPDs (1 point); brief ictal rhythmic discharges (2 points); sporadic epileptiform discharges (1 point); LRDA, LPDs, or BIPDs (1 point); and history of seizures prior connecting to EEG (1 point) [36, 37]. The risks of seizures for each score are 5% (0), 12% (1), 27% (2), 50% (3), 73% (4), 88% (5), and > 95% (≥6) [36, 37].

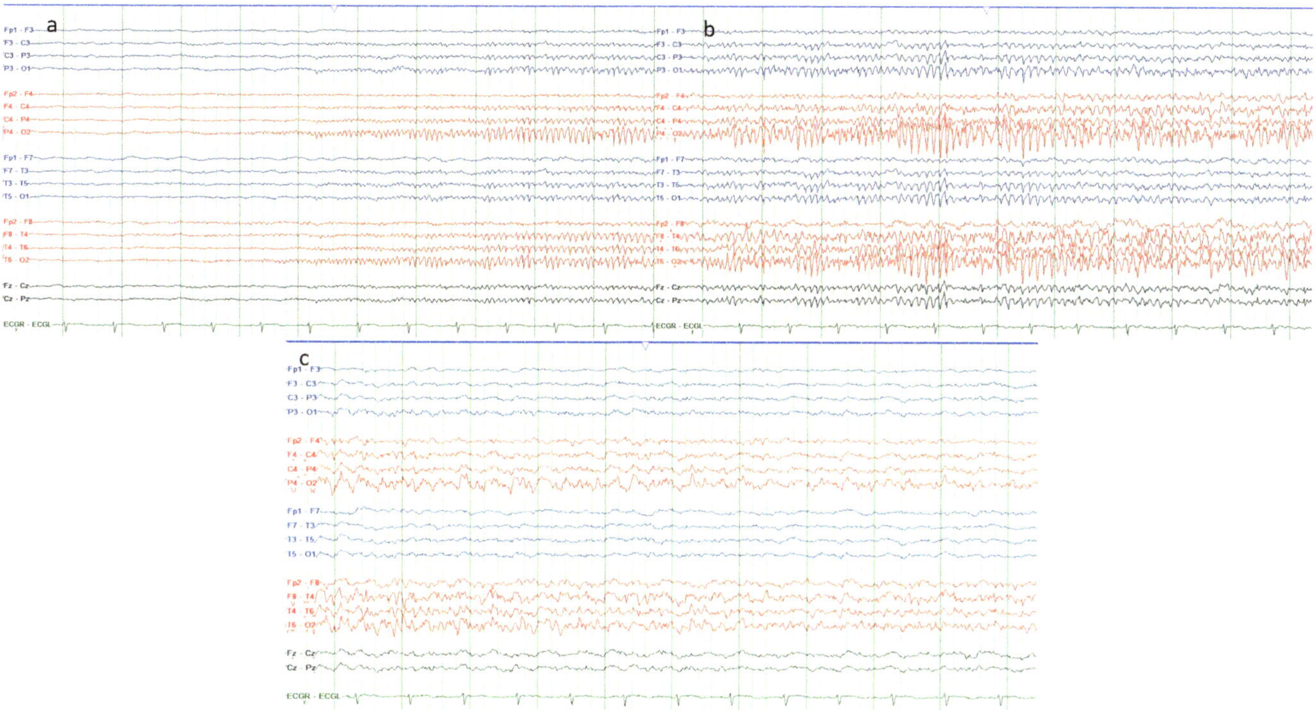

Fig. 6.2 70-year-old female with history of focal epilepsy who was found down with intermittent left eye deviation. (**a**) Bipolar EEG montage showing right posterior quadrant rhythmic sharply contoured alpha activity. (**b**) rhythmic ictal activity increases in amplitude propagating to the temporal and parietal regions. (**c**) ictal activity ends in the right posterior quadrant

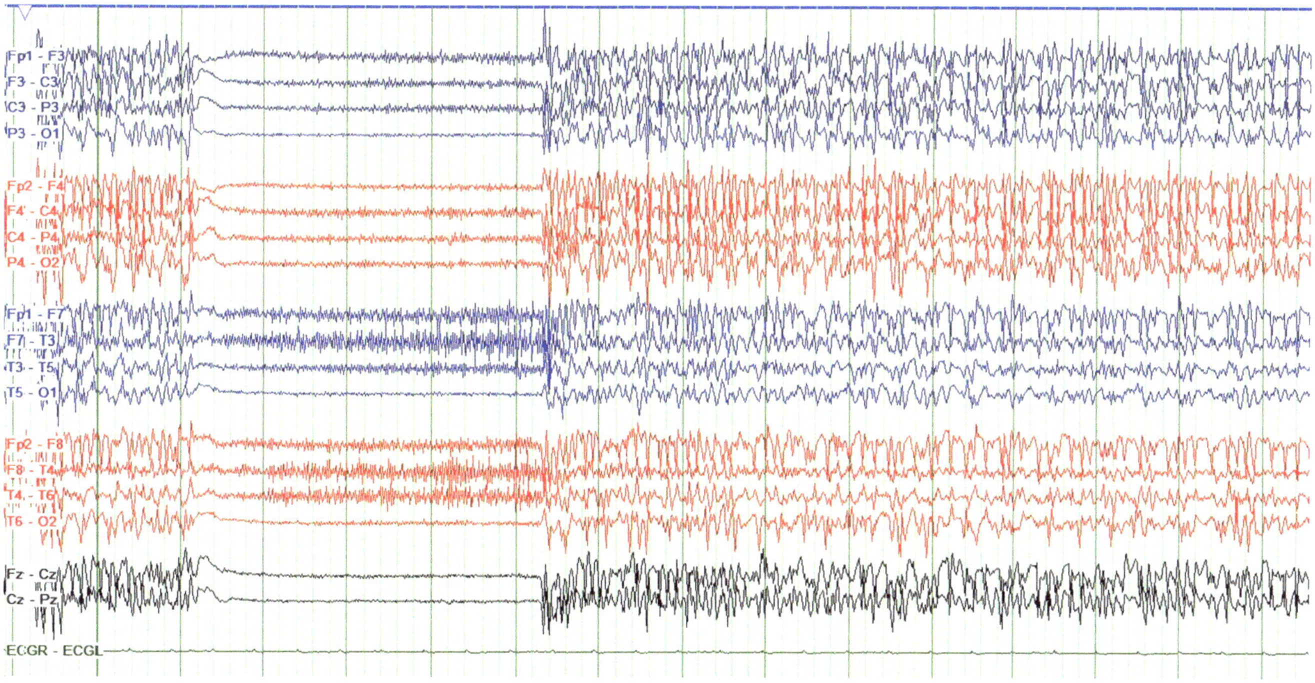

Fig. 6.3 65-year-old woman who presented to the intensive care unit after cardiac arrest. Bipolar montage EEG shows 6–8 Hz bifrontally predominant GPDs with superimposed faster frequencies intermixed with brief periods of suppression lasting 2–4 s without any clinical manifestations. EEG findings are consistent with NCSE

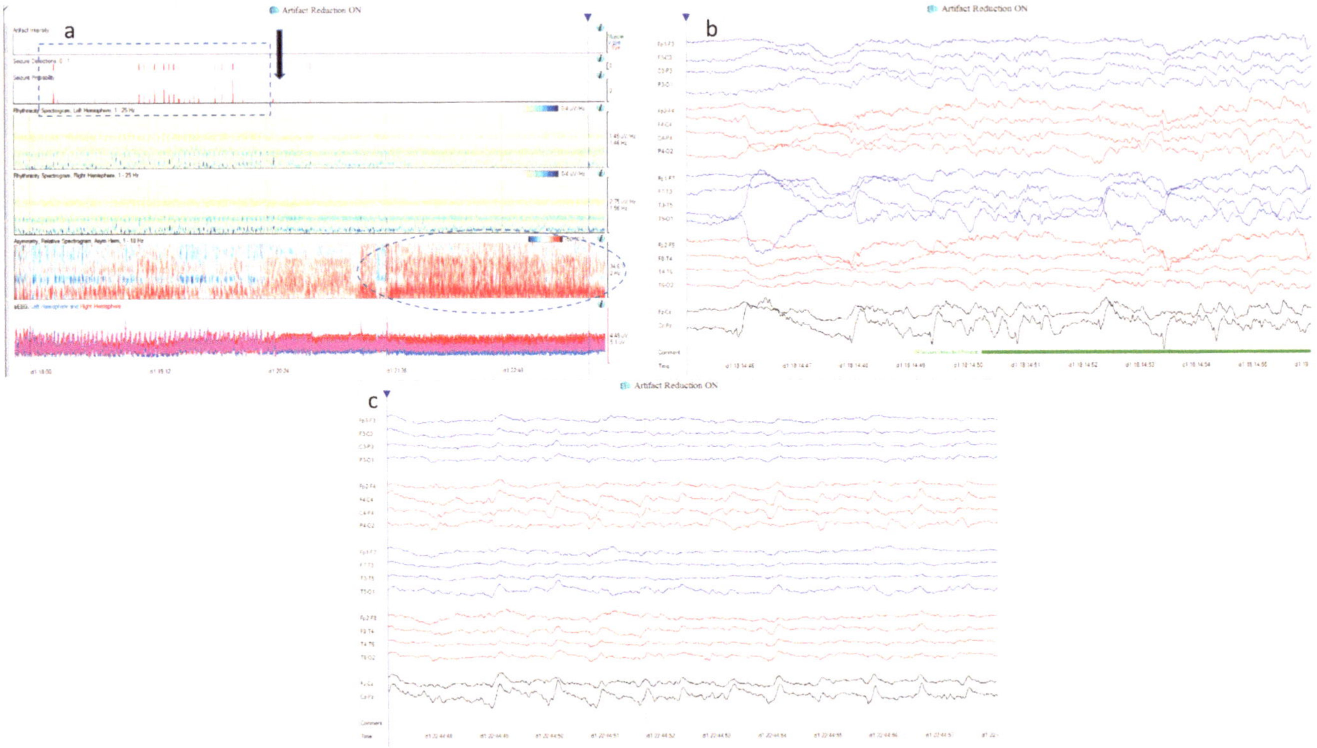

Fig. 6.4 66-year-old male with history of hepatic transplant who presented to the intensive care unit with altered mental status associated with left hand and shoulder clonic movements. (**a**) The seizure detection and probability are shown in a 6-h period of qEEG monitoring showing multiple seizures (12 detections) during the first half of the epoch with improvement after intravenous lacosamide administration (arrow). (**b**) Bipolar montage EEG showing mesial electrodes (Cz-Pz) rhythmic spike and slow wave increasing in frequency rapidly propagating to the frontal regions with superimposed fast frequencies. Seizures correspond to the dashed box shown in Fig. 6.4a. (**c**) Right mesial frontal 0.5–1 Hz lateralized periodic discharges emerging after seizure control. LPDs correspond to the dashed oval shown in Fig. 6.4a. Note the increased red color indicating increased amplitude in the right hemisphere

An important and useful advancement in EEG monitoring has been the development of quantitative EEG (qEEG), which allows for compression of massive amounts of raw data generated by prolonged EEG, thus enabling rapid interpretation. For example, several hours of prolonged EEG can be condensed into a single screen of time–frequency values using a compressed spectral display (Fig. 6.4). Additionally, qEEG may be used by bedside providers (residents, nurses, advance care providers) to quantify seizure burden using the qEEG trend. However, untrained providers may show a high false-positive rate [38].

Challenging EEG Patterns

Although the purpose of this review precludes EEG interpretation, it is essential to highlight some challenging electrographic patterns frequently seen in the ICU to avoid under- or overtreatment. For example, distinguishing generalized patterns with and without a triphasic wave (TW) morphology and the approach to managing these patterns can be challenging [39]. Neurologists are familiar with the non-ictal nature of TWs typically associated with metabolic encephalopathy (hepatic or renal failure, hypoglycemia), drug-induced neurotoxicity (cefepime, baclofen, pregabalin neurotoxicity), and sepsis, among others. See Fig. 6.5. However, seizures can occur in 25% of patients with GPDs with a TW morphology, particularly if EEG focality, interburst suppression, and a history of epilepsy and/or abnormal neuroimaging are present [40, 41]. Studies have demonstrated that TWs have a wide range (kappa = 0.33–0.67) of interrater agreement among proficient electroencephalographers [40–42], thus highlighting the need for better electrographic diagnostic criteria. When present, clinicians should approach TWs in a systematic and dynamic manner with the consultation of the electroencephalographers [43].

The "ictal–interictal continuum (IIC)" represents a "possible" NCS or electrographic SE. The use of this term is still a subject of debate among expert neurophysiologists. It only applies to EEG and does not imply a clinical diagnosis. IIC exemplifies any periodic, spike-wave, or rhythmic delta activity pattern that does not fit into the electrographic seizure or NCSE definition criteria, and there is reasonable chance that it may be conducive to the patient's impaired awareness [44]. (Fig. 6.6).

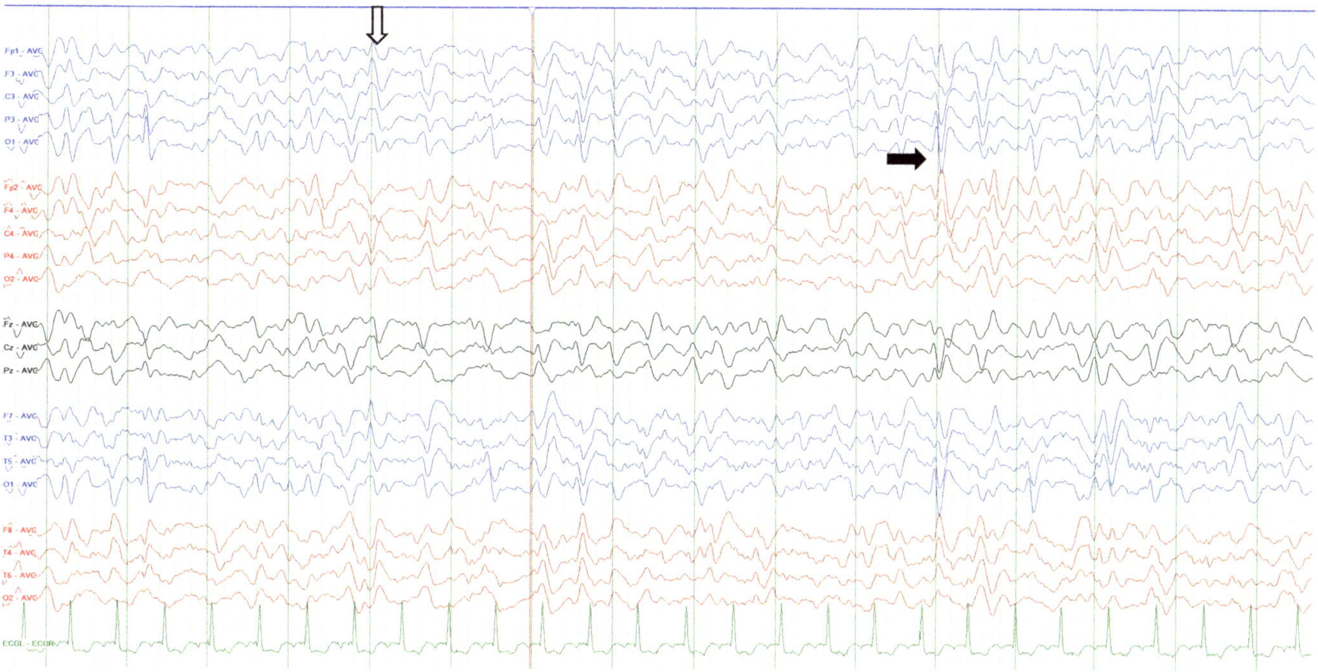

Fig. 6.5 EEG showing triphasic waves. Note the anteriorly predominant blunted discharge with an anterior-to-posterior lag (hollow arrow) and the posteriorly predominant discharge with a posterior-to-anterior lag (solid arrow)

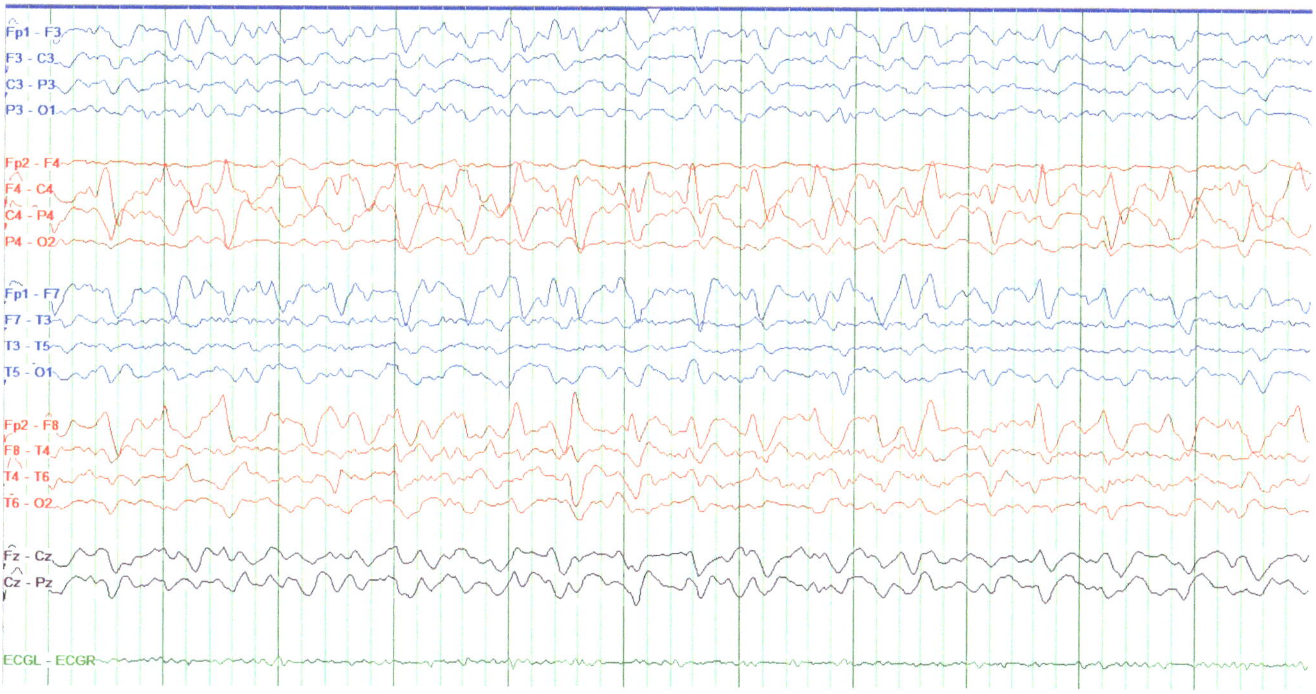

Fig. 6.6 61-year-old male with recent resection of right frontal renal cell carcinoma metastatic lesion who presented to the intensive care unit with altered mental status. Bipolar montage EEG shows right frontocentral 1.5–2 Hz LPDs not meeting criteria for NCS or NCSE, but there a reasonable chance that may be contributing the patient's clinical presentation

When facing a challenging EEG pattern, the analysis should be followed by attempting an ASM or benzodiazepine trial. The trial should be performed in a controlled environment monitoring EEG, blood pressure, oximetry, electrocardiogram, and respiratory status. Sequential small doses of a short-acting drug (e.g., midazolam) are administered to assess for changes on both EEG and clinical improvement. The trial is considered a diagnosis of a NCS or NCSE if there is simultaneous EEG and clinical improvement [45]. In clinical practice, we observe that patients with ictal EEG findings usually require a higher dosage of medications to resolve the pattern. Clinical improvement, although frequently reported, is not commonly seen in clinical practice. More importantly, clinicians should keep in mind when interpreting the trial that lack of improvement or slow improvement can be encountered in both metabolic processes and NCS or NCSE and that both conditions may exist concomitantly [46].

Seizure Etiology

Subarachnoid Hemorrhage (SAH)

Subarachnoid hemorrhage (SAH) is commonly treated in the neuroscience ICU and can occur in the setting of traumatic brain injury or in association with cavernoma, arteriovenous malformation rupture, or aneurysmal subarachnoid hemorrhage (aSAH) [47]. Blood products in proximity to the cortex can act as an irritant and decrease the seizure threshold. NCS and NCSE can occur in 15% and 11%, respectively [48]. Risk factors for the development of seizures in patients with aSAH include intraparenchymal hemorrhage, middle cerebral artery aneurysm, acute hydrocephalus, rebleeding, and thickness of aSAH clot [49]. In patients undergoing aneurysm repair, endovascular coiling was associated with a decreased risk of seizures compared to open craniotomy for clipping [50]. Interestingly, brain injury not only occurs primarily due to the SAH itself but a higher seizure burden is also associated with worse functional and cognitive outcome at 3 months after SAH, thus highlighting the significance of rapid seizure control [51]. In clinical practice, the use of prophylactic ASMs in SAH patients without evidence of clinical or electrographic seizures is commonly seen [52]. The Neurocritical Care Society guidelines recommend a short course (3–7 days) in case prophylaxis is needed [53]. Phenytoin was initially used, but, after the approval of levetiracetam more than two decades ago, clinicians favor the use of levetiracetam over phenytoin due to its good bioavailability, no known drug interactions, lack of level monitoring, and a superior pharmacodynamic and pharmacokinetic profile [54]. However, the current American Stroke Association and American Heart Association guidelines do not recommend the use of prophylactic ASMs [55]. In our practice, we do a short course of ASMs until the aneurysm is secured to avoid the risk of rebleeding if patients have seizures. More recently, Zafar et al. have found that continuing ASMs in patients with aSAH with EEG abnormalities does not improve functional outcomes [56].

Stroke

Acute seizures present a substantial complication in patients with ischemic or hemorrhagic strokes and are associated with prolonged hospitalization and increased morbidity and mortality [57]. Poststroke seizures have been classified into acute and late seizures, with an arbitrarily defined cutoff of 1–2 weeks. Hemorrhagic stroke, stroke severity, and alcohol use are the predisposing factors for acute seizures, whereas cortical involvement and stroke severity are the risk factors for late seizures [58]. Poststroke seizures are more commonly seen in patients with hemorrhagic lesions compared to those with ischemic lesions in 28–30% and 6–10%, respectively [59, 60]. A recent meta-analysis has identified that the incidence of SE was approximately 7 per 1000 strokes, with NCSE being more common [61]. The use of prophylactic ASMs in patients with either ischemic or hemorrhagic stroke is not recommended [62, 63].

Traumatic Brain Injury

Post-traumatic seizures (PTSs) can be a serious complication of moderate-to-severe traumatic brain injury (TBI) with increased mortality in the first days and weeks following trauma [64]. NCSs have been identified in up to 22% of patients after TBI [65]. Early metabolic and neurochemical imbalances seen after acute TBI have been implicated in patient outcomes and are usually coupled with abnormalities seen on EEG [66]. These include an increase in extracellular glutamate and lactate and decreased glucose concentration. Concomitantly, neurons exhibit an increase in the depolarization rate in the setting of altered neurotransmitters, which may spiral into increased metabolic requirements, raised intracranial pressure, cerebral hypoxia, and, ultimately, seizures [67, 68]. The risk factors for PTS include penetrating brain injuries, chronic alcohol use, intracerebral hemorrhage, Glasgow Coma Scale <10, loss of awareness, and younger age [69]. According to the most recent brain trauma foundation guidelines, phenytoin has been recommended for prophylaxis during the first 7 days after TBI [70]. Given levetiracetam's favorable safety profile, it is an alternative to prophylaxis. However, there is not enough evidence to support its use over phenytoin [70]. In our practice, we use levetiracetam for the first 7 days after injury and discontinue prophylaxis after 7 days if there is no evidence of seizures.

Intracranial Tumors

Seizures can occur in cancer patients due to chemotherapy-induced toxicity (e.g., chimeric antigen receptor (CAR) T cells, cisplatin, busulfan, ifosfamide, intrathecal chemotherapy, methotrexate, vincristine, etc.), parenchymal brain lesions, cerebrovascular events, CNS infections, toxic metabolic derangements, and paraneoplastic syndromes [71–74]. Although the frequency is poorly defined, seizures can occur in approximately 13% of all patients with malignancy [75, 76] and in up to 51% of patients with intracranial tumors [77], representing approximately 7% of all causes of adult SE [10]. The risk increases depending on the tumor location with increased epileptogenicity of the frontal, temporal, and insular lobe lesions and with leptomeningeal involvement [78]. Additionally, seizures are more likely to occur in primary brain, low-grade, and dysembryoplastic neuroepithelial tumors [79]. Prophylactic ASMs are not recommended in patients with newly diagnosed primary or metastatic brain lesions [80].

Metabolic Disorders

Sodium Abnormalities

Sodium concentration abnormalities are frequently seen in the inpatient setting affecting approximately 50% of patients, making it the most common electrolyte disturbance in the neurological ICU [81]. Diagnoses associated with hyponatremia include SAH (34%), TBI, brain tumors, meningitis (up to 30%), acute inflammatory demyelinating polyradiculopathy (30%), and neurosurgical procedures [82–84]. Hyponatremia is defined as sodium concentration < 135 mEq/L (more specifically, mild 130–134 mEq/L, moderate 120–129 mEq/L, and severe hyponatremia <120 mEq/L). Clinical signs and symptoms include headaches, depressed level of awareness, vomiting, respiratory depression, seizures, coma, and/or death. These symptoms are more common with acute changes in sodium levels [84]. More importantly, a low serum sodium level may worsen cerebral edema with grave complications. Common causes of hyponatremia include cerebral salt wasting syndrome, gastrointestinal losses, excessive sweating, iatrogenic causes (insufficient volume, use of hypotonic solutions), syndrome of inappropriate secretion of antidiuretic hormone, adrenal insufficiency, hypothyroidism, acute renal failure, and cirrhosis, amongst others [84].

Clinical management should be individualized depending on symptom severity and whether the condition is acute or chronic. Water restriction, furosemide, and hypertonic saline (NaCl 3%) are commonly used in the treatment of hyponatremia depending on the etiology. Rapid correction may induce central pontine or extrapontine myelinolysis. It is recommended not to correct more than 8–12 mmol/L over a 24-h period [85].

Glucose Abnormalities

Extreme glucose variations are associated with an increased risk of seizures, namely, hypoglycemia and nonketotic hyperglycemia, rarely in ketotic hyperglycemia (possibly due to the ketone's protective effects against seizures) [86]. In nonketotic hyperglycemia, seizures can occur in approximately 25% of patients, with approximately 6% presenting as repetitive focal motor seizures or epilepsia partialis continua (EPC) [87].

Calcium Abnormalities

Calcium is an essential mineral for nerve conduction activity, muscle contraction, and bone mineralization. Normal calcium concentration ranges from 8.5 to 10.5 mg/dL. Hypocalcemia is defined as an ionized calcium concentration < 4.0 mg/dL or a plasma calcium level < 8.5 mg/dL. Hypocalcemic disorders are relatively common in clinical practice. Common causes include vitamin D deficiency, parathyroid hormone deficiency, drug-induced complications (bisphosphonates), etc. Symptoms include neuromuscular hyperexcitability, tetany, seizures, and altered mental status, amongst others. Convulsive seizures and focal motor seizures may occur in 20–25% of patients with acute hypocalcemia [88, 89]. Cases of NCSE have been reported as well [90]. Hypocalcemic seizures are treated by prompt calcium replacement. Hyperphosphatemia (>4.5 mg/dL or > 1.46 mmol/L) is commonly seen in hypocalcemia with symptomatology frequently associated with the latter. Frequent causes include renal failure, hypoparathyroidism, and tumor lysis syndrome. Treatment is aimed at restriction of phosphate intake and administration of phosphate-binding antacids, such as calcium carbonate [91].

Hypercalcemia is defined as a calcium level > 10.5 mg/dL and is characterized by gastrointestinal symptoms (e.g., nausea, vomiting, constipation) and disorders of awareness ranging from lethargy to confusion and, in rare case, coma. This disorder usually produces decreased neuronal membrane excitability; hence, seizures rarely occur [92].

Magnesium Abnormalities

Hypomagnesemia (defined as serum magnesium levels <1.5 mEq/L) can be caused by overuse of drugs such as laxatives, loop diuretics, aminoglycosides, or cisplatin, among others. Symptomatic hypomagnesemia is usually seen at levels <1.2 mg/dL and may be characterized by cardiac arrhythmias, neuromuscular irritability, and CNS hyperexcitability. Patients may present with irritability, confusion, hallucinations, or movement disorders (chorea, myoclonus). Convulsive seizures typically occur at levels of <1 mEq/L [88]. Acute symptomatic seizures are treated with 1–2 g of magnesium sulfate over a 5–15-min period, followed by 1–2 g per hour until normal serum levels are reached.

Approximately 10% of patients with eclampsia will continue to experience repetitive seizures if left untreated [93]. Magnesium sulfate is the drug of choice used in the prevention of recurrent seizures [94]. Administration consists of a loading dose of magnesium sulfate of 4–6 g intravenously administered over 15 min, followed by a maintenance dose of 1–3 g per hour [94]. Caution should be exercised in patients with renal failure.

Hypermagnesemia (defined as serum magnesium levels >2.2 mEq/L) is usually seen in the setting of accidental overdose of magnesium-containing drugs (i.e., Epsom salts, magnesium citrate). High levels are characterized by electrocardiographic changes, confusion, lethargy, respiratory depression, and coma. Increased levels are rarely associated with the development of symptomatic seizures [92, 95].

Renal Failure

Seizures and coma are common complications of uremic encephalopathy seen in renal failure. This is typically reflected as an increase in serum creatinine and blood urea nitrogen (BUN), although the laboratory findings can often lag behind clinical manifestations. "Toxic metabolic encephalopathy," a term used broadly by neurologists to denote a nonspecific encephalopathic process, is the result of direct neuronal injury or transmission. Cytotoxic injury can be a consequence of exogenous and/or endogenous drugs or toxins that result from inadequate removal of waste by the kidneys, resulting in altered excitatory–inhibitory neurotransmitters and/or cerebral edema [96]. Patients with uremic toxic metabolic encephalopathy exhibit a wide variety of symptoms, including cognitive decline, behavioral changes, somnolence, obtundation, seizures, coma, and movement disorders such as myoclonus.

Patients requiring dialysis may experience dialysis disequilibrium syndrome, typically caused by rapid removal of urea during the procedure, causing cerebral edema. Symptoms include agitation, disorientation, headaches, asterixis, confusion, seizures, coma, and death. This complication can be reduced if dialysis is performed slowly via continuous veno-venous hemofiltration (CVVH), especially in patients with acute brain injury [97].

Hepatic Failure

Chronic hepatic dysfunction is notoriously known to be related to a myriad of neurological symptoms such as asterixis (i.e., negative myoclonus), movement disorders (chorea), hepatic encephalopathy, confusion, and coma. Hepatic failure has been identified as a risk factor for the development of seizures and/or SE [98, 99] occurring in up to 30% of patients [100]. Interestingly, in a large population-based cohort, liver cirrhosis has been associated with a higher risk of developing SE [98]. Acute seizures might be related to cerebral edema and/or toxic metabolic derangements. Treatment should be focused on addressing the underlying cause of hepatic dysfunction, the use of lactulose, incorporating a low-protein diet, and employing ASMs not metabolized by the liver such as levetiracetam, gabapentin, pregabalin, topiramate, and lacosamide (dose adjustment may be necessary). and status epilepticus in older patients with liver disease. Epilepsia.

2018;59:1392–7.

Alcohol and Other Drug-Induced Seizures

Alcohol-related seizures may occur in up to 10% of patients experiencing alcohol withdrawal, usually described as generalized tonic-clonic seizures occurring 6–48 h after the last alcoholic intake, with approximately 60% chance of experiencing further withdrawal seizures if left untreated [101]. Seizures may occur without any preceding typical symptoms of alcohol withdrawal (tachycardia, agitation, hallucinations, etc.). SE may occur in up to 13% of patients with alcohol withdrawal seizures. Fortunately, these seizures frequently respond to benzodiazepines with good efficacy and tolerability [101, 102].

Seizures may occur in up to 8% of patients that present to the emergency room with acute cocaine intoxication [103]. They can occur immediately after its use without any signs of toxicity. Cocaine acts by blocking dopamine transporters, inhibiting the reuptake of serotonin and norepinephrine, and suppressing GABA inhibition, thus ultimately reducing the seizure threshold [104]. The treatment of choice includes intravenous benzodiazepines to prevent neurological complications; beta-blockers, nitrates, and phentolamine are typically used to counter cardiovascular symptoms. However, caution should be exercised when using beta-blockers in patients with acute cocaine intoxication due to the theoretical concerns of coronary artery vasoconstriction and systemic hypertension, resulting from unopposed alpha-adrenergic stimulation. There is evidence suggesting that mixed alpha/beta-blockers, such as labetalol and carvedilol, may be effective and safe for clinical use [105, 106].

Methamphetamine is a commonly used drug comparable to cocaine. This drug also acts as a sympathomimetic agent, leading to increases in blood pressure, further increasing the risk of myocardial infarction and stroke, especially hemorrhagic strokes [107]. Seizures related to methamphetamines usually occur within hours of use, complemented by other symptoms such as agitation, hypertension, fever, and autonomic instability [104]. Treatment of methamphetamine-induced seizures is similar to that of cocaine-induced seizures. Comorbid polysubstance use and alcohol should always be assessed in patients with suspected drug overdose, as these may also contribute to lowering the seizure threshold. Additional medications associated with lowering the seizure threshold can be seen in Table 6.2 [108, 109].

Table 6.2 Drugs Associated With Lowering the Seizure Threshold

Class	Medications
Antibiotics	Cephalosporins Carbapenems Penicillins Fluoroquinolones Isoniazid
Psychotropics	Bupropion Clozapine Tricyclic antidepressants Venlafaxine Lithium
Analgesics	Meperidine Tramadol
Stimulants	Cocaine Amphetamines Methylphenidate
Withdrawal	Alcohol Benzodiazepines Baclofen Opioids Gabapentin
Miscellaneous	Local anesthetics (lidocaine) Theophylline Organophosphates

Central Nervous System Infections and Sepsis

Infectious meningitis, meningoencephalitis, and/or abscesses can be caused by different organisms, including bacteria, viruses, parasites, and fungi. Common neurological manifestations include encephalopathy, focal neurological signs, venous sinus thrombosis, hydrocephalus, cranial neuropathies, cerebrovascular accidents, and seizures. Patients presenting with fever and neck stiffness should be screened for CNS infections. Acute meningitis and encephalitis are important causes of SE found in approximately 1–3% of patients with 32% mortality [10, 110].

Sepsis is commonly seen across all different types of ICUs. Although the mechanism in which sepsis can induce encephalopathy or reduce the seizure threshold is still not fully understood, it is suspected that this condition may disrupt the blood–brain barrier, damage cerebral endothelial cells, induce cytokine storm, and increase excitatory neurotransmitters [111]. In a retrospective study of 201 patients admitted to the medical ICU who underwent continuous EEG, sepsis was the primary diagnosis in 60% of the cases, followed by metabolic dysfunction (19%), intoxication (11%), and other medical conditions (10%). Sepsis was the only variable found to be associated with the occurrence of seizures of periodic discharges in approximately 32% of patients [112].

Since the arrival of SARS-CoV-2 in late 2019, a growing number of neurological syndromes have been reported, including headaches, myelitis, anosmia, cerebrovascular disease, neuropathy, encephalopathy, and myositis, amongst others [113]. More recently, seizures have been linked to acute SARS-CoV-2 infection, although a direct association has not been demonstrated. Acute symptomatic seizures may be secondary to the direct neurotropic effect of the virus, microvascular ischemia, and/or hypercoagulable state [114]. Additionally, viral infection stimulates pro-inflammatory cytokines such as interleukin-6, interleukin-8, and monocyte chemoattractant protein-1 (MCP-1), thus promoting alteration and breakdown of the blood–brain barrier and cortical irritation [115]. A recent epidemiological study has shown that SE incidence during the pandemic did not differ from the general SE incidence compared to prior years [116]. These data could be underestimated due to the highly contagious nature of the virus limiting EEG access and other diagnostic tests to encephalopathic patients. The treatment of acute symptomatic seizures in patients with SARS-CoV-2 should follow the current recommendations for the management of seizures and status epilepticus.

Unknown Etiology of Seizures

Cryptogenic causes of SE may be encountered in approximately 15–20% of cases, which may lead to delays in treating the underlying cause [117]. Such patients may fall under the umbrella of new-onset refractory status epilepticus (NORSE) or febrile infection-related epilepsy syndrome (FIRES). NORSE is a clinical presentation rather than a diagnosis seen in patients without a history of epileptic seizures or other neurological disorders, presenting with RSE without an inciting event [118]. The culprit is usually attributed to autoimmune encephalitis (paraneoplastic or non-paraneoplastic) seen in up to 37% of cases [119, 120] or viral causes (Epstein–Barr, enterovirus, herpes simplex virus 6 and 7, etc.) [117, 121], usually less commonly seen [120]. If there is no apparent cause, it is then considered cryptogenic NORSE [120]. FIRES is a subcategory of NORSE, characterized by fever starting between 1 and 14 days prior to the onset of RSE, with or without fever at the onset of SE [122]. These two entities are usually regarded as different conditions, with FIRES requiring fever for its diagnosis, mostly affecting male children, and NORSE being devoid of fever in up to 30% of patients, mostly affecting adult women [120, 123]. Prodromal symptoms may precede the onset of NORSE in 60% of affected patients, including memory loss, behavioral and cognitive changes, fatigue, headaches, and confusion [124]. However, they both affect patients without a prior history of seizures with nonspecific laboratory and pathological findings to indicate a different pathophysiological process with increased morbidity and mortality. In terms of treatment, there is no specific therapy or randomized controlled trials for either cryptogenic NORSE or FIRES. An abnormal inflammatory response has been postulated as the underlying pathophysiological process [119], proposing the use of immunosuppressive agents for its treatment. Unfortunately, there are no randomized controlled trials or specific therapies for the treatment of cryptogenic NORSE or FIRES, and standard ASMs or anesthetics may not be sufficient [122]. Intravenous steroids, intravenous immunoglobulins, and plasma exchange are typically used early in the disease course [123, 125]. If there is no clinical improvement, drugs such as rituximab and cyclophosphamide are administered as steroid-sparing agents. More recently, anakinra and tocilizumab have gained attention as potential specific therapies [124]. Table 6.3 includes common dosing or administration of immunosuppressive therapies utilized for cryptogenic SE.

Seizures and Organ Transplantation

Neurological complications may be seen in 10–30% of patients undergoing organ transplantation during their hospitalization, including encephalopathy, cerebrovascular accidents, infection, and seizures, among others [126]. Neurological complications are also related to the type of organ transplanted and postoperative complications. Additionally, neurotoxicity (headaches, paresthesia, tremors, seizures) is commonly seen in association with the use of immunosuppressive agents such as tacrolimus and cyclosporine [127]. Seizures occur in approximately 5–10% of patients undergoing organ transplant, often described as generalized tonic-clonic, typically occurring in the acute postoperative period [128]. The risk is increased in immunosuppressant toxicity, electrolyte disturbances, cerebral infections, and ischemic and/or hemorrhagic lesions [129]. Seizure management in this patient population can be challenging given the altered pharmacokinetic profile. Caution should be exercised when using phenytoin due to its pharmacodynamic properties, including high protein affinity, enzyme-inducing capability, and drug–drug interactions with antibiotics and immunosuppressants, especially in liver transplant recipients. Newer ASMs such as lacosamide and levetiracetam have been increasingly used due to decreased hepatic metabolism and lack of drug–drug interactions.

Table 6.3 Immunosuppressive agents used in cryptogenic Status Epilepticus

First Line	IVMP 1000 mg in 3–5 days. May be followed by oral prednisone 1 mg/kg daily
	IVIG 1 g/kg in 3–5 days
	Plasma exchange 3–5 sessions in alternate days
Second Line	Rituximab 375 mg/m^2 weekly, up to 4 doses
	Cyclophosphamide 500–1000 mg/m^2 monthly
	Anakinra 5 mg/kg twice daily
	Tocilizumab 4–8 mg/kg

IVMP intravenous methylprednisolone, *IVIV* intravenous immunoglobulin

Status Epilepticus, Refractory, and Super-Refractory Status Epilepticus

As previously described, RSE is defined as continuous seizure activity not controlled after first- and second-line ASMs [6], whereas SRSE is defined as continuous seizure activity not controlled after anesthetics [7]. Approximately 10–15% of in-hospital SE patients will progress to SRSE at some point [130]. Risk factors for the development of RSE include an altered level of consciousness, new-onset SE, focal motor seizures, and NCSE at onset [9, 131]. The management of SRSE not only involves seizure control but also managing and preventing long-term complications from prolonged sedation and mechanical ventilation [132]. Some complications of RSE include prolonged immobility (risk of pulmonary embolism), immunosuppression, sepsis, ileus, polypharmacy and drug–drug interactions, pressure ulcers, etc. Although the literature has clearly defined the importance of prompt treatment of status epilepticus, the degree of electrographic suppression (seizure suppression, burst suppression, or complete suppression [isoelectric background]) is still unclear when treating RSE [133, 134]. A meta-analysis of 193 patients with RSE treated with midazolam, propofol, or pentobarbital found that approximately 50% of patients died, concluding that compared to seizure suppression, background suppression was associated with decreased seizure activity at the cost of hypotension with no improvement in mortality [135]. A retrospective study of 107 patients with SE found that outcomes were independent of the specific coma-inducing agents used and the extent of EEG burst suppression, suggesting that the underlying cause represents its main determinant [136]. Another retrospective analysis of 63 consecutive episodes of non-anoxic RSE found that seizure suppression when compared to EEG suppression (burst suppression or isoelectric background) was associated with better functional outcome, and, similar to prior studies, mortality is independent of the choice of the anesthetic agent, the type of SE, and history of epilepsy [137]. Maintaining electrographic suppression or seizure control for 24–48 h, followed by gradual withdrawal of anesthetics, is recommended [138]. Some patients may have recurrent seizures, requiring higher doses of anesthetics for an additional period. Interestingly, a retrospective observational study of 182 patients diagnosed with RSE analyzed the relationship between the duration of therapeutic coma and outcome. The study found that a longer duration of therapeutic coma (>35 h) was independently associated with increased chances of seizure recurrence when attempting to wean off anesthetics but not with functional neurological outcome, in-hospital complications, or mortality. Additionally, higher doses of anesthetics (deeper sedation) were independently associated with fewer in-hospital complications and a short duration of mechanical ventilation, thus suggesting that a shorter duration of therapeutic coma in combination with deeper sedation may be more effective than the currently recommended guidelines of 24–48 h [139].

Status Epilepticus Outcome and Prognosis

Several scores have been developed to prognosticate outcomes in status epilepticus. The Status Epilepticus Severity Score (STESS) is based on age, seizure type, level of consciousness, and history of seizures [140]. The Epidemiology-Based Mortality Score in Status Epilepticus (EMSE) is based on retrospective epidemiological data from factors that have been shown to be predictive of mortality, including age, comorbidities, and EEG findings [141]. The END-IT score (encephalitis, NCSE, diazepam resistance, imaging abnormalities, tracheal intubation) is also an outcome prediction score assigning points to the variables listed [142].

The overall mortality for SE and RSE is approximately 20% and 30–40%, respectively [9, 10, 131, 136, 137, 143]. For SRSE mortality, it is approximately 40–50% [8, 144, 145]. Many variables have been identified as important determinants of poor outcome and mortality such as sex, age, ethnicity, etiology, EEG characteristics, level of consciousness, semiology, and duration. Of these, age, nonconvulsive semiology, prolonged duration of SE, and etiology are among the most important determinants of outcome.

Advanced age (>60 years of age) is an independent factor of death in SE [146]. As such, it has been incorporated in EMSE and STESS. Younger age, however, has been associated with more refractory cases [147].

Seizure etiology is the main outcome determinant, also incorporated in STESS and EMSE scores. In patients with acute hypoxic/anoxic brain injury (e.g., a cardiac arrest) and acute stroke, the prognosis is poor, with increased mortality rates of 50–70% and 33%, respectively [10]. Both are associated with poor functional recovery. In contrast, low ASM levels and alcohol abuse show a more favorable outcome with <10% mortality [148]. TBI is also associated with a more favorable outcome in terms of seizure control [149]. Comorbidities such as pneumonia, sepsis, renal and hepatic failure, valvular heart disease, sodium abnormalities, diabetes mellitus, and extracranial malignancies are usually associated with worse outcomes [150].

Impaired level of consciousness at SE onset is an independent factor of death in SE. In patients presenting with somnolence, stupor, and/or coma, mortality is 33%, compared to 8.2% in patients that are fully awake or awake with reduced cognition [146]. Regarding semiology, prominent motor phenomena are associated with a more favorable outcome compared to worse outcome in NCSE. For example, the case fatality rates for NCSE, nonconvulsive semiology at the end of the semiology sequence, nonconvulsive semiology at the beginning of the sequence, and nonconvulsive semiology at all (only motor phenomena) were 27.6%, 25.6%, 10%, and 3.5%, respectively [146]. Post-arrest myoclonic SE has been associated with poor outcome and increased mortality [151]. However, good outcomes have been reported in selected cases in this patient population [152, 153].

A longer duration of SE has been associated with increased mortality, although it is challenging to identify the onset of SE in some cases [154, 155]. It is important to note that NORSE is associated with prolonged and persistent seizures and many patients may show significant neurological recovery after sustained SE when the culprit is identified and treated accordingly [156].

Certain electrographic findings may aid in prognostication. However, these findings are less substantial than the etiology and duration of SE. The occurrence of burst suppression (excluding sedation) after SE ictal discharges and periodic discharges have been associated with increased mortality. Additionally, EEG reactivity after SE is associated with good outcome [157–159]. In all cases, the management of SE should be treated vigorously following the patient's clinical and electrographic data [160], and treatment should not be stopped unless there is a clear devastating condition.

Pharmacological Treatment

Status epilepticus treatment should be initiated quickly while carefully maximizing therapy to achieve seizure cessation and limiting the adverse effects associated with antiseizure medications (ASMs). A tiered approach has commonly been recommended with different medications being utilized in early, refractory, and super-refractory status epilepticus.

Emergent Initial Therapy

Initial management of status epilepticus with aggressive benzodiazepine therapy is considered the standard of care [138]. Large, prospective, randomized trials comparing benzodiazepines with other ASMs have consistently found intravenous lorazepam to be efficacious for early-status epilepticus [23, 161, 162]. Although intravenous diazepam may also be considered, lorazepam is typically preferred due to its longer duration of the antiepileptic effect. In the setting of status epilepticus without intravenous access, intramuscular midazolam appears to be equally as effective as intravenous lorazepam therapy [162]. When administredred intramuscularly, midazolam is rapidly absorbed into systemic circulation where it can exert its pharmacological effect and may avoid the delay associated with obtaining intravenous access [162, 163]. Additional routes of administration for benzodiazepines for the acute management of status epilepticus include intranasal midazolam and rectal diazepam, with both having an onset of action within 10 min.

The recommended dose for intravenous lorazepam for the cessation of seizure activity is 0.1 mg/kg (with a maximum single dose of 4 mg). A second dose of adequately dosed benzodiazepine therapy may be repeated 5 min following the initial dose. Intramuscular and intranasal midazolam are commonly dosed at 10 mg for patients weighing >40 kg, whereas rectal diazepam is dosed at 0.2 mg/kg (with a maximum single dose of 20 mg) [138, 162].

Urgent Control Therapy

Following emergent initial therapy, urgent control therapy should be rapidly administered with the goal to further aid in cessation of seizure activity and maintain prolonged antiseizure effects. Historically, phenobarbital and phenytoin have been utilized in this setting; however, with significant advancements in ASM therapies since the 1970s, these agents have started to fall out of favor in clinical practice due to their adverse effects and numerous drug interactions.

In 2019, levetiracetam, fosphenytoin, and valproic acid were analyzed in the Established Status Epilepticus Treatment Trial (ESETT) for benzodiazepine-refractory status epilepticus [164]. There was no significant difference in the rates of seizure cessation within 60 min among the three treatment arms, with almost half of all patients responding to the second-line therapy. Intensive care unit admission rates and time to seizure cessation were also similar between groups at approximately 60% and 10 h, respectively. Although fosphenytoin had slightly higher rates of hypotension and endotracheal intubation compared to levetiracetam and valproic acid, the differences were not statistically significant [164].

Levetiracetam

Levetiracetam works by binding to the synaptic vesicle glycoprotein 2A on glutamate-containing vesicles, resulting in decreased neurotransmitter release [165]. For status epilepticus, it is dosed at an initial loading dose of 60 mg/kg up to a maximum of 4.5 g [164]. A therapeutic trough range of 20–40 mcg/mL has been suggested by some; however, with a broad therapeutic window, serum concentrations are not routinely monitored [166]. The most notable adverse effects associated with levetiracetam include CNS depression, somnolence, and psychiatric and behavioral symptoms. While behavioral side effects are more common in children, alternative therapeutic options may be considered in patients with known mood disorders [165].

Fosphenytoin/Phenytoin

Phenytoin works by inhibiting the influx of sodium ions across the cell membrane, thus prolonging its fast inactivated state [165]. Fosphenytoin is the prodrug formulation of phenytoin, which has a lower rate of cardiac adverse effects and infusion reactions when administered intravenously. For status epilepticus, they are most commonly dosed at an initial loading dose of 20 mg phenytoin equivalent/kg [164]. Phenytoin has a narrow therapeutic index with goal total levels of 10–20 mcg/mL and free levels of 1–2 mcg/mL. Total phenytoin levels should be corrected in the setting of hypoalbuminemia given the medication's high protein binding. Additionally, phenytoin exhibits nonlinear or Michaelis–Menten kinetics, meaning that a small increase in dose may result in a large, nonproportional increase in serum levels. Common side effects include cardiac arrhythmias, hypotension, CNS depression, drowsiness, rash, and nystagmus. Phenytoin is also a potent cytochrome inducer that contributes to many drug interactions [165].

Valproic Acid

Valproic acid exerts anticonvulsant effects via multiple pathways, including enhancing GABA and inhibiting sodium channels. It may also work by inhibiting T-type calcium channels and NMDA receptors. For status epilepticus, it is frequently dosed at an initial loading dose of 40 mg/kg up to a maximum of 3 g [164]. Valproic acid requires therapeutic drug monitoring with goal serum concentrations between 50 and 150 mcg/mL, but high protein binding similar to phenytoin free levels may also be monitored [167]. Notable adverse effects of valproic acid include CNS depression, hyperammonemia, hepatotoxicity, pancreatitis, and dose-dependent thrombocytopenia. Valproic acid is a potent cytochrome inhibitor, which may result in supratherapeutic concentrations of concomitant medications metabolized via these pathways [165].

Phenobarbital

Phenobarbital is a $GABA_A$ agonist, which prolongs the opening of the associated chloride channel. F3or status epilepticus, it is dosed at an initial loading dose of 20 mg/kg and the recommended therapeutic range is 20–40 mcg/mL. Phenobarbital's most limiting adverse effects include bradycardia, hypotension, CNS and respiratory depression, and mood changes [165]. It is also formulated with propylene glycol, which carries the additional risk of toxicities such as metabolic acidosis and new-onset renal failure. Like phenytoin, phenobarbital is also a potent cytochrome inducer, resulting in a large number of drug interactions.

Adjunctive ASMs

Lacosamide, topiramate, clobazam, brivaracetam, and perampanel are a few additional ASM options, which may be considered in refractory cases, typically as adjunctive therapy [168, 169]. These newer ASMs tend to have fewer or less severe adverse effects, lower rates of drug interactions, and more favorable pharmacokinetic profiles when compared to older, more traditional ASMs. Unfortunately, there are currently insufficient clinical outcome data associated with these agents for status epilepticus to recommend the use of one over another. Therefore, medication and patient-specific factors often drive adjunctive ASM therapy selection in cases of refractory status epilepticus.

Anesthetic Therapy for RSE and SRSE

Although there are no current, high-quality clinical trials comparing anesthetic therapies for the management of RSE and SRSE, midazolam, propofol, pentobarbital, and ketamine have become the most commonly utilized agents. Based on expert opinion, it is often recommended to achieve 24–48 h of seizure-free activity or therapeutic coma prior to weaning anesthetic therapy for SE [138]. More recent literature, however, has reported a higher risk of seizure recurrence associated with longer durations (>35 h) of therapeutic coma [139]. Therefore, shorter durations of deeper sedation may be beneficial for this patient population. An additional retrospective study assessed the safety and efficacy of early medically induced coma (anesthetics) after first-line (benzodiazepines) treatment instead of using second-line (valproate, levetiracetam, fosphenytoin) medications in 205 patients. This study revealed that early induced coma, or aggressive treatment escalation, was associated with a shorter duration of SE and hospital stay without increasing complications, especially in younger patients presenting with convulsions and more severe SE [170]. More research, ideally in prospective, randomized settings, is needed to determine the most appropriate therapeutic strategies for anesthetic infusions in SE.

Midazolam

Midazolam is a benzodiazepine that works by binding to and potentiating the activity of $GABA_A$ receptors. For refractory status epilepticus, midazolam is dosed as a 0.2 mg/kg intravenous initial bolus and as needed for acute seizure cessation, followed by continuous infusion at a rate of 0.05–2.9 mg/kg/h [138, 171]. Advantages of midazolam include its short half-life and quick onset of action, allowing for easy titration; however, it should be noted that prolonged sedation can occur in the setting of obesity and hepatic or renal impairment due to its high lipophilicity, large proportion of hepatic metabolism, and renal elimination. The most common adverse effects associated with midazolam use in refractory status epilepticus include CNS and respiratory depression, hypotension, and tachyphylaxis [138].

Propofol

Propofol is another potential first-line agent for refractory status epilepticus, which works as a fast-acting anesthetic via GABA potentiation and possible NMDA inhibition [167, 172]. With doses for refractory status epilepticus ranging from 30 to 200 mcg/kg/min, propofol's use for this indication is often limited by its dose-dependent adverse effects [138]. Additionally, due to its extremely rapid onset of action and high risk of adverse cardiovascular events with bolus dosing, loading doses are typically unnecessary and may actually result in unwanted harm. The adverse effects associated with propofol include hypotension, respiratory depression, hypertriglyceridemia, and propofol-related infusion syndrome (PRIS). PRIS often presents as bradycardia, followed by cardiovascular collapse, severe metabolic acidosis, rhabdomyolysis, renal failure, and hepatomegaly, and is associated with extremely high mortality rates [138, 172]. Daily caloric intake should also be adjusted while on high-dose propofol therapy because it is formulated as an intravenous emulsion containing 10% lipid (with 1 mL containing 1.1 kcal [138]. Therefore, dietitian consultation is recommended for patients receiving high-dose propofol therapy in order to optimize nutrition goals.

Ketamine

Ketamine has a unique mechanism of action as an NMDA antagonist in comparison to our other anesthetic therapies, which work via GABA augmentation. With sustained seizure activity, GABA receptor endocytosis and NMDA receptor upregulation occur, thus offering a potential therapeutic advantage for ketamine in refractory status epilepticus [173]. Ketamine is typically dosed as a 1–3 mg/kg intravenous bolus as needed for acute seizure activity cessation, followed by a continuous infusion of 1–10 mg/kg/h [174]. Aside from its mechanism of action, ketamine may also provide a therapeutic advantage with its more favorable adverse effect profile. From a cardiovascular standpoint, it more commonly results in hypertension and tachycardia in comparison to the suppressed cardiovascular effects of alternative anesthetic therapies [172]. Notable side effects of ketamine include cardiac arrhythmias, metabolic acidosis, and an emergence phenomenon upon discontinuation; however, emergence reactions are minimized with the concomitant use of midazolam therapy for status epilepticus. Finally, although the previous literature has reported ketamine use to be linked to increased intracranial pressure, newer evidence has negated this association [175]. In fact, in 11 patients with cerebral multimodal monitoring available, a retrospective study found no significant effect of high doses of ketamine infusion on intracranial pressure, cerebral perfusion pressure, or cerebral blood flow [175].

Pentobarbital

Pentobarbital is a barbiturate that binds to $GABA_A$ receptors enhancing chloride channel opening. It is administered at a loading dose of 5–15 mg/kg followed by a continuous infusion of 0.5–5 mg/kg/h. The main adverse effects associated with pentobarbital use include significant hypotension, cardiac and respiratory depression, paralytic ileus, and metabolic acidosis secondary to its propylene glycol excipient [138]. Withdrawal seizures have also frequently been reported upon weaning therapy. Pentobarbital's use is primarily limited by its noteworthy adverse effect profile and prolonged duration of action; therefore, it is typically reserved for super-refractory status epilepticus uncontrolled by other continuous anesthetics and adjunctive therapies. Pentobarbital also has a half-life of up to 48 h, which can be prolonged when utilized at higher doses or for longer durations, thus making accurate neurological assessments extremely difficult even days after discontinuing therapy.

Non-pharmacological Treatment of Seizures

Certain cases of SE may require non-pharmacological therapies in addition to ASMs. As previously described, immunotherapy should be considered early in cases of NORSE and/or FIRES once infectious or other common causes have been ruled out [176–178]. Neuromodulation techniques include noninvasive transcranial magnetic stimulation [179] and electroconvulsive therapy [180], and invasive techniques such as deep brain stimulation [181] and vagal nerve stimulation [182] have been used in the treatment of SRSE [183]. However, the available neuromodulation knowledge is based on a small number of cases, and some of these publications may be prone to reporting bias.

Hypothermia has been employed after a cardiac arrest, and it has been studied in the treatment of SRSE. A large multicenter study randomized patients to hypothermia (32–34 °C) for 24 h as adjunctive therapy. This intervention was not associated with significantly better 90-day outcomes than standard care alone, and it was associated with other complications such as coagulopathy, infections, hypotension, and paralytic ileus, especially when barbiturates were used concomitantly [184, 185]. Furthermore, seizures can recur in the rewarming period [186]. Resective surgery is a useful option in patients with an identifiable lesion on neuroimaging and concordant scalp EEG ictal onset and semiology [187–189].

Another treatment modality is the use of ketogenic diet (KD) in patients admitted to the ICU [190, 191]. Additionally, KD may be an alternative therapy in patients with NORSE and FIRES [192]. It mimics a fasting state by introducing a high-fat, low-carbohydrate, and low-protein diet. Although the mechanism by which this diet reduces seizure activity is not fully understood, an anti-inflammatory response, ketone-induced metabolic shift toward acidosis reducing neuronal hyperexcitability, glucose restriction, and GABA potentiation, amongst others have been proposed as the possible mechanisms of action [193, 194]. The diet can be administered through a nasogastric tube with the goal of producing ketonuria. Side effects include hypoglycemia, nausea, vomiting, acidosis, and weight loss, amongst others [195].

Conclusions

In patients with an altered level of awareness, the early use of EEG is critical to rule out nonconvulsive seizures. If SE is identified, then prompt treatment with benzodiazepines and ASM therapy should be initiated. If there is no response, then seizures may evolve into RSE or SRSE that requires high doses of anesthetics, which increases the risk of systemic complications. The most important determinant of prognosis remains the underlying cause of SE, with anoxic brain injuries carrying higher risks of mortality and morbidity.

References

1. Park A, et al. EEG utilization in Canadian intensive care units: a multicentre prospective observational study. Seizure. 2016;43:42–7.
2. Sagduyu A, Tarlaci S, Sirin H. Generalized tonic-clonic status epilepticus: causes, treatment, complications and predictors of case fatality. J Neurol. 1998;245(10):640–6.
3. Trinka E, Höfler J, Zerbs A. Causes of status epilepticus. Epilepsia. 2012;53(s4):127–38.
4. Hesdorffer DC, et al. Incidence of status epilepticus in Rochester, Minnesota, 1965-1984. Neurology. 1998;50(3):735–41.
5. Govoni V, et al. Incidence of status epilepticus in southern Europe: a population study in the health district of Ferrara, *Italy*. Eur Neurol. 2008;59(3–4):120–6.

6. Bleck TP. Refractory status epilepticus. Curr Opin Crit Care. 2005;11(2):117–20.
7. Shorvon S, Ferlisi M. The treatment of super-refractory status epilepticus: a critical review of available therapies and a clinical treatment protocol. Brain. 2011;134(Pt 10):2802–18.
8. Delaj L, et al. Refractory and super-refractory status epilepticus in adults: a 9-year cohort study. Acta Neurol Scand. 2017;135(1):92–9.
9. Mayer SA, et al. Refractory status epilepticus: frequency, risk factors, and impact on outcome. Arch Neurol. 2002;59(2):205–10.
10. DeLorenzo RJ, et al. Epidemiology of status epilepticus. J Clin Neurophysiol. 1995;12(4):316–25.
11. Sutter R. Are we prepared to detect subtle and nonconvulsive status epilepticus in critically ill patients? J Clin Neurophysiol. 2016;33(1):25–31.
12. Pandian JD, et al. Digital video-electroencephalographic monitoring in the neurological-neurosurgical intensive care unit: clinical features and outcome. Arch Neurol. 2004;61(7):1090–4.
13. Sutter R, et al. Continuous video-EEG monitoring increases detection rate of nonconvulsive status epilepticus in the ICU. Epilepsia. 2011;52(3):453–7.
14. Claassen J, et al. Detection of electrographic seizures with continuous EEG monitoring in critically ill patients. Neurology. 2004;62(10):1743–8.
15. Wright NMK, et al. Evaluating the utility of rapid response EEG in emergency care. Emerg Med J. 2021;38(12):923–6.
16. Goodkin HP, et al. GABA(a) receptor internalization during seizures. Epilepsia. 2007;48(Suppl 5):109–13.
17. Naylor DE, et al. Rapid surface accumulation of NMDA receptors increases glutamatergic excitation during status epilepticus. Neurobiol Dis. 2013;54:225–38.
18. Jones DM, et al. Characterization of pharmacoresistance to benzodiazepines in the rat Li-pilocarpine model of status epilepticus. Epilepsy Res. 2002;50(3):301–12.
19. Meldrum BS, Horton RW. Physiology of status epilepticus in primates. Arch Neurol. 1973;28(1):1–9.
20. Fisher RS, et al. Epileptic seizures and epilepsy: definitions proposed by the international league against epilepsy (ILAE) and the International Bureau for Epilepsy (IBE). Epilepsia. 2005;46(4):470–2.
21. Trinka E, et al. A definition and classification of status epilepticus--Report of the ILAE Task Force on Classification of Status Epilepticus. Epilepsia. 2015;56(10):1515–23.
22. Trinka E, Kälviäinen R. 25 years of advances in the definition, classification and treatment of status epilepticus. Seizure. 2017;44:65–73.
23. Treiman DM, et al. A comparison of four treatments for generalized convulsive status epilepticus. Veterans affairs status epilepticus cooperative study group. N Engl J Med. 1998;339(12):792–8.
24. DeLorenzo RJ, et al. Persistent nonconvulsive status epilepticus after the control of convulsive status epilepticus. Epilepsia. 1998;39(8):833–40.
25. Kaplan PW. Assessing the outcomes in patients with nonconvulsive status epilepticus: nonconvulsive status epilepticus is underdiagnosed, potentially Overtreated, and confounded by comorbidity. J Clin Neurophysiol. 1999;16(4):341–52.
26. Fernández-Torre JL, et al. Postanoxic alpha, theta or alpha-theta coma: clinical setting and neurological outcome. Resuscitation. 2018;124:118–25.
27. Hirsch LJ, et al. American clinical neurophysiology Society's standardized critical care EEG terminology: 2012 version. J Clin Neurophysiol. 2013;30(1):1–27.
28. Treiman DM, Walton NY, Kendrick C. A progressive sequence of electroencephalographic changes during generalized convulsive status epilepticus. Epilepsy Res. 1990;5(1):49–60.
29. Vespa PM, et al. Early detection of vasospasm after acute subarachnoid hemorrhage using continuous EEG ICU monitoring. Electroencephalogr Clin Neurophysiol. 1997;103(6):607–15.
30. Perera K, et al. EEG patterns and outcomes after hypoxic brain injury: a systematic review and meta-analysis. Neurocrit Care. 2021;36(1):292–301.
31. Kim YJ, et al. Background frequency can enhance the prognostication power of EEG patterns categories in comatose cardiac arrest survivors: a prospective, multicenter, observational cohort study. Crit Care. 2021;25(1):398.
32. Abend NS, et al. Electroencephalographic monitoring in the pediatric intensive care unit. Curr Neurol Neurosci Rep. 2013;13(3):330.
33. Kaplan PW. EEG criteria for nonconvulsive status epilepticus. Epilepsia. 2007;48(Suppl 8):39–41.
34. Beniczky S, et al. Unified EEG terminology and criteria for nonconvulsive status epilepticus. Epilepsia. 2013;54(Suppl 6):28–9.
35. Leitinger M, et al. Salzburg consensus criteria for non-convulsive status epilepticus--approach to clinical application. Epilepsy Behav. 2015;49:158–63.
36. Struck AF, et al. Association of an electroencephalography-based risk score with seizure probability in hospitalized patients. JAMA Neurol. 2017;74(12):1419–24.
37. Moffet EW, et al. Validation of the 2HELPS2B seizure risk score in acute brain injury patients. Neurocrit Care. 2020;33(3):701–7.
38. Alkhachroum A, et al. Quantitative EEG-based seizure estimation in super-refractory status epilepticus. Neurocrit Care. 2021;36(3):897–904.
39. Sutter R, Kaplan PW. Electroencephalographic criteria for nonconvulsive status epilepticus: synopsis and comprehensive survey. Epilepsia. 2012;53(Suppl 3):1–51.
40. Alkhachroum AM, et al. Generalized periodic discharges with and without Triphasic morphology. J Clin Neurophysiol. 2018;35(2):144–50.
41. Foreman B, et al. Generalized periodic discharges and 'triphasic waves': a blinded evaluation of inter-rater agreement and clinical significance. Clin Neurophysiol. 2016;127(2):1073–80.
42. Gaspard N, et al. Interrater agreement for critical care EEG terminology. Epilepsia. 2014;55(9):1366–73.
43. Bicchi MM, Alkhachroum A, Kanner AM. Status Triphasicus versus status epilepticus? J Clin Neurophysiol. 2021;38(5):376–83.
44. Hirsch LJ, et al. American clinical neurophysiology Society's standardized critical care EEG terminology: 2021 version. J Clin Neurophysiol. 2021;38(1):1–29.
45. Friedman D, Claassen J, Hirsch LJ. Continuous electroencephalogram monitoring in the intensive care unit. Anesth Analg. 2009;109(2):506–23.
46. O'Rourke D, et al. Response rates to anticonvulsant trials in patients with Triphasic-wave EEG patterns of uncertain significance. Neurocrit Care. 2016;24(2):233–9.
47. van Gijn J, Kerr RS, Rinkel GJ. Subarachnoid haemorrhage. Lancet. 2007;369(9558):306–18.
48. Claassen J, et al. Prognostic significance of continuous EEG monitoring in patients with poor-grade subarachnoid hemorrhage. Neurocrit Care. 2006;4(2):103–12.
49. Choi KS, et al. Seizures and epilepsy following aneurysmal subarachnoid hemorrhage: incidence and risk factors. J Korean Neurosurg Soc. 2009;46(2):93–8.
50. Molyneux AJ, et al. International subarachnoid aneurysm trial (ISAT) of neurosurgical clipping versus endovascular coiling in 2143 patients with ruptured intracranial aneurysms: a randomised comparison of effects on survival, dependency, seizures, rebleeding, subgroups, and aneurysm occlusion. Lancet. 2005;366(9488):809–17.

51. De Marchis GM, et al. Seizure burden in subarachnoid hemorrhage associated with functional and cognitive outcome. Neurology. 2016;86(3):253–60.
52. Christie C, et al. Effect of newer generation anticonvulsant prophylaxis on seizure incidence after spontaneous intracerebral hemorrhage. World Neurosurg. 2020;141:e461–5.
53. Diringer MN, et al. Critical care management of patients following aneurysmal subarachnoid hemorrhage: recommendations from the Neurocritical care Society's multidisciplinary consensus conference. Neurocrit Care. 2011;15(2):211–40.
54. Kruer RM, et al. Changing trends in the use of seizure prophylaxis after traumatic brain injury: a shift from phenytoin to levetiracetam. J Crit Care. 2013;28(5):883.e9–883.e13.
55. Connolly ES Jr, et al. Guidelines for the management of aneurysmal subarachnoid hemorrhage: a guideline for healthcare professionals from the American Heart Association/american Stroke Association. Stroke. 2012;43(6):1711–37.
56. Zafar SF, et al. Antiseizure medication treatment and outcomes in patients with subarachnoid hemorrhage undergoing continuous EEG monitoring. Neurocrit Care. 2021;36(3):857–67.
57. Huang CW, et al. Influence of seizures on stroke outcomes: a large multicenter study. Neurology. 2014;82(9):768–76.
58. Wang JZ, et al. Incidence and management of seizures after ischemic stroke: systematic review and meta-analysis. Neurology. 2017;89(12):1220–8.
59. Vespa PM, et al. Acute seizures after intracerebral hemorrhage: a factor in progressive midline shift and outcome. Neurology. 2003;60(9):1441–6.
60. Sung CY, Chu NS. Epileptic seizures in intracerebral haemorrhage. J Neurol Neurosurg Psychiatry. 1989;52(11):1273–6.
61. Wang H, et al. Incidence rate and risk factors of status epilepticus after stroke. Seizure. 2021;91:491–8.
62. Jauch EC, et al. Guidelines for the early management of patients with acute ischemic stroke: a guideline for healthcare professionals from the American Heart Association/American Stroke Association. Stroke. 2013;44(3):870–947.
63. Morgenstern LB, et al. Guidelines for the management of spontaneous intracerebral hemorrhage: a guideline for healthcare professionals from the American Heart Association/American Stroke Association. Stroke. 2010;41(9):2108–29.
64. Baguley IJ, et al. Late mortality after severe traumatic brain injury in New South Wales: a multicentre study. Med J Aust. 2012;196(1):40–5.
65. Vespa PM, et al. Increased incidence and impact of nonconvulsive and convulsive seizures after traumatic brain injury as detected by continuous electroencephalographic monitoring. J Neurosurg. 1999;91(5):750–60.
66. da Silva AM, et al. Posttraumatic epilepsy in civilians: clinical and electroencephalographic studies. Acta Neurochir Suppl (Wien). 1992;55:56–63.
67. Nilsson P, et al. Epileptic seizure activity in the acute phase following cortical impact trauma in rat. Brain Res. 1994;637(1–2):227–32.
68. Vespa P, et al. Increase in extracellular glutamate caused by reduced cerebral perfusion pressure and seizures after human traumatic brain injury: a microdialysis study. J Neurosurg. 1998;89(6):971–82.
69. Frey LC. Epidemiology of posttraumatic epilepsy: a critical review. Epilepsia. 2003;44(s10):11–7.
70. Carney N, et al. Guidelines for the Management of Severe Traumatic Brain Injury. Fourth Edition Neurosurgery. 2017;80(1):6–15.
71. Nussbaum ES, et al. Brain metastases. Histology, multiplicity, surgery, and survival. Cancer. 1996;78(8):1781–8.
72. Steeghs N, et al. Cisplatin-induced encephalopathy and seizures. Anti-Cancer Drugs. 2003;14(6):443–6.
73. La Morgia C, et al. Busulfan neurotoxicity and EEG abnormalities: a case report. Neurol Sci. 2004;25(2):95–7.
74. Gultekin SH, et al. Paraneoplastic limbic encephalitis: neurological symptoms, immunological findings and tumour association in 50 patients. Brain. 2000;123(7):1481–94.
75. Singh G, Rees JH, Sander JW. Seizures and epilepsy in oncological practice: causes, course, mechanisms and treatment. J Neurol Neurosurg Psychiatry. 2007;78(4):342–9.
76. Clouston PD, DeAngelis LM, Posner JB. The spectrum of neurological disease in patients with systemic cancer. Ann Neurol. 1992;31(3):268–73.
77. Glantz MJ, et al. Practice parameter: anticonvulsant prophylaxis in patients with newly diagnosed brain tumors. Report of the quality standards Subcommittee of the American Academy of neurology. Neurology. 2000;54(10):1886–93.
78. Englot DJ, Chang EF, Vecht CJ. Epilepsy and brain tumors. Handb Clin Neurol. 2016;134:267–85.
79. van Breemen MS, Wilms EB, Vecht CJ. Epilepsy in patients with brain tumours: epidemiology, mechanisms, and management. Lancet Neurol. 2007;6(5):421–30.
80. Komotar RJ, et al. Prophylactic antiepileptic drug therapy in patients undergoing supratentorial meningioma resection: a systematic analysis of efficacy. J Neurosurg. 2011;115(3):483–90.
81. Human T, et al. Treatment of hyponatremia in patients with acute neurological injury. Neurocrit Care. 2017;27(2):242–8.
82. Hasan D, Wijdicks EF, Vermeulen M. Hyponatremia is associated with cerebral ischemia in patients with aneurysmal subarachnoid hemorrhage. Ann Neurol. 1990;27(1):106–8.
83. Karandanis D, Shulman JA. Recent survey of infectious meningitis in adults: review of laboratory findings in bacterial, tuberculous, and aseptic meningitis. South Med J. 1976;69(4):449–57.
84. Rabinstein AA, Wijdicks EFM. Hyponatremia in critically ill neurological patients. Neurologist. 2003;9(6):290–300.
85. Adrogué HJ, Madias NE. Hyponatremia. N Engl J Med. 2000;342(21):1581–9.
86. Youngson NA, Morris MJ, Ballard JWO. The mechanisms mediating the antiepileptic effects of the ketogenic diet, and potential opportunities for improvement with metabolism-altering drugs. Seizure. 2017;52:15–9.
87. Singh BM, Gupta DR, Strobos RJ. Nonketotic hyperglycemia and Epilepsia Partialis continua. Arch Neurol. 1973;29(3):187–90.
88. Riggs JE. Neurologic manifestations of electrolyte disturbances. Neurol Clin. 2002;20(1):227–39. vii
89. Gupta MM. Medical emergencies associated with disorders of calcium homeostasis. J Assoc Physicians India. 1989;37(10):629–31.
90. Kline CA, et al. Non-convulsive status epilepticus in a patient with hypocalcemia. J Emerg Med. 1998;16(5):715–8.
91. Leung J, Crook M. Disorders of phosphate metabolism. J Clin Pathol. 2019;72(11):741–7.
92. Castilla-Guerra L, et al. Electrolytes disturbances and seizures. Epilepsia. 2006;47(12):1990–8.
93. Pritchard JA, Cunningham FG, Pritchard SA. The parkland memorial hospital protocol for treatment of eclampsia: evaluation of 245 cases. Am J Obstet Gynecol. 1984;148(7):951–63.
94. Sibai BM. Magnesium sulfate prophylaxis in preeclampsia: lessons learned from recent trials. Am J Obstet Gynecol. 2004;190(6):1520–6.
95. Baluarte JH. Neurological complications of renal disease. Semin Pediatr Neurol. 2017;24(1):25–32.
96. Chen R, Young GB. Metabolic encephalopathies. Baillieres Clin Neurol. 1996;5(3):577–98.
97. Arieff AI. Dialysis disequilibrium syndrome: current concepts on pathogenesis and prevention. Kidney Int. 1994;45(3):629–35.
98. Alkhachroum AM, et al. Risk of seizures and status epilepticus in older patients with liver disease. Epilepsia. 2018;59(7):1392–7.

99. Gursky JM, et al. Exacerbation of hepatic cirrhosis may trigger admission for epilepsy and status epilepticus. Epilepsia. 2020;61(3):400–7.
100. Adams RD, Foley JM. The neurological disorder associated with liver disease. Res Publ Assoc Res Nerv Ment Dis. 1953;32:198–237.
101. D'Onofrio G, et al. Lorazepam for the prevention of recurrent seizures related to alcohol. N Engl J Med. 1999;340(12):915–9.
102. Sellers EM, Kalant H. Alcohol intoxication and withdrawal. N Engl J Med. 1976;294(14):757–62.
103. Derlet RW, Albertson TE. Emergency department presentation of cocaine intoxication. Ann Emerg Med. 1989;18(2):182–6.
104. Lappin JM, Sara GE. Psychostimulant use and the brain. Addiction. 2019;114(11):2065–77.
105. Richards JR, et al. Dual cocaine and methamphetamine cardiovascular toxicity: rapid resolution with labetalol. Am J Emerg Med. 2017;35(3):519.e1–4.
106. Banerji D, et al. Carvedilol among patients with heart failure with a cocaine-use disorder. JACC Heart Fail. 2019;7(9):771–8.
107. Huang MC, et al. Risk of cardiovascular diseases and stroke events in methamphetamine users: a 10-year follow-up study. J Clin Psychiatry. 2016;77(10):1396–403.
108. Thundiyil JG, Kearney TE, Olson KR. Evolving epidemiology of drug-induced seizures reported to a poison control center system. J Med Toxicol. 2007;3(1):15–9.
109. Cock HR. Drug-induced status epilepticus. Epilepsy Behav. 2015;49:76–82.
110. Wu YW, et al. Incidence and mortality of generalized convulsive status epilepticus in California. Neurology. 2002;58(7):1070–6.
111. Ebersoldt M, Sharshar T, Annane D. Sepsis-associated delirium. Intensive Care Med. 2007;33(6):941–50.
112. Oddo M, et al. Continuous electroencephalography in the medical intensive care unit*. Crit Care Med. 2009;37(6):2051–6.
113. Mao L, et al. Neurologic manifestations of hospitalized patients with coronavirus disease 2019 in Wuhan. China JAMA Neurol. 2020;77(6):683–90.
114. Pons S, et al. The vascular endothelium: the cornerstone of organ dysfunction in severe SARS-CoV-2 infection. Crit Care. 2020;24(1):353.
115. Li Y, et al. Coronavirus infections in the central nervous system and respiratory tract show distinct features in hospitalized children. Intervirology. 2016;59(3):163–9.
116. Leitinger M, et al. Status epilepticus admissions during the COVID-19 pandemic in Salzburg-a population-based study. Epilepsia. 2020;61(12):e198–203.
117. Watemberg N, Segal G. A suggested approach to the etiologic evaluation of status epilepticus in children: what to seek after the usual causes have been ruled out. J Child Neurol. 2010;25(2):203–11.
118. Hirsch LJ, et al. Proposed consensus definitions for new-onset refractory status epilepticus (NORSE), febrile infection-related epilepsy syndrome (FIRES), and related conditions. Epilepsia. 2018;59(4):739–44.
119. van Baalen A, et al. Febrile infection-related epilepsy syndrome: clinical review and hypotheses of Epileptogenesis. Neuropediatrics. 2017;48(1):5–18.
120. Gaspard N, et al. New-onset refractory status epilepticus. Etiology, clinical features, and outcome. 2015;85(18):1604–13.
121. Jain N, et al. West Nile encephalitis, status epilepticus and West Nile pneumonia in a renal transplant patient. Transpl Int. 2007;20(9):800–3.
122. Gaspard N, et al. New-onset refractory status epilepticus (NORSE) and febrile infection–related epilepsy syndrome (FIRES): state of the art and perspectives. Epilepsia. 2018;59(4):745–52.
123. Kramer U, et al. Febrile infection-related epilepsy syndrome (FIRES): pathogenesis, treatment, and outcome: a multicenter study on 77 children. Epilepsia. 2011;52(11):1956–65.
124. Specchio N, Pietrafusa N. New-onset refractory status epilepticus and febrile infection-related epilepsy syndrome. Developmental Medicine & Child Neurology. 2020;62(8):897–905.
125. Li J, Saldivar C, Maganti RK. Plasma exchange in cryptogenic new onset refractory status epilepticus. Seizure. 2013;22(1):70–3.
126. Senzolo M, Ferronato C, Burra P. Neurologic complications after solid organ transplantation. Transpl Int. 2009;22(3):269–78.
127. Coe CL, Horst SN, Izzy MJ. Neurologic toxicities associated with tumor necrosis factor inhibitors and Calcineurin inhibitors. Neurol Clin. 2020;38(4):937–51.
128. Bronster DJ, et al. Central nervous system complications in liver transplant recipients--incidence, timing, and long-term follow-up. Clin Transpl. 2000;14(1):1–7.
129. Estol CJ, et al. Seizures after liver transplantation: a clinicopathologic study. Neurology. 1989;39(10):1297–301.
130. Cuero MR, Varelas PN. Super-refractory status epilepticus. Curr Neurol Neurosci Rep. 2015;15(11):74.
131. Novy J, Logroscino G, Rossetti AO. Refractory status epilepticus: a prospective observational study. Epilepsia. 2010;51(2):251–6.
132. Hocker S, Wijdicks EF, Rabinstein AA. Refractory status epilepticus: new insights in presentation, treatment, and outcome. Neurol Res. 2013;35(2):163–8.
133. Claassen J, Hirsch LJ, Mayer SA. Treatment of status epilepticus: a survey of neurologists. J Neurol Sci. 2003;211(1–2):37–41.
134. Holtkamp M, et al. The management of refractory generalised convulsive and complex partial status epilepticus in three European countries: a survey among epileptologists and critical care neurologists. J Neurol Neurosurg Psychiatry. 2003;74(8):1095–9.
135. Claassen J, et al. Treatment of refractory status epilepticus with pentobarbital, propofol, or midazolam: a systematic review. Epilepsia. 2002;43(2):146–53.
136. Rossetti AO, Logroscino G, Bromfield EB. Refractory status epilepticus: effect of treatment aggressiveness on prognosis. Arch Neurol. 2005;62(11):1698–702.
137. Hocker SE, et al. Predictors of outcome in refractory status epilepticus. JAMA Neurol. 2013;70(1):72–7.
138. Brophy GM, et al. Guidelines for the evaluation and management of status epilepticus. Neurocrit Care. 2012;17(1):3–23.
139. Muhlhofer WG, et al. Duration of therapeutic coma and outcome of refractory status epilepticus. Epilepsia. 2019;60(5):921–34.
140. Rossetti AO, Logroscino G, Bromfield EB. A clinical score for prognosis of status epilepticus in adults. Neurology. 2006;66(11):1736–8.
141. Leitinger M, et al. Epidemiology-based mortality score in status epilepticus (EMSE). Neurocrit Care. 2015;22(2):273–82.
142. Gao Q, et al. Prediction of functional outcome in patients with convulsive status epilepticus: the END-IT score. Crit Care. 2016;20(1):46.
143. Logroscino G, et al. Short-term mortality after a first episode of status epilepticus. Epilepsia. 1997;38(12):1344–9.
144. Ferlisi M, Shorvon S. The outcome of therapies in refractory and super-refractory convulsive status epilepticus and recommendations for therapy. Brain. 2012;135(Pt 8):2314–28.
145. Strzelczyk A, et al. Costs, length of stay, and mortality of super-refractory status epilepticus: a population-based study from Germany. Epilepsia. 2017;58(9):1533–41.
146. Leitinger M, et al. Epidemiology of status epilepticus in adults: a population-based study on incidence, causes, and outcomes. Epilepsia. 2019;60(1):53–62.
147. Holtkamp M, et al. A "malignant" variant of status epilepticus. Arch Neurol. 2005;62(9):1428–31.
148. Neligan A, Shorvon SD. Frequency and prognosis of convulsive status epilepticus of different causes: a systematic review. Arch Neurol. 2010;67(8):931–40.

149. Koubeissi M, Alshekhlee A. In-hospital mortality of generalized convulsive status epilepticus: a large US sample. Neurology. 2007;69(9):886–93.
150. Belluzzo M, et al. Role of comorbidities and in-hospital complications in short-term status epilepticus outcome. Clin Neurol Neurosurg. 2017;154:13–8.
151. Hui AC, et al. Prognosis following Postanoxic myoclonus status epilepticus. Eur Neurol. 2005;54(1):10–3.
152. Datta S, et al. Post-hypoxic myoclonic status: the prognosis is not always hopeless. Crit Care Resusc. 2009;11(1):39–41.
153. English WA, Giffin NJ, Nolan JP. Myoclonus after cardiac arrest: pitfalls in diagnosis and prognosis. Anaesthesia. 2009;64(8):908–11.
154. Sutter R, et al. Mortality and recovery from refractory status epilepticus in the intensive care unit: a 7-year observational study. Epilepsia. 2013;54(3):502–11.
155. Leitinger M, et al. Predicting outcome of status epilepticus. Epilepsy Behav. 2015;49:126–30.
156. Bausell R, et al. Recovery after severe refractory status epilepticus and 4 months of coma. Neurology. 2011;77(15):1494–5.
157. Nei M, et al. The EEG and prognosis in status epilepticus. Epilepsia. 1999;40(2):157–63.
158. Jaitly R, et al. Prognostic value of EEG monitoring after status epilepticus: a prospective adult study. J Clin Neurophysiol. 1997;14(4):326–34.
159. Kilbride RD, et al. Clinical outcomes following prolonged refractory status epilepticus (PRSE). Neurocrit Care. 2013;18(3):374–85.
160. Rossetti AO, Hirsch LJ, Drislane FW. Nonconvulsive seizures and nonconvulsive status epilepticus in the neuro ICU should or should not be treated aggressively: a debate. Clin Neurophysiol Pract. 2019;4:170–7.
161. Alldredge BK, et al. A comparison of lorazepam, diazepam, and placebo for the treatment of out-of-hospital status epilepticus. N Engl J Med. 2001;345(9):631–7.
162. Silbergleit R, et al. Intramuscular versus intravenous therapy for prehospital status epilepticus. N Engl J Med. 2012;366(7):591–600.
163. Hung OR, et al. Comparative absorption kinetics of intramuscular midazolam and diazepam. Can J Anaesth. 1996;43(5 Pt 1):450–5.
164. Kapur J, et al. Randomized trial of three anticonvulsant medications for status epilepticus. N Engl J Med. 2019;381(22):2103–13.
165. Abou-Khalil BW. Update on antiepileptic drugs 2019. Continuum (Minneap Minn). 2019;25(2):508–36.
166. Jarvie D, Mahmoud SH. Therapeutic drug monitoring of Levetiracetam in select populations. J Pharm Pharm Sci. 2018;21(1s):149s–76s.
167. Vossler DG, et al. Treatment of refractory convulsive status epilepticus: a comprehensive review by the American Epilepsy Society treatments committee. Epilepsy Curr. 2020;20(5):245–64.
168. Fechner A, et al. Treatment of refractory and superrefractory status epilepticus with topiramate: a cohort study of 106 patients and a review of the literature. Epilepsia. 2019;60(12):2448–58.
169. Farrokh S, et al. Use of newer anticonvulsants for the treatment of status epilepticus. Pharmacotherapy. 2019;39(3):297–316.
170. De Stefano P, et al. Safety and efficacy of coma induction following first-line treatment in status epilepticus: a 2-center study. Neurology. 2021;97(6):e564–76.
171. Fernandez A, et al. High-dose midazolam infusion for refractory status epilepticus. Neurology. 2014;82(4):359–65.
172. Prisco L, et al. A pragmatic approach to intravenous anaesthetics and electroencephalographic endpoints for the treatment of refractory and super-refractory status epilepticus in critical care. Seizure. 2020;75:153–64.
173. Hussein O. Acute convulsive seizures: when is it too early to treat? Perm J. 2019;23:18–129.
174. Rosati A, De Masi S, Guerrini R. Ketamine for refractory status epilepticus: a systematic review. CNS Drugs. 2018;32(11):997–1009.
175. Alkhachroum A, et al. Ketamine to treat super-refractory status epilepticus. Neurology. 2020;95(16):e2286–94.
176. Gall CR, Jumma O, Mohanraj R. Five cases of new onset refractory status epilepticus (NORSE) syndrome: outcomes with early immunotherapy. Seizure. 2013;22(3):217–20.
177. Wilder-Smith EP, et al. The NORSE (new-onset refractory status epilepticus) syndrome: defining a disease entity. Ann Acad Med Singap. 2005;34(7):417–20.
178. Khawaja AM, et al. New-onset refractory status epilepticus (NORSE)--The potential role for immunotherapy. Epilepsy Behav. 2015;47:17–23.
179. Rotenberg A, et al. Repetitive transcranial magnetic stimulation in the treatment of epilepsia partialis continua. Epilepsy Behav. 2009;14(1):253–7.
180. Kamel H, et al. Electroconvulsive therapy for refractory status epilepticus: a case series. Neurocrit Care. 2010;12(2):204–10.
181. Stavropoulos I, et al. Low frequency centromedian thalamic nuclei deep brain stimulation for the treatment of super refractory status epilepticus: a case report and a review of the literature. Brain Stimul. 2021;14(2):226–9.
182. De Herdt V, et al. Vagus nerve stimulation for refractory status epilepticus. Eur J Paediatr Neurol. 2009;13(3):286–9.
183. Stavropoulos I, Pak HL, Valentin A. Neuromodulation in super-refractory status epilepticus. J Clin Neurophysiol. 2021;38(6):494–502.
184. Legriel S, et al. Hypothermia for neuroprotection in convulsive status epilepticus. N Engl J Med. 2016;375(25):2457–67.
185. Cereda C, Berger MM, Rossetti AO. Bowel ischemia: a rare complication of thiopental treatment for status epilepticus. Neurocrit Care. 2009;10(3):355–8.
186. Corry JJ, et al. Hypothermia for refractory status epilepticus. Neurocrit Care. 2008;9(2):189–97.
187. Lhatoo SD, Alexopoulos AV. The surgical treatment of status epilepticus. Epilepsia. 2007;48(Suppl 8):61–5.
188. Alexopoulos A, et al. Resective surgery to treat refractory status epilepticus in children with focal epileptogenesis. Neurology. 2005;64(3):567–70.
189. Schrader DV, Steinbok P, Connolly M. Urgent, resective surgery for medically refractory, convulsive status epilepticus. Eur J Paediatr Neurol. 2009;13(1):10–7.
190. Cervenka MC, et al. The ketogenic diet for medically and surgically refractory status epilepticus in the neurocritical care unit. Neurocrit Care. 2011;15(3):519–24.
191. Nam SH, et al. The role of ketogenic diet in the treatment of refractory status epilepticus. Epilepsia. 2011;52(11):e181–4.
192. Nabbout R, et al. Efficacy of ketogenic diet in severe refractory status epilepticus initiating fever induced refractory epileptic encephalopathy in school age children (FIRES). Epilepsia. 2010;51(10):2033–7.
193. Zhang Y, et al. The anticonvulsant effects of ketogenic diet on epileptic seizures and potential mechanisms. Curr Neuropharmacol. 2018;16(1):66–70.
194. Bough KJ, Rho JM. Anticonvulsant mechanisms of the ketogenic diet. Epilepsia. 2007;48(1):43–58.
195. Wusthoff CJ, et al. The ketogenic diet in treatment of two adults with prolonged nonconvulsive status epilepticus. Epilepsia. 2010;51(6):1083–5.

Intracranial Hypertension: Signs, Symptoms, and Management

7

Kara R. Melmed and Ting Zhou

Contents

Abstract

Understanding the physiology of intracranial pressure is critical to developing sound management plans for intracranial hypertension. The principles of treatment are based on a multitude of complex interactions between

K. R. Melmed (✉) · T. Zhou
NYU Langone Health, New York, NY, USA
e-mail: kara.melmed@nyulangone.org; Ting.Zhou@nyulangone.org

E. Mahanna Gabrielli et al. (eds.), *Textbook of Neurointensive Care: Volume 1*, https://doi.org/10.1007/978-3-031-62220-5_7

pathophysiological processes. Molecular, cellular, tissue, and organ pathologies vary according to the primary insult, but management of intracranial hypertension and its causes is crucial for the reduction of further injury, debility, and death.

Chapter Goals

- To define intracranial pressure.
- To define intracranial hypertension, cerebral perfusion pressure, cerebral compliance, and autoregulation.
- To describe the signs and symptoms of intracranial hypertension.
- To review how to measure and monitor ICP.
- To discuss treatment of elevated ICP.

Introduction

Intracranial hypertension is a common neurological emergency. Hence, it is essential that practitioners develop expertise and comfort in the diagnosis and management of this condition. In this chapter, we will discuss the key concepts of cerebral hemodynamics and intracranial pressure (ICP) and its clinical relevance. We will describe conditions that can lead to intracranial hypertension and review in detail the clinical signs and symptoms of elevated intracranial pressure. We will review indications for ICP monitoring and discuss how to interpret an elevated ICP reading. Finally, we will outline and discuss treatment strategies for intracranial hypertension.

Discussion of Concepts

Intracranial Pressure, Intracranial Volume, and Compliance

Intracranial pressure (ICP) is the sum of the pressures exerted by the individual intracranial compartments within the skull: arterial and venous blood volume, brain tissue, and cerebrospinal fluid (CSF). By convention, ICP is measured in millimeters of mercury (mmHg) or centimeter of water (cmH_2O). The relationship between intracranial pressure and intracranial volume is best described by the Monro–Kellie doctrine, which conceptualizes the skull as a fixed-volume container with three noncompressible components: the brain parenchyma, CSF, and blood [1]. As the volume of one component increases, the volume of the other two must decrease to maintain constant ICP (Fig. 7.1). Once this compensatory mechanism is exhausted, the pressure inside the skull will increase exponentially (Fig. 7.1). Diseases that result in an acute increase in the overall brain volume (i.e., hematomas) are more likely to precipitate an ICP crisis than are chronic conditions in which the brain volume rises gradually (such as slow-growing tumors).

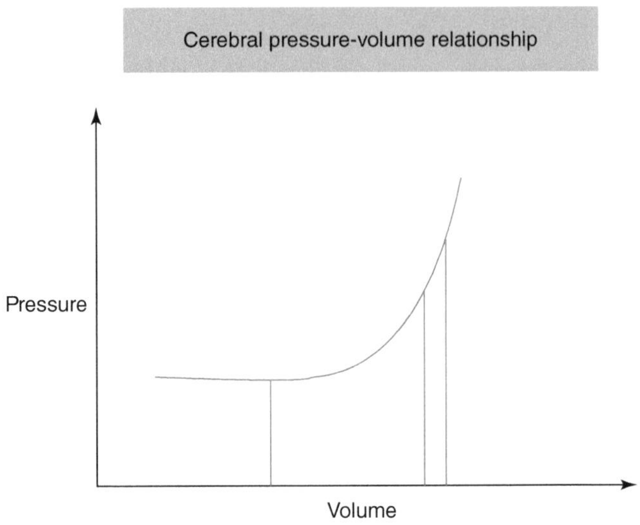

Fig. 7.1 Cerebral pressure-volume relationship. The relationship between intracranial pressure and intracranial volume is described by the Monro-Kellie Doctrine: As the volume of one component increases, the volume of the other two must decrease to maintain constant ICP. Once this compensatory mechanism is exhausted, pressure inside the skull will increase exponentially. A compliant brain is able to accommodate a relatively large increase in volume with a comparatively small rise in pressure (point a). As intracranial volume continues to increase past the accommodative threshold, the brain becomes less compliant and any small change in volume will result in a much larger increase in pressure (point b and c)

Compliance, or the stretch of a material, is another way of expressing the relationship between intracranial volume and pressure. Compliance is defined as the change in volume over the change in pressure (Eq. 7.1).

$$C = \Delta(V/P) \qquad \text{(Eq. 7.1)}$$

A compliant brain is able to accommodate a relatively large increase in volume with a comparatively small rise in pressure (point a, Fig. 7.1). As intracranial volume continues to increase past the accommodative threshold, the brain becomes less compliant and any small change in volume will result in a much larger increase in pressure (points b and c, Fig. 7.1).

Cerebral Blood Flow and Cerebral Autoregulation

Cerebral blood flow (CBF) is the rate at which a certain cerebral blood volume (CBV) transits a certain volume of the brain (Eq. 7.2). CBF is expressed as the quotient of change in cerebral perfusion pressure (CPP) over cerebrovascular resistance (CVR). The average CBF in an adult human is about 50 mL/(100g_{brain}*min) and is regulated by a series of myogenic, neurogenic, and metabolic factors [2].

$$CBF = \text{CPP} / \text{CVR} \tag{Eq. 7.2}$$

Our understanding of the variables that affect CBF can be expressed using Poiseuille's law, which calculates the fluid flow of an idealized Newtonian fluid through a rigid tube (Eq. 7.3). These factors include the length of the vasculature (L), the radius of the blood vessel (r), and the viscosity of the blood (η). However, Poiseuille's law provides merely an approximation of CBF as neither does blood act like a Newtonian fluid nor do arteries behave like rigid tubes. In addition, this equation does not address the role of regional cerebral metabolic demand, to which CBF is tightly coupled.

$$\text{CVR} = 8\eta \text{L} / \pi \text{r4} \tag{Eq. 7.3}$$

Cerebral autoregulation is the mechanism by which the brain maintains adequate blood flow to sustain its high oxygen and metabolic demands in spite of fluctuating systemic blood pressures. Arteriolar radius (r) appears with the fourth power in Poiseuille's law, and, as such, cerebral arteriolar vasodilation and vasoconstriction are believed to be the main drivers of cerebral autoregulation. While the brain may be able to maintain constant CBF across a set range of perfusion pressures, cerebral autoregulation breaks down at the extremes of blood pressures (Fig. 7.2). That is, once CPP rises beyond the upper limit of autoregulation, arterioles passively dilate and CBF will increase proportionally to pressure, causing hyperemic injury. If CPP falls below the lower limit of arteriolar vasodilation, then the vessels will begin to collapse and cause CBF to drop, precipitating cerebral ischemia.

Cerebral arteriolar tone is regulated by partial pressure of carbon dioxide ($PaCO_2$), partial pressure of arterial oxygen (PaO_2), arterial pH, sympathetic nerve activity, cardiac output, and neurohormonal mediators [3]. $PaCO_2$ exerts the strongest effect on cerebral autoregulation. An increase in $PaCO_2$ (hypercarbia) results in cerebral arteriolar vasodilation and a subsequent rise in CBF. A decrease in $PaCO_2$ causes vasoconstriction and a drop in CBF [4].

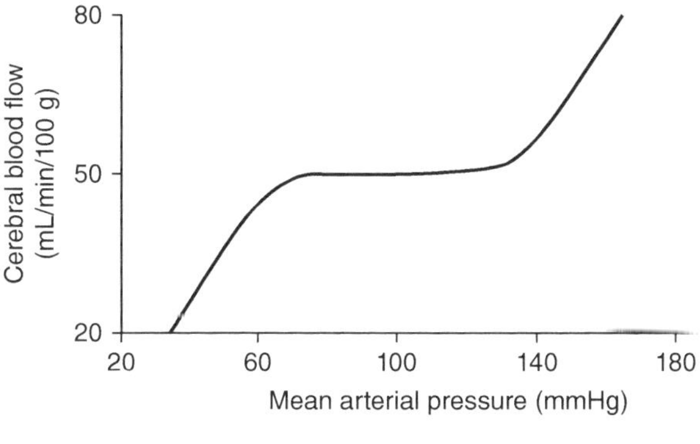

Fig. 7.2 Cerebral autoregulatory curve according to conventional teaching

The modern-day teaching of cerebral autoregulation asserts that the brain is able to maintain constant blood flow across a wide range of mean arterial pressures (MAPs) (from 50 to 150 mmHg) (Fig. 7.2). However, this was based on an erroneous interpretation of the original CBF versus MAP graph, which was based on the average CBF and MAP measurements of different patient groups with various medical conditions rather than within individual readings [4]. Newer studies suggest that the brain's autoregulatory range may be significantly narrower than previously believed and that CBF can fluctuate greatly from even small perturbations in perfusion pressure and other physiological changes [5, 6]. Autoregulatory function also varies substantially in healthy individuals, with autoregulatory patterns ranging from robust to nearly absent [7, 8].

Cerebral Perfusion Pressure

Cerebral perfusion pressure is the pressure gradient between systemic arterial blood pressure and the downstream intracranial pressure that drives blood flow to the brain (Eq. 7.4).

$$\text{CPP} = \text{MAP} - \text{ICP} \tag{Eq. 7.4}$$

CPP is an effector of CBF, and recent studies on cerebral autoregulation have suggested that CBF may be much more sensitive to perturbations in CPP than previously believed. At either extreme of perfusion pressures where autoregulatory function breaks down, or in individuals who have nearly absent cerebral autoregulation, CBF becomes passively dependent on CPP.

Clinical Significance of ICP, CPP, and CBF

CBF is the most clinically relevant parameter in the determination of brain perfusion. However, bedside evaluation of CBF is not always easy or readily available. Measurements of CBF obtained via imaging techniques such as xenon-enhanced computed tomography (CT) or CT or magnetic resonance (MR) perfusion studies provide only temporal snapshots of CBF and are often challenging to obtain in the critically ill population. Invasive CBF probes using thermal diffusion technology provide continuous but regional measurements that are relevant only to the brain area being monitored. As such, CPP is commonly used as a surrogate for global CBF and is derived from measurements of MAP and ICP, which can be easily obtained at the bedside.

Conditions that Cause Intracranial Hypertension

Disorders of the Arterial and Venous Structures

The cerebral vasculature holds about 100–130 mL of blood [9]. An increase in arterial blood volume can be caused by inflammation or infection, an increase in regional or global cerebral metabolic demand driven by fever or seizures, or autoregulatory breakthrough as seen with malignant hypertension or posterior reversible encephalopathy syndrome (Fig. 7.3). Conditions that lead to hypercarbia might also increase arterial blood volume [4]. Venous hypertension can be the result of obstruction in the venous drainage system either due to external compression or venous thrombosis. Medications that cause arterial and venous dilation, such as sodium nitroprusside, can also trigger ICP elevation by increasing cerebral blood volume.

Disorders of CSF Production and Absorption

The average total CSF volume in an adult is approximately 150 mL. CSF is produced at approximately 450 mL/day from the intraventricular choroid plexus and is reabsorbed by the arachnoid granulations [10]. Increased production or decreased absorption can lead to excess CSF volume and intracranial hypertension. Conditions such as traumatic brain injury (TBI) and subarachnoid hemorrhage (SAH) are often associated with impaired CSF reabsorption and hydrocephalus. Tumors or intraventricular hemorrhages can also cause obstructive hydrocephalus due to blockage of the flow of CSF.

Intra-Axial and Extra-Axial Space-Occupying Lesions

The volume of the cranial vault includes the brain parenchyma and epidural, subdural, and subarachnoid compartments [9, 11]. Space-occupying lesions refer to tumors, hemorrhages, infections, or abscesses that develop quickly or slowly in any of these intra- and extra-axial spaces.

Cerebral edema is an excess in intracerebral water content due to either focal or diffuse brain swelling and is often associated with significant morbidity. It is categorized into four subtypes based on its pathophysiology: vasogenic, cytotoxic, osmotic, and hydrostatic. Brain pathologies frequently present with a mix of different types of edemas.

Vasogenic Edema

Vasogenic edema is caused by increased permeability of the blood–brain barrier (BBB) due to dysfunction of the endothelial cells and their tight junctions. Serum proteins such as albumin that would otherwise be confined to the intravascular space extravasate and draw fluid into the brain interstitium, causing expansion in brain volume. Injuries that lead to damage of the BBB include toxins released by microbes, inflammatory responses triggered by immune or

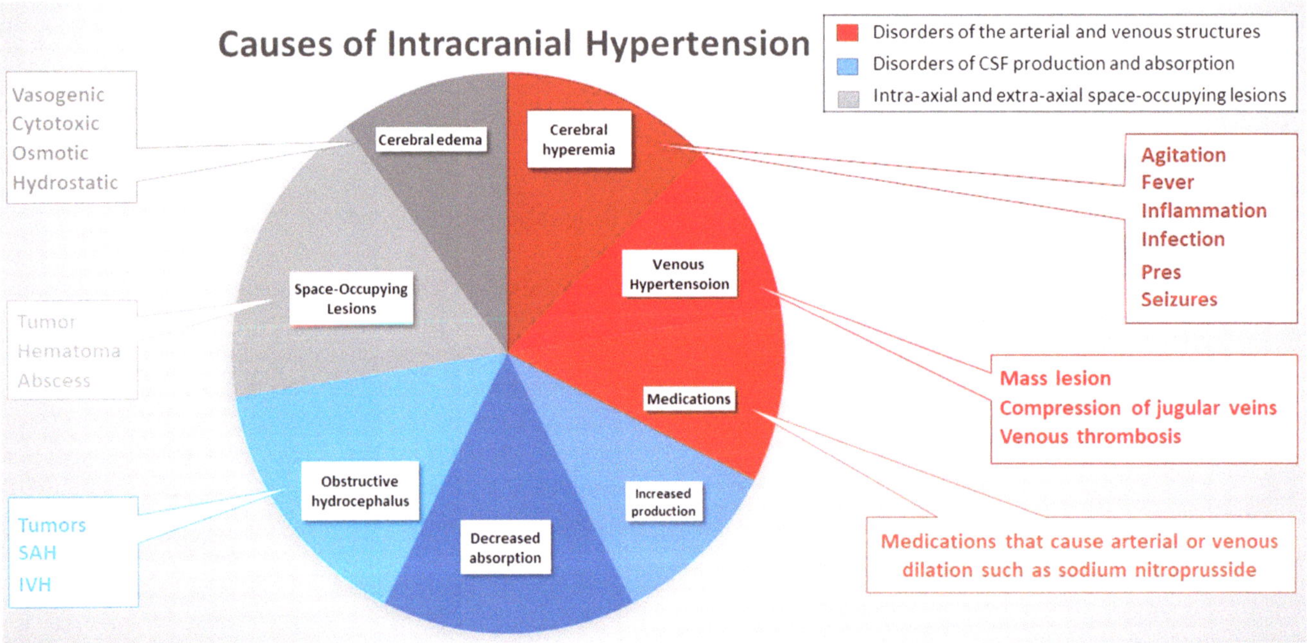

Fig. 7.3 Causes of intracranial hypertension

tumor cells, trauma, and ischemia-induced endothelial damage.

Cytotoxic Edema

Cytotoxic edema refers to increased intracellular fluid content. It is caused by shutdown of the transmembrane adenosine triphosphate (ATP)-mediated ion pumps that maintain intracellular homeostasis. The outcome is an unchecked influx of extracellular ions into the dying brain cells along with water molecules. Cytotoxic edema is most commonly seen with ischemic insults such as arterial or venous strokes and anoxic brain injury following a cardiac arrest. Cytotoxic edema can also be the sequelae of inborn disorders of metabolism, status epilepticus, drug intoxications, and metabolic derangements.

Osmotic Edema

Osmo-active solutes maintain their osmolar gradient across the BBB. The osmolarity of the brain parenchyma is kept in close range to that of the serum in order to achieve an overall net zero flux of water molecules. Brain cells can adapt to gradual changes in the osmolar gradient by adjusting the intracellular concentration of organic osmolytes and electrolytes [12]. However, in scenarios where the serum osmolarity acutely decreases (as in the case of acute hyponatremia, fulminant liver failure, dialysis disequilibrium syndrome, or over rapid correction of severe hyperglycemia), the brain cannot adjust its intracellular osmolarity quickly enough and diffuse cell swelling and cerebral osmotic edema can ensue.

Hydrostatic Edema

Although it has been used in the older literature to describe brain swelling seen in malignant hypertension, hydrostatic edema refers to the fluid buildup in the periventricular brain parenchyma as a consequence of hydrocephalus. The pressure from increased CSF volume pushes fluid across the ependymal lining, from the CSF spaces into the surrounding interstitium. Hydrostatic edema can be seen most prominently around the ventricular horns. This phenomenon is also known as transependymal flow.

Signs and Symptoms of Intracranial Hypertension

Headache, nausea, and vomiting are the common symptoms of raised ICP. Headaches may occur gradually or have sudden "thunderclap"-like onset and may be exacerbated by coughing or Valsalva maneuvers. They also may be positional in nature where the severity is worse when the patient is lying down versus being upright.

Papilledema and cranial nerve VI palsy are two "false localizing" signs of elevated ICP. These occur infrequently in patients who suffer from acute intracranial hypertension. Cranial nerve VI, having the longest intracranial route compared to other cranial nerves, is particularly vulnerable to shear and compressive stress.

Altered mentation is another usual symptom of intracranial hypertension and can manifest as both agitation and lethargy. At first, it may be the consequence of decreased cerebral perfusion from ICP elevation. Later on, downward pressure exerted onto the brain stem structures that modulate arousal, such as the reticular activating system in the upper midbrain and pons, becomes the main cause of obtundation and coma.

Perhaps the most notable sign of elevated ICP is Cushing's reflex [13], which consists of hypertension with widened pulse pressures, bradycardia, and irregular respirations [14, 15]. Patients are more likely to exhibit parts of Cushing's reflex than the whole triad. Harvey Cushing proposed that hypertension is a sympathetic response to medullary ischemia when ICP rapidly surpasses the perfusing blood pressure. In the early phase of brain compression when cerebral perfusion is still preserved, blood pressure and heart rate are both elevated through sympathetic excitation to maintain adequate CPP. The bradycardia seen during the late stages of an ICP crisis is caused by vagal activation from progressive medullary compression and ischemia [15] rather than the response of extracranial baroreceptors to the hypertension [16, 17]. Cushing's reflex is a sign in the late stages of brain compression where herniation and possibly death are imminent.

Herniation Syndromes

The cranial vault is divided into supratentorial and infratentorial compartments by the tentorium cerebelli, and the hemispheres of the brain are separated by the falx cerebri. In the case of an expanding intracranial mass lesion, the brain tissue will be shifted from the higher pressure compartment to the lower pressure compartments. Herniation can occur laterally, downward (through the tentorial notch and the foramen magnum), or upward (Fig. 7.4) [18]. Herniation can lead to further ischemic injury from strangulation of the arterial or venous vasculature or direct damage caused by incarceration of important brain structures.

Subfalcine Herniation

Subfalcine herniation is the most common form of herniation, where a mass lesion causes the ipsilateral cingulate gyrus to protrude underneath the falx cerebri. Subfalcine herniation is often clinically silent but can result in lower extremity weakness and spasticity if the anterior cerebral arteries are compressed.

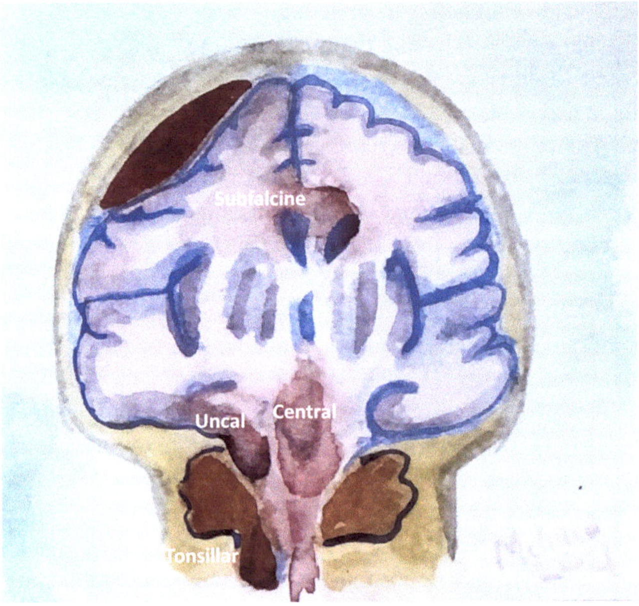

Fig. 7.4 This illustration shows (1) subfalcine herniation, (2) central herniation, (3) uncal herniation, and (4) tonsillar herniation

Uncal Herniation

Symptomatic uncal herniation is the result of a rapidly expanding unilateral hemispheric or temporal lesion [19]. This lesion displaces the medial uncus and hippocampal gyrus over the tentorial incisura, entraps the third nerve and the posterior cerebral artery running through the ambient cistern, and compresses the ipsilateral cerebral peduncle in the midbrain. This first results in a unilateral and usually ipsilateral dilated pupil. Although the patient may retain consciousness at this point, they are often agitated or confused. As herniation progresses, a complete cranial nerve III palsy develops and is accompanied by contralateral weakness, hyperventilation, and progression to stupor and coma. Hemiparesis of the limbs ipsilateral to the side of uncal herniation can occur due to compression of the contralateral cerebral peduncle against Kernohan's notch. In the late stage of herniation, both pupils become midsized (5–6 mm) and fixed, oculomotor functions are either decreased or absent, and the patient develops persistent hyperpnea and bilateral decerebrate rigidity. This is followed by central herniation.

Central Herniation

Central herniation, also known as downward or transtentorial herniation, occurs when the brain is inferiorly displaced along the vertical axis. In so doing, the pontine perforators from the basilar artery can shear and bleed, forming Duret hemorrhages in the pons with fatal consequences. In the early diencephalic phase of central herniation, the patient exhibits decreased alertness, deep sighs, yawns, and brief apneic periods. Their eyes may deviate medially and inferiorly ("sunset eyes") due to pressure on the diencephalon. Pupils tend to be small but reactive. Increased tone and positive Babinski signs are common. In the late diencephalic stage, the patient becomes stuporous and comatose [19]. Cheyne–Stokes respirations can be seen, and motor response devolves to plegia or decorticate posturing. Next, the midbrain–upper pons stage is characterized by bilateral cranial nerve III palsies with mid-position and fixed pupils, hyperventilation, and impaired oculocephalic and oculovestibular reflexes. It is also accompanied by loss of purposeful movement and eventually decerebrate posturing. In the final lower pons–upper medullary stage, the patient's breathing becomes rapid and shallow, oculocephalic and oculovestibular reflexes become absent, tone may be flaccid, and the motor response may be triple flexion or completely absent [19].

Tonsillar Herniation

Increased pressure in the posterior fossa can result in the cerebellar tonsils descending through the foramen magnum. This leads to compression of the medulla, causing cardiac and respiratory irregularities (as described by Cushing's triad) and eventually death [13]. Decorticate or decerebrate posturing may be observed at first, which would then progress to flaccid paralysis.

Upward Herniation

Space-occupying lesions in the cerebellum can also cause upward herniation across the tentorium cerebelli, which results in compression of the midbrain, superior cerebellar arteries, and the deep central draining cerebral veins. When a posterior fossa lesion or cerebellar edema obstructs the fourth ventricle causing obstructive hydrocephalus, a ventriculostomy is often performed to divert the extra CSF. However, care should be taken not to drain CSF overaggressively, as this could create a superiorly directed pressure gradient, leading to upward herniation of the cerebellum [19].

ICP Monitoring

Indications for Monitoring Intracranial Pressure

Intracranial pressure monitoring is indicated when intracranial hypertension is suspected and may lead to significant disability from brain ischemia or herniation or if cerebral physiological goals are needed to titrate ICP-targeted treatments.

Traumatic Brain Injury

Since 1996, the Brain Trauma Foundation (BTF) has put forth guidelines for the management of acute traumatic brain injuries. This included recommendations for ICP monitoring and treatment targets for ICP and CPP, with data to suggest that adherence to the BTF guidelines has significantly reduced mortality in TBI [20, 21]. The most recent 2016 guidelines have recommended ICP monitoring for all salvageable patients with severe TBI (post-resuscitation Glasgow Coma Scale (GCS) 3–8) and an abnormal CT scan (level II recommendation) or for severe TBI patients with a normal head CT and two or more of the following: age > 40 years, motor posturing, or any systolic blood pressure (SBP) measurement <90 mmHg (level III recommendations) [22].

However, the Benchmark Evidence from South American Trials: Treatment of Intracranial Pressure (BEST:TRIP) trial generated controversy over the utility of invasive ICP monitoring for TBI [23]. Conducted in Bolivia and Ecuador, this prospective study randomized patients with severe TBI to a treatment protocol guided by either invasive ICP monitoring or serial neurological and radiographic exams. This study showed no difference in the primary end point of long-term composite functional and cognitive outcomes between the two groups and no difference in 6-month mortality. Responses to the study ranged from criticisms of the trial's lack of generalizability to calls for abandoning invasive ICP monitoring in severe TBI altogether. Consensus-based expert interpretation of the BEST:TRIP asserts that the purpose of the trial is not to study the efficacy of ICP monitoring in TBI but rather to compare two different sets of treatment protocols. In addition, the impact of the results from the trial is meant to generate more research into physiology-oriented treatments and should not change the current practice of ICP monitoring for severe TBI [23].

Subarachnoid Hemorrhage and Intraparenchymal Hemorrhage

Intracranial pressure monitoring with CSF diversion is common practice in patients with a decreased level of consciousness secondary to subarachnoid hemorrhage and intraparenchymal hemorrhage. Due to the high rate of hydrocephalus in these populations, external ventricular drain (EVD) placement is both diagnostic and therapeutic [24, 25]

Cerebral Edema from Acute Liver Failure (ALF)

Cerebral edema is a well-described complication of acute liver failure (ALF) [26]. Hyperammonemia and glutamate-mediated oxidative stress likely play important roles in the complex pathophysiology of brain swelling. Even though ICP monitoring for grade III/IV hepatic encephalopathies is recommended by expert opinion, there is little evidence that ICP monitoring improves the outcome in this population [27]. The high prevalence of coagulopathy associated with liver failure is another deterrent to invasive ICP monitoring, as the risk of intracranial hemorrhage associated with ICP monitor placement ranges from 7% to 20% [28–30]. As a result, invasive monitoring for hepatic encephalopathy has been declining over time [31]. Serial radiographic evaluation and noninvasive modes of ICP measurement may be more attractive options for ALF patients [26].

Other Conditions Causing Elevated ICP

There are no guideline recommendations or strong empiric data to support routine ICP monitoring for diseases such as malignant hemispheric infarction, tumors, inflammatory conditions such as acute demyelinating encephalomyelitis, anoxic brain injury following cardiac arrest, infectious abscesses, meningitis, or encephalitides. The decision to place an ICP monitor in these scenarios should be made on a case-by-case basis.

Modes of Monitoring

ICP can be measured by both invasive and noninvasive means, each with its merits and drawbacks. Invasive monitors such as external ventricular drains (Fig. 7.6) and intraparenchymal monitors provide continuous and direct measurements of ICP but carry risks of hemorrhage and infections. Noninvasive techniques tend to measure qualitative changes in ICP rather than a numeric ICP value and thus indicate whether a state of elevated ICP or cerebral hypoperfusion exists. Noninvasive methods vary greatly in their accuracy and often offer discrete rather than continuous measurements. Detailed description of the various modes of ICP monitoring is covered in another chapter.

Interpreting the ICP Waveform

Components of the ICP Waveform

Besides the numeric value of ICP, the patterns of ICP tracings also provide insights into cerebral physiology. A typical ICP waveform occurs with each cardiac cycle and consists of three peaks: P1 (percussion wave), P2 (tidal wave), and P3 (dicrotic wave) (Fig. 7.5). The P1 peak corresponds to the choroid plexus pulsation and the arterial systolic pressure. P2 represents the rebound pulse waves from the ventricles.

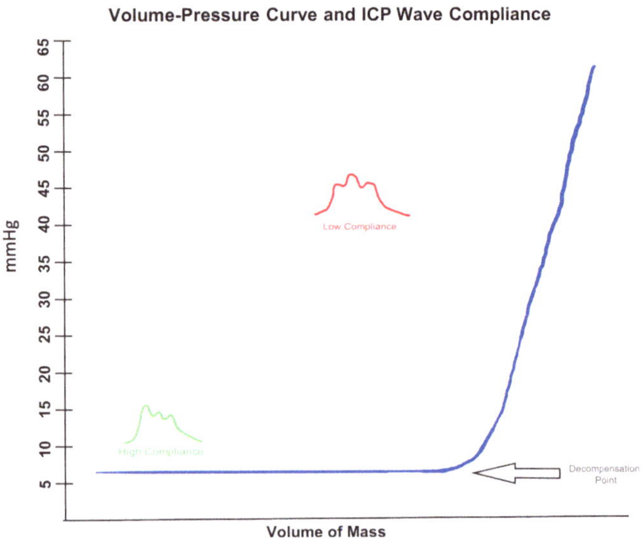

Fig. 7.5 Components of ICP wave, showing compliant (green) and noncompliant (red) patterns

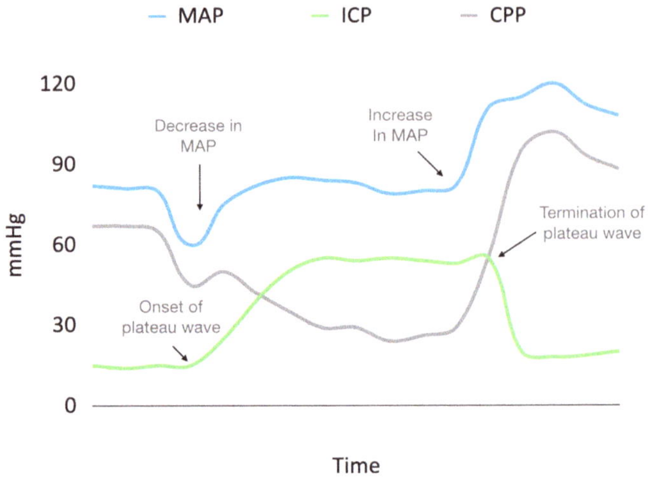

Fig. 7.6 Illustration of the relationship between MAP, CPP and ICP during a plateau wave. The onset of the plateau wave is preceded by a dip in MAP, followed by a sustained rise in ICP. As a result, CPP drops significantly. The plateau wave is sustained until the MAP increases, which improves CPP and ends the plateau wave

P3 is believed to be generated by venous pulsations. In a normal compliant brain, the value of P1 is always the highest compared to those of P2 and P3. When the brain is noncompliant, the waveform will have greater amplitude peaks, particularly of P2 with a prominent upstroke. This is because the pressure waves from the choroid plexus pulsations transmitted via the CSF in the ventricles are mostly reflected, rather than absorbed, by the stiff surrounding brain tissue. Noncompliant ICP waveforms can precede ICP elevation.

ICP waveforms are affected by other cerebral biomechanical processes as well, although their correlations with the waveform patterns are much less understood [32–34].

Time-Dependent Fluctuations in ICP

When examining an extended time series of ICP tracing, one can discover several patterns of spontaneous fluctuations in the ICP value. These are referred to as Lundberg A waves, B waves, and C waves [35]. Lundberg A wave, also known as the "plateau wave," is perhaps the most clinically relevant. Plateau waves are characterized by an abrupt increase in ICP as high as more than 100 mmHg that is sustained up to 20–30 min at a time, followed by a rapid fall back to the baseline (Fig. 7.6). Plateau waves are precipitated by a sudden steep drop in systemic blood pressure. This, in turn, causes vasodilation of the cerebrovasculature to maintain CBF and results in an increase in CBV. This translates to a swift rise in ICP and a net decrease in CPP that further perpetuates the plateau wave. Finally, a spike in MAP restores the CPP, triggering the reverse autoregulatory process and thus concluding the plateau wave [36]. This proposed mechanism behind the Lundberg A wave implies that the brain's autoregulation is preserved and that augmentation of systemic blood pressure (and therefore CPP) may be both an effective diagnosis and therapy for intracranial hypertension.

The clinical significance and the sources of Lundberg B and C waves are much less clear. B waves occur once per minute and tend to have lower amplitudes and coincide with Cheyne–Stokes respirations. C waves (6-per-min waves) are believed to be related to the baroreceptor-mediated oscillations in systemic blood pressure [35].

Management of Intracranial Hypertension

Diagnosing Intracranial Hypertension

The value of "normal" ICP is often cited as <10–15 mmHg, mildly elevated ICP as 15–25 mmHg, 25–40 mmHg as moderately elevated, and severely elevated if >40 mmHg [37]. However, ICP varies between individuals. It also fluctuates throughout the day and can be transiently elevated by actions such as Valsalva maneuver and coughing (Table 7.1). Hence, the diagnosis of intracranial hypertension should not be made solely on the basis of numeric values but, more importantly, on whether it may lead to cerebral circulatory and metabolic compromise. Increased ICP becomes clinically significant and a neurological emergency when it causes drops in CPP and CBF, threatening cerebral ischemia, or creates large enough intracranial pressure gradients that lead to brain herniation. On the other hand, clinicians must not be falsely reassured by a low ICP reading that herniation would not occur, for example, uncal herniation caused by a temporal mass lesion or cerebellar herniation from the posterior fossa pathology is still possible in the setting of "normal" ICP values.

Table 7.1 A systematic approach to diagnosing elevated ICP ensures that all causes are considered

A checklist for troubleshooting a patient with elevated ICP	
Is the EVD (or ICP monitor) properly calibrated? Is the EVD obstructed?	• Examine the ICP waveform on the bedside monitor – A malfunctioning EVD or ICP probe may have dampened or absent waveforms • Ensure the EVD is appropriately leveled and zeroed • Patency of the EVD can be quickly assessed using the "drop test," where the EVD setup is lowered below the bed to see if CSF drains with gravity • If the EVD is not draining, neurosurgery should be notified and the entire EVD setup should be examined closely from the head to the collection system for obstruction • Consider imaging to rule out malpositioning of the monitor
Is the patient positioned in the optimal way?	• Ensure the head of the bed is elevated and the neck in neutral position
Is the patient adequately sedated or in pain?	• Assess the patient and vital signs for evidence of pain or agitation • Rule out urinary retention, which is a common cause of agitation in the ICU that is not always evaluated • Try a push dose of analgesic and sedative and monitor for response in ICP
Is the patient febrile, retaining CO_2, or seizing?	• Obtain a current set of vitals including core temperature and arterial blood gas • Obtain continuous video electroencephalogram monitoring to rule out non-convulsive seizures
Are there certain precipitants of the ICP elevation?	• Review vital sign and clinical trends • If the high ICP value is associated with a plateau wave, sometimes a drop in MAP may be seen just before the ICP spike • Augmenting the MAP with vasopressors or fluids may effectively resolve the episode
Does the patient have worsening hydrocephalus, cerebral edema, expanding hemorrhages, or new infarcts?	• Obtain new brain imaging if the patient is stable • New focal lesions will require further workup and discussion with the neurosurgical team about the need for additional surgical intervention • Worsening diffuse cerebral edema may warrant intensifying hyperosmolar therapy and other edema-targeted treatments

Thresholds for ICP-Lowering Treatment

Much of the data on ICP treatment come from the literature on TBI. The BTF recommends a target ICP of <22 mmHg, as ICP beyond this threshold is associated with increased mortality and should be treated with ICP-lowering therapies (level IIb recommendation). CPP should be controlled between 60 and 70 mmHg to optimize the likelihood of survival and favorable outcome (level Iib), but maintaining a persistent CPP >70 mmHg with fluids and vasopressors is discouraged due to increased rates of acute respiratory distress syndrome and heart failure (level III). There are limitations to these recommended ICP and CPP ranges because they are derived from only a handful of class 2 studies and because optimal ICP and CPP targets may differ across individuals.

Rather than applying a single ICP and CPP goal to all patients, more clinicians are gravitating toward tailoring management to individualized optimal CPP values [38]. One method of finding optimal CPP uses a patient's pressure reactivity index (PRx), which is a calculated value that depicts changes in one's vasomotor tone in response to blood pressure, thus acting as a proxy for cerebral autoregulation. The optimal CPP (CPPopt) is defined as the CPP value that corresponds to the minimum value of PRx [39]. This PRx minimum indicates the point where ICP is least affected by fluctuations in blood pressure or where the autoregulatory responses are most robust. Studies have shown that CPPopt is a stronger predictor of outcomes than ICP in select TBI populations and that patients whose CPP fell below their CPPopt range had higher mortality [40]. Although achieving CPPopt in TBI patients is possible, it is still unknown whether autoregulation-directed CPP management in the TBI population would improve the outcome.

Strategies for ICP Management

Like all emergencies, management of intracranial hypertension begins with the evaluation of airways, breathing, and circulation. Patients who are unable to protect their airways should be endotracheally intubated and those with cardiovascular instability should be immediately stabilized. Treatment of intracranial hypertension deserves the same urgency and attention as those of acute hemorrhage, hypoxia, and shock, which means that clinicians ought to remain at the bedside in order to constantly monitor the patients and reevaluate their treatment response until the ICP crisis has resolved.

One approach to ICP management is a tiered method beginning with the least invasive interventions and escalating from one tier to the next if ICP fails to respond (Fig. 7.7) [41]. Tier 1 management includes keeping the level of the head at least ≥30° and in the neutral position to promote venous and CSF outflow, optimizing sedation/analgesia and treating fever or seizures to decrease metabolic demand, and ensuring normocapnia. Tier 2 involves implementation of hyperosmolar therapies. For patients with an EVD in place, additional CSF may be drained to lower total intracranial volume. Cerebral autoregulation should also be assessed (for example, by calculating the PRx) for more individualized blood pressure management. If the patient is ventilated, then a lower $PaCO_2$ range of 30–35 mmHg may be targeted. A push dose of a neuromuscular blocker can also be administered to assess for ICP response. Tier 3 management includes invasive procedures such as paralysis with continuous infusion of neuromuscular blockers, surgical decompression, therapeutic hypothermia (TH), and barbiturate coma.

Target-oriented ICP management is an alternative strategy, in which the more definitive treatment for the pathology causing intracranial hypertension is prioritized (Fig. 7.8a and b). For example, in a patient who presents with signs of elevated ICP due to a focal mass lesion, surgical evacuation of the lesion may come early in the treatment algorithm before an EVD placement. Or if the cause of intracranial hypertension is driven by extensive cerebral venous sinus thrombosis, then the patient may warrant endovascular thrombectomy and systemic anticoagulation before hyperosmolar therapy.

In practice, clinicians use a combination of the tiered and target-oriented approaches to treating intracranial hypertension.

Techniques for Reducing ICP

Treatments to Reduce Arterial and Venous Blood Volume

Initial efforts at controlling ICP elevations should always include elevating the head of the bed and ensuring that the neck is in a neutral position and is not being compressed. The head of the bed is elevated to 30° to enhance the venous outflow by the aid of gravity. Hard cervical collars may inhibit cerebral venous outflow and should be loosened if appropriate.

Hyperventilation can be used to lower CBV as a temporizing measure to control ICP. One major caveat is the rebound vasodilation and ICP elevation once normocapnia is restored. Unless the pathology for high ICP is cerebral hyperemia, extreme caution should be exercised with hyperventilation as vasoconstriction may precipitate further ischemic injury by reducing CBF. Nonetheless, transient or mild hyperventilation (usually to a target $PaCO_2$ of 30–35 mmHg) is reasonable as a bridge therapy until the patient undergoes a more definitive ICP-lowering procedure [22].

In general, lowering arterial blood pressure to treat ICP is not recommended because of the impact on lowering

Tier Zero (Basic Severe TBI Care - Not ICP Dependent)

Expected Interventions:

- Admission to ICU
- Endotracheal intubation and mechanical ventilation
- Serial evaluations of neurological status and pupillary reactivity
- Elevate HOB 30-45°
- Analgesia to manage signs of pain (not ICP directed)
- Sedation to prevent agitation, ventilator asynchrony, etc. (not ICP directed)
- Temperature management to prevent fever
  - *Measure core temperature*
  - *Treat core temperature above 38 °C*
- Consider anti-seizure medications for 1w only (in the absence of an indication to continue)
- Maintain CPP initially ≥ 60 mmHg
- Maintain Hb > 7g/dL
- Avoid hyponatremia
- Optimize venous return from head (eg. keeping head midline, ensure cervical collars are no too tight)
- Arterial line continuous blood pressure monitoring
- Maintain SpO2 ≥ 94%

Recommended Interventions:

- Insertion of a central line
- End-tidal CO_2 monitoring

Fig. 7.7 Tiered ICP management

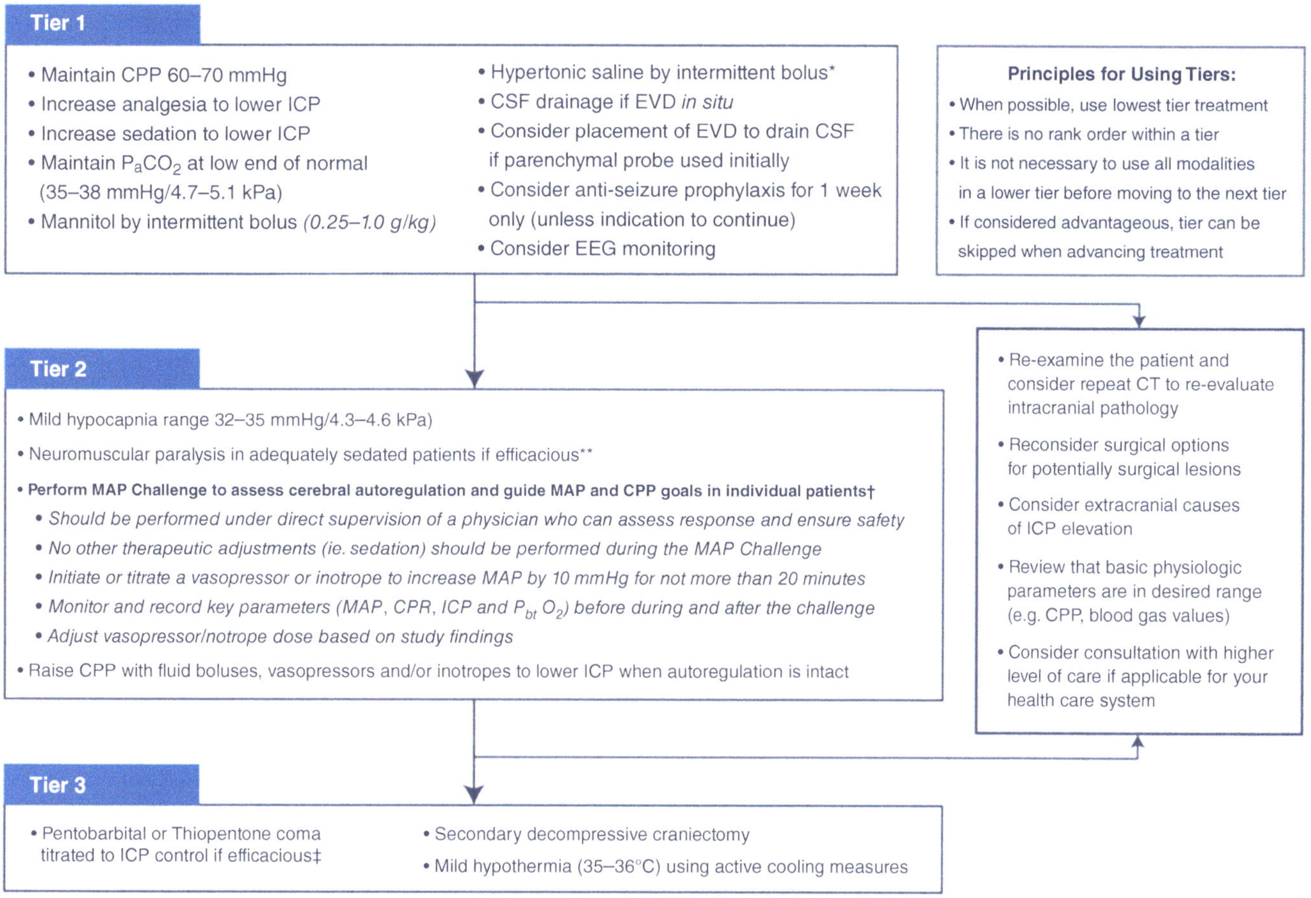

* We recommend using sodium and osmolality limits of 155 mEq/L and of 320 mEq/L respectively as administration limits for both mannitol and hypertonic saline.
** We recommend a trial dose of neuromuscular paralysis and only proceeding to a continuous infusion when efficacy is demonstrated.
† Rosenthal G. et al 2011
‡ Barbiturate administration should only be continued when a beneficial effect on ICP is demonstrated.
Titrate barbiturate to achieve ICP control but do not exceed the dose which achieves burst suppression.
Hypotension must be avoided when barbiturates are administered.

Fig. 7.7 (continued)

CPP. However, decreasing blood pressure may be reasonable to treat patients suffering from luxury perfusion, where CBF exceeds the regional cerebral metabolic requirement (such as posterior reversible encephalopathy syndrome, subacute strokes, and reperfusion syndrome following cerebral artery revascularization).

Treatments to Reduce CSF Volume

CSF diversion via an EVD is the mainstay of treating elevated ICP due to hydrocephalus or intraventricular hemorrhage (Fig. 7.9). EVDs are also frequently placed in TBI patients for the dual purpose of ICP measurement and control. To a lesser extent, lumbar drains have also been utilized in the treatment of hydrocephalus. Diuretics such as acetazolamide and furosemide have been demonstrated to decrease CSF production and CSF volume, but their effect of lowering ICP in the case of acute hydrocephalus is minimal. In addition, diuretics carry the undesirable side effect of hypovolemia, which can compound the risk of cerebral hypoperfusion.

Treatments for Brain Edema

Hyperosmolar therapy is the mainstay of treating cerebral edema. Effective osmolar solutions have tonicities that are higher than that of the brain, and an intact blood–brain barrier is necessary to act as the semipermeable membrane that maintains the osmolar gradient. Hypertonic saline (HTS) and mannitol are the most commonly used hyperosmolar solutions.

Mannitol is a carbohydrate alcohol that is administered intravenously (IV). Its mechanisms of action are twofold [42–44]. First, mannitol exerts a rheological effect by reducing blood viscosity through plasma volume expansion. This increases CBF, microvascular circulation of erythrocytes, and O_2 delivery, which can reduce ICP immediately. Second, mannitol increases serum tonicity, thereby drawing fluid from

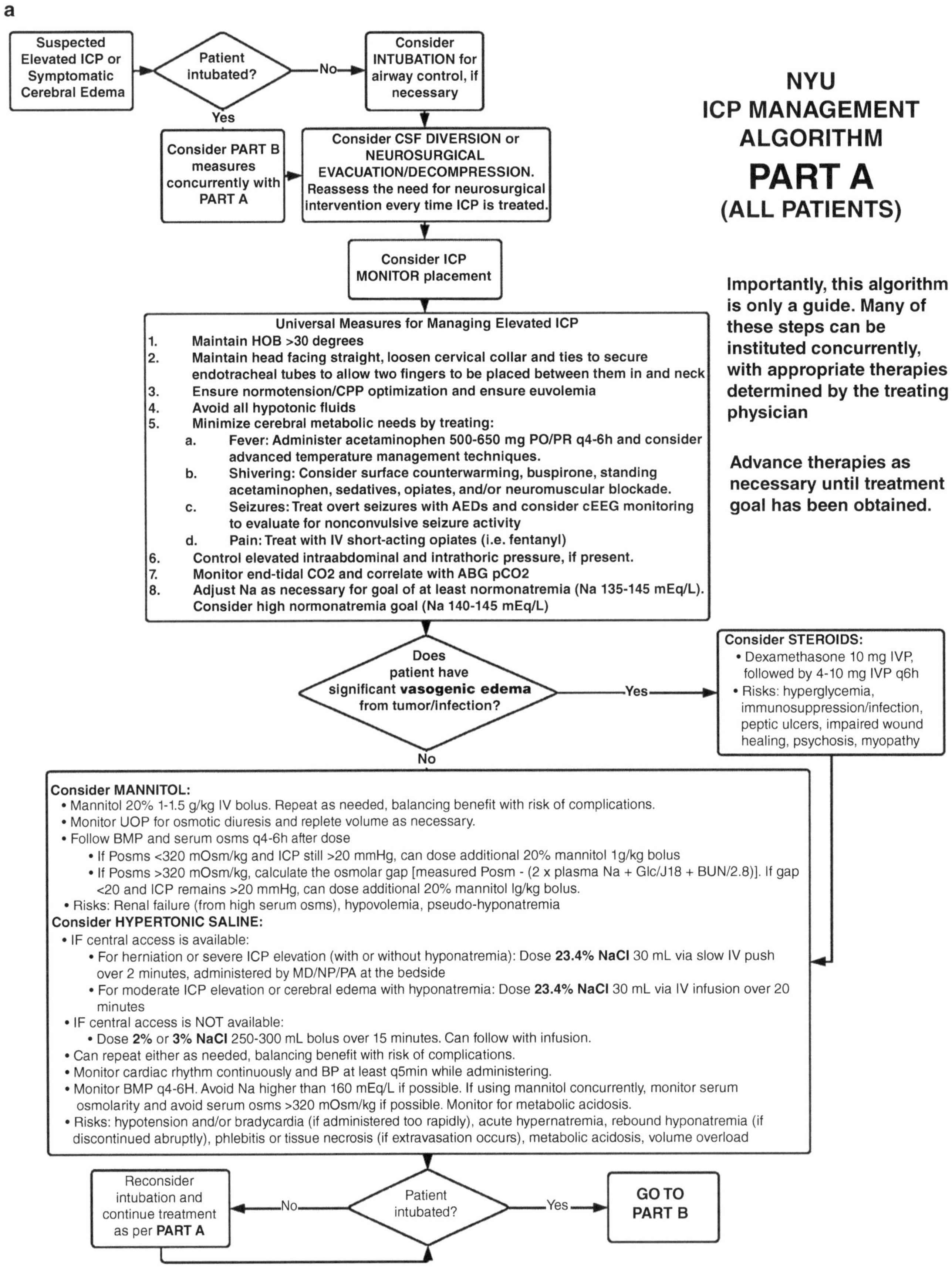

Fig. 7.8 Alternative ICP management strategy, courtesy of Barry Czeisler, MD

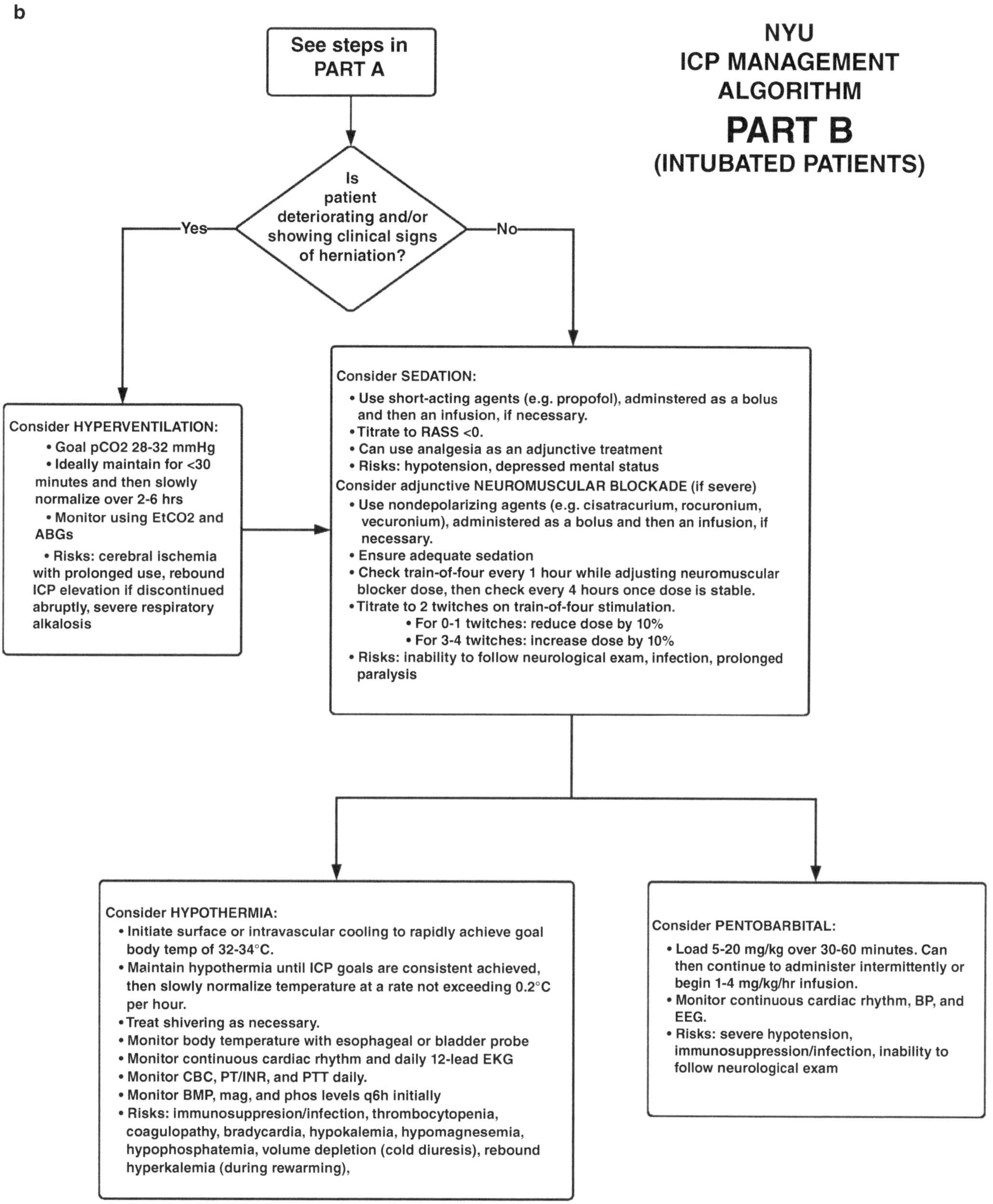

Fig. 7.8 (continued)

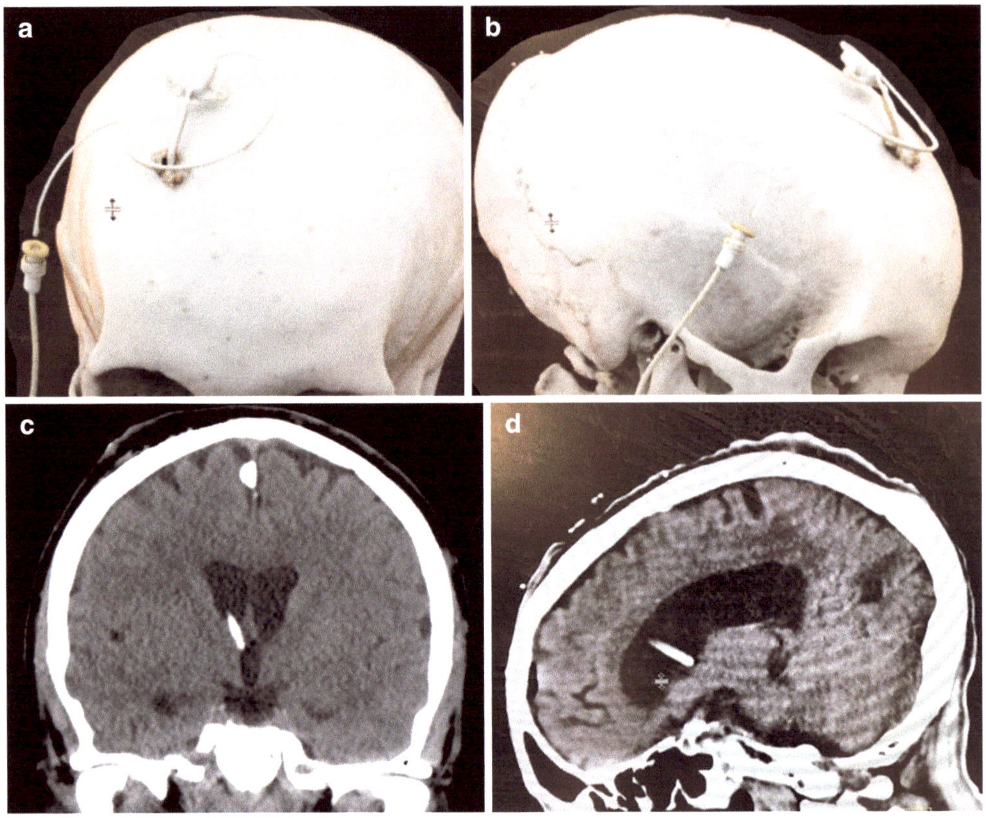

Fig. 7.9 External ventricular drain. (**a** and **b**) With EVD entering through burr hole in skull, (**c**) coronal non-contrast head CT and (**d**) sagittal non-contrast head CT with EVD traversing the lateral ventricles towards the 3rd ventricle

the brain interstitium into the intravascular space. The osmotic effect of mannitol occurs 15–30 min after administration and may last up to 1.5–6 h. Since mannitol is not renally reabsorbed and causes osmotic diuresis, care should be taken to avoid hypovolemia and associated hypotension. This can be mitigated with prompt hydration with isotonic fluid. With prolonged use, mannitol crosses the blood–brain barrier and accumulates in the brain parenchyma. Hence, bolus administration is preferred over a continuous infusion to decrease buildup [45]. Mannitol is administered in bolus doses of 0.25–1.0 g/kg of body weight, and the dosing can be repeated in a standing or as-needed manner. Because mannitol can lead to acute tubular necrosis from volume depletion, volume status and serum osmolar gap should be monitored every 4–6 h. Mannitol may be re-dosed if intravascular volume is adequate and the serum osmolarity is <320 or if the osmolarity is 320–360 and the osmolar gap is <25 [46].

HTS refers to any formulations of sodium chloride with a concentration higher than 0.9%. In the United States, commercially available HTS come in the form of 3%, 5%, and 23.4% solutions, from which other concentrations can be prepared. Unlike mannitol, HTS does not cross the blood–brain barrier and therefore has little risk of accumulating in the brain tissue. HTS can be administered as a bolus or as a continuous infusion. Standard bolus dosing is 30–60 mL of 23.4% or 250–500 mL of the 3% or 5% solution. A continuous infusion of 2% or 3% HTS usually starts at 10–30 mL/h and is titrated to a desired sodium goal. The therapeutic sodium range is not well established and may be different across individuals, but a rise in sodium by 4–6 mEq/L is effective in staving off herniation [47]. At sodium levels above 160 mmol/L, the risks of seizures and renal failure significantly increase. Clinical trials have not found a difference in mortality, neurological outcome, or effect on ICP and CPP between the bolus and continuous infusion strategies. However, continuous HTS infusion is associated with a higher rate of severe hypernatremia (Na >160 mmol/L) and thromboembolic events [48]. In theory, bolus dosing appears to be the more physiological approach. This is because brain cells rapidly adapt to the changing osmotic environment through a complex sequence of regulating transports of electrolytes and organic osmolytes across the cell membrane [12]. Therefore, the osmotic effect of a higher serum osmolarity established by a continuous HTS infusion would be abolished by concomitant changes in intracellular osmolarity. For the same reasons, prophylactic hyperosmolar therapy to prevent cerebral edema is not rationally sound. Prolonged periods of treatment with any hyperosmolar therapy are at risk of rebound cerebral edema, and the treatment should be tapered rather than stopped abruptly. Other adverse events from hypertonic saline administration include volume overload, risk of osmolar demyelination when given to patients with chronic hyponatremia, metabolic acidosis from hyperchloremia, and cardiac arrhythmias.

Since there is no high-level evidence suggesting that one hyperosmolar therapy is more efficacious than another, the choice of treatment is in part steered by its side effect profile. For example, hypertonic saline is favored over mannitol for patients with conditions that cause volume depletion or renal failure. Conversely, mannitol may be the better choice in a patient who is already volume overloaded. In the past, administration of mannitol and hypertonic saline required placement of a central venous access because of the risk of extravasation and tissue injury. However, safety data suggest that both mannitol and 23.4% HTS may be safely administered through a large-bore peripheral IV, along with continuous vigilant monitoring of the infusion site [49, 50].

Steroids do not have a role in the routine treatment of cerebral edema but may be used to treat vasogenic edema caused by brain tumors, whole brain radiation, or select cases of bacterial and fungal infections [46]. Dexamethasone is the standard agent because of its potency and minimal mineralocorticoid activity to promote fluid retention. Steroids are not recommend for TBI, intracerebral hemorrhage, and ischemic stroke due to an increased risk of mortality and infectious complications. [22, 25, 51, 52]

Initial Management to Reduce Cerebral Metabolic Demand

Another tier 1 ICP treatment strategy is to mitigate conditions that increase cerebral metabolic demand, such as pain, agitation, fever, and seizures. Analgesia is an effective treatment for pain-induced intracranial hypertension and should be the first-line therapy for postoperative patients or for those with painful traumatic injuries. Most sedatives and analgesics, especially when used in combination, can lead to significant systemic hypotension and a drop in CPP, which should be promptly corrected.

Propofol is an attractive medication for neurocritical care patients given its short half-life and ease of titration to maintain a sedated yet responsive state, with the added benefit of reducing cerebral oxygen demand and ICP [53]. Vigilant monitoring is necessary for propofol-related infusion syndrome (PRIS), a rare but fatal complication associated with bradycardia, cardiovascular collapse, rhabdomyolysis, metabolic acidosis, and renal failure. Serum triglyceride levels may serve as a biomarker for the risk of PRIS and pancreatitis, and infusion should be discontinued if triglycerides rise above 400–500 mg/dL.

Dexmedetomidine, a centrally acting alpha 2-adrenoreceptor agonist, is another commonly used sedative given its ease of titration. Its efficacy in lowering ICP in an already comatose patient is much less established. However, dexmedetomidine causes little respiratory suppression and therefore is a desirable medication for agitated, non-intubated patients at risk of intracranial hypertension and is preferred over benzodiazepines for intensive care unit (ICU) sedation [54, 55]. The side effects of bradycardia and hypotension often limit the dose of dexmedetomidine infusion.

Benzodiazepines are less desirable due to their unpredictable effects on the neurological exam and drug redistribution, especially with prolonged use, in the elderly and the obese population.. However, benzodiazepines should remain as the first-line treatment for patients with uncontrolled seizures and status epilepticus [56]. Intravenous midazolam is the most appropriate medication for continuous infusion over lorazepam or diazepam, due to the risk of propylene glycol toxicity with the latter two.

Fever is highly common in the brain-injured population and can further exacerbate the ICP crisis [57]. Repeatedly, fever has been associated with poorer neurological outcomes and higher rates of death in a variety of acute brain injuries [58]. However, there is less robust data to support that active or prophylactic fever control will improve outcomes. There is a prospective randomized controlled trial underway that assesses the effect of fever prevention in patients with acute stroke [59]. Nonetheless, most clinicians will still aggressively treat persistent fevers with standing antipyretics or external cooling.

Advanced Treatments to Reduce Cerebral Metabolism

When maximal medical and surgical treatments fail to control recalcitrant ICP, hypothermia and barbiturate coma are salvage therapies that decrease cerebral metabolic demand in order to minimize injuries from mismatch in energy delivery and consumption.

Therapeutic hypothermia (TH) has long been used for neuroprotection. The temperature-dependent neurotoxic cascade that drives secondary brain injury serves as the justification for TH. In vitro and animal models have shown that hypothermia improves neurological recovery through inhibiting apoptotic pathways, mitigating the immune-mediated inflammatory cascade, and decreasing free radical production from reperfusion injury [60, 61]. The most positive data supporting the use of TH have come from the early cardiac arrest literature, where patients who suffered from hypoxic ischemic injury had better neurological outcomes and survival if treated with TH at 32–34 °C [62, 63]. However, larger, more recent clinical studies have called into question whether the survival benefit after a cardiac arrest was indeed due to TH or instead because of aggressive fever control and standardized period of observation before neurological prognostication. Several prospective trials in TBI have demonstrated the efficacy of hypothermia in reducing ICP, but this has not translated into definitive improvements in neurological outcomes [64–66]. A meta-analysis of preclinical studies found evidence that TH decreased perihematomal edema and improved outcomes in nontraumatic intraparenchymal hemorrhage, although data from large clinical trials are still pending at this time [61, 67]. The complications of TH are nontrivial; these include coagulopathy, hyperglycemia, immune suppression, cardiac arrhythmias, electrolyte imbalance, rhabdomyolysis, and side effects related to prolonged sedation and paralysis to treat shivering. Skin breakdown and thermal injury are serious side effects of external cooling devices, and intravascular cooling devices carry the risk of line-associated infections and thromboses. Rewarming from TH must be carried out with caution, as rapid rewarming can lead to hemodynamic instability, severe electrolyte imbalance, rhabdomyolysis, and rebound ICP crisis.

Pentobarbital has long been in use to decrease cerebral metabolic expenditure for treating an ICP crisis [68]. Only one randomized trial showed that pentobarbital was associated with improved ICP control as compared to standard therapy, and patients whose ICP responded to pentobarbital achieved better neurological outcomes than did nonresponders [69]. Nonetheless, a meta-analysis of the randomized control trials on pentobarbital did not demonstrate any outcome benefit [70]. A major drawback of barbiturates is hypotension due to suppression of sympathetic tone, causing peripheral vasodilation and diminished myocardial contractility, and thereby decreasing brain perfusion. Pentobarbital coma requires continuous electroencephalogram (EEG) monitoring to guide appropriate dosing. Pentobarbital has a long half-life of 15–50 h and can significantly confound the neurological exam and mimic brain death by obscuring pupillary light response and other cranial nerve reflexes. As such, pentobarbital poses additional challenges to determining brain death in individuals with neurological demise. A protracted period of time is required for the serum drug level to fall below the therapeutic range before brain death examination can be initiated [71]. Other complications of pentobarbital include ileus, pneumonia, and mucous plugging due to diminished respiratory ciliary cell function and immune suppression, causing higher rates of infections.

Surgical Decompression for Focal Mass Lesions and Intracranial Hemorrhage

Evacuating hematomas and resecting tumors is the logical solution for managing ICP and neurological deterioration caused by these intracranial lesions. Removal of tumors will often result in rapid reduction of the volume occupied by the tumor as well as by the peritumor edema. For evacuation of intracranial hemorrhage, the data are more nuanced. The decision to evacuate various types of traumatic hemorrhages is based on the volume and mass effect of the hematoma, the neurological examination, and the surrounding clinical circumstances [72–75].

Previous studies showed that early evacuation of nontraumatic intracerebral hemorrhages did not improve mortality or functional outcomes as compared to conservative management [76], although a subset of patients with lobar hemorrhages close to the cortical surface and features of poor prognosis may benefit from early surgery [77]. In recent years, several minimally invasive surgical techniques have been developed for evacuating deep subcortical hematomas. The first randomized trial that studied the outcome of stereotactic removal of hematoma, followed by lysis of the residual clot with alteplase, showed no improvement in the mortality or functional outcome associated with surgical evacuation [78]. The low rate of adequate hematoma evacuation, as well as the variable experience among surgeons with this particular technique, may have contributed to this trial's null result. Additional trials are underway to examine the impact of different minimally invasive surgical techniques on nontraumatic intracerebral hemorrhages [79, 80].

Prophylactic bifrontal craniectomy for TBI is no longer routinely performed due to results from the Decompressive Craniectomy (DECRA) trial, in which TBI patients with ICP above 20 mmHg were randomized to either early prophylactic bifrontal craniectomy or continued medical management [81]. The study found that patients who underwent surgery had worse functional outcomes and higher mortality despite having initially fewer incidents of ICP elevation, received less ICP-oriented treatment, and had fewer ICU days. Aside from the possible explanation that bifrontal craniectomy does not confer functional or mortality benefit on patients with TBI-related diffuse cerebral edema, the study also had several design flaws that may have biased the conclusion. For one, the surgical arm had a higher number of patients with bilateral fixed pupils, indicating more severe injury. Two, most surgical patients did not fail medical treatments for high ICP initially as ICP was well controlled in both groups, suggesting that surgical decompression is not superior to medical therapy in the absence of recalcitrant ICP. The Randomized Evaluation of Surgery with Craniectomy for Uncontrollable Elevation of Intracranial Pressure (RESCUEicp) trial addressed some of DECRA's limitations by enrolling patients who demonstrated failure of both tier 1 and tier 2 therapies. Even though the surgical treatment included both hemicraniectomy and bifrontal craniectomy, the majority of the patients who received surgery still underwent bifrontal craniectomies (63%). Patients who received surgery had a higher rate of survival but were more likely to remain in a vegetative state [82]. Synthesizing the findings from DECRA and RESCUEicp, the updated BTF 2020 guidelines on decompressive craniectomy recommend secondary decompressive craniectomy to be performed for late refractory ICP and against decompressive craniectomy for early ICP elevations (<72 h) [83]. As such, craniectomy remains as a salvage therapy for select patients who fail other aggressive medical treatments.

Decompressive hemicraniectomy (DHC) is a common neurosurgical procedure to treat intracranial hypertension in a variety of brain injuries caused by focal mass lesions, including traumatic brain injury with focal contusions or subdural hematomas, ischemic strokes with malignant cerebral edema, and intracranial hemorrhage [84]. An effective DHC requires a large enough area of bone removal to allow for hemispheric decompression as well as an adequate durotomy. DHC is also associated with morbid complications, including derangements in CSF reabsorption and paradoxical brain herniation.

In both the TBI and ischemic stroke literature, DHC has been consistently shown to reduce the mortality associated with intracranial hypertension, but not necessarily improve functional outcomes, with some studies showing even a worse neurological function in the surviving elderly patients [84]. According to a pooled analysis of DHC in ischemic stroke trials separated by age, younger patients (age < 60 years) had a 18% chance of achieving functional independence, whereas none of the older patients regained independence [52]. DHC for strokes with malignant cerebral edema has the highest likelihood of achieving a fair outcome when performed in the first 48 h and in younger patients with a "good" neurological exam. Some practitioners are still dissuaded from offering DHC to patients with dominant hemispheric strokes, citing worse functionality and quality of life caused by aphasia. There is not enough evidence from clinical trials to support that dominant hemispheric strokes indeed have worse quality of life compared to the nondominant ones. Therefore, in order to promote a patient-centered decision-making process about surgery, it is particularly important that providers always clearly communicate expectations of what DHC accomplishes and the likely neurological prognosis.

Conclusions

Intracranial hypertension is a neurological emergency when it causes decreased cerebral perfusion or leads to brain herniation. Diseases that are associated with an increase in the volume of any of the intracranial compartments can precipitate intracranial hypertension. Knowledge of the basics of cerebral hemodynamics is essential to understanding the clinical implications of elevated ICP. Familiarity with the signs and symptoms of elevated ICP and herniation syndromes allows prompt recognition and treatment of intracranial hypertension. Knowing the indications for ICP monitoring is important as is understanding how to interpret the ICP value and waveform in relation to other physiological markers. The decision tree for treating clinical intracranial hypertension or an elevated ICP value should include an assessment of the entire clinical picture, the patient's neurological exam, and the risk of secondary brain injuries if treatment is delayed. ICP is best managed by directly addressing the underlying cause of intracranial hypertension, combined with a systematic and tiered approach of lowering ICP. A thorough understanding of cerebral physiology and the broad array of available treatment strategies and their side effects will enhance the care of the patient with intracranial hypertension.

Acknowledgments The *authors* thank A. Joseph Layon, Andrea Gabrielli, and Shelly D. Timmons for the provision of the chapter on elevated intracranial pressure from the previous editions of this book as guidance.

References

1. Kellie G. An account of the appearances observed in the dissection of two of three individuals presumed to have perished in the storm of the 3d, and whose bodies were discovered in the vicinity of Leith on the morning of the 4th, November 1821; with some reflections on the pathology of the brain: part I. Trans Med Chir Soc Edinb. 1824;1:84–122.
2. Kety SS, Schmidt CF. The nitrous oxide method for the quantitative determination of cerebral blood flow in man: theory, procedure and normal values. J Clin Invest. 1948;27(4):476–83.
3. Lassen NA. Cerebral blood flow and oxygen consumption in man. Physiol Rev. 1959;39(2):183–238.
4. Ainslie PN, Duffin J. Integration of cerebrovascular CO2 reactivity and chemoreflex control of breathing: mechanisms of regulation, measurement, and interpretation. Am J Physiol Regul Integr Comp Physiol. 2009;296(5):R1473–95.
5. Patel PM, Drummond JC, Lemkuil BP. Cerebral physiology and the effects of anethetic drugs. In: Miller RD, editor. Miller's anesthesia. Elsevier Health Sciences; 2019. p. 294–332.
6. Tymko MM, Ainslie PN. To regulate, or not to regulate? The devious history of cerebral blood flow control. J Physiol. 2017;595(16):5407–8.
7. Drummond JC. The lower limit of autoregulation: time to revise our thinking? Anesthesiology. 1997;86(6):1431–3.
8. de Jong DLK, Tarumi T, Liu J, Zhang R, Claassen J. Lack of linear correlation between dynamic and steady-state cerebral autoregulation. J Physiol. 2017;595(16):5623–36.
9. Wilson MH. Monro-Kellie 2.0: the dynamic vascular and venous pathophysiological components of intracranial pressure. J Cereb Blood Flow Metab. 2016;36(8):1338–50.
10. Sakka L, Coll G, Chazal J. Anatomy and physiology of cerebrospinal fluid. Eur Ann Otorhinolaryngol Head Neck Dis. 2011;128(6):309–16.
11. Lyden PD, Zweifler R, Mahdavi Z, Lonzo L. A rapid, reliable, and valid method for measuring infarct and brain compartment volumes from computed tomographic scans. Stroke. 1994;25(12):2421–8.
12. Wilson CS, Mongin AA. Cell volume control in healthy brain and Neuropathologies. Curr Top Membr. 2018;81:385–455.
13. Cushing H. Concerning a definite regulatory mechanism of the vasomotor centers which controls blood pressure during cerebral compression. Bull Johns Hopkins Hosp. 1901;12:290.
14. Schmidt EA, Despas F, Pavy-Le Traon A, Czosnyka Z, Pickard JD, Rahmouni K, et al. Intracranial pressure is a determinant of sympathetic activity. Front Physiol. 2018;9:11.
15. Tsai YH, Lin JY, Huang YY, Wong JM. Cushing response-based warning system for intensive care of brain-injured patients. Clin Neurophysiol. 2018;129(12):2602–12.
16. Lau EO, Lo CY, Yao Y, Mak AF, Jiang L, Huang Y, et al. Aortic baroreceptors display higher Mechanosensitivity than carotid baroreceptors. Front Physiol. 2016;7:384.

17. Pirahanchi Y, Bordoni B. Anatomy, head and neck, carotid baroreceptors. In: StatPearls. Treasure Island (FL): StatPearls Publishing., Copyright © 2021, StatPearls Publishing LLC.; 2021.
18. Adler DE, Milhorat TH. The tentorial notch: anatomical variation, morphometric analysis, and classification in 100 human autopsy cases. J Neurosurg. 2002;96(6):1103–12.
19. Fred P, Jermone P. The diagnosis of stupor and coma. 3rd ed. Philadelphia: Oxford University Press; 1982.
20. Gerber LM, Chiu YL, Carney N, Härtl R, Ghajar J. Marked reduction in mortality in patients with severe traumatic brain injury. J Neurosurg. 2013;119(6):1583–90.
21. Farahvar A, Gerber LM, Chiu YL, Carney N, Härtl R, Ghajar J. Increased mortality in patients with severe traumatic brain injury treated without intracranial pressure monitoring. J Neurosurg. 2012;117(4):729–34.
22. Carney N, Totten AM, O'Reilly C, Ullman JS, Hawryluk GW, Bell MJ, et al. Guidelines for the Management of Severe Traumatic Brain Injury, Fourth Edition. Neurosurgery. 2017;80(1):6–15.
23. Chesnut RM, Bleck TP, Citerio G, Classen J, Cooper DJ, Coplin WM, et al. A consensus-based interpretation of the benchmark evidence from south American trials: treatment of intracranial pressure trial. J Neurotrauma. 2015;32(22):1722–4.
24. Connolly ES Jr, Rabinstein AA, Carhuapoma JR, Derdeyn CP, Dion J, Higashida RT, et al. Guidelines for the management of aneurysmal subarachnoid hemorrhage: a guideline for healthcare professionals from the American Heart Association/american Stroke Association. Stroke. 2012;43(6):1711–37.
25. Hemphill JC, Greenberg SM, Anderson CS, Becker K, Bendok BR, Cushman M, et al. Guidelines for the Management of Spontaneous Intracerebral Hemorrhage: a guideline for healthcare professionals from the American Heart Association/American Stroke Association. Stroke. 2015;46(7):2032–60.
26. Reynolds AS, Brush B, Schiano TD, Reilly KJ, Dangayach NS. Neurological monitoring in acute liver failure. Hepatology. 2019;70(5):1830–5.
27. Stravitz RT, Kramer AH, Davern T, Shaikh AO, Caldwell SH, Mehta RL, et al. Intensive care of patients with acute liver failure: recommendations of the U.S. acute liver failure study group. Crit Care Med. 2007;35(11):2498–508.
28. Karvellas CJ, Fix OK, Battenhouse H, Durkalski V, Sanders C, Lee WM. Outcomes and complications of intracranial pressure monitoring in acute liver failure: a retrospective cohort study. Crit Care Med. 2014;42(5):1157–67.
29. Keays RT, Alexander GJ, Williams R. The safety and value of extradural intracranial pressure monitors in fulminant hepatic failure. J Hepatol. 1993;18(2):205–9.
30. Vaquero J, Fontana RJ, Larson AM, Bass NM, Davern TJ, Shakil AO, et al. Complications and use of intracranial pressure monitoring in patients with acute liver failure and severe encephalopathy. Liver Transpl. 2005;11(12):1581–9.
31. Reuben A, Tillman H, Fontana RJ, Davern T, McGuire B, Stravitz RT, et al. Outcomes in adults with acute liver failure between 1998 and 2013: an observational cohort study. Ann Intern Med. 2016;164(11):724–32.
32. Cardoso ER, Reddy K, Bose D. Effect of subarachnoid hemorrhage on intracranial pulse waves in cats. J Neurosurg. 1988;69(5):712–8.
33. Klassen PA, Cardoso ER, Shwedyk E. Haemodynamic modelling for the arterial pulsatile component of the intracranial pulse wave. Neurol Res. 1991;13(3):194–8.
34. Kirkness CJ, Mitchell PH, Burr RL, March KS, Newell DW. Intracranial pressure waveform analysis: clinical and research implications. J Neurosci Nurs. 2000;32(5):271–7.
35. Lundberg N. Continuous recording and control of ventricular fluid pressure in neurosurgical practice. Acta Psychiatr Scand Suppl. 1960;36(149):1–193.
36. Daley ML, Leffler CW, Czosnyka M, Pickard JD. Plateau waves: changes of cerebrovascular pressure transmission. Acta Neurochir Suppl. 2005;95:327–32.
37. Wijdicks EFM. Lundberg and his waves. Neurocrit Care. 2019;31(3):546–9.
38. Tas J, Beqiri E, van Kaam RC, Czosnyka M, Donnelly J, Haeren RH, et al. Targeting autoregulation-guided cerebral perfusion pressure after traumatic brain injury (COGiTATE): a feasibility randomized controlled clinical trial. J Neurotrauma. 2021;38(20):2790–800.
39. Aries MJ, Czosnyka M, Budohoski KP, Kolias AG, Radolovich DK, Lavinio A, et al. Continuous monitoring of cerebrovascular reactivity using pulse waveform of intracranial pressure. Neurocrit Care. 2012;17(1):67–76.
40. Aries MJ, Czosnyka M, Budohoski KP, Steiner LA, Lavinio A, Kolias AG, et al. Continuous determination of optimal cerebral perfusion pressure in traumatic brain injury. Crit Care Med. 2012;40(8):2456–63.
41. Hawryluk GWJ, Aguilera S, Buki A, Bulger E, Citerio G, Cooper DJ, et al. A management algorithm for patients with intracranial pressure monitoring: the Seattle international severe traumatic brain injury consensus conference (SIBICC). Intensive Care Med. 2019;45(12):1783–94.
42. Barry KG, Berman AR, Mannitol infusion. III. The acute effect of the intravenous infusion of mannitol on blood and plasma volumes. N Engl J Med. 1961;264:1085–8.
43. James HE. Methodology for the control of intracranial pressure with hypertonic mannitol. Acta Neurochir. 1980;51(3–4):161–72.
44. McGraw CP, Howard G. Effect of mannitol on increased intracranial pressure. Neurosurgery. 1983;13(3):269–71.
45. Kaufmann AM, Cardoso ER. Aggravation of vasogenic cerebral edema by multiple-dose mannitol. J Neurosurg. 1992;77(4):584–9.
46. Roberts I, Yates D, Sandercock P, Farrell B, Wasserberg J, Lomas G, et al. Effect of intravenous corticosteroids on death within 14 days in 10008 adults with clinically significant head injury (MRC CRASH trial): randomised placebo-controlled trial. Lancet. 2004;364(9442):1321–8.
47. Sterns RH, Silver SM. Complications and management of hyponatremia. Curr Opin Nephrol Hypertens. 2016;25(2):114–9.
48. Roquilly A, Moyer JD, Huet O, Lasocki S, Cohen B, Dahyot-Fizelier C, et al. Effect of continuous infusion of hypertonic saline vs standard care on 6-month neurological outcomes in patients with traumatic brain injury: the COBI randomized clinical trial. JAMA. 2021;325(20):2056–66.
49. Dillon RC, Merchan C, Altshuler D, Papadopoulos J. Incidence of adverse events during peripheral Administration of Sodium Chloride 3. J Intensive Care Med. 2018;33(1):48–53.
50. Faiver L, Hensler D, Rush SC, Kashlan O, Williamson CA, Rajajee V. Safety and efficacy of 23.4% sodium chloride administered via peripheral venous access for the treatment of cerebral herniation and intracranial pressure elevation. Neurocrit Care. 2021;35(3):845–52.
51. Cook AM, Morgan Jones G, Hawryluk GWJ, Mailloux P, McLaughlin D, Papangelou A, et al. Guidelines for the acute treatment of cerebral edema in Neurocritical care patients. Neurocrit Care. 2020;32(3):647–66.
52. Powers WJ, Rabinstein AA, Ackerson T, Adeoye OM, Bambakidis NC, Becker K, et al. Guidelines for the early Management of Patients with Acute Ischemic Stroke: 2019 update to the 2018 guidelines for the early Management of Acute Ischemic Stroke: a guideline for healthcare professionals from the American Heart Association/American Stroke Association. Stroke. 2019;50(12):e344–418.
53. Kelly DF, Goodale DB, Williams J, Herr DL, Chappell ET, Rosner MJ, et al. Propofol in the treatment of moderate and severe head injury: a randomized, prospective double-blinded pilot trial. J Neurosurg. 1999;90(6):1042–52.

54. Aryan HE, Box KW, Ibrahim D, Desiraju U, Ames CP. Safety and efficacy of dexmedetomidine in neurosurgical patients. Brain Inj. 2006;20(8):791–8.
55. Saver JL, Goyal M, Bonafe A, Diener HC, Levy EI, Pereira VM, et al. Stent-retriever thrombectomy after intravenous t-PA vs. t-PA alone in stroke. N Engl J Med. 2015;372(24):2285–95.
56. Brophy GM, Bell R, Claassen J, Alldredge B, Bleck TP, Glauser T, et al. Guidelines for the evaluation and management of status epilepticus. Neurocrit Care. 2012;17(1):3–23.
57. Kilpatrick MM, Lowry DW, Firlik AD, Yonas H, Marion DW. Hyperthermia in the neurosurgical intensive care unit. Neurosurgery. 2000;47(4):850–5; discussion 5–6.
58. Rincon F, Hunter K, Schorr C, Dellinger RP, Zanotti-Cavazzoni S. The epidemiology of spontaneous fever and hypothermia on admission of brain injury patients to intensive care units: a multicenter cohort study. J Neurosurg. 2014;121(4):950–60.
59. Greer DM, Ritter J, Helbok R, Badjatia N, Ko SB, Guanci M, et al. Impact of fever prevention in brain-injured patients (INTREPID): study protocol for a randomized controlled trial. Neurocrit Care. 2021;35(2):577–89.
60. Polderman K, Lockhart K, Badjatia N. Temperature management in neurological and neurosurgical intensive care units. Ther Hypothermia Temp Manag. 2014;4(2):62–6.
61. Melmed KR, Lyden PD. Meta-analysis of pre-clinical trials of therapeutic hypothermia for intracerebral hemorrhage. Ther Hypothermia Temp Manag. 2017;7(3):141–6.
62. Hypothermia after Cardiac Arrest Study Group. Mild therapeutic hypothermia to improve the neurologic outcome after cardiac arrest. N Engl J Med. 2002;346(8):549–56.
63. Bernard SA, Gray TW, Buist MD, Jones BM, Silvester W, Gutteridge G, et al. Treatment of comatose survivors of out-of-hospital cardiac arrest with induced hypothermia. N Engl J Med. 2002;346(8):557–63.
64. Clifton GL, Valadka A, Zygun D, Coffey CS, Drever P, Fourwinds S, et al. Very early hypothermia induction in patients with severe brain injury (the National Acute Brain Injury Study: hypothermia II): a randomised trial. Lancet Neurol. 2011;10(2):131–9.
65. Andrews PJ, Harris BA, Murray GD. Hypothermia for Intracranial Hypertension after Traumatic Brain Injury. N Engl J Med. 2016;374:1385.
66. Lyden P, Hemmen T, Grotta J, Rapp K, Ernstrom K, Rzesiewicz T, et al. Results of the ICTuS 2 trial (intravascular cooling in the treatment of stroke 2). Stroke. 2016;47(12):2888–95.
67. Dumitrascu OM, Lamb J, Lyden PD. Still cooling after all these years: meta-analysis of pre-clinical trials of therapeutic hypothermia for acute ischemic stroke. J Cereb Blood Flow Metab. 2016;36(7):1157–64.
68. Lyons MK, Meyer FB. Cerebrospinal fluid physiology and the management of increased intracranial pressure. Mayo Clin Proc. 1990;65(5):684–707.
69. Eisenberg HM, Frankowski RF, Contant CF, Marshall LF, Walker MD. High-dose barbiturate control of elevated intracranial pressure in patients with severe head injury. J Neurosurg. 1988;69(1):15–23.
70. Roberts I, Sydenham E. Barbiturates for acute traumatic brain injury. Cochrane Database Syst Rev. 2012;12(12):Cd000033.
71. Wijdicks EF, Varelas PN, Gronseth GS, Greer DM. Evidence-based guideline update: determining brain death in adults: report of the quality standards Subcommittee of the American Academy of neurology. Neurology. 2010;74(23):1911–8.
72. Bullock MR, Chesnut R, Ghajar J, Gordon D, Hartl R, Newell DW, et al. Surgical management of posterior fossa mass lesions. Neurosurgery. 2006;58(3 Suppl):S47–55; discussion Si-iv.
73. Bullock MR, Chesnut R, Ghajar J, Gordon D, Hartl R, Newell DW, et al. Surgical management of traumatic parenchymal lesions. Neurosurgery. 2006;58(3 Suppl):S25–46; discussion Si-iv.
74. Bullock MR, Chesnut R, Ghajar J, Gordon D, Hartl R, Newell DW, et al. Surgical management of acute epidural hematomas. Neurosurgery. 2006;58(3 Suppl):S7–15; discussion Si-iv.
75. Bullock MR, Chesnut R, Ghajar J, Gordon D, Hartl R, Newell DW, et al. Surgical management of acute subdural hematomas. Neurosurgery. 2006;58(3 Suppl):S16–24; discussion Si-iv.
76. Mendelow AD, Gregson BA, Fernandes HM, Murray GD, Teasdale GM, Hope DT, et al. Early surgery versus initial conservative treatment in patients with spontaneous supratentorial intracerebral haematomas in the international surgical trial in intracerebral Haemorrhage (STICH): a randomised trial. Lancet. 2005;365(9457):387–97.
77. Mendelow AD, Gregson BA, Rowan EN, Murray GD, Gholkar A, Mitchell PM, et al. Early surgery versus initial conservative treatment in patients with spontaneous supratentorial lobar intracerebral haematomas (STICH II): a randomised trial. Lancet. 2013;382(9890):397–408.
78. Hanley DF, Thompson RE, Rosenblum M, Yenokyan G, Lane K, McBee N, et al. Efficacy and safety of minimally invasive surgery with thrombolysis in intracerebral haemorrhage evacuation (MISTIE III): a randomised, controlled, open-label, blinded endpoint phase 3 trial. Lancet. 2019;393(10175):1021–32.
79. Kellner CP, Song R, Pan J, Nistal DA, Scaggiante J, Chartrain AG, et al. Long-term functional outcome following minimally invasive endoscopic intracerebral hemorrhage evacuation. J Neurointerv Surg. 2020;12(5):489–94.
80. Kobata H, Ikeda N. Recent updates in neurosurgical interventions for spontaneous intracerebral hemorrhage: minimally invasive surgery to improve surgical performance. Front Neurol. 2021;12:703189.
81. Cooper DJ, Rosenfeld JV, Murray L, Arabi YM, Davies AR, Ponsford J, et al. Patient outcomes at twelve months after early Decompressive Craniectomy for diffuse traumatic brain injury in the randomized DECRA clinical trial. J Neurotrauma. 2020;37(5):810–6.
82. Hutchinson PJ, Kolias AG, Timofeev IS, Corteen EA, Czosnyka M, Timothy J, et al. Trial of Decompressive Craniectomy for traumatic intracranial hypertension. N Engl J Med. 2016;375(12):1119–30.
83. Hawryluk GWJ, Rubiano AM, Totten AM, O'Reilly C, Ullman JS, Bratton SL, et al. Guidelines for the Management of Severe Traumatic Brain Injury: 2020 update of the Decompressive Craniectomy recommendations. Neurosurgery. 2020;87(3):427–34.
84. Lin J, Frontera JA. Decompressive Hemicraniectomy for large hemispheric strokes. Stroke. 2021;52(4):1500–10.

Acute Focal Deficit

8

Jasmine Singh and Rick Gill

Contents

Abstract

Recognizing an acute change in clinical status is critical in patients with neurologic injury. Priority should be given to the patient's airway, breathing, and circulation, and subsequent localization of focal deficits which will guide stabilization and management decisions. Close attention should be paid to the recognition of hemodynamic and respiratory changes that may suggest an acute intracranial process or neurologic emergency. In the case of a clinical emergency, such as brain herniation, stabilization and initial management is often followed by urgent radiographic imaging. Multimodal monitoring may be considered when there is a concern for elevated intracranial pressure (ICP), or alterations in cerebral hemodynamics and metabolism. In the absence of a new identifiable lesion, seizures should be on the differential diagnosis and surface or depth EEG (electroencephalogram) may be considered. Alternative diagnoses such as metabolic disturbances, infections, or toxins may need to be considered in the absence of a primary neurologic cause. In the case of blood pressure variations, various shock classifications should be investigated and treated appropriately.

Introduction

Chapter Goals

- Arousal and cranial nerve assessment.
- How to approach aphasia.
- Understanding various breathing patterns associated with central lesions.
- Understanding cerebrovascular hemodynamics.
- Recognize different herniation syndromes.
- Evaluation of shock.
- When to obtain further imaging and studies.

J. Singh
Neurocritical Care, University of California San Diego Health, San Diego, CA, USA

R. Gill (✉)
Department of Neurology, Loyola University Medical Center, Maywood, IL, USA

E. Mahanna Gabrielli et al. (eds.), *Textbook of Neurointensive Care: Volume 1*, https://doi.org/10.1007/978-3-031-62220-5_8

Key Clinical Questions

The chapter will answer:

- What are the localizing features of pupillary deficits?
- How should aphasia be assessed?
- What exam findings are present in different herniation syndromes?
- What changes in vital signs should be monitored closely as an indication of change in cerebrovascular hemodynamics?

Essential Management Priorities

Early: Immediate and First 24 h

Examination and Localization

The initial assessment of a patient with neurologic injury should include an assessment of the patient's level of arousal as this may indicate dysfunction of the components of the ascending reticular activating system (ARAS), a collection of nuclei in network primarily responsible in the regulation of consciousness. Global cerebral injury such as anoxic brain injury, trauma resulting in diffuse axonal injury or elevated intracranial pressure, seizure and status epilepticus are only a few examples of conditions that can impair the level of consciousness. The ARAS is primarily composed of four main centers: the locus coeruleus, raphe nuclei, the posterior hypothalamus, and the pontine tegmentum. Each of these centers is made up of multiple nuclei which contain many neurotransmitters involved in the neuronal circuits of wakefulness [1]. Changes in the level of arousal may be an early indication of a change in the patient's clinical state. Obtundation is a mild-to-moderate reduction in alertness, whereas stupor is the state when the patient can only be aroused with vigorous and continuous stimulation [2]. Coma occurs when the patient has no meaningful response to even vigorous stimulation and appears in a sleep like state with the eyes closed [2].

If able, language should also be evaluated in its main components of comprehension, fluency, naming, and repetition which will normally localize to the parasylvian regions of the dominant hemisphere, however, these may extend deeper in the thalamus or caudate/putamen (Table 8.1). Fluency and comprehension can be evaluated through conversational evaluation of the patient's ability to understand and follow commands starting with simple and then multistep commands and beginning with central commands with progression to appendicular commands. Patients with nonfluent speech will speak slowly with frequent pauses, have word-finding difficulties, and may omit connecting words in a sentence [3]. In a conduction aphasia, repetition of speech can be impaired and may be evaluated by asking the patient to repeat a short sentence. A conduction aphasia will indicate a lesion in the arcuate fasciculus. Additionally, certain types of language impairments can also affect naming in which patients may make paraphasic errors. All these components should be evaluated when assessing language as a new deficit may indicate a new lesion. A Broca's aphasia will typically present with non-fluent speech and good comprehension and will localize to the inferior frontal gyrus of the dominant hemisphere, typically the left hemisphere. A Wernicke's aphasia will present with fluent speech and poor comprehension which localizes to the superior gyrus of the dominant temporal lobe [3]. The assessment of aphasia is often more complex, and patients often have impairments in more than one domain. Dysarthria or slurred speech should not be confused with aphasia. Dysarthria may by be the sequelae of neuromuscular weakness of the face or oropharynx. Conditions commonly associated with dysarthria vary greatly from amyotrophic lateral sclerosis and myasthenia gravis to acute stroke, alcohol intoxication, and traumatic brain injury.

Table 8.1 Evaluation of Language—Aphasia types and clinical findings in each

Aphasia type	Clinical findings
Expressive (Broca's)	Nonfluent, good comprehension, impaired repetition, and naming
Receptive (Wernicke's)	Fluent, poor comprehension, impaired repetition, and naming
Transcortical motor	Nonfluent, good comprehension, intact repetition, and naming
Transcortical sensory	Fluent, poor comprehension, intact repetition, and naming
Conduction	Fluent, good comprehension, impaired repetition, and naming
Global	Nonfluent, poor comprehension, impaired repetition, and naming

Following an assessment of level of arousal, orientation, and language function, the cranial nerves should be examined as they may offer clues to the presence of a burgeoning neurologic emergency. Physiologic constriction of the pupil is mediated by the parasympathetic nervous system's cholinergic innervation of the pupillary sphincter, whereas the sympathetic nervous system mediates pupillary dilation. Pupillary reaction is facilitated by the optic nerve (cranial nerve [CN] II) receiving input of light which then travels to the superior colliculus followed by the dorsal midbrain to reach the synapse in the olivary pretectal nucleus [4]. Here, the fibers then travel to the Edinger–Westphal nucleus to form the parasympathetic fibers of oculomotor nerve (CN III) to the ciliary ganglion in the orbit which innervate the pupillary constrictors and ciliary muscles. An abnormality in the pupillary light reflex can manifest as an afferent pupillary defect, also known as a relative afferent pupillary defect (RAPD). RAPD occurs when there is a discrepancy in the response of the pupils to light between the two eyes, suggesting a dysfunction in the optic nerve or retina. It is typically observed as a reduced pupillary constriction or even paradoxical dilation of the affected eye when exposed to light. RAPD is often associated with optic nerve disorders, such as optic neuritis or optic nerve compression, and it can be detected using the swinging flashlight test during a neurological examination.

Pupillary dilation is mediated by the sympathetic nervous system, which consists of a three-neuron system. Additionally, this pathway innervates Mueller's muscle (a minor contributor to eyelid elevation) and the sweat glands of the face; impairment of this system results in the triad of miosis, ptosis, and anhidrosis (Horner's syndrome). The first-order neuron is located in the periventricular and arcuate nuclei of the ipsilateral hypothalamus which communicates caudally through the lateral brainstem and cervical spine to synapse on the second-order neurons at the ciliospinal nucleus of Budge which extends from C8 to T2 [4]. The second-order neuron, the preganglionic sympathetic neuron, then exits through the ventral roots of the spinal cord to ascend through the thorax along the common carotid artery to synapse via Type II nicotinic acetylcholine (AcH) receptors onto the superior cervical ganglion [4]. The third-order postganglionic neuron travels from the carotid bulb along the internal carotid artery through the cavernous sinus to follow the ophthalmic artery into the orbit to synapse on the dilator pupillae muscle causing pupillary dilation [4]. Understanding anatomy can assist in the localization when pupillary abnormalities are noted on exam. A monocular constricted pupil can indicate denervation of the sympathetic input to the pupillary dilator. This finding could result from damage to a first-order neuron in the hypothalamus; however, the most common pathologies affecting the first-order neuron include brainstem strokes, such as the lateral medullary infarction (Wallenberg's syndrome) which often is the result of thromboembolism of the vertebral or posterior inferior cerebellar arteries. Associated lower brainstem dysfunction of the Wallenberg's syndrome includes ipsilateral tongue deviation, hoarseness, ipsilateral ataxia, ipsilateral face, and contralateral truncal loss of pain and temperature sensation. In patients under 50 years of age, special attention should be given to vessel wall integrity, as vertebral artery dissection is a common cause of stroke in this population leading to brainstem infarction. The second-order neuron is susceptible to compressive injury from Pancoast tumor and upper chest wall trauma such as stab wounds. The third-order neural plexus surrounding the internal carotid artery may suffer direct injury from carotid dissection resulting in a partial Horner's syndrome that excludes anhidrosis as sweat fibers ascend to the face with the external carotid artery.

If a new monocular dilated pupil is noted on exam, this may indicate disruption of parasympathetic input to the pupillary sphincter. Evaluating for a CN III palsy is important as this can indicate a compressive midbrain lesion such as herniation of the medial temporal lobe (the uncus), global increased intracranial pressure (ICP), upper brainstem hemorrhage, infarction or mass lesions or a posterior communicating artery aneurysm [5, 6]. The clinical importance stems from the proximity of the arousal centers of the ARAS and the risk of progression to coma and death. Signs accompanying a complete third nerve palsy include ptosis from denervation of the levator palpebrae superioris muscle, the major contributor to elevation of the eyelid and somatic extraocular muscle dysfunction of the medial, superior and inferior recti as well as the inferior oblique, leaving the eye in a downward and outward position, with limited adduction and supra- and infraduction.

Assessment of horizontal and vertical gaze may offer insight into the etiology of visual disturbances resulting from impairment of eye movement or a malalignment of the eyes. Horizontal control of eye movement originates in the frontal eye fields, which act as opposing forces pushing the eyes conjugately to the opposite side. The frontal eye fields communicate with the contralateral CN VI nuclei controlling the lateral rectus and paramedian pontine reticular formation which subsequently signals the CN III nucleus via the rostral medial longitudinal fasciculus (rMLF) activating the medial rectus. A lesion affecting the rMLF can lead to an internuclear ophthalmoplegia (INO), characterized by impaired abduction of the eye ipsilateral to the rMLF lesion and a contralateral dissociated horizontal abducting nystagmus. An INO may be the result of a demyelinating lesion or brainstem infarction.

When assessing for pupillary or gaze abnormalities, papilledema should also be assessed for which fundoscopy is an essential tool. Papilledema refers to swelling of the optic disc and often occurs due to increased intracranial pressure. Fundoscopy is a diagnostic procedure used to examine the back of the eye, particularly the retina and the optic disc using an ophthalmoscope. The differential diagnosis of papilledema involves considering other conditions that can mimic its appearance. Some potential causes of optic disc swelling, besides increased intracranial pressure, include optic neuritis, or inflammation of the optic nerve, often associated with multiple sclerosis. Additionally, optic nerve sheath meningiomas, ischemic optic neuropathy, idiopathic intracranial hypertension, space-occupying brain lesion, meningitis, hydrocephalus, and venous sinus thrombosis can all result in papilledema. To determine the underlying cause of papilledema, additional diagnostic tests and evaluations may be necessary, such as visual field testing, imaging studies, and lumbar puncture to measure cerebrospinal fluid pressure.

The corneal reflex offers insight into pontine brainstem function as the afferent limb involved the CN V1 distribution of the trigeminal nerve and the efferent limb is the facial nerve thus assessing a two cranial nerve reflex. Additionally, facial weakness of the upper and lower face (forehead wrinkling, assessment of the nasolabial folds, and smile symmetry) to assess for facial nerve involvement should also be assessed to the best of the examiner's ability as new facial weakness could be indicative of a new acute focal pontine process. Involvement of the upper part of the face, suggesting involvement of the CN VII subnuclei which receive dual cortical innervation or the CN VII through its peripheral route, can help differentiate from the facial weakness of a cortical or upper brainstem lesion. Assessment of the oculocephalic reflex evaluates reflexive horizontal eye movements coordinated by the oculomotor nerve, abducens nerve, as well as the vestibulocochlear nerve. Angular rotation of the head causes endolymph in the horizontal semicircular canals to rotate in the opposite direction of the head to activate the ipsilateral vestibular nerve, which in turn inhibits the contralateral vestibular nucleus. Both vestibular nuclei will then activate both abducens nuclei which in turn will send signals to the contralateral oculomotor nerve via the medial longitudinal fasciculus to activate or inhibit the medial rectus [7]. Thus, this maneuver will produce the "doll's eyes" reflex.

It is important to recognize that false localizing signs can occur in the setting of elevated intracranial pressure. A common false localizing deficit is an abducens nerve (CN VI) palsy as obstructive hydrocephalus may cause compression of the nerve along the base of the skull or stretching of the nerve along its path in the setting of increased intracranial pressure even if the primary lesion is located near the foramen magnum [6]. Additionally, aqueductal enlargement in the setting of hydrocephalus may lead to features of a Perinaud's syndrome consisting of impaired upgaze, bilateral lid retraction, convergence retraction nystagmus, and light-near dissociation [6]. False localizing signs can also present motor findings on examination. If uncal herniation progresses to the point of compressing the contralateral midbrain, the contralateral cerebral peduncle can be affected causing an ipsilateral paralysis to the uncal herniation as in the Kernohan notch phenomenon [8].

In patients who have a depressed mental status, performing a full sensory exam may be difficult, however it should at least be assessed whether the patient is able to localize to or withdraw purposefully from painful stimulus or has a triple flexion response as this can indicate higher cortical function versus a reflexive spinal response respectively.

Painful central or peripheral stimulus may also elicit reflexive responses of the extremities with localizing value. Decerebrate posturing, also known as extensor posturing, is characterized by rigid extension of the arms and legs. The arms are typically adducted and extended, and the legs are extended and internally rotated. The head may be arched backward, and the jaw clenched. Decorticate posturing, also known as flexor posturing, is characterized by rigid flexion of the arms and extension of the legs. The arms are typically adducted and flexed, with the wrists and fingers flexed. The legs may be extended and internally rotated. Decerebrate and decorticate posturing patterns provide clues about the location of brain injury or dysfunction. It is important to note that these posturing patterns are not diagnostic of specific conditions but rather indicative of severe regional brain dysfunction. Decerebrate posturing suggests damage to the brainstem, particularly the midbrain or upper pons. Decorticate posturing suggests damage to the cerebral hemispheres, including the cortex and subcortical structures. Classically the red nucleus represented the border separating injuries leading to decerebrate (below the red nucleus) and decorticate (above the red nucleus) posturing.

A more thorough sensory evaluation in patients who can readily participate in the neurologic examination can be helpful. The assessment of sensation to pain and temperature (transmitted by the spinothalamic tract) and proprioception, vibration, and light touch (transmitted by the dorsal columns) is part of a complete sensory examination and may assist in localization of spinal cord pathology. Assessment of an acutely progressive ascending sensory deficit may indicate an acute peripheral demyelinating or axonal process such as acute inflammatory demyelinating polyneuropathy (AIDP) or the axonal variants. A truncal sensory level can be a hallmark of a spinal cord lesion and indispensable in the clinical localization of spinal cord pathology.

Evaluation of muscle stretch reflexes (MSR) can broadly differentiate upper versus lower motor neuron lesions, with the former presenting with hyperreflexia and the latter hyporeflexia. The evaluation of a patient's reflexes may also offer insight into the progression or improvement of an underlying neuromuscular disease such as AIDP or spinal cord pathology.

Thorough evaluation of motor tone, strength and muscle bulk can also aide in determining whether a lesion affects the upper or lower motor neurons. Muscle strength should be assessed at each major joint in the extremities and graded using the Medical Research Council (MRC) scale of 0 (no movement) to 5 (full strength). A useful point of reference when using this scale is that a grade of 3 represents antigravity strength. Upper motor neuron lesions present with hyperreflexia as well as upgoing toes, whereas lower motor neuron lesions will present with hyporeflexia and there will not be a positive Babinski noted on examination. Additionally, fasciculations and atrophy can be seen in lower motor neuron lesions as well as a decrease in tone. An upper motor neuron lesion indicates a lesion within a pathway above the anterior horn cell such as motor pathways in the cortex, brainstem, and spinal cord. A lower motor neuron lesion will affect the peripheral nerves indicating an interruption in the spinal cord reflex arc, which can also affect the motor root.

Airway, Breathing, Circulation (ABCs)

In any patient presenting with acute neurologic deficits, early attention should be given to to the airway, breathing patterns, and circulation, as progression of a myriad of neurologic injuries may compromise any or all of the ABCs leading to a life-threatening emergency. This is particularly true in patients with an impaired level of consciousness, often a result of a lesion affecting the ARAS, where hypoventilation, apnea, and poor protection of the airway from collapse and aspiration become of paramount importance.

Lesions of the lower midbrain or upper pontine tegmentum can cause central neurogenic hyperventilation, which is characterized by an increase in the depth and rate of respiration to the extent that it causes a respiratory alkalosis [9]. Lower pontine lesions, usually caused by basilar artery occlusions, can lead to apneustic breathing during which a few rapid deep breaths alternate with apnea [9]. Dorsomedial medullary lesions can lead to ataxia of breathing or Biot's breathing which is characterized by each breath varying in depth and rate progressing to prolonged inspiratory gaps followed by apnea [9]. Rarely, in cases of unilateral or bilateral brainstem infarcts, loss of autonomic function during sleep with preserved voluntary breathing during wakefulness can be seen in Ondine's curse, thought to be due to interruption of descending medullocervical pathways that contribute to automatic breathing [10]. Most of these patients will require stabilization with mechanical ventilation in the acute setting.

In patients with neuromuscular disease such as myasthenia gravis, close attention must be paid to objective measure of respiratory performance, including the negative inspiratory force (NIF) and vital capacity (VC). Deterioration in values or falling below established cutoffs of NIF and VC may indicate impending or active respiratory failure. Similar attention should be paid to patients with Guillain–Barre syndrome or AIDP presenting with areflexic paraparesis. These patients may display paradoxical respiration during which the abdominal wall contracts during inspiration due to the failure of the diaphragm to contract [10]. Due to muscular weakness, many of these patients may also display use of accessory respiratory muscles, whereby the patient appears labored and activates muscles other than the diaphragm and intercostal muscles to breath. Rapid shallow breathing can be a sign of respiratory muscle weakness as well as abdominal paradoxical breathing, activation of the scalene, sternocleidomastoid and pectoralis major muscles, and external intercostals.

With stabilization of the airway and recognition of various breathing patterns that may occur, close attention should also be paid to circulation to recognize when a patient may be in shock with secondary effects on cerebrovascular hemodynamics. Patients with an increased ICP may initially have nonspecific symptoms such as a headache, nausea, vomiting, which can quickly progress to decreased level of consciousness. The Cushing triad may be present consisting of hypertension with widened pulse pressure, bradycardia, and irregular respirations. ICP monitoring may be helpful in guiding direct management of ICP crises and indirectly through assessment of cerebrovascular hemodynamics whereby elevated ICP may lead to a decrease in CBF (cerebral blood flow) leading to secondary hypoxic/ischemic injury due to cerebral hypoperfusion. Cerebral perfusion pressure (CPP) is a function of the difference between the mean arterial pressure (MAP)and ICP. In a normal brain, autoregulation of the vasculature will maintain CPP between 60 and 80 mm Hg with minimal fluctuations and a constant CBF. It is critical to maintain normocarbia in patients with brain injury at risk for elevated ICP who may be hypoventilating, as the risk of cerebral vasodilation from hypercarbia may worsen ICP.

In patients with intracranial lesions or injury, cerebrovascular hemodynamic and intracranial pressure monitoring devices may identify abnormal waveform patterns and changes in intracranial compliance and cerebral perfusion which can be intervened upon and augmented with the goal of improving patient outcomes. Intracranial compliance is the change in volume over the change in pressure during which as volume increases, ICP also increases. Once the compensatory mechanisms of intracranial vasculature have reached their limits, a small change in volume will lead to large changes in ICP [10]. With changes in compliance, the ICP waveforms and amplitude will also change.

Many patients with cervical or upper thoracic spinal cord injuries may present with spinal as well as neurogenic shock. Normally, spinal shock will occur after trauma to the spine which may present with varying degrees of loss of neurologic (motor and sensory) and reflex activity below the level of the lesion. Neurogenic shock is a hemodynamic phenomenon which can be considered a type of distributive shock. This presents with loss of sympathetic tone and vasomotor activity leading to hypotension, bradycardia, and poikilothermia as there is loss of systemic vascular resistance. The parasympathetic input is preserved in this state. Hypotension should be avoided in spinal cord injury patients as the spinal cord is susceptible to ischemia which can perpetuate further injury. Spinal cord injury is the most common cause of neurogenic shock; however, other etiologies such as Guillain–Barre syndrome and transverse myelitis should be considered.

In patients with spinal cord injuries who display acute fluctuations in hemodynamics, autonomic dysreflexia must also be considered. There is an episodic sympathetic response to a sensory stimulus applied below the level of the spinal cord lesion, such as a distended bladder or rectum, which provokes a pathologic sympathetic reflex that travels via the paraspinal sympathetic ganglia to cause vasoconstriction below the level of the lesion. Subsequently, the resulting hypertension results in vagal stimulation by the carotid bodies which produces bradycardia and pupillary constriction [11]. Patients who may have underlying comorbidities such as Parkinson's disease, multiple system atrophy (MSA), progressive supranuclear palsy (PSP) may have autonomic dysfunction associated with their disease processes which can lead to cardiovascular dysfunction.

Herniation Syndromes

Clinicians caring for patients with intracranial lesions, particularly those which may expand or compress the brain, should both recognize and anticipate potential clinical examination changes which are suggestive of herniation syndromes. Tentorial herniation (involving the uncus and parahippocampal areas of the temporal lobe) can present with unilateral pupillary dilation and ophthalmoplegia due to CN III involvement as well as decreased consciousness from pressure on the midbrain reticular formation and ipsilateral paralysis. However, it is important to note that this can be a false localizing sign due to Kernohan's notch syndrome in which there is contralateral compression of the cerebral peduncle due to herniation. The Cushing triad as well as hiccups may also occur. In some cases, the posterior cerebral artery can be compressed and lead to an occipital lobe stroke as well. Upward cerebellar herniation can cause similar findings on examination as well.

Subfalcine herniation is a result of the cingulate gyrus migrating below the anterior falx which can lead to compression of the anterior cerebral artery leading to contralateral lower extremity weakness. In central herniation, there is transtentorial herniation which can similarly present as uncal herniation; however, pupils will also be in mid-position, fixed, and may be eventually become dilated. This is an important consideration and potential pitfall prior to pupillary dilation when evaluating the pupils of a patient at risk for central herniation. Patient with central herniation commonly become agitated, and this can be erroneously overlooked as delirium in a patient with a space occupying lesion that is progressing and clinically deteriorating. The stretching and shearing forces can lead to Duret hemorrhages due to tearing of the small vessels in the brainstem. Downward cerebellar tonsillar herniation can occur which through compression of the medulla and cervical spinal cord and presents with cardiac and respiratory dysrhythmia and abnormal extensor posturing due to involvement of the rubrospinal tract.

It is important to note that patients with neurosurgical procedures due to large intracranial pathologies can also have transcalvarial or external herniation. In patients who have had a hemicraniectomy, it is important to note that in the months following they can develop the syndrome of Trephined, also known as sunken flap syndrome. They can present with vague symptoms of mood fluctuation, headache, and focal deficits due to stretching of the dura and underlying cortex due to atmospheric changes. Rarely, this can lead to subfalcine herniation which can be noted on imaging. Rapid improvement following cranioplasty has been observed.

Next Steps

Imaging

When a new acute focal deficit is found, after stabilization of the patient, imaging of the appropriate region of the neuroaxis should be completed. It is imperative that a patient with a tenuous airway or unstable hemodynamics, or the propensity to progress to an unstable clinical state during imaging, have their safety prioritized through a secure airway and ensuring hemodynamic stability. Trivial movements and adjustments in those with elevated ICP can have dire consequences and hypoventilation, and subsequent hypoxia and hypercarbia can worsen intracranial injury and increase intracranial pressure respectively. Magnetic resonance imaging (MRI) offers high resolution and better sensitivity for differentiating edema, hemorrhage, infarction, and various enhancing lesions as well as subtle pathology which may be below the resolution of computed tomography (CT); however, in many situations CT imaging is sufficient as it is less burdensome, shorter in duration, and has a high sensitivity for hemorrhage, infarction after 6–8 h, mass effect, and herniation. Additionally, CT can be helpful in the early detection of cerebral edema and hydrocephalus, and it is the most practical means for obtaining serial imaging to assess for acute progression of intracranial pathology such as hydrocephalus, hemorrhage, or herniation. Vascular imaging may be helpful in diseases such as subarachnoid hemorrhage and intraparenchymal hemorrhage in the assessment of vascular malformations responsible for the hemorrhage and acute ischemic stroke, particularly those eligible for mechanical thrombectomy. Cerebral perfusion imaging has become a useful tool in patient selection for mechanical thrombectomy treatment of ischemic stroke. Empiric treatment for herniation is often initiated when clinical suspicion is high but will almost certainly need confirmation with imaging to guide subsequent management and assess response to treatment. Optic nerve sheath ultrasound can be considered as a novel, noninvasive technique to assess for signs of elevated ICP. While a consensus of normal and abnormal nerve sheath diameter values nor measurement techniques exists, optic nerve sheath measurement offers a data point which may help guide clinical management in patients deemed too unstable to travel for imaging.

Electroencephalogram (EEG)

Patients with intracranial lesions will also be more prone to the development of seizures. It is important to recognize that an abrupt change in mental status could be an indicator of subclinical seizures, particularly if the patients imaging remains stable. Non-convulsive status epilepticus (NCSE) should be considered in patients with mentation changes where no other non-neurologic cause has been determined. Up to 30% of patients admitted to the intensive care unit (ICU) have incidence of NCSE which can be mistaken as encephalopathy; this is a high morbidity condition, but early treatment has the potential for a meaningful improvement in outcomes. In those who may have a new focal deficit, a post ictal (Todd's) paralysis should be considered as a sign of possible previous seizure activity [12]. Routine or continuous EEG is a helpful, noninvasive technique to detect possible seizures and a means to guide subsequent management in patients with seizures. Additionally, in a patient having intermittent ICP crises, seizures should be ruled out as the cause of ICP spikes as they may raise the cerebral metabolic rate leading to transient and potentially harmful increases in ICP.

Electrolyte Disturbances

Patients with increased ICP will often be treated with hyperosmolar agents such as hypertonic saline or mannitol, requiring close electrolyte monitoring. It is important to note that these agents can have side effects such as nephrotoxicity, volume overload, or excess diuresis.

Patients with intracranial pathology may develop electrolyte disturbances due to cerebral salt wasting (CSW), syndrome of inappropriate antidiuretic hormone (SIADH), or central diabetes insipidus (DI) Table 8.2). Cerebral salt wasting can occur in any intracranial insult; however, it is commonly seen in patients with subarachnoid hemorrhage. During this time, the patient's serum sodium will decrease, and their urine output will rapidly increase leading to a hypovolemic hyponatremia. In patients where there is concern for cerebral edema and elevated ICP, this hypovolemic state may have deleterious effects on cerebral perfusion. DI and SIADH can also be seen in patients with intracranial pathology. Central DI is characterized by excessive thirst and excretion of large volumes of diluted urine (>250 cc for consecutive hours, increasing serum sodium, and urine specific gravity <1.006). It is caused by a deficiency in the hormone vasopressin, also known as antidiuretic hormone (ADH), produced by the hypothalamus. SIADH is a euvolemic hyponatremia and is a result of excess release of vasopressin.

These conditions are also seen with relative frequency in those having had pituitary surgery, either in isolation or in a triple phase response in which there is an initial DI with rising serum sodium, increase urine output, and decrease in urine specific gravity due to cerebral dysfunction and initial diminished vasopressin release. This is then followed by SIADH during which time serum sodium will fall, urine output will decrease, and there will be an increase in urine specific gravity, due to release of residual vasopressin stores from cell injury. As these stores deplete, the patient will return to a DI state. Thus, there can be major electrolyte shifts if not monitored closely. In patients with longer standing hyponatremia, there is a risk of developing osmotic demyelination syndrome (ODS) due to rapid correction of hyponatremia; the pontine region of the brainstem is particularly prone and the consequences of ODS can be unresponsiveness and quadriplegia. It is not recommended to correct sodium more than 8–10 mEq/L in a 24-h period. Conversely, the risk of worsening cerebral edema due to a rapid overcorrection of hypernatremia should not be overlooked. Initiation of hemodialysis due to renal failure is a period of particular risk as osmolar shifts can be dramatic and a pragmatic approach would be to begin with slow continuous hemodialysis before transitioning to an intermittent schedule allowing the brain to exit the higher risk acute period of injury. Additionally, it should be noted that some patients may present with SIADH or hyponatremia due to a secondary cause such as lung cancer or liver disease, respectively, for which the underlying pathology should be addressed.

Multimodality Monitoring

If there is concern for elevated intracranial pressure, a variety of intracranial monitors may be considered. One of the most common devices is an external ventricular drain (EVD) which can be placed at the bedside using landmarks and imaging to guide the placement of a drain into the ventricular space terminating in the third ventricle, which also transduces a waveform and ICP and allows for treatment through CSF diversion. This device allows for real-time and rapid monitoring and management and is particularly helpful in patient with hydrocephalus and intraventricular hemorrhage. A subdural bolt may be an option if it is not safe to place a catheter into the ventricular space. When cerebral ischemia is a concern, intraparenchymal oxygenation monitors may be

Table 8.2 Electrolyte disturbances seen with intracranial pathology

Disease	Volume status	Serum Na	Urine Na	Urine osmolarity	Serum osmolarity	Urine output
DI	Hypovolemic	High	Low	Low	High	High
SIADH	Euvolemic	Low	High	High	Low	Low/normal
CSW	Hypovolemic	Low	High	High	Low	High

helpful for regional measurement of brain oxygen tension; for a global measure of cerebral oxygenation a jugular bulb monitor may be considered. Cerebral oxygenation measure may guide hemodynamic and ventilator augmentation maneuvers in a goal-directed approach to patient care. The risk versus benefit of placing intracranial monitors should be, considered as the risks of secondary injury, while small, may still have devastating consequences in those with existing brain injury who may be at heightened risk of procedural complications such as bleeding.

Metabolic Disturbances

When an acute change is noted in a patient with neurologic injury, expedited imaging, EEG monitoring, and evaluation for a central cause are the intuitive first steps in care. When this initial evaluation is not revealing of a cause, we are often left with nonspecific symptoms and metabolic disturbances should be considered. Patients with intracranial disease have a reduced tolerance for toxic, metabolic, and infectious disturbances. This is particularly evident in the elderly with chronic age-related cerebral changes and neurocognitive disorders, where even trivial metabolic derangements or infections can present with disproportionately pronounced clinical signs. Iatrogenic causes of infection should also be considered, and in the ICU, ventilator associated pneumonia, central line-associated blood stream infection, catheter-related urinary tract infections, and device-related infections such as ventriculitis may present as acute neurologic change in our patients. Minimizing invasive lines and devices is a prudent approach in all ICU patients.

Systemic disease can confound the evaluation of patients with primary neurologic injury; worsening renal function may lead to electrolyte derangements, acidemia, or uremia. Hepatic failure leading to hepatic encephalopathy due to hyperammonemia is another consideration, and both hepatic and renal causes of encephalopathy are often difficult to distinguish from convulsive and nonconvulsive seizures. Patients with acute hepatic failure are at an increased risk of developing cerebral edema as well as intracranial hemorrhage due to coagulopathy. A thorough review of medications a patient uses in the outpatient and inpatient setting should be performed; many medications have neurotoxic side effects and may also lower the seizure threshold, including commonly prescribed antibiotics such as cefepime.

One specific type of therapy, CAR-T cell (chimeric antigenic receptor), which is a groundbreaking treatment for certain types of cancers, has known neurotoxic effects such as cerebral edema, encephalopathy, and seizures. It is thought that this therapy produces a robust inflammatory response which drives blood–brain barrier disruption and neuronal injury. Additionally, secondary immunosuppression places these patients at increased risk of central nervous system (CNS) infection, and in any patient on an immune modulating treatment presenting with encephalopathy, consideration should be given for the potential of a CNS infection and treatment decisions should take into consideration the patients heightened risk of atypical and opportunistic infections.

Classic Near Misses

With lesions in the posterior fossa, it is especially important to recognize the utility of serial imaging as expansion is often clinically silent until there is sufficient mass effect to cause symptoms or a secondary process such as herniation or acute obstructive hydrocephalus. New onset nausea, vomiting as well as hiccups can indicate that the area postrema around the fourth ventricle is being affected in the setting of an expansile lesion which becomes concerning for increased ICP.

Additionally, it is important to consider airway protection in patients with neurologic diseases as their mental status may preclude them from being able to protect their airway. Thus, securing their airway should be acted on rapidly to avoid further complications that can arise from prolonged respiratory failure.

It is important to recognize that changes in the clinical status of a patient with neurologic disease should never be assumed to be due to benign or due to non-neurologic causes, particularly in the acute phase of their disease process. A secondary neurologic process such as hydrocephalus or seizures, resulting from the primary disease is not uncommon, and early recognition and intervention is crucial. A prioritized evaluation using the clinical examination, imaging, and EEG can aide a clinician in rapidly recognizing an otherwise elusive etiology of an acute clinical change or new neurologic deficit. Medication effects should not be overlooked as a possible cause of acute changes in this patient population.

Diagnostic Algorithm

(See Diagnostic and Treatment Flow Diagrams).

Take Home Message

Early recognition of acute neurologic deficits in this patient population can impact outcomes. Patient safety and stability with close attention to the airway, breathing, and circulation remains paramount, followed by a focused neurologic examination should serve as the foundational approach for all patients with acute neurologic injury. Early recognition of acute intervenable neurologic diseases allows for rapid treatment particularly when time windows for treatment may be limited. Subtle symptom complexes that may be indicative of focal neurologic injury such as patterns of brain herniation signs, reflexive posturing, pupillary changes as well as pathologic breathing pattern variations or vital sign changes may be understated signs of acute focal neurologic injury. Additional testing, including imaging, EEG, and CSF analysis, will often confirm the pathologic process from a clinicians refined differential and guide subsequent treatment.

Diagnostic Flow Diagram

Approach to Acute Focal Deficit

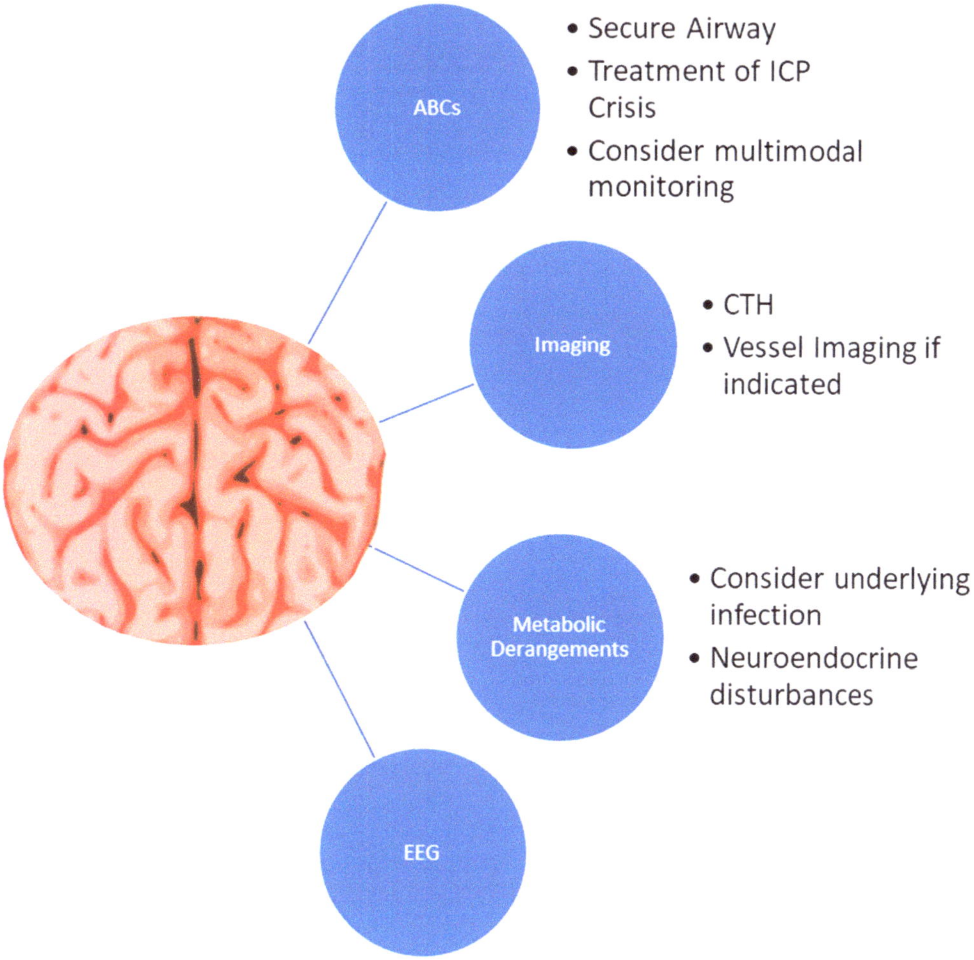

Treatment Flow Diagram

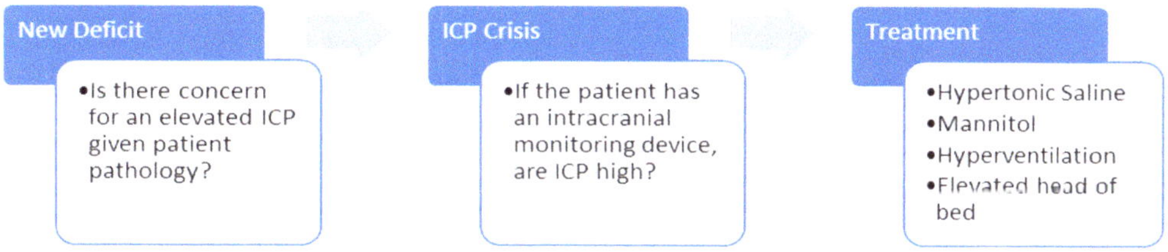

Key Clinical Questions

Immediate/Early Priorities Checklist &/or table

- Is there a change in the patient's exam? If so, where is the lesion?
  - Are they stable enough to obtain imaging?
  - Consider EEG
- Are they protecting their airway?
  - Consider intubation
- What are their vital signs?
  - Consider vasopressors
  - Consider anti-hypertensive agents
- Is there concern for an ICP crisis?
  - Consider hyperosmolar therapy
  - Hyperventilation
  - Elevated head of bed

Diagnostic Pearls Tables

Treatment Pearls Tables (*Table 8.3*)

Table 8.3 Treatment "Pearls" for selected problems

Problem	Treatment	Imaging
Elevated ICP	Hyperosmolar therapy	CTH
New focal deficit	Localize	CTH Consider MRI Consider EEG
Change in mental status	Consider intubation if not protecting airway	CTH
Elevated blood pressure	Anti-hypertensive agents if appropriate	Consider vessel imaging
Low blood pressure	Resuscitation	Consider further imaging depending on type of shock

References

1. Arguinchona JH, Tadi P. Neuroanatomy, reticular activating system. National Center for Biotechnology Information; 2022.
2. Posner JB, Plum F, Plum F. Plum and Posner's diagnosis of stupor and coma. Oxford University Press; 2007.
3. Biller J, Gruener G, Brazis PW. The patient's mental status and higher cerebral functions. In: DeMyer's the neurologic examination: a programmed text, 7e. McGraw Hill; 2016.
4. Szabadi E. Functional Organization of the Sympathetic Pathways Controlling the pupil: light-inhibited and light-stimulated pathways. Front Neurol. 2018;9:1069.
5. Martin TJ, Corbett JJ. Ocular motility disorders: cranial nerve palsies. In: Practical Neuroopthalmology. 1st ed. McGraw Hill; 2013.
6. Biller J, Gruener G, Brazis PW. A synopsis of the neurologic investigation and formulary of Neurodiagnosis. In: DeMyer's the neurologic examination: a programmed text, 7e. McGraw Hill; 2016.
7. Kandel ER, Koester JD, Mack SH, Siegelbaum SA. The vestibular system. Principles of Neural Science: McGraw Hill; 2021.
8. Berkowitz AL. Disorders of intracranial pressure. In: Clinical neurology and neuroanatomy: a localization-based approach. McGraw Hill; 2016.
9. Ropper AH, Samuela MA, Klein JP, Prasad S. Disorders of the autonomic nervous system. In: Adams and Victor's principles of neurology, 11e. McGraw Hill; 2019.
10. Lee K, Mayer SA. Management of increased intracranial pressure. In: The NeuroICU book, 2e. McGraw Hill; 2017.
11. Amthor FR, Theibert AB, Standaert DG, Roberson ED. Neurotrauma. In: Modern Neuroscience. McGraw Hill; 2020.
12. Ascoli M, Ferlazzo E. Epidemiology and outcomes of status epilepticus. Int J Gen Med. 2021;14:2965–73.

Further Reading

Biller J, Gruener G, Brazis PW. A synopsis of the neurologic investigation and formulary of neurodiagnosis. Demyer's the neurologic examination: a programmed text, 7e. McGraw Hill; 2016.

Posner JB, Plum F, Plum F. Plum and Posner's diagnosis of stupor and coma. Oxford University Press; 2007.

Ropper AH, Samuela MA, Klein JP, Prasad S. Disorders of the Autonomic Nervous System. Adams and Victor's Principles of Neurology, 11e. McGraw Hill; 2019.

Dyspnea and Respiratory Distress in the Neuro ICU

9

Samuel M. Cohen, Kevin W. Hatton, and Maurizio Cereda

Contents

S. M. Cohen
Department of Anesthesiology and Critical Care Medicine, University of Pennsylvania, Philadelphia, PA, USA

K. W. Hatton
Department of Anesthesiology, University of Kentucky, Lexington, KY, USA

M. Cereda (✉)
Massachusetts General Hospital, Harvard Medical School, Boston, MA, USA
e-mail: mcereda@mgh.harvard.edu

E. Mahanna Gabrielli et al. (eds.), *Textbook of Neurointensive Care: Volume 1*, https://doi.org/10.1007/978-3-031-62220-5_9

Abstract

Dyspnea, a sensation of breathlessness, is a common occurrence in the intensive care unit. The differential diagnosis of dyspnea is innumerable and can be related to multiple organ systems. The clinical importance of recognizing and evaluating dyspnea is that it can be a harbinger of acute respiratory decompensation and potential cardiopulmonary collapse. For patients in the neurological and neurosurgical ICU, underlying neurological diseases can make them more prone to dyspnea and respiratory distress.

Respiratory distress and concomitant respiratory failure can be due to various factors causing problems with oxygenation and ventilation. The biomechanics and neurochemical regulation of breathing is a complex system. Patients in the neuro ICU can suffer from disease processes affecting one or multiple aspects of the respiratory system, that is, central or peripheral neurological regulation of respiration, respiratory muscle weakness, or primary lung pathology. Altered mentation and bulbar dysfunction cause high secretion burdens and potential aspiration pneumonia. Neurogenic pulmonary edema and neuromuscular diseases in patients in the neuro ICU also contribute to the risk of respiratory failure. Understanding the role of early and deliberate use of noninvasive ventilatory support such as high-flow nasal cannula and BiPAP to improve oxygenation and ventilation can stabilize patients and prevent further decompensation. Frequent reassessment of patients at risk for respiratory failure and timely initiation of invasive ventilation remains the hallmark of successful management.

Introduction

Goals of This Chapter

- Summarize basic respiratory pathophysiology and causes of gas exchange impairment, dyspnea, and acute respiratory failure.
- Describe the diagnostic of acute respiratory compromise in the hospital and the ICU environment.
- List specific considerations in treating of respiratory failure in neurological patients.
- Discuss the acute management of the patient with acute respiratory failure.
- Summarize the current standard of care for invasive and noninvasive respiratory support, including lung protective strategies, positional therapy, and ventilator liberation.
- List advanced respiratory support strategies such as inhaled vasodilation and extracorporeal assist.

This chapter addresses how to manage the neurologically injured patient with dyspnea and acute respiratory failure. We are using a structured, evidence-based, and physiology-based approach. The chapter will also address specific issues encountered when respiratory compromise complicates neurological and neurosurgical conditions.

The Respiratory System

The respiratory system is a network of conducting airways, delicate capillary beds, muscles, and complex central and peripheral neural signaling pathways. The lungs are responsible for gas exchange, metabolism, and filtration. In sequence, the respiratory tract runs from the nasopharynx to the oropharynx, past the vocal cords, down the trachea to the bronchi, lobar bronchi, segmental, terminal, and finally, the respiratory bronchioles to the alveoli, the functional unit of the lung where gas exchange occurs. In an estimated, 500 million alveoli with a combined volume of approximately 4 L, inspired air (with varying concentrations of oxygen) diffuses across a thin blood–gas barrier and is taken up into the capillary blood following partial pressure gradients [1, 2].

Airways that do not participate in gas exchange (e.g., the upper airway, trachea, and bronchi) are collectively known as anatomic dead space and amount to approximately 150 mL. The separation between gas exchanging and nonexchanging airspaces is functional, rather than anatomically demarcated, and its position varies with respiratory pattern [3] (Fig. 9.1).

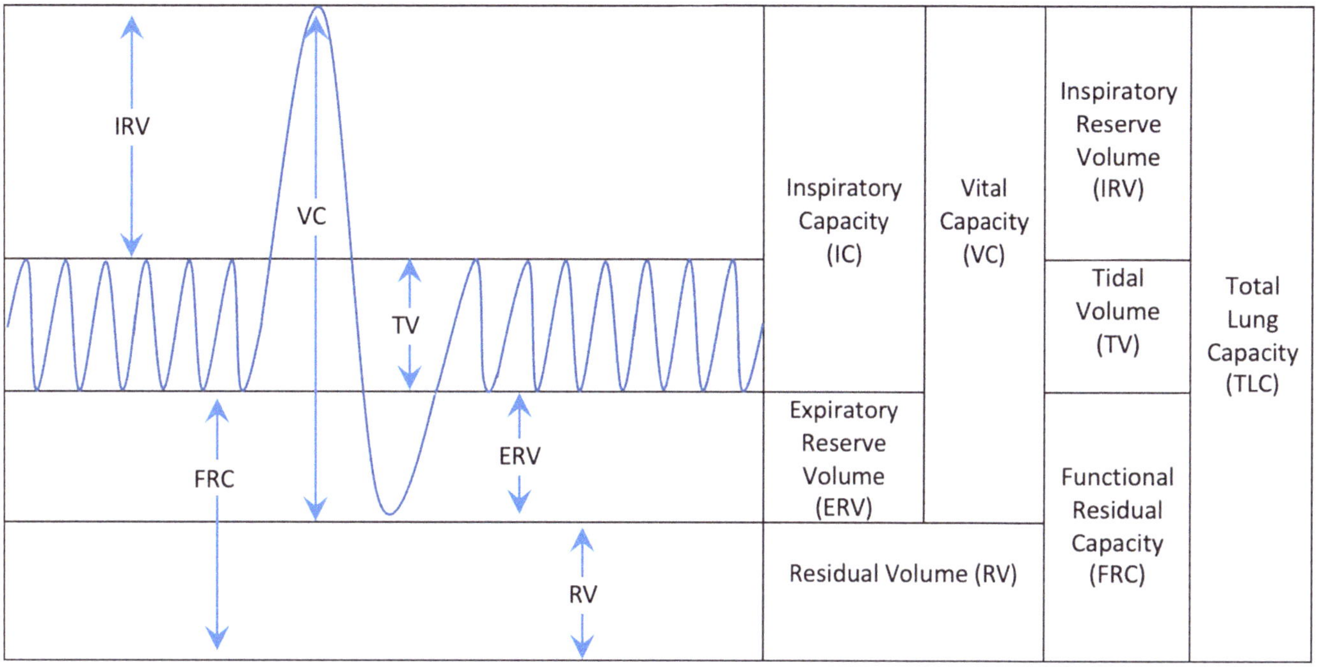

Fig. 9.1 Lung volumes

Respiratory Mechanics

From a mechanical point of view, the respiratory system is composed of the lungs, the chest wall, and the abdomen. All compartments are intrinsically elastic and require pressure and mechanical work generated by the inspiratory muscles to increase their volume (Table 9.1). The primary muscle responsible for inspiration is the diaphragm. Secondary muscles of inspiration include the external intercostal muscles, as that raise the ribs and expand the chest cavity up and forward, and the scalene and sternocleidomastoid muscles. During inspiration, the pressure in the pleura and within the alveoli decreases, creating a pressure gradient driving air into the lungs. As the lungs and chest wall distend during inspiration, they accumulate potential energy, creating a recoil pressure in the alveoli that drives gas out during expiration. This is passive at rest, but it is facilitated by abdominal wall musculature and internal intercostal muscles during exercise or in case of tachypnea.

The elastic impedances of the whole respiratory system and its pulmonary and chest wall compartments are quantified by their compliance values (Table 9.2) [5]. Chest wall and pulmonary compliances are roughly equivalent in normal health, but in disease, they variably contribute to increased work of breathing. Each contribution depends on the clinical picture (e.g., restrictive lung disease vs. abdominal compartment syndrome) and body habitus (e.g., obesity). Additionally, the airways present a resistive impedance, quantified as resistance (Table 9.2), which is low in healthy subjects but increases considerably, raising the work of breathing in obstructive lung diseases [6].

Table 9.1 Approximate normal values for various lung volumes in spontaneously breathing patients [4]

	Men (mL)	Women (mL)
Residual volume	1250	1000
Expiratory reserve volume	1000	750
Tidal volume	500	500
Inspiratory reserve volume	3500	2000
Functional residual capacity	2250	1750
Vital capacity	5000	3250
Total lung capacity	6250	4250

Table 9.2 Formulas

	Formula	
Resistance	$R = \frac{\Delta P}{\Delta Q}$	Resistance = Peak Pressure - Plateau Pressure/Flow (in Liters per second)
Resistance of Respiratory System	$R_{rs} = R_t + K_1 + K_2\dot{V}$	R_{rs}: resistance of the respiratory system, R_t: resistance from deformation of the lungs and chest wall, K_1: empirical constant representing gas viscosity K_2: empirical constant representing gas density and airway geometry $\dot{V}$: flow as volume per unit time
	Normal = 1 to 8 $cmH_2O/L/s$ COPD, Asthma = 15 $cmH_2O/L/s$	
Compliance	$\text{Compliance} = \frac{\Delta V}{\Delta P}$	V = volume, P = pressure
Compliance of the respiratory system	$\frac{1}{C_{rs}} = \frac{1}{C_l} + \frac{1}{C_{cw}}$	C_{rs} = compliance respiratory system, C_l = compliance of lung, C_{cw} = compliance of chest wall
	$\text{Normal} = 50\text{–}100 \text{ mL/cm } H_2O$ $\text{COPD/Asthma} = 60 \text{ mL/cm } H_2O$ $\text{ARDS} = 20\text{–}40 \text{ mL/cm } H_2O$	
Dynamic Compliance	$C_{dyn} = V_T/\text{PIP} - \text{PEEP}$	V_T: tidal volume PIP: peak inspiratory pressure, PEEP: positive end respiratory pressure
Static compliance	$C_{Stat} = V_T/P_{PLAT} - \text{PEEP}$	V_T: tidal volume P_{Plat}: Plateau pressure; PEEP: positive end respiratory pressure
Fick's Law for Diffusion	$\dot{V}_{gas} = \frac{A \times D \times (P_1 - P_2)}{T}$	V_{gas}: volume of gas diffusing through the tissue barrier per time (ml/min); A: surface area available for diffusion; D: diffusion coefficient of the gas; P_1 and $P2$: partial pressures of gas across the barrier; T: thickness of barrier
Alveolar ventilation	$V_A = [V_T - V_D] \times RR$	V_T: tidal volume, V_D = dead space volume; RR: respiratory rate
Alveolar oxygen equation	$P_AO_2 = [F_iO_2\, x(P_{bar} - P_{H_2O})] - [P_aCO_2/RQ]$	FiO_2: fraction of inspired oxygen, P_{bar}: barometric pressure, PH_2O: water vapor pressure, $PaCO_2$: partial pressure of carbon dioxide, RQ: respiratory quotient (0.8)
A-a gradient	$P_AO_2 - P_aO_2$ Normal = < 15 mmHg	P_AO_2: alveolar partial pressure of oxygen, P_aO_2: arterial partial pressure of oxygen
Arterial blood oxygen content	$C_aO_2 = (1.34 \times [Hb] \times S_aO_2) + (0.003 \times P_aO_2)$	C_aO_2 = arterial oxygen content of arterial blood (mL/dL), 1.34: volume of oxygen bound to 1 g of saturated hemoglobin (mL/g), [Hb]: concentration of hemoglobin (g/L), S_aO_2: percent of hemoglobin fully saturated with oxygen (%), 0.03: solubility coefficient of oxygen in plasma, P_aO_2: partial pressure of oxygen dissolved in arterial blood
Oxygen delivery equation	$DO_2 = CO \times \{(1.34 \times Hb \times S_aO_2) + (P_aO_2 \times 0.003)\}$	DO_2: oxygen delivery (mL/min), CO: cardiac output (heart rate x stroke volume) (L/min), 1.34: maximal oxygen carrying capacity of hemoglobin (mL/g), Hb: hemoglobin, S_aO_2: percent of hemoglobin fully saturated with oxygen (%),P_aO_2: partial pressure of oxygen dissolved in arterial blood, 0.003: solubility constant for blood
Shunt fraction	$Q_s/Q_t = C_CO_2 - C_aO_2/C_CO_2 - C_vO_2$	Q_s: blood flow through shunt, Q_t: total cardiac output, C_CO_2 = pulmonary alveolar capillary content of oxygen = $(1.34 \times [Hb] \text{ x } S_AO_2 + (0.003 \times P_AO_2)$ $C_VO_2 = (1.34 \times [Hb] \times S_VO_2 + (0.003 \times P_VO_2)$
Minute ventilation	$\dot{V}_E = V_T \times f$	V_E: minute ventilation, V_T: tidal volume, f: respiratory rate
Dead space equation	$V_D/V_T = P_aCO_2 - P_{et}CO_2/P_aCO_2$	Where: V_D = physiological dead space, V_T = tidal volume, P_aCO_2 = arterial partial pressure of carbon dioxide, $P_{et}CO_2$ = end tidal partial pressure of carbon dioxide. The result is given as a percentage; normal should not exceed 0.3 (30%)

Pulmonary Perfusion

The pulmonary vasculature is a low-pressure, low-resistance system, which allows it to accommodate all of the cardiac output at rest as well as during exercise. Mean pulmonary artery pressure is approximately one-sixth of systemic arterial pressure at rest. Abnormally high pulmonary vascular resistance, due to parenchymal or vascular disease, results in pulmonary hypertension and, if acute or severe enough, right ventricular failure. The alveolar–capillary membranes are sensitive to pressure swings, and the transmural pressure in the alveolar capillaries depends on both intravascular and alveolar pressure. Pathology that causes pressure back up in the pulmonary veins (e.g., excessive left ventricular afterload or left-sided heart failure) causes congestion in the thin capillaries. When capillary pressure is greater than interstitial hydrostatic pressure, and lymphatic drainage is overwhelmed, low-protein fluid leaks into the interstitial space and the alveoli (hydrostatic edema). Finally, acute inflammatory lung conditions increase vascular permeability and leakage of protein-rich fluid in the absence of high intravascular pressure (non-hydrostatic edema), typically observed in acute respiratory distress syndrome (ARDS).

Pulmonary blood flow is somewhat heterogeneous throughout the lungs and this distribution is partly affected by body position and exercise. Classic studies suggested vertical (gravitational) gradients of lung perfusion, with increasing values from apex to base when standing and from ventral to dorsal when supine. However, changing position from supine to prone attenuates but does not invert perfusion gradients [7]. More recent studies showed that gravity explains only a small fraction of perfusion distribution in the lungs, with more significant contributions from anatomical factors [8, 9].

An important physiologic feature of the pulmonary vasculature is hypoxic pulmonary vasoconstriction (HPV), a compensatory response to hypoxia that directs blood flow away from hypoventilated or non-ventilated lung units. The endothelial cells release thromboxane A_2 and endothelin-1, potent vasoconstrictors, which increase pulmonary vascular resistance. Conversely, pulmonary arteriolar dilation occurs via nitric oxide, generated from endothelial nitric oxidase synthase, which increases cyclic GMP to decrease sarcoplasmic reticulum calcium allowing for vasodilation. Inhaled nitric oxide and epoprostenol cause pulmonary vasodilation in ventilated lung regions, improving ventilation-perfusion match, gas exchange, and reducing pulmonary hypertension.

Hypoxemia

Arterial partial pressure of oxygen (PaO_2) and carbon dioxide ($PaCO_2$) are tightly regulated by several homeostatic control mechanisms. The alveolar partial pressure of oxygen (PAO_2) can be determined from the alveolar air equation (Table 9.2), assuming CO_2 has identical alveolar and arterial partial pressures. In cases of hypoventilation, PaO_2 decreases comparably to the increase in $PaCO_2$, but the normal PAO_2–PaO_2 gradient is preserved (Table 9.2). Oxygen therapy corrects hypoxemia during hypoventilation, but hypercapnia persists and, if untreated (e.g., by inspiratory support), may reach life-threatening levels.

The flux of oxygen and carbon dioxide across the alveolar–capillary membrane is proportional to its area and gas solubility and inversely proportional to barrier thickness [1, 10]. This transfer is highly efficient and is rarely compromised in the acute setting [11]. To calculate oxygen carried in the blood, one needs to account for the oxygen bound to hemoglobin and its physically dissolved portion (Table 9.2). Because the latter quantity is minimal, arterial oxygen content—and oxygen delivery to tissues—heavily relies on hemoglobin concentration and function, hence the importance of treating anemia in severely hypoxemic patients.

Once hypoventilation is ruled out or corrected, hypoxemia is most often due to abnormally scattered distribution of ventilation and perfusion, causing arterial O_2 contents to be lower than at the capillary level. At the lowest end, loss of ventilated airspaces due to collapse (atelectasis) or flooding of perfused alveoli causes intrapulmonary shunt, typical of ARDS. This shunt fraction is quantified as the portion of cardiac output perfusing non-ventilated lung tissue (Table 9.2). Adequate oxygenation of ventilated alveolar–capillary units does not adequately compensate for elevated shunt, due to the sigmoid shape of the O_2–hemoglobin dissociation curve limiting oxygen uptake by blood. When the shunt fraction is higher than approximately 30%, oxygen therapy alone cannot restore normal PaO_2: alveolar recruitment (e.g., by positive airway pressure) is then necessary to restore gas exchange. Patients with obstructive lung disease can be hypoxemic but still respond to oxygen because ventilation of perfused airspaces is decreased but not abolished [12].

Hypercapnia

Hypercapnia occurs when carbon dioxide is unable to be cleared by respiration. Several disease states such as chronic obstructive lung disease (COPD), severe obstructive sleep apnea (OSA), neuromuscular disorders, obesity hypoventilation syndrome (OHS), and respiratory depressant drug overdose can cause hypercapnia through hypoventilation. In contrast, *hyper*ventilation is observed in hypoxemia, anxiety, and neurological injuries.

Minute ventilation (MV) is the amount of gas inspired or expired each minute (Table 9.2) and averages 5–8 L per min in healthy subjects. Subtracting dead space (calculated through the Bohr equation, Table 9.2) from MV yields alveolar ventilation, the fraction that participates in CO_2 exchange. Arterial CO_2 content and alveolar ventilation are inversely proportional, which implies that to maintain normal $PaCO_2$, minute volume needs to be increased in the presence of dead space [11]. In addition to natural airways, artificial airways, tubing extensions, and heat-moisture exchangers increase dead space ("apparatus dead space"). Finally, alveolar dead space, composed of ventilated alveoli but not perfused, hinders CO_2 elimination in diseased lungs. This can be due to pulmonary embolism and emphysema. In ARDS, a larger dead space complicates ventilator management and predicts higher mortality [13]. Alveolar dead space increases the difference between expired and arterial CO_2 partial pressures, complicating the clinical use of capnometry to monitor P_aCO_2.

Neurologic Control of Respiration

Central and peripheral chemoreceptors sense blood O_2, CO_2, and pH. These receptors feedback information to the brainstem and regulate respiration. Subconscious breathing starts in the brainstem with rhythmic breathing controlled in the medulla. Anatomically, the medullary respiratory center sits on either side of the reticular formation beneath the floor of the fourth ventricle. The medulla is broken down into the dorsal and ventral medullary respiratory groups (DRG/VRG). The DRG is responsible for inspiration and receives input from peripheral chemoreceptors via the vagus and glossopharyngeal nerves. The VRG (pre-Bötzinger complex) generates respiratory rhythm and is responsible for expiration. Central chemoreceptors detect changes in $PaCO_2$ and pH, but not PaO_2. Peripheral chemoreceptors at carotid bodies and bifurcation of common carotid arteries and in aortic bodies respond to CO_2, O_2, and pH changes—but the most vital stimulus to breathe is $PaCO_2$ [14]. The upper and lower pons both have specific tasks. The apneustic center in the lower pons is responsible for the stimulation of inspiratory muscles, while the pneumotaxic center in the upper pons sends an inhibitory transmission to the inspiratory center. Voluntary respiratory control comes from cortical signaling can force hyperventilation and with more difficulty, hypoventilation. The limbic system and hypothalamus, heavily involved in emotional and pain processing, also control breathing patterns. This is significant since there is an emotional component to dyspnea [15], often seen in anxiety.

Diseases affecting the nervous system can cripple the respiratory system anywhere along the path from the central respiratory control center to the muscles of respiration. Increased intracranial pressure (ICP), stroke, trauma, and structural issues such as neoplasms affect central neural control centers and connections. Upper motor neurons can be damaged by trauma with a profound impact on respiratory function depending on location. This can be seen in complete lesions above C3/4 affect phrenic (diaphragmatic) innervation, while trauma to the lower cervical vertebrae will cause loss of intercostal respiratory muscles. A classic example of neurologic disease affecting respiration is poliomyelitis affecting the anterior horn cells causing total paralysis of respiratory muscles. Lastly, conditions affecting the muscles or neuromuscular junction, such as botulism, myasthenia gravis, Lamber Eaton syndrome, nerve gas, and organophosphate poisoning, can cause acute respiratory failure (Fig. 9.2).

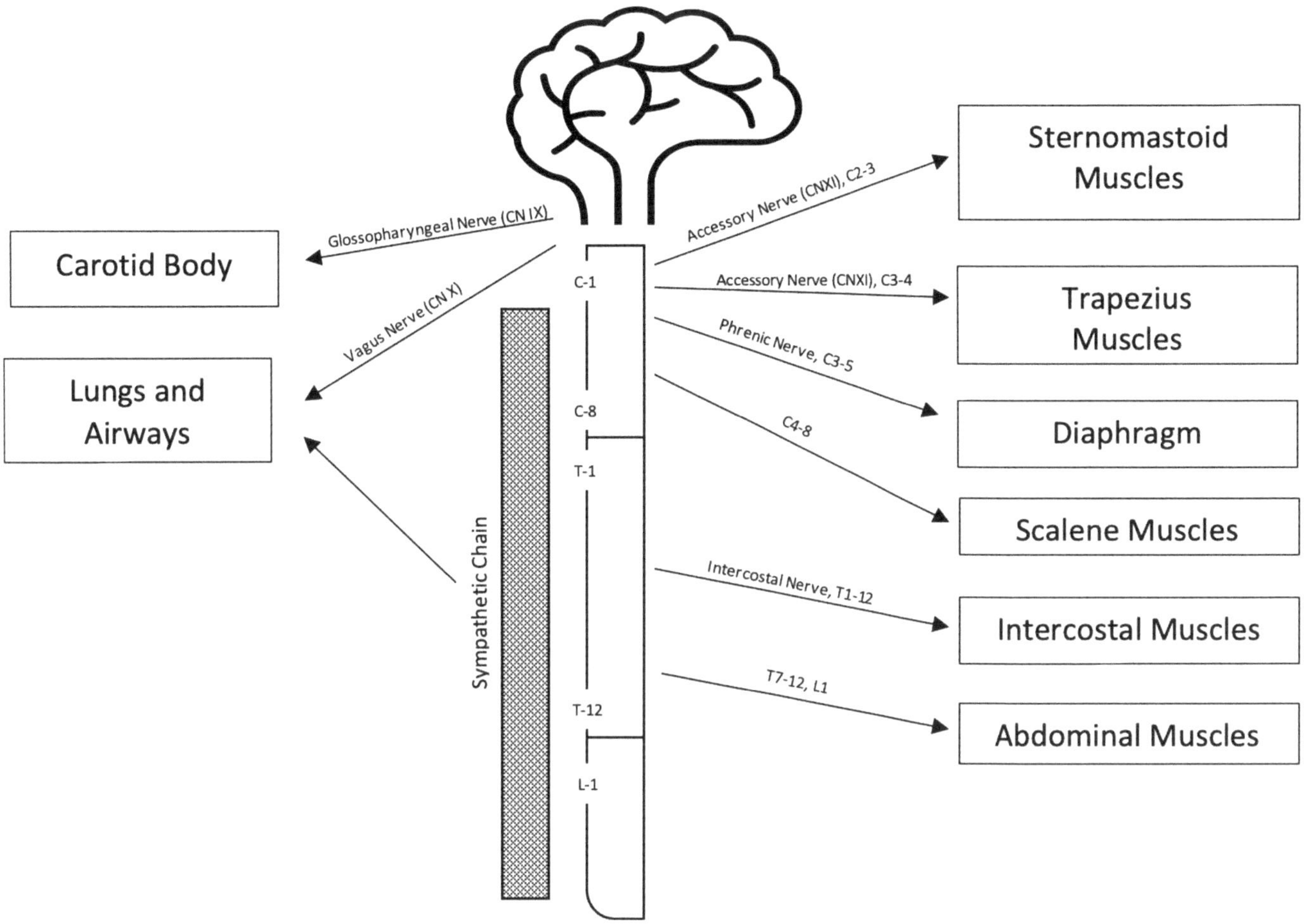

Fig. 9.2 Schematic of innervation of different respiratory. Adopted from Tobin' [16]

Dyspnea

One of the first descriptions of dyspnea was by Sir James Parkinson in his 1817 "An essay on the shaking palsy" describing a patient "fetching his breath rather hard" [17]. Dyspnea is a subjective feeling of breathing discomfort or breathlessness that subjects both healthy and ill feel, and often called "air hunger" [16]. As described by a patient with lung cancer: it feels "you're going to die because you're not getting enough air" [18]. The sensation of dyspnea is not a direct sensation or reaction to hypoxemia or hypercarbia but rather a reaction to the muscle ventilatory response. Some patients are more aware of dyspnea than others. This has been shown in polio patients with grossly abnormal ABGs who do not feel dyspnea since respiratory paralysis prevents a compensatory rescue breathing pattern. As discussed earlier, the amygdala and hippocampus are involved in the neural control of breathing, and functional MRI studies have localized cortical areas activated by dyspnea close to those activated by pain, suggesting there is both an emotional and psychological component to dyspnea [15]. Dyspnea neural inputs range from the airway vagal receptors, pulmonary stretch receptors, irritant receptors, and local C fibers to respiratory muscle and chest wall sensory receptors. These inputs all synapse in the central nervous system to create the sensation of dyspnea [15].

Respiratory Failure

Respiratory failure results from an imbalance between load and capacity that leads to muscle fatigue secondary to excessive work of breathing (e.g., due to abnormal lung or chest wall mechanics) relative to the patient's muscle strength and endurance, which can be expected at first or pathologically decreased. Respiratory failure is typically associated with increased respiratory rate, rapid shallow breathing, and ultimately hypoventilation with failure to maintain acceptable blood gases and sustain life. While low PaO_2 alerts to the severity of the respiratory failure, it is the $PaCO_2$ changes that allow diagnosing of impending fatigue. When this happens, PaO_2 changes more rapidly than $PaCO_2$ since oxygen body stores are small. Neurogenic causes of respiratory failure can be broken into central and peripheral causes. Any neurologic insult—from toxic, metabolic, infectious or inflammatory, to traumatic brain injury (TBI), spinal cord injury (SCI), or central nervous system (CNS), degeneration can trigger respiratory failure if not treated. Peripheral causes such as spinal cord trauma, nerve injury from surgery (i.e., phrenic nerve damage during cardiothoracic surgery), or chronic neuromuscular disease (NMD) can set the stage for respiratory failure.

Essential Management Priorities

General Work Up of Dyspnea

Before working up dyspnea, the first question to answer is whether the patient requires acute management and support (e.g., intubation) of their acute respiratory failure. Key clinical signs such as tachypnea, tachycardia, staccato speech, cyanosis, sweating, weak voice, accessory muscle use, and obtundation suggest impending respiratory collapse and can be rapidly observed. Paradoxical breathing, an ominous hallmark of impending exhaustion, is seen in patients with out-of-phase chest wall and abdominal movements during respiration (Table 9.3).

If time allows, investigating for obvious cardiac and pulmonary signs such as chest pain, palpitations, murmurs, wheezes, and rales is the first step of dyspnea workup. In the acute setting, chest radiography and bedside point-of-care ultrasound can quickly diagnose or exclude causes of acute respiratory and cardiovascular issues such as pneumonia, pleural effusion, pneumothorax, valvular problems, and cardiogenic shock [19, 20]. Exertional dyspnea, orthopnea from left ventricular failure and diaphragm weakness, platypnea in hepatopulmonary syndrome, and dyspnea from depression or anxiety must also be excluded [15].

Some neurologic patients have "sensory dyspnea" meaning they complain of shortness of breath, but have no obvious signs of respiratory failure and normal laboratory and imaging evaluation [21]. Furthermore, the immediate subjective perception and sensation of dyspnea due to impending respiratory failure will often times provoke anxiety and panic, worsening the symptoms as the drive to breath is not matched by adequate ventilatory response.

The incidence of deep vein thrombosis (DVT) and pulmonary embolism (PE) in neurosurgical patients is estimated to be as high as 25%, with PE mortality rate up to 50% [21]. Many chronic neurologic patients are bed-bound and are at risk for these complications, which can present as dyspnea and anxiety. Moreover, thromboembolic risk in surgical ICU patients is increased by limited mobility, malignancies, dehydration, and coagulopathies. It has been suggested that "neuromedical" patients have less incidence of DVT/PE, likely due to earlier DVT prophylaxis, less gross inflammatory response, and ability to mobilize [21, 22].

For patients who do not need emergent invasive support, several strategies can improve dyspnea, such as conventional oxygen therapy, various forms of noninvasive respiratory support, and in selected cases, opioids or anxiolytics. These strategies can reduce both the drive to breathe and dyspneic symptoms. Sometimes reassurance can be helpful. Yet, a high vigilance and suspicion for respiratory fatigue or depression is vital.

Table 9.3 Clinical exam findings of neuromuscular respiratory failure

Bedside exam findings of neuromuscular respiratory failure	
Restlessness	Staccato speech
Diaphoresis	Accessory muscle use
Tachycardia	Weak cough
Tachypnea	Abdominal paradoxical breathing

Prevention of Dyspnea and Respiratory Failure

Respiratory therapists, occupational therapists, and physical therapists can all contribute to prevent the setup for respiratory failure. A common characteristic shared by patients with neuromuscular diseases is challenging secretion management by decrease awareness or airway reflexes. Uncontrolled secretions can cause microaspiration, hypoxia, hypercapnia, and dyspnea leading to respiratory failure. Humidifying all supplemental air and breathing treatments, exercising to increase minute ventilation and open airways by spirometry, and using medications such as hypertonic saline nebulization, scopolamine, and bronchodilators are all tools to prevent a significant secretion burden. Patients with severe bulbar involvement, for example, can be managed with atropine drops or botulinum toxin B to minimize secretions and improve tolerance to noninvasive treatment [23]. Implementing aggressive trachea bronchial pulmonary toilet, chest physiotherapy, patient mobilization and repositioning, devices such as incentive spirometers, vibratory oscillatory devices, cough assist, CPAP, and intrapulmonary percussive ventilation (IPV) can prevent atelectasis and improve patient's respiratory trajectory.

Acute Management of Respiratory Failure

The first-line treatment for hypoxemia is supplemental oxygen. While this is the fastest and most efficient way to correct hypoxemia, the underlying causes should be understood and treated. For example, oxygen therapy alone will not correct ventilatory failure nor resolve atelectasis. Depending on the clinical scenario, the next step is to support inspiration, improve respiratory mechanics, and reopen collapsed airspaces using one of the various forms of noninvasive respiratory support.

Noninvasive Respiratory Support

The term noninvasive respiratory support encompasses various forms of noninvasive ventilation (NIV), continuous positive airway pressure (CPAP), and High Flow Nasal Cannula (HFNC) oxygen therapy. Investigation for noninvasive support began in neurological diseases such as GBS, to support respiratory drive and maintain oxygenation. COPD and COPD exacerabtions are a more classic indication for BIPAP. CPAP is now an established treatment for OSA, and it is often used for cardiogenic pulmonary edema [24, 25]. The role noninvasive support in acute hypoxemic respiratory failure continues to be investigated [26–28]. A 2020 meta-analysis looked at 21 separate trials to evaluate the utility of NIV as treatment in acute hypoxemic respiratory failure compared with standard oxygen therapies. Their results showed that treatment with NIV compared to standard oxygen therapy was associated with a lower risk of death and endotracheal intubation [29]. Their review showed no clear mortality benefit when comparing HFNC and nasal cannula.

NIV by BIPAP delivers inspiratory assist and reduces work of breathing and muscle fatigue while providing positive end expiratory pressure (PEEP) to reduce atelectasis and shunt. CPAP does not provide inspiratory support and is used when the work of breathing is not excessive or can be reduced by rapidly improving lung recruitment and compliance. The advantage of CPAP is that it can be delivered by simplified systems that do not require a ventilator. NIV and CPAP are delivered through face mask. Although mask design has improved tolerance, it still can cause skin damage and breakdown, claustrophobia, and discomfort. Furthermore, the mask interface is often associated with leaks in patients who are edentulous, have sunken faces, have nasogastric tubes, or facial hair.

High flow nasal cannula (HFNC) has proved a reliable treatment for patients developing acute hypoxic respiratory failure. HFNC can run heated and humidified oxygen flows up to 60 L/min and can generate above 5 cm H_2O pressure in the upper airway [30–32]. In contrast to conventional oxygen therapy, HFNC is effective in washing out anatomic dead space, reducing tidal volume, work of breathing, and dyspnea [33]. A more tolerable patient interface may explain the success of HFNC over NIV in the treatment of acute hypoxemic respiratory failure. The FLORALI trial compared patients with acute hypoxemic respiratory failure without hypercapnia managed with HFNC and those treated with nasal cannula or NIV. They found ICU and 90-day mortality significantly reduced in the HFNC group (with no difference in intubation rates) [34]. Recently, HFNC has been shown to help lower reintubation rates when used after extubation [33]. HFNC has been extensively used during COVID-19 where it was superior to conventional oxygen [35]. Combining awake prone positioning and HFNC has greatly reduced intubation rates in acute hypoxemic failure due to COVID-19 [36].

The helmet system is an interface for NIV and CPAP delivery where the patient wears a sealed helmet that provides pressure around the head and neck, sparing facial skin from pressure. The volume of a helmet system is about 10 L and while there is some degree of CO_2 rebreathing, the improved tolerance outweighs this limitation. Studies showed some superiority of helmet over mask in acute hypoxemic respiratory failure and over HFNC in severely hypoxemic respiratory failure [37, 38]. Despite a widespread use of the helmet in Europe, it has not been yet adopted in North America.

Noninvasive support should not be used in patients with profoundly altered mentation (encephalopathic, GCS <10), hemodynamic instability, severe upper gastrointestinal bleeding, upper airway obstruction, high aspiration risk or severe dysphagia, high secretion burden, multi-organ failure, and cardiac or respiratory arrest (Table 9.4). In patients who mildly encephalopathic from hypercapnia rather than hypoxia, NIV has been effective in stabilizing them if successfully reducing $PaCO_2$, but constant reevaluation must happen to ensure ETI is not delayed [39]. The success of noninvasive support should be evaluated shortly after initiation (1–2 h). If gas exchange has not improved, a decision to intubate and establish an invasive airway should be made to avoid further deterioration.

Invasive Mechanical Ventilation

Detailed ventilator management is out of scope for this chapter, but the essential concepts are summarized. A ventilator delivers gas flow at a desired pressure (pressure control) or volume (volume control) or a combination of both. Pressure and volume can be delivered to completely support breathing when the patient has no respiratory activity (total ventilator support) or to aid spontaneous breathing (partial ventilator support). Each patient breath can be supported with more or less pressure as in pressure support ventilation (PSV) or by delivering a set amount of machine breaths as in synchronized intermittent mandatory ventilation (SIMV). Airway pressure release ventilation (APRV) is a ventilation mode where the patient is maintained at a

Table 9.4 Contraindications to noninvasive ventilation

Contraindications to NIV	
Uncooperative patient Reduced level of consciousness Delirium with restlessness or agitation Undrained pneumothorax	Severe dysphagia Excessive secretions Severe hypoxemia (PAO_2 <600 mmHg with FiO_2 >0.6) Coexistence of two other organ failures

high upper airway pressure and then released to a lower airway pressure. At the higher pressure, the spontaneously breathing patient can take small breaths at or above the high pressure.

The choice of ventilator modalities is highly individualized and depends on patient physiology, as there is no data clearly supporting the superiority of an approach over others.

The complications of mechanical ventilation include barotrauma when extremely high pressures are applied and ventilator-induced injury (VILI), an inflammatory condition due to excessive stretch/strain of ventilated airspaces. The relevance of VILI in patients who do not have ARDS is still debated.

Significantly, dyspnea can impact even mechanically ventilated patients. It has been reported that dyspnea affects up to half of ventilated patients, and it often goes unrecognized by clinicians due to communication issues [40–42]. As mentioned previously, the neural pathways of dyspnea share much in common with fear and pain, and detecting dyspnea in mechanically ventilated patients can be done using different scales incorporating heart rate, facial expressions of fear, respiratory rate, and accessory muscles or paradoxical abdominal movement during breathing [40].

Acute Respiratory Distress Syndrome (ARDS)

Acute respiratory distress syndrome (ARDS) is clinically defined based on consensus criteria that include severity of hypoxemia, chest radiography, and low suspicion that heart failure is the primary cause of respiratory decompensation [43]. ARDS can evolve from a multitude of disease processes, and it must be recognized early to expedite appropriate treatment measures. In the neurological ICU, nosocomial pneumonia, gastric aspiration, non-pulmonary sepsis, shock, concomitant trauma, and drug overdose can all lead to ARDS [44]. Up to one-third of brain damaged patients develop ARDS, due to increased sympathetic tone and activity leading to neurogenic pulmonary edema, a systemic inflammatory response with pro-inflammatory cytokines [45]. ARDS lungs are stiff, noncompliant, and filled with fluid due to leaky capillaries. However, ventilated residual healthy lung "baby lung" with normal mechanical characteristics persists, although in a grossly decreased quantity. As ARDS progresses, functionally viable baby lung further declines, and ventilated airspaces receive excessive mechanical stress for each breath, promoting iatrogenic VILI. The only accepted approach to prevent or reduce VILI—and improve ARDS survival—is lung-protective ventilation with a low tidal volume, ideally of 6 mL/kg predicted body weight and PEEP adjusted to guarantee acceptable oxygenation [46]. This strategy requires the abandonment of normalized blood gases as therapeutic targets, with tolerance of relatively low PaO_2 and higher $PaCO_2$ than normal (permissive hypercapnia). This can be problematic in neurological patients with borderline brain ischemia and/or high ICP, and often an added cause of mortality.

Approaches to decrease VILI by improving regional stretch near atelectatic tissue (atelectrauma) with higher PEEP failed despite strong preclinical evidence. Prone positioning improves ARDS survival, which might be related to attenuation of regional stretch. Inhaled vasodilators improve gas exchange but beneficial long-term outcome effects have yet to be demonstrated. Overall, the ideal management of ARDS remains elusive, and increasing evidence supports an individualized approach based on detailed characterization of patient biology and physiology rather than protocoled adoption of standardized ventilator strategies.

Extracorporeal Membrane Oxygenation (ECMO)

If mechanical ventilation and maximal medical therapy fail to oxygenate the patient and or clear carbon dioxide, venovenous Extra Corporeal Membranous Oxygenation (VV ECMO) can be employed. ECMO takes the patient's blood out of the body, oxygenates it, delivers it back to the circulation, and allows the diseased lungs to rest. VV ECMO specifically, accesses only the patient's venous system and relies on a working circulatory system to pump newly oxygenated blood throughout the body.

VV ECMO is not without risk, ranging from cannulation complications, to arterial embolization, and venous thrombosis. Absolute contraindications to ECMO include severe multi-organ system failure, intracranial hemorrhage, and poor short-term prognosis (cancer) to name a few [47, 48].

It is unclear whether the early use of ECMO modifies the trajectory of lung injury. In the current age, ECMO remains a rescue form of life-supporting treatment, as clinical trial results do not unambiguously support its use of ECMO. When a better survival is observed, it is partially due to timing and or decreasing incidence of VALI since on ECMO, by the ability to reduce their tidal volumes, PEEP, and driving pressures [47, 49, 50].

Specific Concerns in the Neurological ICU

Implications of Comorbid Conditions

General medical comorbidities can affect patients in the neuro ICU and can cause dyspnea and respiratory failure such as COPD, sepsis, and heart failure. Other concurrent diseases that affect the chest wall or lung tissue itself (pulmonary fibrosis, acute lung injury, empyema) and chest wall deformities such as kyphoscoliosis, or severe burns that constrict the chest wall all can cause dyspnea. Septic patients demand a high level of oxygen to support organ systems during acute illness. If the patients have underlying respiratory muscle weakness, they are more prone to respiratory distress.

Great care must be taken when inducing and or intubating a patient in the neuro ICU. During neurologic crisis, such as an acute SAH, global myocardial dysfuntion (up to 30% of patients with SAH) leads to unstable and challenging hemodynamic management during induction and positive pressure ventilation [51]. Similarly, patients with Duchenne muscular dystrophy (DMD) not only have chronic respiratory failure but frequently have present with ventricular dysfunction due to cardiomyocyte hypertrophy and fibrosis leading to ventricular failure and arrythmias [52]. Neurogenically induced and reversible cardiomyopathies can also be seen with ischemic strokes, GBS, status epilepticus, acute hydrocephalus, acute spinal cord infarction, and emotional stress. Intubation and skill of manual ventilation, careful selection of induction agents and pharmacological support, and troubleshooting the effect of PPV on the cardiovascular system further hemodynamic deterioration can be limited.

Optimizing Ventilation in Acute Brain Injury

After an acute brain injury, there is often a combination of increase in ICP and a sympathetic and catecholamine surge from neuroinflammation. This combination can induce increased capillary permeability, venous pressure, and capillary alveolar damage. Massive brain injuries can cause autonomic dysfunction, increased PVR and pulmonary edema, leading to ARDS [53, 54]. Additionally, secondary injuries associated with TBI can also aggravate the respiratory failure such as pneumonia, pulmonary contusion, transfusion-related acute lung injury, chest wall damage, flail chest, and hemothorax.

For example, about a third of TBI patients will have developed respiratory failure by the end of their acute hospitalization. Patients with TBI are not necessarily in respiratory distress or failure on presentation, but are at risk of losing their protective reflexes, having an impaired cough, and changing their breathing control.

There are competing physiologic interests when managing a TBI patient. One is to preserve the integrity of the brain and one is facilitate oxygenation and end organ perfusion. The keys to TBI management include optimizing cerebral perfusion pressure, lowering the cerebral metabolic rate of oxygen, controlling the CO_2 effect on cerebrovascular tone, reducing nosocomial pneumonia by head elevation, using lower PEEP to allow for cerebral venous drainage, and limiting paralysis and sedation to allow frequent neuroevaluations. Most of these clinical managements are in contrast with mechanical ventilation optimization in ARDS. Fulminant neurogenic pulmonary edema complicate the clinical picture even further. The key to a successful clinical management is avoid a dogmatic approach to mechanical ventilation guidelines and to prioritize key principles of neuroprotection.

A 2021 systematic review and meta-analysis on TBI and mechanical ventilation illustrates this point. The incidence of ARDS following TBI has been estimated to be about 20% of patients with a median time of 3 days for presentation [55]. To optimize management, it is recommended to achieve normocarbia with a PaO_2 over 110 mmHg, maintain a PEEP less than or equal to 12 cm H_2O, titrate PEEP based on ICP measurements, and consider hyperosmolar therapy before proning. If the patient is eligible for ECMO, the use anticoagulation and the site of venous cannulation [53] need to be strategically discussed in view of the neurological risk of secondary injuries.

Acute and Chronic Respiratory Failure in Neuromuscular Diseases

Chronic neuromuscular diseases such as Guillen–Barre Syndrome (GBS), Amyotrophic Lateral Sclerosis (ALS), Myasthenia Gravis (MG), Smooth Muscle Atrophy (SMA), Duchenne Muscular Dystrophy (DMD), polymyositis, and dermatomyositis can evolve to progressive respiratory dysfunction from muscular weakness (Table 9.4). The respiratory weakness includes bulbar musculature, diaphragm, intercostals, and expiratory muscles causing respiratory emergencies due to oropharyngeal dysfunction, low minute ventilation with hypercapnia, and pulmonary aspiration. Knowing a patient's medical history and comorbidities can significantly help anticipate problems. The most common neuromuscular diseases requiring aggressive respiratory care include myasthenic crisis, GBS, myopathies, and ALS [56]. Many patients with neurological diseases have problems with dysphagia and gastric and esophageal dysmotility (Table 9.5).

Table 9.5 Respiratory failure in neuromuscular diseases, Adopted from "Practical Approaches to Respiratory Emergencies" [57]

Rate of occurrence of respiratory failure	Diseases
Unavoidable	Duchenne muscular dystrophy (DMD) amyotrophic lateral sclerosis (ALS)
Frequent	Guillain–Barré syndrome (GBS) Spinal muscular atrophy type 2 (SMA2) Myasthenia gravis (MG) Myotonic dystrophy type 1 (DM1)
Occasional	Becker muscular dystrophy (BMD) Some types of Charcot–Marie–tooth disease Some mitochondrial diseases
Rare	Oculopharyngeal muscular dystrophy Carchot-Marie-tooth

Swallowing is a complex mechanism involving over 50 muscles and neuronal connections to include the cortex, afferent connections, brainstem swallowing centers, cranial nerves V, VII, IX, X, XII, and spinal nerves C1–3. Any issue with these connections can impact a patient's respiratory status [58]. Frequently bulbar and expiratory muscle dysfunction leads to inadequate cough, pooling of secretions, aspiration, pneumonia, and ultimately to respiratory failure, which is why multimodal therapies to prevent and optimize patients with this medical history is so important. In the acute setting, clinicians need to constantly evaluate for neuromuscular respiratory failure. Patients with acute GBS flairs, can present with tachypnea and distress, but patients with chronic weakness like ALS can appear comfortable even if on the verge of respiratory failure [56]. A quick bedside test to predict the need for ventilatory support is using a spirometer to measure a vital capacity (VC) breath. If the VC is less than 20 cc/kg worsening respiratory function from weakness is likely, and the patient should be immediately considered for noninvasive or invasive ventilatory support.

Outside of bedside spirometry and VC, it is challenging to identify respiratory muscle weakness in patients with neuromuscular disease. Compiling and tracking bedside evaluations, spirometry, physical exams, and arterial blood gas can prevent aspiration events and acute decompensation needing emergent intubation. More sophisticated tests of muscle weakness such as phrenic nerve conduction studies or enteric electric stimulation of swallowing are still technology in progress and rarely practical in neurological injured patients [58].

GBS

It is estimated that 25% of patients with GBS suffer from respiratory failure due to weakness of the respiratory muscles. Management of GBS patients who are admitted with dyspnea include mechanical ventilation, as their clinical status will continue to decline to hypercapnic respiratory failure. In GBS, it is recommended to perform bedside spirometry every 6 h during the acute phase of the illness. GBS patients cannot be safely supported on NIV and often show signs of severe or rapidly progressing weakness, bulbar weakness, and early ventilatory compromise [56].

GBS is associated with cardiovascular dysautonomia, and they can develop malignant tachy and brady arrhythmias during intubation or early stages of mechanical ventilation [56]. Values that indicate impending respiratory failure include VC less than 20 mm, MIV <−30 cm H_2O, MEP <40 mmHg, or decrease in VC of more than 30% over 24 h. These patients should be mechanically ventilated [56]. An example of managing a GBS patient is illustrated in Fig. 9.3.

Myasthenia Gravis

Myasthenic crisis affects 20% of MG patients, and causes a pseudo upper airway obstruction, leading to hypoventilation from bulbar and inspiratory muscle weakness and furthermore, can cause significant atelectasis and potentially aspiration. For patients in myasthenic crisis, NIV BiPAP trials can stave off an intubation, except in the setting of high secretion burden or severe blood gas abnormalities. In patients requiring intubation for over a week, a tracheostomy is often necessary, since the failure rate of extubation is approximately 25% [56].

Parkinson's Disease

Patients with Parkinson's Disease may present to the ICU with a restrictive lung pattern on pulmonary function tests due to respiratory muscle rigidity and a degree of kyphoscoliosis. The combination of these factors causes the patients to be unable to accommodate a high respiratory demand, like during a respiratory infection. PD patients can also develop upper airway obstruction symptoms, diaphragmatic weakness, and can succumb to the effects of their dopamine agonists resulting in acute respiratory decompensation [15].

Central Nervous System Pathology

Autonomic nervous system disruption can cause carotid and aortic sinus transmission dysfunction, a drop in vagal tone, prevent bronchodilation, and cause a blunted response to hypoxia and hypercarbia. Stroke patients present a mixed bag of respiratory issues ranging from central nervous system damage from primary or secondary insult at respiratory control centers, cerebral edema, resultant muscle weakness, and changes in chest wall mechanics. It is estimated that a third of stroke patients will develop a pneumonia and have three times the risk of death in the first 30 days. In the acute phase of stroke management, many suggest using supplemental oxygen if the SPO_2 is less than 94% [59]. Failure to appreciate respiratory distress and promptly establish an airway can lead to secondary neuronal injury [59]. Unfortunately, the mortality rate of a stroke patient being intubated is 40–80% with only 50% surviving 30 days, and 38% surviving 1 year. To assess stroke patients, breathing patterns can be diagnostic aids. For example, clustered or ataxic breathing patterns are seen in brainstem syndrome, and recurrent apneic episodes ties into basilar artery occlusion. After a massive stroke, patients often develop Cheyne Stokes breathing with cycles of hyperpnea and apnea.

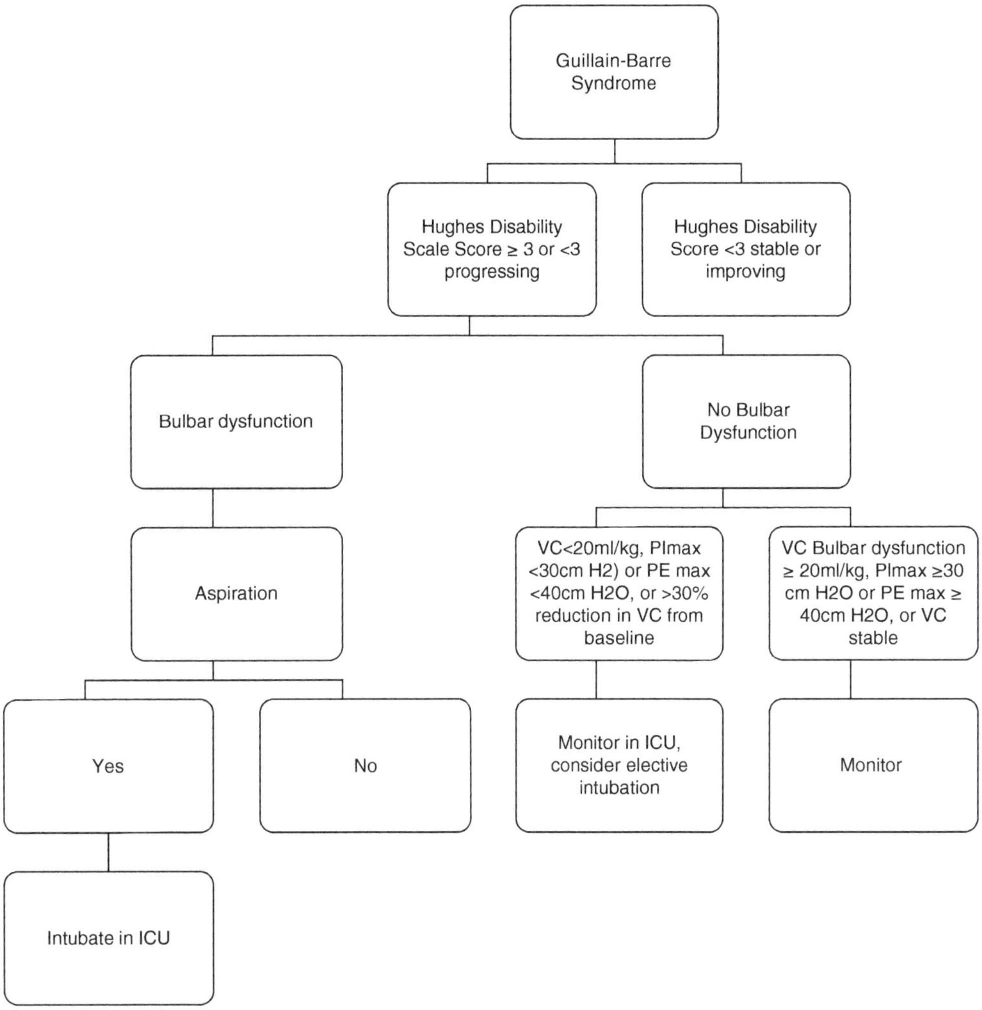

Fig. 9.3 Decision tree to manage respiratory distress in Guillain-Barre, Adapted from "Warning signs of imminent respiratory failure in neurological patients" [14]

SCI

One of the major causes of morbidity and mortality for SCI patients is respiratory failure with an incidence roughly ranging from 30% to 80%. The severity of respiratory distress is directly a result of spinal level injured. A full lesion to C2–4, will cause 100% vent dependence, while injury to C3–5 may impact the phrenic nerve only partially and depending on degree of injury, will impair the diaphragm. Damage to C5–8 will cause weakness or paralysis of intercostals or abdominal musculature. Even injury below the level of C8 by reducing the sympathetic outflow can cause increased secretions, bronchospasm, decrease in surfactant production and hinder effective coughs. Any of these injuries can decrease the efficiency of the ventilatory muscle, leading to atelectasis, increased secretion burden, pneumonia, and ventilatory failure [57].

Long-Term Ventilator Management

Ventilator Weaning

The goal of mechanical ventilation is to support the patients while the cause of their respiratory failure is identified, managed, and treated to the point that they can once again breathe on their own. Ventilator liberation is a protocolized, structured approach to free patients from the ventilator. Unfortunately, many patients are unable to liberate from mechanical ventilation and become ventilator dependent. Studies in the 1990s showed that a structured approach to liberation with protocols was better than a more subjective approach [60]. The first step is to identify patients that meet certain eligibility criteria for liberation. This criterion includes a low F_iO_2, low PEEP, hemodynamic stability, and resolution of the cause of respiratory failure (e.g., pneumonia). The eligible patients undergo a spontaneous breathing

Fig. 9.4 Ventilator weaning parameters

Parameter	Values to predict weaning outcome
Minute Ventilation	≤ 15 L/min
Respiratory Rate	≤ 35 breath/min
Tidal Volume	≥ 5ml/kg body weight
Negative Inspiratory Force	≤ -20 cm H2O
Rapid Shallow Breathing Index	≤ 105 breaths/min/L

Fig. 9.5 SBT readiness criteria for a Neuro ICU patient

Parameter	Threshold Values for Readiness
Glasgow Coma Scale	≥ 8
Airway Reflexes	Intact reflexes (good cough with suctioning)
Tracheal Suctioning	≤ 2 times / hour
Serum sodium concentration	135-145 mEq/L
Core temperature	< 38.5°C over the last 8 hours
PaO2/FiO2	≥ 200
PEEP	Reasonable for ETT size and lung pathology
PaCO2	≤ 50 mmHg
Heart Rate	≤ 125 BPM
Systolic Blood Pressure	≥ 90 mmHg

trial (SBT), which lasts at least 30 min. During SBTs, the patient is placed on minimal to no support and allowed to breathe spontaneously. Anxiety, fatigue, hypoxia, and apnea are common causes of SBT failures. Passing the SBT is a reflection of the patient's ability to breathe without mechanical support—it does not guarantee they will be able to be extubated safely and successfully. The "extubatability" of a patient is reflected in their neurologic status, predicted ability to protect the airway, and absence of airway swelling, as a few examples. The neurointensivist evaluation of *all* these factors ultimately dictates the strategy of extubation. If the patients pass their SBT and meet extubation criteria by airway maintenance criteria, they are extubated. The level of consciousness is of course important but not always interfering with a safe extubation. Patients who fail the SBT several times or are reintubated undergo *ventilator weaning*, which is the process of gradually decreasing inspiratory support with a goal toward liberation (Fig. 9.4).

There is limited evidence to guide weaning. Physiological assessment of respiratory muscle strength and endurance can be performed using negative inspiratory force (NIF), rapid shallow breathing index (RSBI), or even diaphragm ultrasound to measure thickness of the diaphragm, which has recently been shown to be a good predictor of failure and respiratory muscle weakness. Unfortunately, many time the neurologically injured patient is unable to cooperate with the respiratory therapist to perform such maneuvers effectively. The consequences of prolonged ventilation with an endotracheal tube include pneumonia, vocal cord paralysis, tracheomalacia, tracheal erosion, and tracheal stenosis—not to mention patient discomfort. To improve comfort and avoid many of these complications, tracheostomy is often performed in neurological patient failing extubation multiple times. Tracheostomy facilitates weaning, pulmonary hygiene, and transition to long-term care facility, but the optimal time to perform the procedure in neurologically impaired patients has not been clearly established [61] (Fig. 9.5).

Once extubated, neurologically injured patients can have difficulty with secretions, weakness, and level of consciousness; constant evaluation and pulmonary toilet is necessary to prevent reintubation. The U.K.'s 2019 Breathe Trial RCT investigated weaning strategies for patients who failed SBTs comparing extubating to NIV versus gradual reductions in pressure support with daily SBTs. While early extubation to NIV did not significantly improve the overall time to pure vent liberation, the patients who were extubated to NIV received less sedation and antibiotics [62]. NIV should be considered as a bridge to full liberation in neurological patients with mild upper airway obstruction, as long as able to clear secretions.

Conclusions

Effectively evaluating, managing, and treating a neurological patient with dyspnea is a complex task, and objective evaluation of pulmonary function is not always possible. Furthermore, dyspnea is all but uncommon in critical care units and uncovering its etiology can be complex, but as Dr. Tobin stated, "[while] there is no universally accepted definition of dyspnea…everybody has experienced the sensation and thus has an intuitive understanding of the phenomenon" [16]. At its core, the acute management of dyspnea in the neuro ICU is timely optimize both ventilation and oxygenation. Both hypercapnia and hypoxemia can aggravate the injury and impact on outcome. The heavy reliance on noninvasive ventilation strategies such as high flow nasal canula, BiPAP, and the helmet during the COVID-19 pandemic has proven them to be powerful tools in the management of acute respiratory failure in ICU, and it have been progressively introduced in the neuroICU for more selective indications. The key takeaways of improving outcome in patients with respiratory insufficiency are early identification of patients who are at risk of respiratory failure, integrating all members of the critical care team to optimize bronchopulmonary hygiene (e.g., respiratory therapist, physical therapists), and tailoring all respiratory support to the patient's specific underlying pathology.

References

1. West JB. Respiratory physiology : the essentials. Philadelphia: Wolters Kluwer Health/Lippincott Williams & Wilkins; 2012.
2. Ochs M, et al. The number of alveoli in the human lung. Am J Respir Crit Care Med. 2004;169(1):120–4.
3. Butler JP, Tsuda A. Transport of gases between the environment and alveoli--theoretical foundations. Compr Physiol. 2011;1(3):1301–16.
4. Stocks J, Quanjer PH. Reference values for residual volume, functional residual capacity and total lung capacity. ATS workshop on lung volume measurements. Official statement of the European Respiratory Society. Eur Respir J. 1995;8(3):492–506.
5. Robatto F, Bates J. Respiratory mechanics in anaesthesia. Br J Anaesth. 1990;65:4–12.
6. Urbankowski T, Przybyłowski T. Methods of airway resistance assessment. Pneumonol Alergol Pol. 2016;84(2):134–41.
7. Richter T, et al. Effect of prone position on regional shunt, aeration, and perfusion in experimental acute lung injury. Am J Respir Crit Care Med. 2005;172(4):480–7.
8. Hopkins SR, et al. Vertical gradients in regional lung density and perfusion in the supine human lung: the Slinky effect. J Appl Physiol. 2007;103(1):240–8.
9. Glenny R, Robertson HT. Distribution of perfusion. Compr Physiol. 2011;1(1):245–62.
10. Elliott M, Ghosh D. Respiratory failure and non-invasive ventilation. In: Hart S, Greenstone M, editors. Foundations of respiratory medicine. Cham: Springer International Publishing; 2018. p. 153–64.
11. Wagner PD. The physiological basis of pulmonary gas exchange: implications for clinical interpretation of arterial blood gases. Eur Respir J. 2015;45(1):227–43.
12. Santos C, et al. Pulmonary gas exchange response to oxygen breathing in acute lung injury. Am J Respir Crit Care Med. 2000;161(1):26–31.
13. Nuckton TJ, et al. Pulmonary dead-space fraction as a risk factor for death in the acute respiratory distress syndrome. N Engl J Med. 2002;346(17):1281–6.
14. Rabinstein AA, Wijdicks EF. Warning signs of imminent respiratory failure in neurological patients. Semin Neurol. 2003;23(1):97–104.
15. Vijayan S, et al. Dyspnea in Parkinson's disease: an approach to diagnosis and management. Expert Rev Neurother. 2020;20(6):619–26.
16. Tobin MJ, Dyspnea. Pathophysiologic basis, clinical presentation, and management. Arch Intern Med. 1990;150(8):1604–13.
17. Parkinson J. An essay on the shaking palsy. 1817. J Neuropsychiatry Clin Neurosci. 2002;14(2):223–36; discussion 222.
18. O'Driscoll M, Corner J, Bailey C. The experience of breathlessness in lung cancer. Eur J Cancer Care (Engl). 1999;8(1):37–43.
19. Gartlehner G, et al. Point-of-care ultrasonography in patients with acute dyspnea: an evidence report for a clinical practice guideline by the American College of Physicians. Ann Intern Med. 2021;174(7):967–76.
20. Qaseem A, Etxeandia-Ikobaltzeta I, Mustafa RA, Kansagara D, Fitterman N, Wilt TJ, Clinical Guidelines Committee of the American College of Physicians, Batur P, Cooney TG, Crandall CJ, Hicks LA, Lin JS, Maroto M, Tice J, Tufte JE, Vijan S, Williams JW Jr. Appropriate use of point-of-care ultrasonography in patients with acute Dyspnea in emergency department or inpatient settings: a clinical guideline from the American College of Physicians. Ann Intern Med. 2021;174(7):985–93.
21. Behera SS, et al. Incidence of deep vein thrombosis in neurointensive care unit patients-does prophylaxis modality make any difference? Indian J Crit Care Med. 2019;23(1):43–6.
22. Dubinski D, et al. Pulmonary embolism in neurocritical care-introduction of a novel grading system for risk stratification: the Frankfurt AMBOS score. Neurosurg Rev. 2021;44(2):1165–71.
23. Dorst J, Ludolph AC. Non-invasive ventilation in amyotrophic lateral sclerosis. Ther Adv Neurol Disord. 2019;12:1756286419857040.
24. Brochard L, et al. Noninvasive ventilation for acute exacerbations of chronic obstructive pulmonary disease. N Engl J Med. 1995;333(13):817–22.
25. Demoule A, et al. How to ventilate obstructive and asthmatic patients. Intensive Care Med. 2020;46(12):2436–49.
26. Motley HL, Cournand A, et al. Intermittent positive pressure breathing; a means of administering artificial respiration in man. JAMA J Am Med Assoc. 1948;137(4):370–82.
27. Pierson DJ. History and epidemiology of noninvasive ventilation in the acute-care setting. Respir Care. 2009;54(1):40–52.
28. Annunziata A, et al. Daytime alternatives for non-invasive mechanical ventilation in neuromuscular disorders. Acta Myol. 2021;40(1):51–60.
29. Ferreyro BL, et al. Association of noninvasive oxygenation strategies with all-cause mortality in adults with acute hypoxemic respiratory failure: a systematic review and meta-analysis. JAMA. 2020;324(1):57–67.
30. Chertoff J. High-flow oxygen, positive end-expiratory pressure, and the Berlin definition of acute respiratory distress syndrome: are they mutually exclusive? Am J Respir Crit Care Med. 2017;196(3):396–7.
31. Papazian L, et al. Use of high-flow nasal cannula oxygenation in ICU adults: a narrative review. Intensive Care Med. 2016;42(9):1336–49.
32. Groves N, Tobin A. High flow nasal oxygen generates positive airway pressure in adult volunteers. Aust Crit Care. 2007;20(4):126–31.
33. Raoof S, et al. High-flow, noninvasive ventilation and awake (nonintubation) proning in patients with coronavirus disease 2019 with respiratory failure. Chest. 2020;158(5):1992–2002.
34. Frat JP, et al. High-flow oxygen through nasal cannula in acute hypoxemic respiratory failure. N Engl J Med. 2015;372(23):2185–96.
35. Ospina-Tascon GA, et al. Effect of high-flow oxygen therapy vs conventional oxygen therapy on invasive mechanical ventilation and clinical recovery in patients with severe COVID-19: a randomized clinical trial. JAMA. 2021;326(21):2161–71.
36. Ehrmann S, et al. Awake prone positioning for COVID-19 acute hypoxaemic respiratory failure: a randomised, controlled, multinational, open-label meta-trial. Lancet Respir Med. 2021;9(12):1387–95.
37. Grieco DL, et al. Effect of helmet noninvasive ventilation vs high-flow nasal oxygen on days free of respiratory support in patients with COVID-19 and moderate to severe hypoxemic respiratory failure: the HENIVOT randomized clinical trial. JAMA. 2021;325(17):1731–43.

38. Patel BK, et al. Effect of noninvasive ventilation delivered by helmet vs face mask on the rate of endotracheal intubation in patients with acute respiratory distress syndrome: a randomized clinical trial. JAMA. 2016;315(22):2435–41.
39. Goncalves G, et al. Non-invasive ventilation in patients with an altered level of consciousness. A clinical review and practical insights. Adv Respir Med. 2020;88(3):233–44.
40. Decavele M, Similowski T, Demoule A. Detection and management of dyspnea in mechanically ventilated patients. Curr Opin Crit Care. 2019;25(1):86–94.
41. Haugdahl HS, et al. Underestimation of patient breathlessness by nurses and physicians during a spontaneous breathing trial. Am J Respir Crit Care Med. 2015;192(12):1440–8.
42. Binks AP, Desjardin S, Riker R. ICU clinicians underestimate breathing discomfort in ventilated subjects. Respir Care. 2017;62(2):150–5.
43. Force ADT, et al. Acute respiratory distress syndrome: the Berlin definition. JAMA. 2012;307(23):2526–33.
44. Meyer NJ, Gattinoni L, Calfee CS. Acute respiratory distress syndrome. Lancet. 2021;398(10300):622–37.
45. Koutsoukou A, et al. Respiratory mechanics in brain injury: a review. World J Crit Care Med. 2016;5(1):65–73.
46. Ventilation with lower tidal volumes as compared with traditional tidal volumes for acute lung injury and the acute respiratory distress syndrome. N Engl J Med. 2000;342(18):1301–8.
47. Combes A, et al. Extracorporeal life support for adults with acute respiratory distress syndrome. Intensive Care Med. 2020;46(12):2464–76.
48. Quintel M, et al. Extracorporeal membrane oxygenation for respiratory failure. Anesthesiology. 2020;132(5):1257–76.
49. Combes A, et al. Extracorporeal membrane oxygenation for severe acute respiratory distress syndrome. N Engl J Med. 2018;378(21):1965–75.
50. Sameed M, Meng Z, Marciniak ET. EOLIA trial: the future of extracorporeal membrane oxygenation in acute respiratory distress syndrome therapy? Breathe (Sheff). 2019;15(3):244–6.
51. Kerro A, Woods T, Chang JJ. Neurogenic stunned myocardium in subarachnoid hemorrhage. J Crit Care. 2017;38:27–34.
52. Mavrogeni S, et al. Cardiac involvement in Duchenne and Becker muscular dystrophy. World J Cardiol. 2015;7(7):410–4.
53. Kim JA, et al. Focused management of patients with severe acute brain injury and ARDS. Chest. 2022;161(1):140–51.
54. Oddo M, Citerio G. ARDS in the brain-injured patient: what's different? Intensive Care Med. 2016;42(5):790–3.
55. Fan TH, et al. Prevalence and outcome of acute respiratory distress syndrome in traumatic brain injury: a systematic review and meta-analysis. Lung. 2021;199(6):603–10.
56. Hocker S. Primary acute neuromuscular respiratory failure. Neurol Clin. 2017;35(4):707–21.
57. Racca F, Vianello A, Mongini T, Ruggeri P, Antonio Versaci GLV, Vita G. Practical approach to respiratory emergencies in neurological diseases. Neurol Sci. 2020;41:497–508.
58. Zuercher P, et al. Dysphagia in the intensive care unit: epidemiology, mechanisms, and clinical management. Crit Care. 2019;23(1):103.
59. Herpich F, Rincon F. Management of acute ischemic stroke. Crit Care Med. 2020;48(11):1654–63.
60. Ely EW, et al. Effect on the duration of mechanical ventilation of identifying patients capable of breathing spontaneously. N Engl J Med. 1996;335(25):1864–9.
61. Schonenberger S, et al. Early tracheostomy in ventilated stroke patients: study protocol of the international multicentre randomized trial SETPOINT2 (stroke-related early tracheostomy vs. prolonged orotracheal intubation in neurocritical care trial 2). Int J Stroke. 2016;11(3):368–79.
62. Perkins GD, et al. Protocolised non-invasive compared with invasive weaning from mechanical ventilation for adults in intensive care: the breathe RCT. Health Technol Assess. 2019;23(48):1–114.

Hypotension and Shock

10

Alexander C. Fort, I. Cordoba Torres, and R. Parker

Contents

A. C. Fort (✉) · I. Cordoba Torres
Department of Anesthesiology, Perioperative Medicine and Pain Management, University of Miami Miller School of Medicine, Miami, FL, USA
e-mail: acfort@med.miami.edu

R. Parker
Department of Anesthesiology, University of Florida College of Medicine, Gainesville, FL, USA

E. Mahanna Gabrielli et al. (eds.), *Textbook of Neurointensive Care: Volume 1*, https://doi.org/10.1007/978-3-031-62220-5_10

Abstract

Shock is a common finding in critical illness that can lead to significant morbidity and mortality. Shock results from inadequate delivery of oxygen leading to tissue hypoxia and end-organ damage. Through prompt diagnostic evaluation and appropriate therapies that also aim to minimize secondary injury, poor outcomes in the setting of shock can be minimized. Shock in the setting of central nervous system (CNS) injury results in unique challenges to the clinician. Pathophysiologic responses unique to the CNS must be understood in order to properly treat a wide spectrum of CNS pathology—this pathophysiology is particularly key in minimizing further injuries in the CNS-injured patient. The appropriate treatment of hypotension and shock can help maintain adequate CNS physiologic functions and lead to better outcomes.

Introduction

Within the Intensive Care Unit (ICU) setting, shock is a commonly encountered finding requiring prompt diagnosis and treatment in order to prevent irreversible organ damage. There is a broad range of etiologies leading to shock. A thorough understanding of pathophysiology, diagnostic workup, and treatment is required to adequately treat a patient in shock. Timely treatment is necessary as initially reversible causes of shock may lead to organ damage, multiorgan failure (MOF), and death.

The broad categories of shock include distributive, hypovolemic, cardiogenic, and obstructive. Within each of these categories exist a number of diagnoses, each with unique clinical characteristics and specific therapeutic strategies. (Fig. 10.1) Shock states do not exclusively fall into one of the four broad categories—patients may have etiologies from more than one group. In specific settings, such as trauma, when the etiology of shock is unclear both evaluation and treatment should occur simultaneously.

Injuries of the central nervous system (CNS) can lead to profound physiologic disturbance including shock and result in end-organ damage. Given the wide spectrum of CNS injuries, a thorough understanding of pathophysiologic principles is needed to provide appropriate therapies. Given the significant morbidity and mortality that can accompany CNS injury, these insults must be addressed appropriately to ensure avoid morbidity and mortality.

There are a number of etiologies of CNS injury, which can be divided into injuries of the brain and spinal cord. Blood pressure management is key in preserving these organs and avoiding secondary injury, one of the key principles in the care of the CNS injured patient. Importantly, non-CNS etiologies of shock must be considered when evaluating the hypotensive CNS injured patient. In the setting of trauma, hemorrhagic shock often co-exists with Traumatic Brain Injury (TBI) due to either cranial injuries themselves or additional traumatic injuries. Appropriate resuscitation is critical in preventing secondary injuries of the CNS in the poly-trauma patient.

Goals of This Chapter

- Review the epidemiology of shock in critically ill populations.
- Understand the definition of shock.
- Describe the pathophysiology of shock states with emphasis on the relationship between the central system and shock.
- Review the primary monitoring techniques used in the evaluation and management of shock.
- Describe the four major categories of shock and review specific goals and management strategies with respect to common etiologies of shock.

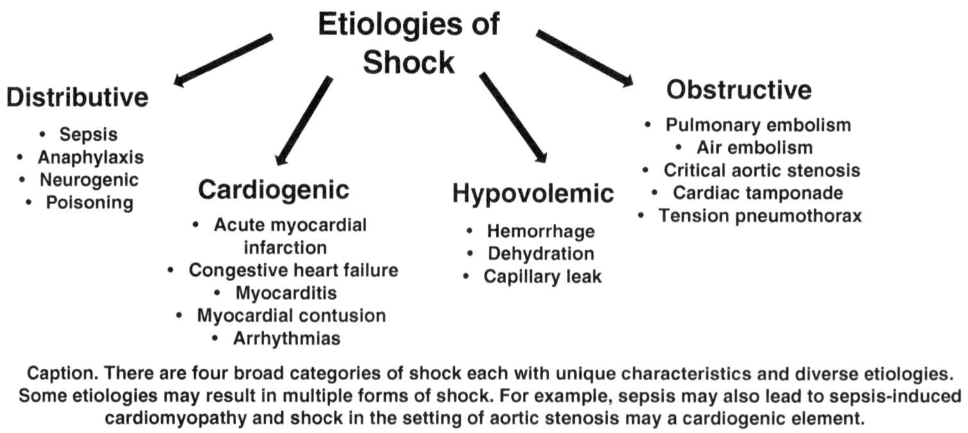

Fig. 10.1 *Etiologies of shock.* There are four broad categories of shock each with unique characteristics and diverse etiologies. Some etiologies may result in multiple forms of shock. For example, sepsis may also lead to sepsis-induced cardiomyopathy and shock in the setting of aortic stenosis may a cardiogenic element

Key Clinical Questions

- How does shock affect outcomes in the neurocritical care populations?
- What is the pathophysiologic relationship between shock and neurocritical illness?
- What advanced monitoring techniques can be used in shock to improve diagnostic accuracy and facilitate treatment?
- What are the clinical features of the four categories of shock states?
- How does the clinician accurately diagnose a specific shock state at the bedside?
- What are the specific treatment goals with of the most common shock states?

Epidemiology

Although less than 1% of patients presenting to the emergency department meet clinical criteria for shock, the diagnosis carries significant morbidity and mortality [1]. Among patients ultimately hospitalized with critical illness, shock occurs at much higher rates with roughly one-third of patients meeting clinical criteria [2]. The most commonly encountered form of shock in the ICU is septic, accounting for roughly two-thirds of cases, followed by cardiogenic and hypovolemic [3]. In contrast, among emergency department patients septic shock accounts for roughly one-third of cases with higher rates of hypovolemic and cardiogenic shock roughly equal to that of septic depending on the patient cohort [4–6].

With respect to the CNS injured patient, hypotension and shock are commonly encountered and may be the result from a number of etiologies. In the setting of TBI, roughly 35% of patients exhibit hypotension (SBP <90 mmHg) in the prehospital setting [7]. In the TBI population, systolic blood pressure (SBP) readings below 80 mmHg correlate with morbidity and mortality [8]. When compared to hypothermia and hypoxia, hypotension in the setting of TBI has the strongest negative prognostic effect [9]. The effect on mortality is particularly dramatic for TBI patients, with a 150% increase in mortality when hypotension (SBP <90 mmHg) occurs in the prehospital setting [7].

Unique to patients with CNS injuries is neurogenic shock, a form shock that may include elements of distributive and cardiogenic shock. Among patients with spinal cord injuries, reported incidences range between 19.3% and 31% [10, 11].

Current guidelines recommend specific blood pressure targets for TBI populations [12]. Although these guidelines should be considered in caring for these patients, the degree of hypotension that leads to secondary injury may be patient specific and a true blood pressure inflection point under which mortality increases may not exist [13].

Shock Definition

Shock is defined as hemodynamic collapse resulting in tissue hypoxia and eventual dysfunction. At the cellular level, hypoxia can result from reduced oxygen delivery, increased oxygen consumption, or the inefficient oxygen transport into cells, but varying degrees of each are often present. Hypoxia forces cells to generate energy through inefficient anaerobic pathways that result in energy deficits. While reduced energy production creates a metabolic challenge for all tissues, cells with high metabolic demand, such as the brain, heart, and kidneys are especially vulnerable. The cellular dysfunction in shock is initially reversable with early treatment but if prolonged will eventually lead to MOF. Because of the high metabolic demand of the brain and the relative hypoxia associated with shock, timely treatment is essential in the neurointensive care setting.

Pathophysiology

Under normal conditions, cells meet their metabolic requirements by utilizing oxygen and aerobic metabolism to generate adenosine triphosphate (ATP). The first step of energy production is glycolysis, an anaerobic process that converts glucose to pyruvate and nets two ATP molecules and two molecules of nicotinamide adenine dinucleotide (NADH). Under normal conditions with adequate oxygen delivery, pyruvate enters the tricarboxylic acid (TCA) cycle, and oxygen is utilized to generate 36 ATP molecules via oxidative phosphorylation. ATP is generated through the oxygen-dependent electron transport chain, and the inadequate delivery of oxygen encountered in states of shock renders the TCA cycle and specifically the electron transport chain ineffective. Under these conditions, pyruvate is shunted away from the TCA cycle and converted anaerobically to lactate [14]. Without the TCA cycle and oxidative phosphorylation, cells experience energy deficits and the accumulation of lactate. If cellular hypoxia persists, irreversible cellular damage occurs.

Shock States

The metabolic derangements found in shock result from tissue hypoxia and inadequate oxygen delivery at the cellular level. The delivery of oxygen (DO_2) is characterized by the following equation: $DO_2 = CO \times (SaO_2 \times [Hgb] \times 1.39) + (PaO_2 \times 0.03)$. As such, most forms of shock result from one or more derangements of the DO_2 equation. Shock is broadly categorized as either hypovolemic, cardiogenic, obstructive, or distributive. Hypovolemic shock alters DO_2 in several ways. Most notably, cardiac output (CO) is reduced as a result of decreased preload in the setting of hypovolemia. Additionally, hypovolemic shock resulting from hemorrhage reduces hemoglobin levels and further reduces DO_2. Both cardiogenic and obstructive shock primarily reduces DO_2 by direct reductions in CO. Distributive shock, which is associated with systemic vasodilation, is unique in that DO_2 can be normal or even elevated with increased CO. However, capillary dilation and rapid transport of red blood cells through the capillary system prevents effective oxygen transfer from hemoglobin to cells. As such, delivery to the cell may be relatively normal but reduced uptake to the cell results in hypoxia. Whether distributive, obstructive, cardiogenic, or hypovolemic, all forms of shock impede oxygen delivery to cells and potentially result in irreversible metabolic derangements.

Neural Mechanisms of Blood Pressure Control

The regulation and modulation of the circulatory system is determined by neural and humoral elements. The neural elements include cardiovascular control centers, vasomotor tone, the autonomic nervous system, and reflexes. Humoral elements include catecholamines, the renin–angiotensin-aldosterone system, and nitric oxide.

The product of CO and systemic vascular resistance (SVR) determines blood pressure. Cardiac output is determined by stroke volume (SV) and heart rate (HR). A number of CNS-mediated processes effect these determinants of blood pressure. In the setting of CNS injury, neurohormonal functions can be activated or attenuated, and through specific neural pathways lead to hemodynamic changes.

Neurogenic shock, which can occur following cranial or spinal cord injury, can lead to circulatory failure via several mechanisms. Importantly, neurogenic and spinal shock are two distinct entities that both result from spinal cord injury, with the latter having no hemodynamic sequelae (Fig. 10.2). In the setting of spinal cord injury (SCI), loss of vasomotor tone results from attenuated excitatory input to preganglionic alpha-sympathetic neurons, thereby contributing to hypotension [15, 16]. Secondly, loss of sympathetic activity resulting in relative parasympathetic dominance may lead to bradycardia and bradyarrhythmia's [15]. Finally, loss of sympathetic activity may reduce myocardial beta-adrenergic receptor input thereby leading to reduced contractility [15]. In sum, these three elements—reduced systemic vascular resistance, bradycardia, and reduced myocardial contractility—contribute in varying degrees to the hypotension that can be seen following SCI.

Neurogenic shock as a result of intracranial injury has less clear pathophysiologic mechanisms. Classic teaching suggests brain injury alone is not a cause for hypotension unless in the setting of medullary failure from brainstem death [17]. However, some evidence including an animal model does suggest intracranial injury can be a primary cause of hypotension [18–20]. The medulla appears to be critically important in the regulation of blood pressure through tonic discharge that maintains activity of spinal vasoconstrictor neurons [16]. Although global medullary failure, such as in the setting of brain death, is known to cause hypotension, even small lesions within the medulla can lead to significant arterial hypotension [21]. Additionally, particularly in the setting of hemorrhagic shock, injuries of the brain may lead to central sympathoadrenal failure or a failure of vasomotor responses to shock [18, 22, 23]. Lastly, catecholamine surge may lead to myocardial damage and cardiogenic shock, which may contribute to hypotension after TBI. Levels of catecholamines have been shown to be elevated in intracranial injury and these levels are postulated

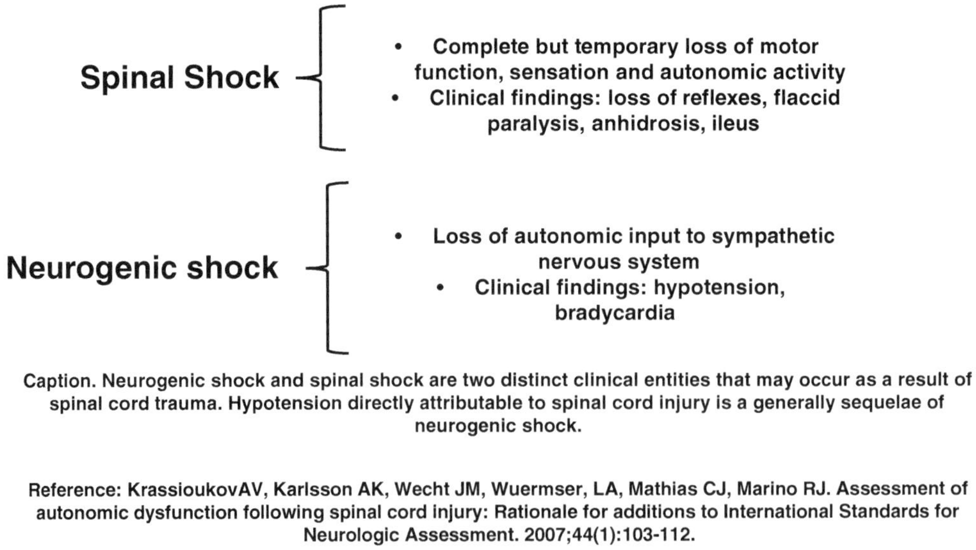

Fig. 10.2 *Comparison of spinal shock and neurogenic shock.* Neurogenic shock and spinal shock are two distinct clinical entities that may occur as a result of spinal cord trauma. Hypotension directly attributable to spinal cord injury is a generally sequelae of neurogenic shock. *Reference:* Krassioukov AV, Karlsson AK, Wecht JM, Wuermser, LA, Mathias CJ, Marino RJ. Assessment of autonomic dysfunction following spinal cord injury: Rationale for additions to International Standards for Neurologic Assessment. 2007;44 (1):103–112

to cause myocardial ischemia and damage leading to reduced cardiac contractility [24–27].

Cerebral Autoregulation

Autoregulatory processes unique to the CNS are key in the preservation of cerebral blood flow. The ability of the brain to maintain a constant cerebral blood flow (CBF) despite changes in blood pressure is referred to as cerebral autoregulation. Maintenance of CBF generally occurs between mean arterial pressures (MAPs) of 60 and 150 mmHg [28–30]. These blood pressure limits are shifted upward in patients with chronic hypertension [28]. In the setting of TBI and stroke, there may be absence or impairment of cerebral autoregulation [31, 32]. Therefore, in areas of injured brain with impaired autoregulation, the relationship between cerebral perfusion and blood pressure may be linear.

In the setting of shock, changes in the limits of cerebral autoregulation, such as in the setting of chronic hypertension, may lead to relative brain hypoperfusion despite seemingly appropriate blood pressures. Adjustment of blood pressure goals to higher values may be appropriate to maintain adequate brain perfusion.

Cerebral Perfusion Pressure and Intracranial Pressure

Cerebral perfusion pressure (CPP) is defined as the difference between the MAP and the intracranial pressure (ICP). In cases where the central venous pressure (CVP) is greater than the ICP, the CVP replaces ICP for the calculation. The most recent guidelines from the Brain Trauma Foundation recommend treating ICP values >22 mmHg and maintaining CPP values between 60 and 70 mmHg [12].

In the setting of shock, regardless of the etiology, maintenance of an adequate MAP is important in providing adequate organ perfusion, and with respect to the brain avoiding cerebral ischemic injury. When intracranial pathology exists, such as intracranial hemorrhage or cerebral edema, intracranial pressures can often be elevated—in these settings, maintaining normal or even supranormal MAP is critical to ensuring adequate CPP.

Monitoring Techniques

Shock occurs when hemodynamic abnormalities prevent efficient oxygen delivery to tissue, and hemodynamic monitoring facilitates the diagnosis and treatment of shock. Selection of the appropriate techniques and proper understanding of the strengths and limitations is important to effectively treat shock. In general, all modalities have limitations—data obtained in aggregate among several devices are more useful and trends are often more valuable than individual numbers. Three common hemodynamic indices used to evaluate and treat shock are the blood pressure, CVP, SVR, and CO. Together, these values help differentiate the etiology of shock and help guide treatment (Table 10.1).

Table 10.1 Hemodynamic indices in shock

	Blood pressure	Central venous pressure	Cardiac output	Systemic vascular resistance
Hypovolemic	↓	↓	↓	↑
Distributive	↓	↓	↑	↓
Cardiogenic	↓	↑	↓	↑
Obstructive	↓	↑	↓	↑

Characteristics of blood pressure, central venous pressure, cardiac output and systemic vascular resistance can help differentiate different forms of shock

Reference: Adapted from Marino P. The ICU Book. 4th Ed. Philadelphia, PA: Lippincott Williams and Wilkins; 2014

Arterial Line

Invasive blood pressure monitoring is useful when assessing the hemodynamic instability associated with shock because it offers the advantages of continuous beat-to-beat blood pressure monitoring, more accurate readings at low blood pressures, and easy access to laboratory draws. In the neurocritical care setting, arterial lines provide a continuous MAP for calculating CPP, and the visible representation of the blood pressure tracing allows the use of other dynamic indices, such as pulse pressure variation (PPV), stroke volume variation (SVV), and CO monitoring when combined with additional systems. The major disadvantage of invasive blood pressure monitoring is the potential for arterial thrombus, but this is mitigated by utilizing short, narrow catheters made of specialized materials. Also, common use of the radial artery mitigates this risk because of abundant collateral blood flow to the hand.

Understanding of the basic components is important for proper interpretation and troubleshooting of an arterial line system. The basic system consists of an arterial catheter to directly sample arterial blood, pressure filled tubing to couple the arterial blood to a transducer, and a pressure transducer to convert the arterial pressure to an electrical signal for visible display. To give an accurate reading, the transducer is zeroed to open air and leveled to the heart. Movement of the transducer down will produce falsely elevated blood pressure readings, while improper elevation of the transducer will result in falsely low blood pressure readings.

Central Venous Pressure

Measuring the CVP via central venous access provides another hemodynamic data point in shock patients, and when interpreted correctly, can provide useful diagnostic information in the acutely unstable patient and after resuscitation is complete. CVP has the advantage of being an easily attainable parameter with a transducer similar to the arterial line. The major disadvantage of CVP measurements is the degree to which readings are altered by external variables, such as elevation of the patient's head, positive pressure ventilation, and infusions going through the central venous catheter, among others. When these variables are accounted for, CVP is a surrogate of right ventricular and to a lesser extent, left ventricular preload. In the acute stages of shock, CVP values are beneficial in differentiating obstructive and cardiogenic shock from hypovolemic and distributive shock and are useful in guiding resuscitation in the treatment of shock. Because of the many variables that effect CVP, its usefulness as a sole measurement to guide fluid resuscitation is limited, but extreme CVP measurements (<8 mmHg) do effectively predict fluid responsiveness [33, 34]. Furthermore, after resuscitation is complete, targeting lower CVP values after stabilization is useful for avoiding hypervolemia and its associated organ dysfunction [35]. When combined with other monitoring techniques, CVP values can be useful in the diagnosis and management of shock.

Cardiac Output

Cardiac output monitoring is available in both invasive and non-invasive modalities, and in the appropriate patient, CO monitoring can be both diagnostic and help guide therapy. Classically, Swan-Ganz catheters inserted in the pulmonary artery provide pulmonary artery pressures and cardiac output readings through thermodilution, and newer devices have the option for continuous cardiac output monitoring and continuous mixed venous oxygen (SvO_2) measurements. Multiple trials have shown higher complication rates and no improved outcomes with the use of PA catheters, but with the appropriate patient selection and well-trained provider, PA catheters provide valuable diagnostic information [36–38]. Several less invasive devices are available that utilize arterial wave form analysis to calculate SV and subsequently generate CO readings (CO = HR × SV). These devices also calculate SVV and PPV to guide fluid responsiveness [39]. Stroke volume variation works under the premise that changes in SV occur in fluid-responsive individuals with respiratory variations, and in the appropriate patient, high SVV predicts fluid responsiveness [40, 41]. Generally, this means that patients need to be in a regular rhythm and intubated with at least 8 cc/kg of tidal volume [40]. When used appropriately, SVV provides additional diagnostic data to help manage the hemodynamic derangements of shock by providing CO and predicting fluid responsiveness.

Etiologies and Management of Shock States

Immediate Management and Diagnostic Strategies

The management of shock requires a timely response to prevent reversible and ultimately irreversible organ damage. Although specific treatment strategies differ depending on the underlying etiology, there are four common phases to the treatment of shock (Table 10.2). The goal of immediate essential management in all forms of shock is to minimize morbidity and mortality and accurately diagnose the etiology (Table 10.3). In these early phases of shock, both the diagnosis and treatment occur simultaneously, particularly in patients in extremis. A practical diagnostic approach using

Table 10.2 Phases of treatment of shock

Salvage	Optimization	Stabilization	De-escalation
Achieve acceptable blood pressure	Provide adequate tissue perfusion	Provide multiorgan organ support	Wean hemodynamic support
Perform emergent lifesaving maneuvers	Optimize cardiac output	Minimize and manage post-resuscitation complications	De-resuscitate: Achieve negative fluid balance with diuresis

There are four described phases of treatment of shock including salvage, optimization, stabilization, and de-escalation. Under each heading are goals unique to each phase

Reference: Adapted from Vincent JL, De Backer D. Circulatory Shock. N Engl J Med. 2013;369 (18):1726–34

Table 10.3 Salvage phase—immediate management priorities

	Recommendation	Specific examples
ABC's	Assess airway, breathing and circulation.	Airway/breathing ➔ invasive or noninvasive ventilation Circulation ➔ ACLS, vasopressors/inotropes
Vital signs and hemodynamic monitoring	Place the patient on a continuous monitor that includes HR, BP and SpO_2. Consider invasive hemodynamic monitoring.	Arterial blood pressure monitoring for refractory or worsening hypotenson.
Venous access	Establish intravenous access either peripherally or centrally.	Large bore access for hemorrhagic shock or central venous access for vasopressors.
H + P	Perform a focused history and physical.	Important early PE components ➔ capillary refill, extremity warmth, pulse exam, lung and heart auscultation, abdominal exam, mental status assessment
ECG/CXR/US	Depending on the patient scenario consider ECG, CXR and US to search of immediately reversible causes of shock.	ECG ➔ myocardial ischemia or arrythmias CXR ➔ pneumothorax US ➔ cardiac, thoracic, abdominal pathologies
Labs	Early labs should be sent as part of the diagnostic workup.	Lactate, troponin, ABG, BNP, CBC, BMP, Type and Cross

There are a number of essential management priorities common to all patients in shock. Quickly addressing these priorities will minimize morbidity and mortality. The overall goal is stabilization of the patient while quickly finding and correcting underlying emergent causes of shock

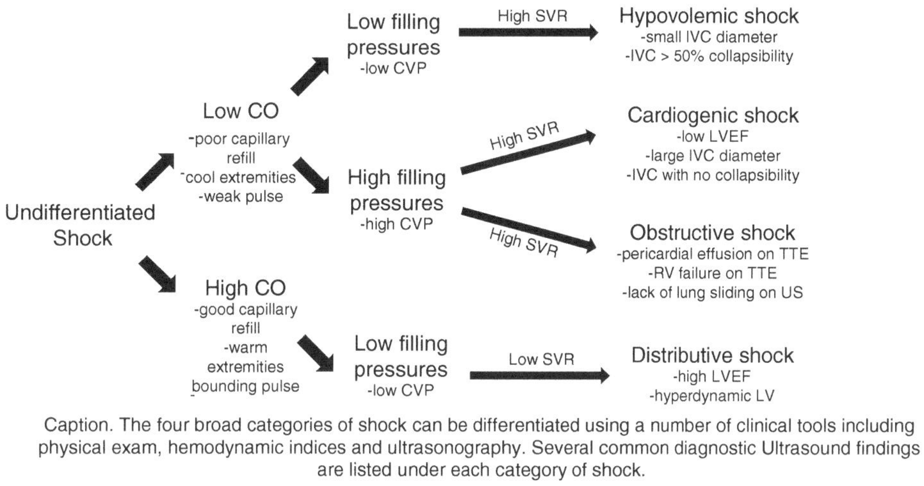

Fig. 10.3 *A practical diagnostic algorithm for shock*. The four broad categories of shock can be differentiated using a number of clinical tools including physical exam, hemodynamic indices and ultrasonography. Several common diagnostic Ultrasound findings are listed under each category of shock

clinical tools including physical exam, hemodynamic indices and ultrasonography is shown in Fig. 10.3.

Hypovolemic Shock

Hypovolemic shock occurs when intravascular volume depletion reduces CO and impedes oxygen delivery to tissues. Broadly characterized as hemorrhagic and non-hemorrhagic, both result in depleted intravascular volume that disrupts oxygen delivery to cells and undermines aerobic metabolism. The associated oxygen debt can lead to cellular death and tissue dysfunction if intravascular volume is not restored. Prompt treatment of the hypotension associated with hypovolemic shock and restoration of both DO_2 and CPP is essential in the setting of CNS injuries. While volume resuscitation with either crystalloid or colloid fluids is the treatment for hypovolemic shock, the temporary use of vasoactive medications may be needed during early resuscitation to maintain CPP.

Non-hemorrhagic Hypovolemic Shock

Non-hemorrhagic hypovolemic shock is the most common form of shock in children and is usually the result of diarrheal illnesses in the developing world, although elderly patients with less physiologic reserve are more susceptible [42]. Common etiologies include GI losses, renal losses, excessive sweating, and third space losses. Hemodynamic parameters commonly associated with more severe stages of hypovolemic shock are a low CVP, high heart rate, low blood pressure, and a low CO. Diagnosis on strict physical findings is often difficult in the early stages of volume depletion because the body has both local and global mechanisms to maintain O_2 delivery in the early stages of shock. This concept, known as compensatory reserve, is more robust in younger patients, and the physical findings are often masked until later stages of shock [43]. Additional electrolyte and metabolic derangements may also be present depending on the source of hypovolemia.

Hemorrhagic Shock

Hemorrhage results in close to 2 million worldwide deaths annually [44]. More than three quarters of those are the result of trauma, but other forms of hemorrhage are GI bleeding, peripartum hemorrhage, and perioperative hemorrhage [45]. While identifying hemorrhage in the trauma patient is sometimes obvious, occult bleeding can be difficult to diagnose with the compensatory mechanisms often seen in younger patients, and hypotension may not develop until approximately 30% of the blood volume is lost [45]. Sights of occult bleeding, such as the retroperitoneum and proximal thigh, are sometimes able to hold large volumes of blood and are not always seen on physical exam. In general, hemorrhagic shock falls into four stages depending on blood loss (Table 10.4). In more severe stages, typical hemodynamic findings would be a reduced CVP, tachycardia, and hypotension with a narrow pulse pressure. In addition to physical findings, laboratory values of assessing volume status (base deficit) and the degree of anaerobic metabolism (lactate) are useful.

Treatment of hemorrhagic shock has improved dramatically in the last two decades. Early interventions include hemorrhage control at compressible sites and identification of occult sources of bleeding with ultrasound (FAST Exam) or imaging. After hemorrhage control, immediate resuscitation is the treatment of choice for hemorrhagic shock. Multiple trials have shown no benefit to resuscitation with hypertonic saline, plasma volume expanders, and albumin, and while there is no definitive evidence for specific component therapy ratios, a balanced resuscitation with packed red blood cells, plasma, and platelets is generally agreed upon when whole blood is unavailable [45, 46]. During ongoing resuscitation, it is important to actively treat the acidosis, hypothermia, and coagulopathy commonly associated with hemorrhagic shock. In addition to restoring DO_2 and aerobic metabolism with resuscitation, patients should be kept warm and blood products should be warmed for infusion. Guided component therapy with viscoelastic assays of hemostasis is also useful to treat coagulopathy.

Table 10.4 Stages of hemorrhagic shock

	I	II	III	IV
Blood Loss	<15%	15–30%	30–40%	>40%
Heart Rate	60–100	100–120	120–140	>140
Blood Pressure	Normal	Normal	Low	Low
Mental Status	Alert	Anxious	Confused	Lethargic

Traditional Advanced Trauma Life Support teaching categorizes hemorrhagic shock into four general categories based on hemodynamics and clinical exam

Reference: Adapted from American College of Surgeons' Committee on Trauma. Advanced Trauma Life Support. Chicago: American College of Surgeons; 2018

Burn Shock

Burn shock is a subset of hypovolemic shock that deserves unique attention. Burn trauma is associated with a 3–8% mortality that correlates with the size of the burn and the age of the patient [47]. Larger percentage of total body surface area with full thickness burns and older patients have higher mortality [48]. Burn shock represents a unique form of intravascular hypovolemic shock with total body hypervolemia. The pathophysiology of burn shock is related to a systemic inflammatory response that occurs after thermal injury and results in widespread endothelial dysfunction, capillary leak, and fluid shifts from the intravascular to extracellular space. In general, full thickness burns covering more than 20% of the total body surface area require large volume resuscitation to treat the resulting hypovolemic shock, but continual extravasation occurs in the presence of continued capillary leak. As such specialized formulas, such as the Parkland Formula, exist to guide the continuous need for resuscitation [49, 50]. The Parkland Formula, and others like it, attempt to replace adequate intravascular volume and avoid the complications of hypervolemia, such as abdominal compartment syndrome and pulmonary edema.

Distributive Shock

Distributive shock is characterized by relative hypovolemia, a pathological redistribution of intravascular volume that results from a loss of vascular tone and/or disordered vascular permeability. Hemodynamically, it is characterized by a decrease in SVR. Main subtypes of distributive shock include septic, anaphylactic, and neurogenic etiologies while less common etiologies include pancreatitis and toxins or poisonings.

Septic Shock

According to current Sepsis-3 criteria, sepsis is defined as a dysregulated response by the body to an infection resulting in life-threatening organ dysfunction [51]. These organ dysfunctions are characterized and quantified by an increase in Sequential Organ Failure Assessment (SOFA) scores [52]. Septic shock is present in a subset of patients with sepsis with a lactate value above 2 mmol/L and persistent hypotension requiring the administration of vasopressors to keep MAP above 65 mmHg [53].

Patients with septic shock may present with a number of pathologies including hypovolemia, vasodilation, impaired cardiac function, and mitochondrial dysfunction. From a pathophysiology standpoint, several processes may occur simultaneously. Generally, an initial state of endothelial dysfunction is described that leads to dysregulation in vascular tone causing decreased SVR, altered distribution of circulation, and increased vascular permeability [54, 55]. Some patients will develop impaired myocardial function in the form of septic cardiomyopathy, which can increase mortality [56].

The treatment of septic shock is time sensitive. Critical early components of management include the circulatory support with infusion of balanced crystalloids solutions, administration of vasopressors (e.g., norepinephrine or vasopressin) and inotropic support if needed [52, 54]. The initiation of antibiotic therapy should be done as soon as possible. One of the pillars of treatment consists of timely source control. In the CNS injured patient, fever in the setting of sepsis or septic shock should be addressed. Secondary insults due to the increase in metabolic demands may cause secondary CNS injuries.

Anaphylactic Shock

Anaphylactic shock is an acute medical emergency with high risk of morbidity and mortality without proper treatment. It is described as an allergic hypersensitivity reaction mediated by IgE and is characterized by massive histamine-mediated vasodilation and fluid shifts from the intravascular to extravascular compartment.

Characteristic hemodynamic findings in anaphylactic shock include hypotension, decrease in SVR, and relative hypovolemia. Associated findings include skin manifestations, abdominal symptoms, and/or respiratory symptoms. It can lead to cardiovascular collapse, arrhythmias, ventricular dysfunction, and death [57].

The treatment for anaphylactic shock consists of eliminating the offending agent, when possible, early administration of epinephrine and fluid replacement [58]. In addition, initiation of systemic glucocorticoids, such as methylprednisolone is indicated, as well as the use of antihistamines. Some authors advocate for the administration of H1 and H2 blockers [58]. In the case of bronchospasm, the use of inhaled beta agonists can be beneficial [58].

Neurogenic Shock

Neurogenic shock is a state of imbalance between sympathetic and parasympathetic tone. It is characterized by the sudden drop of SBP to <100 mmHg and heart rate to <60/min. Systemic venous pressure decreases significantly [59]. Any injury that disrupts the circulatory regulation and sympathetic/parasympathetic balance can cause neurogenic shock. Direct injury to circulatory regulation centers can be secondary to brainstem compression (e.g., traumatic brain injury, brainstem trauma, herniation), ischemia (e.g., basilar artery thrombosis), or drugs.

High spinal cord injuries account for the most frequent cases of neurogenic shock [60]. Other causes of neurogenic shock include surgical intervention in the lumbar region, cerebral ischemia, traumatic brain injury, subarachnoid hemorrhage, meningitis, rapid onset of Guillain–Barré syndrome, and cerebral herniation.

Hypotension and bradycardia occur due to the interruption of autonomic pathways. Administration of balanced crystalloids, vasopressors, and inotropic or chronotropic agents with direct or indirect sympathomimetic effects are therapeutic options [61]. Bradycardia may require administration of parasympatholytics and external pacing.

In patients with spinal cord injury and patients with TBI, maintaining adequate blood pressure leads to adequate perfusion limiting secondary ischemic injury. Current recommendations in TBI suggest maintaining SBP >100 mmHg for patients 50–69 years old and >110 mmHg for patients 15–49 or >70 years old [12]. In the setting of spinal cord injury, current guidelines recommend a MAP of at least 85–90 mmHg for 7 days post-injury [62].

Shock Due to Endocrinopathies

The clinical findings in Addisonian crisis occur due to glucocorticoid and mineralocorticoid deficiency. Deficiency in these hormones leads to vasodilatation through altered vascular tone and hypovolemia secondary to aldosterone deficiency. Hormone supplementation is lifesaving. Hydrocortisone is the ideal steroid for treatment as it has both glucocorticoid and mineralocorticoid properties.

Clinical findings in myxedema coma occur due to thyroid hormone deficiency. Although the mechanisms by which thyroid deficiency leads to shock a less well elucidated, it is believed that marked vasodilation is a key pathophysiologic process. Additional findings may include myocardial depression and pericardial effusions. Treatment consists of intravenous hormone supplementation and hemodynamic support with vasopressors and fluids.

In the patient with CNS injury, maintaining higher blood pressure goals to maintain adequate perfusion is critical. When weighing risks and benefits of administering systemic steroids, although systemic steroids have been associated with worse outcomes in TBI populations, patients with Addisonian crisis will likely benefit from steroid supplementation [63]. Patients with cervical spinal cord injury can present with adrenal suppression and Addisonian crisis may ensue. The true incidence is unknown, but adrenal insufficiency is suspected when shock persists despite ongoing resuscitation and hemodynamic support [60]. Steroids may lead to disturbances in glucose homeostasis—avoiding hypoglycemia and hyperglycemia will also decrease the risk of a second insults in the CNS injured patient.

Cardiogenic Shock

A disorder of cardiac function causes cardiogenic shock. Pump failure can be secondary to systolic or diastolic dysfunction. The pillars of diagnosis are echocardiography and invasive monitoring. Cardiogenic shock is defined by SBP <90 mmHg or MAP of 30 mmHg below the baseline value and cardiac index (CI) <1.8 L/min/m^2 without pharmacologic or mechanical support or <2.0 L/min/m^2 with support [64].

Pump failure can be secondary several causes including structural, arrhythmogenic, and mechanical.

- Structural: The most frequent cause of pump failure secondary to myocardial disease is acute coronary syndrome (ACS)/myocardial infarction. Other causes of cardiomyopathies include myocarditis, takotsubo (stress induced) cardiomyopathy, pharmacotoxicity, and blunt trauma to the heart.
- Arrhythmogenic: Both tachyarrhythmias and bradyarrhythmias may result in pump failure, reduced cardiac output, hypoperfusion, and shock. Identifying the cause of arrhythmia, administering antiarrhythmics, providing defibrillation, cardioversion, and/or pacing when warranted can result in resolution of shock.
- Mechanical: Advanced acute and chronic valvular disease, including mechanical complications after myocardial infarction, and the presence of intracavitary structures that impede flow.

Similar to other forms of shock, the main goal of treatment is addressing the underlying cause of shock in a timely manner. This is particularly important in the setting of myocardial infarction, where revascularization procedures are often warranted. Coronary reperfusion in ACS is recommended to be performed as early as possible. Revascularization can be done via percutaneous coronary intervention (bare-metal stents or drug-eluting stents) and/or coronary artery bypass in multivessel coronary disease [64, 65]. When interventional revascularization is not feasible, thrombolytics can be lifesaving. Other causes of cardiomyopathies, such as myocarditis and stress cardiomyopathy (a diagnosis of exclusion characterized by apical ballooning), generally require supportive treatment only.

Mechanical causes of obstruction can be addressed surgically or via interventional treatments (e.g., mitral clip for severe mitral regurgitation). Consulting interventionists and cardiothoracic surgeons early is recommended. Supportive treatment with the use of vasopressors, inotropes, and chronotropes will likely be necessary with the aim of improving hemodynamics and end-organ perfusion.

Other support devices include intra-aortic balloon counterpulsation, surgical and percutaneous implantable ventricular support systems, and extracorporeal membrane oxygenation. These options are usually only available in tertiary care centers.

Obstructive Shock

Obstructive shock is characterized by circulatory obstruction of the heart or great vessels. Hemodynamic findings may resemble cardiogenic shock. A common characteristic to most causes of obstructive shock is the sudden decrease in blood pressure, cardiac output, and end-tidal CO_2. Early diagnosis of obstructive shock is necessary as the treatment is the relief of the obstruction.

Obstructive shock can be classified according to the location of the obstruction.

- Impaired diastolic filling: Examples include vena cava compression syndrome, cardiac tamponade, tension pneumothorax, and high-PEEP ventilation. These cause a decrease in right ventricular preload and decrease in left ventricular preload.
- Obstruction to pulmonary flow: Examples include pulmonary embolism, air embolism, fat embolism, amniotic fluid embolism, mediastinal space-occupying mass. These cause an increase in right ventricular afterload and decrease in left ventricular preload.
- Obstruction of the aortic flow: Examples include aortoiliac occlusive disease and critical aortic valve stenosis. These cause an increase in left ventricular afterload.

Obstructive shock can progress very quickly and can lead to cardiovascular collapse and cardiocirculatory arrest [66]. History and clinical examination (including auscultation, percussion, and the use of echocardiography) are essential.

The use of point-of-care ultrasonography (POCUS) and formal echocardiography plays a role in conjunction with the patient's symptomatology in promptly identifying the causes of obstructive shock. Point-of-care ultrasound become a key tool for bedside diagnosis. Several studies have shown the role of echocardiographic monitoring in guiding therapy for pulmonary emboli and pericardial effusions [67]. For example, the clinical signs of shock and the presence of pericardial fluid can suggest the diagnosis of cardiac tamponade. The presence of shock, subcutaneous emphysema, jugular venous distention, deviation of the trachea, and absence of lung sliding is considered diagnostic for tension pneumothorax. In the setting of a sitting craniotomy with sudden hypotension, the presence of air bubbles, interventricular flattening, and a dilated right ventricle suggests air emboli syndrome.

In addition to providing hemodynamic support, the treatment of obstructive shock generally requires emergent interventions. Tension pneumothorax and cardiac tamponade are relieved by immediate drainage via needle decompression or chest tube placement and pericardiocentesis or a pericardial window. Pulmonary thromboembolism with hypotension requires advanced interventions such as thrombectomy, catheter-directed thrombolysis, or systemic thrombolysis. Leriche syndrome or aortoiliac occlusive disease is treated by surgical embolectomy. On occasion, simple measures may suffice to relieve the obstruction, such as changing the position of a patient with caval compression syndrome or suspected air embolism.

Near Misses

There are a number of conditions that may confound to the clinician with respect to the diagnosis and management of shock. These "near misses" should always be considered when patients are not responding to therapies in an expected or timely manner (Table 10.5). With respect to patients presenting with shock in the setting of traumatic neurologic injuries, care should be taken to evaluate for additional sources of shock including hemorrhagic and cardiogenic.

Table 10.5 Near misses in shock

Near miss	Clinical scenario	Recommendation
Anaphylaxis	Anaphylaxis can mask as a number of different diagnoses especially sepsis.	Perform a thorough physical exam on each patient looking for stigmata of anaphylaxis.
Polytrauma	Polytrauma patients can have occult injuries contributing to or causing shock.	Consider alternative diagnoses in polytrauma patients including myocardial injury, neurogenic shock and hemorrhage from occult injuries.
Myocardial injury in TBI	Myocardial injury can lead to cardiogenic shock in TBI.	Consider myocardial shock in the setting of TBI particularly in the setting of refractory hypotension.
Auto-PEEP	Auto-PEEP can lead to an obstructive form of shock.	In mechanically ventilated patients with shock review the expiratory flow waveform to evaluate for auto-PEEP. A trial of disconnection for mechanical ventilatory circuit can be diagnostic and therapeutic.
Adrenal insufficiency	Adrenal insufficiency can be a primary or secondary source of shock, particularly in critically ill patients.	Perform a thorough medication review and history to evaluate for steroid use. Consider a trial of empiric steroids when home steroid dose or duration is unknown.
Preoperative ACEI use	ACEI use in the preoperative setting can lead to refractory intraoperative hypotension.	Perform a thorough medication review in patients with intraoperative or postoperative hypotension. Vasopressin is the vasopressor of choice in this setting.

Near misses in shock can lead to significant morbidity and mortality. It is essential to thoroughly evaluate patients with special focus on the history and physical exam

Conclusion

Shock is a dynamic condition requiring prompt recognition and treatment to minimize morbidity and mortality. Understanding the pathophysiologic principles of the four main subtypes of shock is critical, particularly in the setting of CNS injury, where secondary insults play a crucial role in outcomes. The CNS injured patient poses unique challenges—a thorough understanding of the relationship between circulatory failure and neurologic pathology can improve outcomes in this patient population. Using new diagnostic tools, such as dynamic physiologic parameters and POCUS, the contemporary ICU clinician has the ability to more effectively identify and treat the patient in shock.

References

1. Holler JG, Henriksen DP, Mikkelsen S, Rasmussen LM, Pedersen C, Lassen AT. Shock in the emergency department; a 12 year population based cohort study. Scand J Trauma Resusc Emerg Med. 2016;24:87.
2. Sakr Y, Reinhart K, Vincent JL, Sprung CL, Moreno R, Ranieri VM, et al. Does dopamine administration in shock influence outcome? Results of the sepsis occurrence in acutely ill patients (SOAP) study. Crit Care Med. 2006;34(3):589–97.
3. De Backer D, Biston P, Devriendt J, Madl C, Chochrad D, Aldecoa C, et al. Comparison of dopamine and norepinephrine in the treatment of shock. N Engl J Med. 2010;362(9):779–89.
4. Jones AE, Tayal VS, Sullivan DM, Kline JA. Randomized, controlled trial of immediate versus delayed goal-directed ultrasound to identify the cause of nontraumatic hypotension in emergency department patients. Crit Care Med. 2004;32(8):1703–8.
5. Arendts G, Stone SF, Fatovich DM, van Eeden P, MacDonald E, Brown SG. Critical illness in the emergency department: lessons learnt from the first 12 months of enrolments in the Critical Illness and Shock Study. Emerg Med Australas. 2012;24(1):31–6.
6. Kheng CP, Rahman NH. The use of end-tidal carbon dioxide monitoring in patients with hypotension in the emergency department. Int J Emerg Med. 2012;5(1):31.
7. Chesnut RM, Marshall LF, Klauber MR, Blunt BA, Baldwin N, Eisenberg HM, et al. The role of secondary brain injury in determining outcome from severe head injury. J Trauma. 1993;34(2):216–22.
8. Marmarou A, Anderson RL, Ward D, Choi S, Young HF, Eisenberg HM, et al. Impact of ICP instability and hypotension on outcome in patients with severe head trauma. J Neurosurg. 1991;75(Supplement):S59–66.
9. McHugh GS, Engel DC, Butcher I, Steyerberg EW, Lu J, Mushkudiani N, et al. Prognostic value of secondary insults in traumatic brain injury: results from the IMPACT study. J Neurotrauma. 2007;24(2):287–93.
10. Guly HR, Bouamra O, Lecky FE, Trauma A, Research N. The incidence of neurogenic shock in patients with isolated spinal cord injury in the emergency department. Resuscitation. 2008;76(1):57–62.

11. Bilello JF, Davis JW, Cunningham MA, Groom TF, Lemaster D, Sue LP. Cervical spinal cord injury and the need for cardiovascular intervention. Arch Surg. 2003;138(10):1127–9.
12. Carney N, Totten AM, O'Reilly C, Ullman JS, Hawryluk GW, Bell MJ, et al. Guidelines for the management of severe traumatic brain injury, fourth edition. Neurosurgery. 2017;80(1):6–15.
13. Spaite DW, Hu C, Bobrow BJ, Chikani V, Sherrill D, Barnhart B, et al. Mortality and prehospital blood pressure in patients with major traumatic brain injury: implications for the hypotension threshold. JAMA Surg. 2017;152(4):360–8.
14. Marino P. The ICU book. 4th ed. Philidelphia, PA: Lippincott Williams and Wilkins; 2014.
15. Tibbs PA, Young B, McAllister RG, Brooks WH, Tackett L. Studies of experimental cervical spinal cord transection. Part I: hemodynamic changes after acute cervical spinal cord transection. J Neurosurg. 1978;49(4):558–62.
16. Calaresu FR, Yardley CP. Medullary basal sympathetic tone. Annu Rev Physiol. 1988;50:511–24.
17. American College of Surgeons' Committee on Trauma. Advanced trauma life support. Chicago: American College of Surgeons; 2018.
18. Fulton RL, Flynn WJ, Mancino M, Bowles D, Cryer HM. Brain injury causes loss of cardiovascular response to hemorrhagic shock. J Investig Surg. 1993;6(2):117–31.
19. Chesnut RM, Gautille T, Blunt BA, Klauber MR, Marshall LF. Neurogenic hypotension in patients with severe head injuries. J Trauma. 1998;44(6):958–63; discussion 63–4.
20. Mahoney EJ, Biffl WL, Harrington DT, Cioffi WG. Isolated brain injury as a cause of hypotension in the blunt trauma patient. J Trauma. 2003;55(6):1065–9.
21. Guertzenstein PG, Silver A. Fall in blood pressure produced from discrete regions of the ventral surface of the medulla by glycine and lesions. J Physiol. 1974;242(2):489–503.
22. Law MM, Hovda DA, Cryer HG. Fluid-percussion brain injury adversely affects control of vascular tone during hemorrhagic shock. Shock. 1996;6(3):213–7.
23. Chen B, Mutschler M, Yuan Y, Neugebauer E, Huang Q, Maegele M. Superimposed traumatic brain injury modulates vasomotor responses in third-order vessels after hemorrhagic shock. Scand J Trauma Resusc Emerg Med. 2013;21:77.
24. Beckman DL, Iams SG. Circulating catecholamines in cats before and after lethal head injury. Proc Soc Exp Biol Med. 1979;160(2):200–2.
25. Pilati CF, Clark RS, Gilloteaux J, Bosso FJ, Holcomb P, Maron MB. Excessive sympathetic nervous system activity decreases myocardial contractility. Proc Soc Exp Biol Med. 1990;193(3):225–31.
26. Rosner MJ, Newsome HH, Becker DP. Mechanical brain injury: the sympathoadrenal response. J Neurosurg. 1984;61(1):76–86.
27. Yuan XQ, Wade CE, Clifford CB. Suppression by traumatic brain injury of spontaneous hemodynamic recovery from hemorrhagic shock in rats. J Neurosurg. 1991;75(3):408–14.
28. Lassen NA. Cerebral blood flow and oxygen consumption in man. Physiol Rev. 1959;39(2):183–238.
29. Strandgaard S, Olesen J, Skinhoj E, Lassen NA. Autoregulation of brain circulation in severe arterial hypertension. Br Med J. 1973;1(5852):507–10.
30. Paulson OB, Strandgaard S, Edvinsson L. Cerebral autoregulation. Cerebrovasc Brain Metab Rev. 1990;2(2):161–92.
31. Bouma GJ, Muizelaar JP, Bandoh K, Marmarou A. Blood pressure and intracranial pressure-volume dynamics in severe head injury: relationship with cerebral blood flow. J Neurosurg. 1992;77(1):15–9.
32. Markus HS. Cerebral perfusion and stroke. J Neurol Neurosurg Psychiatry. 2004;75(3):353–61.
33. Gottlieb M, Hunter B. Utility of central venous pressure as a predictor of fluid responsiveness. Ann Emerg Med. 2016;68(1):114–6.
34. Eskesen TG, Wetterslev M, Perner A. Systematic review including re-analyses of 1148 individual data sets of central venous pressure as a predictor of fluid responsiveness. Intensive Care Med. 2016;42(3):324–32.
35. De Backer D, Vincent JL. Should we measure the central venous pressure to guide fluid management? Ten answers to 10 questions. Crit Care. 2018;22(1):43.
36. Sandham JD, Hull RD, Brant RF, Knox L, Pineo GF, Doig CJ, et al. A randomized, controlled trial of the use of pulmonary-artery catheters in high-risk surgical patients. N Engl J Med. 2003;348(1):5–14.
37. Payen D, Gayat E. Which general intensive care unit patients can benefit from placement of the pulmonary artery catheter? Crit Care. 2006;10(Suppl 3):S7.
38. Chatterjee K. The swan-Ganz catheters: past, present, and future. A viewpoint. Circulation. 2009;119(1):147–52.
39. Augusto JF, Teboul JL, Radermacher P, Asfar P. Interpretation of blood pressure signal: physiological bases, clinical relevance, and objectives during shock states. Intensive Care Med. 2011;37(3):411–9.
40. Kobe J, Mishra N, Arya VK, Al-Moustadi W, Nates W, Kumar B. Cardiac output monitoring: technology and choice. Ann Card Anaesth. 2019;22(1):6–17.
41. Khwannimit B, Bhurayanontachai R. Prediction of fluid responsiveness in septic shock patients: comparing stroke volume variation by FloTrac/Vigileo and automated pulse pressure variation. Eur J Anaesthesiol. 2012;29(2):64–9.
42. Thomas NJ, Carcillo JA. Hypovolemic shock in pediatric patients. New Horiz. 1998;6(2):120–9.
43. Suresh MR, Chung KK, Schiller AM, Holley AB, Howard JT, Convertino VA. Unmasking the hypovolemic shock continuum: the compensatory reserve. J Intensive Care Med. 2019;34(9):696–706.
44. Lozano R, Naghavi M, Foreman K, Lim S, Shibuya K, Aboyans V, et al. Global and regional mortality from 235 causes of death for 20 age groups in 1990 and 2010: a systematic analysis for the Global Burden of Disease Study 2010. Lancet. 2012;380(9859):2095–128.
45. Cannon JW. Hemorrhagic shock. N Engl J Med. 2018;378(4):370–9.
46. Annane D, Siami S, Jaber S, Martin C, Elatrous S, Declère AD, et al. Effects of fluid resuscitation with colloids vs crystalloids on mortality in critically ill patients presenting with hypovolemic shock: the CRISTAL randomized trial. JAMA. 2013;310(17):1809–17.
47. Rae L, Fidler P, Gibran N. The physiologic basis of burn shock and the need for aggressive fluid resuscitation. Crit Care Clin. 2016;32(4):491–505.
48. Christofides C, Moore R, Nel M. Baux score as a predictor of mortality at the CHBAH adult burns unit. J Surg Res. 2020;251:53–62.
49. Baxter CR, Shires T. Physiological response to crystalloid resuscitation of severe burns. Ann N Y Acad Sci. 1968;150(3):874–94.
50. Guilabert P, Usúa G, Martín N, Abarca L, Barret JP, Colomina MJ. Fluid resuscitation management in patients with burns: update. Br J Anaesth. 2016;117(3):284–96.
51. Singer M, Deutschman CS, Seymour CW, Shankar-Hari M, Annane D, Bauer M, et al. The third international consensus definitions for sepsis and septic shock (Sepsis-3). JAMA. 2016;315(8):801–10.
52. Rhodes A, Evans LE, Alhazzani W, Levy MM, Antonelli M, Ferrer R, et al. Surviving sepsis campaign: international guidelines for management of sepsis and septic shock: 2016. Intensive Care Med. 2017;43(3):304–77.
53. Shankar-Hari M, Phillips GS, Levy ML, Seymour CW, Liu VX, Deutschman CS, et al. Developing a new definition and assessing new clinical criteria for septic shock: for the third international consensus definitions for sepsis and septic shock (Sepsis-3). JAMA. 2016;315(8):775–87.
54. Gotts JE, Matthay MA. Sepsis: pathophysiology and clinical management. BMJ. 2016;353:i1585.

55. Vincent JL, De Backer D. Circulatory shock. N Engl J Med. 2013;369(18):1726–34.
56. Antonucci E, Fiaccadori E, Donadello K, Taccone FS, Franchi F, Scolletta S. Myocardial depression in sepsis: from pathogenesis to clinical manifestations and treatment. J Crit Care. 2014;29(4):500–11.
57. Triggiani M, Montagni M, Parente R, Ridolo E. Anaphylaxis and cardiovascular diseases: a dangerous liaison. Curr Opin Allergy Clin Immunol. 2014;14(4):309–15.
58. Ring J, Beyer K, Biedermann T, Bircher A, Fischer M, Fuchs T, et al. Guideline (S2k) on acute therapy and management of anaphylaxis: 2021 update: S2k-guideline of the German Society for Allergology and Clinical Immunology (DGAKI), the Medical Association of German Allergologists (AeDA), the Society of Pediatric Allergology and Environmental Medicine (GPA), the German Academy of Allergology and Environmental Medicine (DAAU), the German Professional Association of Pediatricians (BVKJ), the Society for Neonatology and Pediatric Intensive Care (GNPI), the German Society of Dermatology (DDG), the Austrian Society for Allergology and Immunology (OGAI), the Swiss Society for Allergy and Immunology (SGAI), the German Society of Anaesthesiology and Intensive Care Medicine (DGAI), the German Society of Pharmacology (DGP), the German Respiratory Society (DGP), the patient organization German Allergy and Asthma Association (DAAB), the German Working Group of Anaphylaxis Training and Education (AGATE). Allergo J Int. 2021;30(1):1–25.
59. Summers RL, Baker SD, Sterling SA, Porter JM, Jones AE. Characterization of the spectrum of hemodynamic profiles in trauma patients with acute neurogenic shock. J Crit Care. 2013;28(4):531 e1–5.
60. Pastrana EA, Saavedra FM, Murray G, Estronza S, Rolston JD, Rodriguez-Vega G. Acute adrenal insufficiency in cervical spinal cord injury. World Neurosurg. 2012;77(3–4):561–3.
61. Wood GC, Boucher AB, Johnson JL, Wisniewski JN, Magnotti LJ, Croce MA, et al. Effectiveness of pseudoephedrine as adjunctive therapy for neurogenic shock after acute spinal cord injury: a case series. Pharmacotherapy. 2014;34(1):89–93.
62. Walters BC, Hadley MN, Hurlbert RJ, Aarabi B, Dhall SS, Gelb DE, et al. Guidelines for the management of acute cervical spine and spinal cord injuries: 2013 update. Neurosurgery. 2013;60(CN_suppl_1):82–91.
63. Alderson P, Roberts I. Corticosteroids for acute traumatic brain injury. Cochrane Database Syst Rev. 2005;2005(1):CD000196.
64. Furer A, Wessler J, Burkhoff D. Hemodynamics of cardiogenic shock. Interv Cardiol Clin. 2017;6(3):359–71.
65. Nuding S, Werdan K, Prondzinsky R. Optimal course of treatment in acute cardiogenic shock complicating myocardial infarction. Expert Rev Cardiovasc Ther. 2018;16(2):99–112.
66. Soar J, Nolan JP, Bottiger BW, Perkins GD, Lott C, Carli P, et al. European resuscitation council guidelines for resuscitation 2015: section 3. Adult advanced life support. Resuscitation. 2015;95:100–47.
67. Porter TR, Shillcutt SK, Adams MS, Desjardins G, Glas KE, Olson JJ, et al. Guidelines for the use of echocardiography as a monitor for therapeutic intervention in adults: a report from the American Society of Echocardiography. J Am Soc Echocardiogr. 2015;28(1):40–56.

Uncontrolled Hypertension

11

Alexis Alvarado Arias, Aleksandra V. Ferreira, Matthew Imm, and Mohan Kottapally

Contents

A. A. Arias (✉)
Department of Neurology, University of Mississippi Medical Center, Jackson, MS, USA

A. V. Ferreira
Department of Neurology, Las Vegas Neurology Center, Las Vegas, NV, USA

M. Imm
Department of Medicine, University of Miami Miller School of Medicine, Miami, FL, USA

M. Kottapally
Department of Neurology, University of Miami Miller School of Medicine, Miami, FL, USA

E. Mahanna Gabrielli et al. (eds.), *Textbook of Neurointensive Care: Volume 1*, https://doi.org/10.1007/978-3-031-62220-5_11

Abstract

Uncontrolled hypertension can lead to the onset of cardiovascular, renovascular, and cerebrovascular end-organ damage and is often found in patients with primary central nervous system injury. Several pathophysiologic mechanisms have been proposed for the development of hypertension and its progression to hypertensive urgencies and emergencies. Short-acting and rapid-onset vasoactive agents are often needed for acute management while avoiding subsequent hypotension and end-organ ischemia. A review of uncontrolled hypertension, its pathophysiology, mechanisms of onset, and organ-specific injuries with treatment considerations is provided.

Chapter Objectives

- Outline the epidemiology and pathophysiology of blood pressure homeostasis and hypertension
- Review complications of uncontrolled hypertension
- Review the pathophysiology of end-organ hypertensive emergencies, as well as recognition of clinical symptoms
- Review management principles and antihypertensive agents utilized in the management of uncontrolled hypertension

Introduction

Hypertension, recognized as a systolic blood pressure (SBP) of ≥130 mmHg and diastolic blood pressure (DBP) of ≥80 mmHg [1], is a significant risk factor for the development of cardiovascular, renovascular, and cerebrovascular disease [1, 2]. With an estimated prevalence of nearly 50% within the general population [3], the prompt recognition and management of hypertension in the inpatient and critical care environments is important to avoid such complications and disease [4, 5].

Uncontrolled hypertension is commonly found amongst hospitalized patients, especially those with central nervous system (CNS) injury [6–8]. The prevalence of hypertension in acute ischemic stroke, for example, has risen to 79% in recent years [9]. Extremes of blood pressure are also associated with higher morbidity and mortality across different CNS diseases, including ischemic and hemorrhagic stroke [10–14], traumatic brain injury (TBI) [15], and cardiac arrest [16]. While autoregulatory mechanisms may contribute to hypertension to preserve cerebral blood flow to injured tissues [17], the risk of injury from sustained hypertension must be mitigated against the risk of ischemia from aggressive blood pressure reduction [18]. A thorough understanding of the physiologic control of arterial blood pressure, end-organ perfusion pressure, and the mechanisms of blood pressure regulation in both homeostasis and disease is therefore essential in optimizing patient care. Admission to either an intermediate care unit (IMCU) or intensive care unit (ICU) is often required for careful, targeted blood pressure control with titration of short- and long-acting vasoactive agents and close monitoring [18–20].

This chapter focuses on the epidemiology, pathophysiology, and complications associated with uncontrolled hypertension, with special attention to the neurocritically injured patient. Areas of emphasis are the recognition of hypertensive end-organ emergencies and the ICU management of hypertension.

Epidemiology

National surveys estimate the prevalence of hypertension at 45% of the U.S population [21], with approximately 53% of hypertensive patients having poor outpatient blood pressure control [2].

Several patient-related factors have been associated with the development of uncontrolled blood pressure [22]. Age, sex, obesity, and lack of exercise not only constitute risk factors for hypertension but have been described as likely contributors to difficult blood pressure control [23–26]. Race has also been identified as a strong risk factor, with Hispanics and Blacks having the lowest rate of successful blood pressure control [27]. Access to healthcare and socioeconomic status have been previously associated with uncontrolled hypertension [28, 29]; however, based on the National Health and Nutrition Examination Survey (NHANES) data, no definitive association has been observed [24]. In specific high-risk populations such as those with diabetes, chronic kidney disease, and coronary artery disease, the rates of uncontrolled hypertension remain high [30–33].

Hypertensive Emergency Versus Urgency

Hypertensive emergency, defined as uncontrolled hypertension leading to end-organ damage or failure, is a true medical emergency requiring rapid intervention and management [1, 34]. However, clear blood pressure thresholds for such emergencies may vary from patient to patient due to numerous factors such as average baseline blood pressure, rate of rise in blood pressure, and absolute peak in blood pressure values [35–37]. A famous example is the case of President Franklin D. Roosevelt who, after having severe uncontrolled hypertension (with systolic blood pressures between 200 and 230 mmHg) for over a year, eventually succumbed to an acute intracranial hemorrhage when his blood pressure reached an estimated 350/195 mmHg [38]. As such, severe uncontrolled hypertension recognized as blood pressure greater than 180/120 mmHg often prompts acute evaluation and treatment, even in the absence of end-organ damage or symptoms (a condition known as hypertensive urgency) [39].

Hypertensive emergency is seen in approximately 1%–2% of all patients with hypertension [27, 40], with approximately 1% of this population presenting with a cerebrovascular injury such as ischemic stroke, ICH, or hypertensive encephalopathy [41]. In addition, mortality rates can be four times higher in patients with CNS injury and acute hypertension [42, 43]. Thus, careful and timely blood pressure control is paramount in preventing progression, end-organ damage, and subsequent morbidity and mortality [42].

Physiology of Blood Pressure Homeostasis

Blood pressure homeostasis relies on the direct autonomic regulation of myocardial contractility and systemic vascular resistance, as well as the neurohormonal regulation of renal sodium and free water retention. Arterial blood pressure is directly determined by cardiac output (CO), a product of heart rate (HR) and stroke volume (SV), and peripheral vascular resistance (PVR). SV itself is further affected by myocardial contractility and intravascular preload volume.

Autonomic Feedback

Moment-to-moment blood pressure homeostasis is largely a function of the autonomic nervous system [44–46]. Changes in mean arterial pressure (MAP) are detected by baroreceptors within the carotid sinus and aortic arch, which upon sensing arterial wall luminal stretch trigger afferent signals through the glossopharyngeal and vagus nerves to the nucleus tractus solitarii (NTS) in the dorsal medulla [47]. Excitatory glutamatergic fibers from the NTS then project to the caudal ventrolateral medulla, sending GABAergic inhibitory fibers toward the rostral ventrolateral medulla. This causes downregulation of the sympathetic activity of the rostral ventrolateral medulla [48–51], a decline in activity of sympathetic cell bodies within the intermediolateral spinal cord and paraspinal sympathetic chain ganglia, and subsequent decreased sympathetic tone within the heart and peripheral vasculature resulting in a reduction of MAP [48–51]. Declining MAP, conversely, results in less baroreceptor stimulation, leading to sympathetic activation, increased myocardial contractility, and vasoconstriction causing a rise in blood pressure [48–51].

Increased sympathetic activity raises CO by two main pathways: (1) increasing HR and cardiac contractility through beta-1 receptor stimulation and (2) increasing PVR through alpha-1 mediated peripheral vasoconstriction [44–46, 52–54].

Intravascular Volume Regulation

Intravascular volume control via the Renin–Angiotensin-Aldosterone System (RAAS) is the predominant factor affecting long-term blood pressure variation [46, 55, 56]. The juxtaglomerular apparatus (JGA) is a sensory organ located at the confluence of the vascular pole of the glomerulus and the distal convoluted tubule. It is made up of three types of cells: juxtaglomerular cells, the macula densa, and extraglomerular mesangial cells [57].

Juxtaglomerular cells function as baroreceptors within the tunica media of the afferent glomerular arteriole, secreting renin in response to decreased luminal stretch. Stimulation of sympathetic activity through beta-1 receptors also promotes renin release from juxtaglomerular cells [46, 55, 56]. The macula densa, in response to decrease sodium delivery to the distal convoluted tubule, can further signal juxtaglomerular cells to secrete renin through beta adrenergic stimulation [58, 59].

Circulating renin converts angiotensinogen to angiotensin I, which is then subsequently activated to angiotensin II through the action of angiotensin-converting enzyme (ACE) located within vascular endothelium [46, 55, 56]. Angiotensin II acts to increase MAP both directly and indirectly through a number of mechanisms and feedback loops. Angiotensin II directly induces smooth muscle contraction leading to vasoconstriction, increasing PVR, and blood pressure elevation [46, 55, 56]. In addition, angiotensin II stimulates the release of aldosterone from the adrenal glomerulus, promoting sodium reabsorption from the proximal tubule, increasing circulating blood volume and increasing blood pressure [46, 55, 56]. Angiotensin II also has direct action on the hypothalamus, increasing antidiuretic hormone secretion leading to thirst, and free water absorption by the kidney. The continued circulation of angiotensin II further triggers a feedback loop to inhibit renin secretion and downregulate the RAAS [60].

Physiology of Hypertension

Dysregulations of the homeostatic mechanisms outlined above are implicated in the development and maintenance of pathologic hypertension. Renal and vascular adaptations to sustained elevations of blood pressure lead in turn to structural changes in the kidney, heart, and peripheral vasculature which can perpetuate and maintain hypertension [61].

Sympathetic Dysregulation

Over-activation of the sympathetic nervous system is one contributing mechanism in the pathophysiology of hypertension [62]. The purest example of this is pheochromocytoma, in which catecholamine production by neoplastic neuroendocrine cells leads to sustained and often critical elevations of blood pressure. Excision of the tumor is curative, illustrating the role catecholamines play in hypertension. Increased sympathetic tone can also be seen in obstructive sleep apnea and obesity, suggesting it may have an important etiologic risk factor for the development of hypertension in these diseases [63–67].

Vascular and Endothelial Dysfunction

Sustained periods of vasoconstriction may promote vascular remodeling through mechanisms related to endothelial dysfunction, smooth muscle proliferation, and arterial stiffness, thus further contributing to the cycle of hypertension [46, 52, 68, 69]. Angiotensin II, for example, is a potent mitogen and can lead to smooth vascular muscle growth and resultant arterial narrowing [70]. Because vascular resistance varies inversely with the fourth power of the radius, minute changes in vessel cross-section may have dramatic consequences for PVR systemically. Vascular compliance also declines over periods of sustained hypertension [71, 72]. This leads to relatively disproportionate increases in pressure with modest increases in circulating volume when comparing hypertensive to non-hypertensive patients.

Imbalance of vasoactive metabolites and endothelium dysfunction has also been implicated in developing hypertension [55]. In healthy vasculature, the endothelium produces several vasoactive metabolites (see Table 11.1) such as nitric oxide (a powerful vasodilator) and endothelin (for vasoconstriction) to regulate vascular tone [73–76].

Table 11.1 Vasoactive metabolites involve in vasodilation and vasoconstriction

Vasodilating metabolites	Vasoconstricting metabolites
Nitric oxide (NO)	Endothelin 1 (ET-1)
Prostacyclin	Angiotensin II
Calcitonin gene related peptide	Tromboxane A2
Adrenomedullin	Prostaglandin A2.
Substance P	
Glucagon-like peptide-1 (GLP-1)	

Adapted from [73–76]

Endothelial dysfunction can arise following stressors such as shearing injury, local oxidative stress, and chronic high salt ingestion [46, 55, 77, 78]. This dysfunction decreases nitric oxide bioavailability, leading to an imbalance of vasoactive metabolites favoring vasoconstriction and promoting hypertension [55, 76, 77].

Sodium Chloride Imbalance

When sodium intake surpasses the renal capacity for excretion, intravascular volume rises causing an increase in CO and MAP [79]. This increased CO will transiently increase blood flow to distal vascular beds. Many organs autoregulate perfusion set points to maintain constant blood flow, and in response to increased MAP their vascular beds will vasoconstrict to regulate appropriate perfusion pressures [80]. If sustained over time, this autoregulatory set point may reset to a higher level of blood pressure, even as cardiac output normalizes [81].

Uncontrolled Hypertension and Cerebral Autoregulation

Variations in blood pressure affect cerebral blood volume (CBV), cerebral perfusion pressure (CPP), and brain tissue oxygenation [43, 82, 83]. A cerebrovascular autoregulatory mechanism exists to ensure a constant cerebral blood flow (CBF) that allows a steady CBV and adequate CPP despite variations in the MAP [43, 84].

During elevations in intracranial blood pressure, neuromyogenic changes in the precapillary arteriolar diameter induce cerebral vasoconstriction, decreasing CBF, and maintaining a steady CBV, ICP, and CPP [82]. Under extreme elevations of blood pressure, and beyond the limits of autoregulation, this mechanism may fail and lead to a hyperperfusive CBF state causing endothelial injury, blood–brain barrier breakdown, and cerebral edema [85]. Moreover, dysfunction of this auto-regulatory mechanism can occur after an acute CNS injury, either due to the injury itself or as a result of a neurohumoral protective response mechanism to augment cerebral blood flow and prevent further injury [43].

Once failure of cerebral auto-regulation occurs, prompt management of uncontrolled hypertension is needed to maintain appropriate CBV, CBF, and CPP and prevent further hyperperfusive injury from hypertension. Targeted and careful lowering of blood pressure is required to avoid subsequent cerebral ischemia from aggressive blood pressure control [18, 20, 86, 87].

Autonomic Receptors

Alpha and beta receptors are adrenoceptors located throughout the body that mediate blood pressure control through their effects on CO and PVR [88–90].

Alpha-1 Receptors

Alpha-1 receptors are activated by norepinephrine released from sympathetic nerve terminals and by epinephrine released from the adrenal medulla [88, 89]. These receptors are mainly found within smooth muscle, having varying effects depending on its location [88, 89]. In the peripheral vasculature, stimulation of alpha-1 receptors in the vascular smooth muscle causes arterial and venous constriction, increasing PVR and venous preload return, ultimately increasing CO and elevating blood pressure [44, 88, 89].

Alpha-2 Receptors

These receptors are located in pre- and post-synaptic neurons, mediating an inhibitory role in the central and peripheral sympathetic nervous systems [88, 89]. Stimulation results in a net hyperpolarization of pre-synaptic noradrenergic neurons, decreasing the release of norepinephrine [88, 89]. This leads to a decrease in HR, TPR, and MAP [44, 88, 89]. In addition, alpha-2 receptor stimulation of the kidneys causes a decreased release of renin, suppressing the RAAS pathway and reducing blood pressure [88, 89].

Other effects of alpha-2 stimulation include anxiolysis by decreasing the activity of the ascending noradrenergic pathway. In the dorsal horn of the spinal cord, alpha-2 activation causes a reduction in the release of substance P, inhibiting nociceptive neuronal signal and having an analgesic effect [89, 91].

Beta Receptors

Beta receptors have two main subtypes, beta-1 and beta-2, with different characteristics based on location and subtype [88, 89, 92, 93].

Beta-1 receptors are found in the myocardium throughout the sinoatrial node, atrium, atrioventricular node, ventricles, and Purkinje system [88, 89]. Stimulation leads to chronotropic and inotropic effects, promoting cardiac muscle contractility and cardiac conduction, increasing HR and blood pressure [88, 91]. Systemically, beta-1 stimulation promotes blood pressure elevation through the secretion of renin from the kidneys, the release of antidiuretic hormone from the posterior pituitary, and release of norepinephrine from the pre-synaptic sympathetic terminal [88, 89].

Beta-2 receptors are located in vascular smooth muscle, inducing vasodilation by smooth muscle relaxation when stimulated. This leads to a decrease in PVR and lowering of MAP [44, 88, 91].

Pharmacological Management of Uncontrolled Hypertension

In the acute management of severe uncontrolled hypertension, blood pressure control requires careful titration of vasoactive medication to prevent further end-organ ischemia and hypoperperfusion-related injuries. Many agents may be utilized to accomplish this goal (see Table 11.2) [43, 94]. As noted earlier, extremes of blood pressure in either direction have been associated with poor outcomes [42]. Similarly, patient comorbidities and side effect profiles must be taken into consideration when selecting a proper agent [43]. The cerebral venous vasodilatory effects of IV nitroprusside, for example, may potentially worsen elevated ICP crises in patients with an intracranial mass lesion [95]. An appropriate strategy is to therefore choose first-line agents with short half-lives and easy titratability so that changes in patient condition can be closely monitored while achieving optimal blood pressure control in a safe and targeted manner.

Table 11.2 Parenteral vasoactive agents in neurological emergencies: preferred antihypertensives

Drug	Mechanism	Dose	Onset	Duration	Common adverse effects	Cautions
Antihypertensives						
Labetalol	α1, β1, β2 antagonist	20–80 mg bolus every 10 min, up to max 300 mg; 0.5–2 mg/min infusion	5–10 min	3–6 h	Bradycardia (heart block), dizziness, nausea, vomiting, scalp tingling, bronchospasm, orthostatic hypotension, orthostatic hypotension, hepatic injury	Asthma, COPD, LV failure, second or third-degree AV block
Esmolol	β1 antagonist	500 μg/kg bolus, 50–300 μg/kg/min infusion	1–2 min	10–30 min	Bradycardia (heart block), hypotension, nausea, bronchospasm	Asthma, LV failure, second or third-degree AV block, COPD
Nicardipine	L-type CCB (dihydropyridine)	5–15 mg/h infusion	5–10 min	30 min–4 h	Reflex tachycardia, headache, nausea, flushing, local phlebitis	LV failure, severe AS, cardiac ischemia
Enalaprilat	ACE inhibitor	0.625 mg bolus, then 1.25–5 mg every 6 h	15–30 min	6–12 h	Variable response, precipitous fall in BP in high-renin states, headache, cough	Acute MI, h/o hypersensitivity
Fenoldopam	DA-1 agonist	0.1–0.3 μg/kg/min infusion	5–15 min	30 min–4 h	Tachycardia, headache, nausea, dizziness, flushing	Glaucoma, liver disease (cirrhosis with portal HTN)
Clevidipine	L-type CCB (dihydropyridine)	1–2 mg/h infusion	2–4 min	5–15 min	Headache, nausea, vomit	Soybean allergy
Nitroprusside[a]	Nitrovasodilator (arterial and venous)	0.25–10 μg/kg/min infusion	Immediate	1–4 min	Nausea, vomiting, muscle twitching, sweating, thiocyanate and cyanide intoxication	Coronary artery disease, elevated ICP

Adapted with kind permission of Springer Nature from Rose and Mayer [43, 94]

Abbreviations: *COPD* Chronic obstructive pulmonary disease, *LV* Left ventricle, *AV* Atrioventricular, *AS* Aortic stenosis, *CCB* Calcium channel blocker, *ACE* Angiotensin-converting enzyme, *MI* Myocardial infarction, *CAD* Coronary artery disease, *PVC* Premature ventricular contraction, *HCM* Hypertrophic cardiomyopathy

[a]Nitroprusside is becoming less favored for use in neurological emergencies

Organ-Specific Hypertensive Emergencies

Neurologic Emergencies

Ischemic Stroke

Acute ischemic stroke results from diminished cerebral perfusion. Symptoms such as facial droop, unilateral weakness or numbness, aphasia, gaze deviation, and unsteadiness of gait may be seen. Hypertension, and the subsequent formation of atherosclerotic lesions, is the most common and important treatable risk factor in acute ischemic stroke (AIS), with a rising prevalence of 79% in the U.S. population [9, 96–98]. The presence of hypertension is further associated with an increased likelihood of subclinical or silent stroke, elevating the risk for future recurrent strokes and vascular dementia [99–101]. In the acute setting, patients presenting with AIS and a history of hypertension tend to present with higher blood pressure than those without a previous diagnosis of hypertension [102].

In AIS, special considerations apply to blood pressure targets for patients eligible to receive intravenous (IV) thrombolytic therapy. Prior to initiation of thrombolytics, it is recommended to treat hypertension to a systolic pressure ≤185 mmHg and diastolic blood pressure ≤110 mmHg [19]. Further blood pressure goals for patients undergoing mechanical thrombectomy may vary on an individual basis [103]. Following acute stroke, blood pressure tends to decrease spontaneously by 20 mmHg systolic and 10 mmHg diastolic within the first 10 days of onset of injury [46].

Spontaneous Intracerebral Hemorrhage

Poorly controlled hypertension is the most common etiology [104] and important risk factor for the development of spontaneous intracerebral hemorrhage (ICH) [105, 106]. Nearly 60% of intracranial hemorrhages are estimated to be due to rupture of small arterioles secondary to hypertension [107]. ICH most often presents with an acute focal neurological abnormality including headache, severe hypertension, and decreased level of consciousness [107]. Immediate neuroimaging with non-contrast head computed tomography (CT) scan is required to confirm diagnosis [108].

Immediate control of blood pressure is the primary mainstay of treatment for ICH. Several studies have investigated optimal blood pressure goals in this setting [109–111]. According to recent data and per guidelines from American

Heart Association (AHA) and American Stroke Association (ASA), achieving an early and smooth blood pressure control, targeting a systolic blood pressure <140 mmHg, is safe and might be associated with favorable outcomes [20, 102, 109–112]. However, careful attention and monitoring for signs of systemic hypoperfusion, including renal impairment, must be taken into account during early intervention [110]. Acute treatment further involves airway protection, reversal of underlying coagulopathies and close neuromonitoring in the event that surgical interventions are required [113].

Hypertensive Encephalopathy

Hypertensive encephalopathy, frequently described as Posterior Reversible Encephalopathy Syndrome (PRES), is a condition characterized by rapidly evolving neurologic symptoms including headache, confusion, and seizures in the setting of hypertensive emergency [114]. It is attributed to dysfunctional cerebral autoregulation in the setting of persistent hypertension [115]. Failure of cerebrovascular autoregulation in this manner leads to inappropriate cerebral vasodilation and hyperperfusion injuries, causing breakdown of the blood–brain barrier with resultant cerebral edema [115]. Symptom resolution usually occurs once blood pressure is lowered toward normotensive goals. A safe approach is to target blood pressure lowering by 10–20% over the first hour of treatment, with additional lowering toward normotensive goals as best tolerated over the remainder of a 24-h period.

Hypertensive Retinopathy

The retina is the only part of the vasculature that can be visualized non-invasively. Fundoscopic examination is therefore a key element in evaluating the hypertensive patient. Persistently elevated blood pressure can lead to microvascular retinal changes such as arteriolar thickening, narrowing, or opacification. Papilledema, microaneurysms, and hemorrhage may result [116].

Evidence suggests a link between hypertensive retinopathy and systemic vascular disease including stroke, coronary heart disease, and kidney damage [117–123]. Retinopathy can regress with adequate blood pressure management, making this a useful physical examination finding to track in determining successful long-term hypertension management [124].

Cardiac Emergencies

The most common cardiac disorders in the setting of hypertensive emergency are acute systolic heart failure (often with left ventricular dysfunction and pulmonary edema) [125] and acute coronary syndrome [126].

Acute Heart Failure

In the setting of acute heart failure, careful attention should be paid to the presence of hypertension, respiratory distress, and pulmonary edema. Chest radiography, electrocardiography, pulse oximetry, and transthoracic echocardiography help with establishing the diagnosis [125]. Pulmonary edema is likely attributable to multiple factors including hyperactivity of the RAAS, excessive imbalance of endothelin to nitric oxide, impaired cardiac contractility, increased pulmonary capillary permeability, and a surplus of circulating catecholamines [127]. Once identified, patients with left ventricular dysfunction and pulmonary edema often respond well to loop diuretics. Short-acting and titratable vasodilators such as IV nitroprusside and nitroglycerin are often utilized for afterload reduction [128]. Drugs such as nonselective beta-blockers that impair cardiac contractility should be avoided [129], with the goal of treatment being reductions in afterload, circulating volume and blood pressure with improvement in pulmonary edema and respiratory distress [128].

Acute Coronary Syndrome

Uncontrolled hypertension contributes significantly to coronary artery disease and acute coronary events. Extreme elevations in blood pressure are often noted in ST-segment and non-ST-segment elevation myocardial infarction, as well as unstable angina [130]. Blood pressure levels above 180/110 mmHg are also associated with acute heart damage [130]. Dyspnea, chest pain, and anxiety are frequently observed in such cases [131]. Management often involves acute treatment of anxiety and pain, afterload reduction with IV agents such as nitroglycerin, and utilization of beta-blockers for reduction of myocardial oxygen consumption [132]. Further sub-specialty management with cardiology consultation may be indicated.

Vascular Emergencies

Acute Aortic Dissection

In response to severe hypertension, the layers of the aortic wall may separate due to an intimal tear, allowing blood to enter the intima-media space. Persistent hypertension can then continue to propagate and worsen this disease [133]. Dissecting tears are common in the ascending aorta but can occur in the aortic arch and descending thoracic aorta as well [134]. Some population-based studies suggest the incidence of aortic dissection to be approximately 3/100,000 per year [135]. This condition carries a high short-term morbidity, with medical management aimed at achieving a lower systolic blood pressure target of <120 mmHg in a rapid period of 20 min or less [136]. Antihypertensive treatment should target reducing the velocity of left ventricular contraction thus decreasing vascular shear stress and progression of dissection [137]. Rapid onset IV agents such as esmolol that affect both cardiac contractility and heart rate are beneficial in this setting. While observational studies suggest that lowering blood pressure does reduce rate of progression of disease [138, 139], further subspecialty surgical consultation may be required for continued management.

Renal Emergencies

Acute Hypertensive Nephrosclerosis

Acute hypertensive nephrosclerosis is a condition characterized by hematuria and elevated serum creatinine and is found in 75% of patients with hypertensive emergencies [140]. Common pathologic findings include intimal thickening of small renal arteries and glomerular arterioles, deposition of hyaline-like material into arteriolar walls, and glomerulosclerosis [141–143]. Subsequent renal interstitial changes may occur and can be severe. Proteinuria may start off mild, but progression into severe proteinuria can occur [144].

In patients with proteinuric chronic kidney disease and hypertension, ACE inhibitors and angiontensin II receptor blockers are the antihypertensive agents of choice [145]. Ideal blood pressure targets may vary based on other underlying co-morbidities, though high-risk patients with cardiac risk factors may benefit from lower systolic blood pressure goals <120 mmHg [146, 147]. In addition, further therapies including intermittent hemodialysis or continuous renal replacement therapies may be indicated. Long-term improvement in kidney function is observed in a minority of patients with hypertensive nephrosclerosis, though younger patients with lower protein-to-creatinine ratios may have more favorable resolution of disease [148].

Obstetric Emergencies

Pregnancy, Pre-eclampsia & Eclampsia

The American College of Obstetricians and Gynecologists defines hypertensive emergency in pregnancy as an acute and persistent SBP >160 or DBP >110 mmHg in the setting of pre-eclampsia or eclampsia [149] and is thought to be a product of abnormal placental vascular development [131]. Pre-eclampsia is a multisystem disorder characterized by hypertension and proteinuria, affecting mothers in the last half of pregnancy or post-partum.

Hypertension plays a central role in the progression of pre-eclampsia to eclampsia. Extreme elevations in blood pressure can cause dysfunction of cerebrovascular autoregulation, endothelial dysfunction, tissue hyperperfusion, and subsequent cerebral edema in a manner similar to PRES [150, 151]. Seizures and intracranial hemorrhage may result and are recognized as global leading causes of maternal and perinatal morbidity and mortality [131].

Eclampsia is characterized as a generalized grand mal seizure in the pregnant patient with pre-eclampsia. The most common antecedent signs and symptoms before seizure onset include hypertension, headache, visual disturbances, and right upper quadrant or epigastric pain [152]. Physical examination findings may include clonus, visual deficits, altered mental status as well as cranial nerve palsies [153, 154]. Treatment is often emergent, as once seizures occur, the utmost priority is airway protection, maternal oxygenation, and prevention of inadvertent injuries during the ictal event. The mainstay of treatment involves acute blood pressure management, seizure control, and delivery of the child [155].

Emergent blood pressure control should be initiated with fast-acting and titratable medications such as IV labetalol, nicardipine, or hydralazine, aiming to reduce MAP no more than 25% over 2 h for a target of SBP 130–150 mmHg and DBP 80–100 mmHg. Aggressively lower blood pressure targets below 120/80 mmHg should be avoided to prevent uteroplacental hypoperfusion [156]. The antiepileptic agent of choice for seizure control is magnesium sulfate [157]. Careful monitoring of fetal heart rate should be maintained throughout hospitalization, and abnormal heart rate tracings persisting 10–15 min despite aggressive interventional therapies should prompt consideration for emergency delivery [155].

Sympathetic Dysregulation

Sympathomimetic Agents

Ingestion of sympathomimetic agents such as amphetamine, cocaine, or tyramine-containing foods when taking a chronic monoamine oxidase inhibitors can lead to sympathetic hyperactivity and precipitate a hypertensive crisis [158, 159]. This process may occur through several mechanisms including activation of RAAS, central alpha-2 receptor antagonism, central alpha-2 agonist withdrawal, peripheral alpha-adrenergic agonism, nicotinic receptor agonism, gamma aminobutyric acid (GABA)-A and -B withdrawal, prostaglandin synthesis, mineralocorticoid excess, and nitric oxide inhibition [160].

General management is largely supportive. Hyperthermia should be swiftly recognized and aggressively managed with direct cooling devices [161]. While drug-induced hypertension frequently responds well to sedation with benzodiazepines, hypertensive emergencies should be treated accordingly based on specific symptomatic end-organ considerations [160, 162].

Dysautonomia

Neurogenic Essential Hypertension

There is evidence to suggest that patients with chronic untreated essential hypertension may have increased levels of norepinephrine and subsequent sympathetic hyperactivity in skeletal muscle vasculature [163–168]. This chronic sympathetic nervous system over activation perpetuates hypertension by directly stimulating the heart, the peripheral vasculature as well as augmenting renin secretion and reabsorption of sodium in the kidneys [163–168].

Treatment of neurogenic essential hypertension involves targeting the sympathoadrenal system (SAS). The agents of choice are alpha- and beta-adrenergic receptor blockers, central alpha agonists, and older agents such as reserpine, guanethidine, guanadrel, and imidazoline receptor agonists. Of the agents listed above, alpha- and beta-adrenergic receptor blockers remain the most popular secondary to widespread availability and favorable side effect profile [169]. Blocking both alpha- and beta-receptors by dual therapy reduces SAS-mediated blood pressure elevation thus blunting blood pressure reactivity. Monotherapy with agents such as ACE inhibitors or diuretics does not seem to provide equal effect [170–178].

Withdrawal of Anti-Hypertensive Agents

Antihypertensive agent withdrawal, in particular withdrawal from short-acting agents such as clonidine and propranolol, can be associated with severe hypertension. These withdrawal symptoms are often attributed to a rapid return of catecholamine secretion or adrenoreceptor sensitivity that had been previously suppressed during antihypertensive therapy [179–182]. Sympathetic hyperactivity is therefore dependent on both the rate at which each antihypertensive agent wears off as well as the rate of adrenoreceptor downregulation (with adrenoreceptor half-lives ranging from 24 to 36 h) [183].

An important distinction should be made between clonidine and beta blocker withdrawal. While abrupt cessation of these agents can cause acute rebound hypertension [179], beta blockade withdrawal in patients with underlying coronary artery disease can be concomitantly associated with angina, myocardial infarction, or sudden death [179, 180, 184–186].

These hypertensive crises can at times be mistaken for symptoms of pheochromocytoma. Symptom resolution can often be obtained by reinitiating the discontinued drug. A safe strategy to avoid withdrawal symptoms in drug cessation is slow discontinuation of the antihypertensive agent over a 6- to 10-day interval, cutting the dose in half every 2–3 days [179, 186]. If symptoms of withdrawal recur, reinstitution of the antihypertensive agent should alleviate symptoms while a modified tapering schedule is considered.

Autonomic Dysreflexia Following Spinal Cord Injury

Autonomic dysreflexia (AD) is a subacute to chronic phenomenon of paroxysmal bouts of severe hypertension following traumatic spinal cord injury (SCI), attributed to compensatory autonomic nervous system mechanisms that arise during the recovery phase [187]. AD, often triggered by noxious stimulation below the level of SCI (such as distension of the pelvic viscera), results from a loss of coordinated autonomic cardiovascular responses to afferent stimuli [187–189].

Occurring in both incomplete and complete SCI above the level of T6, with an incidence of up to 70% after complete SCI [190], this condition is manifested by debilitating hypertension with reflexive bradycardia, often accompanied by episodes of dizziness, sweating, and nausea [190–192]. The severity of these attacks can range from asymptomatic hypertension to hypertensive crisis, intracranial hemorrhage, and cardiac arrest [193], requiring careful clinical recognition and symptomatic management accordingly. In addition, AD-related admissions and their associated complications can lead to extended hospitalizations, further driving up the overall lifetime costs per patient [194].

The hallmark features associated with AD include life-threatening hypertension with flushing, headache, and nausea similar to attacks of hypertensive urgency and emergency. The hypertensive component is due to sympathetic-mediated peripheral vasoconstriction in response to noxious stimuli, limited to vasculature below the level of SCI [188, 189, 195]. SBP elevations can be as high as 300 mmHg [193] and can occur up to 41 times/day (average 11 times/day) in the majority of patients with chronic SCI above the T6 level [196]. Paradoxically, as carotid baroreceptors experience these elevated tensile and shearing forces, blood vessels above the level of SCI undergo parasympathetic-mediated vasodilation with subsequent clinical symptoms of flushing, nausea, and vomiting [195]. Bradycardia is also common, due once again to this parasympathetic component [195].

Early treatment for AD is targeted toward quick relief of noxious stimuli and targeted symptom management. Bowel and bladder decompression strategies, removal of tight-fitting clothing, treatment of spasticity, and bed repositioning are common first steps [197]. Most medical therapies are symptomatic, and ideally should be rapid-acting and short-onset given the paroxysmal nature of hypertensive episodes of AD [197]. Nitrates are the most commonly used treatment for acute hypertensive episodes due to their direct relaxing effect on vascular smooth muscle [195]. The application of 1–2 inches of nitroglycerin paste above the level of the lesion is effective and can be wiped off once blood pressure normalizes [198]. Nitrates should be avoided, however, in patients known to be taking sildenafil for erectile dysfunction due to their combined interactions and effects of profound hypotension [197]. Rapid onset IV antihypertensive therapies such as hydralazine and labetalol are often frequently utilized [197, 199]. Acute treatment with oral antihypertensives such as immediate-release nifedipine can be considered, as nifedipine acts on both RAAS and alpha-adrenergic receptors [195, 200]. Caution is warranted, though, for its associated side effects of hypotension, dizziness, fatigue, and weakness [197, 201].

Guillain Barre Syndrome

Guillain Barre Syndrome (GBS) is an acute inflammatory demyelinating polyneuropathy that affects peripheral nerves, usually presenting as a symmetric progressively ascending weakness with areflexia and various sensory symptoms [202, 203]. Cardiovascular symptoms are common, including paroxysmal blood pressure fluctuation, tachy-and brady-arrythmias, and at times even heart failure [202]. Episodes of hypertension are believed secondary to transient rises in catecholamine levels as well as dysregulation of baroreceptor reflexes [202], attributable to demyelination of pre-ganglionic sympathetic axons and degeneration of post-ganglionic axons, leading to an altered feedback control mechanism [204]. These paroxysmal episodes may be seen in up to 24% of patients with GBS, with one study suggesting 3% of patients having sustained hypertension [205]. If left untreated, sudden death can occur [204]. Acute antihypertensive therapy includes use of IV labetalol, nicardipine, clevidipine, or nitroprusside [206, 207], though care must be taken to adjust medication dosage given the risk of possible denervation hypersensitivity [206].

Neurodegenerative Disorders

Orthostatic hypotension remains the most frequent clinical symptom of cardiovascular autonomic failure in patients with Parkinson's disease and Multiple System Atrophy [208, 209]. Supine hypertension, however, may arise in association with left ventricular hypertrophy [210] and is a negative prognostic factor for survival and cognitive decline in these patients [211–215]. This hypertension can occasionally lead to a true hypertensive crisis [216]. The pathophysiology is thought to be due to an increase in PVR due to residual sympathetic tone. Avoidance of supine position is useful during the day, while at night transdermal nitroglycerin can be effective [217]. Risks and benefits of treatment should be weighed carefully for each patient given individual blood pressure lability.

Catecholamine-Secreting Neoplasms

Catecholamine-secreting neoplasms originating from the chromaffin cells of the adrenal medulla and the sympathetic ganglia are a rare cause of hypertensive emergency [218], being recognized as "pheochromocytomas" and "catecholamine-secreting paragangliomas" respectively. While many clinicians utilize the term "pheochromocytoma" to refer to either of these neoplasms, distinction is important to aid in diagnostic workup and management.

Catecholamine-secreting tumors are rare, occurring in 0.2% of patients with hypertension [219, 220]. Although these neoplasms are reported to have an annual incidence of 0.8 per 100,000 person-years, this figure may be underestimated as one 50-year autopsy series found 54 autopsy-proven cases of pheochromocytoma [221]. While these neoplasms may arise at any age, they are most common in the fourth to fifth decade and are equally common amongst males and females [222].

Catecholamine over-secretion from these neoplasms can promote sympathetic hyperactivity and lead to a potentially lethal hypertensive crisis [218]. The classic triad of symptoms includes episodic headache, sweating, and tachycardia [219, 223]. While paroxysmal or sustained hypertension is the most common feature of pheochromocytoma, approximately 5%–15% of patients may present with normal blood pressure [223].

A 24-h urine collection measuring fractionated catecholamines and metanephrines is the most reliable method for identifying catecholamine-secreting neoplasms [224] and should be pursued for patient with a low suspicion for pheochromocytoma or paraganglioma. Higher suspicion (family history of pheochromocytoma, genetic syndrome, previous history of pheochromoxytoma, etc) prompts evaluation including measuring plasma fractionated metanephrines (high sensitivity 96%–100%, lower specificity 85%–89%) [224, 225]. Biochemical confirmation of the diagnosis should be followed by further imaging workup [219, 223], not the other way around. Computed tomography (CT) or magnetic resonance imaging (MRI) are often utilized, and coordination with Endocrinology and surgical subspecialties may help in determining optimal imaging approach.

Once diagnosis is made, surgical resection of pheochromocytoma is indicated. Careful pre-operative medical preparation is often required. Agents such as glucagon, beta-adrenergic blockade in the absence of alpha-adrenergic blockade, dopamine D2 receptor antagonists such as metoclopramide, and opioid analgesics should be avoided as these may provoke a paroxysmal catecholamine surge [226]. Alpha-adrenergic blockade for at least 7 days preoperatively is utilized to normalize blood pressure and expand the vascular space, with phenoxybenzamine being the drug of choice [226]. Beta-adrenergic blockade is initiated only after sufficient alpha-adrenergic blockade is achieved, normally 2–3 days preoperatively [226]. In the setting of hypertensive crisis, many fast acting agents can be utilized such as IV sodium nitroprusside, phentolamine, and nicardipine to achieve blood pressure stabilization [227].

Conclusion

In conclusion, uncontrolled hypertension may arise through a variety of mechanisms and can manifest widely in multi-system end-organ damage. Prevention, early recognition, and appropriate treatment of hypertensive urgencies and emergencies are paramount in optimizing acute patient care.

References

1. Whelton PK, Carey RM, Aronow WS, Casey DE, Collins KJ, Dennison Himmelfarb C, et al. 2017 ACC/AHA/AAPA/ABC/ACPM/AGS/APhA/ASH/ASPC/NMA/PCNA guideline for the prevention, detection, evaluation, and management of high blood pressure in adults: a report of the American College of Cardiology/American Heart Association task force on clinical practice guidelines. Hypertension. 2018;71(6):e13–115.
2. Valderrama A, Gillespie C, King S, George M, Hong Y. Vital signs: awareness and treatment of uncontrolled hypertension among adults—United States, 2003–2010. MMWR Morb Mortal Wkly Rep. 2012;61
3. Chobufo MD, Gayam V, Soluny J, Rahman EU, Enoru S, Foryoung JB, et al. Prevalence and control rates of hypertension in the USA: 2017-2018. Int J Cardiol Hypertens. 2020;6:100044.
4. Chobanian AV, Bakris GL, Black HR, Cushman WC, Green LA, Izzo JL, et al. Seventh report of the joint National Committee on prevention, detection, evaluation, and treatment of high blood pressure. Hypertens Dallas Tex 1979. 2003;42(6):1206–52.
5. Gu Q, Dillon CF, Burt VL, Gillum RF. Association of hypertension treatment and control with all-cause and cardiovascular disease mortality among US adults with hypertension. Am J Hypertens. 2010;23(1):38–45.
6. Krishnamoorthy V, Chaikittisilpa N, Kiatchai T, Vavilala M. Hypertension after severe traumatic brain injury: friend or foe? J Neurosurg Anesthesiol. 2017 Oct;29(4):382–7.
7. Krishnamoorthy V, Mackensen GB, Gibbons EF, Vavilala MS. Cardiac dysfunction after neurologic injury: what do we know and where are we going? Chest. 2016 May;149(5):1325–31.
8. Oppenheimer SM. Neurogenic cardiac effects of cerebrovascular disease. Curr Opin Neurol. 1994 Feb;7(1):20–4.
9. Otite FO, Liaw N, Khandelwal P, Malik AM, Romano JG, Rundek T, et al. Increasing prevalence of vascular risk factors in patients with stroke: a call to action. Neurology. 2017;89(19):1985–94.
10. Carlberg B, Asplund K, Hägg E. The prognostic value of admission blood pressure in patients with acute stroke. Stroke. 1993 Sep;24(9):1372–5.
11. Vemmos KN, Tsivgoulis G, Spengos K, Zakopoulos N, Synetos A, Manios E, et al. U-shaped relationship between mortality and admission blood pressure in patients with acute stroke. J Intern Med. 2004 Feb;255(2):257–65.
12. Willmot M, Leonardi-Bee J, Bath PMW. High blood pressure in acute stroke and subsequent outcome: a systematic review. Hypertens Dallas Tex 1979. 2004 Jan;43(1):18–24.
13. Zhang Y, Reilly KH, Tong W, Xu T, Chen J, Bazzano LA, et al. Blood pressure and clinical outcome among patients with acute stroke in Inner Mongolia, China. J Hypertens. 2008 Jul;26(7):1446–52.
14. Dandapani BK, Suzuki S, Kelley RE, Reyes-Iglesias Y, Duncan RC. Relation between blood pressure and outcome in intracerebral hemorrhage. Stroke. 1995 Jan;26(1):21–4.
15. Cooper DJ, Myles PS, McDermott FT, Murray LJ, Laidlaw J, Cooper G, et al. Prehospital hypertonic saline resuscitation of patients with hypotension and severe traumatic brain injury: a randomized controlled trial. JAMA. 2004;291(11):1350–7.
16. Kilgannon JH, Roberts BW, Reihl LR, Chansky ME, Jones AE, Dellinger RP, et al. Early arterial hypotension is common in the post-cardiac arrest syndrome and associated with increased in-hospital mortality. Resuscitation. 2008 Dec;79(3):410–6.
17. Waltz AG. Effect of blood pressure on blood flow in ischemic and in nonischemic cerebral cortex. Neurology. 1968;18(7):613.
18. Jain V, Choudhary J, Pandit R. Blood pressure target in acute brain injury. Indian J Crit Care Med Peer-Rev Off Publ Indian Soc Crit Care Med. 2019;23(Suppl 2):S136–9.
19. Powers WJ, Rabinstein AA, Ackerson T, Adeoye OM, Bambakidis NC, Becker K, et al. Guidelines for the early management of patients with acute ischemic stroke: 2019 update to the 2018 guidelines for the early management of acute ischemic stroke: a guideline for healthcare professionals from the American Heart Association/American Stroke Association. Stroke. 2019;50(12):e344–418.
20. Hemphill JC, Greenberg SM, Anderson CS, Becker K, Bendok BR, Cushman M, et al. Guidelines for the management of spontaneous intracerebral hemorrhage. Stroke. 2015;46(7):2032–60.
21. Ostchega Y, Fryar CD, Nwankwo T, Nguyen DT. Hypertension prevalence among adults aged 18 and over: United States, 2017-2018. NCHS Data Brief. 2020 Apr;364:1–8.
22. Wang TJ, Vasan RS. Epidemiology of uncontrolled hypertension in the United States. Circulation. 2005;112(11):1651–62.
23. Lloyd-Jones DM, Evans JC, Larson MG, O'Donnell CJ, Roccella EJ, Levy D. Differential control of systolic and diastolic blood pressure: factors associated with lack of blood pressure control in the community. Hypertens Dallas Tex 1979. 2000 Oct;36(4):594–9.
24. Hyman DJ, Pavlik VN. Characteristics of patients with uncontrolled hypertension in the United States. N Engl J Med. 2001;345(7):479–86.
25. He J, Muntner P, Chen J, Roccella EJ, Streiffer RH, Whelton PK. Factors associated with hypertension control in the general population of the United States. Arch Intern Med. 2002;162(9):1051–8.
26. Burt VL, Whelton P, Roccella EJ, Brown C, Cutler JA, Higgins M, et al. Prevalence of hypertension in the US adult population. Results from the Third National Health and Nutrition Examination Survey, 1988–1991. Hypertens Dallas Tex 1979. 1995;25(3):305–13.
27. Hajjar I, Kotchen TA. Trends in prevalence, awareness, treatment, and control of hypertension in the United States, 1988-2000. JAMA. 2003;290(2):199–206.
28. Shea S, Misra D, Ehrlich MH, Field L, Francis CK. Predisposing factors for severe, uncontrolled hypertension in an inner-city minority population. N Engl J Med. 1992;327(11):776–81.
29. Bone LR, Hill MN, Stallings R, Gelber AC, Barker A, Baylor I, et al. Community health survey in an urban African-American

neighborhood: distribution and correlates of elevated blood pressure. Ethn Dis. 2000;10(1):87–95.
30. Coresh J, Wei GL, McQuillan G, Brancati FL, Levey AS, Jones C, et al. Prevalence of high blood pressure and elevated serum creatinine level in the United States: findings from the third National Health and nutrition examination survey (1988-1994). Arch Intern Med. 2001;161(9):1207–16.
31. Agarwal R, Nissenson AR, Batlle D, Coyne DW, Trout JR, Warnock DG. Prevalence, treatment, and control of hypertension in chronic hemodialysis patients in the United States. Am J Med. 2003;115(4):291–7.
32. Geiss LS, Rolka DB, Engelgau MM. Elevated blood pressure among U.S. adults with diabetes, 1988-1994. Am J Prev Med. 2002;22(1):42–8.
33. Ho PM, Masoudi FA, Peterson ED, Grunwald GK, Sales AE, Hammermeister KE, et al. Cardiology management improves secondary prevention measures among patients with coronary artery disease. J Am Coll Cardiol. 2004;43(9):1517–23.
34. van den Born BJH, Lip GYH, Brguljan-Hitij J, Cremer A, Segura J, Morales E, et al. ESC Council on hypertension position document on the management of hypertensive emergencies. Eur Heart J Cardiovasc Pharmacother. 2019;5(1):37–46.
35. Marik PE, Varon J. Hypertensive crises: challenges and management. Chest. 2007;131(6):1949–62.
36. Varon J, Marik PE. The diagnosis and management of hypertensive crises. Chest. 2000;118(1):214–27.
37. Rey E, LeLorier J, Burgess E, Lange IR, Leduc L. Report of the Canadian hypertension society consensus conference: 3. Pharmacologic treatment of hypertensive disorders in pregnancy. CMAJ Can Med Assoc J J Assoc Medicale Can. 1997;157(9):1245–54.
38. Bruenn HG. Clinical notes on the illness and death of President Franklin D. Roosevelt Ann Intern Med. 1970;72(4):579–91.
39. Mancia G, Fagard R, Narkiewicz K, Redón J, Zanchetti A, Böhm M, et al. 2013 ESH/ESC guidelines for the management of arterial hypertension: the task force for the management of arterial hypertension of the European Society of Hypertension (ESH) and of the European Society of Cardiology (ESC). J Hypertens. 2013;31(7):1281–357.
40. Rosamond W, Flegal K, Friday G, Furie K, Go A, Greenlund K, et al. Heart disease and stroke statistics—2007 update: a report from the American Heart Association Statistics Committee and Stroke Statistics Subcommittee. Circulation. 2007;115(5):e69–171.
41. Janke AT, McNaughton CD, Brody AM, Welch RD, Levy PD. Trends in the incidence of hypertensive emergencies in US emergency departments from 2006 to 2013. J Am Heart Assoc. 2016;5(12):e004511.
42. Mayer SA, Kurtz P, Wyman A, Sung GY, Multz AS, Varon J, et al. Clinical practices, complications, and mortality in neurological patients with acute severe hypertension: the studying the treatment of acute hyperTension registry. Crit Care Med. 2011 Oct;39(10):2330–6.
43. Rose JC, Mayer SA. Optimizing blood pressure in neurological emergencies. Neurocrit Care. 2004;1(3):287–99.
44. Bruss ZS, Raja A. Physiology, stroke volume. In: StatPearls [internet]. Treasure Island (FL): StatPearls Publishing; 2021 [cited 2021 Nov 30]. http://www.ncbi.nlm.nih.gov/books/NBK547686/
45. Vincent JL. Understanding cardiac output. Crit Care Lond Engl. 2008;12(4):174.
46. Beevers G, Lip GY, O'Brien E. ABC of hypertension: the pathophysiology of hypertension. BMJ. 2001;322(7291):912–6.
47. Armstrong M, Kerndt CC, Moore RA. Physiology, baroreceptors. In: StatPearls [Internet]. Treasure Island (FL): StatPearls Publishing; 2021 [cited 2022 Jan 11]. http://www.ncbi.nlm.nih.gov/books/NBK538172/
48. Persson P, Ehmke H, Kirchheim H, Seller H. Effect of sino-aortic denervation in comparison to cardiopulmonary deafferentiation on long-term blood pressure in conscious dogs. Pflugers Arch. 1988;411(2):160–6.
49. Kougias P, Weakley SM, Yao Q, Lin PH, Chen C. Arterial baroreceptors in the management of systemic hypertension. Med Sci Monit Int Med J Exp Clin Res. 2010;16(1):RA1–8.
50. Willette RN, Punnen S, Krieger AJ, Sapru HN. Interdependence of rostral and caudal ventrolateral medullary areas in the control of blood pressure. Brain Res. 1984;321(1):169–74.
51. Suarez-Roca H, Klinger RY, Podgoreanu MV, Ji RR, Sigurdsson MI, Waldron N, et al. Contribution of baroreceptor function to pain perception and perioperative outcomes. Anesthesiology. 2019;130(4):634–50.
52. Grassi G, Mark A, Esler M. The sympathetic nervous system alterations in human hypertension. Circ Res. 2015;116(6):976–90.
53. Alhayek S, Preuss CV. Beta 1 receptors. In: StatPearls [Internet]. Treasure Island (FL): StatPearls Publishing; 2022 [cited 2022 Jan 12]. http://www.ncbi.nlm.nih.gov/books/NBK532904/
54. Thiele RH, Nemergut EC, Lynch C. The clinical implications of isolated alpha(1) adrenergic stimulation. Anesth Analg. 2011;113(2):297–304.
55. Oparil S, Acelajado MC, Bakris GL, Berlowitz DR, Cífková R, Dominiczak AF, et al. Hypertension. Nat Rev Dis Primer. 2018;(4):18014–4.
56. Hall ME, Hall JE. 5—Pathogenesis of hypertension. In: Bakris GL, Sorrentino MJ, editors. Hypertension: a companion to Braunwald's heart disease (3rd ed) [Internet]. Elsevier; 2018. p. 33–51. https://www.sciencedirect.com/science/article/pii/B9780323429733000056
57. Kriz W, Elger M. Renal anatomy. Compr Clin Nephrol 3rd Ed Phila. 2010:1–11.
58. Schweda F, Friis U, Wagner C, Skott O, Kurtz A. Renin release. Physiol Bethesda Md. 2007;22:310–9.
59. Peti-Peterdi J, Harris RC. Macula densa sensing and signaling mechanisms of renin release. J Am Soc Nephrol JASN. 2010;21:1093–6.
60. Bonjour J, Malvin R. Stimulation of ADH release by the renin-angiotensin system. Am J Physiol-Leg Content. 1970;218(6):1555–9.
61. Weller RO. Vascular pathology in hypertension. Age Ageing. 1979;8(2):99–103.
62. DeQuattro V, Lee DD. Blood pressure reactivity and sympathetic hyperactivity. Predictors of hypertension. Am J Hypertens. 1991;4(11):624S–8S.
63. Lavie P, Ben-Yosef R, Rubin AE. Prevalence of sleep apnea syndrome among patients with essential hypertension. Am Heart J. 1984;108(2):373–6.
64. Kales A, Bixler EO, Cadieux RJ, Schneck DW, Shaw LC, Locke TW, et al. Sleep apnoea in a hypertensive population. Lancet Lond Engl. 1984;2(8410):1005–8.
65. Fletcher EC, DeBehnke RD, Lovoi MS, Gorin AB. Undiagnosed sleep apnea in patients with essential hypertension. Ann Intern Med. 1985;103(2):190–5.
66. Williams AJ, Houston D, Finberg S, Lam C, Kinney JL, Santiago S. Sleep apnea syndrome and essential hypertension. Am J Cardiol. 1985;55(8):1019–22.
67. Lambert EA, Esler MD, Schlaich MP, Dixon J, Eikelis N, Lambert GW. Obesity-associated organ damage and sympathetic nervous activity. Hypertension. 2019;73(6):1150–9.
68. Fujita T. Mechanism of salt-sensitive hypertension: focus on adrenal and sympathetic nervous systems. J Am Soc Nephrol. 2014;25(6):1148–55.
69. Lacolley P, Regnault V, Segers P, Laurent S. Vascular smooth muscle cells and arterial stiffening: relevance in development, aging, and disease. Physiol Rev. 2017;97(4):1555–617.

70. Ushio-Fukai M, Alexander RW, Akers M, Griendling KK. p38 mitogen-activated protein kinase is a critical component of the redox-sensitive signaling pathways activated by angiotensin II: ROLE IN VASCULAR SMOOTH MUSCLE CELL HYPERTROPHY*. J Biol Chem. 1998;273(24):15022–9.
71. Walsh JA, Hyman C, Maronde RF. Venous distensibility in essential hypertension. Cardiovasc Res. 1969;3(3):338–49.
72. Gribbin B, Pickering TG, Sleight P. Arterial distensibility in normal and hypertensive man. Clin Sci Lond Engl 1979;56(5):413–7.
73. Khaddaj Mallat R, Mathew John C, Kendrick DJ, Braun AP. The vascular endothelium: a regulator of arterial tone and interface for the immune system. Crit Rev Clin Lab Sci. 2017;54(7–8):458–70.
74. Sandoo A, van Zanten JJCSV, Metsios GS, Carroll D, Kitas GD. The endothelium and its role in regulating vascular tone. Open Cardiovasc Med J. 2010;4:302–12.
75. Kohan DE, Barton M. Endothelin and endothelin antagonists in chronic kidney disease. Kidney Int. 2014;86(5):896–904.
76. Spieker LE, Flammer AJ, Lüscher TF. The vascular endothelium in hypertension. Handb Exp Pharmacol. 2006;176(Pt 2):249–83.
77. Panza JA, Casino PR, Badar DM, Quyyumi AA. Effect of increased availability of endothelium-derived nitric oxide precursor on endothelium-dependent vascular relaxation in normal subjects and in patients with essential hypertension. Circulation. 1993;87(5):1475–81.
78. Popolo A, Autore G, Pinto A, Marzocco S. Oxidative stress in patients with cardiovascular disease and chronic renal failure. Free Radic Res. 2013;47(5):346–56.
79. Hall JE, Guyton AC, Coleman TG, Mizelle HL, Woods LL. Regulation of arterial pressure: role of pressure natriuresis and diuresis. Fed Proc. 1986;45(13):2897–903.
80. Coleman TG, Granger HJ, Guyton AC. Whole-body circulatory autoregulation and hypertension. Circ Res. 1971;28(5_suppl_2):II–76.
81. Raven PB, Chapleau MW. Blood pressure regulation XI: overview and future research directions. Eur J Appl Physiol. 2014;114(3):579–86.
82. Mount CA, M Das J. Cerebral Perfusion Pressure. In: StatPearls [Internet]. Treasure Island (FL): StatPearls Publishing; 2021 [cited 2021 Dec 15]. http://www.ncbi.nlm.nih.gov/books/NBK537271/
83. Baron JC. Perfusion thresholds in human cerebral ischemia: historical perspective and therapeutic implications. Cerebrovasc Dis Basel Switz. 2001;11(Suppl 1):2–8.
84. Qureshi AI. Acute hypertensive response in patients with stroke. Circulation. 2008;118(2):176–87.
85. Jordan JD, Powers WJ. Cerebral autoregulation and acute ischemic stroke. Am J Hypertens. 2012;25(9):946–50.
86. Castillo J, Leira R, García MM, Serena J, Blanco M, Dávalos A. Blood pressure decrease during the acute phase of ischemic stroke is associated with brain injury and poor stroke outcome. Stroke. 2004;35(2):520–6.
87. Owens WB. Blood pressure control in acute cerebrovascular disease. J Clin Hypertens Greenwich Conn. 2011;13(3):205–11.
88. Vidt DG, Bakst AW, Graham RM. Adrenergic receptors: structure and function. Cleve Clin J Med. 1990;57(5):481–91.
89. Hieble JP. Adrenergic Receptors. In: Squire LR, editor. Encyclopedia of neuroscience [internet]. Oxford: Academic Press; 2009. p. 135–9. https://www.sciencedirect.com/science/article/pii/B978008045046900694X.
90. Ahlquist RP. A study of the adrenotropic receptors. Am J Phys. 1948;153(3):586–600.
91. Giovannitti JA Jr, Thoms SM, Crawford JJ. Alpha-2 adrenergic receptor agonists: a review of current clinical applications. Anesth Prog. 2015;62(1).31–9.
92. Lands AM, Arnold A, McAuliff JP, Luduena FP, Brown TG. Differentiation of receptor systems activated by sympathomimetic amines. Nature. 1967;214(5088):597–8.
93. Furchgott RF. The pharmacological differentiation of adrenergic receptors. Ann N Y Acad Sci. 1967;139(3):553–70.
94. Rincon F, Rose JC, Mayer SA. Blood pressure management after central nervous system injury. In: Layon AJ, Gabrielli A, Friedman WA, editors. Textbook of Neurointensive care [internet]. London: Springer; 2013. [cited 2022 Jan 25]. p. 241–54. https://doi.org/10.1007/978-1-4471-5226-2_12.
95. Cottrell JE, Patel K, Turndorf H, Ransohoff J. Intracranial pressure changes induced by sodium nitroprusside in patients with intracranial mass lesions. J Neurosurg. 1978;48(3):329–31.
96. O'Donnell MJ, Chin SL, Rangarajan S, Xavier D, Liu L, Zhang H, et al. Global and regional effects of potentially modifiable risk factors associated with acute stroke in 32 countries (INTERSTROKE): a case-control study. Lancet Lond Engl. 2016;388(10046):761–75.
97. Prevention of stroke by antihypertensive drug treatment in older persons with isolated systolic hypertension: final results of the systolic hypertension in the elderly program (SHEP). JAMA. 1991;265(24):3255–64.
98. Collins R, Peto R, MacMahon S, Hebert P, Fiebach NH, Eberlein KA, et al. Blood pressure, stroke, and coronary heart disease. Part 2, short-term reductions in blood pressure: overview of randomised drug trials in their epidemiological context. Lancet Lond Engl. 1990;335(8693):827–38.
99. Vermeer SE, Longstreth WT, Koudstaal PJ. Silent brain infarcts: a systematic review. Lancet Neurol. 2007;6(7):611–9.
100. Prabhakaran S, Wright CB, Yoshita M, Delapaz R, Brown T, DeCarli C, et al. Prevalence and determinants of subclinical brain infarction: the northern Manhattan study. Neurology. 2008;70(6):425–30.
101. Das RR, Seshadri S, Beiser AS, Kelly-Hayes M, Au R, Himali JJ, et al. Prevalence and correlates of silent cerebral infarcts in the Framingham offspring study. Stroke. 2008;39(11):2929–35.
102. Anderson CS, Selim MH, Molina CA, Qureshi AI. Intensive blood pressure lowering in intracerebral hemorrhage. Stroke. 2017;48(7):2034–7.
103. Anadani M, Arthur AS, Tsivgoulis G, Simpson KN, Alawieh A, Orabi Y, et al. Blood pressure goals and clinical outcomes after successful endovascular therapy: a multicenter study. Ann Neurol. 2020;87(6):830–9.
104. Poon MTC, Bell SM, Al-Shahi SR. Epidemiology of intracerebral Haemorrhage. Front Neurol Neurosci. 2015;37:1–12.
105. Woo D, Sauerbeck LR, Kissela BM, Khoury JC, Szaflarski JP, Gebel J, et al. Genetic and environmental risk factors for intracerebral hemorrhage: preliminary results of a population-based study. Stroke. 2002;33(5):1190–5.
106. Woo D, Haverbusch M, Sekar P, Kissela B, Khoury J, Schneider A, et al. Effect of untreated hypertension on hemorrhagic stroke. Stroke. 2004;35(7):1703–8.
107. Claude Hemphill J, Lam A. Emergency neurological life support: intracerebral hemorrhage. Neurocrit Care. 2017;27(Suppl 1):89–101.
108. Elliott J, Smith M. The acute management of intracerebral hemorrhage: a clinical review. Anesth Analg [Internet]. 2010;110(5). https://journals.lww.com/anesthesia-analgesia/Fulltext/2010/05000/The_Acute_Management_of_Intracerebral_Hemorrhage_.28.aspx
109. Anderson CS, Heeley E, Huang Y, Wang J, Stapf C, Delcourt C, et al. Rapid blood-pressure lowering in patients with acute intracerebral hemorrhage. N Engl J Med. 2013;368(25):2355–65.
110. Qureshi AI, Palesch YY, Barsan WG, Hanley DF, Hsu CY, Martin RL, et al. Intensive blood-pressure lowering in patients with acute cerebral hemorrhage. N Engl J Med. 2016;375(11):1033–43.
111. Butcher KS, Jeerakathil T, Hill M, Demchuk AM, Dowlatshahi D, Coutts SB, et al. The intracerebral hemorrhage acutely decreasing arterial pressure trial. Stroke. 2013;44(3):620–6.

112. Moullaali TJ, Wang X, Martin RH, Shipes VB, Robinson TG, Chalmers J, et al. Blood pressure control and clinical outcomes in acute intracerebral haemorrhage: a preplanned pooled analysis of individual participant data. Lancet Neurol. 2019;18(9):857–64.
113. Delgado MG, Bogousslavsky J. Cerebral Hyperperfusion syndrome and related conditions. Eur Neurol. 2020;83(5):453–7.
114. Schwartz RB, Jones KM, Kalina P, Bajakian RL, Mantello MT, Garada B, et al. Hypertensive encephalopathy: findings on CT, MR imaging, and SPECT imaging in 14 cases. Am J Roentgenol. 1992;159(2):379–83.
115. Vaughan CJ, Delanty N. Hypertensive emergencies. Lancet. 2000;356(9227):411–7.
116. Walsh JB. Hypertensive retinopathy. Description, classification, and prognosis. Ophthalmology. 1982;89(10):1127–31.
117. Wong TY, Klein R, Sharrett AR, Duncan BB, Couper DJ, Klein BEK, et al. Retinal arteriolar diameter and risk for hypertension. Ann Intern Med. 2004;140(4):248–55.
118. Wong TY, Klein R, Couper DJ, Cooper LS, Shahar E, Hubbard LD, et al. Retinal microvascular abnormalities and incident stroke: the atherosclerosis risk in communities study. Lancet Lond Engl. 2001;358(9288):1134–40.
119. Ong YT, Wong TY, Klein R, Klein BEK, Mitchell P, Sharrett AR, et al. Hypertensive retinopathy and risk of stroke. Hypertension. 2013;62(4):706–11.
120. Wong TY, Klein R, Sharrett AR, Duncan BB, Couper DJ, Tielsch JM, et al. Retinal arteriolar narrowing and risk of coronary heart disease in men and women. The atherosclerosis risk in communities study. JAMA. 2002;287(9):1153–9.
121. Cheung N, Bluemke DA, Klein R, Sharrett AR, Islam FMA, Cotch MF, et al. Retinal arteriolar narrowing and left ventricular remodeling: the multi-ethnic study of atherosclerosis. J Am Coll Cardiol. 2007;50(1):48–55.
122. Wong TY, Coresh J, Klein R, Muntner P, Couper DJ, Sharrett AR, et al. Retinal microvascular abnormalities and renal dysfunction: the atherosclerosis risk in communities study. J Am Soc Nephrol JASN. 2004;15(9):2469–76.
123. Shantha GPS, Kumar AA, Bhaskar E, Sivagnanam K, Srinivasan D, Sundaresan M, et al. Hypertensive retinal changes, a screening tool to predict microalbuminuria in hypertensive patients: a cross-sectional study. Nephrol Dial Transplant. 2010;25(6):1839–45.
124. Bock KD. Regression of retinal vascular changes by antihypertensive therapy. Hypertens Dallas Tex 1979. 1984;6(6 Pt 2):III158–62.
125. Endorsed by the European Society of Intensive Care Medicine. Executive summary of the guidelines on the diagnosis and treatment of acute heart failure: the task force on acute heart failure of the European Society of Cardiology. Eur Heart J. 2005;26(4):384–416.
126. Nadar SK, Tayebjee MH, Messerli F, Lip GYH. Target organ damage in hypertension: pathophysiology and implications for drug therapy. Curr Pharm Des. 2006;12(13):1581–92.
127. Rimoldi SF, Yuzefpolskaya M, Allemann Y, Messerli F. Flash pulmonary edema. Symp Renov Dis. 2009;52(3):249–59.
128. Yancy CW, Jessup M, Bozkurt B, Butler J, Casey DE, Drazner MH, et al. 2013 ACCF/AHA guideline for the management of heart failure. Circulation. 2013;128(16):e240–327.
129. Alexander P, Alkhawam L, Curry J, Levy P, Pang PS, Storrow AB, et al. Lack of evidence for intravenous vasodilators in ED patients with acute heart failure: a systematic review. Am J Emerg Med. 2015 Feb;33(2):133–41.
130. Tocci G, Figliuzzi I, Presta V, Miceli F, Citoni B, Coluccia R, et al. Therapeutic approach to hypertension urgencies and emergencies during acute coronary syndrome. High Blood Press Cardiovasc Prev Off J Ital Soc Hypertens. 2018;25(3):253–9.
131. Mahendra V, Clark SL, Suresh MS. Neuropathophysiology of preeclampsia and eclampsia: a review of cerebral hemodynamic principles in hypertensive disorders of pregnancy. Pregnancy Hypertens. 2021;23:104–11.
132. Lau J, Antman EM, Jimenez-Silva J, Kupelnick B, Mosteller F, Chalmers TC. Cumulative meta-analysis of therapeutic trials for myocardial infarction. N Engl J Med. 1992;327(4):248–54.
133. Hagan PG, Nienaber CA, Isselbacher EM, Bruckman D, Karavite DJ, Russman PL, et al. The international registry of acute aortic dissection (IRAD)new insights into an old disease. JAMA. 2000;283(7):897–903.
134. Kouchoukos NT, Dougenis D. Surgery of the thoracic aorta. N Engl J Med. 1997;336(26):1876–89.
135. Mészáros I, Mórocz J, Szlávi J, Schmidt J, Tornóci L, Nagy L, et al. Epidemiology and clinicopathology of aortic dissection. Chest. 2000;117(5):1271–8.
136. Miller JB, Suchdev K, Jayaprakash N, Hrabec D, Sood A, Sharma S, et al. New developments in hypertensive encephalopathy. Curr Hypertens Rep. 2018;20(2):13.
137. Di Eusanio M, Trimarchi S, Patel HJ, Hutchison S, Suzuki T, Peterson MD, et al. Clinical presentation, management, and short-term outcome of patients with type a acute dissection complicated by mesenteric malperfusion: observations from the international registry of acute aortic dissection. J Thorac Cardiovasc Surg. 2013;145(2):385–390.e1.
138. Hiratzka LF, Bakris GL, Beckman JA, Bersin RM, Carr VF, Casey DE, et al. 2010 ACCF/AHA/AATS/ACR/ASA/SCA/SCAI/SIR/STS/SVM guidelines for the diagnosis and management of patients with thoracic aortic disease: a report of the American College of Cardiology Foundation/American Heart Association task force on practice guidelines, American Association for Thoracic Surgery, American College of Radiology, American Stroke Association, Society of Cardiovascular Anesthesiologists, Society for Cardiovascular Angiography and Interventions, Society of Interventional Radiology, Society of Thoracic Surgeons, and Society for Vascular Medicine. Circulation. 2010;121(13):e266–369.
139. van Bogerijen GHW, Tolenaar JL, Rampoldi V, Moll FL, van Herwaarden JA, Jonker FHW, et al. Predictors of aortic growth in uncomplicated type B aortic dissection. J Vasc Surg. 2014;59(4):1134–43.
140. Elliott WJ, Weber RR, Nelson KS, Oliner CM, Fumo MT, Gretler DD, et al. Renal and hemodynamic effects of intravenous fenoldopam versus nitroprusside in severe hypertension. Circulation. 1990;81(3):970–7.
141. Zucchelli P, Zuccalà A. Primary hypertension—how does it cause renal failure? Nephrol Dial Transplant Off Publ Eur Dial Transpl Assoc Eur Ren Assoc. 1994;9(3):223–5.
142. Harvey JM, Beevers DG, Howie AJ, Lee SJ, Newbold KM, Adu D, et al. Renal biopsy findings in hypertensive patients with proteinuria. Lancet. 1992;340(8833):1435–6.
143. Marcantoni C, Ma LJ, Federspiel C, Fogo AB. Hypertensive nephrosclerosis in African Americans versus Caucasians. Kidney Int. 2002;62(1):172–80.
144. Mujais SK, Emmanouel DS, Kasinath BS, Spargo BH. Marked proteinuria in hypertensive nephrosclerosis. Am J Nephrol. 1985;5(3):190–5.
145. Jafar TH, Stark PC, Schmid CH, Landa M, Maschio G, de Jong PE, et al. Progression of chronic kidney disease: the role of blood pressure control, proteinuria, and angiotensin-converting enzyme inhibition: a patient-level meta-analysis. Ann Intern Med. 2003;139(4):244–52.
146. SPRINT Research Group, Lewis CE, Fine LJ, Beddhu S, Cheung AK, Cushman WC, et al. Final report of a trial of intensive versus standard blood-pressure control. N Engl J Med. 2021;384(20):1921–30.
147. SPRINT Research Group, Wright JT, Williamson JD, Whelton PK, Snyder JK, Sink KM, et al. A randomized trial of inten-

sive versus standard blood-pressure control. N Engl J Med. 2015;373(22):2103–16.
148. Hu B, Gadegbeku C, Lipkowitz MS, Rostand S, Lewis J, Wright JT, et al. Kidney function can improve in patients with hypertensive CKD. J Am Soc Nephrol JASN. 2012;23(4):706–13.
149. Committee Opinion no. 514: emergent therapy for acute-onset, severe hypertension with preeclampsia or eclampsia. Obstet Gynecol. 2011;118(6):1465–8.
150. Marra A, Vargas M, Striano P, Del Guercio L, Buonanno P, Servillo G. Posterior reversible encephalopathy syndrome: the endothelial hypotheses. Med Hypotheses. 2014;82(5):619–22.
151. Johnson AC, Tremble SM, Chan SL, Moseley J, LaMarca B, Nagle KJ, et al. Magnesium sulfate treatment reverses seizure susceptibility and decreases neuroinflammation in a rat model of severe preeclampsia. PLoS One. 2014;9(11):e113670.
152. Berhan Y, Berhan A. Should magnesium sulfate be administered to women with mild pre-eclampsia? A systematic review of published reports on eclampsia. J Obstet Gynaecol Res. 2015;41(6):831–42.
153. Chuan FS, Charles BG, Boyle RK, Rasiah RL. Population pharmacokinetics of magnesium in preeclampsia. Am J Obstet Gynecol. 2001;185(3):593–9.
154. Shah AK, Rajamani K, Whitty JE. Eclampsia: a neurological perspective. J Neurol Sci. 2008;271(1–2):158–67.
155. Sibai BM. Diagnosis, prevention, and management of eclampsia. Obstet Gynecol. 2005;105(2):402–10.
156. Visintin C, Mugglestone MA, Almerie MQ, Nherera LM, James D, Walkinshaw S, et al. Management of hypertensive disorders during pregnancy: summary of NICE guidance. BMJ. 2010;341:c2207.
157. Sibai BM. Magnesium sulfate prophylaxis in preeclampsia: lessons learned from recent trials. Am J Obstet Gynecol. 2004;190(6):1520–6.
158. Goldstein S, Richards JR. Sympathomimetic toxicity. In: StatPearls [Internet]. Treasure Island (FL): StatPearls Publishing; 2022 [cited 2022 Jan 13]. http://www.ncbi.nlm.nih.gov/books/NBK430757/
159. Baumann BM, Pescatore RM. 27—Hypertensive emergencies. In: Brown DL, editor. Cardiac intensive care (third edition) [internet]. Philadelphia: Elsevier; 2019. p. 275–291.e5. https://www.sciencedirect.com/science/article/pii/B9780323529938000278.
160. King A, Dimovska M, Bisoski L. Sympathomimetic toxidromes and other pharmacological causes of acute hypertension. Curr Hypertens Rep. 2018;20(1):8.
161. Rosenberg J, Pentel P, Pond S, Benowitz N, Olson K. Hyperthermia associated with drug intoxication. Crit Care Med. 1986;14(11):964–9.
162. Levy P, Compton S, Welch R, Delgado G, Jennett A, Penugonda N, et al. Treatment of severe decompensated heart failure with high-dose intravenous nitroglycerin: a feasibility and outcome analysis. Ann Emerg Med. 2007;50(2):144–52.
163. Greenwood JP, Stoker JB, Mary DASG. Single-unit sympathetic discharge. Circulation. 1999;100(12):1305–10.
164. Grassi G, Colombo M, Seravalle G, Spaziani D, Mancia G. Dissociation between muscle and skin sympathetic nerve activity in essential hypertension, obesity, and congestive heart failure. Hypertension. 1998;31(1):64–7.
165. Shannon JR, Flattem NL, Jordan J, Jacob G, Black BK, Biaggioni I, et al. Orthostatic intolerance and tachycardia associated with norepinephrine-transporter deficiency. N Engl J Med. 2000;342(8):541–9.
166. Goldstein DS, Robertson D, Esler M, Straus SE, Eisenhofer G. Dysautonomias: clinical disorders of the Autonomic nervous system. Ann Intern Med. 2002;137(9):753–63.
167. Esler M, Julius S, Zweifler A, Randall O, Harburg E, Gardiner H, et al. Mild high-renin essential hypertension. N Engl J Med. 1977;296(8):405–11.
168. S J. Changing role of the autonomic nervous system in human hypertension. J Hypertens Suppl Off J Int Soc Hypertens. 1990;8(7):S59–65.
169. Mann SJ. Neurogenic essential hypertension revisited: the case for increased clinical and research attention. Am J Hypertens. 2003;16(10):881–8.
170. Julius S. The blood pressure seeking properties of the central nervous system. J Hypertens. 1988;6(3):177–85.
171. Maconochie JG, Richards DA, Woodings EP. Modification of pressor responses induced by "cold" [proceedings]. Br J Clin Pharmacol. 1977;4(3):389P.
172. Pandhi P, Sharma PL, Sharma BK, Wahi PL. Comparative effect of propranolol and labetalol on isometric exercise and cold stress induced increase in arterial blood pressure. Int J Clin Pharmacol. 1986;24(5):249–53.
173. Anand MP, Dattani KK, Datey KK. Effect of isometric exercise and mental stress on blood pressure--comparative effects of propranolol and labetalol. Indian Heart J. 1984;36(1):4–7.
174. Mills PJ, Dimsdale JE. Cardiovascular reactivity to psychosocial stressors. A review of the effects of beta-blockade. Psychosomatics. 1991;32(2):209–20.
175. Dimsdale JE, Mills P, Ziegler M, Leitz K, Nelesen R. Converting enzyme inhibition and blood pressure reactivity to psychological stressors. Hypertens Dallas Tex 1979. 1992;20(2):210–3.
176. Shapiro AP. Pressor responses to noxious stimuli in hypertensive patients. Circulation. 1962;26(2):242–50.
177. Niarchos AP, Pickering TG, Morganti A, Laragh JH. Plasma catecholamines and cardiovascular responses during converting enzyme inhibition in normotensive and hypertensive man. Clin Exp Hypertens A. 1982;4(4–5):761–89.
178. Mann SJ, Pickering TG, Alderman MH, Laragh JH. Assessment of the effects of alpha- and beta-blockade in hypertensive patients who smoke cigarettes. Am J Med. 1989;86(1B):79–81.
179. Houston MC. Abrupt cessation of treatment in hypertension: consideration of clinical features, mechanisms, prevention and management of the discontinuation syndrome. Am Heart J. 1981;102(3 Pt 1):415–30.
180. Lefkowitz RJ, Caron MG, Stiles GL. Mechanisms of membrane-receptor regulation. Biochemical, physiological, and clinical insights derived from studies of the adrenergic receptors. N Engl J Med. 1984;310(24):1570–9.
181. Vanholder R, Carpentier J, Schurgers M, Clement DL. Rebound phenomenon during gradual withdrawal of clonidine. Br Med J. 1977;1(6069):1138.
182. Metz S, Klein C, Morton N. Rebound hypertension after discontinuation of transdermal clonidine therapy. Am J Med. 1987;82(1):17–9.
183. Frishman WH, Klein N, Strom J, Cohen MN, Shamoon H, Willens H, et al. Comparative effects of abrupt withdrawal of propranolol and verapamil in angina pectoris. Am J Cardiol. 1982;50(5):1191–5.
184. Psaty BM, Koepsell TD, Wagner EH, LoGerfo JP, Inui TS. The relative risk of incident coronary heart disease associated with recently stopping the use of β-blockers. JAMA. 1990;263(12):1653–7.
185. Miller RR, Olson HG, Amsterdam EA, Mason DT. Propranolol-withdrawal rebound phenomenon. Exacerbation of coronary events after abrupt cessation of antianginal therapy. N Engl J Med. 1975;293(9):416–8.
186. Rangno RE, Nattel S, Lutterodt A. Prevention of propranolol withdrawal mechanism by prolonged small dose propranolol schedule. Am J Cardiol. 1982;49(4):828–33.
187. Cowan H, Lakra C, Desai M. Autonomic dysreflexia in spinal cord injury. BMJ. 2020;371:m3596.
188. Krassioukov AV, Johns DG, Schramm LP. Sensitivity of sympathetically correlated spinal interneurons, renal sympathetic nerve activity, and arterial pressure to somatic and visceral stimuli after chronic spinal injury. J Neurotrauma. 2002;19(12):1521–9.

189. Mathias CJ. The cardiovascular system in tetraplegia and paraplegia. Handb Clin Neurol. 1992:435–56.
190. Snow JC, Sideropoulos HP, Kripke BJ, Freed MM, Shah NK, Schlesinger RM. Autonomic hyperreflexia during cystoscopy in patients with high spinal cord injuries. Spinal Cord. 1978;15(4):327–32.
191. Karlsson AK. Autonomic dysreflexia. Spinal Cord. 1999;37(6):383–91.
192. Lindan R, Joiner E, Freehafer AA, Hazel C. Incidence and clinical features of autonomic dysreflexia in patients with spinal cord injury. Paraplegia. 1980;18(5):285–92.
193. Wan D, Krassioukov AV. Life-threatening outcomes associated with autonomic dysreflexia: a clinical review. J Spinal Cord Med. 2014;37(1):2–10.
194. Spinal cord injury facts and figures at a glance. J Spinal Cord Med. 2012;35(4):197–8.
195. Blackmer J. Rehabilitation medicine: 1. Autonomic dysreflexia. CMAJ. 2003;169(9):931–5.
196. Squair JW, West CR, Krassioukov AV. Neuroprotection, plasticity manipulation, and regenerative strategies to improve cardiovascular function following spinal cord injury. J Neurotrauma. 2015;32(9):609–21.
197. Bycroft J, Shergill IS, Chung EAL, Arya N, Shah PJR. Autonomic dysreflexia: a medical emergency. Postgrad Med J. 2005;81(954):232–5.
198. Ginsberg DA, Boone TB, Cameron AP, Gousse A, Kaufman MR, Keays E, et al. The AUA/SUFU guideline on adult neurogenic lower urinary tract dysfunction: diagnosis and evaluation. J Urol. 2021;206(5):1097–105.
199. Wecht JM. Management of blood pressure disorders in individuals with spinal cord injury. Curr Opin Pharmacol. 2021;62:60–3.
200. Braddom RL, Rocco JF, Autonomic dysreflexia. A survey of current treatment. Am J Phys Med Rehabil. 1991;70(5):234–41.
201. Kirshblum SC, Priebe MM, Ho CH, Scelza WM, Chiodo AE, Wuermser LA. Spinal cord injury medicine. 3. Rehabilitation phase after acute spinal cord injury. Arch Phys Med Rehabil. 2007;88(3 Suppl 1):S62–70.
202. Mukerji S, Aloka F, Farooq MU, Kassab MY, Abela GS. Cardiovascular complications of the Guillain-Barré syndrome. Am J Cardiol. 2009;104(10):1452–5.
203. Koeppen S, Kraywinkel K, Wessendorf TE, Ehrenfeld CE, Schürks M, Diener HC, et al. Long-term outcome of Guillain-Barré syndrome. Neurocrit Care. 2006;5(3):235–42.
204. Zochodne DW. Autonomic involvement in Guillain–Barre syndrome: a review. Muscle Nerve. 1994;17(10):1145–55.
205. Lyu RK, Tang LM, Hsu WC, Chen ST, Chang HS, Wu YR. A longitudinal cardiovascular Autonomic function study in mild Guillain-Barré syndrome. Eur Neurol. 2002;47(2):79–84.
206. Ropper AH, Gress DR, Diringer MN, Green DM, Mayer SA, Bleck TP. Neurological and neurosurgical intensive care. 4th ed. Lippincott Williams & Wilkins (LWW); 2003. 403 pp.
207. Truax BT. Autonomic disturbances in the Guillain-Barré syndrome. Thieme Medical Publishers; 1984. p. 462–8.
208. Barone P, Antonini A, Colosimo C, Marconi R, Morgante L, Avarello TP, et al. The PRIAMO study: a multicenter assessment of nonmotor symptoms and their impact on quality of life in Parkinson's disease. Mov Disord Off J Mov Disord Soc. 2009;24(11):1641–9.
209. Köllensperger M, Geser F, Ndayisaba JP, Boesch S, Seppi K, Ostergaard K, et al. Presentation, diagnosis, and management of multiple system atrophy in Europe: final analysis of the European multiple system atrophy registry. Mov Disord. 2010;25(15):2604–12.
210. Vagaonescu TD, Saadia D, Tuhrim S, Phillips RA, Kaufmann H. Hypertensive cardiovascular damage in patients with primary autonomic failure. Lancet Lond Engl. 2000;355(9205):725–6.
211. Fanciulli A, Strano S, Ndayisaba JP, Goebel G, Gioffrè L, Rizzo M, et al. Detecting nocturnal hypertension in Parkinson's disease and multiple system atrophy: proposal of a decision-support algorithm. J Neurol. 2014 Jul;261(7):1291–9.
212. Fanciulli A, Jordan J, Biaggioni I, Calandra-Buonaura G, Cheshire WP, Cortelli P, et al. Consensus statement on the definition of neurogenic supine hypertension in cardiovascular autonomic failure by the American Autonomic Society (AAS) and the European Federation of Autonomic Societies (EFAS): Endorsed by the European Academy of Neurology (EAN) and the European Society of Hypertension (ESH). Clin Auton Res Off J Clin Auton Res Soc. 2018 Aug;28(4):355–62.
213. Plaschke M, Trenkwalder P, Dahlheim H, Lechner C, Trenkwalder C. Twenty-four-hour blood pressure profile and blood pressure responses to head-up tilt tests in Parkinson's disease and multiple system atrophy. J Hypertens. 1998 Oct;16(10):1433–41.
214. Jordan J, Shannon JR, Pohar B, Paranjape SY, Robertson D, Robertson RM, et al. Contrasting effects of vasodilators on blood pressure and sodium balance in the hypertension of autonomic failure. J Am Soc Nephrol JASN. 1999 Jan;10(1):35–42.
215. Low PA, Reich SG, Jankovic J, Shults CW, Stern MB, Novak P, et al. Natural history of multiple system atrophy in the USA: a prospective cohort study. Lancet Neurol. 2015 Jul;14(7):710–9.
216. Robottom BJ, Weiner WJ, Factor SA. Movement disorders emergencies. Part 1: Hypokinetic disorders. Arch Neurol. 2011 May;68(5):567–72.
217. Jordan J, Biaggioni I. Diagnosis and treatment of supine hypertension in autonomic failure patients with orthostatic hypotension. J Clin Hypertens Greenwich Conn. 2002 Apr;4(2):139–45.
218. Mazza A, Armigliato M, Marzola MC, Schiavon L, Montemurro D, Vescovo G, et al. Anti-hypertensive treatment in pheochromocytoma and paraganglioma: current management and therapeutic features. Endocrine. 2014;45(3):469–78.
219. Stein PP, Black HR. A simplified diagnostic approach to pheochromocytoma. A review of the literature and report of one institution's experience. Medicine (Baltimore). 1991 Jan;70(1):46–66.
220. Pacak K, Linehan WM, Eisenhofer G, Walther MM, Goldstein DS. Recent advances in genetics, diagnosis, localization, and treatment of pheochromocytoma. Ann Intern Med. 2001;134(4):315–29.
221. Sutton MG, Sheps SG, Lie JT. Prevalence of clinically unsuspected pheochromocytoma. Review of a 50-year autopsy series. Mayo Clin Proc. 1981 Jun;56(6):354–60.
222. Guerrero MA, Schreinemakers JMJ, Vriens MR, Suh I, Hwang J, Shen WT, et al. Clinical spectrum of pheochromocytoma. J Am Coll Surg. 2009 Dec;209(6):727–32.
223. Bravo EL. Pheochromocytoma: new concepts and future trends. Kidney Int. 1991 Sep;40(3):544–56.
224. Sawka AM, Jaeschke R, Singh RJ, Young WF. A comparison of biochemical tests for pheochromocytoma: measurement of fractionated plasma metanephrines compared with the combination of 24-hour urinary metanephrines and catecholamines. J Clin Endocrinol Metab. 2003 Feb;88(2):553–8.
225. Lenders JWM, Pacak K, Walther MM, Linehan WM, Mannelli M, Friberg P, etal. Biochemical diagnosis of PheochromocytomaWhich test is best? JAMA. 2002;287(11):1427–34.
226. Lenders JWM, Duh QY, Eisenhofer G, Gimenez-Roqueplo AP, Grebe SKG, Murad MH, et al. Pheochromocytoma and paraganglioma: an endocrine society clinical practice guideline. J Clin Endocrinol Metab. 2014 Jun;99(6):1915–42.
227. Pappachan JM, Raskauskiene D, Sriraman R, Edavalath M, Hanna FW. Diagnosis and management of pheochromocytoma: a practical guide to clinicians. Curr Hypertens Rep. 2014 Jul;16(7):442.

Chest Pain and Arrhythmias in the Neurointensive Care Unit

12

Jorge Penalver, Neal Olarte, Chaitra Mohan, and Litsa Lambrakos

Contents

Abstract

There are common cardiac presentations of neurologic disease including chest pain and arrhythmias that are seen in the neurointensive care unit. Cardiac causes of chest pain include myocardial infarction, hypertensive emergency/urgency, and aortic dissection. Cardiac chest pain is frequently provoked by neurologic injury, a consequence of the brain–heart interaction. Acute neurologic chest pain in the neurointensive care unit can also have a noncardiac origin. There are ECG changes that are frequently seen with neurologic emergencies, including repolarization abnormalities and dysrhythmias, such as bradyarrhythmias and tachyarrhythmias.

J. Penalver · N. Olarte · C. Mohan
Cardiology, University of Miami/Jackson Memorial Hospital, Miami, FL, USA
e-mail: Jorge.penalver@jhsmiami.org; neal.olarte@jhsmiami.org; Chaitra.Mohan@jhsmiami.org

L. Lambrakos (✉)
Cardiology/Clinical Cardiac Electrophysiology, University of Miami Miller School of Medicine, Miami, FL, USA
e-mail: llambrakos@med.miami.edu

Introduction

In the neurointensive care unit, understanding and troubleshooting the causes of acute chest pain and arrhythmias can be challenging as underlying causes are frequently complex and multifactorial. Cardiovascular complications can be serious, frequently require intervention, and impact the neuro-

E. Mahanna Gabrielli et al. (eds.), *Textbook of Neurointensive Care: Volume 1*, https://doi.org/10.1007/978-3-031-62220-5_12

logical outcome and prognosis of the patient. There may be primary cardiac causes of chest pain that will need cardiac workup; alternatively, there may be cardiac sequela of primary neurological insults. Additionally, there are noncardiac causes of chest pain. Cardiac arrhythmias are commonly seen in the critically ill. These may occur de novo or may be secondary to a primary cardiac etiology. They may also occur because of medical intervention. These include tachyarrhythmias such as supraventricular and ventricular tachycardias, as well as bradyarrhythmias. The goal of this chapter will be to examine important chest pain and arrhythmia presentations in the neurointensive care unit that impact the comprehensive treatment of these critically ill patients.

Key Clinical Questions

- What is the differential for cardiac and noncardiac causes of chest pain?
- What is the pathophysiology of the Stroke-Heart-Syndrome and clinical phenotypes associated with this?
- What are some of the findings that may indicate neurogenic stunned myocardium/neurogenic stress cardiomyopathy over an acute coronary syndrome?
- How does injury to the insular cortex affect cardiac function and rhythm?
- When should temporary pacing be considered in bradyarrhythmias?
- What are the diagnostic and treatment algorithms for supraventricular tachycardias and wide complex tachycardias?
- How is atrial fibrillation in the setting of stroke managed? What is AFDAS?

Cardiac Causes of Chest Pain

Chest pain is one of the most common causes of medical consultation in the general population. After traumatic injuries, chest pain is the second most common reason for adults to present to the emergency department (ED) in the United States and accounts for >6.5 million visits, which is 4.7% of all ED visits [1]. Although the cause of chest pain is often noncardiac, coronary artery disease (CAD) affects >18.2 million adults in the United States and remains the first cause of death for men and women [2]. Hence, distinguishing between life-threatening conditions from more benign causes of chest pain is crucial. The most common etiologies of noncardiac chest pain are respiratory, gastrointestinal, musculoskeletal, and psychogenic disorders [3]. Neurologic conditions can also be implicated in the development of chest pain.

Chest pain has been traditionally classified as "typical," "atypical," and noncardiac types [4]. Chest pain that is more likely associated with coronary ischemia (typical) consists of (1) substernal chest discomfort, (2) provoked by physical or emotional stress, and (3) relieved by rest or nitroglycerin. The atypical chest pain term has been used to indicate angina without typical chest symptoms (classically meeting two of the aforementioned criteria). Noncardiac chest pain meets one or none of the criteria. The new 2021 consensus guidelines for chest pain [4] recommend the use of "cardiac" (3/3 criteria), "possible cardiac" (2/3 criteria), and "noncardiac" (1 or 0/3 criteria) to describe the suspected cause of chest pain.

Cardiovascular causes of Chest pain	
Stable atherosclerosis	Chronic stable atherosclerotic heart disease (stable angina)
Acute coronary syndrome (ACS)	1-unstable angina, 2-nonST elevation ACS or traditionally nonST elevation myocardial infarction or NSTEMI, 3-ST-elevation myocardial infarction or STEMI
Coronary spasm	Prinzmetal angina
Structural heart disease	Valvular disease. Regurgitant or stenotic valvular lesions
Inflammatory	Pericarditis Myocarditis

Reference: Adapted from Zipes DP, Libby P, Bonow RO, Mann DL, Tomaselli GF, Braunwald E. Braunwald's heart disease: a textbook of cardiovascular medicine. 11th ed. Philadelphia, PA: Elsevier; 2019

Noncardiac causes of chest pain	
Neurologic	Migraines, central poststroke pain, epilepsy, herpes zoster/post-herpetic neuralgia, spinal cord disorders, Guillain–Barré syndrome, complex regional pain syndrome, multiple sclerosis, among others.
Gastrointestinal	Gastroesophageal reflux disease Peptic ulcer disease Gastritis Esophagitis Esophageal motility disorders
Pulmonary	Pleural effusion Pneumothorax Pneumonia Malignancy
Vascular	Aortic dissection Pulmonary embolism
Musculoskeletal	Costochondritis Trauma Rib fractures Muscle strain
Psychogenic	Panic attacks Major depressive disorder Post-traumatic stress disorder Generalized anxiety disorder

Reference: Adapted from Smith, Lane M., and Simon A. Mahler. "Chest pain." *Tintinalli's emergency medicine: a comprehensive study guide. 9th ed. McGraw-Hill* (2020)

There are multiple causes of chest pain caused by diseases of the neurological system, both acute and chronic—migraines, central poststroke pain, epilepsy, herpes zoster/

postherpetic neuralgia, spinal cord disorders, Guillain–Barré syndrome, complex regional pain syndrome, multiple sclerosis, among others. The pathophysiology of chest pain in these conditions remains poorly understood and involves multiple mechanisms. Peripheral nerve or root trauma or inflammation, peripheral and central sensitization, alterations of thalamic activity, excitability of the ganglionic or spinal cord neurons have been some of the proposed processes [5]. These causes must be distinguished from cardiovascular chest pain.

Myocardial Infarction in Neurologic Patients

Acute neurological conditions can trigger acute cardiac pathology and, more commonly, cardiac pathology such as acute myocardial infarction (MI) can cause neurological complications such as acute ischemic strokes. Neurologic events can cause cardiac abnormalities ranging from arrhythmias, ventricular dysfunction, myocardial infarction, and sudden cardiac death. In one study, approximately 13% of patients had an associated acute myocardial infarction within 3 days of a cerebrovascular accident [6]. During the first month after a stroke, cardiac events are the most common non-neurologic cause of mortality [7]. Within 5 years after a stroke, there is still a 2% annual risk of myocardial infarction [8]. The ischemic stroke and acute MI association has been noted for decades and it is associated with poor outcomes. The risk of ischemic stroke in patients presenting with MI has declined (to 1–2%) since thrombolytic or anticoagulant therapy has been implemented [9]. Ischemic strokes in the setting of MI are multifactorial, including processes such as systemic inflammation, vulnerable cerebrovascular and cardiovascular atherosclerotic plaque, and cardioembolic phenomena [10, 11].

Myocardial infarction is defined as the presence of myocardial necrosis recognized by elevation of cardiac biomarkers in the blood (above the assay-specific 99th percentile upper reference limit) and can be accompanied by ECG changes suggestive of ischemia [12]. There are multiple pathophysiological processes that can lead to myocardial ischemia and infarction, but two of the most important ones are (1) ischemia from atherosclerotic plaque rupture (Type 1 MI) and (2) oxygen supply-demand mismatch from various conditions or Type 2 MI (anemia, hypertension, hypotension, arrhythmias, coronary artery spasm, coronary artery embolism, among others). Hypertensive crisis and tachyarrhythmia are important causes of type 2 myocardial infarction that have to be considered and treated [13]. The incidence of AMI after a stroke is about 1.7%/year [14]. An acute myocardial infarction from coronary atherosclerotic plaque rupture, thrombus formation, and limited myocardial blood flow will present with various combinations of chest, upper extremity, mandibular, or epigastric discomfort during exertion or at rest, or an ischemic equivalent such as dyspnea or fatigue. Frequently, the discomfort is diffuse [12]. Diagnosis of AMI in the context of an acute stroke is made with the clinical presentation, ischemic ECG changes (T wave inversions, ST segment depressions or elevations), a rising and falling pattern of troponin levels, new ischemic regional wall-motion abnormalities on cardiac imaging, and/or an acute coronary thrombus on coronary angiography [12].

In cases of nonischemic acute myocardial injury after a stroke, cardiac troponin elevation occurs in the absence of typical coronary symptoms (such as chest pain, dyspnea), ST-segment elevations, or wall motion abnormalities on echocardiogram [15]. It is important to distinguish acute from chronic myocardial injury by applying serial measurements of troponin levels [16]. Acute myocardial injury manifests with a rising and/or falling pattern of troponin levels, whereas in chronic myocardial injury due to clinically stable structural heart disease there is no such pattern. This distinction matter because acute myocardial injury is related to worse outcomes [17].

Distinguishing myocardial injury caused by a neurologic event from an ACS is challenging. Patients with acute neurologic illness frequently manifest ECG changes suggestive of cardiac injury. The classic ECG changes of deep T-wave inversion were described in patients with subarachnoid hemorrhage, thromboembolic strokes, intracranial masses, and meningitis [18]. Cardiac troponin is a biomarker that has been used to confirm the presence of myocardial injury in complex clinical situations. Myocardial damage and elevation of cardiac troponin have been observed in patients with acute neurological insults such as intracranial hemorrhages, trauma, ischemic strokes, seizures [19, 20]. In acute neurological pathology, the concomitant cardiac injury might be an important predictor of poor outcomes [18]. The mechanism for myocardial injury in this setting is unclear but autonomic dysfunction, catecholamine surge, and hemodynamic changes have been proposed. The elevated troponin levels in patients with seizures may be related to increased oxygen requirements, diffuse cerebral stimulation, edema, respiratory and metabolic acidosis. A relevant form of neurogenic myocardial injury is the neurogenic stunned myocardium (NSM) or neurogenic stress cardiomyopathy (NSC). This is a cardiac insult that occurs after a neurologic event (i.e., ischemic stroke, subarachnoid hemorrhage, or seizures) due to dysregulation of the autonomic nervous system and catecholamine surge [21]. The clinical manifestations of the NSM can be diverse but it often resembles an ACS, presenting with chest pain, ischemic ECG changes, elevated cardiac biomarkers, impaired ventricular function [22]. Patient with NSM do not necessarily have obstructive atherosclerosis or spams of the coronary arteries to manifest myocardial necrosis, left ventricular wall motion abnormalities or ECG changes [23, 24]. The absence of preexistent heart disease, left ventricular dysfunction without ischemic ECG changes, ventricular wall motion abnormalities that do not follow a coronary distribution, cardiac troponin <2.8 ng/mL in the presence of LVEF <40% are some of the suggested findings that indicate NSM/NSC over ACS [25]. However, patients with acute ischemic stroke often have concomitant coronary atherosclerosis and differentiating ACS from a pure neuromediated cardiac insult remains difficult.

It is recommended that patients with acute ischemic stroke or TIA undergo cardiovascular risk assessment and aggressive risk factor modification [26]. The American Heart Association/American Stroke Association also recommends that patients with elevated cardiovascular risks (Framingham 10-year risk of ≥20%) should be considered for noninvasive coronary artery disease testing. Patients with fewer cardiovascular risk factors who do not have significant carotid artery disease or who present with stroke subtypes not clearly related to atherosclerosis are at lower risk for coronary events, and routine coronary testing is not recommended. The decision to treat acute ischemic heart disease medically or invasively in the setting of neurological disease will depend on the patient's clinical profile. However, a strong clinical suspicion of plaque rupture or ACS may still warrant coronary angiography [23]. The diagnostic and therapeutic workflow is complex when caring for cardiac pathology after a stroke and it is recommended to obtain an early cardiology consultation.

In patients with a recent stroke, there are no clear guidelines regarding the safety of percutaneous coronary intervention (PCI) or coronary artery bypass graft surgery (CABG). Timing of coronary revascularization (PCI or CABG) after a recent stroke is controversial. The risk of recurrent ischemic stroke or the occurrence of hemorrhagic conversion (potentiated by using intraprocedural anticoagulation) during PCI or CABG are important factors to consider. It has been described that prior ischemic stroke increases the risk of post-PCI CVA by over twofold [27]. There is also a 50% increase in the risk of intracranial hemorrhage post-PCI with previous history of ischemic stroke and >fourfold increase with previous history of hemorrhagic stroke [28]. Cardiac catheterization has been typically delayed 6 weeks after an acute ischemic stroke, but there is no good evidence that dictates this practice. Extrapolation has been made from the anticoagulation guidelines for arrhythmias in the setting of stroke guidelines from the American Heart Association/American Stroke Association that state that it is reasonable to start anticoagulation 4–14 days after an acute ischemic stroke in the setting of atrial fibrillation [29]. It has been proposed that the larger the infarct size, the higher the risk of hemorrhagic conversion when anticoagulation is introduced, and it seems safer to wait longer in patient with larger infarcts [30]. Similarly, patients with a history of a recent stroke are at higher risk of recurrent stroke after noncardiac and cardiac surgery. This is relevant as some critically ill neuro patients must undergo urgent surgeries for management of acute comorbidities or complications. Guidelines suggest that elective cardiac surgery should be delayed if a patient has experienced a stroke within 6–9 months of the planned procedure. [31]

Hypertensive Emergencies in the Neurological Patient

According to the International Society of Hypertension, the definition of hypertension is a blood pressure of ≥140/90 mmHg following repeated examination [32]. However, the latest report of the ACC/AHA Task Force now defines hypertension as a BP higher 130/80 mmHg and by considering normal BP as values lower than 120/80 mmHg [33]. Hypertension-mediated organ damage is defined as the alteration of the arterial vasculature and/or the organs it supplies that is caused by elevated blood pressure. Hypertension is the main risk factor for cardiac and cerebrovascular diseases and is associated with adverse clinical outcomes. Epidemiological data show that less than 20% of patients with arterial hypertension achieve adequate blood pressure control [34]. Control of chronic hypertension and avoidance, recognition, and early treatment of acute hypertensive states are very important strategies to prevent and treat neurological pathology.

Hypertensive crises are divided in hypertensive emergencies and urgencies. Hypertensive emergencies are characterized by severe elevations in BP (>180/120 mmHg) complicated by evidence of impending or progressive target organ damage. Examples include hypertensive encephalopathy, intracerebral hemorrhage, acute myocardial infarction, acute left ventricular failure with pulmonary edema, unstable angina pectoris, dissecting aortic aneurysm, or eclampsia. Hypertensive urgencies have severe elevations in BP without progressive target organ dysfunction [35]. Symptoms of hypertensive crises include chest pain, nausea and vomiting, headache, epistaxis, blurred vision, anxiety, dyspnea, heart failure, seizures, confusion and altered mentation [36].

Patients with a hypertensive emergency should be admitted to an intensive care unit for continuous monitoring of BP and parenteral administration of therapies. The initial goal of therapy in hypertensive emergencies is to reduce mean arterial BP by no more than 25% (within minutes to 1 h), then, if stable, to 160/100 to 110 mmHg within the next 2–6 h [37]. Excessive falls in pressure, which may precipitate renal, cerebral, or coronary ischemia, should be avoided. However, patients with an ischemic stroke are exceptions to this recommendation since there is no clear evidence supporting the use of immediate antihypertensive treatment.

Prevention of acute BP elevations helps prevent acute neurological conditions. Similarly, acute ischemic and hemorrhagic strokes can trigger acute hypertension and adequate BP management in the neurological ICU is associated with clinical outcomes. In ischemic strokes, international guidelines recommend that the BP should be lowered and maintained at lower than 180/105 mmHg for at least the first 24 h after thrombolysis [38]. However, the benefit of brisk BP reduction in patients with acute ischemic stroke who do not receive IV thrombolysis is less clear. Drastic drop in BP in ischemic stroke is associated to poor prognosis in terms of neurological deterioration, infarct volume, neurological outcome, and mortality [39]. Rapid and aggressive lowering of BP is usually not recommended due to the detrimental effects on cerebral perfusion in the ischemic penumbral areas [40]. In patients with intracranial hemorrhage, an acute hypertensive response is observed in up to 75% of patients [41]. In intracranial hemorrhage (ICH), a BP target <180 mmHg SBP is practiced with optimal targets lower than 160/90 mmHg because effective and early reductions in BP may reduce the risk of neurological deterioration and hematoma growth [42]. In patients with ICH, several trials have demonstrated either a small benefit or no benefit with intensive SBP reduction (Below 120 mmHg SBP) compared with modest (<160 mmHg SBP) or standard BP reduction [43–45]. The current recommendation for ICH is targeting a SBP <140 mmHg.

The current AHA/ASA guidelines for BP management in acute ischemic stroke recommend [38]

Clinical situation	Recommendation	Class of recommendation and level of evidence
tPA candidate	Should have their SBP <185 mmHg and DBP <110 mmHg before thrombolytic therapy is initiated	Class IB
Not a tPA candidate	Lower BP by 15% during the first 24 h after onset of stroke. The exact level of BP is not known, but medical therapy is recommended if the BP is >220/120 mmHg	Class IC
Mechanical thrombectomy candidate	It is reasonable to maintain BP ≤185/110 mmHg before the procedure	Class IIa
Poststroke	Restarting antihypertensive medications after the first 24 h in patients who have preexisting hypertension and are neurologically stable, unless a specific contraindication to restarting treatment is known	

In patients otherwise eligible for emergency reperfusion therapy but the BP is >185/110 mmHg, treatment options are intravenous beta blockers, calcium channel blockers, hydralazine, among others. If BP is not ≤185/110 mmHg then alteplase should not be given. During or after alteplase administration, the BP should be monitored every 15 min for 2 h, then every 30 min for 6 h, and then every hour for 16 h. If the BP is 180–230/105–120 mmHg, IV sodium nitroprusside can be considered [38].

In patients that present with hypertensive crises that need to undergo mechanical thrombectomy for ischemic stroke, there is less data that guides BP management. Mechanical thrombectomy is the standard of care for patients who present with an acute ischemic stroke within 6 h of symptom onset and up to 24 h in some cases. The optimal BP management is unclear given the impaired autoregulatory mechanisms of the re-perfused tissue and the risk of intraprocedural hypotension. Permissive HTN in these patients (between 180–220/105–120 mmHg) may be harmful after successful thrombectomy. BP control <160/90 mmHg has been associated with improved mortality after thrombectomy [46].

Aortic Dissection

Aortic dissection is the most common life-threatening disorder affecting the aorta [47]. Aortic dissection is precipitated by a tear in the aortic intima through which blood surges into the aortic media, separating the intima from the adventitia [48]. In the Stanford classification system, dissections occurring in the ascending aorta are classified as type A dissections and dissections occurring in the descending aorta are classified as type B dissections. Several risk factors are associated with aortic dissections, such as hypertension, genetic disorders affecting the blood vessel wall, atherosclerosis, cocaine use, and trauma [49].

The immediate mortality rate in aortic dissection is as high as 1% per hour over the first several hours; thus, early diagnosis and intervention is critical. Most patients with acute dissection present with sudden, severe chest, back or abdominal pain [50]. However, the symptoms of aortic dissection may be highly variable, and one must have a high index of suspicion for the disease. Transient or permanent neurologic symptoms at onset of aortic dissection are frequent, reported to occur in 17–40% of patients [51]. These symptoms may mask the underlying disease. Neurological symptoms occur because of occlusion of arteries—carotid, vertebral, spinal and vasa nervorum of peripheral nerves—and because of hypotension with a consequent cerebral perfusion defect [52].

The majority of patients (86.1%) present with initial chest or back pain [52]. Pain in the head or neck may also be a complaint. Chest pain, although the most common presentation, is not an obligatory symptom of aortic dissection, with 5–15% of patients with aortic dissection presenting without pain. However, about one-third of patients may not complain of significant pain but have other neurologic clinical manifestations such as persistent or transient ischemic stroke, spinal cord ischemia, ischemic neuropathy, hypoxic encephalopathy, syncope, seizures, and transient global amnesia [50, 51]. Neurologic symptoms associated with aortic disease are often dramatic and in critically ill patients, frequently underestimated. Symptoms frequently appear at or shortly after the onset of dissection and may be transient. Aortic dissection should be suspected in patients presenting with an unusual combinations of neurologic symptoms such as involvement of central and peripheral nervous system or simultaneous occurrence of syncope, seizure, and cerebral, spinal, or peripheral nerve ischemia [52]. It is unclear that the presence of neurologic symptoms is an independent predictor of worsened outcomes as there has been conflicting evidence from different investigations [51, 53, 54].

In the setting of chest pain, an ECG is obtained in the initial evaluation. Aortic dissection that does not involve coronary ostia can usually be distinguished from acute coronary syndrome by the nature of the chest pain and the absence of ECG changes characteristic of ischemia. However, involvement of a coronary artery in an aortic dissection may not manifest changes in the electrocardiogram. ECG findings are usually nonspecific. In the International Registry of Acute Aortic Dissection (IRAD) series, the ECG showed nonspecific ST and T-wave changes in 42% (commonly, left ventricular hypertrophy and strain patterns associated with hypertension), ischemic changes in 15%, and evidence of an acute myocardial infarction in 5% of type A AAD (see Fig. 12.1). It is not surprising that an abnormal ECG can lead to a delay in diagnosis because clinicians often pursue coronary disease as a primary diagnosis since it is so much more prevalent [55]. In one retrospective study, cases with ST depression or T-wave changes had a higher incidence of shock and cardiac tamponade compared with those without changes [56].

The chest X-ray may show an enlarged aorta and widened mediastinum. However, both the ECG and chest X-ray may be completely normal in aortic dissection and cannot diagnose or exclude aortic dissection [49].

When neurological symptoms are present, they can confound the diagnosis. Depending on the extent of aortic dissection extension, it may cause various organ impairments and clinical symptoms; about 6% of aortic dissection patients have concomitant ischemic stroke or transient ischemic attack (TIA) due to extension to the cervicocerebral arteries or emboli from the site of dissection. Major brain injury at the onset of dissection can be a complication in approximately 10% of type A acute aortic dissections. This includes coma or stroke, typically implicates arch vessel involvement, and generally portends an increased mortality [55].

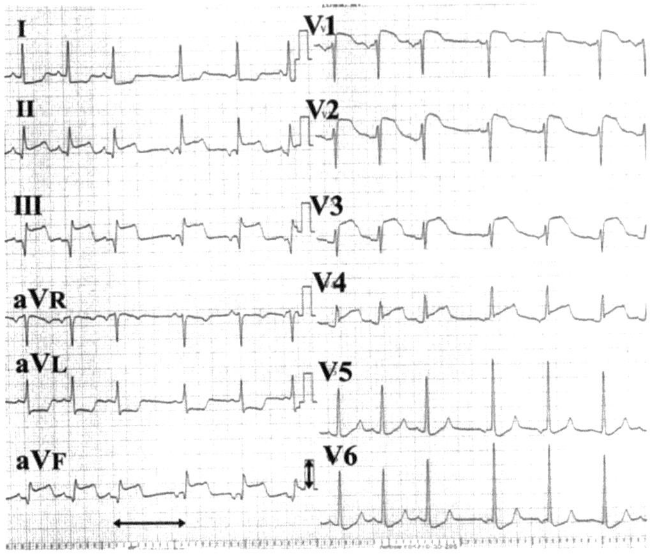

Fig. 12.1 ECG in a patient with Type A Aortic Dissection and Cardiac Tamponade. From Hirata et al. Electrocardiographic changes in patients with type A acute aortic dissection: Incidence, patterns and underlying mechanisms in 159 cases. J Cardiol. 2010

In the setting of stroke, approximately 1.7% of patients have an acute Type A dissection. Patients presenting with ischemic stroke may not make the typical complaints of back and chest pain because of cortical symptoms such as amnesia, aphasia, or conscious disturbance secondary to the stroke. Since the advent of rt-PA and the use of thrombolytics in acute ischemic stroke, there have been reports in the literature that caution against the potential presence of acute aortic dissection as the cause of ischemic stroke since this can lead to inappropriate thrombolytic therapy (frequently fatal) and a delay in appropriate surgical treatment [57]. When assessing suspected stroke patients, one must keep in mind the possibility of aortic dissection albeit relatively uncommon.

In the patient assessment, it is important to evaluate for cardiac symptoms, upper limb blood pressures, and changes in consciousness that could affect reporting of symptomatology. If an acute Type A aortic dissection in the setting of ischemic stroke is suspected, a CXR and contrast chest CT in addition to a head CT or MRI should be performed. Carotid ultrasonography or contrast CT can be helpful to detect extension of the aortic dissection to the common carotid artery (commonly, the right side) or blood flow obstruction due to obstruction of blood flow to the cervicocerebral arteries by the aortic dissection [57]. If diagnosed, surgical treatment should be initiated as soon as possible. The complication of ischemic stroke has been considered a predictor of a poor prognosis; however, with early diagnosis and appropriate surgical treatment, concomitant neurological symptoms have been reported to be associated with no increase in mortality [53, 55].

Initial management of aortic dissection needs high clinical suspicion and imaging, which can include transesophageal echocardiography or contrast CT of the chest. When a patient is diagnosed with an aortic dissection, the goals are to control the tear, determine whether repairing the tear would benefit the patient, and treat any complications. To control the tear, blood pressure is reduced as much as possible. Surgery is considered, and any complications are treated [49]. Urgent surgical resection of the ascending aorta is standard management of type A dissection, whereas management of a type B dissection includes medical therapy with strict control of blood pressure and possible intervention for complicated patients in whom aortic rupture is suspected or shown. However, some physicians favor stent-graft placement to cover the aortic dissection [58].

In-hospital mortality rates for aortic dissection are very high and are reported between 9% and 36% but as high as 60%–70% in some studies [51]. In the International Registry of Aortic Dissection (IRAD), independent preoperative predictors of mortality were age >70 years, previous cardiac surgery, hypotension or shock at presentation, migrating pain, cardiac tamponade, any pulse deficit, and an ECG showing findings of myocardial ischemia or infarction [47].

Cardiac Chest Pain as a Result of Neurologic Injury: The Brain–Heart Interaction

The interaction between the heart and the brain is complex. There is a central autonomic network (CAN) that consists of interconnected areas throughout the neuroaxis and the brain, which regulates the sympathetic and parasympathetic outflow to the heart, including the cardiac conduction system and the myocardium. In the setting of an acute neurologic event, there is a physiological interplay between the neurological and cardiovascular systems, such that a patient who presents with a cerebrovascular insult is also at risk for a cardiac event. There are also converging risk factors for cardiovascular and cerebrovascular disease including hypertension, diabetes mellitus, and hyperlipidemia [59]. This presents challenges in triaging, diagnosing, and treating cardiac sequela of neurologic disease.

Acute cerebral insults and stroke (ischemic stroke, brain hemorrhage, and subarachnoid hemorrhage) may induce cardiac changes in patients even without coronary disease [60, 61]. The insular cortex plays a critical role in the autonomic control of cardiovascular function, and strokes in this area are associated with adverse cardiac outcomes including repolarization abnormalities, arrhythmias, neurogenic cardiac damage, heart failure, and sudden death [62–65]. In stroke, specifically, the downstream cardiac effects of cerebral injury is called "stroke-induced heart injury" or SIHI, which describes the series of pathophysiological processes that in turn lead to the "Stroke-heart syndrome" (SHS), the resultant cardiovascular effects of the injury [66]. Cardiac events seen in in this syndrome include: (1) poststroke acute myocardial infarction, (2) ischemic and nonischemic acute myocardial injury presenting with elevated cardiac troponin, (3) left ventricular dysfunction, takotsubo (stress-induced) syndrome, (4) poststroke arrhythmias, commonly atrial fibrillation, and (5) poststroke neurogenic sudden cardiac death [66]. A history of heart failure, high baseline serum creatinine, stroke severity, and prolonged corrected QT interval (QTc) or ventricular extrasystole has been shown in studies to be independent risk factors for serious cardiac events [67]. As such, it is important to determine whether the cardiac dysfunction seen is triggered by a neurological insult, the underlying cause, or an unrelated complication.

The pathogenesis of myocyte damage in acute neuronal injury is thought to be neurally mediated through abnormal autonomic activity or sympathetic overactivity and abnormally enhanced systemic inflammation [66]. For example, activation of the hypothalamic–pituitary–adrenal axis after ischemic stroke causes a surge in circulating catecholamines and massive catecholamine release from myocardial nerve endings [68]. The myocardium adjacent to the nerve is damaged. One mechanism of cardiac injury results from small foci of subendocardial hemorrhage or swollen myocytes surrounding epicardial nerves. This phenomenon called myocytolysis is different than the coagulation necrosis seen in myocardial ischemia—it is acute cardiac muscle fiber stress and is often not associated with ECG abnormalities [60]. Catecholamine surge can also cause cardiac hypertrophy or myocardial ischemia [59]. Catecholamines act on the beta receptors of the heart, which leads to an increase in cytosolic cyclic AMP (cAMP) and ultimately mitochondrial calcium overload, triggering oxidative stress and myocyte cell death (see Fig. 12.2). Catecholamine-mediated myocardial injury is believed to be multifactorial—tachycardia, coronary spasm and vasoconstriction, toxic effects on cardiac myocytes, and an increased intracellular concentration of calcium [25].

Elevations in cardiac enzyme levels such as cardiac troponins and NT-proBNP are frequently seen after an acute neurologic event and have both ischemic and nonischemic triggers. There is a spectrum of presentation from asymptomatic troponin elevation to Type I acute coronary syndromes. Serum troponin I (cTnI) or troponin T (cTnT) levels after neurologic injury are indicators of cardiac damage. Elevation of serum myocardial enzymes is reported in 11%–21% of SAH patients and in 1%–17% of ischemic stroke patients and elevated cardiac enzymes may predict new onset atrial fibrillation in ischemic stroke patients [69]. Relatively silent cardiac injury occurs in up to 6% of all

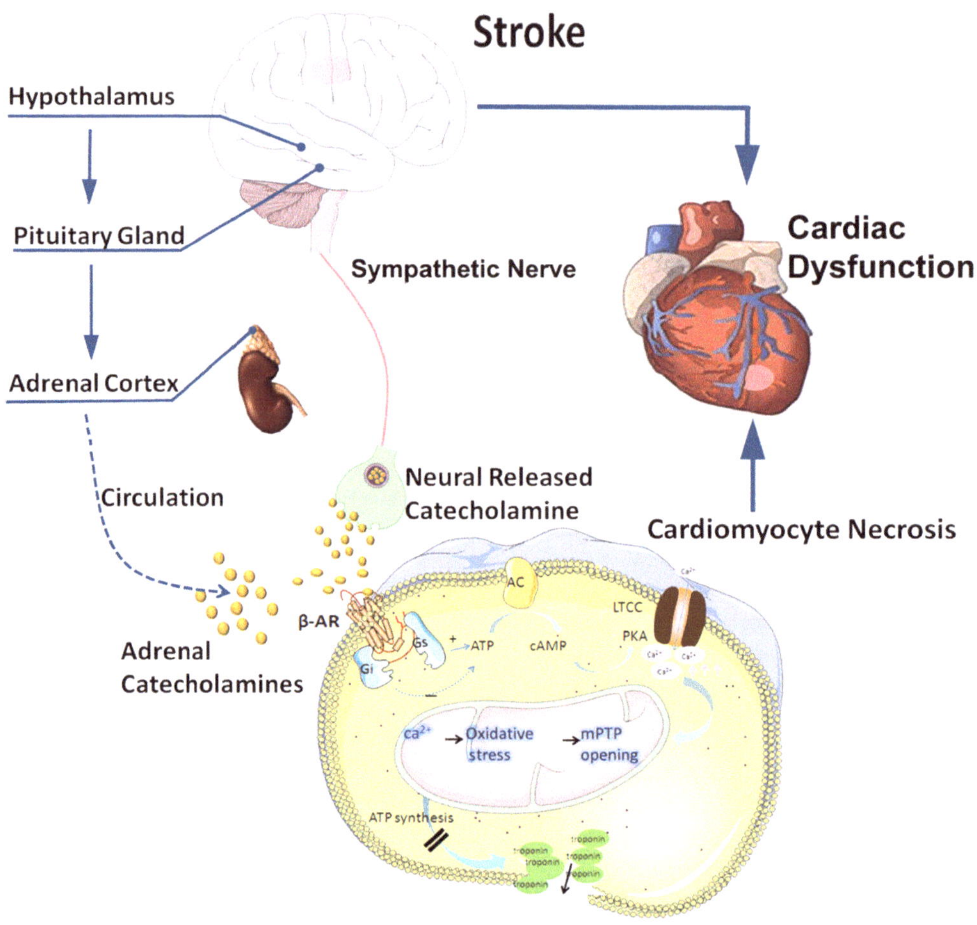

Fig. 12.2 Myocyte damage in acute neuronal injury. The hypothalamic–pituitary–adrenal (HPA) axis, catecholamine surge, and sympathetic and parasympathetic regulation mediate cardiac dysfunction after stroke. Catecholamines act on β receptors, β receptors increase cytosolic cAMP. cAMP leads to downstream mitochondrial Ca2+ overload. Mitochondrial Ca2+ overload triggers oxidative stress and the subsequent opening of their inner membrane permeability transition pore with ensuing osmotic swelling, and loss of ATP synthesis leads to myocardial cell death. From Chen et al. Brain–Heart Interaction: Cardiac Complications After Stroke. Circ Res. 2017

stroke patients [60]. In subarachnoid hemorrhage, elevated cardiac troponin I levels are associated with an increased risk of left ventricular diastolic dysfunction and in-hospital morbidity and mortality. In ischemic stroke, cTnI is an independent predictor of stroke prognosis. Levels of cardiac markers are associated with poorer long-term outcomes in SAH patients and increased stroke severity, mortality, and worse functional outcome in ischemic stroke. The location of the stroke influences the degree of myocardial damage—lesions within the right anterior insular cortex, which plays an important role within the central autonomic network, are associated with high rates of post-stroke acute myocardial injury [65].

Differentiating myocardial infarction from reversible neurogenic cardiac injury is critical for early intervention of the neurological insult and initiation of appropriate therapies [25]. In SAH, patient can have ECG ventricular repolarization disturbances such as ST segment elevation and T-wave inversion that mimic acute MI [70]. Seventy-five percent of stroke patients have some ECG abnormalities [59]. In hemorrhagic cerebrovascular events, prolonged QT intervals, large, usually inverted T waves and frequent U waves are seen [71]. Overall, ECG changes in ICH or SAH (40–70%) are more common than ischemic stroke (15%–40%).

In one study that looked at cardiac dysfunction in SAH, the following criteria were used to distinguish between acute myocardial infarction and reversibly stunned myocardium with high sensitivity and specificity: (1) no history of cardiac problems, (2) new onset of abnormal cardiac function (EF <40%), (3) cardiac wall motion abnormalities on echocardiogram that did not correlate with the coronary vascular distribution noted on ECGs, and (4) cTnT values less than 2.8 ng/mL in patients with an EF less than 40% [25]. Chest pain may be the best indicator of a true coronary ischemic event and its absence suggests that the cardiac enzyme elevations are from cardiac stress, not coronary occlusion. Coronary angiography can be performed to exclude an acute plaque rupture and obstructive coronary artery disease. The higher the levels of cTn and their rise or fall, the greater the odds that the cause is an AMI [17].

In neurologic injury, there is also a downstream phenomenon of LV dysfunction that can cause heart failure. This has been termed neurogenic stunned myocardium (NSM) or neurogenic stress cardiomyopathy (NSC) and is a cause of reversible left ventricular dysfunction after a serious neurologic insult. It meets all the diagnostic criteria of Takotsubo cardiomyopathy. Whereas a distinction between Takotsubo syndrome (TTS) and NSC was made in the past, this is now felt to be the same clinical entity. It is diagnosed by reduced left ventricular (LV) ejection fraction, ventricular wall motion abnormalities, elevated serum cardiac enzymes, and ECG changes [59]. Importantly, there is an absence of angiographic evidence of obstructive coronary disease or acute plaque rupture. The myocardial dysfunction seen is presumed to be related to the stress of catecholamine excess. In both subarachnoid hemorrhage (SAH) and ischemic stroke, symptoms of neurogenic cardiomyopathy can be seen, which include dyspnea and chest pain, with ECG abnormalities including ST-elevation, T wave inversion, and prolonged QT and left ventricular dysfunction with echocardiographic wall motion abnormalities. Left ventricular diastolic dysfunction can also be seen in patients, which can result in pulmonary edema. The degree of cardiac dysfunction increases with the severity of stroke or hemorrhage. This reversible cardiac dysfunction is more common in SAH and ischemic stroke but has also been described after other acute neurological events including intracerebral hemorrhage, seizures/status epilepticus, migraine, traumatic brain injury, and Guillain–Barré syndrome. [72]

ECG changes seen in acute neuronal injury frequently do not represent ischemic heart disease but are merely a manifestation of autonomic dysregulation, possibly caused by a lesion that affected the cortical representation of the autonomic nervous system [71]. A wide variety of electrocardiographic changes can be seen in acute neuronal injury as previously mentioned [67]. Dysrhythmias and repolarization changes are the two major categories. ECG abnormalities that are commonly seen include deep T wave inversions or peaked T waves with QT prolongation, ST elevations across multiple precordial leads, Q waves, and nonspecific ST-segment and T wave changes [73]. The rapid appearance and disappearance of the ST changes argue against macrovascular factors and in favor of neural factors [74].

The American Stroke Association recommends a baseline ECG and troponin assessment in the initial evaluation of cardiac symptomatology as well as >24-h cardiac rhythm monitoring and an echocardiogram. If a cardiovascular insult is suspected, is important to assess cardiac function with serial troponin levels (to assess trends), serial ECGs, NT-proBNP level, in addition to echocardiography [38]. If the cardiac event is assessed to be myocardial dysfunction and stunning and not a primary ACS, then it would be important to prioritize stabilization of the patient in relation to the neurologic injury over prioritizing the treatment of the cardiac dysfunction such as pursuing a coronary angiography. Secondary complications of neurocardiogenic injury, including vasospasm, delayed cerebral ischemia, and pulmonary edema and other heart failure symptoms should be addressed. Drugs that decrease sympathetic tone such as beta blockers and central sympatholytics may have a role in treatment of neurogenic stress cardiomyopathy/Takotsubo Syndrome. Beta blockers and angiotensin-converting enzyme inhibitors have been suggested, but data are limited to make strong recommendations about their true clinical value [66]. Supportive care of LV dysfunction and heart failure management is indicated. In rare circumstances, in patients with life-threatening acute LV failure, intra-aortic balloon pump and ventricular assist devices may also be necessary. Prolonged and intensive cardiovascular monitoring is recommended in patients manifesting cerebrogenic cardiovascular disturbances and in high-risk patients with insular involvement, right-sided stroke, advancing age, coexisting hypertensive or coronary artery disease, or intense emotional stress. Severely affected patients should be evaluated by a cardiologist before the initiation of appropriate therapy [62]. There are also anesthetic considerations in the care of neurologically critically ill patients with cardiac co-morbidities since anesthesia medications can influence myocardial stunning and impact the autonomic nervous system.

Acute Noncardiac Neurologic Chest Pain

The Guillain–Barré syndrome (GBS) is the most common cause of acute flaccid paralysis and an important cause of admission to intensive care units [75]. It is an acute inflammatory demyelinating polyneuropathy and is characterized by symmetrical progressive ascending weakness with areflexia and variable sensory complaints. The neurologic manifestations of immune mediated disorders such as Guillain–Barré are variable—it affects motor, sensory, and autonomic fibers—frequently causing pain. Truncal pain was the least common pain presentation but occurred in 11% of those with pain preceding weakness and 12% of individuals with pain in the acute phase [5]. This frequently manifests as chest pain. Evaluation of pain should include assessment for cardiac causes with a screening ECG and possible cardiac markers if true cardiac pain is suspected. Cardiovascular abnormalities can be seen in the GBS and are attributed to autonomic neuropathy [75].

Cardiovascular symptoms, including chest pain, may be associated with epileptic seizures. Chest pain has been reported to precede as well as accompany seizure activity. Multiple cases of episodic chest pain resembling angina have been described [76]. Chest pain in this setting has been found to respond well to anti-epileptics. The pathophysiology of chest pain in epilepsy has not been well elucidated; however, the hypothalamus, cingulate cortex, parietal lobe, and insula have all been implicated as contributing to the clinical presentation [5].

Arrhythmias in the Neurointensive Care Unit

Abnormal ECGs Associated with Neurologic Emergencies

The bidirectional relationship between the brain and heart is well established [59, 77, 78]. As previously discussed, the acute neurovascular pathology that leads to catecholamine surge and enhanced sympathetic activity can in turn lead to secondary cardiotoxicity, cardiomyocyte necrosis, and tachyarrhythmias [59, 77, 79]. Simultaneously, there is enhanced parasympathetic activity which can lead to bradyarrhythmias, atrioventricular delay, and dysfunction in cardiac contractility [77]. Tachyarrhythmias, prolonged QTc interval, and left bundle-branch block (LBBB) are seen in strokes of the right insular cortex [59, 77, 78, 80]. Right-sided strokes in general are associated with cardiac arrhythmias [77]. A history of heart failure, hypertension, cardiac disease, and arrhythmia, and the severity of the stroke influences the risk of ECG abnormalities and poststroke cardiac events [59, 77, 81]. Additionally, neuroleptics and antiepileptics commonly used in the ICU may prolong the QTc interval, which may increase the risk of arrhythmia [77]. In this context, ECG abnormalities and arrhythmias following any brain injury, even in the absence of preexisting cardiac disease, [59, 82] are commonly encountered and may affect ICU and in-hospital outcomes [59, 77, 79, 81].

Electrocardiographic changes occur in 60%–90% of ischemic strokes, 7.8%–71% of hemorrhagic strokes, and 40%–100% of subarachnoid hemorrhages (SAH) [59, 77, 82–85]. Among ischemic stroke patients, the most common ECG abnormalities observed are T wave inversion ("cerebral T waves"), ST segment abnormalities (with or without troponin elevation), prolonged QTc interval, and U waves [77, 79, 80]. Among patients with hemorrhagic stroke or SAH, ECG abnormalities are similar, although there is much higher incidence of ST depression and T wave inversion among hemorrhagic stroke patients compared to either ischemic stroke or SAH [82]. The presence of ECG abnormalities may not always be accompanied with echocardiographic abnormalities. Among SAH patients, echocardiographic changes are found predominately in patients with higher clinical severity, while ECG changes are seen at lower grades [59]. Myocardial injury or infarct, systolic or diastolic dysfunction, Takotsubo, or neurogenic stress cardiomyopathy frequently occur independent of any ECG changes [59, 77]. Echocardiographic cardiac dysfunction regardless of ECG abnormalities is independently associated with adverse poststroke outcomes [59].

For any brain injury or stroke subtype, the most common arrhythmias encountered are sinus tachycardia (ST), premature atrial or ventricular contractions (PACs or PVCs), and atrial fibrillation (AF) [77, 80]. Other supraventricular or ventricular arrhythmia may also occur with varying incidence, although malignant arrhythmias are rare [77, 80]. Approximately 25% of patients with acute ischemic stroke will have a new arrhythmia [79]. In the presence of increased intracranial pressure, Cushing's triad of hypertension, bradycardia, and irregular respirations may also be present [86] (Fig. 12.3).

Bradyarrhythmias in the Neuro ICU

Bradycardia is defined as a heart rate less than 60 beats per minute and is commonly observed in the ICU setting. Bradycardia in the critical care setting is typically transient and is often secondary to enhanced vagal tone or other reversible causes. For example, the "Cushing's triad," classified by hypertension, bradycardia, and bradypnea, is often seen secondary to increased intracranial pressure (ICP), such as in subdural hematomas, which can compress or stretch the brainstem. Bradycardia alone without the associated hypertension or bradypnea is usually the first manifestation of increased ICP. Classically, the "Cushing's triad" is generally observed in patients with impending herniation, and thus, the observation of one of the signs of the triad, such as bradycardia, is important in identifying the need for potential expedient surgical intervention [88].

Dysautonomia is a common complication in various neurological conditions, such as Guillain–Barré syndrome and multiple sclerosis, which can lead to bradyarrhythmias. Serious bradyarrhythmias necessitating the administration of atropine or pacemaker placement, including atrioventricular block and asystole, have been reported in up to 34% of patients with Guillain–Barré syndrome, and thus, early recognition of this dysrhythmia is of utmost importance in both prevention and management of the sequela [75, 89]. Aggressive correction of associated factors such as hypoxia, medication side effects, and metabolic abnormalities may help mitigate the bradycardic events. Similarly, bradycardia is commonly seen in patients with spinal cord injuries, specifically, severe cervical cord injury, but less so in thoracolumbar injury. The mechanism of this phenomenon is thought to be secondary to the acute autonomic imbalance caused by the disruption of the sympathetic pathway located in the cervical spinal cord with preservation of the parasympathetic pathway, leading to hypotension and bradycardia [90]. Most bradyarrhythmias do not necessitate temporary pacing; however, temporary transvenous pacing should be considered in critically ill patients when symptoms or hemodynamic compromise are noted. In general, supportive care, including management of the underlying illness, withholding of rate-lowering medications, and support of the blood pressure, is sufficient (Fig. 12.4).

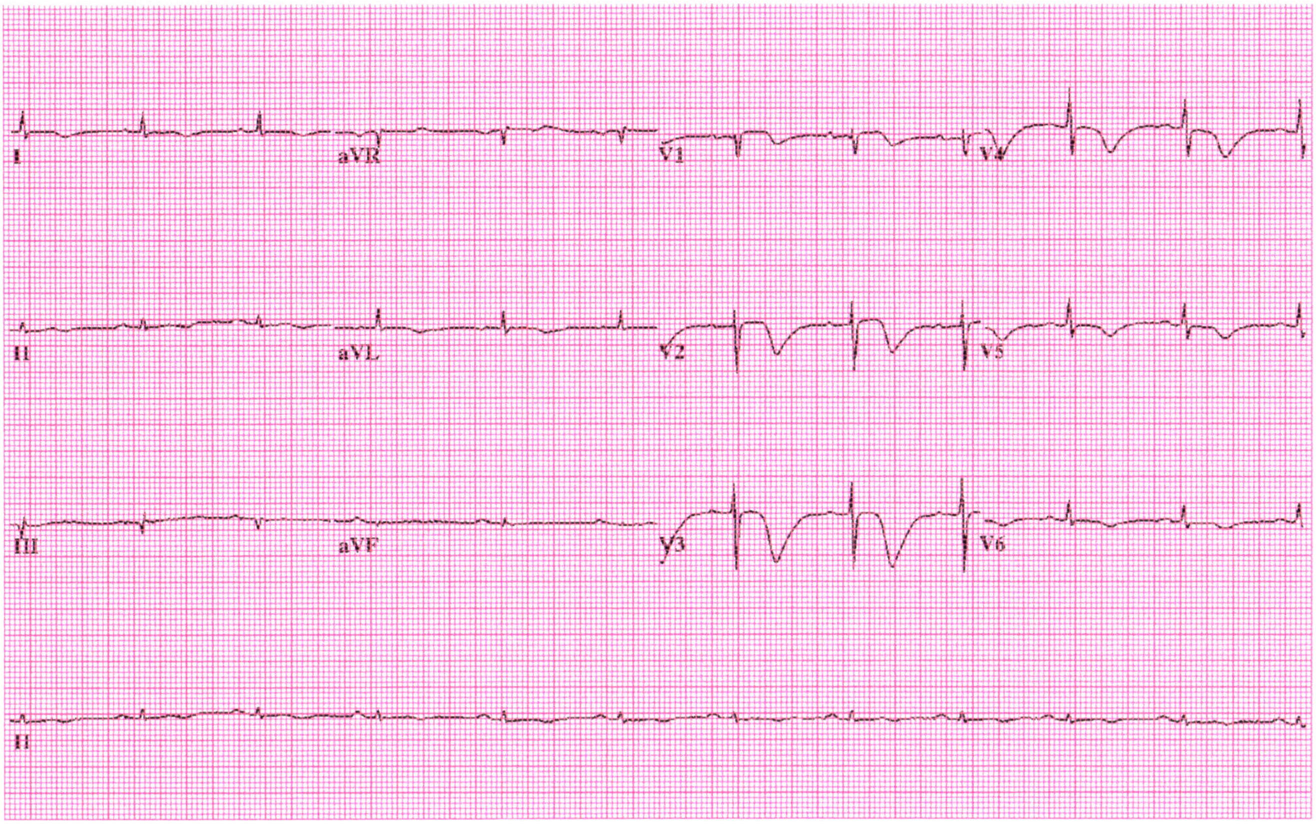

Fig. 12.3 ECG taken from a patient with a new onset neurological deficit, demonstrating several of the acute ECG derangements that can be seen following an acute central neurological event including deep T wave inversions ("cerebral T waves") and a prolonged QT interval. Image taken from O'Keefe et al., *The Complete Guide to ECGs*, third edition [87]

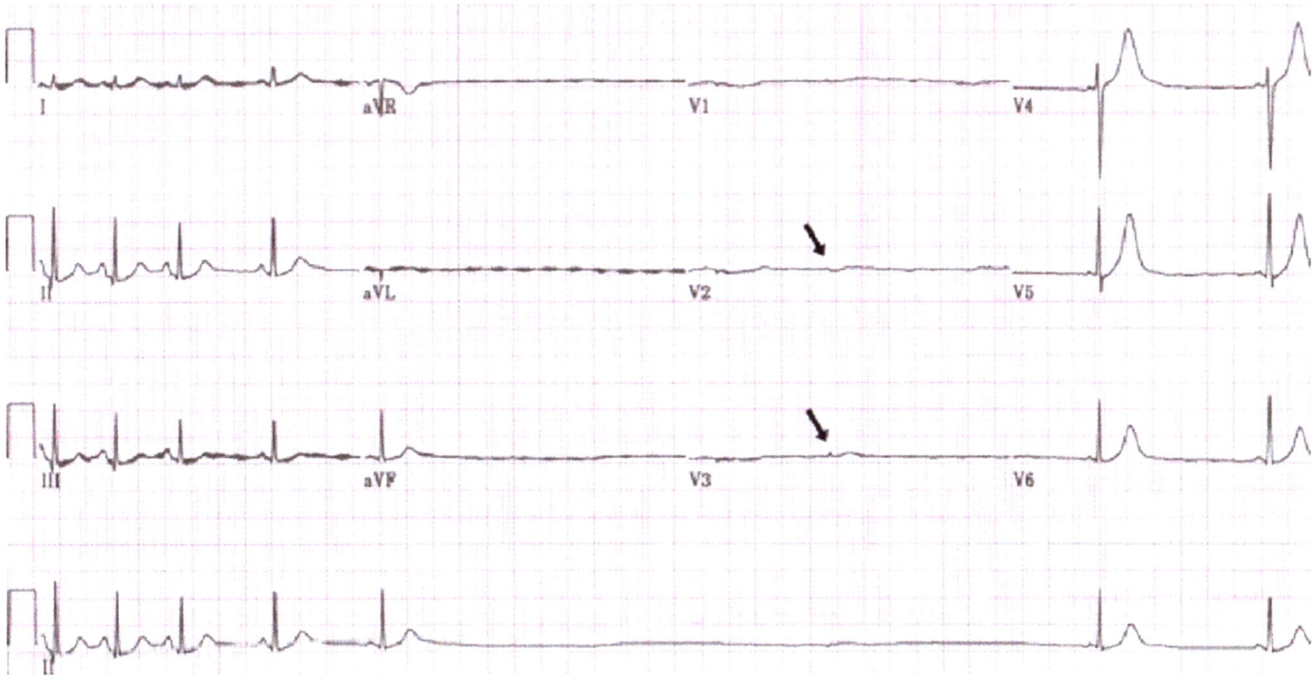

Fig. 12.4 Electrocardiogram of a patient with GBS demonstrating severe bradyarrhythmias and prolonged asystole. From Mukerji et al. Cardiovascular Complications of the Guillain-Barré Syndrome. Am J Cardiol. 2009

Tachyarrhythmias in the Neuro ICU

Tachyarrhythmias are common in the critically ill patient, of which sinus tachycardia and atrial fibrillation are the most common. We will discuss the presentation of the most common tachyarrhythmias below.

Sinus Tachycardia

Sinus tachycardia occurs when the sinus rate exceeds 100 bpm and is a physiological response to acute metabolic stressors; in rare cases, sinus tachycardia may be inappropriate, that is unexplained by physiological demands at rest [91], but this is uncommon in the critical care setting. The most common etiologies of sinus tachycardia in the ICU setting are due to underlying causes of acute illness such as infection, hypoxemia, and electrolyte imbalances. However, given the complexity of ICU patients, the etiology of sinus tachycardia is often multifactorial. A higher heart rate for >72 h has been observed to be associated with a longer ICU stay and is an independent predictor of mortality in a critically ill patient. Therefore, addressing the underlying pathology is imperative in the management of sinus tachycardia in the ICU setting [92].

Paroxysmal sympathetic hyperactivity (PSH) has been described in patients with a history of traumatic brain injury (TBI) and intracranial hemorrhage (ICH) and involves a dysregulation of the sympathetic nervous system. Clinical findings may include tachycardia, hypertension, hyperthermia, diaphoresis, tachypnea, and dystonia. The prevalence of PSH occurs around 33% of patients with TBI and is frequently underrecognized. Treatment of PSH include both pharmacological and non-pharmacological therapies. Pharmacotherapies include beta blockers, alpha2 receptor agonists, opioids, muscle relaxants, and GABA receptor agonists, whereas non-pharmacotherapies include supportive therapy with nutrition, hydration, and correction of electrolyte imbalances. An understanding of the clinical features and recognition of PSH is necessary given its complexity and prevalence in patients with TBI. [93]

Supraventricular Tachycardia

Supraventricular tachycardias (SVT) are narrow complex (QRS duration <120 ms) tachyarrhythmias, excluding AF, occurring at rest, and originating from above or within the His bundle [91, 94]. The differential diagnosis includes unifocal or multifocal atrial tachycardia (AT), sinus node reentry tachycardia (SNRT), macro-reentrant AT (including atrial flutter [AFL]), junctional tachycardia (JT), atrioventricular nodal reentrant tachycardia (AVNRT), and various forms of accessory pathway-mediated reentrant tachycardias, including atrioventricular reentrant tachycardia (AVRT). SVTs can usually be differentiated from ST by their abrupt onset and offset and changes in P wave morphology. An ECG should be obtained during normal sinus rhythm and during the arrhythmia as it can give clues to the mechanism of the arrhythmia and distinguish aberrant conduction [91, 94]. During the event, the tachyarrhythmia should be identified as regular or irregular as each has their own differential diagnoses: irregular arrhythmias include MAT, AF, or AFL with variable AV block while most other SVTs (particularly reentrant arrhythmias involving the AV node) are regular [91, 94]. JT can be regular or irregular [91]. The P wave morphology and proximity to the preceding QRS (RP interval) may also help identify the arrhythmia. Focal and multifocal AT demonstrate aberrant P wave morphologies. Regular SVTs with P waves that follow closely behind the preceding QRS (within 80 ms) are "short-RP" tachycardias, the differential of which includes typical AVNRT and AVRT, while "long-RP" tachycardias include ST, AT, JT, and atypical AVNRT or AVRT [91]. The duration of the arrhythmia is also helpful as re-entrant arrhythmias tend to last longer and recur more frequently [94]. AVNRT, the most common SVT, second to AF, is a macro-reentrant, "short-RP" tachycardia, with 1:1 conduction between the ventricles and atria, composed of two distinct and separate conduction pathways ("slow" and "fast") within the AV node [91, 95]. AVRT is a reentrant tachycardia involving the native AV conduction system and an accessory AV pathway; preexcitation, or a "delta wave," may be present on the ECG during normal sinus rhythm but its presence is unnecessary for making the diagnosis [95]. JT is a non-reentrant SVT originating from within the AV node or His bundle caused by ectopic foci or by enhanced automaticity [91, 94, 95]. A regular, WCT (QRS duration >120 ms) may either be ventricular tachycardia (VT) or SVT with aberrant conduction (i.e., BBB) which may be rate-related, preexistent during sinus rhythm, or due to preexcitation from an accessory pathway [91] (Fig. 12.5).

Treatment of acute SVT depends on the rhythm and relative stability of the patient. Vagal maneuvers should be attempted first, or adenosine given if vagal maneuvers fail or are infeasible, to re-establish sinus rhythm and/or identify the underlying rhythm [91]. Synchronized cardioversion is recommended for patients who are hemodynamically unstable, severely symptomatic, or when pharmacotherapy (non-dihydropyridine calcium channel blockers [CCB] or beta blockers [BB]) fails. CCBs should be avoided in patients who have systolic heart failure or are hemodynamically unstable, have VT, or pre-excited AF [91]. AADs including Class IC antiarrhythmic agents (flecainide, propafenone) and Class III antiarrhythmic agents such as amiodarone and sotalol can be used acutely for SVTs. However, in cases of pre-excited AF, digoxin, amiodarone, CCB, and BB are

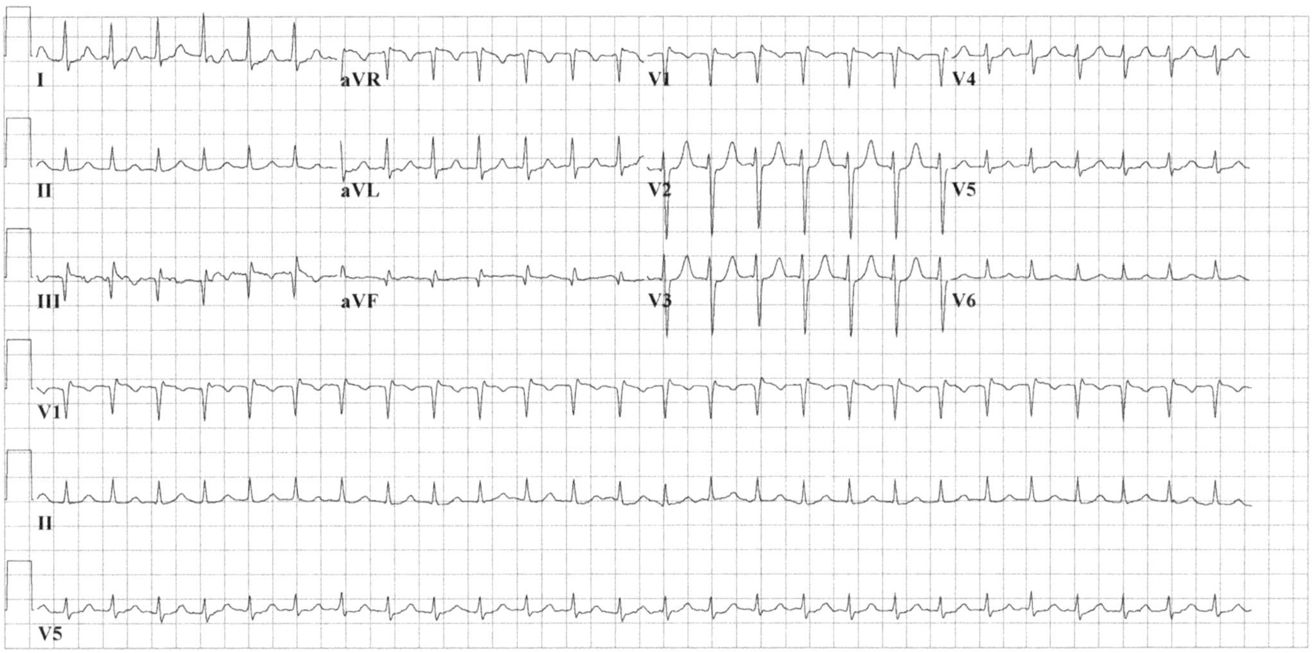

Fig. 12.5 An example of atrioventricular nodal reentrant tachycardia (AVNRT). Note the rSR' in lead V1 which is characteristic of this short R-P tachycardia

absolutely contraindicated as these agents may precipitate life-threatening ventricular arrhythmias (VA) by blocking the AV node and allowing for rapid conduction down the accessory pathway [91]. In this instance, ibutilide or IV procainamide can be used for rate or rhythm control and only in hemodynamically stable patients [91].

Atrial tachycardia encompasses unifocal AT, multifocal atrial tachycardia (MAT), and sinus node reentry tachycardia (SNRT). Unifocal AT is a regular tachyarrhythmia originating from potentially any atrial tissue away from the sinus node; thus, while the ECG demonstrates a P wave before every QRS, the morphology differs from that of sinus rhythm. At onset ("warm-up") and offset ("warm-down"), AT may appear irregular [91, 94]. The atrial rate can be between 100 and 250 bpm and may be sustained or nonsustained [91]. MAT is an irregular SVT, usually accompanying another primary process such as pulmonary, cardiac, or valvular disease, characterized by ≥3 distinct P wave morphologies at different rates [91]. The rhythm is always irregular and may be difficult to distinguish from AF, thus a 12-lead ECG is usually needed to confirm the diagnosis—the presence of a flat or stable isoelectric period (the TP interval) between P waves almost universally excludes the AF. The first-line treatment of MAT is to treat the underlying primary pathology. Magnesium administration may be helpful while cardioversion is not; the use of antiarrhythmic agents is limited, with some evidence to suggest that verapamil, followed by metoprolol, may be the most useful agents [91].

Atrial flutter is a macro-reentrant arrhythmia that originates within the right atrium and is typically dependent on the cavotricuspid isthmus (CTI) for re-entry [91, 94]. Rarely, AFL may not rely on the CTI or may originate outside of the right atrium. On ECG, there is a constant P wave morphology ("flutter waves") at a regular rate, usually >250 bpm [91]. Flutter waves appear inverted without an isoelectric TP interval, giving the classic "sawtooth" appearance that is best appreciated in the inferior leads [96]. The ratio of flutter waves to QRS complexes is usually fixed at an even number (e.g., 2:1); although, AFL with variable block can occur [96]. Fixed, odd-numbered AV conduction ratios are uncommon, while ratios >4:1 may indicate concomitant AV block, as can be seen with digoxin toxicity [91, 96]. AFL frequently coexists with AF as the two share common risk factors; similarly, the two arrhythmias have the same risk for thromboembolism and medical management is the same [91, 94] (Fig. 12.6).

Atrial fibrillation is the most common adult arrhythmia and one of the most common arrhythmias observed in critically ill patients [97]. The anatomical substrate of AF is presumed to be underlying myocardial fibrosis, secondary to systemic inflammation, which leads to alteration of left atrial electrical activity [97]. The hallmark of AF is irregular atrial activity with an absence of distinct P waves and random oscillation of the baseline interval. Similarly, the RR interval is irregularly irregular. At faster rates, AF may appear regular and be mistaken for SVT, but careful scrutiny of the ventricular rhythm may reveal subtle irregularity [87] (Fig. 12.7).

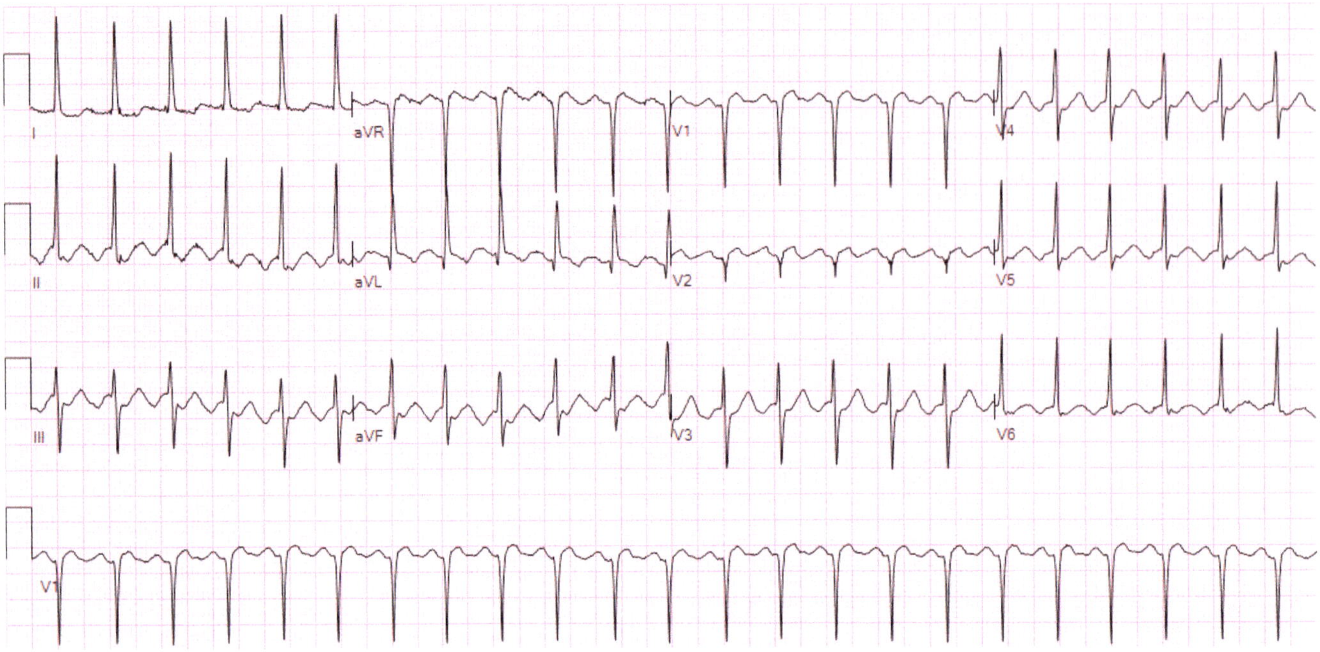

Fig. 12.6 An example of atrial flutter with 2:1 AV block

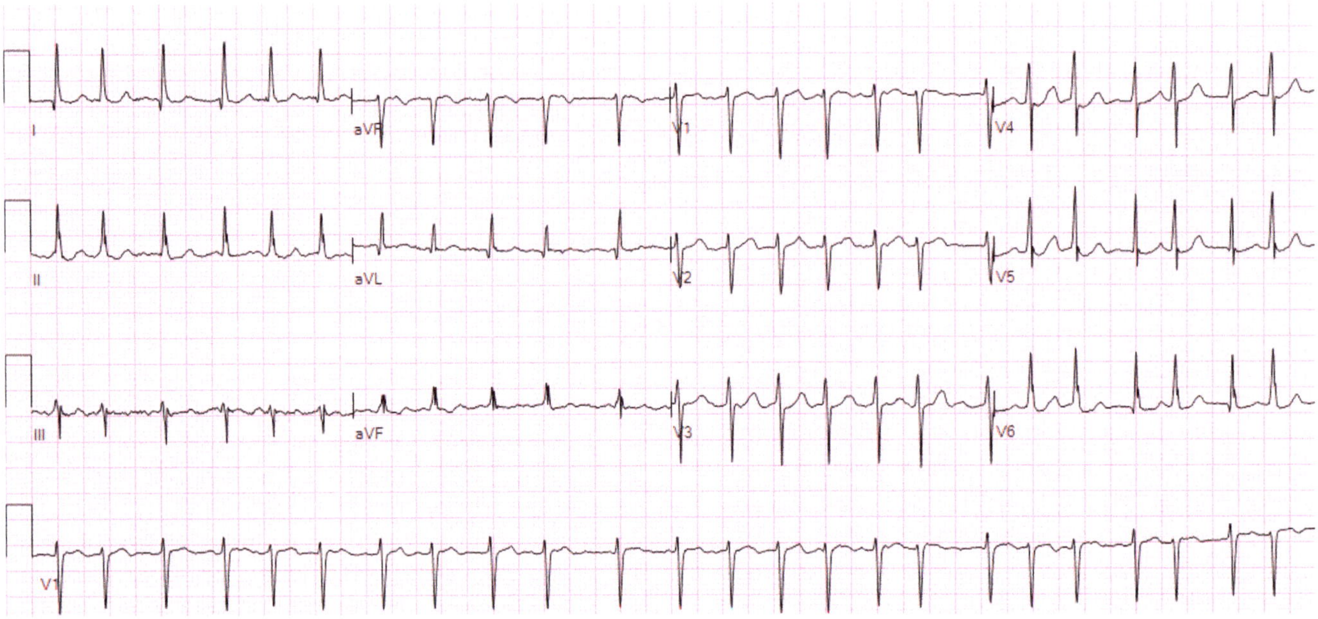

Fig. 12.7 An example of atrial fibrillation with rapid ventricular response

AF is associated with a five-fold increased risk of ischemic stroke [59, 97] as blood stagnates within the left atrium, particularly within the left atrial appendage, which increases the risk for thrombus formation and thromboembolic events [77]. New or recurrent AF is common following an acute stroke [77, 81, 82] but has not been shown in and of itself to negatively affect prognosis [77]. The incidence of atrial fibrillation is eight times higher among patients with acute ischemic stroke. Atrial fibrillation detected after stroke (AFDAS) is a recently described clinical entity which accounts for either preexisting AF or AF triggered by the stroke. The etiology of AFDAS is comprised of cardiogenic factors, neurogenic, or a mixture of both, and the pathophysiology appears to differ from AF known prior to a stroke. Autonomic dysregulation and inflammation have been identified as the neurogenic mechanisms of AFDAS [66]. In clinical studies, AFDAS is characteristically low burden, with over 50% of documented paroxysms lasting <30 s. Thus, it is not clear that the associated risk of recurrent stroke is as high as that of AF known before the cerebrovascular event. If diagnosed, long-term cardiac monitoring is recommended upon hospital discharge.

Management of AF/AFL is similar to SVT but with the additional caveat of assessing the need for anticoagulation to minimize thromboembolic risk [98, 99]. The CHA2DS2-VASc score has been validated for assessing stroke risk in AF/AFL [91, 98, 99] but is reserved for non-valvular AF (i.e., patients without mitral valvular disease such as moderate mitral stenosis or history of a mechanical mitral valve or rheumatic heart disease). For patients with mechanical valves or significant mitral stenosis, current guidelines recommend anticoagulation with warfarin [99]. In non-valvular AF, anticoagulation with heparin products (acutely) or a direct oral anticoagulant (DOAC) is recommended for patients with a CHA2DS2-VASc score of ≥2 if male and ≥3 if female [99]. For patients on dialysis, warfarin or apixaban at a reduced dose may be used, and for patients with advanced chronic kidney disease not on dialysis, anticoagulation options include most DOACs at reduced doses [99]. The use of anticoagulation in the acute setting must be balanced against the underlying issue and the risk of bleeding from anticoagulation. Certain neurological diagnoses will preclude the use of anticoagulation even in the setting of AF/AFL.

For patients who present with hemodynamically unstable rapid AF/AFL, synchronized cardioversion is recommended. If the duration of AF has been >48 h, a transesophageal echocardiogram (TEE) is unnecessary if the patient has been receiving anticoagulation for at least 3 weeks prior to cardioversion [99]. Otherwise, a TEE is recommended to evaluate the left atrium for thrombus immediately prior to cardioversion, and anticoagulation should be initiated as soon as possible and continued for at least 4 weeks afterwards regardless of the patient's CHA2DS2-VASc score [99]. For patients who present with acute ischemic stroke and AF, the decision to begin anticoagulation should be carefully balanced against the risk of a hemorrhagic conversion of the primary stroke.

For patients who are symptomatic or have left ventricular (LV) dysfunction, rate control to a goal of <80 bpm is recommended [98]. Lenient rate control to a goal of <110 bpm is acceptable for patients who are asymptomatic and have preserved LV function [98]. Rate control medication options include BB or CCB in the absence of preexcitation, and LV systolic dysfunction should be evaluated for prior to starting the latter [98, 99]. Amiodarone may be cautiously used as an adjunctive agent in patients without preexcitation [98] but caution should be used as there is a risk of chemical cardioversion into a normal sinus rhythm which may increase the risk of cardioembolic stroke among patients who have not been anticoagulated.

Wide Complex Tachycardia

Wide complex tachycardias (WCTs) are tachyarrhythmias in which the QRS duration exceeds 120 ms [100]. The differential diagnosis includes VT, SVT with pre-existing bundle-branch block, SVT with rate-related aberrant conduction due to tachycardia (normal QRS when in sinus rhythm), SVT with wide QRS related to drugs, electrolyte or metabolic disorder, SVT with conduction over an accessory pathway (pre-excitation), paced rhythm, or artifact [91, 94, 100]. During an SVT episode, there is usually evidence of 1:1 atrial to ventricular association since the arrhythmia originates from above the His bundle [100]. AV dissociation, where there is less than a 1:1 ratio of P waves to QRS (i.e., ventricular rate faster than atrial rate), has near 100% specificity for VT [100]. However, 1:1 AV conduction does not completely exclude VT [100]. Capture complexes (narrow QRS complexes that resemble the native sinus QRS due to atrial activity conducting down the His–Purkinje system) are further evidence of AV dissociation and are pathognomonic for VT [91, 94, 100]. Similarly, a hybrid QRS known as a "fusion complex" is also strongly suggestive of VT and may occur due to simultaneous ventricular activation from both ventricular and atrial sources, thus the fused QRS resembles a combination of the native and ventricular QRS [100]. ECG findings that are specific, but not sensitive, for VT include: QRS duration >140 ms if right BBB (RBBB) or >160 ms if LBBB morphology; axis change or extreme axis deviation; and chest lead concordance such that precordial QRS complexes are either all positive or negative, with the latter having a greater specificity for VT [91, 94]. Distinguishing SVT from VT with aberrancy is critical as inappropriate treatment of VT can prove fatal [101]. In cases of monomorphic, regular, and hemodynamically tolerated WCT, adenosine may be used to convert the rhythm to sinus and aid in the diagnosis [91]. However, WCT should be assumed to be VT until proven otherwise, particularly in patients with a history of ischemic heart disease [91, 94] (Fig. 12.8).

Ventricular arrhythmia (VA) is a spectrum of disease encompassing PVCs, both sustained and non-sustained VT, and ventricular fibrillation (VF) [101]. VA, particularly PVCs, is common in the acute period following stroke and are associated with increased mortality [77, 102, 103]. The pathophysiology of ventricular arrhythmogenesis is primarily reliant on the insular cortex, autonomic imbalance, and increased sympathetic activity [103]. Damage to the insular cortex may lead to increased sympathetic activity to the heart, which in turn leads to continuous cardiomyocyte beta-adrenergic activation, continuous calcium influx, an inability for the calcium channels to close, failure to sequester the excess calcium, and impaired cardiomyocyte relaxation; the accumulation of the aforementioned insults leads to cardiomyocyte death [103]. The His–Purkinje system is particu-

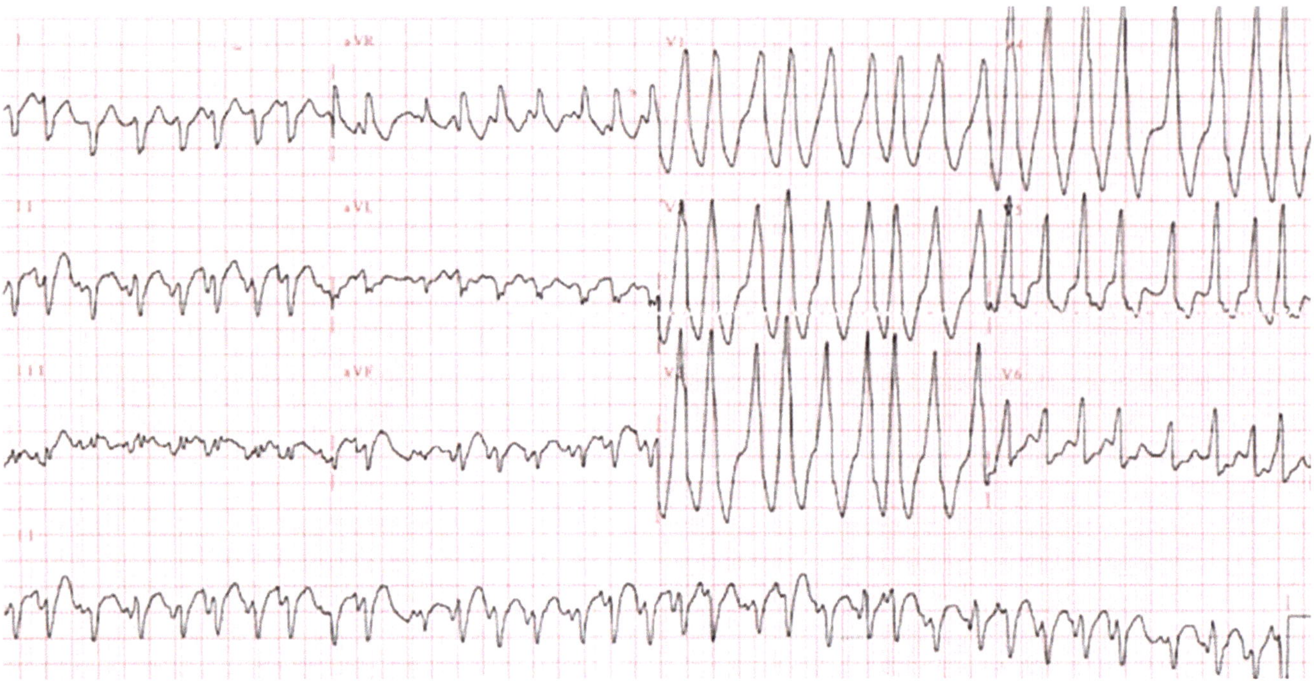

Fig. 12.8 An example of atrial fibrillation with preexcitation (i.e., Wolff–Parkinson-White)

larly vulnerable to sympathetic hyperactivity as myofibrillar degeneration is predominantly subendocardial. Additionally, sympathetic hyperactivity may also lead to hypokalemia and hypomagnesemia, which are both associated with VA [103]. On the surface ECG, catecholamine surge presents as QTc prolongation and PVCs. Catecholamine surge can also precipitate Takotsubo cardiomyopathy, which may also increase risk of VA [103]. Predictors of VA following stroke include ischemic stroke, stroke severity, age, female sex, preexisting cardiac disease, prolonged QTc, hypertension, and diabetes [103, 104]. Angiotensin-converting enzyme inhibitors and angiotensin II receptor antagonists are protective against VA [101, 103]. Mechanisms of malignant VA include reentry, derangement in automaticity, and triggered activity induced by early or late afterdepolarizations [101].

Ventricular tachycardia (VT) is defined as ≥3 consecutive ventricular QRS complexes at >100 bpm and can further be stratified based on QRS morphology and duration of the arrhythmia. Sustained VT is when the arrhythmia is >30 s or requires early termination due to hemodynamic instability. NSVT lasts <30 s and terminates spontaneously. VT/VF storm is defined by ≥3 episodes of sustained VT or VF within a 24-h period. Monomorphic VT demonstrates a stable, single QRS morphology throughout the arrhythmia, while polymorphic VT has a multiform QRS. The morphology of the QRS is an important distinction as it can give clues as to the etiology of the arrhythmia—polymorphic VT is often seen in acute cardiac ischemic events, channelopathies, iatrogenic QT prolongation (such as from medications), or idiopathic. Sustained monomorphic VT is often scar-related or in the absence of structural heart disease, due to an automatic focus within the ventricles, and may furthermore degenerate to VF [101] (Fig. 12.9).

Torsade de Pointes (TdP) is a specific type of polymorphic VT that occurs in the setting of a prolonged QT interval and is characterized by a waxing and waning QRS amplitude, that is the pathognomonic twisting of the QRS, which may or may not always be present [101]. TdP is often preceded by a long RR interval followed by a short RR interval initiating sequence, which is exacerbated in the setting of bradycardia, and usually a result of an underlying acquired QT prolongation. Assessment of QT prolonging medications and electrolyte abnormalities should be undertaken. Electrolyte repletion, including magnesium and potassium, as well as isoproterenol or cardiac pacing to increase the heart rate, may be beneficial to prevent TdP recurrence [101]. For medication-induced arrhythmias (as in the case of iatrogenic QT prolongation), the offending medication should be stopped.

Ventricular fibrillation (VF) is characterized by rapid and irregular ventricular activity with marked variability in the QRS at a rate usually >300 bpm [101] (Fig. 12.10).

The evaluation of new onset VA should prioritize assessing whether or not the patient is stable followed by assessing for LV dysfunction or ischemic or structural heart disease [101, 105]. Acutely, patients who present with a new WCT should be presumed to have VA until proven otherwise [91, 101]. The patient assessment should include evaluating for preexisting cardiac disease, risk factors for cardiovascular disease, and potential offending medications (e.g., stimu-

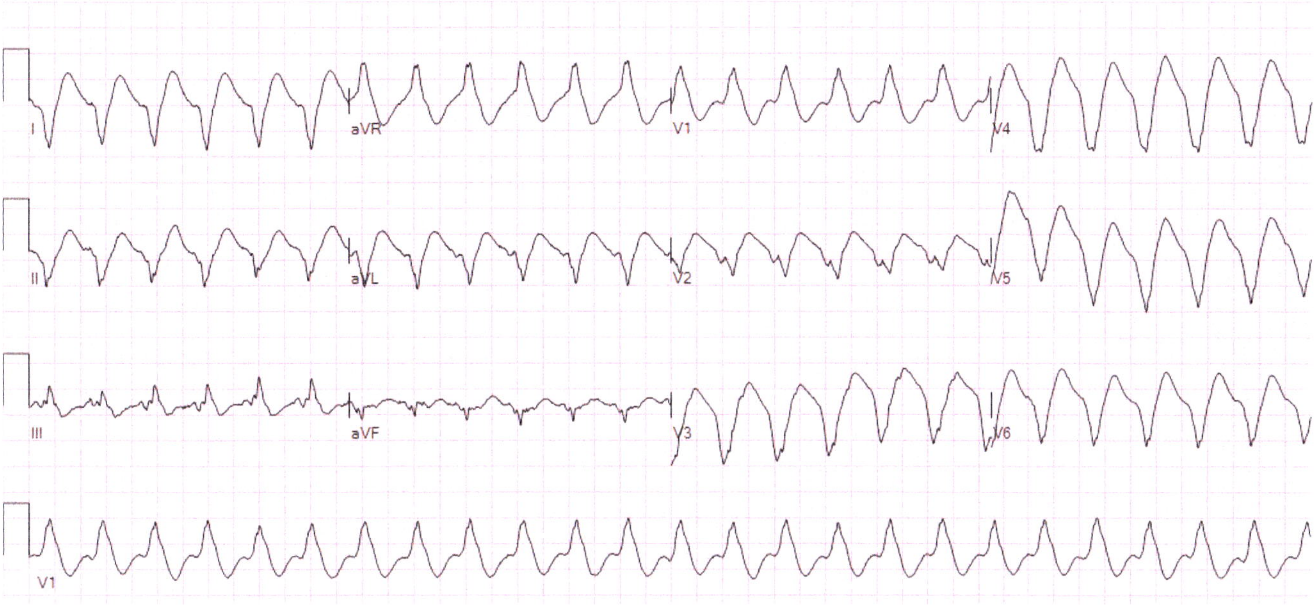

Fig. 12.9 An example of monomorphic ventricular tachycardia

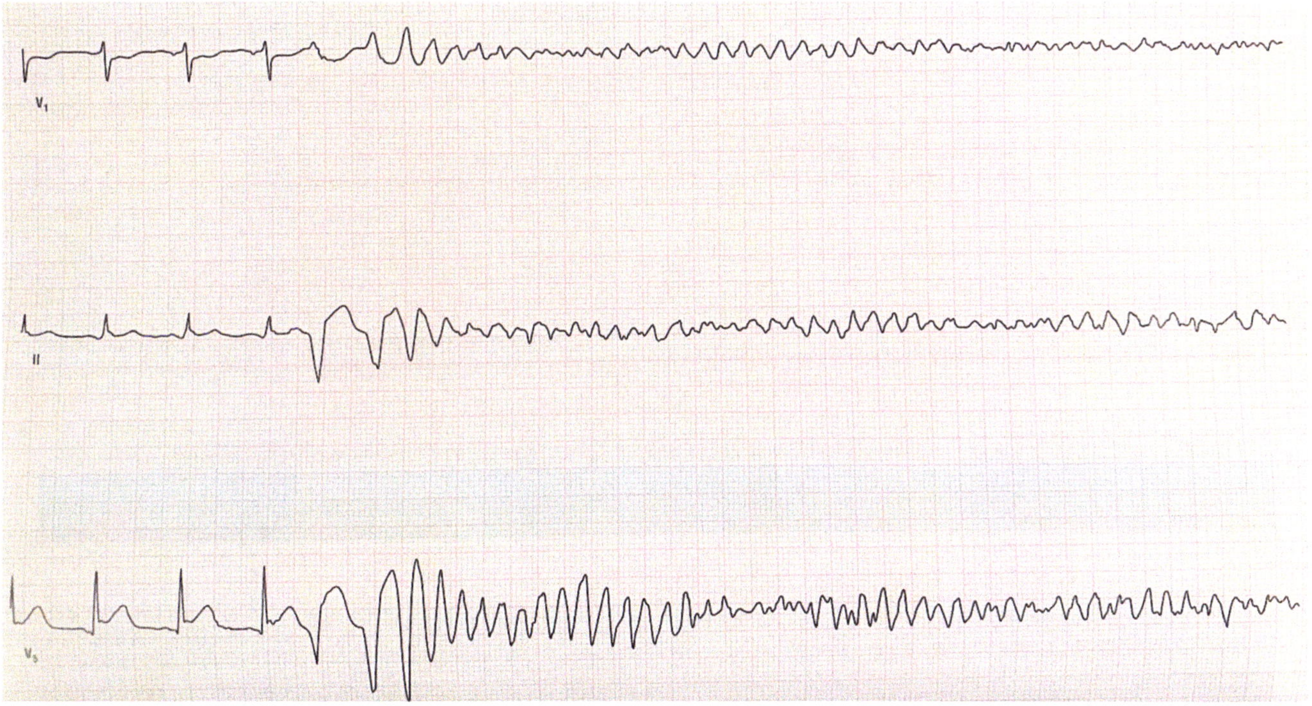

Fig. 12.10 Sinus rhythm degenerating into ventricular arrhythmia. The first four beats are sinus tachycardia before the rhythm degenerates into polymorphic VT/Torsade de Pointes which then degenerates further into ventricular fibrillation. Note the ST elevation in V5, indicating acute cardiac ischemia. Image taken from O'Keefe et al., *The Complete Guide to ECGs*, 3rd edition [87]

lants and QT prolonging medications) [101, 105]. A 12-lead ECG during the arrhythmia and during sinus rhythm is vitally important to assess for evidence of cardiac structural abnormalities and to help differentiate between VA versus SVT with aberrancy [91, 101, 105]. Furthermore, an echocardiogram is mandatory and additional noninvasive cardiac imaging may be helpful on a case-by-case basis. Cardiac biomarkers (BNP and troponin) should also be obtained to assess for prognosis and risk for sudden cardiac death or arrest [101].

Patients who are hemodynamically unstable should undergo immediate direct current cardioversion/defibrillation [101, 105] and if unsuccessful, amiodarone intravenously should be administered [101]. In cases of VF or polymorphic VT, lidocaine intravenously may also be given [101]. If hemodynamically stable, intravenous amiodarone, sotalol, or procainamide can be used to attempt to terminate VT [101]. VA in the setting of Type I ST-elevation myocardial infarction should be given intravenous beta blocker and undergo emergent cardiac revascularization if not otherwise contraindicated [101, 105]. Patients with sustained VA or who survive cardiac arrest should otherwise undergo cardiac ischemic evaluation and be considered for coronary angiography [101, 105].

Beta blockers are foundational to treating and preventing VA. Additional antiarrhythmic agents may be indicated in consultation with a cardiologist. Furthermore, in patients with systolic LV dysfunction, guideline-directed heart failure medications should be initiated to reduce the risk of sudden cardiac death [101, 105]. Patients who have sustained VT not due to reversible causes, or have hemodynamically unstable VT, or have survived sudden cardiac death should be evaluated in the long-term for placement of an automatic implantable cardioverter-defibrillator for secondary prevention of recurrent VA [101].

Near Misses in Patients with Chest Pain or Arrhythmia

- Differentiating between acute coronary syndrome (ACS) and neurogenic stunned myocardium/neurogenic stress cardiomyopathy (NSM/NSC)
  - NSM is favored when there is an absence of preexisting heart disease, there are lack of ischemic changes on ECG, wall motion abnormalities on echocardiogram do not follow a coronary distribution, and cardiac troponin levels are relatively low and do not trend upward significantly.
- Detection of aortic dissection
  - Chest pain is a common complaint. However, many patients may present only with neurologic manifestations including ischemic stroke, spinal cord ischemia, ischemic neuropathy, hypoxic encephalopathy, syncope, seizures, and transient global amnesia. Symptoms may be transient thus impeding the diagnosis.
- Underestimation of the severity of bradyarrhythmias in Guillain–Barré syndrome
  - Serious bradyarrhythmias requiring IV medications or pacemaker placement are common in this syndrome and require early recognition as aggressive management of associated hypoxia and metabolic abnormalities may mitigate the severity.
- Misdiagnosis of a wide complex tachycardia (WCT) as a supraventricular tachycardia
  - Patients with a new WCT should be presumed to have a ventricular arrhythmia (VA) until proven otherwise. Assessment of preexisting cardiac disease, cardiac risk factors, potential offending medications (e.g., possible QT prolonging meds) is imperative. An ECG can help differentiate between VA and SVT with aberrancy. Hemodynamically unstable patients should undergo immediate electric cardioversion/defibrillation irrespective of the etiology of the arrhythmia.

Conclusion

The neurological and cardiovascular systems are intricately intertwined with multiple manifestations of neurocardiogenic disease presenting in the neurointensive care unit. Familiarity with clinical presentations of chest pain and arrhythmias allows for optimal management of these critically ill patients.

References

1. Rui P, Kang K. National Hospital Ambulatory Medical Care Survey: 2017 emergency department summary tables. National Center for Health Statistics; 2017.
2. Tsao CW, Aday AW, Almarzooq ZI, Alonso A, Beaton AZ, Bittencourt MS, et al. Heart disease and stroke Statistics-2022 update: a report from the American Heart Association. Circulation. 2022;145(8):e153–639.
3. Frieling T. Non-cardiac chest pain. Visc Med. 2018;34(2): 92–6.
4. Writing Committee M, Gulati M, Levy PD, Mukherjee D, Amsterdam E, Bhatt DL, et al. 2021 AHA/ACC/ASE/CHEST/SAEM/SCCT/SCMR guideline for the evaluation and diagnosis of CHEST Pain: a report of the American College of Cardiology/American Heart Association Joint Committee on clinical practice guidelines. J Am Coll Cardiol. 2021;78(22):e187–285.
5. Khan U, Robbins MS. Neurological causes of chest Pain. Curr Pain Headache Rep. 2021;25(5):32.
6. Chin PL, Kaminski J, Rout M. Myocardial infarction coincident with cerebrovascular accidents in the elderly. Age Ageing. 1977;6(1):29–37.
7. Silver FL, Norris JW, Lewis AJ, Hachinski VC. Early mortality following stroke: a prospective review. Stroke. 1984;15(3):492–6.
8. Touze E, Varenne O, Chatellier G, Peyrard S, Rothwell PM, Mas JL. Risk of myocardial infarction and vascular death after transient ischemic attack and ischemic stroke: a systematic review and meta-analysis. Stroke. 2005;36(12):2748–55.
9. Hurlen M, Abdelnoor M, Smith P, Erikssen J, Arnesen H. Warfarin, aspirin, or both after myocardial infarction. N Engl J Med. 2002;347(13):969–74.
10. Lombardo A, Biasucci LM, Lanza GA, Coli S, Silvestri P, Cianflone D, et al. Inflammation as a possible link between coronary and carotid plaque instability. Circulation. 2004;109(25):3158–63.
11. Komrad MS, Coffey CE, Coffey KS, McKinnis R, Massey EW, Califf RM. Myocardial infarction and stroke. Neurology. 1984;34(11):1403–9.

12. Thygesen K, Alpert JS, White HD, Joint ESCAAHAWHFTFftRoMI. Universal definition of myocardial infarction. J Am Coll Cardiol. 2007;50(22):2173–95.
13. Scheitz JF, Nolte CH, Doehner W, Hachinski V, Endres M. Stroke-heart syndrome: clinical presentation and underlying mechanisms. Lancet Neurol. 2018;17(12):1109–20.
14. Boulanger M, Bejot Y, Rothwell PM, Touze E. Long-term risk of myocardial infarction compared to recurrent stroke after transient ischemic attack and ischemic stroke: systematic review and meta-analysis. J Am Heart Assoc. 2018;7(2)
15. Ahn SH, Kim YH, Shin CH, Lee JS, Kim BJ, Kim YJ, et al. Cardiac vulnerability to Cerebrogenic stress as a possible cause of troponin elevation in stroke. J Am Heart Assoc. 2016;5(10)
16. DeFilippis AP, Chapman AR, Mills NL, de Lemos JA, Arbab-Zadeh A, Newby LK, et al. Assessment and treatment of patients with type 2 myocardial infarction and acute nonischemic myocardial injury. Circulation. 2019;140(20):1661–78.
17. Scheitz JF, Mochmann HC, Erdur H, Tutuncu S, Haeusler KG, Grittner U, et al. Prognostic relevance of cardiac troponin T levels and their dynamic changes measured with a high-sensitivity assay in acute ischaemic stroke: analyses from the TRELAS cohort. Int J Cardiol. 2014;177(3):886–93.
18. Dixit S, Castle M, Velu RP, Swisher L, Hodge C, Jaffe AS. Cardiac involvement in patients with acute neurologic disease: confirmation with cardiac troponin I. Arch Intern Med. 2000;160(20):3153–8.
19. Horowitz MB, Willet D, Keffer J. The use of cardiac troponin-I (cTnI) to determine the incidence of myocardial ischemia and injury in patients with aneurysmal and presumed aneurysmal subarachnoid hemorrhage. Acta Neurochir. 1998;140:87–93.
20. Kolin A, Norris JW. Myocardial damage from acute cerebral lesions. Stroke. 1984;15(6):990–3.
21. Nguyen H, Zaroff JG. Neurogenic stunned myocardium. Curr Neurol Neurosci Rep. 2009;9(6):486–91.
22. Aminoff MJ, Josephson SA. Aminoff's neurology and general medicine. Amsterdam: Academic Press; 2021. https://www.sciencedirect.com/science/book/9780128193068
23. Kono T, Morita H, Kuroiwa T, Onaka H, Takatsuka H, Fujiwara A. Left ventricular wall motion abnormalities in patients with subarachnoid hemorrhage: neurogenic stunned myocardium. J Am Coll Cardiol. 1994;24(3):636–40.
24. Shams YH. Acute cardiac sympathetic disruption in the pathogenesis of the takotsubo syndrome: a systematic review of the literature to date. Cardiovasc Revasc Med. 2014;15(1):35–42.
25. Bulsara KR, McGirt MJ, Liao L, Villavicencio AT, Borel C, Alexander MJ, et al. Use of the peak troponin value to differentiate myocardial infarction from reversible neurogenic left ventricular dysfunction associated with aneurysmal subarachnoid hemorrhage. J Neurosurg. 2003;98(3):524–8.
26. Adams RJ, Chimowitz MI, Alpert JS, Awad IA, Cerqueria MD, Fayad P, et al. Coronary risk evaluation in patients with transient ischemic attack and ischemic stroke: a scientific statement for healthcare professionals from the stroke council and the council on clinical cardiology of the American Heart Association/American Stroke Association. Circulation. 2003;108(10):1278–90.
27. Xu JJ, Song Y, Jiang P, Gao Z, Li JX, Chen J, et al. Effect of prior stroke on long-term outcomes of percutaneous coronary interventions in Chinese patients: a large single-center study. Catheter Cardiovasc Interv. 2019;93(2):E75–80.
28. Natsuaki M, Morimoto T, Watanabe H, Nakagawa Y, Furukawa Y, Kadota K, et al. Ischemic and bleeding risk after percutaneous coronary intervention in patients with prior ischemic and hemorrhagic stroke. J Am Heart Assoc. 2019;8(22):e013356.
29. Warner JJ, Harrington RA, Sacco RL, Elkind MSV. Guidelines for the early management of patients with acute ischemic stroke: 2019 update to the 2018 guidelines for the early management of acute ischemic stroke. Stroke. 2019;50(12):3331–2.
30. Kirchhof P, Benussi S, Kotecha D, Ahlsson A, Atar D, Casadei B, et al. 2016 ESC guidelines for the management of atrial fibrillation developed in collaboration with EACTS. Europace. 2016;18(11):1609–78.
31. Gaudino M, Benesch C, Bakaeen F, DeAnda A, Fremes SE, Glance L, et al. Considerations for reduction of risk of perioperative stroke in adult patients undergoing Cardiac and thoracic aortic operations: a scientific statement from the American Heart Association. Circulation. 2020;142(14):e193–209.
32. Unger T, Borghi C, Charchar F, Khan NA, Poulter NR, Prabhakaran D, et al. 2020 International Society of Hypertension global hypertension practice guidelines. J Hypertens. 2020;38(6):982–1004.
33. Reboussin DM, Allen NB, Griswold ME, Guallar E, Hong Y, Lackland DT, et al. Systematic review for the 2017 ACC/AHA/AAPA/ABC/ACPM/AGS/APhA/ASH/ASPC/NMA/PCNA guideline for the prevention, detection, evaluation, and Management of High Blood Pressure in adults: a report of the American College of Cardiology/American Heart Association task force on clinical practice guidelines. Circulation. 2018;138(17):e595–616.
34. Ettehad D, Emdin CA, Kiran A, Anderson SG, Callender T, Emberson J, et al. Blood pressure lowering for prevention of cardiovascular disease and death: a systematic review and meta-analysis. Lancet. 2016;387(10022):957–67.
35. National High Blood Pressure Education Program. The seventh report of the Joint National Committee on Prevention, Detection, Evaluation, and Treatment of High Blood Pressure; 2004.
36. Agarwal AK, Rees CJ, Pollack CV. Chapter 52—Hypertensive crisis. 4th ed.; 2014, pp 371–9.
37. Vaughan CJ, Delanty N. Hypertensive emergencies. Lancet. 2000;356(9227):411–7.
38. Powers WJ, Rabinstein AA, Ackerson T, Adeoye OM, Bambakidis NC, Becker K, et al. Guidelines for the early management of patients with acute ischemic stroke: 2019 update to the 2018 guidelines for the early management of acute ischemic stroke: a guideline for healthcare professionals from the American Heart Association/American Stroke Association. Stroke. 2019;50(12):e344–418.
39. Castillo J, Leira R, Garcia MM, Serena J, Blanco M, Davalos A. Blood pressure decrease during the acute phase of ischemic stroke is associated with brain injury and poor stroke outcome. Stroke. 2004;35(2):520–6.
40. Jeong HG, Kim BJ, Kim H, Jung C, Han MK, Liebeskind DS, et al. Blood pressure drop and penumbral tissue loss in nonrecanalized emergent large vessel occlusion. Stroke. 2019;50(10):2677–84.
41. Anderson CS, Huang Y, Wang JG, Arima H, Neal B, Peng B, et al. Intensive blood pressure reduction in acute cerebral haemorrhage trial (INTERACT): a randomised pilot trial. Lancet Neurol. 2008;7(5):391–9.
42. Anderson CS, Huang Y, Arima H, Heeley E, Skulina C, Parsons MW, et al. Effects of early intensive blood pressure-lowering treatment on the growth of hematoma and perihematomal edema in acute intracerebral hemorrhage: the Intensive Blood Pressure Reduction in Acute Cerebral Haemorrhage Trial (INTERACT). Stroke. 2010;41(2):307–12.
43. Investigators TET. Efficacy of nitric oxide, with or without continuing antihypertensive treatment, for management of high blood pressure in acute stroke (ENOS): a partial-factorial randomised controlled trial. Lancet. 2015;385(9968):617–28.
44. Anderson CS, Heeley E, Huang Y, Wang J, Stapf C, Delcourt C, et al. Rapid blood-pressure lowering in patients with acute intracerebral hemorrhage. N Engl J Med. 2013;368(25):2355–65.

45. Qureshi AI, Palesch YY, Barsan WG, Hanley DF, Hsu CY, Martin RL, et al. Intensive blood-pressure lowering in patients with acute cerebral hemorrhage. N Engl J Med. 2016;375(11):1033–43.
46. Blech B, Chong BW, Sands KA, Wingerchuk DM, Jackson WT, Marks LA, et al. Are postprocedural blood pressure goals associated with clinical outcome after mechanical thrombectomy for acute ischemic stroke? Neurologist. 2019;24(1):44–7.
47. Hagan PG, Nienaber CA, Isselbacher EM, Bruckman D, Karavite DJ, Russman PL, et al. The international registry of acute aortic dissection (IRAD): new insights into an old disease. JAMA. 2000;283(7):897–903.
48. DeSanctis RW, Doroghazi RM, Austen WG, Buckley MJ. Aortic dissection. N Engl J Med. 1987;317(17):1060–7.
49. Juang D, Braverman AC, Eagle K. Cardiology patient pages. Aortic dissection. Circulation. 2008;118(14):e507–10.
50. Braverman AC. Acute aortic dissection: clinician update. Circulation. 2010;122(2):184–8.
51. Gaul C, Dietrich W, Erbguth FJ. Neurological symptoms in aortic dissection: a challenge for neurologists. Cerebrovasc Dis. 2008;26(1):1–8.
52. Gaul C, Dietrich W, Friedrich I, Sirch J, Erbguth FJ. Neurological symptoms in type a aortic dissections. Stroke. 2007;38(2):292–7.
53. Ehrlich MP, Ergin MA, McCullough JN, Lansman SL, Galla JD, Bodian CA, et al. Results of immediate surgical treatment of all acute type a dissections. Circulation. 2000;102:III248–52. (19 Suppl 3).
54. Chirillo F, Marchiori MC, Andriolo L, Razzolini R, Mazzucco A, Gallucci V, et al. Outcome of 290 patients with aortic dissection. A 12-year multicentre experience. Eur Heart J. 1990;11(4):311–9.
55. Evangelista A, Isselbacher EM, Bossone E, Gleason TG, Eusanio MD, Sechtem U, et al. Insights from the international registry of acute aortic dissection: a 20-year experience of collaborative clinical research. Circulation. 2018;137(17):1846–60.
56. Hirata K, Wake M, Kyushima M, Takahashi T, Nakazato J, Mototake H, et al. Electrocardiographic changes in patients with type a acute aortic dissection. Incidence, patterns and underlying mechanisms in 159 cases. J Cardiol. 2010;56(2):147–53.
57. Koga M, Iguchi Y, Ohara T, Tahara Y, Fukuda T, Noguchi T, et al. Acute ischemic stroke as a complication of Stanford type a acute aortic dissection: a review and proposed clinical recommendations for urgent diagnosis. Gen Thorac Cardiovasc Surg. 2018;66(8):439–45.
58. Golledge J, Eagle KA. Acute aortic dissection. Lancet. 2008;372(9632):55–66.
59. Chen Z, Venkat P, Seyfried D, Chopp M, Yan T, Chen J. Brain-heart interaction: Cardiac complications after stroke. Circ Res. 2017;121(4):451–68.
60. Julio A, Chalela MAE, Davis L, Warach S. Myocardial injury in acute stroke. Neurocrit Care. 2004;1:343–6.
61. Oppenheimer SM, Hachinski VC. The cardiac consequences of stroke. Neurol Clin. 1992;10(1):167–76.
62. Cheung RT, Hachinski V. Cardiac effects of stroke. Curr Treat Options Cardiovasc Med. 2004;6(3):199–207.
63. Laowattana S, Zeger SL, Lima JA, Goodman SN, Wittstein IS, Oppenheimer SM. Left insular stroke is associated with adverse cardiac outcome. Neurology. 2006;66(4):477–83; discussion 63.
64. Abboud H, Berroir S, Labreuche J, Orjuela K, Amarenco P, Investigators G. Insular involvement in brain infarction increases risk for cardiac arrhythmia and death. Ann Neurol. 2006;59(4):691–9.
65. Ay H, Koroshetz WJ, Benner T, Vangel MG, Melinosky C, Arsava EM, et al. Neuroanatomic correlates of stroke-related myocardial injury. Neurology. 2006;66(9):1325–9.
66. Sposato LA, Hilz MJ, Aspberg S, Murthy SB, Bahit MC, Hsieh CY, et al. Post-stroke cardiovascular complications and neurogenic Cardiac injury: JACC state-of-the-art review. J Am Coll Cardiol. 2020;76(23):2768–85.
67. Gopinath R, Ayya SS. Neurogenic stress cardiomyopathy: what do we need to know. Ann Card Anaesth. 2018;21(3):228–34.
68. Jacob WA, Van Bogaert A, De Groodt-Lasseel MH. Myocardial ultrastructure and haemodynamic reactions during experimental subarachnoid haemorrhage. J Mol Cell Cardiol. 1972;4(4):287–98.
69. Bugnicourt JM, Rogez V, Guillaumont MP, Rogez JC, Canaple S, Godefroy O. Troponin levels help predict new-onset atrial fibrillation in ischaemic stroke patients: a retrospective study. Eur Neurol. 2010;63(1):24–8.
70. Wybraniec MT, Mizia-Stec K, Krzych L. Neurocardiogenic injury in subarachnoid hemorrhage: a wide spectrum of catecholamin-mediated brain-heart interactions. Cardiol J. 2014;21(3):220–8.
71. Samuels MA. The brain-heart connection. Circulation. 2007;116(1):77–84.
72. Morris NA, Chatterjee A, Adejumo OL, Chen M, Merkler AE, Murthy SB, et al. The risk of Takotsubo cardiomyopathy in acute neurological disease. Neurocrit Care. 2019;30(1):171–6.
73. Kenigsberg BB, Barnett CF, Mai JC, Chang JJ. Neurogenic stunned myocardium in severe neurological injury. Curr Neurol Neurosci Rep. 2019;19(11):90.
74. Chua HC, Sen S, Cosgriff RF, Gerstenblith G, Beauchamp NJ Jr, Oppenheimer SM. Neurogenic ST depression in stroke. Clin Neurol Neurosurg. 1999;101(1):44–8.
75. Mukerji S, Aloka F, Farooq MU, Kassab MY, Abela GS. Cardiovascular complications of the Guillain-Barre syndrome. Am J Cardiol. 2009;104(10):1452–5.
76. Devinsky O, Price BH, Cohen SI. Cardiac manifestations of complex partial seizures. Am J Med. 1986;80(2):195–202.
77. Battaglini D, Robba C, Lopes da Silva A, Dos Santos SC, Leme Silva P, Dal Pizzol F, et al. Brain-heart interaction after acute ischemic stroke. Crit Care. 2020;24(1):163.
78. Meloux A, Bejot Y, Rochette L, Cottin Y, Vergely C. Brain-heart interactions during ischemic processes: clinical and experimental evidences. Stroke. 2020;51(2):679–86.
79. Gregory T, Smith M. Cardiovascular complications of brain injury. Continu Educ Anaesth Crit Care Pain. 2012;12(2):67–71.
80. Zazulia A. Critical care management of acute ischeic stroke. Continuum Lifelong Learn Neurol. 2009;15:68–82.
81. Frontera JA, Parra A, Shimbo D, Fernandez A, Schmidt JM, Peter P, et al. Cardiac arrhythmias after subarachnoid hemorrhage: risk factors and impact on outcome. Cerebrovasc Dis. 2008;26(1):71–8.
82. Togha M, Sharifpour A, Ashraf H, Moghadam M, Sahraian MA. Electrocardiographic abnormalities in acute cerebrovascular events in patients with/without cardiovascular disease. Ann Indian Acad Neurol. 2013;16(1):66–71.
83. Daniele OCG, Fierro B, Natalè E. Stroke and cardiac arrhythmias. J Stroke Cerebrovasc Dis. 2002;11(1):28–33.
84. Kallmunzer B, Breuer L, Kahl N, Bobinger T, Raaz-Schrauder D, Huttner HB, et al. Serious cardiac arrhythmias after stroke: incidence, time course, and predictors—a systematic, prospective analysis. Stroke. 2012;43(11):2892–7.
85. Ruthirago D, Julayanont P, Tantrachoti P, Kim J, Nugent K. Cardiac arrhythmias and abnormal electrocardiograms after acute stroke. Am J Med Sci. 2016;351(1):112–8.
86. Cushing H, Concerning A. Definite regulatory mechanism of the Vaso-motor Centre which controls blood pressure during cerebral compression. Bull Johns Hopkins Hosp. 1901;12:290–2.
87. O'Keefe JH, Hammill SC, Freed MS, Pogwizd SM. The complete guide to ECGs. 3rd ed. Sudbury, MA: Physcians' Press; 2008. p. 556.
88. Faried A, Sendjaja AN, Melia R, Arifin MZ. Bradycardia without hypertension and bradypnea in acute traumatic subdural hema-

toma is a sensitive predictor of the Cushing triad: 3 case reports. Interdiscip Neurosurg. 2016;6:84–6.

89. Flachenecker P. Autonomic dysfunction in Guillain-Barre syndrome and multiple sclerosis. J Neurol. 2007;254(Suppl 2):II96–101.
90. Lehmann KG, Lane JG, Peipmeier JM, Batsford WP. Cardiovascular abnormalities accompanying acute spinal cord injury in humans: incidence, time course and severity. J Am Coll Cardiol. 1987;10:46.
91. Page R, Joglar J, Caldwell M, et al. 2015 ACC/AHA/HRS guideline for the Management of Adult Patients with Supraventricular Tachycardia. J Am Coll Cardiol. 2016;67(13):e27–e115.
92. Park S, Kim DG, Suh GY, Park WJ, Jang SH, Hwang YI, et al. Significance of new-onset prolonged sinus tachycardia in a medical intensive care unit: a prospective observational study. J Crit Care. 2011;26(5):534 e1–8.
93. Zheng RZ, Lei ZQ, Yang RZ, Huang GH, Zhang GM. Identification and management of paroxysmal sympathetic hyperactivity after traumatic brain injury. Front Neurol. 2020;11:81.
94. Brugada J, Katritsis DG, Arbelo E, Arribas F, Bax JJ, Blomstrom-Lundqvist C, et al. 2019 ESC guidelines for the management of patients with supraventricular tachycardia The task force for the management of patients with supraventricular tachycardia of the European Society of Cardiology (ESC). Eur Heart J. 2020;41(5):655–720.
95. Ganz L, Friedman P. Supraventricular tachycardia. N Engl J Med. 1995;332(3):162–73.
96. O'Keefe JH, Hammill SC, Freed MS. The complete guide to ECGs. 4th ed. Burlington, MA: Jones & Bartlett Learning; 2016. p. 615.
97. Kornej J, Borschel CS, Benjamin EJ, Schnabel RB. Epidemiology of atrial fibrillation in the 21st century: novel methods and new insights. Circ Res. 2020;127(1):4–20.
98. January CT, Wann LS, Alpert JS, Calkins H, Cigarroa JE, Cleveland JC Jr, et al. 2014 AHA/ACC/HRS guideline for the management of patients with atrial fibrillation: a report of the American College of Cardiology/American Heart Association task force on practice guidelines and the Heart Rhythm Society. Circulation. 2014;130(23):e199–267.
99. January CT, Wann LS, Calkins H, Chen LY, Cigarroa JE, Cleveland JC Jr, et al. 2019 AHA/ACC/HRS focused update of the 2014 AHA/ACC/HRS guideline for the management of patients with atrial fibrillation: a report of the American College of Cardiology/American Heart Association task force on clinical practice guidelines and the Heart Rhythm Society in collaboration with the Society of Thoracic Surgeons. Circulation. 2019;140(2):e125–e51.
100. Ding WY, Mahida S. Wide complex tachycardia: differentiating ventricular tachycardia from supraventricular tachycardia. Heart. 2021;107(24):1995–2003.
101. Al-Khatib SM, Stevenson WG, Ackerman MJ, Bryant WJ, Callans DJ, Curtis AB, et al. 2017 AHA/ACC/HRS guideline for management of patients with ventricular arrhythmias and the prevention of sudden cardiac death: a report of the American College of Cardiology/American Heart Association task force on clinical practice guidelines and the Heart Rhythm Society. Heart Rhythm. 2018;15(10):e73–e189.
102. Colivicchi F, Bassi A, Santini M, Caltagirone C. Prognostic implications of right-sided insular damage, Cardiac autonomic derangement, and arrhythmias after acute ischemic stroke. Stroke. 2005;36(8):1710–5.
103. Koppikar S, Baranchuk A, Guzman JC, Morillo CA. Stroke and ventricular arrhythmias. Int J Cardiol. 2013;168(2):653–9.
104. Garzon ME, Fuhrmann KM, McLouth CJ, Vachharajani VT, Datar SV. Predictors of ventricular dysrhythmias in neurology intensive care unit patients with prolonged QTc. Neurocrit Care. 2020;33(3):769–75.
105. Priori SG, Blomstrom-Lundqvist C, Mazzanti A, Blom N, Borggrefe M, Camm J, et al. 2015 ESC guidelines for the management of patients with ventricular arrhythmias and the prevention of sudden cardiac death: the task force for the management of patients with ventricular arrhythmias and the prevention of sudden cardiac death of the European Society of Cardiology (ESC). Endorsed by: Association for European Paediatric and Congenital Cardiology (AEPC). Eur Heart J. 2015;36(41):2793–867.

Bodily Water and Electrolyte Abnormalities in Neurological Disease

13

Olanrewaju Olaoye, Gajapathiraju Chamarthi, Maryam Rahman, and Azra Bihorac

Contents

Abstract

Bodily water and electrolyte abnormalities can significantly impact the clinical course of patients with neurological diseases. Specifically, hypo- and hypernatremia are common in this subset of patients and the understanding of the pathophysiology involved in each case, and its optimal management, determine the outcome of the individual patients. The diagnosis and treatment algorithms for the

O. Olaoye · G. Chamarthi · A. Bihorac (✉)
Division of Nephrology, Hypertension and Renal Transplantation, Department of Medicine, College of Medicine, University of Florida, Gainesville, FL, USA
e-mail: abihorac@ufl.edu

M. Rahman
Department of Neurological Surgery, University of Florida College of Medicine, Gainesville, FL, USA

E. Mahanna Gabrielli et al. (eds.), *Textbook of Neurointensive Care: Volume 1*, https://doi.org/10.1007/978-3-031-62220-5_13

management of bodily water and sodium disturbances in patients with neurological diseases are discussed in this chapter. Also included are disorders of potassium, calcium, phosphorus, and magnesium homeostasis.

Goals of This Chapter

- To review the homeostasis of bodily water, serum osmolality, and plasma sodium.
- To enumerate the pathophysiology of these regulatory mechanisms leading to bodily water and sodium disorders.
- To define the proneness of patients with central nervous system disorders, or brain trauma, leading to disruption of these homeostatic mechanisms.
- To diagnose and systematically manage the most common dyselectrolytemia encountered in critical care medicine (Hyponatremia and Hypernatremia) in regard to under versus excessive correction and the potential complications.
- To recognize the life-threatening cardiac manifestations of potassium disorders and their management.
- To manage magnesium, calcium, and phosphorus disorders in the critical care setting.

Introduction

Dyselectrolytemias may develop rapidly in patients in the neurointensive care unit (neuro-ICU) and can significantly impact their disease course. Primary or secondary injuries, diseases, or surgery, affecting the anatomical component(s) of the hypothalamic-pituitary-adrenal (HPA) axis, play significant roles in leading to the pathophysiologic mechanisms underlying the manifestations of fluid and electrolyte abnormalities, typically encountered in neuro-ICU patients. The disturbance of sodium and water homeostasis can have grave consequences for patients with neurological problems. In this chapter, we will discuss the basic elements that maintain homeostasis and then address specific electrolyte abnormalities, their management, and potential outcomes. Clinical scenarios will be used to emphasize certain clinical points.

Pathophysiology of Bodily Water and Sodium Balance

Disorders of bodily water homeostasis, biochemically recognized as abnormalities of plasma sodium concentration, mostly hyponatremia, and to a lesser extent hypernatremia, are the most common fluid and electrolyte disorder worldwide [1]. Hyponatremia, even when mild, is associated with increased mortality [2] and potentially poses a grave impact on neurological and neurosurgical patients. The homeostatic processes are recruited to correct bodily water imbalance, determine plasma sodium concentration, and the understanding of these mechanisms is critical to clinical diagnosis of sodium disorders. Water constitutes between 50 and 60% of total body weight depending on age and gender. Total body water (TBW) is divided into two major compartments within the body: 2/3 in the intracellular space (ICS) and 1/3 in the extracellular space (ECS). The ECS fluid is further divided into the intravascular compartment (1/3), and the interstitium (2/3) (Fig. 13.1).

Water moves between the ICS and the ECS in response to osmotic forces exerted across the semipermeable cellular membrane, which are determined by the concentration of solute particles in the fluid. The osmotic activity of the solutes is usually measured as serum osmolality defined as the number of solutes per kilogram of water (mOsm/kg H_2O). The major solutes determining plasma osmolality are sodium (mMol/L), blood urea nitrogen/ BUN (mg/dL), and glucose (mg/dL). The calculated serum osmolality can differ from the actual or directly measured osmolality due to other osmotically active exogenous solutes, such as alcohol, resulting in "osmolar gap." The equation to calculate estimated serum osmolality is:

$$\text{Serum Osmolality}\,(\text{mOsm}/\text{kg}\,\text{H}_2\text{O}) = 2(\text{Na}) + \text{BUN}/2.8 + \text{glucose}/18$$

The differences in osmolality between the ICS and ECS separated by semipermeable cellular membrane, create an osmotic gradient. The *osmotic gradient* contributes to the effective osmolality or tonicity and dictates fluid shifts between compartments. *Sodium* in the ICS and ECS (Fig. 13.1b) is the major determinant of tonicity since it cannot freely diffuse across the cellular membrane. Conversely, BUN diffuses easily through the cell membrane and will rapidly equilibrate between the ICS and ECS, even in the face of azotemia (Fig. 13.1c). Given that the total plasma sodium content is the principal determinant of the relative volumes of the ICS and ECS, mechanisms aimed at regulating effective circulating volumes are involved in the maintenance of stable plasma sodium concentration. On the other hand, mechanisms aimed at the regulation of water balance, maintain a relatively constant plasma tonicity. Bodily water and sodium balance are regulated through different systems. Osmoreceptors and hypothalamic-

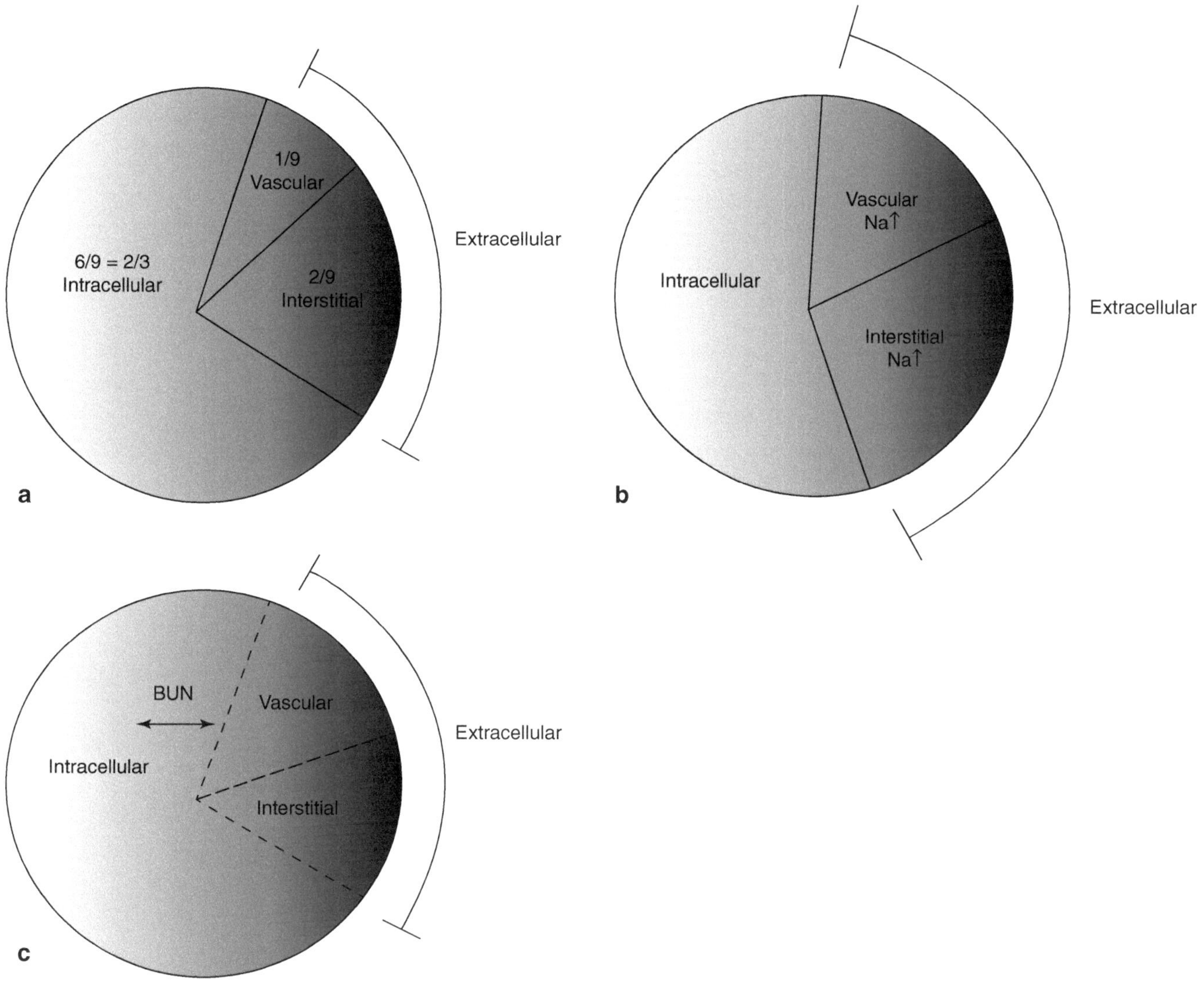

Fig. 13.1 Total body water: (**a**) Total body water can be divided into the intracellular and extracellular fluid compartments. The extracellular fluid compartment can be further divided into the vascular and interstitial compartments. Sodium cannot freely diffuse across the cell membrane and is a major determinant of tonicity (**b**). Therefore, as extracellular Na increases,the water content in the extracellular space increases as well. (**c**) Because blood urea nitrogen (BUN) diffuses easily through the cell membrane, it allows for equilibration between the intracellular and extracellular compartments if the extracellular Na increases or decreases; Adapted from our previously authored chapter in the last edition of this book

pituitary axis control plasma tonicity, while baroreceptors, in conjunction with multiple vasopressors, hormones, vascular system, and kidneys, constitute short and long-term responses to changes in effective circulating volumes through sodium conservation and excretion.

Plasma tonicity is strictly regulated by water intake and loss, primarily by thirst and the ability of renal tubules to conserve or excrete water. Water loss that cannot be controlled physiologically includes "insensible losses" through the skin and lungs, as well as some losses through the gastrointestinal tract. The losses can add up; a normal 70-kg person loses approximately 1.5 L/day of water. If this volume is not offset by at least the same volume of water, plasma tonicity increases. Osmolality of ECS fluid (ECF), including plasma, is tightly regulated between 280 and 290 mOsm/kg. Changes in ECF osmolality can cause water to flow across cell membranes to equilibrate the osmolality of the cytoplasm with that of the ECF potentially leading through alteration of cell volume and intracellular ionic strength to cell death. Hence, in response to changes in plasma osmolality, humans promptly engage in a myriad of physiological responses that actively oppose osmotic perturbations and serve to restore ECF osmolality towards a seemingly fixed osmotic "set point" near 300 mOsm/kg [3]. An increase in ECF osmolality stimulates the sense of thirst, to promote water intake, and release of vasopressin (VP; also known as antidiuretic hormone, ADH), to enhance water reabsorption in the kidney. In contrast, ECF hypo-osmolality suppresses basal VP secretion in humans [4, 5]. Because renal reabsorption is partly stimulated by VP levels at rest [4], this inhibition of VP release effectively stimulates diuresis. This osmoregulatory response is initiated by the peripheral and central osmoreceptors that provide a sensory mechanism that can detect osmotic perturbations in the ECF. Peripheral osmoreceptors exist along the upper regions of the alimentary tract and in the blood vessels that collect solutes absorbed from the intestines, including the oropharyngeal cavity [6], the gastrointestinal tract [7], the splanchnic mesentery [8], the hepatic portal vein, and the liver [9].

The primary central osmoreceptors that modulate thirst and VP release are located in regions of the brain that are devoid of a blood–brain barrier, such as the hypothalamus and circumventricular organs [10, 11], and the neurons in the *organum vasculosum laminae terminalis* (OVLT) and subfornical organ, as well as magnocellular neurosecretory cells (MNCs) in the hypothalamic supraoptic nucleus (SON) [12, 13], have been proposed to serve as primary osmoreceptors in humans [14, 15].

Information derived from peripheral and cerebral osmoreceptors is transmitted to a subset of MNCs located in the paraventricular nucleus (PVN) and hypothalamic SON, which are involved in the synthesis of a nine amino acid peptide hormone arginine vasopressin (AVP), a major regulator of free water excretion by the kidney (Fig. 13.2).

The firing rate of MNCs that prevails under resting conditions (~1–3 Hz) mediates basal VP secretion, whereas

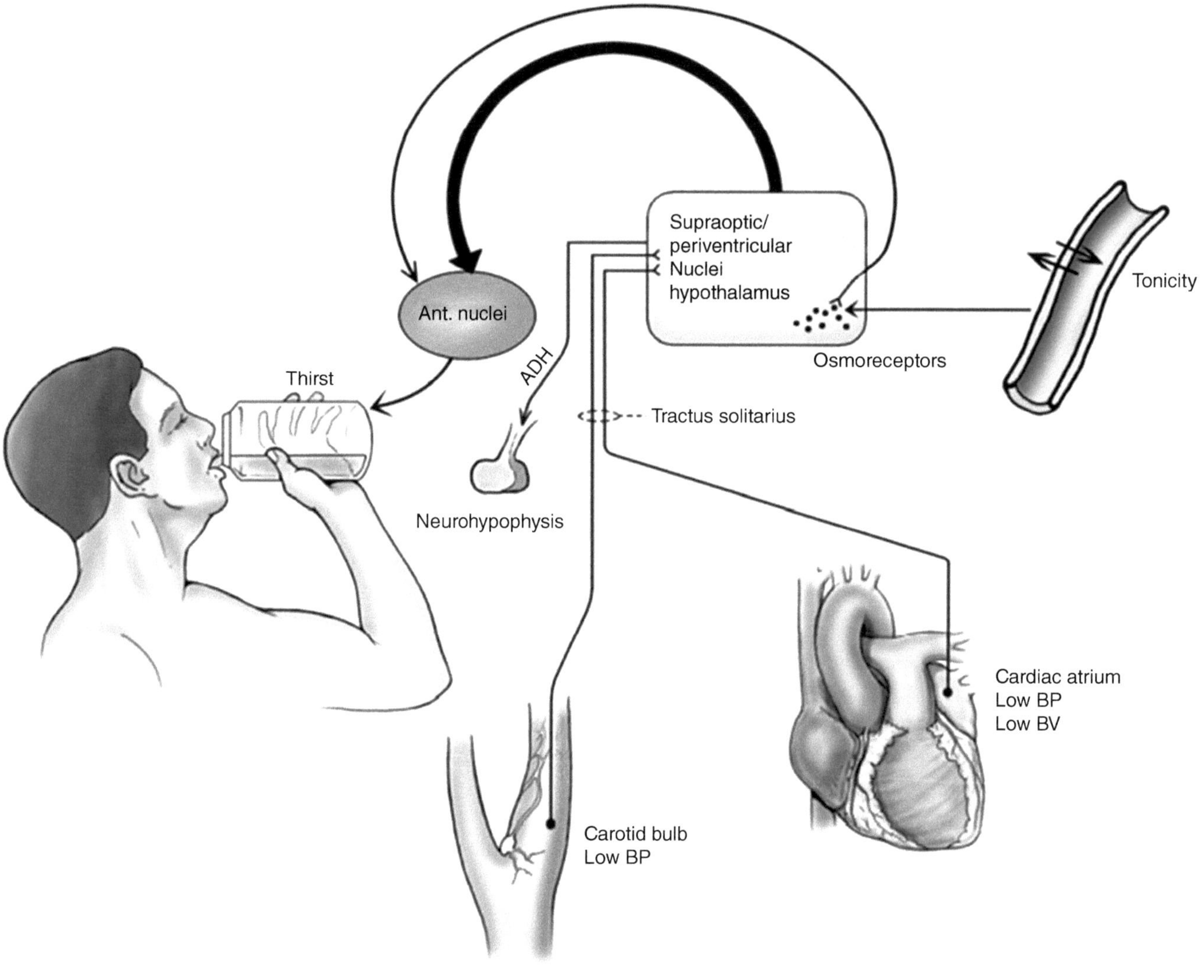

Fig. 13.2 Sodium physiology: Osmoreceptors in the hypothalamus and circumventricular organs sense increases in plasma tonicity as well as decreases in circulating volume, either because of true volume loss or a low perfusion state such as cardiac failure. These osmoreceptors induce thirst via the anterior nucleus of the thalamus to increase water intake. They also send efferents to the supraoptic and paraventricular hypothalamic nuclei. These neurons produce antidiuretic hormone (ADH), which is transported to the neurohypophysis and secreted to take its effect in the kidney for water retention; Ant nuclei anterior nucleus of the thalamus, BP blood pressure, BV blood volume (Used with permission of David Peace, Medical Illustrator, University of Florida School of Medicine, Department of Neurosurgery)

decreases/increases in firing frequency inhibit/enhance hormone release during ECF hypotonicity/hypertonicity, respectively [16]. The synthesized peptide is enzymatically cleaved from its prohormone and is stored within neurosecretory granules. The increase in plasma osmolality causes the secretion of AVP into the bloodstream, leading to the activation of AVP V2 receptors in the kidney and insertion of aquaporin-2 water channels into the apical membranes of collecting tubule principal cells [17]. As a result, the increase in water permeability of the collecting duct allows free water conservation and restores the plasma osmolality set point towards normal limits.

Regulation of Sodium and Effective Plasma Volume

Maintenance of sodium (Na^+) homeostasis theoretically requires a balance between intake and excretion of Na^+ but the challenges posed by the infeasible tight regulation of sodium intake, place emphasis on the renal excretion of Na^+ as the main mechanism to ensure its homeostasis [18]. Since Na^+ ensures maintenance of the ECS volume and directly supports blood pressure, the mechanisms for renal excretion of sodium are numerous and substantially more complex than those involved in the regulation of water balance. Renal Na^+ excretion varies directly with the effective circulating volume from urine Na^+ concentration, which is as low as 1 mMol/L with effective volume expansion [19]. The changes in renal Na^+ excretion can result from alterations in the filtered load, determined by the glomerular filtration rate (GFR) and in tubular reabsorption, which is affected by multiple factors including the renin-angiotensin-aldosterone system (RAAS) and natriuretic hormones, i.e., atrial natriuretic peptide (ANP) and urodilatin [20]. Low effective circulating volume also induces release of renin and norepinephrine. Renin leads to the conversion of angiotensin I to angiotensin II, which increases sodium reabsorption at the proximal tubule. The resulting aldosterone release causes reabsorption of sodium by the distal tubule and collecting duct. The norepinephrine causes a decrease in GFR and stimulates sodium reabsorption at the proximal tubule. All these mechanisms lead to increased sodium and water retention with resultant increase in circulating volume. In contrast, expansion of the ECS volume results in an appropriate increase in urinary Na^+ excretion induced by suppression of RAAS, a small elevation in GFR, and an effect of natriuretic hormones. ANP is primarily released from the atria in response volume expansion, which appears to be sensed as an increase in atrial stretch [21]. It causes an increase in GFR without raising renal blood flow, directly reduces sodium reabsorption in the inner medullary collecting duct by closing the Na^+ channels, and diminishes sodium reabsorption in the proximal tubule through the local release of dopamine.

Hyponatremia

Hyponatremia is the most common electrolyte disorder encountered in clinical medicine [22]. Approximately 1 million hospitalizations per year in the USA have a principal or secondary diagnosis of hyponatremia. The annual cost of managing patients with hyponatremia has been estimated at $3.6 billion [22]. In addition to monetary costs, hyponatremia is associated with adverse outcomes for patients. Specifically, the mortality rates are significantly higher in hyponatremic patients across a broad range of primary disorders [23]. In some disease states, such as congestive heart failure, hyponatremia is an independent risk factor for increased mortality [24, 25].

The prevalence of hyponatremia in the neurosurgical population has been reported as high as 50% [26–28]. Due to the cerebral effects of hyponatremia, neurosurgical patients are at increased risk for complications such as severe cerebral edema, mental status changes, seizures, vasospasm, and death. Unfortunately, these complications may also arise from the inappropriate treatment of hyponatremia. Correction of hyponatremia that is too slow or too fast can lead to cerebral edema, seizures, osmotic demyelinating syndrome, or death [29, 30].

Despite the costs and complications associated with hyponatremia in the neurosurgical population, few randomized studies have been completed, describing when hyponatremia becomes clinically significant and how it should be treated. The evaluation and treatment are left to the discretion of the individual healthcare provider or treatment team. This lack of standardized treatment approach contributes to variable outcomes.

Evaluation/Diagnostic Workup of Hyponatremia

Hyponatremia is classically defined as serum sodium (sNa) of less than 135 mMol/L meanwhile clinically significant hyponatremia has not been clearly defined [22, 31]. Hyponatremia is associated with increased mortality [32, 33]. Hyponatremia in patients with subarachnoid hemorrhage (SAH) has a clear association with increased morbidity. Increased rates of cerebral ischemia have been documented in SAH patients with hyponatremia [34, 35]. Through our literature review of the symptomatology of hyponatremia in the last edition of this book, we observed that the evidence indicating clinically significant sNa level varies. Based on our experience, we recommended a diagnostic workup in neurosurgical patients with sNa of less than 131 mMol/L. Going forward, we still stand by that recommendation.

Diagnostic workup for hyponatremia should be guided by the suspected cause(s), which traditionally have been categorized by body fluid status. There is no standard reference test for hyponatremia evaluation, and this often leads to inadequate diagnostic workup including failure to check plasma osmolality (P_{osm}), urine Na (uNa), and urine osmolality (U_{osm}). In a retrospective study of 104 patients with a sNa of less than 125 mMol/L, osmolality was measured in only 26% of patients. Mortality was higher in the group with inadequate workup and management (41% versus 20%, $p = 0.002$) [36]. Most experts have previously proposed a combination of physical exam (PE) findings and laboratory tests to distinguish between the etiologies of hyponatremia [27, 29, 31, 37–39]. This approach has been described to be important in distinguishing between hyponatremic etiologies like syndrome of inappropriate antidiuresis (SIAD; *changed from "syndrome of inappropriate ADH secretion-SIADH" based on the evolved understanding of the pathophysiology*) and cerebral salt wasting (CSW).

In our practice, we continue to find another tool, *point-of-care ultrasound* (POCUS) exams, very resourceful in buttressing physical exam findings in the evaluation of fluid status of neurological patients. With other centers sharing the same experience [40], we hereby recommend incorporating POCUS volume status exams as part of complete evaluation of hyponatremic neurological patients.

Neurosurgery patients often develop hyponatremia in the setting of natriuresis. *Hyponatremia with natriuresis* is caused by either SIAD or CSW once diuretic use has been excluded. Criteria for SIAD proposed by Janicic et al. include P_{osm} less than 275 mOsm/kg, inappropriate urinary concentration (U_{osm} greater than 100 mOsm/kg), clinical euvolemia (absence of orthostasis, tachycardia, decreased skin turgor, dry mucous membranes, or edema/ascites), elevated urinary Na excretion with normal salt and water intake, and absence of other causes of euvolemic hypo-osmolality (hypothyroidism, hypocortisolism). However, these criteria have proven to be inadequate in distinguishing between SIAD and CSW. Ten of 12 neurosurgery patients in a prospective study who met the lab criteria for SIAD (serum Na <135 mMol/L, P_{osm} <280 mOsm/kg, uNa >25 mMol/L, and U_{osm} >than P_{osm}) had low blood cell mass, plasma volume, and total blood volume compared to controls [41]. ECF status is the key to distinguishing between SIAD and CSW [37, 41–44]. The determination of ECF status using a physical exam alone has been shown to be inaccurate [43, 45]. A prospective study of 35 patients with a sNa less than 130 mMol/L was divided into four groups (those who had received diuretics, polydipsic patients, saline responders, and saline nonresponders). Saline responders were patients who had a sustained increase in sNa of at least 5 mMol/L. All patients were initially determined to be hypo- or normo-volemic based on PE findings (mucosal hydration, skin tugor, jugular vein distention), orthostatic changes in pulse (increase of 10% upright compared to supine), and systolic blood pressure (decrease of 10% upright compared to supine). The saline responders and those who had received diuretics were considered the true hypovolemic patients. Clinical determination of ECF status using PE finding parameters had a sensitivity of 41.1% and a specificity of 80%.

We propose that *the absence*, or *the presence*, of POCUS findings *like hyperdynamic left ventricle, collapsible inferior vena cava* (IVC), and supportive *venous excess ultrasonographic* (VExUS) *score*, will further distinguish between *neurological hyponatremic SIAD* or *CSW*, respectively.

Based on several studies about hyponatremia evaluation, a uNa of less than 30 mMol/L has a positive predictive value of 71%–100% for an infusion of 0.9% saline to increase the sNa level [44, 46]. Uric acid has also been used to distinguish SIAD from other etiologies of hyponatremia. In the study of saline responsiveness in hyponatremia patients, the polydipsic and nonresponsive patients tended to have lower plasma urea and uric acid compared to the other two groups [46]. A serum uric acid level of less than 4 mg/dL (in the presence of hyponatremia) has been shown to have a positive predictive value for SIAD of 73%–100%. However, the definitions for SIAD used in these studies were broad and most likely included patients with CSW [47].

To distinguish between SIAD and CSW, central venous pressure (CVP) can also be used to determine intravascular volume status. Damaraju et al. treated hyponatremia based on CVP values (<5 cm H_2O; 6–10 cm H_2O; >10 cm H_2O). Hypovolemic patients (CVP <5 cm H_2O) were given normal saline (50 mL/kg/day) and salt (12 g/d). Normovolemic patients (CVP 6–10 cm H_2O) were given normal saline with 12 g of salt per day. In addition, patients with anemia (hematocrit <27%) were administered whole blood. No patients were found to be hypervolemic (CVP >10 cm H_2O). Seventy-three percent of patients corrected their sNa within 72 hours, and 12% more within the following 24–48 hours. The patients included three nonresponders, and two of these were found to have severe dehydration on blood volume measurements [43].

The treatment of hyponatremia in SAH has generated controversy given the association of fluid restriction or dehydration with symptomatic vasospasm [35, 36]. Traditionally, hyponatremia in SAH patients has been attributed to SIAD

[27]. However, more recent studies show that hyponatremic SAH patients often demonstrate a negative Na balance (loss of Na in urine >Na intake per day) and lower ECF [34].

A general approach to the evaluation of hyponatremia is shown (Fig. 13.3 and Table 13.1). Using the evaluation paradigm, a sNa value of less than 131 mMol/L should prompt a workup that includes measuring serum and urine osmolarity, urine electrolytes, and an evaluation of ECF volume status. A normal or high serum osmolality may result from lab error, or pseudohyponatremia, e.g., hyperglycemia or hypertriglyceridemia. Hypotonic hyponatremia is categorized by ECF volume status. Volume status can be determined based on the criteria listed in Table 13.1. Hypovolemia results from extrarenal loss or intrarenal loss such as CSW, diuretics, or adrenal insufficiency. In normovolemic patients, thyroid disease, hypocortisolism, and polydipsia should be ruled out before a diagnosis of SIAD is given. Moreover, hypervolemic hyponatremia is less common in neurological patients, and the treatment team should rule out cirrhosis, congestive heart failure, and renal failure.

Table 13.1 Diagnostic criteria for CSW versus SIAD

	CSW	SIAD
S Na (mmol/L[a])	<135	<135
S Osm (mOsm/kg[a])	<285	<285
U Osm (mOsm/kg[a])	>200	>200
U Na (mmol/L)	>25	>25
Weight	↓	↑
Fluid balance	↓	↑
JVD	–	+
Hct	↑	↓
BUN	↓	↓
Cre	↑	↓
Uric acid	–↓	↓
Bicarb	↑	↓
CVP cm H_2O	<6	≥6
Pulm wedge pressure mmHg	<8	≥8

S Na Serum, *S Osm* Serum osmolality, *U Osm* Urine osmolality, *U Na* Urine sodium, *JVD* Jugular venous distension, *Hct* Hematocrit, *BUN* Blood urea nitrogen, *Cre* Creatinine, *Bicarb* Bicarbonate, *CVP* Central venous pressure, *pulm* Pulmonary
Adapted from our previously authored chapter in the last edition of this book
[a]Must have starred criteria and at least three of the non-starred criteria for diagnosis

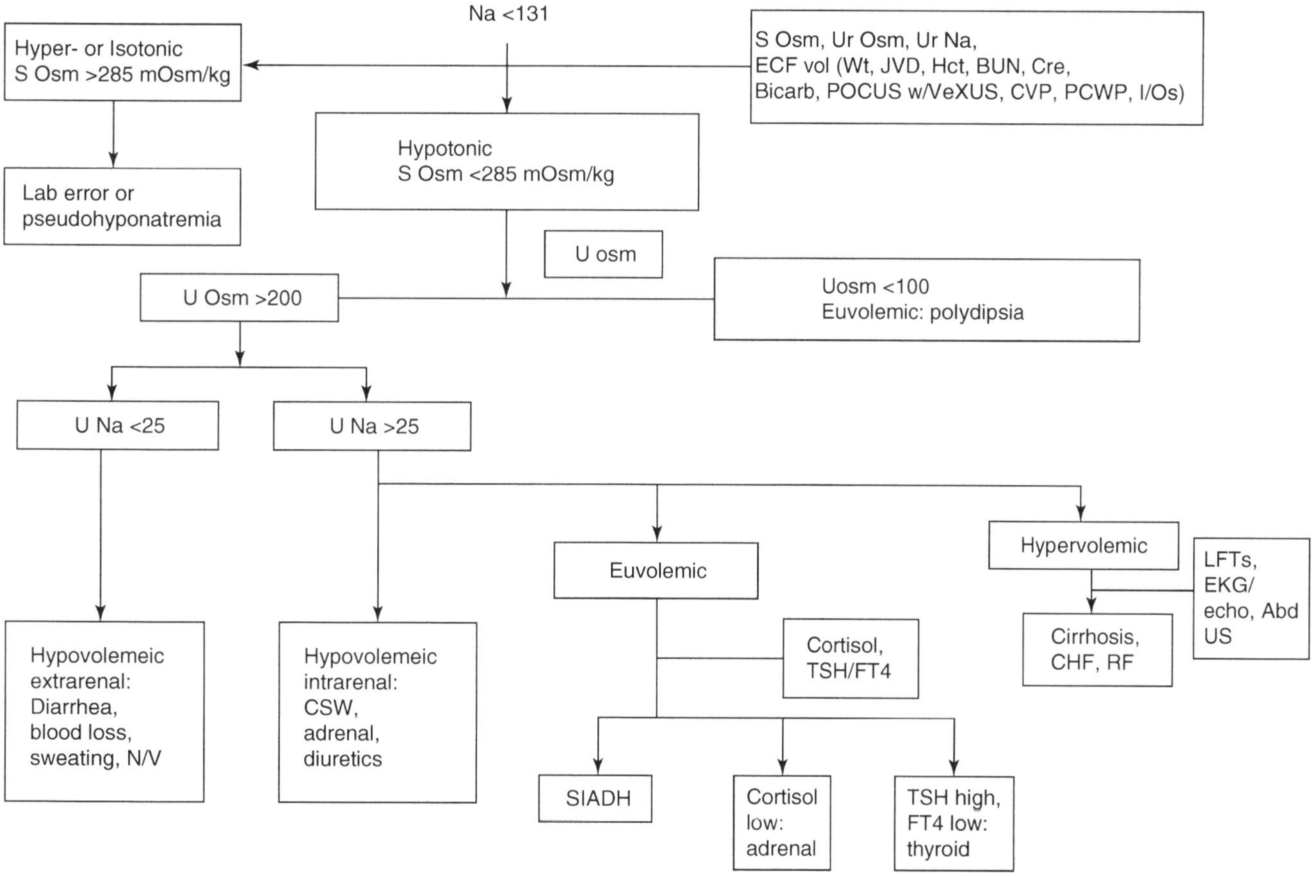

Fig. 13.3 Hyponatremia diagnostic protocol: Hyponatremic patients should undergo a workup including lab values and physical exam findings. Hypotonic hyponatremia can be categorized by volume status. *S* Serum, *Osm* Osmolarity, *Ur* Urine, *ECF* Extracellular fluid, *vol* Volume, *Wt* Weight, *JVD* Jugular venous distension, *Hct* Hematocrit, *BUN* Blood urea nitrogen, *Cre* Creatinine, *bicarb* Bicarbonate, *CVP* Central venous pressure, *PCWP* Pulmonary catheter wedge pressure, *I/Os* In and out, *N/V* Nausea and vomiting, *CSW* Cerebral salt wasting, adrenal insufficiency, *TSH* Thyroid stimulating hormone, *FT4* Free T4, *LFTs* Liver function tests, *EKG* Electrocardiogram, echo echocardiogram, *Abd* US abdominal ultrasound, *CHF* Congestive heart failure, *RF* Renal failure; Adapted from our previously authored chapter in the last edition of this book

Treatment of Hyponatremia (Figs. 13.4 and 13.5)

Generally, the rate of correction of hyponatremia is determined by the severity of symptoms and rapidity of onset. Studies have shown that the severity of hyponatremia symptoms correlates with the magnitude of hyponatremia and the rate of onset [23, 28]. Given the significant morbidity/mortality associated with severely symptomatic hyponatremia, evidence exists to correct symptomatic severe hyponatremia aggressively with hypertonic saline. This approach is based loosely on the idea that acute hyponatremia tends to be more symptomatic and that treatment complications happen in the setting of chronic hyponatremia [48, 49].

Central pontine myelinosis or osmotic demyelinating syndrome (ODS) is the most frequently cited complication in the treatment of hyponatremia. This entity was first described in the 1970s [50]. ODS is more likely to occur with correction of serum Na greater than 12 mMol/L/day and in the setting of chronic hyponatremia (>48 h) [30]. In a retrospective study of patients with ODS, all patients had chronic hyponatremia (prior to hospitalization) and a serum Na less than 110 mMol/L. All of the patients had their Na corrected faster than 12 mMol/L/day [51]. A review of the literature found that all of the patients with severe hyponatremia (Na <106 mMol/L) and Na correction greater than 12 mMol/L/day developed some type of neurological complication. No neurological complications developed in those who were corrected more slowly [51].

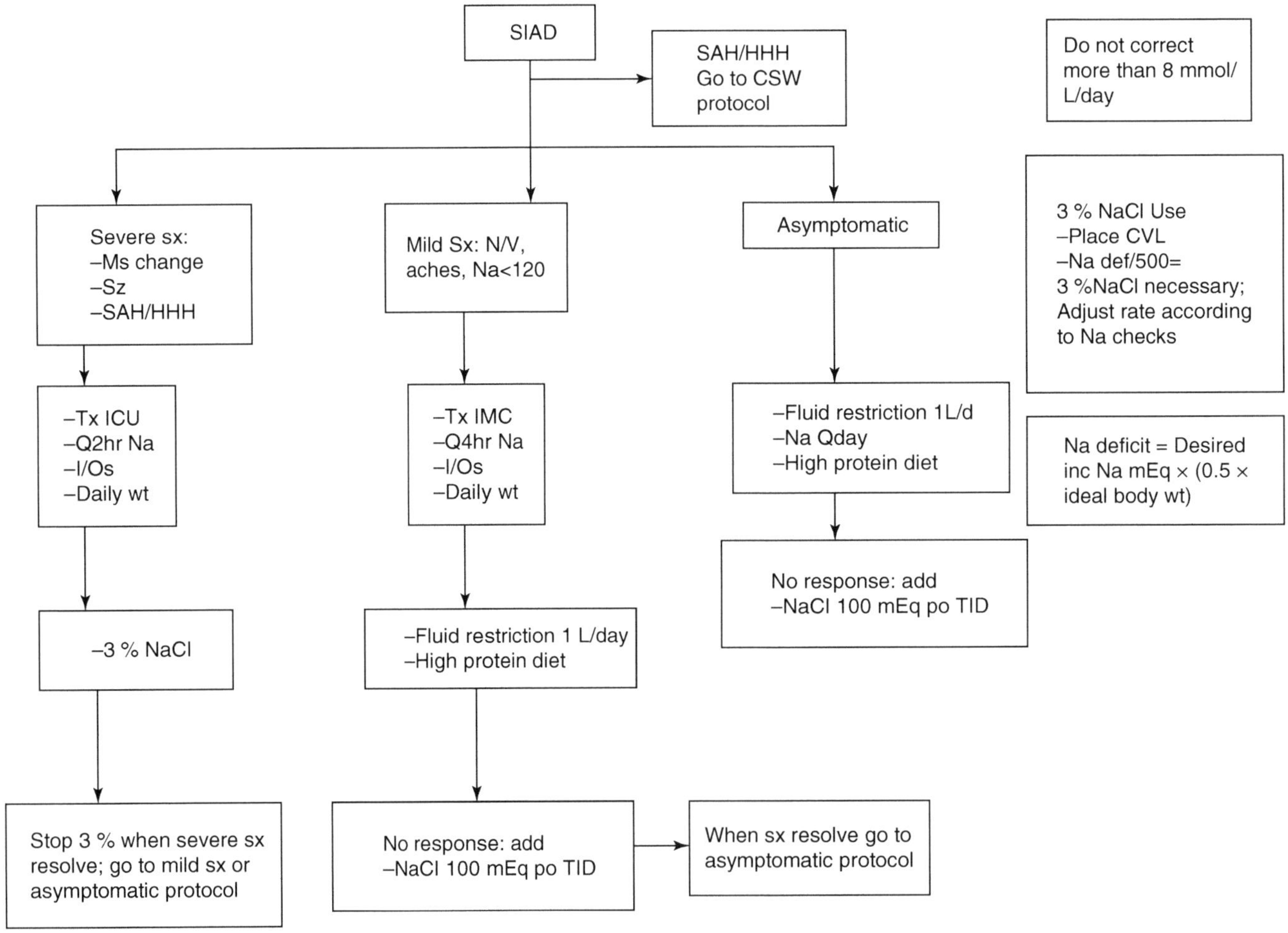

Fig. 13.4 Treatment of SIAD: Symptoms are used to guide the treatment of SIAD. Patients with severe symptoms or SAH at risk for vasospasm will receive hypertonic saline; otherwise, the cornerstone of treatment for SIAD is fluid restriction. Acute hyponatremia and/or severe symptoms should have 6 mmol/L corrected over 6 hours or until severe symptoms improve. The total correction of Na should not exceed 8 mmol/L over 24 hours. Therefore, if 6 mmol/L is corrected in 6 h, the Na should not be increased more than 2 mmol/L in the following 18 hours. The total correction of Na is based on the Na deficit which is calculated conservatively with the formula depicted. With improvement of symptoms, the patients can be moved to the less aggressive treatments in the algorithm, until Na reaches 131 mmol/L. *MS* Mental status, *sx* Symptoms, *sz* Seizure, *tx* Transfer, *ICU* Intensive care unit, *I/Os* In and out, *wt* Weight, *N/V* Nausea and vomiting, *IMC* Intermediate care unit, *CVL* Central venous line, *def* Deficit, *inc* Increase; Adapted from our previously authored chapter in the last edition of this book

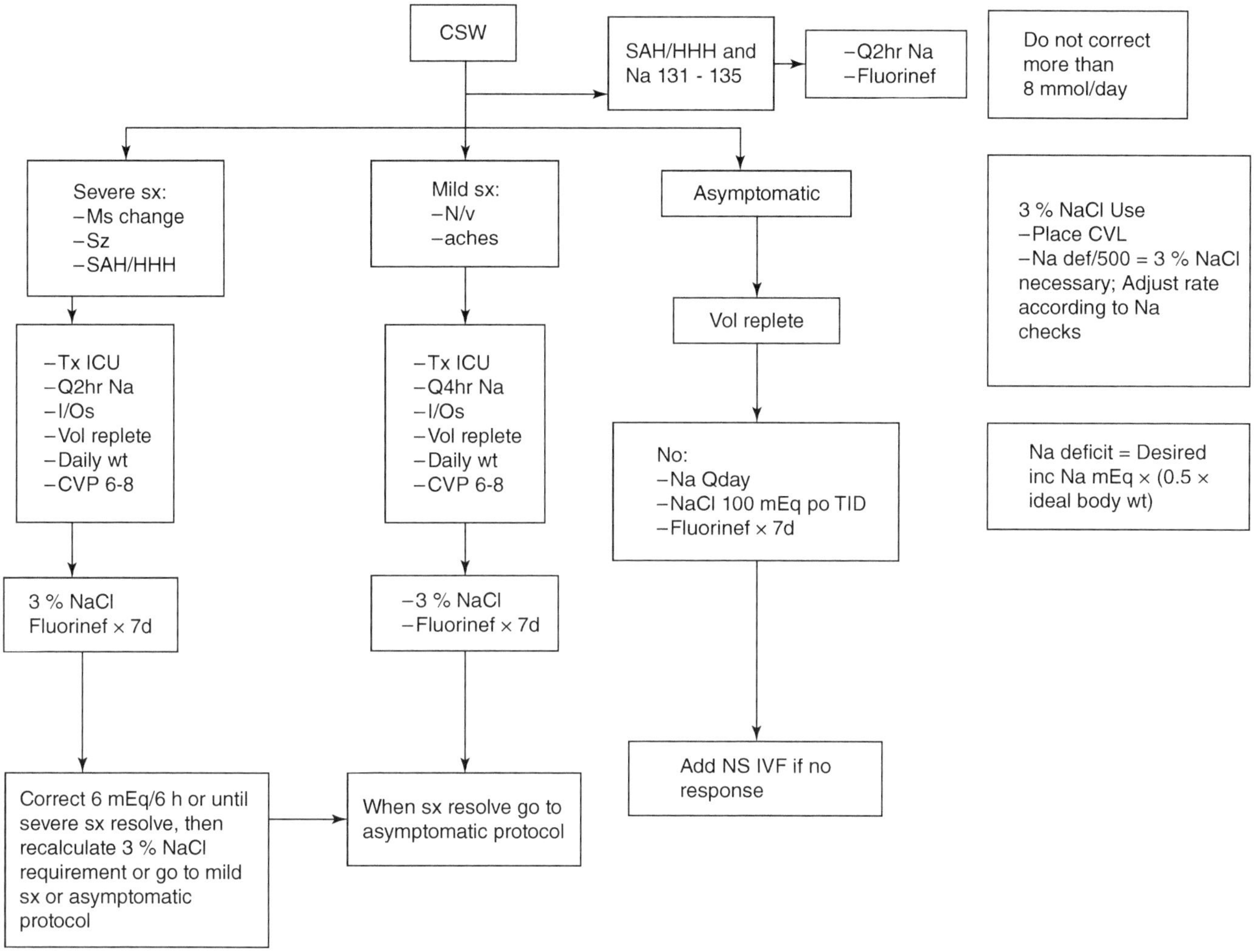

Fig. 13.5 Treatment of CSW: Once a diagnosis of CSW is confirmed, treatment is based on symptoms. Patients with severe symptoms should be treated in the ICU with hypertonic saline and fludrocortisone. Acute hyponatremia and/or severe symptoms should have 6 mmol/L corrected over 6 h or until severe symptoms improve. The total correction of Na should not exceed 8 mmol/L over 24 hours. Therefore, if 6 mmol/L is corrected in 6 hours, the Na should not be increased by more than 2 mmol/L in the following 18 hours. The total correction of Na is based on the Na deficit which is calculated conservatively with the formula depicted. With the improvement of symptoms, patients can be moved to the less aggressive treatments in the algorithm, until Na reaches 131 mmol/L. SAH patients are an exception and receive treatment even for a serum Na of 131–135 mmol/L. *HHH* Hypervolemia, hypertension, hemodilution, *sx* Symptoms, *MS* Mental status, *sz* Seizure, *Tx* Transfer, *ICU* Intensive care unit, *IMC* Intermediate care unit, *hr* Hour, *I/Os* In and out, *vol* Volume, *wt* Weight, *N/V* Nausea and vomiting, *U* Urine, *CVL* Central venous line, *def* Deficit, *inc* Increase, *NS* Normal saline, *IVF* Intravenous fluids; Adapted from our previously authored chapter in the last edition of this book

A prospective study of 33 medical patients with symptomatic hyponatremia (mean sNa of 108 mMol/L) showed no episodes of ODS despite an increase in mean sNa to 126 mMol/L within 48 hours [45]. The authors evaluated a group of 12 patients retrospectively, all of whom had evidence of cerebral demyelinating lesions at autopsy. The rate of correction of their hyponatremia was similar to the prospectively evaluated patients. However, they all had one of four characteristics: an increase in sNa to normal or hypernatremic levels within 48 h, a sNa change of more than 25 mMol/L within 48 hours, a hypoxic episode and/or hepatic encephalopathy [45]. Based on case reports and animal data, the development of ODS is associated with the rate and magnitude of Na correction in chronic hyponatremia (>48 hours), with hypokalemia, and with malnourished states (e.g. alcoholism, cirrhosis, burns) [50]. Chronic hyponatremia should not be rapidly corrected.

Generally, rapid correction at a rate of over 1 mMol/L/h should be reserved for severely symptomatic and/or acute hyponatremia (<48 h). Severe symptoms (e.g., seizures, coma) indicate cerebral edema and should trigger prompt treatment [50, 51]. A retrospective study of inpatients with sNa greater than 115 mMol/L demonstrated an increase in mortality in patients who had slower correction of their hyponatremia. The sNa after 48 hours of treatment was 127.1 mMol/L in survivors versus 118.8 mMol/L in patients who died (p = 0.0016) [25]. A general protocol for the treatment of SIADH and CSW in acute hyponatremia is provided (Figs. 13.4 and 13.5).

Hypernatremia

Hypernatremia, defined as a rise in the serum sodium concentration above 145 mMol/L, is a common electrolyte disorder that almost always results from a deficit of water in relation to total body sodium stores [52]. The water deficit occurs as a consequence of net water loss or a hypertonic sodium gain. The presence of hypernatremia does not signify that there is an excess of sodium content in the body as sodium stores may be either normal (in cases of pure water loss) or decreased (in cases of hypotonic fluids losses such as vomiting or diarrhea) [52].

Since sustained severe hypernatremia can only occur when thirst mechanisms or access to water are impaired, patients with altered mental status, intubated patients, infants, and elderly persons are at the highest risk for hypernatremia. Critically ill patients, particularly those in neurocritical care units frequently meet these conditions and are at the highest risk. Additionally, problems encountered with the patients' thirst mechanism including hypodipsia may be a part of neurological impairment. Furthermore, these patients may have excessive diaphoresis from agitation or fever, which can further exacerbate hypotonic fluid losses.

The effects of hypernatremia on the brain tissue cause the induction of a series of compensatory responses aimed at restoring brain volume. These involve the generation of osmotically active substances known as idiogenic osmoles or organic brain osmoles [53, 54]; this process is not immediate but occurs over hours to days [55]. Through the generation of the idiogenic osmoles, the brain becomes capable of maintaining volume at hyperosmolar states. Rapid overcorrection of hypernatremia, greater than 12 mMol/L/day, especially in the presence of chronic hyperosmolality, can render the brain incapable of eliminating the accumulated osmoles promptly enough, resulting in cerebral edema, generalized tonic-clonic seizures, coma, and death [56].

Assessment of the patients with hypernatremia should begin with an evaluation of the extracellular fluid volume. Attention should be focused on recent changes in body weight, the presence of peripheral edema, pulse rate, access to free water, hourly intake and output, intraoperative fluids, colloids, or blood products given, orthostatic changes in blood pressure, jugular venous distention, and POCUS with VeXUS findings. Initial assessment of hypernatremia should be evaluated with basic laboratory analysis, including sNa and serum osmolality, as well as uNa and urine osmolality, and specific gravity.

A low uNa concentration of less than 10 mMol/L, in addition to other clinical signs of hypervolemia, would suggest decreased extracellular fluid volume. A fractional excretion of sodium (FeNa) lower than 1% is suggestive of volume depletion in non-edematous patients.

Hypernatremia with low extracellular fluid volume implies a loss of hypotonic fluids and usually implies that major route of water loss in extrarenal. Excessive diuresis, vomiting, and diarrhea are the usual suspects in these situations. Hypernatremia with normal extracellular fluid volume indicates a loss of free water. Diabetes insipidus should be excluded and the appropriateness of the tonicity of fluids for ongoing replacement reassessed [57]. Hypernatremia with high extracellular fluid volume results from a gain of hypertonic fluids. It is usually iatrogenic, secondary to the use of hypertonic NaCl and $NaHCO_3$ solutions or hypertonic feeding associated with osmotic diuresis, but it can also occur in cases of mineralocorticoid excess.

Clinical Manifestation of Hypernatremia

Hypernatremia usually becomes symptomatic only when the sNa concentration exceeds 160 mMol/L [58]. However, the rapidity of the elevation of sNa levels is equally important. With rapid elevation, stupor emerges more frequently. The signs and symptoms of hypernatremia mostly reflect central nervous system dysfunction caused by the reduction of intracellular fluid volume in the brain. These symptoms may remain undetected in patients with other, more obvious causes for the neurological symptoms, such as extensive and prolonged brain injuries. Decreased levels of consciousness and confusion are the most common manifestations, with the level of consciousness correlating with the severity of the hypernatremia. Generalized tonic–clonic seizures can occur, but rapid progression to deep levels of coma is rare and should prompt additional tests for other possible causes [48]. Hypernatremia may initially present as intense thirst but may disappear with the progression of the disorder. Absence of thirst in a patient with pronounced hypernatremia and a preserved level of consciousness should raise suspicion for hypothalamic dysfunction. Finally, neuromuscular manifestations are uncommon, but rhabdomyolysis has been reported in a series of anecdotal cases [59].

Common Causes of Hypernatremia in the Neurointensive Care Unit

Hypernatremia in the neurointensive care unit is most commonly due to net free water loss, often related to a defective central release of vasopressin (VP) or antidiuretic hormone (ADH) or induced osmotic diuresis. Acute severe hypernatremia is most often iatrogenic and produced by the administration of hypertonic saline solutions (e.g., 2, 3, or 23.4% NaCl) given as a treatment for increased intracranial pressure, or as hypervolemic therapy in patients with subarachnoid hemorrhage diagnosed with symptomatic vasospasm, or sodium bicarbonate solutions for the correction of lactic acidosis [60]. Less commonly, acute hypernatremia can be caused by nutritional formulas or repeated use of hypertonic saline enemas.

Hyperosmolar therapy is often utilized in the treatment of critically ill neurological and neurosurgical patients presenting with cerebral edema. Although to a lesser degree than hypertonic saline infusion, mannitol is expected to cause hypernatremia from free water loss. Serum osmolality must be monitored and should not exceed 320 mOsm/kg because the dehydrated state correlates with the risk of renal failure [61]. Tromethamine (THAM), an alkalinizing agent, can represent a useful therapeutic alternative to mannitol in patients with increased intracranial pressure and hypernatremia [62, 63].

Diabetes Insipidus

Diabetes insipidus (DI) is most commonly encountered among patients undergoing pituitary surgery or with craniopharyngiomas [64]; however, it is theoretically a risk factor for patients with head injuries, primary or metastatic brain neoplasms, global anoxic brain damage, meningitis or encephalitis, massive cerebral edema, and diencephalic herniation syndromes [65]. It is almost obligatory for patients fulfilling brain death criteria.

DI is classically diagnosed in patients with an elevated sNa level (>145 mMol/L), an elevated urine output (>30 mL/kg/day), and a low urine specific gravity (<1.003) [66]. DI in the neuro-ICU is most often secondary to hypothalamic/pituitary dysfunction leading to ADH deficiency (central or hypothalamic DI). Clinically, significant free water loss and polyuria do not occur until more than three-fourths of the ADH-producing neurons are destroyed. DI may also be encountered as a consequence of renal unresponsiveness to ADH. Nephrogenic DI occurs in critically ill patients most commonly secondary to acute kidney injury (e.g., iodinated contrast dye or the polyuric phase of tubular necrosis); however, it may also be encountered in patients with preexisting conditions (lithium use, aminoglycosides, or amphotericin B) [67].

The clinical hallmarks of DI are polyuria and polydipsia, especially in patients with intact thirst mechanisms; nocturia is normally present. DI in the neuro-ICU frequently shows an abrupt onset. In patients with a reduced level of consciousness, impaired access to water, or without intact thirst mechanisms, hypernatremia may ensue. In fact, patients with intact thirst mechanisms who have central or nephrogenic DI may be able to regulate their osmolality through oral intake of free water. In addition to hypertonic encephalopathy and circulatory collapse, the "washout" effect induced by polyuria leads to hypomagnesemia, hypocalcemia, hypokalemia, and hypophosphatemia [68].

Unless the hypothalamic damage is severe and irreversible, the disruption of ADH secretion may be partial and temporary. This is often the case in patients following pituitary surgery or head trauma. In more than half of those cases, normal osmoregulation returns after 3–5 days. A study of 881 patients undergoing transsphenoidal microneurosurgery found that persistent DI was present only in 12.4% of cases. In addition, independent risk factors included CSF leak (33.3% transient, 4.4% persistent), Rathke cleft cyst (38.7%), Cushing's disease (22.2%), and craniopharyngioma (62.1%) [64]. In such patients, the return of normal hypothalamic function needs to be anticipated and monitored to avoid excessive treatment with fluid fluids or overcorrection with free water leading to hyponatremia and central pontine myelinosis.

Brain death is a common cause of DI in the neurointensive care unit. Occasionally, it may precede the diagnosis of brain death in patients with severe diencephalic herniation causing compression of the pituitary stalk against the *diaphragma sellae*. In patients who are clinically "brain dead," the death of the neurosecretory neurons of the hypothalamus is rapidly followed by a sudden decrease in blood pressure often preceded by massive diuresis. In cases where organ donation may be considered, this situation calls for a very aggressive treatment with intravenous fluid replacement and intravenous vasopressin to avoid hypoperfusion to those organs [65, 69].

The Approach to the Hypernatremic Patient

When treating the hypernatremic patient, the first priority is to assess the patient's volume status and to treat hypovolemia if present [70, 71]. Volume replacement with crystalloids (0.9% NaCl) normally suffices to maintain cardiac output and adequate perfusion pressures. However, severe cases may require the use of colloids such as hetastarch or 5% albumin solutions.

Following the stabilization of hemodynamic status, attention should be focused on correcting the patient's free water deficit. The calculation relies on the assumption that the total body water (TBW) and serum Na (sNa) are always constant.

Hence,

$$\text{Current TBW} \times \text{Current sNa} = \text{Normal TBW} \times \text{Normal sNa}$$

Therefore, assuming that a normal sNa is 140 mMol/L, the current TBW may be calculated as follows:

$$\text{Current TBW} = \text{Normal TBW} \times \left(140 / \text{Current sNa}\right)$$

Normal TBW in liters usually accounts for 60% of lean body weight in kilograms for men and 50% in women. The proportion of TBW decreases with age, representing 50% in elderly men and 45% in elderly women [72]. The free water deficit can then be calculated through the difference between normal and current TBW:

$$\text{Free water deficit} = \text{Normal TBW} - \text{Current TBW}$$

The actual volume of replacement fluid needed to correct the free water deficit will depend on the sodium concentration present in the replacement fluid chosen. Hypotonic solutions are preferred in these situations. The volume of the replacement fluid can be calculated using the following formula:

$$\text{Replacement fluid volume}\left(\text{liters}\right) = \text{Free water deficit} \times \left(1/1 - X\right)$$

where X = replacement fluid Na divided the isotonic fluid Na.

When hypernatremia develops over a period of hours, rapid correction of water deficit is safe, because the accumulated electrolytes can be rapidly eliminated from the brain cells [54]. A reduction of sNa by 1 mMol/L/h is appropriate for these patients.

However, the approach to correcting hypernatremia in patients with hypernatremia of longer or unknown duration must be exercised with caution. In these cases, it is prudent to assume that accumulated organic brain osmoles (idiogenic osmoles) have already occurred. This creates an equilibrium between the osmolality of brain cells and the surrounding interstitial fluid. The process of eradication of these osmoles will take several days to be completed. Therefore, the rate of correction of hyponatremia in these patients needs to be slower to avoid the risk of cerebral edema. A maximal rate of 0.5 mMol/L/h or 10 mMol/L/day is usually recommended [54, 73].

Traditionally, half of the total volume is given over the first 24 hours while carefully monitoring the decline in serum sodium level.

It is always necessary to compensate for ongoing fluid losses (obligatory or incidental, measurable, and insensible) while correcting the existing water deficit. Therefore, an average of 1.5 L/day will be required in addition to the volume given to correct the deficit. This amount may vary according to individual cases, and it may be much greater in patients with profuse continuous losses (e.g., diabetes insipidus, gastric suctioning, excessive sweating). Close monitoring of electrolyte concentrations (2–6 hours) and fluid balance (hourly) is the best way to ensure safe and adequate correction of hypernatremia.

Obviously, the underlying cause of hypernatremia needs to be addressed. Often, the hypernatremia cannot be fully corrected until its cause is identified and treated. Furthermore, mild cases of hypernatremia can be fully reversed by managing the underlying cause, such as stopping gastrointestinal fluid losses, controlling fever, avoiding glucosuria, and changing a nutritional formula. Management is particularly essential in polyuric patients with possible diabetes insipidus. The general management approach for polyuric patient is illustrated in Fig. 13.6.

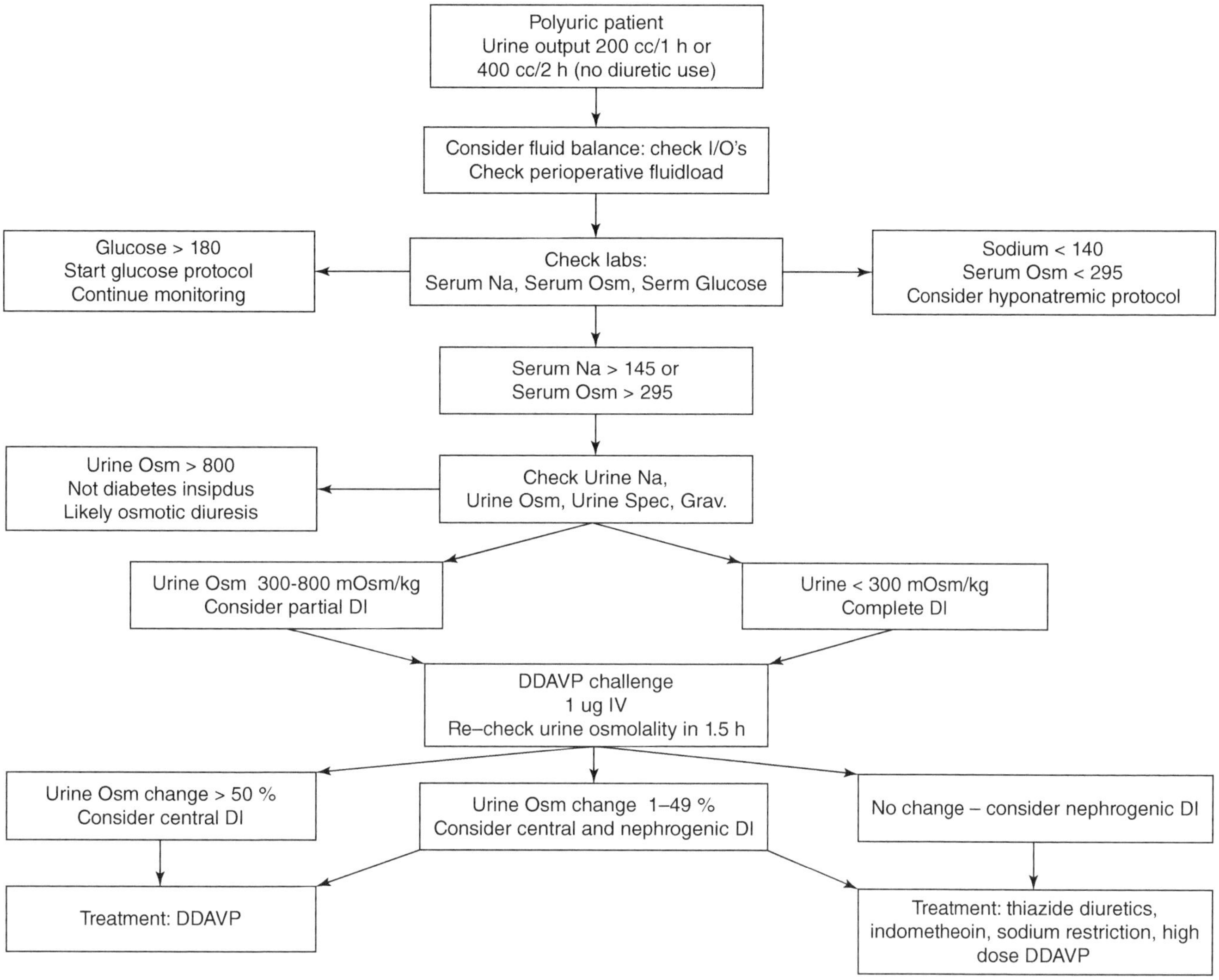

Fig. 13.6 Management of the polyuric patient (Adapted from our previously authored chapter in the last edition of this book)

Potassium Disturbances

Potassium is an important intracellular cation and is vital for maintaining cell function. 98% of total potassium is in the intracellular compartment. Only 2% of the potassium stores are found in the extracellular compartment with a serum concentration of 3.5–5 mEq/L. Thus, serum potassium concentrations are poor indicators of total body potassium stores [74, 75].

In response to a dietary potassium load, the kidney can eliminate the excess potassium. However, this process can occur over 6–12 h; therefore, buffering by transcellular shifts of potassium between the extracellular and intracellular compartments plays an important role in preventing dangerous swings of the serum potassium levels.

Hyperkalemia

Hyperkalemia is usually defined as a serum potassium concentration exceeding 5.5 mEq/L. Hyperkalemia is rarely seen in patients with normal renal function. Pseudohyperkalemia can occur secondary to hemolysis during venipuncture and in patients with severe thrombocytosis or leukocytosis. The unexpected finding of hyperkalemia in an asymptomatic patient should always prompt a repeat measurement before any therapeutic measures are taken.

Cases of hyperkalemia in the neuro-ICU usually share the same causes as those in any other ICU (Table 13.2). However, trauma patients are particularly at risk due to rhabdomyolysis and a higher incidence of prerenal insufficiency and blood

Table 13.2 Common causes of hyperkalemia in the neuro-ICU

Pseudohyperkalemia (fist clenching, hemolysis, thrombocytosis, leukocytosis)
Renal insufficiency (acute or chronic kidney disease)
Hypoadrenalism, Hypoaldosteronism
Diabetes ketoacidosis (insulin deficiency)
Obstructive uropathy
Drugs
Drugs affecting renin-angiotensin-aldosterone pathway Decrease renin release (NSAIDs, β-blockers, cyclosporine, tacrolimus) Direct Renin inhibitors (aliskiren) ACE inhibitors (lisinopril, enalapril) Angiotensin receptor blockers (losartan, valsartan) Decrease aldosterone synthesis (heparin, ketoconazole) Mineralocorticoid receptor blockers (spironolactone)
Potassium sparing diuretics (amiloride, triamterene)
Potassium containing drugs like potassium chloride, potassium penicillin
Modulation of Na^+- K^+ – ATPase (β blockers, digoxin)
THAM
Succinylcholine
In trauma patients
Rhabdomyolysis
Rewarming after (induced) hypothermia
Massive blood transfusions

ACE Angiotensin-converting enzyme, *THAM* Tromethamine, Adapted from last edition; our previously authored chapter, after initial reproduction by Rahman et-al [100] following permission from Rabinstein and Wijdicks

transfusions. In addition, when hypothermia is induced in patients with head trauma and increased intracranial pressure, hyperkalemia can occur during the rewarming phase and exacerbate the risk of cardiac arrhythmia. Several drugs have been associated with the development of hyperkalemia, but more pertinent to the neuro-ICU are THAM(tromethamine) and succinylcholine [76, 77].

Clinical Manifestations of Hyperkalemia

The most dangerous consequences of hyperkalemia are cardiac conduction abnormalities due to changes in the electrical excitability of cellular membranes. Electrocardiograph(ECG) findings include initial "peaking" of the T waves (tall, tented T waves best seen in precordial leads) followed by diminished amplitude of P waves and progressive widening of the PR interval and QRS complexes. Eventually, ventricular fibrillation and asystole ensue [76].

Neurological manifestations may include proximal limb weakness and burning dysesthesias. Progression to generalized paralysis with respiratory compromise has been reported but is rare. Weakness should recover within hours of reversal of the hyperkalemia; failure to recover shortly after treatment should suggest that other causes are responsible for the weakness [78, 79].

Management of Hyperkalemia

Early: Immediate and first 24 hours: Acute management of hyperkalemia should be focused on avoiding life-threatening cardiac arrhythmias.

(a) In cases of severe hyperkalemia with ECG changes, calcium salts (gluconate or chloride) should be administered immediately to antagonize the actions of potassium on the cellular membrane excitability. Intravenous calcium gluconate (10 mL of 10%) can be given over 3–5 minutes while monitoring the ECG changes. The dose can be repeated once after 5 minutes if ECG changes are persistent. The response to calcium will last for approximately 20–30 min and allow time for the administration of other therapies to enhance potassium clearance from the body [80, 81].
(b) The transcellular shift of potassium from extracellular to the intracellular compartment is achieved by insulin and inhaled β_2 agonists. The mechanisms for enhancing potassium uptake into the cell are different and thus can be synergistic for promoting potassium uptake into the cells. Regular insulin of 10 units is administered along with one ampule of dextrose 50% (50 mL) followed by glucose infusion in the event of hypoglycemia. The effect of insulin on potassium redistribution is seen within 10–20 minutes and can last for 4–6 hours. Patients should be monitored for hypoglycemia [82]. Inhaled β_2 agonists such as albuterol (20 mg) or salbutamol (20 mg) can facilitate potassium intake into the cells and provide additive benefits in addition to insulin. The dose is typically higher than that given in regular bronchodilatation, and the onset of action is within 30 minutes and lasts for 4–6 hours.
(c) Removal of potassium from the body is achieved using diuretics, hemodialysis, and cation-exchange resins.

Diuretics such as furosemide and chlorothiazide can increase urinary potassium excretion if renal function is adequate. Acute hemodialysis may be indispensable for patients with renal failure and is the primary modality for removing potassium in life-threatening situations. Cation exchange resins such as polystyrene sulfonate, patiromer, or sodium zirconium increase the gastrointestinal clearance of potassium by exchanging potassium for cations such as sodium or calcium in the gut. The rate of potassium removal is slow and can be unpredictable. These resins also interfere with drug absorptions and need to be spaced out and hence typically not the first-line medications in acute life-threatening situations [83, 84].

Hypokalemia

Hypokalemia is generally defined as serum potassium less than 3.5 mMeq/L. Sustained hypokalemia typically occurs as a result of insufficient intake or excessive gastrointestinal and renal losses. Although well tolerated in many patients, hypokalemia is associated with increased mortality and morbidity, especially in patients with underlying cardiac disease [85].

Factors such as osmotic and loop diuretics administration in patients with raised intracranial pressure or high doses of corticosteroids in acute spinal cord injury, iatrogenic hyperventilation, and therapeutic hypothermia can result in hypokalemia in the neuro-ICU [86]. Hypomagnesemia is a common electrolyte disturbance seen in chronic alcoholic patients and can contribute to resistant hypokalemia if magnesium is not corrected promptly [87]. Measuring urine potassium in a steady state can help distinguish between the renal and extrarenal causes of potassium losses(Table 13.3).

Table 13.3 Common causes of hypokalemia in the neuro-ICU

Decreased potassium intake (Malnutrition)
Potassium shift into cells
Alkalosis
β-adrenergic agonists(e.g., albuterol)
Increased sympathetic activity: head injury, myocardial infarction
Insulin administration
(Induced) hypothermia
Hypokalemic periodic paralysis
Extra renal potassium losses (potassium loss <20 mmol/24 h Sin urine)
Vomiting or nasogastric suctioning
Diarrhea
Laxative abuse
Renal potassium losses (potassium loss >20 mmol/24 h in uirne)
Potassium-wasting diuretics (loop diuretics, thiazides)
Osmotic diuresis(e.g., hyperglycemia)
Mineralocorticocoid excess (e.g., aldosteronism, renal artery stenosis)
Renal tubular acidosis
Hypomagnesemia
Other drugs (amphotericin B, penicillin derivatives)

Adapted from Rahman [100]

Clinical Manifestations of Hypokalemia

Severe hypokalemia causes hyperpolarisation of the membrane and causes muscle weakness. Hypokalemia can lead to muscle weakness, cramping, and in severe cases, result in rhabdomyolysis. The muscle weakness induced by hypokalemia can be profound and, in extreme cases, can result in flaccid quadriplegia and neuromuscular respiratory failure [88]. Cardiac arrhythmias can occur in patients with hypokalemia, especially in those with underlying heart disease. ECG abnormalities include a depressed ST segment, prominent U waves, flattening and inversion of T waves, and prolongation of the QT interval. Hypokalemia can predispose patients to ventricular arrhythmias resulting in cardiac death. Other manifestations include polyuria, ileus, insulin resistance, and worsening hepatic encephalopathy [74, 88, 89].

Management of Hypokalemia

Potassium replacement, either orally or intravenously, along with addressing the etiology is the cornerstone management of hypokalemia. Overcorrection of hypokalemia can result in hyperkalemia, resulting in cardiac arrhythmias; hence, oral supplementation with frequent monitoring is preferred. The intravenous route administration is usually reserved for life-threatening complications necessitating urgent replacement. On average, serum potassium concentration decreases by 0.3 meq/L for each 100 meq reduction in total body stores in the absence of transcellular shifts. Oral potassium chloride 20–60 meq 2–3 times/day can be given depending on the severity of hypokalemia. The recommended dose of intravenous KCl administration is 10–20 meq per hour. Intravenous potassium should be delivered in dextrose-free solutions as dextrose can stimulate insulin release resulting in intracellular uptake of potassium. Since the redistribution of potassium is difficult to predict, serial measurements of potassium and ECG become essential if a higher rate of intravenous KCl is administered. Measuring serum magnesium levels is recommended in patients with refractory hypokalemia since correction of hypokalemia may not occur unless magnesium is corrected [74, 80, 85, 89].

Disorders of Calcium, Phosphorus, and Magnesium Homeostasis

Calcium Disorders

Calcium is predominantly stored in bone, with only 1% is present in intracellular and extracellular spaces. Calcium is an important cation and plays a vital role in nerve conduction, muscle contraction, blood coagulation, and hormone secretion [90]. The average calcium levels are usually 8.5–10.5 mg/dL. The free or ionized calcium represents 40% of the total calcium and is tightly regulated by PTH and Vitamin D hormones.

Hypercalcemia

Malignancy and primary hyperparathyroidism account for the majority of the cases in adults; (Table 13.4). Clinical manifestations depend on the severity of hypercalcemia. Typical neuropsychiatric clinical features include confusion, lethargy, inability to concentrate, depression, and increased sleepiness. Severe cases can lead to psychosis, obtundation, and even coma. Gastrointestinal symptoms include nausea, vomiting, pancreatitis, and peptic ulcers. Polyuria, polydipsia, and acute kidney injury are common renal manifestations. Nephrocalcinosis and nephrolithiasis can be seen in chronic cases of hypercalcemia. ECG changes include short QT and ST-segment elevation(coving of ST wave) [91, 92].

Management of Hypercalcemia

Correction of the underlying cause is the mainstay of hypercalcemia management. Rapid correction is needed in symptomatic patients with severe hypercalcemia. Volume expansion with isotonic saline to correct volume depletion and facilitate calcium excretion through the kidneys is the most important step in managing hypercalcemia. Loop diuretics can be used only if the patient is deemed euvolemic to avoid worsening hypovolemia and hypercalcemia. Pharmacological agents such as bisphosphonates(e.g., zoledronic acid, pamidronate), calcitonin, denosumab, and glucocorticoids can be used to reduce serum calcium levels. Hemodialysis may be necessary for patients with renal insufficiency [93, 94].

Hypocalcemia

True hypocalcemia(decreased ionized calcium) is often encountered in critical care units. Common causes include hypoparathyroidism (a risk factor after neck surgery), sepsis, blood transfusions, alkalosis, and drugs. Hyperventilation can cause respiratory alkalosis, which can result in acute drop in ionized calcium levels. Neuromuscular manifestations include weakness, paresthesias, irritability, cramping, tetany, and seizures. Laryngeal and bronchospasm can occur in severe cases of hypocalcemia. Cardiovascular manifestations include hypotension, heart failure, bradycardia, and QT prolongation on ECG [95]. Intravenous calcium replacement is often required in cases of severe or symptomatic hypocalcemia. Calcium gluconate 10% (90 mg of calcium /10 mL ampule) is preferred over calcium chloride (273 mg of calcium /10 mL ampule), as calcium chloride is associated with venous sclerosis and skin necrosis in case of extravasation and is usually reserved for cardiopulmonary resuscitation. Hypomagnesemia should be treated. Long-term management of hypocalcemia should be directed towards the underlying etiology and often consists of oral calcium and vitamin D supplementation [94, 95].

Phosphorus Disorders

Phosphate is a critical element required for cell structure, cell signaling, energy production, and skeletal development. Normal serum phosphorus levels are usually 2.5–4.5 mg/dL and are mainly regulated by the hormones PTH and FGF23 (Table 13.5).

Table 13.4 Common causes calcium imbalance in the neuro-ICU

Hypercalcemia
Malignancy
Hyperparathyroidism
Prolonged immobilization
Drugs (e.g., calcium and vitamin D supplements)
Granulomatous disorders
Hypocalcemia
Sepsis
Pancreatitis
Rhabdomyolysis
Renal insufficiency
Neck surgery (transient or permanent hypoparathyroidism)
Hypomagnesemia
Alkalosis
Vitamin D deficiency
Drugs (phenytoin, phenobarbital, cimetidine, aminoglycosides)

Adapted from Rahman [100]

Table 13.5 Common causes phosphorus imbalance in the neuro-ICU

Hyperphosphatemia
Renal insufficiency
Sepsis
Rhabdomyolysis
Multiple trauma with widespread cell necrosis
Tumor lysis syndrome
Medications(phosphate-containing laxatives, vitamin D intoxication, fosphenytoin)
Hypophosphatemia
Head trauma (especially after fluid resuscitation)
Sepsis
Nasogastric suctioning, vomiting
Acid base disorders(respiratory alkalosis, metabolic acidosis)
Refeeding syndrome
Chronic alcoholism
Drugs (diuretics, steroids, β-adrenergic agonists, insulin)

Adapted from Rahman [100]

Hyperphosphatemia

Hyperphosphatemia is defined as serum phosphorus concentration exceeding 4.5 mg/dL (1.45 mMol/L). Hyperphosphatemia is usually seen in patients with renal insufficiency (acute kidney injury or chronic kidney disease) secondary to decreased renal clearance of phosphate. Increased tissue release of phosphorus is commonly seen in conditions such as rhabdomyolysis, trauma, tumor lysis syndrome. Symptoms are most related to a concomitant reduction in serum calcium levels. Phosphate-containing bowel preparations (e.g., sodium phosphate) should be avoided in patients with renal insufficiency. Treatment is based on eliminating the underlying cause and promoting phosphorus clearance by volume resuscitation. Hemodialysis may be warranted in patients with rhabdomyolysis or tumor lysis syndrome and who have concurrent renal insufficiency. Long-term management includes a restricted phosphate diet, and phosphate binders (e.g., calcium acetate, sevelamer) to decrease phosphorus absorption from the gut in patients with chronic kidney disease [96].

Hypophosphatemia

Hypophosphatemia is defined as a serum phosphorus concentration below 2.5 mg/dL (0.8 mMol/L). Hypophosphatemia is a common electrolyte disturbance noted in critically ill patients.. Common causes in the ICU setting include nasogastric suctioning and refeeding syndrome. Most patients are asymptomatic with mild hypophosphatemia, but as the severity of hypophosphatemia ensues, cellular energy production is impaired, and tissue hypoxia(by depletion of 2,3 diphosphoglycerate) can occur. Clinical features include muscle weakness resulting in respiratory insufficiency, failure to wean ventilated patients, decreased myocardial contractility, and skeletal muscle weakness resulting in rhabdomyolysis. Neurological symptoms may include ataxia, tremor, confusion, irritability, and seizures. Appropriate management of hypophosphatemia requires treating the underlying cause, correcting other electrolyte derangements, and replacing phosphorus. Oral phosphate supplementation is the preferred route to restore phosphorus levels in asymptomatic patients. Milk products (1000 mg/quart of skim milk) or phosphate salts(250 mg/capsule of Neutra-Phos K) are typically used for replacement. Intravenous phosphate replacement should be reserved for patients who have severe hypophosphatemia(<1 mg/dL) and are symptomatic. When administering phosphorus intravenously (usually as potassium phosphate), it is necessary to be cautious because it may induce hypocalcemia and calcium phosphate precipitation in the blood and tissues [94, 96, 97].

Magnesium Disorders

Magnesium is the second most abundant intracellular cation in the organism after potassium. Magnesium is crucial in DNA and protein synthesis, mitochondrial function and energy metabolism, neuromuscular function, and cardiac excitability. Normal magnesium levels are maintained between 1.4 and 2.2 mg/dL (0.7–1.1 mMol/L), and the kidneys play an important role in maintaining homeostasis [90] (Table 13.6).

Hypermagnesemia

Hypermagnesemia is defined as a serum magnesium concentration exceeding 2.4 mg/dL. Common causes include renal failure, excessive magnesium intake (antiacids, parenteral nutrition, supplements), and adrenal insufficiency. Hypermagnesemia is usually well tolerated, but extreme levels can impair neuromuscular transmission leading to areflexic paralysis and respiratory failure. It can also cause vasodilatation, hypotension, heart block, and even cardiac arrest. Treatment in patients with preserved renal function should be directed at stopping the magnesium supplements, and reducing magnesium levels can be accomplished by infusing saline and furosemide if necessary to increase urinary excretion. In cases of severe life-threatening conditions, treatment must focus on antagonizing the neuromuscular and cardiac effects by administering intravenous calcium (1–2 g of calcium gluconate 10% over 5–10 minutes). Hemodialysis may be required in patients with renal insufficiency.

Hypomagnesemia

Hypomagnesemia is defined as serum magnesium concentration below 1.7 mg/dL (0.65 mMol/L). It is a common electrolyte derangement in ICU settings. It is usually secondary to gastrointestinal or renal losses. Some of

Table 13.6 Common causes magnesium imbalance in the neuro-ICU

Hypermagnesemia
Renal failure
Excessive magnesium intake (supplements, parenteral nutrition)
Adrenal insufficiency
Hypomagnesemia
Head trauma (especially after fluid resuscitation)
Nasogastric suctioning
Chronic alcoholism
Refeeding syndrome
Diabetic ketoacidosis
Pancreatitis
Drugs (diuretics, aminoglycosides, amphotericin B, proton pump inhibitors)

Adapted from Rahman [100]

the more common causes frequently seen include nasogastric suction, malnutrition, diarrhea, refeeding syndrome, chronic ethanol ingestion, diabetic ketoacidosis, pancreatitis, and drugs. Hypomagnesemia can result in hypokalemia and hypocalcemia, and it is common to find concurrent derangements in these electrolytes [98]. Cardiac abnormalities include prolonged PR, QT prolongation, widened QRS complexes, and *torsades de pointes*. Neurological manifestations include hyperreflexia, muscle weakness, and paresthesias. Severe depletion can result in ataxia, confusion, nystagmus, spasms, tetany, and seizure. Intravenous magnesium sulfate (1–2 g over 15–30 minutes followed by slow infusion over the next 24 hours) should be administered in severely symptomatic patients. Caution should be exercised while repleting magnesium in patients with renal insufficiency as you can overshoot magnesium levels and result in hypermagnesemia. Oral magnesium supplements can be administrated for patients who are asymptomatic [94, 99].

Key Points: Potassium Disorders

- Potassium is the most abundant cation in the ICF. A large potassium gradient between ECF and ICF is necessary to maintain membrane potential, which is crucial for nervous and muscular tissue excitability.
- The kidney primarily maintains potassium homeostasis by excreting excess potassium.
- Oral potassium replacement is preferred for hypokalemia. Intravenous potassium replacement at rates greater than 20 meq/hr requires close clinical and ECG monitoring.
- Check for magnesium levels as hypomagnesemia can cause hypokalemia. Hypokalemia will not be corrected unless magnesium is replaced.
- Acute management of life-threatening hyperkalemia should consist of cardiac stabilization(calcium salts), potassium transfer from ECF to ICF(insulin, β agonists), and potassium removal from the body(diuretics, potassium binders, hemodialysis).

Key Points: Calcium, Magnesium, and Phosphorus Disorders

- Calcium, magnesium and phosphate are essential for cellular functions. Intestinal absorption is balanced by renal excretion in a steady state. Correction of the underlying cause is the mainstay of managing these disorders.
- Check for ionized calcium when evaluating patients with calcium disorders and hypoalbuminemia. Malignancy and Primary Hyperparathyroid disorders account for the majority of hypercalcemia cases in adults.
- Intravenous hydration followed by diuretics is the initial step in the management of symptomatic hypercalcemia. Bone resorptive therapies(bisphosphonates, calcitonin, denosumab) can be utilized for hypercalcemia of malignancy.
- Hyperphosphatemia and Hypermagnesemia are uncommon in patients with adequate renal function.
- Severe hypophosphatemia can result in respiratory failure, failure to wean ventilated patients, seizures, and rhabdomyolysis.
- Hypomagnesemia can cause hypokalemia and hypocalcemia. Correcting magnesium is important for correcting other electrolyte disorders.

References

1. Burst V. Etiology and epidemiology of hyponatremia. Front Horm Res. 2019;52:24–35. https://doi.org/10.1159/000493234.
2. Waikar SS, Mount DB, Curhan GC. Mortality after hospitalization with mild, moderate, and severe hyponatremia. Am J Med. 2009;122(9):857–65. https://doi.org/10.1016/j.amjmed.2009.01.027.
3. Bourque CW. Central mechanisms of osmosensation and systemic osmoregulation. Nat Rev Neurosci. 2008;9(7):519–31. https://doi.org/10.1038/nrn2400.
4. Robertson GL, Shelton RL, Athar S. The osmoregulation of vasopressin. Kidney Int. 1976;10(1):25–37. https://doi.org/10.1038/ki.1976.76.
5. Claybaugh JR, Sato AK, Crosswhite LK, Hassell LH. Effects of time of day, gender, and menstrual cycle phase on the human response to a water load. Am J Physiol Regul Integr Comp Physiol. 2000;279(3):R966–73. https://doi.org/10.1152/ajpregu.2000.279.3.R966.
6. Kuramochi G, Kobayashi I. Regulation of the urine concentration mechanism by the oropharyngeal afferent pathway in man. Am J Nephrol. 2000;20(1):42–7. https://doi.org/10.1159/000013554.
7. Andersen LJ, Jensen TU, Bestle MH, Bie P. Gastrointestinal osmoreceptors and renal sodium excretion in humans. Am J Physiol Regul Integr Comp Physiol. 2000;278(2):R287–94. https://doi.org/10.1152/ajpregu.2000.278.2.R287.
8. Choi-Kwon S, Baertschi AJ. Splanchnic osmosensation and vasopressin: mechanisms and neural pathways. Am J Phys. 1991;261(1 Pt 1):E18–25. https://doi.org/10.1152/ajpendo.1991.261.1.E18.
9. Adachi A. Thermosensitive and osmoreceptive afferent fibers in the hepatic branch of the vagus nerve. J Auton Nerv Syst. 1984;10(3–4):269–73. https://doi.org/10.1016/0165-1838(84)90023-7.
10. McKinley MJ, McAllen RM, Davern P, Giles ME, Penschow J, Sunn N, et al. The sensory circumventricular organs of the mammalian brain. Adv Anat Embryol Cell Biol. 2003;172:III–XII, 1–122, back cover. https://doi.org/10.1007/978-3-642-55532-9.
11. Thrasher TN, Brown CJ, Keil LC, Ramsay DJ. Thirst and vasopressin release in the dog: an osmoreceptor or sodium receptor mechanism? Am J Phys. 1980;238(5):R333–9. https://doi.org/10.1152/ajpregu.1980.238.5.R333.
12. Oliet SH, Bourque CW. Properties of supraoptic magnocellular neurones isolated from the adult rat. J Physiol. 1992;455:291–306. https://doi.org/10.1113/jphysiol.1992.sp019302.

13. Oliet SH, Bourque CW. Mechanosensitive channels transduce osmosensitivity in supraoptic neurons. Nature. 1993;364(6435):341–3. https://doi.org/10.1038/364341a0.
14. Ciura S, Bourque CW. Transient receptor potential vanilloid 1 is required for intrinsic osmoreception in organum vasculosum lamina terminalis neurons and for normal thirst responses to systemic hyperosmolality. J Neurosci. 2006;26(35):9069–75. https://doi.org/10.1523/jneurosci.0877-06.2006.
15. Morita H, Ogino T, Fujiki N, Tanaka K, Gotoh TM, Seo Y, et al. Sequence of forebrain activation induced by intraventricular injection of hypertonic NaCl detected by Mn2+ contrasted T1-weighted MRI. Auton Neurosci. 2004;113(1–2):43–54. https://doi.org/10.1016/j.autneu.2004.05.005.
16. Bourque CW. Osmoregulation of vasopressin neurons: a synergy of intrinsic and synaptic processes. Prog Brain Res. 1998;119:59–76. https://doi.org/10.1016/s0079-6123(08)61562-9.
17. Knepper MA. Molecular physiology of urinary concentrating mechanism: regulation of aquaporin water channels by vasopressin. Am J Phys. 1997;272(1 Pt 2):F3–12. https://doi.org/10.1152/ajprenal.1997.272.1.F3.
18. Verbalis JG. Disorders of body water homeostasis. Best Pract Res Clin Endocrinol Metab. 2003;17(4):471–503. https://doi.org/10.1016/s1521-690x(03)00049-6.
19. Rose BDPT. Clinical physiology of acid base and electrolyte disorders. 6th ed. NewYork: McGraw-Hill; 2006.
20. Colbert HA, Smith TL, Bargmann CI. OSM-9, a novel protein with structural similarity to channels, is required for olfaction, mechanosensation, and olfactory adaptation in Caenorhabditis elegans. J Neurosci. 1997;17(21):8259–69. https://doi.org/10.1523/jneurosci.17-21-08259.1997.
21. Weidmann P, Hasler L, Gnädinger MP, Lang RE, Uehlinger DE, Shaw S, et al. Blood levels and renal effects of atrial natriuretic peptide in normal man. J Clin Invest. 1986;77(3):734–42. https://doi.org/10.1172/jci112368.
22. Boscoe A, Paramore C, Verbalis JG. Cost of illness of hyponatremia in the United States. Cost Eff Resour Alloc. 2006;4:10. https://doi.org/10.1186/1478-7547-4-10.
23. Anderson RJ, Chung HM, Kluge R, Schrier RW. Hyponatremia: a prospective analysis of its epidemiology and the pathogenetic role of vasopressin. Ann Intern Med. 1985;102(2):164–8. https://doi.org/10.7326/0003-4819-102-2-164.
24. Bennani SL, Abouqal R, Zeggwagh AA, Madani N, Abidi K, Zekraoui A, et al. Incidence, causes and prognostic factors of hyponatremia in intensive care. Rev Med Interne. 2003;24(4):224–9. https://doi.org/10.1016/s0248-8663(02)00811-1.
25. Nzerue CM, Baffoe-Bonnie H, You W, Falana B, Dai S. Predictors of outcome in hospitalized patients with severe hyponatremia. J Natl Med Assoc. 2003;95(5):335–43.
26. Peruzzi WT, Shapiro BA, Meyer PR Jr, Krumlovsky F, Seo BW. Hyponatremia in acute spinal cord injury. Crit Care Med. 1994;22(2):252–8. https://doi.org/10.1097/00003246-199402000-00016.
27. Sherlock M, O'Sullivan E, Agha A, Behan LA, Rawluk D, Brennan P, et al. The incidence and pathophysiology of hyponatraemia after subarachnoid haemorrhage. Clin Endocrinol. 2006;64(3):250–4. https://doi.org/10.1111/j.1365-2265.2006.02432.x.
28. Sata A, Hizuka N, Kawamata T, Hori T, Takano K. Hyponatremia after transsphenoidal surgery for hypothalamo-pituitary tumors. Neuroendocrinology. 2006;83(2):117–22. https://doi.org/10.1159/000094725.
29. Diringer MN, Zazulia AR. Hyponatremia in neurologic patients: consequences and approaches to treatment. Neurologist. 2006;12(3):117–26. https://doi.org/10.1097/01.nrl.0000215741.01699.77.
30. Adrogué HJ. Consequences of inadequate management of hyponatremia. Am J Nephrol. 2005;25(3):240–9. https://doi.org/10.1159/000086019.
31. Janicic N, Verbalis JG. Evaluation and management of hypo-osmolality in hospitalized patients. Endocrinol Metab Clin N Am. 2003;32(2):459–81, vii. https://doi.org/10.1016/s0889-8529(03)00004-5.
32. Beukhof CM, Hoorn EJ, Lindemans J, Zietse R. Novel risk factors for hospital-acquired hyponatraemia: a matched case-control study. Clin Endocrinol. 2007;66(3):367–72. https://doi.org/10.1111/j.1365-2265.2007.02741.x.
33. Gill G, Huda B, Boyd A, Skagen K, Wile D, Watson I, et al. Characteristics and mortality of severe hyponatraemia—a hospital-based study. Clin Endocrinol. 2006;65(2):246–9. https://doi.org/10.1111/j.1365-2265.2006.02583.x.
34. Kurokawa Y, Uede T, Ishiguro M, Honda O, Honmou O, Kato T, et al. Pathogenesis of hyponatremia following subarachnoid hemorrhage due to ruptured cerebral aneurysm. Surg Neurol. 1996;46(5):500–7; discussion 7–8. https://doi.org/10.1016/s0090-3019(96)00034-1.
35. Wijdicks EF, Vermeulen M, Hijdra A, van Gijn J. Hyponatremia and cerebral infarction in patients with ruptured intracranial aneurysms: is fluid restriction harmful? Ann Neurol. 1985;17(2):137–40. https://doi.org/10.1002/ana.410170206.
36. Hasan D, Wijdicks EF, Vermeulen M. Hyponatremia is associated with cerebral ischemia in patients with aneurysmal subarachnoid hemorrhage. Ann Neurol. 1990;27(1):106–8. https://doi.org/10.1002/ana.410270118.
37. Palmer BF. Hyponatremia in patients with central nervous system disease: SIADH versus CSW. Trends Endocrinol Metab. 2003;14(4):182–7. https://doi.org/10.1016/s1043-2760(03)00048-1.
38. Maesaka JK, Gupta S, Fishbane S. Cerebral salt-wasting syndrome: does it exist? Nephron. 1999;82(2):100–9. https://doi.org/10.1159/000045384.
39. Vingerhoets F, de Tribolet N. Hyponatremia hypo-osmolarity in neurosurgical patients. "appropriate secretion of ADH" and "cerebral salt wasting syndrome". Acta Neurochir. 1988;91(1–2):50–4. https://doi.org/10.1007/bf01400528.
40. Evins C, Rao A. Point-of-care ultrasound to evaluate volume status in severe hyponatremia. BMJ Case Rep. 2020;13(6) https://doi.org/10.1136/bcr-2020-235304.
41. Nelson PB, Seif SM, Maroon JC, Robinson AG. Hyponatremia in intracranial disease: perhaps not the syndrome of inappropriate secretion of antidiuretic hormone (SIADH). J Neurosurg. 1981;55(6):938–41. https://doi.org/10.3171/jns.1981.55.6.0938.
42. Betjes MG. Hyponatremia in acute brain disease: the cerebral salt wasting syndrome. Eur J Intern Med. 2002;13(1):9–14. https://doi.org/10.1016/s0953-6205(01)00192-3.
43. Damaraju SC, Rajshekhar V, Chandy MJ. Validation study of a central venous pressure-based protocol for the management of neurosurgical patients with hyponatremia and natriuresis. Neurosurgery. 1997;40(2):312–6; discussion 6–7. https://doi.org/10.1097/00006123-199702000-00015.
44. Chung HM, Kluge R, Schrier RW, Anderson RJ. Clinical assessment of extracellular fluid volume in hyponatremia. Am J Med. 1987;83(5):905–8. https://doi.org/10.1016/0002-9343(87)90649-8.
45. Ayus JC, Krothapalli RK, Arieff AI. Treatment of symptomatic hyponatremia and its relation to brain damage. A prospective study. N Engl J Med. 1987;317(19):1190–5. https://doi.org/10.1056/nejm198711053171905.
46. Musch W, Thimpont J, Vandervelde D, Verhaeverbeke I, Berghmans T, Decaux G. Combined fractional excretion of

sodium and urea better predicts response to saline in hyponatremia than do usual clinical and biochemical parameters. Am J Med. 1995;99(4):348–55. https://doi.org/10.1016/s0002-9343(99)80180-6.
47. Beck LH. Hypouricemia in the syndrome of inappropriate secretion of antidiuretic hormone. N Engl J Med. 1979;301(10):528–30. https://doi.org/10.1056/nejm197909063011005.
48. Arieff AI, Llach F, Massry SG. Neurological manifestations and morbidity of hyponatremia: correlation with brain water and electrolytes. Medicine (Baltimore). 1976;55(2):121–9. https://doi.org/10.1097/00005792-197603000-00002.
49. Fraser JF, Stieg PE. Hyponatremia in the neurosurgical patient: epidemiology, pathophysiology, diagnosis, and management. Neurosurgery. 2006;59(2):222–9; discussion -9. https://doi.org/10.1227/01.neu.0000223440.35642.6e.
50. Decaux G, Soupart A. Treatment of symptomatic hyponatremia. Am J Med Sci. 2003;326(1):25–30. https://doi.org/10.1097/00000441-200307000-00004.
51. Sterns RH, Riggs JE, Schochet SS Jr. Osmotic demyelination syndrome following correction of hyponatremia. N Engl J Med. 1986;314(24):1535–42. https://doi.org/10.1056/nejm198606123142402.
52. Adrogué HJ, Madias NE. Hypernatremia. N Engl J Med. 2000;342(20):1493–9. https://doi.org/10.1056/nejm200005183422006.
53. Lien YH, Shapiro JI, Chan L. Effects of hypernatremia on organic brain osmoles. J Clin Invest. 1990;85(5):1427–35. https://doi.org/10.1172/jci114587.
54. Gullans SR, Verbalis JG. Control of brain volume during hyperosmolar and hypoosmolar conditions. Annu Rev Med. 1993;44:289–301. https://doi.org/10.1146/annurev.me.44.020193.001445.
55. Pollock AS, Arieff AI. Abnormalities of cell volume regulation and their functional consequences. Am J Phys. 1980;239(3):F195–205. https://doi.org/10.1152/ajprenal.1980.239.3.F195.
56. Mohmand HK, Issa D, Ahmad Z, Cappuccio JD, Kouides RW, Sterns RH. Hypertonic saline for hyponatremia: risk of inadvertent overcorrection. Clin J Am Soc Nephrol. 2007;2(6):1110–7. https://doi.org/10.2215/cjn.00910207.
57. Tisdall M, Crocker M, Watkiss J, Smith M. Disturbances of sodium in critically ill adult neurologic patients: a clinical review. J Neurosurg Anesthesiol. 2006;18(1):57–63. https://doi.org/10.1097/01.ana.0000191280.05170.0f.
58. Riggs JE. Neurologic manifestations of fluid and electrolyte disturbances. Neurol Clin. 1989;7(3):509–23.
59. Abramovici MI, Singhal PC, Trachtman H. Hypernatremia and rhabdomyolysis. J Med. 1992;23(1):17–28.
60. Gipstein RM, Boyle JD. Hypernatremia complicating prolonged mannitol diuresis. N Engl J Med. 1965;272:1116–7. https://doi.org/10.1056/nejm196505272722109.
61. Rosner MJ, Coley I. Cerebral perfusion pressure: a hemodynamic mechanism of mannitol and the postmannitol hemogram. Neurosurgery. 1987;21(2):147–56. https://doi.org/10.1227/00006123-198708000-00003.
62. Yoshida K, Corwin F, Marmarou A. Effect of THAM on brain oedema in experimental brain injury. Acta Neurochir Suppl (Wien). 1990;51:317–9. https://doi.org/10.1007/978-3-7091-9115-6_107.
63. Wolf AL, Levi L, Marmarou A, Ward JD, Muizelaar PJ, Choi S, et al. Effect of THAM upon outcome in severe head injury: a randomized prospective clinical trial. J Neurosurg. 1993;78(1):54–9. https://doi.org/10.3171/jns.1993.78.1.0054.
64. Nemergut EC, Zuo Z, Jane JA Jr, Laws ER Jr. Predictors of diabetes insipidus after transsphenoidal surgery: a review of 881 patients. J Neurosurg. 2005;103(3):448–54. https://doi.org/10.3171/jns.2005.103.3.0448.
65. Wijdicks EFM. Acid–base disorders, hypertonic and hypotonic states. In: The clinical practice of critical care neurology. Philadelphia: Lippincott-Raven; 1997.
66. Dumont AS, Nemergut EC 2nd, Jane JA Jr, Laws ER Jr. Postoperative care following pituitary surgery. J Intensive Care Med. 2005;20(3):127–40. https://doi.org/10.1177/0885066605275247.
67. Sands JM, Bichet DG. Nephrogenic diabetes insipidus. Ann Intern Med. 2006;144(3):186–94. https://doi.org/10.7326/0003-4819-144-3-200602070-00007.
68. Power BM, Van Heerden PV. The physiological changes associated with brain death—current concepts and implications for treatment of the brain dead organ donor. Anaesth Intensive Care. 1995;23(1):26–36. https://doi.org/10.1177/0310057x9502300107.
69. Wijdicks EAJ. Pathophysiologic responses to brain death. In: Wijdicks E, editor. Brain death. Philadelphia: Lippincot, Williams & Wilkins; 2001.
70. Marino P. Hypertonic and hypotonic syndromes. In: Marino P, editor. The ICU book. Baltimore: Williams & Wilkins; 1998.
71. Ayus JCC. Sodium and potassium disorders. In: Shoemaker W, Ayres S, Grenvik A, Holbrook P, editors. Textbook of critical care. Philadelphia: WB Saunders; 2000.
72. Oh MCH. Regulation of intracellular and extracellular volume. In: Arieff A, DeFronzo R, editors. Fluid and electrolyte, and acid–base disorders. New York: Churchill Livingstone; 1995. p. 1–28.
73. Bagshaw SM, Townsend DR, McDermid RC. Disorders of sodium and water balance in hospitalized patients. Can J Anaesth. 2009;56(2):151–67. https://doi.org/10.1007/s12630-008-9017-2.
74. Weiner DI, Linas SL, Wingo CS. Disorders of potassium metabolism. 6th ed. Comprehensive clinial nephrology. Elsevier; 2019.
75. Gumz ML, Rabinowitz L, Wingo CS. An integrated view of potassium homeostasis. N Engl J Med. 2015;373(1):60–72. https://doi.org/10.1056/nejmra1313341.
76. Montague BT, Ouellette JR, Buller GK. Retrospective review of the frequency of ECG changes in hyperkalemia. Clin J Am Soc Nephrol. 2008;3(2):324–30. https://doi.org/10.2215/cjn.04611007.
77. Martyn JAJ, Richtsfeld M, Warner DO. Succinylcholine-induced hyperkalemia in acquired pathologic states. Anesthesiology. 2006;104(1):158–69. https://doi.org/10.1097/00000542-200601000-00022.
78. Hunter RW, Bailey MA. Hyperkalemia: pathophysiology, risk factors and consequences. Nephrol Dialysis Transpl. 2019;34(Suppl_3):iii2–iii11. https://doi.org/10.1093/ndt/gfz206.
79. Palmer BF, Clegg DJ. Diagnosis and treatment of hyperkalemia. Cleve Clin J Med. 2017;84(12):934–42. https://doi.org/10.3949/ccjm.84a.17056.
80. Palmer BF, Clegg DJ. Physiology and pathophysiology of potassium homeostasis: Core curriculum 2019. Am J Kidney Dis. 2019;74(5):682–95. https://doi.org/10.1053/j.ajkd.2019.03.427.
81. Dépret F, Peacock WF, Liu KD, Rafique Z, Rossignol P, Legrand M. Management of hyperkalemia in the acutely ill patient. Ann Intensive Care. 2019;9(1):32. https://doi.org/10.1186/s13613-019-0509-8.
82. Harel Z, Kamel KS. Optimal dose and method of administration of intravenous insulin in the management of emergency hyperkalemia: a systematic review. PLoS One. 2016;11(5):e0154963. https://doi.org/10.1371/journal.pone.0154963.
83. Packham DK, Rasmussen HS, Lavin PT, El-Shahawy MA, Roger SD, Block G, et al. Sodium zirconium cyclosilicate in hyperkalemia. N Engl J Med. 2015;372(3):222–31. https://doi.org/10.1056/nejmoa1411487.
84. Palmer BF. Potassium binders for hyperkalemia in chronic kidney disease—diet, renin-angiotensin-aldosterone system inhibitor

therapy, and hemodialysis. Mayo Clin Proc. 2020;95(2):339–54. https://doi.org/10.1016/j.mayocp.2019.05.019.
85. Gennari FJ. Hypokalemia. N Engl J Med. 1998;339(7):451–8. https://doi.org/10.1056/nejm199808133390707.
86. Arango MF, Andrews PJD. Systemic complications of neurologic diseases. Curr Opin Crit Care. 2001;7(2):61–7.
87. Palmer BF, Clegg DJ. Electrolyte disturbances in patients with chronic alcohol-use disorder. N Engl J Med. 2017;377(14): 1368–77. https://doi.org/10.1056/nejmra1704724.
88. Palmer BF, Clegg DJ. Physiology and pathophysiology of potassium homeostasis. Adv Physiol Educ. 2016;40(4):480–90. https://doi.org/10.1152/advan.00121.2016.
89. Weiner ID, Wingo CS. Hypokalemia—consequences, causes, and correction. J Am Soc Nephrol. 1997;8(7):1179–88. https://doi.org/10.1681/asn.v871179.
90. Blaine J, Chonchol M, Levi M. Renal control of calcium, phosphate, and magnesium homeostasis. Clin J Am Soc Nephrol. 2015;10(7):1257–72. https://doi.org/10.2215/cjn.09750913.
91. Kleeman CR. Metabolic coma. Kidney Int. 1989;36(6):1142–58. https://doi.org/10.1038/ki.1989.313.
92. Mousseaux C, Dupont A, Rafat C, Ekpe K, Ghrenassia E, Kerhuel L, et al. Epidemiology, clinical features, and management of severe hypercalcemia in critically ill patients. Ann Intensive Care. 2019;9(1):133. https://doi.org/10.1186/s13613-019-0606-8.
93. Maier JD, Levine SN. Hypercalcemia in the intensive care unit. J Intensive Care Med. 2015;30(5):235–52. https://doi.org/10.1177/0885066613507530.
94. Kestenbaum B, Houillier P. Disorders of calcium, phosphate, and magnesium metabolism. 6th ed. Comprehensive clinical nephrology. Philadelphia: Elsevier; 2019.
95. Kelly A, Levine MA. Hypocalcemia in the critically ill patient. J Intensive Care Med. 2013;28(3):166–77. https://doi.org/10.1177/0885066611411543.
96. Wadsworth R, Siddiqui S. Phosphate homeostasis in critical care. BJA Educ. 2016;16(9):305–9. https://doi.org/10.1093/bjaed/mkw033.
97. Geerse DA, Bindels AJ, Kuiper MA, Roos AN, Spronk PE, Schultz MJ. Treatment of hypophosphatemia in the intensive care unit: a review. Crit Care. 2010;14(4):R147. https://doi.org/10.1186/cc9215.
98. Polderman KH, Bloemers FW, Peerdeman SM, Girbes ARJ. Hypomagnesemia and hypophosphatemia at admission in patients with severe head injury. Crit Care Med. 2000;28(6): 2022–5.
99. Lee JW. Fluid and electrolyte disturbances in critically ill patients. Electrolytes Blood Pressure. 2010;8(2):72. https://doi.org/10.5049/ebp.2010.8.2.72.
100. Rahman M, Kohler N, Bihorac A. Water and electrolyte management in neurological disorder. 2nd ed. Textbook of neurointensive care. London: Springer; 2013.

Oliguria, Acute Kidney Injury, and Principles of Blood Purification

14

Gonzalo Ramírez-Guerrero, Thiago Reis, Faeq Husain-Syed, Monica Zanella, and Claudio Ronco

Contents

G. Ramírez-Guerrero (✉)
Critical Care Unit, Carlos Van Buren Hospital, Valparaíso, Chile

Nephrology and Dialysis Unit, Carlos Van Buren Hospital, Valparaíso, Chile

Department of Medicine, Universidad de Valparaíso, Valparaíso, Chile

T. Reis
Laboratory of Molecular Pharmacology, Faculty of Health Sciences, University of Brasilia, Sao Paulo, Brazil

Hospital Sirio-Libanes, Sao Paulo, Brazil

F. Husain-Syed
Department of Internal Medicine II, University Hospital Giessen and Marburg, Justus-Liebig-University Giessen, Giessen, Germany

M. Zanella
Department of Nephrology, Dialysis and Kidney Transplantation, San Bortolo Hospital, Vicenza, Italy

International Renal Research Institute of Vicenza, Vicenza, Italy

C. Ronco
Department of Nephrology, Dialysis and Kidney Transplantation, San Bortolo Hospital, Vicenza, Italy

International Renal Research Institute of Vicenza, Vicenza, Italy

Department of Medicine, Università degli Studi di Padova, Vicenza, Italy

E. Mahanna Gabrielli et al. (eds.), *Textbook of Neurointensive Care: Volume 1*, https://doi.org/10.1007/978-3-031-62220-5_14

Abstract

Acute kidney injury (AKI), is defined by a rapid increase in serum creatinine, decrease in urine output, or both. Its incidence in intensive care has been reported in more than 50% of patients. In neurocritical patients, non-neurological complications such as AKI are independent predictors of worse clinical outcomes. Different research groups have reported an AKI incidence in neurocritical care patients of 11.6% with an incidence of Kidney Disease: Improving Global Outcomes (KDIGO) stage 3 AKI that requires dialysis ranging from 3% to 12%.

Trauma-induced AKI, sepsis, sympathetic overstimulation, tubular epitheliopathy, hyperchloremia, use of nephrotoxic drugs, and renal hypoperfusion are the most common causes of AKI in neurocritical patients. AKI is the result of a sum of events, though the mechanisms underlying many of them remain uncertain.

This review will focus on AKI in neurocritical care patients. Specifically, it will be discussed AKI epidemiology, causes, associated mechanisms, and physiological relationship between brain and kidney or physiological brain–kidney connection. Additionally, we will review, the principles, logistics, and risks of extracorporeal therapies for blood purification in this group of patients.

Introduction

Acute kidney injury (AKI) has traditionally been defined as a rapid deterioration (from hours to weeks) of the glomerular filtration rate (GFR) that is usually reversible [1]. AKI is a complex clinical syndrome rather than a single disease and is an important complication in patients hospitalized in intensive care units (ICU), where its prevalence exceeds 50% [2, 3].

The minimalist vision of anatomical AKI categories (prerenal, intrinsic, and postrenal) has evolved to specific syndromes mainly characterized by their pathophysiology and treatments, all contributing to the clinical spectrum of AKI syndrome. Cardiorenal syndrome, hepatorenal syndrome, perioperative AKI, and sepsis-associated AKI are also all relevant clinical entities with specific managing AKI logistics related to their cause [3].

AKI in patients with neurological diseases has not been extensively described. Neurocritical care advancements in recent decades, and new neuromonitoring techniques, and therapies, have allowed successful treatments of [4] very complex neurological patients require a multidisciplinary approach where the role of the nephrologist is essential [5].

Consensus Definitions and Oliguria

AKI includes a group of conditions classified under acute kidney disease and spanning from mild, self-limiting AKI to severe, persistent AKI [6].

The current diagnosis of AKI is based on the recognition of acute deterioration in GFR, reflected by an increase in serum creatinine levels and/or a deterioration in diuresis. Even small increases in creatinine are associated with an increase in mortality [7]. The international consensus criteria define AKI according to the Kidney Disease: Improving Global Outcomes (KDIGO) guidelines, as shown in Table 14.1 [8]. This classification has superseded the former definitions based on Risk, Injury, Failure, Loss, and End-stage renal disease (RIFLE) and on the AKI Network (AKIN) [9]. By maintaining the basal creatinine of the RIFLE definition and the small increases in creatinine of the AKIN criteria, the KDIGO definition allows for greater sensitivity when diagnosing AKI [10].

Oliguria has been defined in the literature as urine output of less than 200–500 mL in 24 h. KDIGO guidelines have standardized the concept of oliguria as diuresis of <0.5 mL/

Table 14.1 Acute kidney injury and acute kidney disease definition

	Timing	Definition	Threshold	
Acute kidney injury	≤7 days	Creatinine ≥1.5 times baseline (or increase of ≥0.3 mg/dL within any 48 h period)	Urine volume <0.5 mL/kg for ≥6 h	Short and long-term risk of death or RRT is greatest for patients who meet both criteria [86]
– Transient	<48 h	–	–	Transient AKI associated with better outcomes than persistent AKI [86]
– Persistent	>48 h	–	–	
Acute kidney disease [86]	>7 days, <90 days	Creatinine ≥1.5 times baseline (or increase of ≥0.3 mg/dL within any 48 h period)	eGFR <90 mL per min (with damage marker) eGFR mL per min per 1.73 m^2 <60 mL per min	AKD can include AKI and extends through recovery or worsening until for CKD are reached

kg/h for 6 h [8, 11]. One study, including urine output in the diagnosis of AKI precisely, has increased the detection of AKI from 8% to 60% [12].

Urine output is influenced by hemodynamic parameters, intravascular hypovolemia/hypervolemia, and levels of hormones such as aldosterone and antidiuretic hormone (the latter of which is released through various stimuli in neurocritical patients). Therefore, urine output may be an unspecific marker of renal function, and reduced urine output is associated with worse outcomes in critical patients, including greater mortality, ICU admission, and hospitalization in patients with AKI. The risk of mortality of low urine output and increased creatinine increases 2.84 (1.41–5.70) to 7.85 (2.76–22.33) times when combined with a diagnosis of AKI [12–14].

Major surgery is the second most common cause of AKI in ICU patients [15]. There is controversy on oliguria during the intraoperative period (defined as urine output <0.5 mL/kg/h for at least 1 h), as weak predictor of postoperative AKI. One study showed that more than half of postoperative AKI events occurred in patients without intraoperative oliguria [16]. Nevertheless, Shiba et al. and Mizota et al. demonstrated that periods of intraoperative oliguria that last longer than 120 min or a threshold of <0.3 mL/kg/h are associated with a greater risk of developing AKI [17, 18]. These data suggest that the threshold of intraoperative oliguria and its presence must be interpreted on an individual basis according to the patient's condition.

Epidemiology and Outcomes of AKI in Neurocritical Pathologies

AKI is a systemic disease that is one of the most frequent and severe complications in critically ill patients due to its high morbidity and mortality and economic impact [7, 19]. The increased mortality associated with it is even higher when it is present along with dysfunction of another organ; in this case, mortality may be as high as 60%–80% [20]. Reports of additional organ dysfunction apart from central nervous system are up to 81% of patients [21].

Non-neurological complications in neurocritical patients are known to be independent predictors of worse clinical outcomes [22]. Different research groups have reported an AKI incidence of 11.6% in neurocritical patients in general, with rates that vary according to the specific pathology: an incidence of 9.2% has been reported in patients with traumatic brain injury (TBI) [23], 14.5%–20.9% in patients with acute ischemic stroke (AIS), 19%–59.8% in patients with intracerebral hemorrhage (ICH), and 12%–43.3% in patients with subarachnoid hemorrhage (SAH) [5, 24–30] (Table 14.2).

Neurocritical patients tend to be younger, have less comorbidity, and have a different risk profile given the diagnostic and therapeutic procedures. In these patients, AKI can result in an up to a fivefold increase in mortality in direct relation to its severity, lead to poorer functional recovery, and increase the possibility of moderate-to-severe disability at hospital discharge [24, 26, 31, 32]. An incidence of

Table 14.2 Studies showing incidence of AKI in neurological diseases

Study	Year published	Patients *n*	Diseases	Incidence	Diagnosis criteria
Tsagalis [7]	2009	1350	Stroke	14.29%	AKIN
Corral [8]	2012	224	TBI	8%	RIFLE
Zacharia [9]	2009	787	SAH	23.1%	RIFLE
Moore [10]	2010	207	TBI	9.2%	RIFLE
Covic [11]	2008	1090	Stroke	14.5%	RIFLE
Büttner [12]	2020	681	All[a]	11.6%	AKIN
Zorrilla-Vaca [13][b]	2017	5,147,754/615,623	Stroke/ICH	12.9%/19%	AKIN
Tujjar [14]	2017	202	SAH	12%	AKIN
Wang [15]	2018	647	Stroke	20.9%	KDIGO
LI [16]	2011	136	TBI	23%	AKIN
Kong [30]	2017	724	All[a]	43%	KDIGO
Sadan [55]	2017	1267	SAH	16.7%	KDIGO
Eagles	2019	413	SAH	38%	KDIGO

[a]Neurologic autoimmune disorder, Intracranial Hemorrhage, Infection of the CNS, Ischemic stroke, Tumor, Others
[b]Meta-analysis

3%–12% of KDIGO stage 3 AKI that requires dialysis has been reported; this is linked to higher mortality rates (50%–70%) and severe disability due to a less opportunity for hospital rehabilitation in this subgroup of patients [5, 26, 33].

Risk Factors of AKI in Neurocritical Care Unit Patients

AKI risk prediction is fundamental for planning diagnostic and therapeutic procedures in neurocritical patients. Observational studies have identified risk factors associated with the onset of AKI. Many of them are not modifiable, but they do allow us to identify patients at greater risk in order to implement diagnostic and corrective measures. Despite the presence of multiple kidney severity scores, only one is validated for the neurocritical population with a model's predictive accuracy measured by receiver operator characteristic (ROC) at 0.87, one being the best measure of prediction.

This score includes the Glasgow Coma Scale classification; hypertension; coronary disease; pneumonia and heart failure in the first 7 days of hospitalization; and use of furosemide, torsemide, dopamine, and norepinephrine [34]. Nevertheless, one of the most commonly reported factors associated with the onset of AKI in the ICU is the presence of chronic kidney disease. This factor is included among the risk factors along with old age and type of AIS [25, 26].

Physiopathology of AKI in Nerocritical Care Unit Patients

The Brain–Kidney Connection

The brain and kidneys share complex crosstalk in order to maintain homeostasis [5]. AKI can generate anatomical, functional, and biochemical changes in the brain, such as changes in the concentration of neurotransmitters and cytokines, acid–base homeostasis, and drug metabolism; this can cause direct and indirect injuries (Fig. 14.1) [35]. Concomitantly, efferent impulses from the CNS can increase renal sympathetic activity, triggering renin secretion, increasing tubular sodium absorption, and decreasing renal blood flow [36].

Inflammation

Experimental evidence from animal models of AKI has shown that high levels of inflammatory cytokines in the brain, cellular inflammation in astrocytes and microglia, and anatomic and functional injuries increased blood–brain barrier (BBB) permeability and pyknosis in neuronal cells [37]. AKI increases proinflammatory cytokines and decreases their clearance thus increasing the inflammatory response [38]. Only in AKI models—not in other models of systemic inflammation—has an increase been observed in the cerebral cortex and corpus callosum of keratinocyte-derived chemo attractants and granulocyte colony-stimulating factor, along with specific markers of brain inflammation and extravasation of Evans blue dye in the brain [37]. A direct effect of TNF-alpha and an indirect effect of the upregulation of matrix metalloproteinase 9 (MMP-9) have been demonstrated, which can alter endothelial tight junctions with water and protein extravasation, resulting in vasogenic edema [39, 40]. Kidney disease increases the expression of aquaporins-4 to 2.5 times higher than normal values, worsening cerebral edema [5, 41].

This inflammatory state is also triggered from the brain to the kidney. Following brain injury, cellular damage leads to the release of molecular products that trigger inflammation. A breakdown in the BBB leads to leakage of cytokines into the systemic circulation [42, 43]. Evidence from brain-dead kidney donors has shown greater renal inflammation, with infiltration of T-lymphocytes and macrophages. After perfusing these kidneys, cytokine release was observed, which is a stimulating factor of granulocyte colonies, IL-6, IL-9, and MCP-1 [44]

Blood Flow Dysregulation

The brain and kidney have a vascular autoregulation mechanism that maintains blood flow constant despite variations in blood pressure; there is a hemodynamic parallelism between the vascular beds of both organs to ensure adequate perfusion [5, 45, 46].

This cerebrovascular and renal regulation is altered in neurocritical patients. Sustained cerebral autoregulation in patients with neurocritical pathology is associated with renal hyperfiltration and augmented renal clearance with implications on drug pharmacokinetics. The loss of cerebral autoregulation may contribute to kidney autoregulation impairment, generating a decline in creatinine clearance and increasing the susceptibility of developing AKI and poor neurological outcomes [47–51].

Neurotransmitter Alteration

The balance of neurotransmitters is fundamental for normal brain function. AKI and its associated complications, such as metabolic acidosis, generate an imbalance among excitatory and inhibitory neurotransmitters due to an alteration in transport across the BBB and the traffic of neurotransmitters between astrocytes and neurons [52, 53].

The accumulation of guanidine compounds in the brain generates inhibitory effects on gamma-aminobutyric

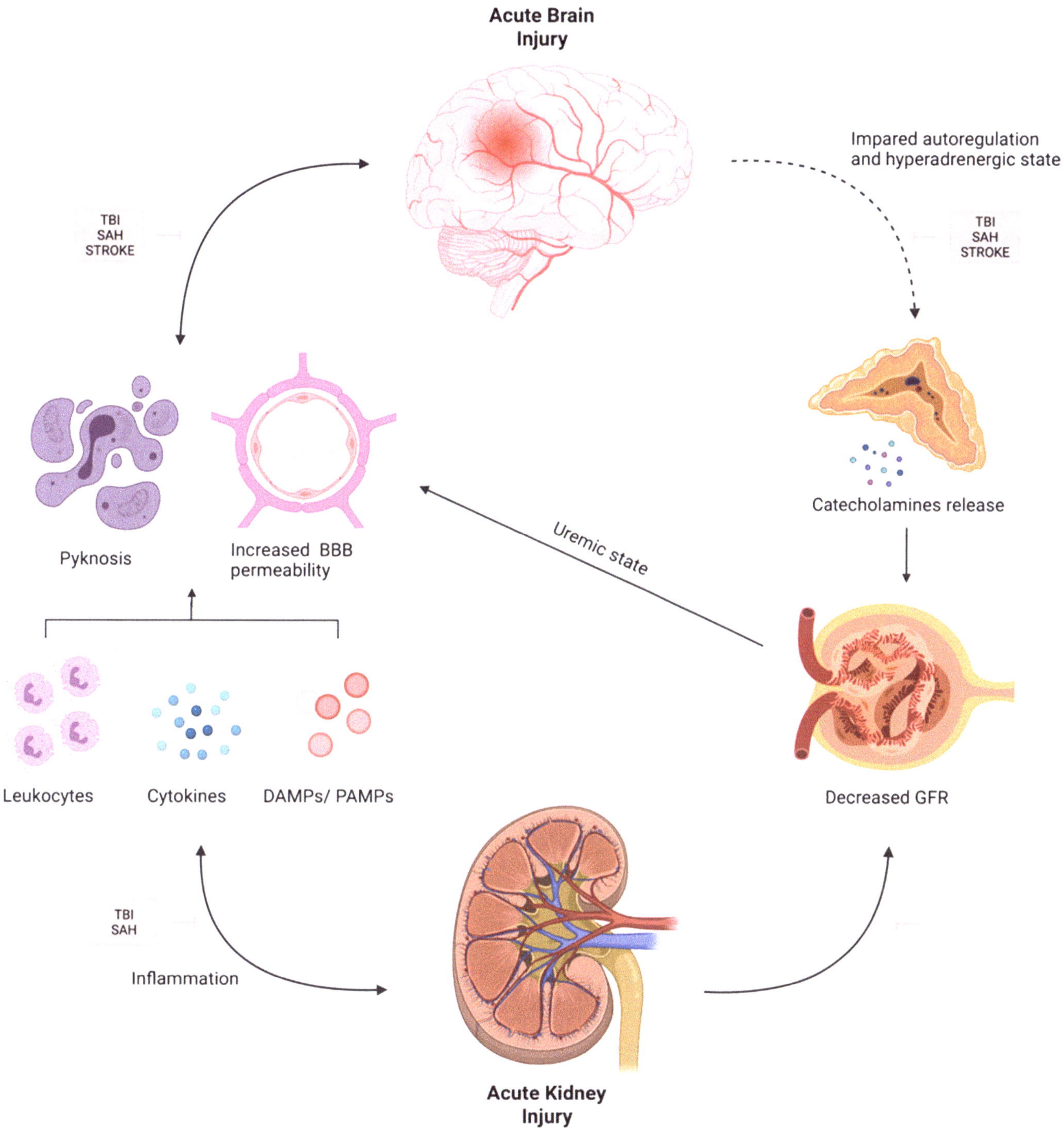

Fig. 14.1 Kidney–brain axis interaction. Role of acute kidney injury and acute brain injury in inflammation, sympathetic nervous system, uremic state, and diseases related to these mechanisms. *DAMPs* Damage-associated molecular patterns, *GFR* Glomerular filtration rate, *PAMPs* Pathogen-associated molecular patterns, *SAH* Subarachnoid hemorrhage, *TBI* Traumatic brain injury. From "Acute kidney injury at the neurocritical care unit" by Ramírez-Guerrero G, Baghetti R and Ronco C, 2021, Neurocritical Care, published ahead of print

receptors and stimulates N-methyl-D-aspartate receptors [54]. Along with the above, AKI interferes with Na+-independent cationic amino acid transporters (CAT1/SLC7A1), generating an accumulation and/or depletion of neurotransmitters in the CNS such as glutamate, glycine, and gamma-aminobutyric acid, which must be strictly regulated in order to maintain a low concentration in the brain tissue [5, 55].

Cell acidification increases the oxidative deamination of glutamate by glutamate dehydrogenase, generating an excess of ammonia and, in consequence, altering the cycle of neurotransmitters [52, 53].

Cause of AKI in Neurocritical Care Unit Patients

Traumatic Brain Injury-Induced Acute Kidney Injury (TBI-iAKI)

AKI is frequently associated with TBI. Following brain injury, several mechanisms are involved in its development (Table 14.3) that are independent of severe episodes of systemic hypoperfusion and nephrotoxin exposure [5, 56].

1. Activation of the brain–kidney axis:
   (a) Sympathetic renal stimulation by sympathetic efferents and activation of the hypothalamic–pituitary–adrenal (HPA) axis induces the release of noradrenaline and adrenaline by the adrenal gland. Catecholamines stimulate beta 1 adrenergic receptors, increasing renin secretion by the juxtaglomerular cells, which increases Na^+ and water reabsorption in addition to producing a vasopressor effect. Catecholamines also stimulate alpha 1 adrenergic receptors in the kidney vasculature, decreasing renal blood flow, GFR, and urine output [5, 57].

   An imbalance in the parasympathetic and sympathetic pathway in patients with severe TBI results in hyperactivity of the sympathetic nervous system, causing a hyperadrenergic state or paroxysmal sympathetic hyperactivity (PSH), as this clinical condition is known. This hyperactive state aims at ensuring adequate oxygen delivery to damaged tissues. However, this state can be maladaptive, leading to intense renal vasoconstriction, decreased renal perfusion, and a lowered glomerular filtration rate [42]. Any anatomical injury to areas that control the autonomic nervous system and modulate renal hemodynamics can result in autonomic dysregulation (hypothalamus, nucleus of the solitary tract, areas A1 to A5 of the medulla, and sublimbic system). Electrical stimulation of these areas in rats leads to changes in visceromotor function, including a reduction in renal blood flow [42, 43] and activation of the renin-angiotensin-aldosterone system (RAAS), which is another factor that leads to AKI by stimulating the development of inflammatory pathways.
2. Functional alterations and apoptosis of renal tubular epithelial cells secondary to a systemic inflammatory reaction in severe brain injury:
   (a) The increase of RAAS and molecular products secondary to cellular damage after brain injury triggers the discharge of inflammatory factors (IL-6, IL-1b, reactive oxygen species (ROS), tumor necrosis factor-a, matrix metalloproteinase-9, MCP-1, MIP1 beta, and IL-33) which are involved in neutrophil adhesion to tubular epithelial cells. ROS injures the epithelium through the disassembly of tight junctions and the degradation of elastases and matrix metalloproteinases [43, 56], increased proteinuria, and plasma NGAL. These markers of tubular damage correlated with inflammatory mediators, suggesting that acute brain damage generates tubular injury [5, 56].

Table 14.3 Relevant mechanisms in Acute Kidney Injury (AKI)

AKI in TBI	AKI in SAH	AKI in AIS and ICH
Sepsis-associated AKI	Sepsis-associated AKI	Sepsis-associated AKI
Trauma-related AKI – Haemorrhagic shock – Rhabdomyolysis – Oxidative stress – DAMPs/ PAMPs	Induced hydroelectrolytic disorders – *Hypernatremia* – *Hyperchloremia*	Renal hypoperfusion
Sympathetic hyperstimulation – *Hyperactivity of SNS* – *Activation of HPA axis*	Contrast-induced AKI	Contrast-associated AKI
Tubular epitheliopathy	Osmotic nephrosis	Osmotic nephrosis
Osmotic nephrosis	Drug-induced AIN: – Levetiracetam – Phenytoin	Drug-induced AIN: – Levetiracetam – Phenytoin
Drug-induced AIN: – Levetiracetam – Phenytoin		

TBI Traumatic brain injury, *SAH* Subarachnoid hemorrhage, *ICH* Intracerebral hemorrhage, *AIS* Acute ischemic Stroke, *HPA* Hypothalamic–pituitary–adrenal axis, *SNS* Sympathetic nervous system, *AIN* Acute interstitial Nephritis. From "Acute kidney injury at the neurocritical care unit" by Ramírez-Guerrero G, Baghetti R and Ronco C, 2021, Neurocritical Care, published ahead of print

Acute Kidney Injury in Subarachnoid Hemorrhage

In contrast to TBI-iAKI, SAH is not an early complication. Most episodes occur more than 1 week after ICU admission due to ICU-specific interventions and medical management strategies, such as the use of hyperosmolar therapy and potential exposure to nephrotoxic agents such as intravenous contrast media [5, 28, 58].

1. Hypernatremia and hyperchloremia due to the use of hypertonic saline therapy:
   (a) Hypertonic saline therapy is often used to control intracranial hypertension and hyponatremia. Hypernatremia and hyperchloremia produce intravascular dehydration and vasoconstriction either directly or through tubule glomerular feedback mechanisms [58]. Hyperchloremia caused by prolonged exposure to hypertonic saline increases the chloride levels within the lumen of the kidney's distal tubule. The increased delivery of sodium chloride to macula densa initiates a signaling cascade that results in reduced GFR via two main mechanisms: afferent arteriole vasoconstriction, mediated by decreased prostaglandin secretion, and vasodilation of efferent arteriole from reduced renin and angiotensin II release [59]. Additionally, kidney volume expansion as a result of large volumes of NaCl may cause decreased pressure gradients across the renal arterioles, resulting in reduced renal blood flow [60].
   (b) A randomized trial comparing a low-chloride (NaCl/Na-acetate) versus high-chloride hypertonic solution (NaCl) for patients who required hyperosmolar therapy for SAH revealed that the rate of AKI was higher in the NaCl group (53.3% vs 11.8%, $p = 0.01$) and suggested that patients with a chloride level of 109 mmol/L or above are those at highest risk for AKI [5, 61, 62].
2. Contrast-induced acute kidney injury (Ci-AKI):
   (a) Patients with SAH have an increased risk of contrast-induced nephropathy through multiple exposures to high doses of contrast agents such as when exposed to CT angiography and coil embolization [5, 63].

Acute Kidney Injury in Acute Ischemic Stroke and Intracerebral Hemorrhage

The proposed mechanisms are the following:

1. Intensive reduction of systolic blood pressure (SBP) in ICH:
   (a) As recommended by current guidelines, an acute reduction of systolic blood pressure to a "safer" limit of 140–160 mmHg can improve functional outcomes in patients with ICH [64], but it is strongly associated with AKI [65]. Lowering SBP by more than 90 mmHg was associated with an increased risk of AKI. It is recommended to keep SBP above 110 mmHg [66].
2. Contrast-associated acute kidney injury (CA-AKI) in endovascular procedures:
   (a) Additional exposure to contrast media in addition to what is received during diagnostic imaging techniques along with use of intra-arterial contrast increase the risk of CA-AKI. It occurs in 1 out of 30 patients [5, 67]
3. Infusion rate of mannitol used to decrease intracranial pressure in patients with ICH:
   (a) Mannitol accumulation in the extracellular space causes an increase in local renal osmolality and osmotic nephrosis, renal vasoconstriction, and deterioration of the GFR [68]

Principles of Blood Purification in the Neurocritical Care Unit

Renal replacement therapy (RRT) has evolved over time to ensure its safe, easy use. Controversy still remains regarding the optimal time to start blood purification therapies and the specific type of technique; a choice must be made based on a pathophysiological basis [6, 69]. Along with RRT, different membranes and adsorption cartridges are available to expand blood purification techniques to hemodynamic support, associated with removing inflammatory mediators in critical patients.

Mechanisms of Solute and Fluid Transport

Solute transport mainly occurs through two mechanisms: convection and diffusion. When the solute removal rate is normalized by the concentration of plasma/blood that enters the filter, the correct term is "solute clearance," expressed in mL/min, which describes the volume of blood that is purified of solute over a unit of time [70].

Ultrafiltration and Convection

Ultrafiltration (UF) describes the transport of plasma water through a semipermeable membrane generated by a pressure gradient between the blood compartment and the dialysate/ultrafiltration compartment. Convection is the process by which solutes pass through the membrane's pores, dragged by the movement of the fluids [70]. This technique allows for controlling solutes of greater molecular weight [71].

UF can be used alone (volume control), as part of hemofiltration (partially or entirely replacing ultrafiltration, achieving control of volume and solutes), or combined with diffusion as hemodialysis/hemodiafiltration.

Hemofiltration exclusively uses UF/convection through high-flow membranes in the absence of dialysis fluid and is associated with the partial or total infusion of replacement solution to the blood tubing line, which can be administered prefilter or postfilter, with the latter being more efficient for solute clearance [70].

Diffusion

Diffusion is the process by which molecules move through semipermeable membranes. The movement of solutes occurs from an area of higher concentration to an area of lower concentration. The concentration gradient is the driving force. Diffusion is greater for molecules of lower molecular weight [72].
Diffusion is the main mechanism of solute removal in hemodialysis. It involves a hemodialyzer in which blood circulates countercurrent from a dialysate solution, maintaining the concentration gradient through the entirety of the dialyzer [70].

Adsorption

Adsorption is when molecules in the plasma or blood bind to the membrane or other adsorbent substances such as resins or gel. This binding depends on the characteristics of each molecule (size, load, and structure) and of each membrane (porosity, composition, surface potential) [70].

Renal Replacement Therapy in Neurocritical Care

Despite the undisputed benefit of RRT in encephalopathy due to retention of nitrogen products and toxic drugs, metabolic acidosis, and sodium and water balance, these therapies may pose a risk to neurocritical patients. They may cause dialysis-associated neurovascular injury and affect the treatment prescribed by the rest of the neurocritical unit team, regardless of the type of therapy used (Fig. 14.2) [5].

Intermittent and continuous therapies have been found to be equally effective in regard to mortality and/or dialysis dependence, but reports have shown significant differences in neurocritical patients [73]. The mechanism and speed at which blood purification occurs is the major difference between the two types of therapies: the goal of removing uremic solutes through diffusion is achieved in a short period of time in the case of intermittent therapies [74] and even in hybrid therapies such as Sustained Low-Efficiency Dialysis (SLED), with a significant increase in perihematomal edema in patients with ICH and worse clinical outcomes reported [5, 75].

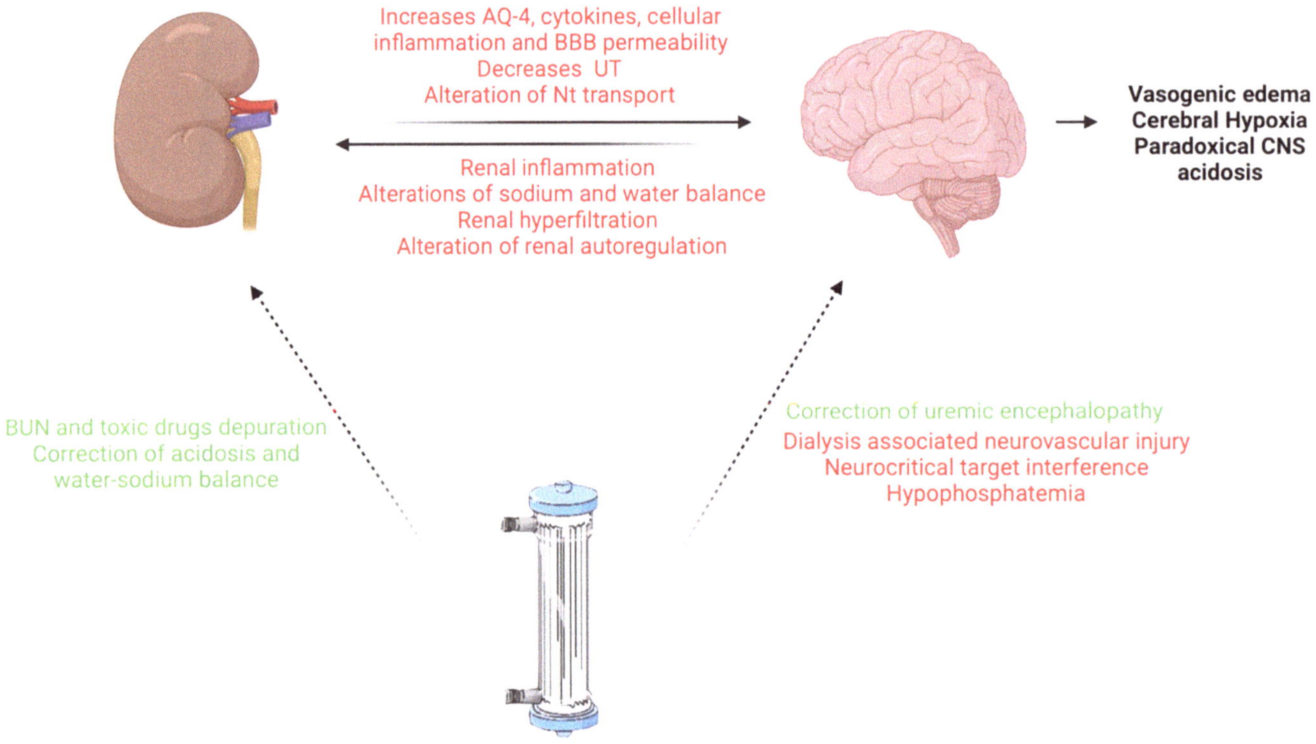

Fig. 14.2 Kidney–brain axis interaction and renal replacement therapy. AQ-4, aquaporin 4, BBB, blood–brain barrier, BUN, blood urea nitrogen, CNS, central nervous system, Nt, neurotransmitters, UT, urea transporter. From "Acute kidney injury at the neurocritical care unit" by Ramírez-Guerrero G, Baghetti R and Ronco C, 2021, Neurocritical Care, published ahead of print

The neurological consequences include de novo cerebral edema or an increase in existing edema up to full herniation, and death; thus, neurocritical patients merit special consideration when planning RRT [5]. Continuous renal replacement therapy (CRRT) has proven to be associated with better mean blood pressure, cardiac output, and oxygen delivery outcomes compared to intermittent hemodialysis (IHD). It offers a better hemodynamic profile and, therefore, better cerebral perfusion pressure (CPP) and cerebral blood flow (CBF) control, which is associated with better neurological outcomes [76, 77].

Significant changes in the density of white and gray matter have been observed after an IHD session in all patients with increased water content in the brain, but these changes were not observed after CRRT [78]. IHD has also been shown to decreased circulating blood volume and decreased CBF, as demonstrated by transcranial Doppler imaging. Furthermore, the absolute brain tissue oxygen tension level was lower during IHD [79, 80] and hypotension was more frequently reported as a complication of IHD compared to CRRT [81]. Possible explanations are increased oxygen consumption secondary to ICP surges (associated with brain hypermetabolism and increased oxygen consumption) and limited brain oxygen diffusion due to increased brain water content [82], secondary to the rapid removal of urea, sodium, and other osmoles from the vascular compartment and compartmentalization of these osmoles at the intracranial level (Fig. 14.3) [5]. CRRT should be the first option in these patients (Table 14.4). Concerning the type of technique, unlike continuous hemodialysis, hemofiltration has been shown to produce a smaller increase in ICP, a smaller decrease in MBP, and stable CPP [77, 83].

The choice of anticoagulation may contribute to effective neuroprotection. It has been suggested that citrate may provide neuroprotection by attenuating hypoxic brain injury through its effects on astrocytes and oxidative phosphorylation [5, 84].

If only IHD is available, the initial decline in osmolality should be moderated by slower dialysate and blood flows coupled with a smaller dialyzer surface, a high dialysate sodium content, planning daily treatments to reduce changes in serum urea [85].

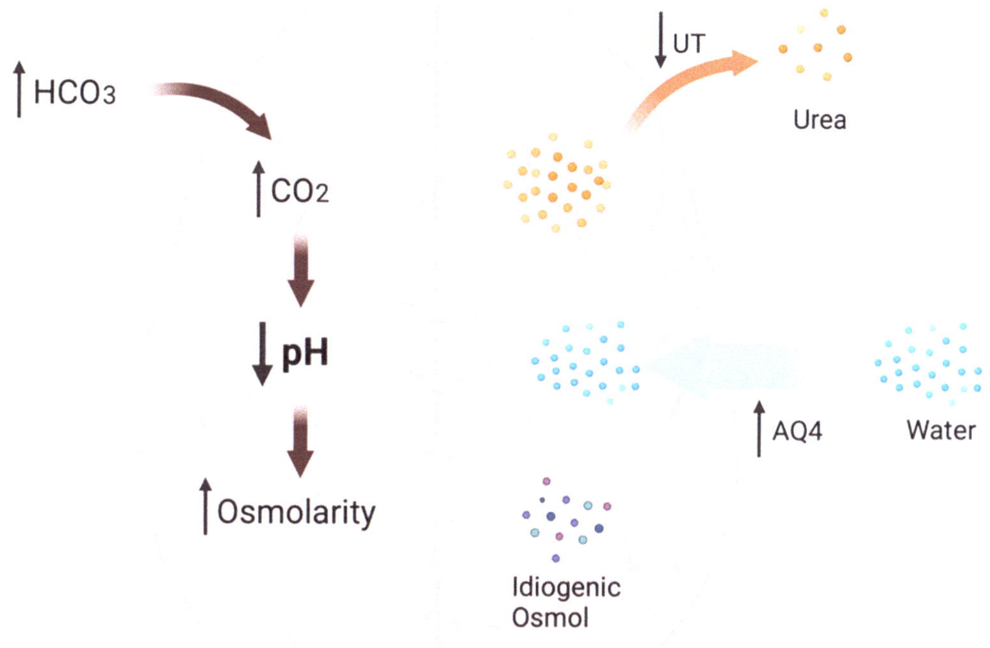

Fig. 14.3 Dialysis disequilibrium syndrome and cerebral vasogenic edemaThe reverse urea effect occurs, which is slower removal of urea from cerebrospinal fluid than from the blood during IHD, causing an osmotic gradient. Urea transporters are downregulated in uremic states and aquaporin channels are overregulated, increasing water entry into the brain. A second mechanism may be due to idiogenic osmoles, in which osmotically active molecules contribute to cerebral edema. A third mechanism is a paradoxical CNS acidosis. The decreased brain pH produced by the elevated bicarbonate concentrations in the dialysate generates an osmotic gradient through the release of intracellular protein-bound sodium and potassium*UT* Urea transporter, *AQ4* Aquaporin-4

Table 14.4 Central nervous system effects of CRRT vs IHD

Intermittent hemodialysis	Continuous renal replacement therapy
Decreased circulatory blood volume	Prefixed sodium
Decreased CBF	Hypophosphatemia-induced hypoxia due to high affinity
Decreased PbtO2	Anticoagulation
Increased ICP	
Cerebral vasodilation	
Changes in density of white and grey matter	
DDS/DANI	

CBF Cerebral blood flow, *PbtO2* Brain tissue oxygenation, *ICP* Intracranial pressure, *DDS* Dialysis disequilibrium syndrome, *DANI* Dialysis-associated neurovascular injury. From "Acute kidney injury at the neurocritical care unit" by Ramírez-Guerrero G, Baghetti R and Ronco C, 2021, Neurocritical Care, published ahead of print

Conclusions

AKI is a frequent complication in neurocritical patients that involves different pathologies such as TBI, SAH, and stroke. Its presence in these patients is associated with worse clinical outcomes that directly affect morbidity, mortality, and functional dependence.

AKI in neurocritical patients is the result of a sum of events, though the mechanisms which underlie most of them remain uncertain. AKI as well as specific diagnostic and therapeutic modalities to improve neurological outcome can significant alter the physiological brain–kidney connection.

Acknowledgements The authors thank Anita Zurita Poza for her excellent technical assistance. GRG thanks Biorender for the design of the figures.

Authors' Contributions All authors contributed equally to literature revision. All authors approved the final version of the manuscript.

Funding Sources None

References

1. Lameire N, Van Biesen W, Vanholder R. Acute renal failure. Lancet. 2005;365(9457):417–30.
2. Hoste EA, Bagshaw SM, Bellomo R, et al. Epidemiology of acute kidney injury in critically ill patients: the multinational AKI-EPI study. Intensive Care Med. 2015;41:1411–23.
3. Ronco C, Bellomo R, Kellum JA. Acute kidney injury. Lancet. 2019;394(10212):1949–64.
4. Van der Schaaf I, Algra A, Wemer M, et al. Endovascular coiling versus neurosurgical clipping for patients with aneurysmal subarachnoid haemorrhage. Cochrane Database Syst Rev. 2005;19(4):CD003085.
5. Ramírez-Guerrero G, Baghetti-Hernandez R, Ronco C. Acute kidney injury at the neurocritical care unit. Neurocrit Care. 2021. [Online ahead of print].;36:640.
6. Kellum JA, Romagnani P, Ashuntantang G, et al. Acute kidney injury. Nat Rev Dis Primers. 2021;7(1):52.
7. Chertow GM, Burdick E, Honour M, et al. Acute kidney injury, mortality, length of stay, and costs in hospitalized patients. J Am Soc Nephrol. 2005;16:3365–70.
8. KDIGO Clinical practice guideline for acute kidney injury. Notice. Kidney Int. 2012;2:1–141.
9. Thomas ME, Blaine C, Dawnay A, et al. The definition of acute kidney injury and its use in practice. Kidney Int. 2015;87(1):62–73.
10. Luo X, Jiang L, Du B, et al. A comparison of different diagnostic criteria of acute kidney injury in critically ill patients. Crit Care. 2014;18(4):R144.
11. Ronco C, Grammaticopoulos S, Rosner M, et al. Oliguria, creatinine and other biomarkers of acute kidney injury. Contrib Nephrol. 2010;164:118–27.
12. Quan S, Pannu N, Wilson T, et al. Prognostic implications of adding urine output to serum creatinine measurements for staging of acute kidney injury after major surgery: a cohort study. Nephrol Dial Trasplant. 2016;31:2049–56.
13. Kellum JA, Sileanu FE, Murugan R, et al. AKI by urine output versus serum creatinine level. J Am Soc Nephrol. 2015;26:2231–8.
14. Mizota T, Minamisawa S, Imanaka Y, Fukuda K. Oliguria without serum creatinine increase after living donor liver transplantation is associated with adverse post-operative outcomes. Acta Anaesthesiol Scand. 2016;60:874–81.
15. Zarbock A, Koyner J, Hoste E, Kellum JA. Update on perioperative acute kidney injury. Anesth Analg. 2018;127(5):1236–45.
16. Myles PS, Bellomo R, Wallace S. Importance of intra-operative oliguria during major abdominal surgery:findings of the RELIEF trial. Br J Anaesth. 2019;122(6):726–33.
17. Shiba A, Uchino S, Fujii T, Takinami M, Uezono S. Association between intraoperative oliguria and acute kidney injury after major noncardiac surgery. Anesth Analg. 2018;127:1229–35.
18. Mizota T, Yamamoto Y, Hamada M, Matsukawa S, Shimizu S, Kai S. Intraoperative oliguria predicts acute kidney injury after major abdominal surgery. Br J Anaesth. 2017;119:1127–34.
19. Uchino S, Kellum JA, Bellomo R, et al. Acute renal failure in critically ill patients: a multinational, multicenter study. JAMA. 2005;294:813–8.
20. Chertow GM, Christiansen CL, Cleary PD, et al. Prognostic stratification in critically ill patients with acute renal failure requiring dialysis. Arch Intern Med. 1995;155:1505–11.
21. Gruber A, Reinprecht A, Illievich UM, et al. Extracerebral organ dysfunction and neurologic outcome after aneurysmal subarachnoid hemorrhage. Crit Care Med. 1999;27:505–14.
22. Zygun D. Non-neurological organ dysfunction in neurocritical care: impact on outcome and etiological considerations. Curr Opin Crit Care. 2005;11(2):139–43.
23. Moore EM, Bellomo R, Nichol A, Harley N, Macisaac C, Cooper DJ. The incidence of acute kidney injury in patients with traumatic brain injury. Ren Fail. 2010;32(9):1060–5.
24. Zacharia BE. Renal dysfunction as an independent predictor of outcome after aneurysmal subarachnoid hemorrhage: a single-center cohort study. Stroke. 2009;40(7):2375–81.
25. Covic A, Schiller A, Mardare NG, et al. The impact of acute kidney injury on short-term survival in an Eastern European population with stroke. Nephrol Dial Transplant. 2008;23(7):2228–34.
26. Buttner S, Stadler A, Mayer C, et al. Incidence, risk factors, and outcome of acute kidney injury in neurocritical care. J Intensive Care Med. 2020;35(4):338–46.
27. Zorrilla-Vaca A, Ziai W, Sander E, Geocadin R, Thompson R, Rivera-lara L. Acute kidney injury following acute ischemic stroke

and intracerebral hemorrhage: a meta-analysis of prevalence rate and mortality risk. Cerebrovasc Dic. 2017;45:1–9.
28. Tujjar O, Belloni I, Hougardy JM, et al. Acute kidney injury after subarachnoid hemorrhage. J Neurosurg Anesthesiol. 2017;29(2):140–9.
29. Wang D, Guo Y, Zhang Y, Li Z, Li A, Luo Y. Epidemiology of acute kidney injury in patients with stroke: a retrospective analysis from the neurology ICU. Intern Emerg Med. 2018;13(1):17–25.
30. Kong HHY, Shum HP, Yan WW. 013 Acute kidney injury in neurocritical patients—incidence, clinical characteristics, and outcome. Kidney Int Reports. 2017;2(4):S1.
31. Li N, Zhao WG, Zhang WF. Acute kidney injury in patients with severe traumatic brain injury: implementation of the acute kidney injury network stage system. Neurocrit Care. 2011;14:377–81.
32. Saeed F, Adil MM, Khursheed F, et al. Acute renal failure is associated with higher death and disability in patients with acute ischemic stroke: analysis of nationwide inpatient sample. Stroke. 2014;45:1478–80.
33. Nadkarni G, Patel A, Konstantinidis I, et al. Dialysis requiring acute kidney injury in acute cerebrovascular accident hospitalizations. Stroke. 2015;46(11):3226–31.
34. An S, Luo H, Wang J, et al. An acute kidney injury prediction nomogram based on neurosurgical intensive care unit profiles. Ann Transl Med. 2020;8(5):194.
35. Palkovits M, Sebekova K, Gallatz K, et al. Neuronal activation in the CNS during different forms of acute renal failure in rats. Neuroscience. 2009;159:862–82.
36. DiBona GF. Physiology in perspective: the wisdom of the body. Neural control of the kidney. Am J Physiol Regul Integr Comp Physiol. 2005;289:R633–41.
37. Liu M, Liang Y, Chigurupati S, et al. Acute kidney injury leads to inflammation and functional changes in the brain. J Am Soc Nephrol. 2008;19(7):1360–70.
38. Andres-Hernando A, Dursun B, Altmann C, et al. Cytokine production increases and cytokine clearance decreases in mice with bilateral nepherectomy. Nephrol Dial Transplant. 2012;27:4339–47.
39. Tsao N, Hsu HP, Wu CM, Liu CC, Lei HY. Tumor necrosis factor-alpha causes an increase in blood-brain barrier permeability during sepsis. J Med Microbiol. 2001;50:812–21.
40. Wiggins-Dohlvik K, Merriman M, Ca S, et al. Tumor necrosis factor-alpha disruption of brain endothelial cell barrier is mediated through matrix metalloproteinase-9. Am J Surg. 2014;208:954–60.
41. Trinh-Trang-Tan MM, Cartron JP, Bankir L. Molecular basis for the dialysis disequilibrium syndrome: altered aquaporin and urea transporter expression in the brain. Nephrol Dial. 2005;20:1984–8.
42. Khalid F, Yang GL, McGuire JL, et al. Autonomic dysfunction following traumatic brain injury: translational insights. Neurosurg Focus. 2019;47:E8.
43. Zhao Q, Yan T, Chopp M, Venkat P, Chen J. Brain-kidney interaction: renal dysfunction following ischemic stroke. J Cereb Blood Flow Metab. 2020;40:246–62.
44. de Vries DK, Lindeman JH, Ringers J, et al. Donor brain death predisposes human kidney grafts to a proinflammatory reaction after transplantation. Am J Transplant. 2011;11:1064–70.
45. Lassen NA. Autoregulation of cerebral blood flow. Circ Res. 1964;15(suppl):201–4.
46. Just A. Mechanisms of renal blood flow autoregulation: dynamics and contributions. Am J Physiol Regul Integr Comp Physiol. 2007;292:R1–17.
47. Dias C, Gaio R, Monteiro E, et al. Kidney-brain link in traumatic brain injury patients? A preliminary report. Neurocrit Care. 2015;22(2):192–201.
48. Castro P, Azevedo E, Rocha I, Sorond F, Serrador JM. Chronic kidney disease and poor outcomes in ischemic stroke: is impaired cerebral autoregulation the missing link? BMC Neurol. 2018;18(1):21.
49. Udy A, Boots R, Senthuran S, et al. Augmented creatinine clearance in traumatic brain injury. Anesth Analg. 2010;111:1505–10.
50. Minville V, Asehnoune K, Ruiz S, et al. Increased creatinine clearance in polytrauma patients with normal serum creatinine: a retrospective observational study. Crit Care. 2011;15:R49.
51. Spencer DD, Jacobi J, Juenke JM, Fleck JD, Kays MB. Steady-state pharmacokinetics of intravenous levetiracetam in neurocritical care patients. Pharmacotherapy. 2011;31:934–41.
52. Zaganas I, Pajecka K, Wender C, Schousboe A, Waagepetersen HS, Plaitakis A. The effect of pH and ADP on ammonia affinity for human glutamate dehydrogenases. Metab Brain Dis. 2013;28(2):127–31.
53. Rothman D, De Feyter HM, Maciejewski PK, Behar KL. Is there in vivo evidence for amino acid shuttles carrying ammonia from neurons to astrocytes? Neurochem Res. 2012;37(11):2597–612.
54. De Deyn PP, Macdonald RL. Guanidino compounds that are increased in cerebrospinal fluid and brain of uremic patients inhibit GABA and glycine responses on mouse neurons in cell culture. Ann Neurol. 1990;28(5):627–33.
55. O'Kane RL, Vina JR, Simpson I, Zaragoza R, Mokashi A, Hawkins RA. Cationic amino acid transport across the blood-brain barrier is mediated exclusively by system y+. Am J Physiol Endocrinol Metab. 2006;291:412–9.
56. Civiletti F, Assenzio B, Mazzeo AT, et al. Acute tubular injury is associated with severe traumatic brain injury: in vitro study on human tubular epithelial cells. Sci Rep. 2019;9(1):6090.
57. Messerer DAC, Halbgebauer R, Nilsson B, Pavenstädt H, Radermacher P, Huber-Lang M. Immunopathophysiology of trauma-related acute kidney injury. Nat Rev Nephrol. 2021;17(2):91–111.
58. Kumar AB, Shi Y, Shotwell MS, Richards J, Ehrenfeld JM. Hypernatremia is a significant risk factor for acute kidney injury after subarachnoid hemorrhage: a retrospective analysis. Neurocrit Care. 2015;22(2):184–91.
59. Rein JL, Coca SG. "I don't get no respect": the role of chloride in acute kidney injury. Am J Physiol Renal Physiol. 2019;316(3):F587–605.
60. Chowdhury AH, Cox EF, Francis ST, Lobo DN. A randomized, controlled, double blind crossover study on the effects of 2-L infusions of 0,9% saline and Plasma-Lyte 148 on renal blood flow velocity and renal cortical tissue perfusion in healthy volunteers. Ann Surg. 2012;1:18–24.
61. Sadan O, Singbartl K, Kraft J, et al. Low-chloride-versus high-chloride-containing hypertonic solution for the treatment of subarachnoid hemorrhage-related complications: the ACETatE (A low ChloriE hyperTonic solution for brain Edema) randomized trial. J Intensive Care. 2020;4(8):32.
62. Sadan O, Singbartl K, Kandiah PA, Martin KS, Samuels OB. Hyperchloremia is associated with acute kidney injury in patients with subarachnoid hemorrhage. Crit Care Med. 2017;45(8):1382–8.
63. Lee HG, Kim WK, Yeon JY. Contrast-induced acute kidney injury after coil embolization for aneurysmal subarachnoid hemorrhage. Yonsei Med J. 2018;59(1):107–12.
64. Hemphill JC 3rd, Greenberg SM, Anderson CS, et al. American Heart Association Stroke Council; Council on Cardiovascular and Stroke Nursing; Council on Clinical Cardiology. Guidelines for the management of spontaneous intracerebral hemorrhage: a guideline for healthcare professionals from the American Heart Association/American Stroke Association. Stroke. 2015;46:2032–60.
65. Qureshi AI, Palesch YY, Martin R, et al. Antihypertensive Treatment of Acute Cerebral Hemorrhage Investigators. Systolic blood pressure reduction and risk of acute renal injury in patients with intracerebral hemorrhage. Am J Med. 2012;125(7):718. e1–6.
66. Qureshi A, Huang W, Lobanova I, Barsan W, Hanley D, Hsu C, et al. Outcomes of intensive systolic blood pressure reduction in patients with intracerebral hemorrhage and excessively high initial

systolic blood pressure: post hoc analysis of a randomized clinical trial. JAMA Neurol. 2020;77(11):1355–65.
67. Diprose WK, Sutherland LJ, Wang MTM, Barber PA. Contrast-associated acute kidney injury in endovascular thrombectomy patients with and without baseline renal impairment. Stroke. 2019;50(12):3527–31.
68. Kim MY, Park JH, Kang NR, et al. Increased risk of acute kidney injury associated with higher infusion rate of mannitol in patients with intracranial hemorrhage. J Neurosurg. 2014;120(6):1340–8.
69. Karkar A, Ronco C. Prescription of CRRT: a pathway to optimize therapy. Ann Intensive Care. 2020;10(1):32.
70. Neri M, Villa G, Garzotto F, Bagshaw S, Bellomo R, Cerda J, et al. Nomenclature for renal replacement therapy in acute kidney injury: basic principles. Crit Care. 2016;20:318.
71. Ronco C, Ghezzi PM, Brendolan A, Crepaldi C, La Greca G. The haemodialysis system: basic mechanisms of water and solute transport in extracorporeal renal replacement therapies. Nephrol Dial Transplant. 1998;13(Suppl 6):3–9.
72. Leonard E. The bases of mass separation processes. In: Ronco C, Bellomo R, Kellum J, editors. Critical care nephrology. Saunders Elsevier; 2009. p. 1131–5.
73. Ghahramani N, Shadrou S, Hollenbeak C. A systematic review of continuous renal replacement therapy and intermittent haemodialysis in management of patients with acute renal failure. Nephrology. 2008;13:570–8.
74. Patel P, Nandwani V, McCarthy P, Conrad S, Scott LK. Continuous renal replacement therapies: a brief primer for the neurointensivist. Neurocrit Care. 2010;13:286–94.
75. Shirazian A, Peralta-Cuervo AF, Aguilera-Pena MP, et al. Sustained low-efficiency dialysis is associated with worsening cerebral edema and outcomes in intracerebral hemorrhage. Neurocrit Care. 2021;35:221–31.
76. Donnelly J, Budohoski KP, Smielewski P, Czosnyka M. Regulation of the cerebral circulation: bedside assessment and clinical implications. Crit Care. 2016;20(1):129.
77. Davenport A, Will EJ, Davidson AM. Improved cardiovascular stability during continuous modes of renal replacement therapy in critically ill patients with acute hepatic and renal failure. Crit Care Med. 1993;21(2):328–38.
78. Ronco C, Bellomo R, Brendolan A, Pinna V, La Greca G. Brain density changes during renal replacement in critically ill patients with acute renal failure. Continuous hemofiltration versus intermittent hemodialysis. J Nephrol. 1999;12(3):173–8.
79. Hata R, Matsumoto M, Handa N, Terakawa H, Sugitani Y, Kamada T. Effects of hemodialysis on cerebral circulation evaluated by transcranial Doppler ultrasonography. Stroke. 1994;25:408–12.
80. Ko S, Choi HA, Gilmore E, Schmidt JM, Claassen J, Lee K. Pearls & Oyster: the effects of renal replacement therapy on cerebral autoregulation. Neurology. 2012;78(6):e36–8.
81. Uchino S, Bellomo R, Kellum JA. Patients and kidney survival by dialysis modality in critically ill patients with acute kidney injury. Int J Artif Organs. 2007;30(4):281–92.
82. Bucci MN, Dechert RE, Arnoldi DK, Campbell J, McGillicyddu JE, Bartlett RH. Elevated intracranial pressure associated with hypermetabolism in isolated head trauma. Acta Neurochir. 1988;93(3–4):133–6.
83. Davenport A, Will EJ, Davison AM. Continuous vs. intermittent forms of haemofiltration and/or dialysis in the management of acute renal failure in patients with defective cerebral autoregulation at risk of cerebral oedema. Contrib Nephrol. 1991;93:225–33.
84. Keller JA, Chan TY, Chan PH, Gregory GA. Protection of astrocytes by fructose 1,6 bisphosphate and citrate ameliorates neuronal injury under hypoxic conditions. Brain Res. 1996;726:167–73.
85. Davenport A. Management of acute kidney injury in neurotrauma. Hemodial Int. 2010;14(1):S27–31.
86. Chawla LS, Bellomo R, Bihorac A, et al. Acute kidney disease and renal recovery: consensus report of the acute disease quality initiative (ADQI) 16 Workgroup. Nat Rev Nephrol. 2017;13(4):241–57.

Acid and Base Abnormalities

15

Tandis Soltani and Darwin Ang

Contents

Abstract

Understanding acid–base physiology is necessary for the management of all critically ill patients. Patients with conditions that predispose them to altered mental status and multi-organ dysfunction will be prone to acid–base disturbances. These disturbances in the patient's normal physiologic pH are a result of pathology either due to the loss of compensatory mechanisms within the body's buffer system or the body being overwhelmed by an exogenous insult such as shock. Timely identification and management of these physiologic disturbances will lead to better clinical outcomes for the patient and may even lead to improved neurological outcomes and survival.

In this chapter, we will review the basic concepts of acid–base physiology as it relates to critically ill patients and describe how to identify and manage abnormalities. We will also outline a simple step-by-step guide to identifying acid–base abnormalities that can be present in each critically ill patient. Finally, this chapter will include a list of differential diagnoses for respiratory acidosis and alkalosis as well as metabolic acidosis and alkalosis.

T. Soltani · D. Ang (✉)
University of Central Florida—College of Medicine, Orlando, FL, USA

Ocala Health, Ocala, FL, USA

University of South Florida, Tampa, FL, USA

Introduction

Whether a patient has either acid or base disturbances it is first identified by simply starting with the patient's pH via arterial blood gas. While there are compensatory mechanisms that can normalize the pH in the setting of disturbances in the patient's acid–base status, for the most part, abnormal or marginal pH values are a good way to screen for initial pathology. Since the body rarely overcompensates in the opposite direction, the direction of the pH determines whether is primarily an acid or base disorder (Table 15.1).

Acidosis can either be due to metabolic or respiratory causes. In severely ill or critically injured patients, a combined respiratory and metabolic acidosis can occur. Metabolic acidosis can be due to loss of sodium bicarbonate ($NaHCO_3$), increases in organic anions such as lactate or ketone bodies, or from external or iatrogenic sources [1]. Metabolic acidosis can be further categorized into gap and non-gap acidosis (Table 15.2). Respiratory acidosis occurs when there is inad-

E. Mahanna Gabrielli et al. (eds.), *Textbook of Neurointensive Care: Volume 1*, https://doi.org/10.1007/978-3-031-62220-5_15

Table 15.1 An overview of the framework and types of questions the provider should ask themselves to determine the processes at hand

Key Clinical Questions:	
Questions to think about	**Descriptions**
What is the primary process?	Use Fig. 15.1 to help determine this. The primary process will be respiratory or metabolic acidosis or alkalosis.
Is there compensation?	If you've identified the primary process, then determine if the other system is providing a balance to return the pH closer to normal. To determine whether there is an appropriate amount of compensation, consider using equations such as Winter's formula depending on the primary and compensatory process.
Is there a secondary process?	Is there two different causes creating acidosis or alkalosis by through the respiratory and metabolic systems?
Early Priorities Checklist	
☐	If there is a respiratory process at hand, whether it is primary or compensatory, determine the need to intubate.
☐	Once the patient is mechanically ventilated, utilize the ventilator in creating a respiratory compensation to drive the pH toward normal.
☐	If there is metabolic process at hand, parse out the specific process as detailed in the algorithms in Figs. 15.1 and 15.2.
☐	Based on this, develop a differential diagnosis and treat the cause.

equate elimination of carbon dioxide (CO_2), relative to CO_2 production as a byproduct of cellular respiration. Recall that CO_2 is produced as a byproduct of the breakdown of carbohydrates for the production of adenosine triphosphate (ATP) at the cellular level. As mentioned earlier, respiratory acidosis is often associated with metabolic acidosis as CO_2 builds up in tissues. Normal $PaCO_2$ values range between 35 and 45 mmHg. However, in chronic CO_2 retention such as with patients who have COPD, this value may be much higher. Patients with respiratory acidosis with chronic CO_2 retention may require compensatory respiratory care (ventilation) directed toward the patient's baseline PCO_2 value.

Metabolic alkalosis is due to either a loss of anions or retention of cations. These strong ion differences must be corrected to normalize the pH. Examples of strong ion differences leading to alkalosis include chloride depletion from gastrointestinal losses (nasogastric tube on suction or loop diuretics) or excess of exogenous cations such as sodium (Table 15.2). Respiratory alkalosis is a result of any process which increases the patient's minute ventilation. Specifically, respiratory alkalosis may be caused either by an increase in respiratory rate or tidal volume leading to hypocapnia. Treatment is directed at the cause driving the increased minute ventilation. For patients who have altered mental status, intubation, sedation, and mechanical ventilation may be necessary to prevent hypoxia and respiratory failure, as well as control the respiratory drive and the work of breathing.

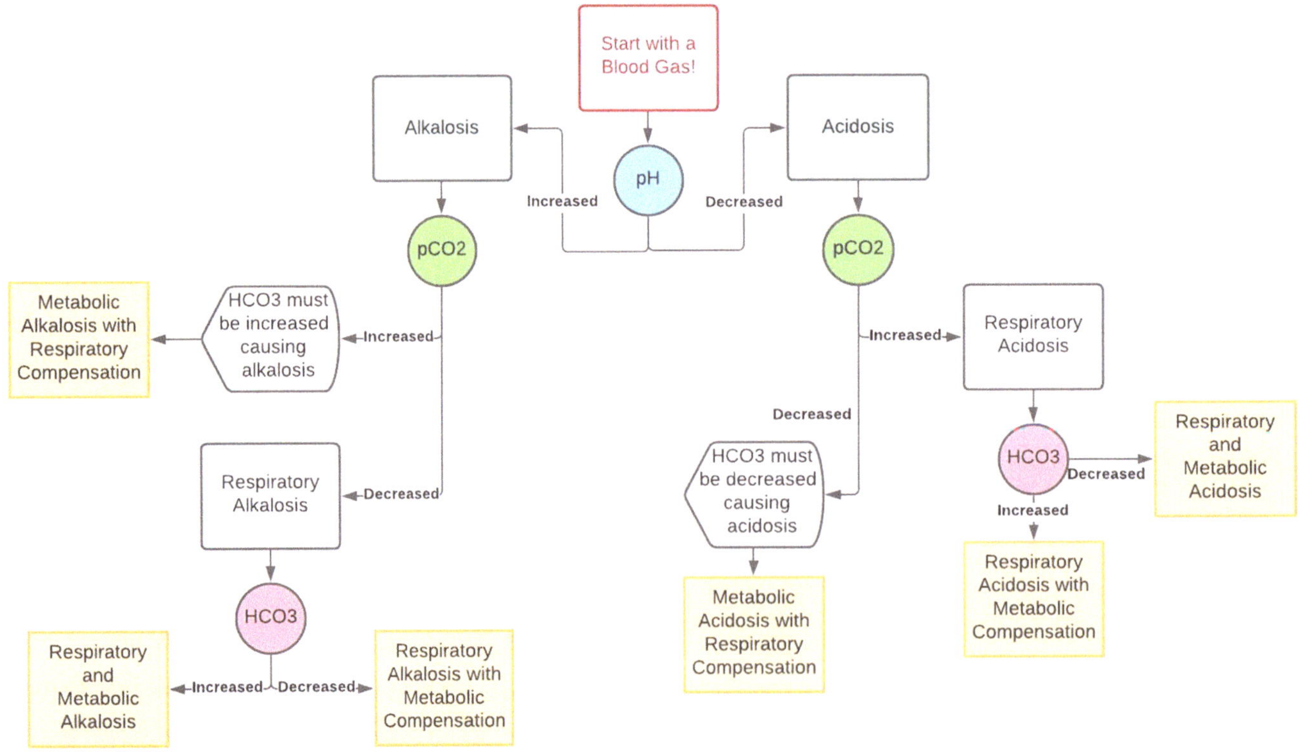

Fig. 15.1 *Diagnostic flow diagram.* Start with an arterial blood gas and follow the algorithm to determine which primary process you have and whether there is a secondary process present or if there is compensation

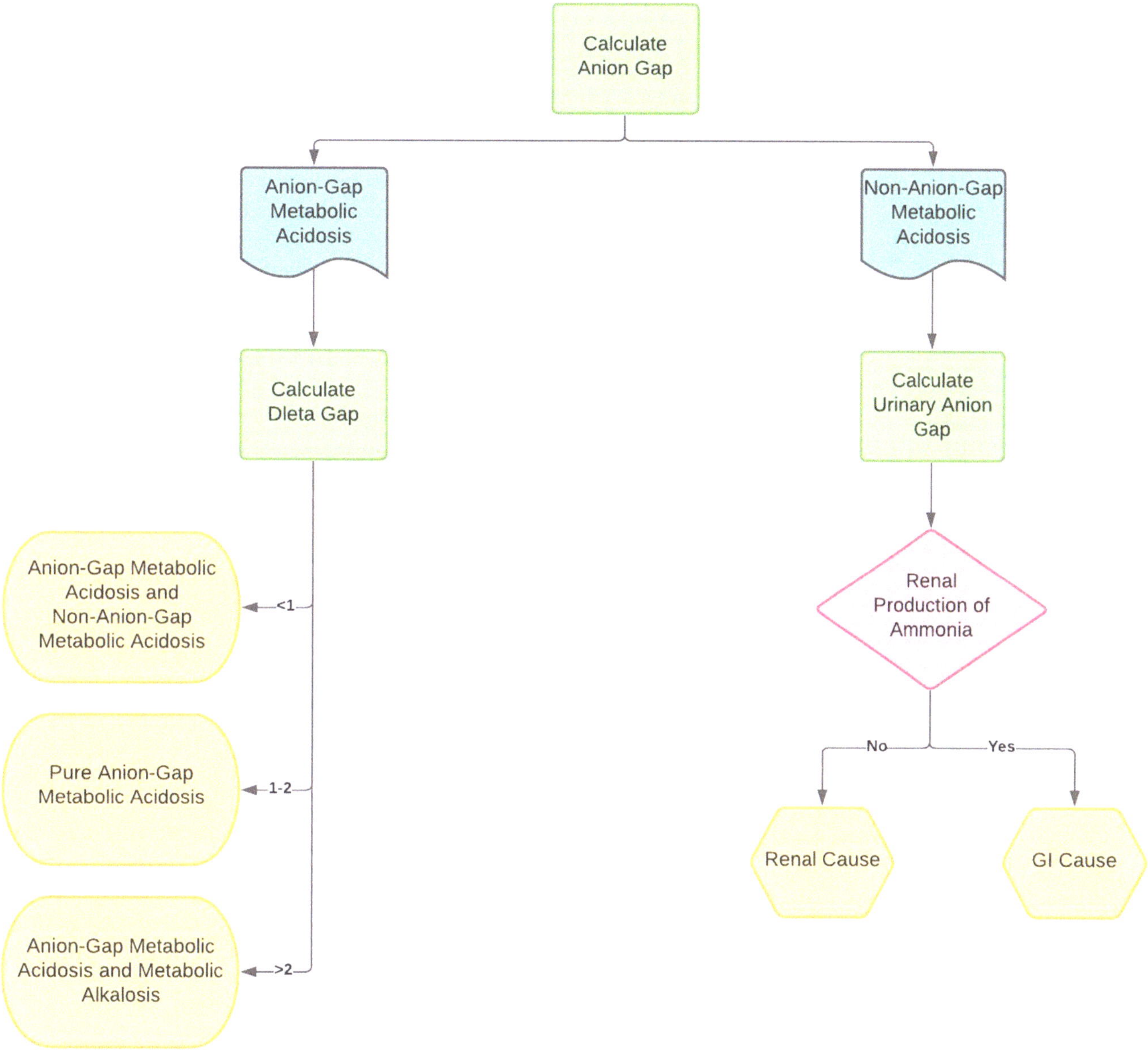

Fig. 15.2 *Diagnostic flow diagram.* Use this algorithm to determine the different metabolic acidosis processes at hand to help with developing your differential and determining the etiology of the metabolic acidosis

In this chapter, we will continue our discussion of acid–base balance and disorders that may be present in critical illness. We will discuss the priorities of management and provide useful diagnostic and treatment algorithms.

Chapter Goals

- Provide an algorithm to determine the primary acid–base disorders present.
- Determine whether the identified acidosis or alkalosis is the primary or compensatory mechanism.
- Distinguish between multiple metabolic acidosis processes.
- Develop a differential diagnosis based on acid–base disturbance type.
- Discuss the effects of acid–base disturbances on cerebral blood flow.

Key Clinical Questions

- How do determine the primary acid–base disorders present in a critically ill patient?
- How do identify whether a compensatory process is present?

Table 15.2 Differential diagnoses of metabolic acidosis and alkalosis

Diagnostic Pearls Tables:	
Process	Differential diagnoses
Metabolic Acidosis	Anion Gap Lactic acidosis Ketoacidosis Renal Failure Toxins (methanol, ethylene glycol, salicylates, paradehydes) Non-Anion Gap Renal Tubular Acidosis GI losses of bicarbonate (GI sources) Iatrogenic (NaCl)
Metabolic Alkalosis	Anion Depletion Chloride Responsive GI losses Vomiting Diarrhea Chloride wasting Chloride Unresponsive Mineralcorticoid excess Hyperaldosteronism Cushing syndrome Exogenous corticoids Excessive licorice intake Cation administration Sodium acetate or citrate administration Massive blood transfusions Parenteral nutrition Plasma volume expanders Sodium lactate (Ringers)
Treatment Pearls Tables	
☐	Does the pH need to be corrected in order for the drugs I am administering to function?
☐	Can the ventilator help with creating compensatory mechanisms?

- How do discover two concurrent metabolic acidosis processes?
- What is the differential diagnosis to keep in mind with each of these disorders?
- How do acid–base disturbances affect cerebral blood flow?

Essential Management Priorities

Early: Immediate and First 24 h

In the first 24 h of the development of an acid–base disorder, the body will attempt to compensate. Respiratory processes may provide rapid compensation for a metabolic process. However, it takes longer for a metabolic process to compensate for respiratory acidosis or alkalosis.

Respiratory Acidosis: This occurs as a result of an increase in pCO_2 resulting in an overall decrease in pH. This occurs frequently in patients who are somnolent from altered mental status decreasing ventilatory drive. It is recommended to secure the airway when patients have a Glasgow coma scale (GCS) is 8 or less. Airway reflex protection and ventilatory drive are usually severely altered in these patients.

Respiratory Alkalosis: This occurs when the patient's minute ventilation is high. This can either be from a high respiratory rate or high tidal volume. Clinically, this could represent compensation for a metabolic acidosis process or more commonly in the neuro ICU an increased ventilatory drive from brainstem disinhibition. In this case, the patient should be monitored closely as they may fatigue and proceed to respiratory failure. Intubation and mechanical ventilation may be required in these situations.

Metabolic Acidosis: Determine the etiology of the acidosis. For both anion gap and non-gap acidosis, volume repletion may be the initial step. However, the choice of fluids may differ [2, 3]. Refer to Fig. 15.2 to determine which metabolic acidosis process is present.

Metabolic Alkalosis: Identify the cause of metabolic acidosis. Table 15.2 provides a differential diagnosis of the causes of this process and treats the underlying cause.

Intermediate Term

If a metabolic process is left untreated, often the patient will fatigue and the attempt to compensate for the metabolic process will eventually lead to respiratory failure.

Classic Near Misses

The presence of non-anion gap acidosis and metabolic alkalosis, in addition to anion gap metabolic acidosis, can often be overlooked. Without calculating the delta gap, one can easily miss two concurrent processes contributing to metabolic acidosis.

Diagnostic Algorithm

Although other values can be used to help identify the presence or absence of acid–base disturbances, in the critically ill patient the most accurate way to study acid–base disorders is to start with an arterial blood gas. The clinician determines whether there is a respiratory or metabolic acid–base disturbance present by identifying whether the pH, partial pressure of carbon dioxide, or bicarbonate are increased or decreased relative to normal. It is important to note that these variables can be obtained from an arterial or a venous blood gas.

The Henderson–Hasselbalch equation defines pH as follows:

$$pH = pK \times \log\left[HCO_3^- / \left(0.03 \times pCO_2\right)\right]$$

This formula helps us identify whether the pH we are looking at is driven primarily by the change in pCO_2 or HCO_3^-. This method helps identify the etiology of the acid–base disorder.

See Fig. 15.1 for an overview of how the values obtained from an arterial blood gas can be used to determine primary and compensatory mechanisms and potential secondary mechanisms.

Respiratory Alkalosis and Acidosis

If the pCO_2 is lower than normal, then we expect pH to be higher, since according to the equation, the two variables have an inverse relationship. If this is the case, then we suspect a *respiratory alkalosis*. Alternatively, if pCO_2 is higher than normal and pH is lower than normal, then we suspect that there is *respiratory acidosis*.

Metabolic Alkalosis and Acidosis

If we find that HCO_3^- is elevated and pH is elevated, given these two variables are proportional according to the Henderson–Hasselbalch equation, we suspect that the increased pH is being driven at least in part by the increase in HCO_3^- and thus, *metabolic alkalosis* is present. We then look at the value of pCO_2 in order to determine whether there is a concomitant respiratory alkalosis or if there is compensation present.

If we find that the pCO_2 is in fact lower than normal, but pH is also lower than normal, we must suspect that this is being driven by a decrease in HCO_3^-. This would be consistent with *primarily metabolic acidosis*, where the respiratory system is attempting to compensate and correct the pH (in this example, by hyperventilation and lowering the pCO_2 in order to bring up the pH). In the case of metabolic acidosis, in order to determine the expected change in pCO_2 as a compensatory mechanism, the following equation, known as the Winter's formula, can be used:

$$pCO_2 = \left(1.5 \times HCO_3^-\right) + 8 \pm 5$$

In the case of metabolic acidosis, there is yet another branching point in the algorithm. In order to narrow the differential diagnosis for this particular set of processes, we must first calculate the anion gap using the equation below:

$$\text{Anion Gap} = \left[Na^+\right] - \left(\left[Cl^-\right] + \left[HCO_3^-\right]\right)$$

While there are other cations and anions present not included in the simplified equation. Unmeasured anions contributing to metabolic acidosis ranged from 37% to 98%. Lactate as the major contributing ion had an even wider distribution, from almost 10%–85%.

However, the above equation is a practical way to estimate the anion gap at the bedside. If the anion gap is elevated relative to normal, then there is an *anion gap metabolic acidosis* present. If the anion gap is not elevated, then there is a *non-anion gap metabolic acidosis* present.

In the case of the non-anion gap metabolic acidosis, in order to determine whether the loss of bicarbonate is from the renal system or the gastrointestinal system, one can calculate the urine anion gap and determine whether there is ammonia production present within the kidneys [4]. If the kidneys are attempting to compensate for the acidosis and thus produce ammonia, then the cause is likely from the gastrointestinal tract. If not, then it is likely renal in origin. See Fig. 15.2 for a flow chart to follow.

As mentioned before, there may be several metabolic processes present affecting the anion gap. This is where calculating the delta gap comes in. The delta gap is really an assessment of whether the change in anion gap relative to normal is proportional to the change in bicarbonate, which would be consistent with a *pure anion gap metabolic acidosis*, or if there are other processes present.

$$\text{Delta gap} = \Delta\text{AnionGap} / \Delta HCO_3^-$$

If the delta gap is elevated, then some bicarbonate is retained by the body and there is also a *metabolic alkalosis* present. If the delta gap is lower than 1, then there is an additional *non-anion gap metabolic acidosis* present.

See Fig. 15.3 for an overview of how to proceed after a metabolic acidosis process has been identified.

Acid–Base Balance and Cerebral Blood Flow

For clinicians caring for patients with neurologic insults, it is particularly important to keep in mind the effect of these acid–base disturbances on the brain. Interestingly, physiologic pre-clinical studies suggest that in acute metabolic alkalosis, cerebral blood flow is regulated by pCO_2 rather than arterial pH. Furthermore, independent of PCO_2 level, HCO_3^- has been shown to have a direct vasodilatory influence [5]. This further highlights the importance of paying close attention to the individual processes at hand and the magnitude of compensation by respiratory or metabolic efforts.

Take-Home Message

- The acid balance of fluids within the body is determined by the partial pressure of carbon dioxide, the concentration of bicarbonate, strong ion difference, and total weak acid concentration.
- Although the patient may be acidemic or alkalemic, meaning the pH of the blood may be decreased or increased relative to normal, there may be underlying acidosis or alkalosis present. Even when the plasma pH is normal, there may be underlying acidosis or alkalosis processes that are developing with compensation.
- The clinician may be required to correct the pH balance of blood in order for pharmaceuticals to function, the primary goal should be directed at determining the various

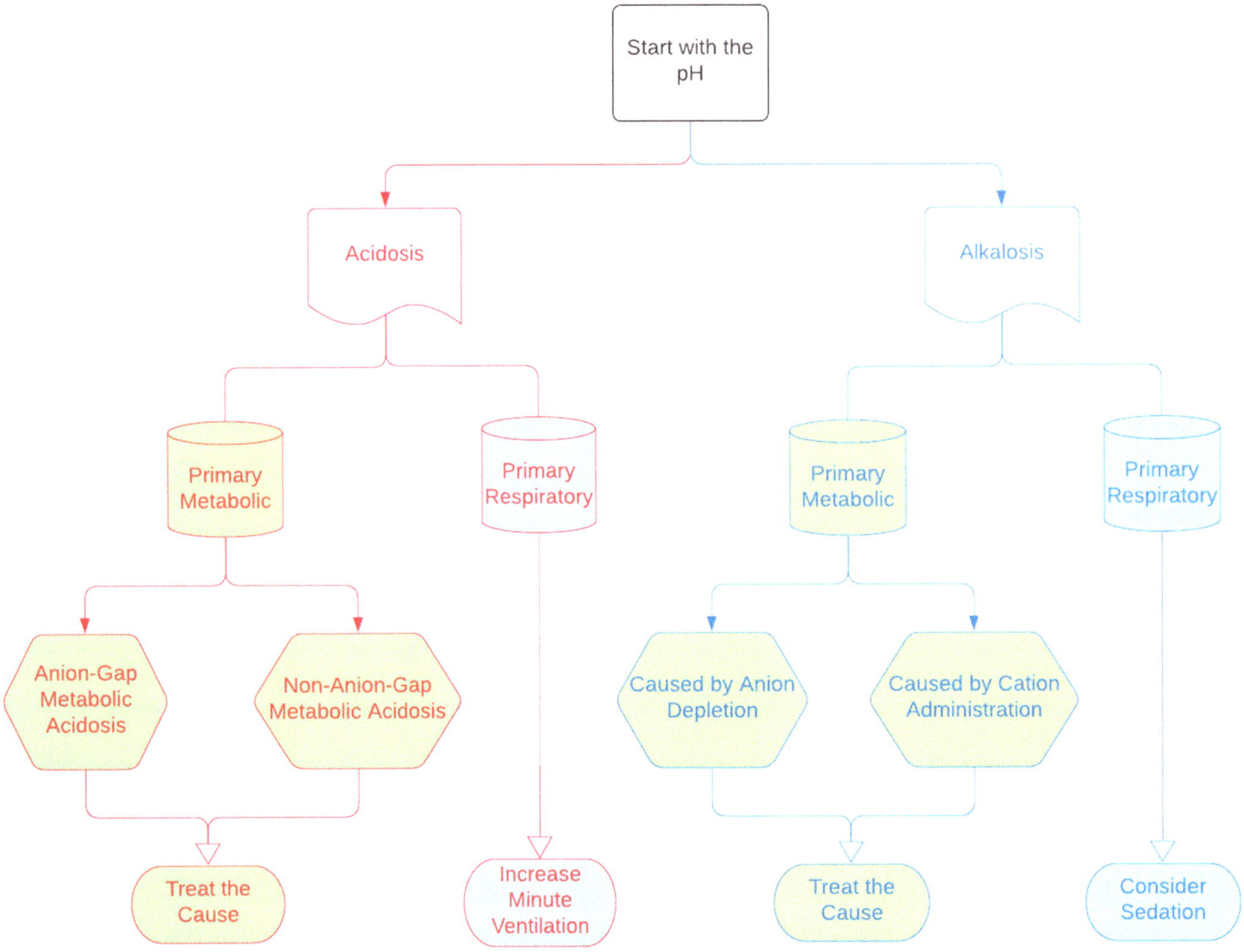

Fig. 15.3 *Treatment flow diagram.* Use this figure as an overview to determine your treatment strategy

acidosis and alkalosis processes in place in order to treat their etiology. However, the traditional approach illustrated may underestimate the severity of the acid–base derangement, the predominant cause, and the contributing unaccounted anions, all factors that may contribute to the outcome if uncorrected.

References

1. Kellum JA. Determinants of blood pH in health and disease. Crit Care. 2000;4:6.
2. Jaber S, Paugam C, Futier E, et al. Sodium bicarbonate therapy for patients with severe metabolic acidaemia in the intensive care unit (BICAR-ICU): a multicentre, open-label, randomised controlled, phase 3 trial. Lancet. 2018;392(10141):31–40.
3. Jung B, Rimmele T, Le Goff C, et al. Severe metabolic or mixed acidemia on intensive care unit admission: incidence, prognosis and administration of buffer therapy. A prospective, multiple-center study. Crit Care. 2011;15(5):R238.
4. Kraut JA, Madias NE. Differential diagnosis of nongap metabolic acidosis: value of a systematic approach. Clin J Am Soc Nephrol. 2012;7(4):671–9.
5. Caldwell HG, Howe CA, Chalifoux CJ, Hoiland RL, Carr JMJR, Brown CV, Patrician A, Tremblay JC, Panerai RB, Robinson TG, Minhas JS, Ainslie PN. Arterial carbon dioxide and bicarbonate rather than pH regulate cerebral blood flow in the setting of acute experimental metabolic alkalosis. J Physiol. 2021;599(5):1439–57. https://doi.org/10.1113/JP280682. Epub 2021 Jan 18.

Dysfunctional Hemostasis

16

Michael McAree and Jennifer A. Frontera

Contents

Abstract

This book chapter provides an overview of hemostasis, with a focus on dysfunctional hemostasis. Hemostasis is a cascade of processes that occur in response to tissue damage to form a clot and prevent excessive bleeding. Primary hemostasis involves platelet activation and the formation of a loosely bound platelet plug. Secondary hemostasis strengthens the platelet plug through the conversion of fibrinogen to fibrin. The intrinsic and extrinsic pathways of the coagulation cascade are discussed, along with the important role of vitamin K in the synthesis of coagulation factors. Evaluation of hemostasis through various tests, such as activated partial thromboplastin time (aPTT) and prothrombin time (PT), is also explored. The chapter concludes with an overview of platelet function testing using light transmission aggregometry and the VerifyNow-P2Y12 assay.

M. McAree · J. A. Frontera (✉)
New York University Grossman School of Medicine, New York, NY, USA
e-mail: michael.mcaree@nyulangone.org; jennifer.frontera@nyulangone.org

Normal Hemostasis

Primary Hemostasis

Primary hemostasis is a series of steps leading to platelet activation and the formation of a loosely bound platelet plug. In response to tissue damage, associated blood vessels undergo endothelin-mediated vasoconstriction. Damage also exposes subendothelial collagen and von Willebrand factor (vWF), a compound synthesized by the Weibel–Palade bodies of the endothelium. Endothelial injury leads to a release of inflammatory mediators, such as thromboxane A2 (TXA2), that help to facilitate platelet activation and adhesion. Vasoconstriction increases the proximity between platelets and the vessel wall. The rolling of platelets along the damaged vessel walls leads to interaction between platelet GPIB proteins and subendothelial vWF. Once bound to the vessel wall, platelets undergo conformational changes and release intracellular contents from their secretory granules. Alpha granules and dense granules release serotonin and ADP into the local environment. ADP binds to P2Y1 and P2Y12 receptors on platelets, increasing the expression of

E. Mahanna Gabrielli et al. (eds.), *Textbook of Neurointensive Care: Volume 1*, https://doi.org/10.1007/978-3-031-62220-5_16

GPIIB/IIIA receptors on platelet surfaces. Nearby thrombin in the bloodstream attaches to protease-activating receptor 1 (PAR-1) receptors and contributes to this cascade of events. Platelets proceed to loosely aggregate with one another by forming bridges between GPIIB/IIIA receptors with fibrinogen residing in the circulation. These interactions lead to the formation of a weak platelet plug that will be strengthened during secondary hemostasis [1]. See Fig. 16.1 for a graphic representation of this process.

Secondary Hemostasis

Secondary hemostasis is the process that strengthens the platelet plug formed in primary hemostasis via the conversion of fibrinogen to fibrin. The conversion of fibrinogen to fibrin is facilitated by thrombin, which is activated by coagulation factor X in the bloodstream. There are two routes by which factor X may be activated: the intrinsic and extrinsic pathways of the coagulation cascade. The intrinsic pathway of the clotting cascade begins with the activation of coagulation factor XII, which in sequence leads to the activation of factors XI, IX, and VIII with calcium as a cofactor. Factor VIII then activates Factor X leading to downstream conversion of fibrinogen to fibrin. Alternatively, the extrinsic pathway begins with the release of tissue factor (TF), a compound found in highly vascular areas. The tissue factor activates factor VII, which then activates factor X. Similarly, this leads to the conversion of fibrinogen to fibrin. The summation of these steps, ultimately leading to the conversion of fibrinogen to fibrin and stabilization of the platelet plug, is often referred to as the coagulation cascade [2].

Additionally, it should be noted that the synthesis of specific coagulation factors, such as factors X, IX, VII, and II, and anticoagulant proteins C and S require vitamin K for their synthesis in the liver. Most clotting factors are synthesized by hepatocytes (factors II, V, VII, IX, X, XI, XII, protein C and S, and fibrinogen), while factor VIII and vWF are generated by endothelial cells. This can help determine whether a coagulopathy is due to hepatic dysfunction versus some other cause. See Fig. 16.2 for a graphic representation of this process.

Evaluation of Hemostasis

Evaluation of the intrinsic pathway of the coagulation cascade can be done by obtaining an activated partial thromboplastin time (aPTT). Evaluation of the extrinsic pathway can be done by obtaining a prothrombin time (PT) level and associated international normalized ratio (INR).

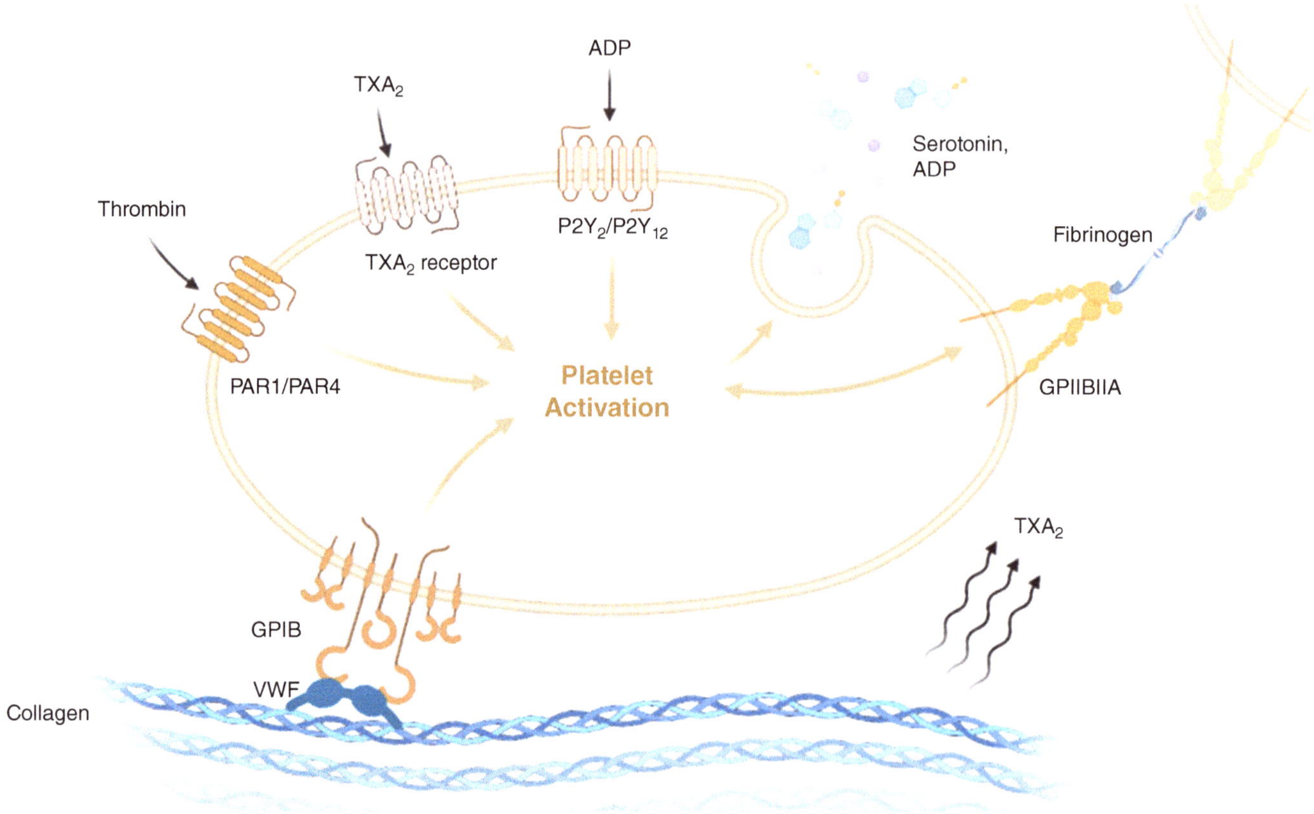

Fig. 16.1 Primary hemostasis. Created with BioRender.com

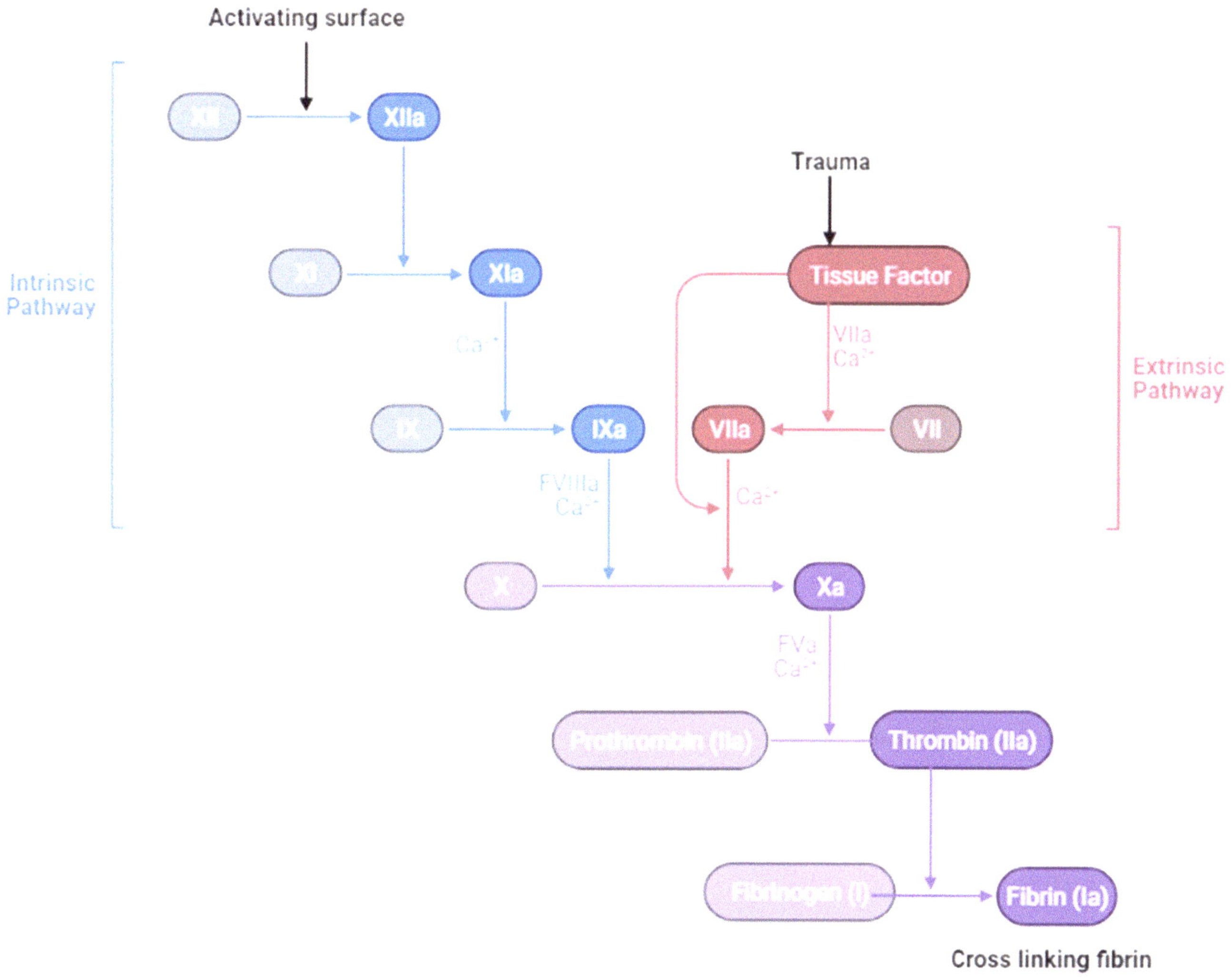

Fig. 16.2 Secondary hemostasis. Created with BioRender.com

The bleeding time was the first in vivo test of platelet function. The test involves making an incision, collecting blood from a patient, and recording the time it takes for blood to coagulate. This test can help identify patients with severe hemostatic defects such as von Willebrand disease and Glanzmann thrombasthenia. While inexpensive, the test is rarely used because it is poorly reproducible, time-consuming, and can lead to scarring at the incision site [3].

Light transmission aggregometry (LTA) also known as optical aggregometry is considered the gold standard for platelet function testing. Aggregometry quantifies platelet response to a variety of agonists, including collagen, adenosine diphosphate (ADP), epinephrine, ristocetin, and arachidonic acid. It is typically performed in a 96 well plate tray so that various agonist concentrations may be assessed. Traditionally, the technique is performed on samples of platelet-rich plasma. As varying concentrations of agonists are added to the samples, light transmission through each sample is measured. Aggregation decreases turbidity of the samples and therefore increases light transmission, and this change in light transmission is quantified. Aggregometry may also be measured on whole blood, but this technique utilizes electrical impedance to quantify platelet activity rather than light [4].

A modified aggregometry technique is the VerifyNow-P2Y12 assay. This assay was created to address limitations of conventional optical aggregation techniques. This technique utilizes a combination of ADP and prostaglandin E1 to measure effects of clopidogrel on the P2Y12 receptor. Addition of ADP activates platelets by saturating the P2Y12 and P2Y1 receptors, while prostaglandin E1 is added to suppress P2Y1 calcium release, and therefore increase test sensitivity for P2Y12 mediated activation [5].

Thromboelastography (TEG) is a novel technique that uses whole blood to collect detailed information about platelet function, clot strength, and fibrinolytic activity. TEG is a viscoelastic, mechanical analysis that uses a sinusoidal force to quantify the strain response over time. In this analysis, a mechanical transducing pin is submerged in a sample of whole blood. The blood is heated to body temperature and oscillates. As the sample oscillates, blood products form clot and adhere to the pin. As more clot forms, the oscillation amplitudes increase. As the clot breaks down, oscillation amplitudes decrease. It follows that the degree of oscillation of the pin is proportional to clot strength. As this process continues, a tracing is generated that provides a visual representation of clot formation and breakdown from start to finish. Below is an example of a TEG run and descriptions of the variables one may obtain from a TEG tracing report. The values on the tracing can be broken down into those that represent clot initiation, clot strength, and clot stability [6]. See Table 16.1 and Fig. 16.3 for variables on a TEG tracing.

Rotational thromboelastometry (ROTEM) is a commercial variant of TEG in which the sample of whole blood remains stationary, and the pin rotates within the sample. This feature presumably makes the sample less susceptible to external vibration. Unlike TEG, ROTEM analyzes whole blood in four channels. A reagent is added to each channel to model various conditions within primary or secondary hemostasis. In the first channel, EXTEM, tissue factor (TF) is added for extrinsic activation of the sample, similar to PT/INR. In the second channel, INTEM, ellagic acid is added for intrinsic activation of the sample, similar to aPTT. In the third channel, FIBTEM, cytochalasian D is added which inhibits platelet contribution to the sample. The resulting clot is only depending on fibrin formation and fibrin polymerization. In the fourth channel, APTEM/HEPEM, aprotinin, and/or heparinase are added to model the addition of either tranexamic acid (TXA) or protamine. The comparison of EXTEM and APTEM allows for rapid detection of fibrinolysis. Furthermore, APTEM enables the estimation if an antifibrinolytic therapy alone normalized the coagulation or if additional measures have to be taken, such as administration of fibrinogen. In HEPTEM, coagulation is activated as in INTEM. The addition of a heparinase in the reagent degrades the presence of heparin in the sample and allows the ROTEM analysis in heparinized samples. The viscoelastic curves generated from each of these channels are similar to the TEG

Table 16.1 Variables on a TEG tracing

Phase of Clot formation	Variable	Definition	Clinical significance
Clot Initiation	Reaction time (R)	Time to initiate first measurable clot, average time from 5 to 10 min	If prolonged, consider anticoagulation reversal or giving FFP
Clot Strength/ Coagulation	Kinetics (K)	Time to achieve 20 mm of clot strength, dependent on fibrinogen levels, average time from 1 to 3 min	If prolonged, consider giving CCP given high fibrinogen content
	Alpha angle (a)	Slope between clot initiation and 20 mm strength point, proportional to rate of clot formation, represents fibrin formation, typical angle from 50° to 70°	If decreased, consider CCP given high fibrinogen content
	Maximum Amplitude (MA)	Represents maximum strength of clot formation, dependent on platelet function	If decreased, consider giving platelets or DDAVP
Clot Stability	LY30	Represents percentage of clot lysis 30 min after MA, quantified clot fibrinolysis, average value is 0%–8%	If increased, consider antifibrinolytic such as tranexamic acid

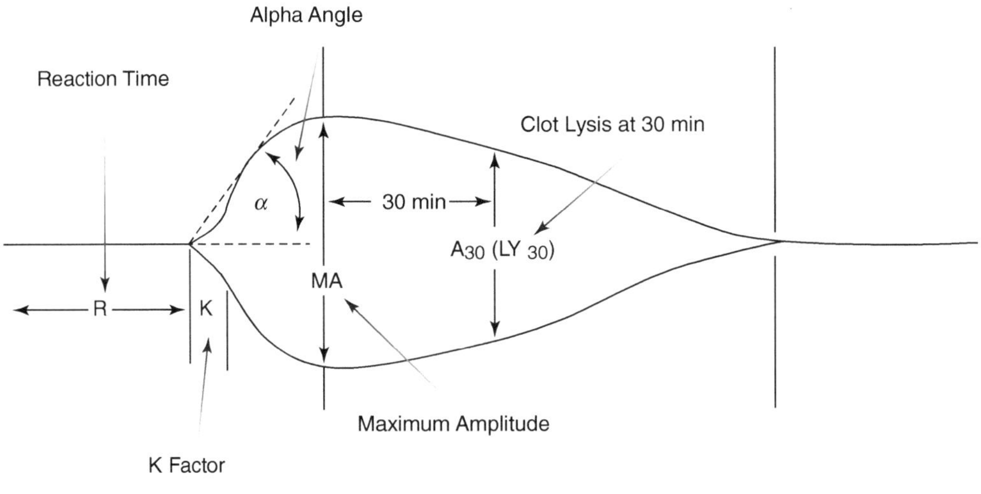

Fig. 16.3 TEG tracing. Created with BioRender.com

Table 16.2 Variables used in ROTEM

Variable	Definition
CT (Clotting time)	Time until the start of clot formation
CFT (Clot formation time)	Time from start of clot formation until 20 mm clot formation achieved
MCF (Maximum clot firmness)	Maximum firmness of clot
ML (Maximum lysis)	Reduction of clot firmness after MCF

tracing but use different variable nomenclature for interpretation given ROTEM is a commercial variant [7]. See Table 16.2 for variables used in ROTEM.

Disorders of Hemostasis—Intrinsic Mechanisms

Disorders of Primary Hemostasis

Disorders of primary hemostasis include quantitative and qualitative disturbances of platelet function. Patients with these disorders may present with ecchymosis, spontaneous bleeding from mucous membranes such as epistaxis, gingival bleeding, hematuria, hemoptysis, and hematemesis. Menorrhagia and excess bleeding are common after trauma, such as surgical trauma and dental extraction. Of note, spontaneous skin petechiae are characteristic of severely decreased platelet count.

Quantitative Platelet Disorders

Thrombocytopenia

Thrombocytopenia is defined as a platelet count of less than 150,000/microL [8]. Thrombocytopenia is not an immediate indication for platelet transfusion. Prophylactic platelet transfusions should be performed in patients with platelet count <10,000/microL that have concern for bone marrow suppression [9]. Beyond this threshold, there is no evidence to support platelet transfusion with higher platelet counts, though in neuraxial bleeding or neurosurgical intervention, it is common to transfuse to maintain a platelet count >50,000/microL–100,000/microL.

Thrombocytopenias can be categorized into disorders of platelet distribution, deficient platelet production, and increased platelet destruction. Understanding disorders of platelet distribution requires an understanding that 30% of total platelets are stored in the spleen. In the setting of infection, inflammation, liver disease, and hematologic disease, splenomegaly may occur, in which up to 90% of platelets become sequestered in the spleen [10]. Deficient production of platelets involves a failure of bone marrow to produce and deliver platelets to peripheral blood. Radiation, drug side effects, aplastic anemia, or myelodysplastic syndromes may lead to bone marrow suppression, hypoplasia of megakaryocytes, and platelet underproduction. Select disorders that lead to the destruction of platelets include heparin-induced thrombocytopenia (HIT), vaccine-induced thrombotic thrombocytopenia (VITT), disseminated intravascular coagulation (DIC), trauma-induced coagulopathy (TIC), thrombotic thrombocytopenic purpura (TTP), and immune thrombocytopenic purpura (ITP) [11].

Heparin-Induced Thrombocytopenia (HIT) is a decrease in the platelet count associated with administration of heparin products. HIT can be divided into type I and type II. Type I HIT is also known as heparin-associated thrombocytopenia (HAT). It is a non-immune-mediated reaction that can occur within the first day of heparin use. It is a direct interaction between heparin and circulating platelets, leading to transient platelet aggregation and sequestration [12]. It is typically mild and may resolve even if heparin is continued [13]. Type II HIT is an immune-mediated hypersensitivity reaction to platelet factor 4 (PF4)/heparin complex. PF4 is a heparin-binding protein found naturally in platelet α granules, which undergoes a conformational change once bound to heparin. Of note, patients are more likely to develop type II HIT with exposure to unfractionated heparin (UFH) compared to low molecular weight heparin (LMWH). Given that it takes time for the body to generate antibodies to the PF4/heparin complex, type II HIT should be suspected if there is a 50% decrease in platelets between days 5 and 14 of initiations of heparin therapy. The mortality rate associated with type II HIT ranges between 10 and 20% [14]. Venous thrombosis is the most common manifestation, with lower limb deep vein thrombosis (DVT) predominating.

One valuable tool for ruling out the possibility of type II HIT is the 4 T score [15]. The 4 T score uses four metrics, including percent platelet decrease, the timing of platelet decrease, the presence of thrombosis, and the possibility of other sources of thrombocytopenia, to develop a predictive score for the presence of HIT. The 4 T score has been shown to have a sensitivity of 97.7%, a specificity of 32.9%, a positive predictive value of 20.1% and a negative predictive value of 98.8%, making it a valuable tool for ruling out HIT [16]. An approach to patients with suspected or confirmed HIT includes discontinuation of all heparin products and administering alternative nonheparin anticoagulation, such as argatroban or bivalirudin. Evaluating for HIT includes obtaining an anti-PF4/heparin antibody level and, if positive, a serotonin release assay (SRA) to confirm the diagnosis. Two studies that assessed the frequency of HIT [17, 18] found that a small minority of patients with thrombocytopenia receiving UFH had HIT. The PF4/heparin-reactive antibodies were more likely to be detected by ELISA than by SRA, suggesting a possible overdiagnosis due to a high false-positive rate by ELISA. Although the duration of therapeutic anticoagulation for a patient with HIT has not been strictly defined in any prospective study, it is suggested that patients with HIT continue anticoagulation with a non-heparin anticoagulant for at least 4 weeks in the absence of a thrombotic event and for at least 3 months if a thrombotic event has occurred.

Similar to HIT, a novel condition known as vaccine-induced immune thrombocytopenia with thrombosis (VITT) has been described. It is a syndrome of thrombosis and thrombocytopenia associated with adenovirus vaccination. While this condition is associated with an antibody response to PF4, the recognized epitope is unique from that of HIT. The antibodies that form are not heparin-dependent. One suspected mechanism of antibody formation is that vaccine components, such as the adenoviral hexon proteins bind to PF4, form a neoantigen, and induce an inflammatory response [19]. These antibodies subsequently activate platelets, coagulation factors, monocytes, and endothelial cells, leading to downstream thrombosis. VITT often presents with thromboses in uncommon sites, such as cerebral venous thrombosis, mesenteric and portal vein thrombosis but may also present with deep vein thrombosis (DVT) and pulmonary emboli. Pan activation of cell lines and coagulation factors may lead to a clinical picture similar to DIC. In patients with VITT, full-dose anticoagulation should be initiated, preferably with a non-heparin-based agent if HIT is in the differential, and patients should also receive immune-modulating treatment with IVIG or plasma exchange. Therapeutic anticoagulation is the primary treatment for VITT unless there is a contraindication such as expanding intracerebral hemorrhage. While anticoagulant choice depends on the patient's clinical status, the preferred choice is DOAC. While the appropriate duration of anticoagulation is not known, a reasonable approach for VITT with thrombosis is to continue anticoagulation for 3 months after normalization of platelet count.

Disseminated Intravascular Coagulation (DIC) is a consumptive coagulopathy involving primary hemostasis, secondary hemostasis, and fibrinolysis. The sequence of events begins with procoagulant exposure, such as the release of TF from bacterial products, sepsis, cancer procoagulants, or trauma to vascular endothelium. The release of TF leads to a dramatic increase in coagulation cascade activity, consumption of coagulation factors, and platelets that lead to micro thrombi accumulation in the microvasculature. At the site of thrombi formation, fibrin degradation products accumulate, leading to simultaneous fibrinolysis of micro thrombi and inhibition of platelet aggregation [20].

DIC may occur in the acute or chronic setting. In acute DIC, frequently seen in sepsis, trauma, and leukemia, the blood is exposed to a large volume of TF in a short time. This leads to a consumption of coagulation factors that far exceeds production. As stated previously, fibrin degradation products then disrupt fibrin polymerization and fibrinogen binding to platelet surfaces via GPIIA/IIIA receptors. High levels of fibrin degradation products may lead to increased bleeding diathesis. Chronic DIC may be seen in cases of advanced malignancy, such as pancreatic, gastric, ovarian, and brain tumors. In these cases, there is intermittent exposure to TF. In this situation, coagulation factors are consumed, but the liver can compensate with its ability to clear fibrin degradation products. Given this pathophysiology, thrombosis predominates over bleeding diathesis. This contributes to the hypercoagulable state associated with malignancy [20]. Treatment of DIC involves addressing the underlying cause. Transfusions may be considered if patients are actively bleeding or at high risk. Fresh frozen plasma (FFP) may be administered to correct coagulation factor levels. Heparin may be necessary in the event a patient experiences a thrombotic event.

Trauma-Induced Coagulopathy (TIC) is a multifactorial response to trauma mediated by dysregulated coagulation, altered fibrinolysis, and endothelial dysfunction. One study demonstrated that 73 min after trauma, approximately 25% of patients were coagulopathic. Furthermore, patients without coagulopathy had approximately 11% risk of death versus patients with coagulopathy, who had almost 50% risk of death [21]. The mechanism behind TIC is complex, and it has historically been worsened by interventions to treat it. Initially, trauma triggers the release of TF, a catecholamine surge, endothelial activation, and hemorrhage. Hypo perfusion from bleeding and endothelial activation is thought to increase activity of protein C increasing anticoagulant activity. Simultaneously, hypo perfusion increases systemic tissue plasminogen activator (tPA), leading to systemic hyper fibrinolysis. The catecholamine surge associated with trauma compromises the blood vessel endothelium and results in the shedding of the endothelial glycocalyx. Glycocalyx shedding leads to increased endothelial permeability and auto-heparinization, further reducing coagulation factor activity [22].

The hypercoagulable state from trauma is thought to be exacerbated by an entity termed the "lethal triad of trauma" comprised of worsening coagulopathy, metabolic acidosis, and hypothermia. Hypoperfusion results in a worsening lactic acidosis, which impairs cardiac performance [23, 24]. This worsens hypoperfusion, the resulting coagulopathy, and continues the cycle. Until recently, treating TIC involved giving large amounts of crystalloids to maintain blood pressure and preserve perfusion. Literature has demonstrated that this may worsen outcomes. Studies in animal models have shown that a more judicious and less aggressive use of crystalloids improves outcomes [25]. An analysis of the Glue Grant database demonstrated that aggressive, early crystalloid resuscitation adversely affected outcomes in trauma patients [26]. The analysis demonstrated that aggressive crystalloid resuscitation resulted in more frequent acute respiratory distress syndrome cases, multi-organ failure, surgical site infection, and abdominal compartment syndrome. This is thought to be because, in the setting of TIC, the compromised glycocalyx layer of the endothelium permits excess fluid to pass into the interstitium, worsening localized hypoxia, lactic acidosis, and exacerbating the lethal triad. Additionally, the SAFE study addressed whether or not fluid resuscitation with albumin compared to saline affected mortality in critically ill patients. It demonstrated no difference when 4% albumin was used for fluid resuscitation compared to normal saline and that 4% albumin should be avoided [27]. A more recent approach to treating patients with TIC involves maintaining normothermia, minimizing crystalloid use, and addressing underlying causes of shock [28].

Of particular interest to neurocritical care physicians is TIC associated with traumatic brain injury (TBI). The brain is very rich in TF. In TBI, the significant release in TF leads to rapid consumption of coagulation factors, leading to the rapid expansion of associated intracranial hemorrhage (ICH) [29]. As with TIC, the trauma leads to downstream disruption of endogenous coagulation, endothelial function, and hyperfibrinolysis. Given the presence of hyperfibrinolysis in trauma, studies evaluating the efficacy of antifibrinolytic agents in the setting of TBI have been performed. Of note, the CRASH-3 assessed the effects of tranexamic acid on head injury-related to death, disability, and adverse events in patients with TBI. Patients were randomly assigned within 3 h of injury. The study did not demonstrate that tranexamic acid reduced mortality from head injury-related death at 28 days. The risk of death related to head injury was reduced for a specific, narrow subgroup of patients seen within 3 hours with mild to moderate head injury and intracranial hemorrhage (ICH) [30].

TBI is typically associated with cerebrovascular damage leading to blood–brain barrier (BBB) breakdown and resultant hemorrhagic contusions. While hemorrhagic complications are common in TBI, ischemic complications may also occur. One mechanism behind post-traumatic cerebral ischemia associated with TBI is intravascular micro thrombosis (IMT) [31]. Diffusion-weighted magnetic resonance imaging (DW-MRI) has demonstrated that IMT is one of the first histological changes in the peri contusion cortex. Additionally, fibrin deposition on endothelial surfaces within the brain may impair oxygen exchange without occluding vessel lumens [32]. See Fig. 16.4 for a suggested mechanism of trauma-induced coagulopathy in CNS injury.

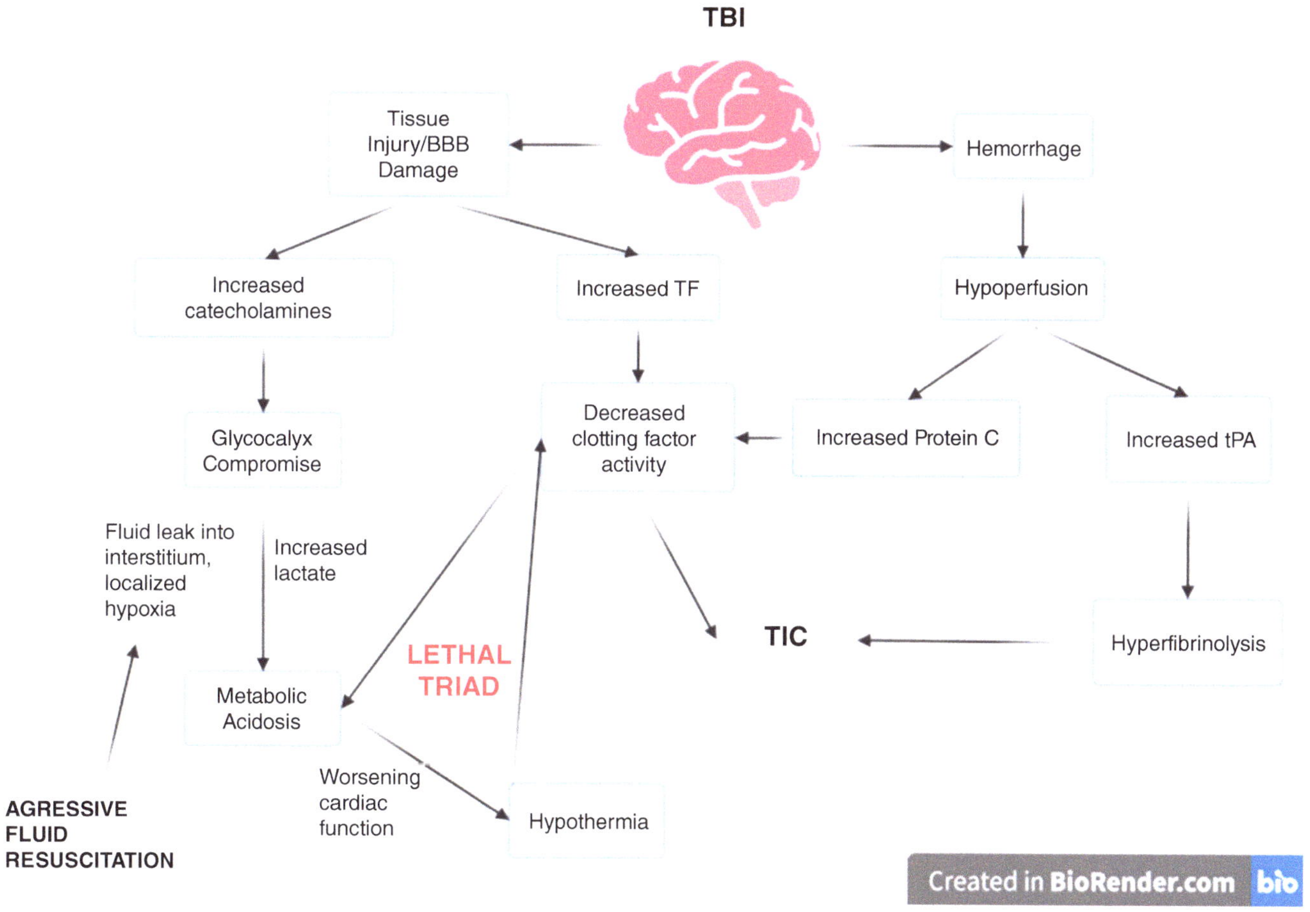

Fig. 16.4 Suggested mechanism of trauma induced coagulopathy in CNS injury. Created with BioRender.com

Thrombotic thrombocytopenic Purpura (TTP) is a disorder of dysfunctional platelet aggregation in the microvasculature. It is often caused by low levels of a specific metalloprotease (ADAMTS13) that rapidly cleaves multimers of vWF [33]. The deficiency of this metalloprotease activity can be inherited or acquired due to autoantibodies. In a small subset of TTP patients, these antibodies can be triggered by drugs: ticlopidine, clopidogrel, mitomycin C, quinine, cyclosporine, FK506 (tacrolimus), and some chemotherapeutic drugs. Typical findings in TTP include a low platelet count, intravascular hemolysis, and a high LDH level. TTP and its closely related disorders—hemolytic uremic syndrome (HUS), thrombotic microangiopathy (TMA), and peripartum HELLP (hemolysis, elevated liver enzymes, and low platelets) syndrome—may be catastrophic and rapidly fatal. TTP can be further described as a pentad of abnormalities: thrombocytopenia from increased platelet destruction, microangiopathic hemolytic anemia caused by mechanical damage to red cells due to vascular lesions, neurologic abnormalities, renal abnormalities, and fever. Many fluctuating neurologic abnormalities may be present, including seizures, altered consciousness, delirium, and paresis. Renal abnormalities may include uremia, hematuria, and proteinuria.

The reasons for fever are unclear. Besides thrombocytopenia, laboratory abnormalities include increased lactate dehydrogenase, absent or low haptoglobin levels, low ADAMTS13 levels, fragmented red blood cells (schistocytes), and reticulocytosis. The threshold for urgent plasma exchange is low because fatality rates in untreated TTP approach 50%. Only thrombocytopenia and microangiopathic hemolytic anemia are needed to begin plasmapheresis. Plasma exchange has dramatically changed TTP prognosis and outcome. Plasma infusion is less effective in adults, but it could be adequate in congenital TTP. Long durations, up to several months, may be required in patients with repeated relapses. Patients with autoantibodies may also require immunosuppressive therapy [34].

Immune Thrombocytopenic Purpura (ITP) is a clinical condition where autoantibodies form toward the host platelet. This may occur in the setting of infection, severe illness, or drug exposure. Autoantibodies bind to platelets in the peripheral circulation; these complexes are sequestered in the spleen and taken in by phagocytes. Laboratory tests that may help with this diagnosis include the Coombs assay, which tests for autoantibodies in the circulation. ITP is primarily a diagnosis of exclusion. Treatment for ITP includes corticosteroids, splenectomy, and rituximab [35].

Thrombocytosis

Disorders of thrombocytosis typically occur when more than 20 platelets per 100 × oil immersion field are present on a peripheral smear. Etiologies include increased production—not platelet lifespan—by the bone marrow, primary disorders occurring from myeloproliferative disorders, and secondary disorders occurring from another disease or source [35].

Essential Thrombocytosis

Primary thrombocytosis is a persistent elevation in platelet count due to clonal thrombopoiesis, occurring in myeloproliferative disorders such as essential thrombocytosis (ET) and polycythemia vera (PV). ET has been associated with small and large vessel ischemic stroke and microvessel vascular occlusive events [36]. Factors that predispose to ET include age, history of thrombosis, and JAK2 allele burden. Patients with JAK2 mutations, specifically JAK2 V617F, are more likely to develop (PV) [37]. Treatment for ET is based on the risk of thrombosis, bleeding, and degree of vasomotor symptoms [38]. Patients older than 60 with a history of thromboembolism and a platelet count greater than 1500×10^3 cells/μL should receive platelet-lowering agents such as hydroxyurea, anagrelide, or IFN-a. Hydroxyurea is recommended in patients older than 60, while IFN-a is recommended in childbearing women. Low-dose aspirin may be added to relieve vasomotor symptoms. Heparin, thrombolytic agents, and plateletpheresis may be used in cases complicated by arterial and venous thrombosis. The goal platelet level should be less than 400×10^3 cells/μL. Certain patients with uncontrolled thrombocytosis have been found to have a defect in vWF, accompanied by an increased risk of bleeding. For this reason, DDAVP or cryoprecipitate may be used to treat hemorrhage in these patients [39].

Qualitative Platelet Disorders

Qualitative platelet disorders present clinically similar to quantitative platelet disorders, including ecchymosis and bleeding diathesis. Mechanistically speaking, qualitative platelet disorders are disorders of platelet adhesion. Disorders of platelet and vessel wall adhesion include von Willebrand Disease—a condition in which ADAMTS13 proteinase activity is reduced, and therefore activated vWF levels are low, decreasing GPIB binding to the endothelium—and Bernard Soulier syndrome. In this condition, there is a defect in the GPIB receptor itself, rendering it unable to bind to vWF and adhere to the endothelium. Additionally, there are disorders of platelet-to-platelet aggregation, one example being Glanzmann's thrombasthenia, a condition where there is a defect in the GPIIB/IIIA receptor, rendering platelets unable to bind to one another via fibrinogen [40].

Uremia—Impaired kidney function and associated uremia can be a source of platelet dysfunction in critically ill patients. While the exact mechanism of platelet dysfunction is not entirely clear, it may be a combination of both intrinsic dysfunction and disrupted platelet endothelial interaction. Uremic toxins may also lead to an impaired release of ADP and serotonin from alpha granules, decreased thromboxane generation, and compromised platelet cytoskeletal assembly. Uremic plasma may lead to dysfunction and poor expression of GPIIB/IIIA rendering platelets unable to aggregate via fibrinogen [41, 42]. Given that platelet function has been shown to improve after dialysis in uremic patients, it suggests that there is a component of plasma contributing to this. While there is no association between urea and bleeding time in patients with kidney failure [43], there is literature suggesting that guanidino succinic acid and methyl guanidine found in uremic plasma may lead to platelet dysfunction via the upregulation of nitric oxide, which is a known inhibitor of platelet aggregation [44, 45]. Nitric oxide also upregulates the cGMP signal transduction cascade, leading to the downregulation of thromboxane and ADP, which may be another mechanism of decreased platelet activity.

Liver Disease—Mechanisms of thrombocytopenia in patients with liver disease include decreased production of thrombopoietin, bone marrow suppression from hepatitis or alcohol use, or sequestration of platelets in the spleen secondary to portal hypertension [46]. Additionally, hepatocytes are responsible for producing various coagulation factors, including fibrinogen, thrombin, and factors V, VII, IX, and XI. Hepatocytes are also responsible for glycosylation and gamma-carboxylation needed to activate certain factors, notably X, IX, VII, and II. Hyper fibrinolysis may be present in patients with liver disease, particularly in decompensated cirrhosis [47, 48]. This mechanism is similar to DIC and is termed accelerated intravascular coagulation and fibrinolysis (AICF) [49].

Hepatocytes and Kupffer cells in the liver also aid in the clearance of coagulation factors and products of fibrinolysis. In patients with liver failure, limited clearance of these products may lead to upregulation of circulating tPA, which can generate plasmin, decrease levels of alpha two antiplasmins, fibrin degradation produces, and increase the fibrinolytic activity of ascitic fluid [50]. Additionally, the production of endogenous inhibitors to coagulation is reduced, such as protein C, protein S, and antithrombin. This places the patient in a prothrombotic state. Whole blood assays of the entire coagulation cascade, such as TEG, may provide better insight than individual coagulation studies into pro-coagulant or anticoagulant states in liver failure.

Disorders of Secondary Hemostasis

While primary hemostasis disorders include platelet function and quantity disorders, secondary hemostasis encompasses dysfunction of the coagulation cascade and associated coagulation factors. Compared to disorders of primary hemostasis—which present typically with petechiae and mucosal bleeding, symptoms of disorders of secondary hemostasis can encompass deeper bleeds—such as hemarthrosis, bleeding into joints, and muscle hematomas. While various disorders of secondary hemostasis exist, the most common inherited disorders are defects in genes that synthesize factors of the intrinsic pathway—Factors VIII, IX, and XI [51].

Factor VIII deficiency, also known as Hemophilia A, is an X-linked recessive disorder in which the function of factor VIII is decreased or absent. Males are primarily affected and typically receive the gene from the maternal transmission. Females are typically asymptomatic carriers. Symptoms of Hemophilia A vary by severity of disease but can include spontaneous hematoma in subcutaneous tissues, hemarthrosis, hemorrhagic body cavity effusions, and excess hemorrhage during trauma. Given that it is a component of the intrinsic pathway, laboratory findings are significant for a prolonged aPTT and decreased factor VIII-coagulant activity. Coagulant activity less than 20% is diagnostic for mild disease, 6%–20% for moderate, and less than 2% for severe disease. Treatments vary depending on severity but may include repeated transfusion of fresh frozen plasma or cryoprecipitate multiple times per day until bleeding is controlled. Additionally, products used to treat hemophilia A include factor VIII replacement products such as concentrates from plasma, recombinant products, as well as emicizumab. Emicizumab is a monoclonal antibody that binds to both factor IXa and factor X, substituting for the role of factor VIII in hemostasis. The HAVEN 3 trial demonstrates that emicizumab has improved efficacy and reduced adverse effects compared with factor VIII products [52].

Factor IX deficiency, also known as Hemophilia B, is clinically similar to Hemophilia A. Factor IX products are used to treat hemophilia B. Previously used sources of factor IX such as PCC are not considered first-line therapy due to an increased risk of thrombosis. Various plasma-derived and recombinant factor IX products exist to treat hemophilia B.

Factor XI deficiency, also known as Hemophilia C, is unique because the bleeding is associated with excessive fibrinolysis. Under normal conditions, thrombin-associated coagulation is upregulated by factor XI. Under normal conditions, a small amount of thrombin generated by tissue factor is enough to activate fibrinolytic inhibitors. The lack of fibrinolytic inhibitors in patients with this disorder leads to delayed hemorrhage in trauma and surgery [51]. Options for factor XI replacement include FFP or high-purity factor XI concentrate derived from human plasma. Factor XI concentrate was provided through an expanded access program in the United States but is no longer available.

Disorders of Fibrinolysis

Increased plasminogen activator activity, such as tPA, may occur in endothelial injury or exposure to pathogens and may increase the conversion of plasminogen to plasmin. A deficiency in inhibitors, such as plasminogen activator inhibitor 1 (PAI-1), can lead to the upregulation of tPA activity. Elevated protein C may also lead to hyper fibrinolysis in trauma patients. In contrast, impaired fibrinolysis may occur in the setting of increased PAI-1 because of trauma and endotoxemia. This is a major contributing factor to the thrombotic phase of DIC [53].

Disorders of Hemostasis—Extrinsic Mechanisms and Antithrombotic Agents

Risk of Intracranial Hemorrhage in Patients on Antithrombotic Agents

The primary risk of intracranial hemorrhage is higher in patients receiving antithrombotic agents compare to those who are not. The baseline risk of intracranial hemorrhage in the general population not on antithrombotic agents is estimated at 0.15% per/year. Rates of intracranial hemorrhage vary based on the antithrombotic agent: dabigatran 0.11%/year, edoxaban 0.21%/year, apixaban 0.32%/year, aspiring 0.40%/year, rivaroxaban 0.50%/year, and warfarin 0.49%/year [54–59].

Among patients with intracerebral hemorrhage, the risk of hemorrhage expansion is higher and occurs over a longer duration of time in anticoagulated patients compared to non-anticoagulated patients. In patients not taking antithrombotics, 25% will have ≥33% increase in ICH volume during the first 24 hours, compared approximately 40% of anticoagulated patients [60–62]. Anticoagulation is associated with higher mortality rates and worse functional outcomes in ICH patients [63]. Among anticoagulated patients, ICH expansion by ≥33% doubles the risk of poor 12-month outcomes [64]. Taking measures to reduce hematoma expansion, such as reversing antithrombotic agents, improves patient outcomes. Lack of antithrombotic reversal doubles the risk of death at 30 days [65]. Indeed, rapid reversal of anticoagulants is imperative as studies have demonstrated that the risk of ICH expansion more than doubles among patients taking warfarin if the INR remains >1.3 at 2–4 h post presentation [64, 66].

Based on recent guidelines for the reversal of antithrombotics in intracranial hemorrhage patients, practitioners should prioritize the reversal of coagulopathy in acute intracranial hemorrhage irrespective of the indication for antithrombotic agents. Patients with mechanical valves, ventricular assist devices, or other high-risk features should receive reversal agents in a similar fashion as lower risk individuals since the immediate intracranial hemorrhage expansion risk outweighs the theoretical increased thrombotic risk. However, in cases of intracranial hemorrhage due to cerebral venous thrombosis, reversal agents should be withheld. In circumstances of concomitant life-threatening thrombosis and hemorrhage (as can occur in DIC), the risks and benefits of coagulopathy reversal should be weighed [67].

Management of Coagulopathy Associated with Liver Failure, Uremia, and Ethanol Use

Liver Failure

The liver is responsible for synthesizing coagulation factors II, V, VII, IX, X, XI, XII, protein C and S, fibrinogen and antithrombin, while factor VIII and vWF are synthesized in human endothelial cells throughout the body, including liver sinusoidal endothelial cells. Viscoelastic testing such as TEG or ROTEM may assist in identifying the most likely mechanism of bleeding in liver failure patients. One study demonstrated that in cirrhosis with coagulopathy, TEG-guided transfusion resulted in lower use of blood products than transfusion guided by INR and platelet count [68]. In the setting of liver failure with active bleeding, vitamin K along with PCC and FFP can be considered. Note that repletion of factor V is essential in controlling hemorrhage related to liver failure, and PCC does not contain factor V. Hence, if PCC is used, FFP should be utilized as well, though in a lower dose than if given without PCC. Because volume overload is frequently an issue with liver failure patients, the combination of PCC and lower dose FFP may be optimal. In cases where fibrinogen levels are also low, cryoprecipitate is considered [69]. After the transfusion, fibrinogen should be monitored for a value greater than 100–150 mg/dL and based on this, a decision to administer more may be made [70]. Note that both FFP and cryoprecipitate contain low levels of factor VIII. Recombinant factor VIII concentrates can be used in cases of hemophilia A or von Willebrand's Disease.

Uremia

The approach to coagulopathy associated with kidney failure is multifaceted. It may include dialysis, DDAVP administration, anemia correction, or cryoprecipitate. Dialysis is the preferred means to correct this coagulopathy in the setting of an active bleed. DDAVP administration is helpful in a situation where rapid correction is needed. However, while DDAVP has shown to increase vWF and associated factor VIII dimers and improve platelet function in vitro [71], its clinical utility in the management of uremic coagulopathy remains uncertain.

Alcohol Use

While mechanisms behind thrombocytopenia associated with alcohol use are not entirely understood, a few potential causes include direct toxicity of alcohol to megakaryocytes and reduced thrombopoietin in the setting of liver disease. The approach to thrombocytopenia associated with alcohol use includes abstinence and potentially a thrombopoietin receptor agonist therapy [72]. Of note, patients with a history of alcohol use disorder are at an increased risk of hematoma expansion due to the impact of alcohol on platelet aggregation. Studies have been done on desmopressin (DDAVP) in these patients. One study found no significant difference in hematoma expansion between DDAVP and non-DDAVP groups (OR 0.63, 95% CI 0.1–3.3) [73]. Overall, evidence regarding the utility of DDAVP in alcohol use related to ICH is limited.

Resumption of Antithrombotic

While the decision to resume antithrombotics after ICH is challenging, evidence suggests that patients who resume anticoagulation may have improved outcomes [74]. In one study, 25 out of 108 with a high risk of thromboembolic events were restarted on anticoagulation after resolution of ICH. No new thromboembolic events occurred in these 25 patients. Although ICH recurred in 7% of patients in the study, these occurred prior to resumption of anticoagulation [75]. Another study found that resumption of anticoagulation after ICH was associated with a reduction in ischemic stroke and all-cause mortality (hazard ratio 0.55, 95% CI 0.39–0.78) without increased risk of recurrent hemorrhage (hazard ratio 0.91, 95% CI 0.56–1.49), also compared to antiplatelet resumption (hazard ratio 0.6, 95% CI 0.37–1.03) [76]. A meta-analysis of eight trials found that resuming anticoagulation after ICH was associated with fewer thromboembolic events (relative risk 0.34, 95% CI 0.25–0.45) without an increased risk of recurrent hemorrhage [77]. While the results of these studies are encouraging, there is inherent bias by indication in observational studies.

There have been some randomized trials addressing resumption of antithrombotics after ICH. The RESTART trial randomized patients with antithrombotic-associated intracerebral hemorrhage to start or avoid antiplatelet therapy [65]. Over 2 years of follow-up, recurrent ICH occurred in 4% of patients who resumed antiplatelet therapy (in a median of 76 days from ICH), compared to 9% of patients allocated to avoid antiplatelets ($P = 0.060$). Major hemorrhage occurred in 7% of antiplatelet patients compared to 9% of patients who avoided antiplatelets ($P = 0.27$). Major occlusive vascular events occurred in 15% of those on antiplatelets compared to 14% of those not on antiplatelets ($P = 0.92$). Overall, antiplatelet therapy appeared to be safe following ICH when resumed in a delayed fashion (median 76 days from ICH).

The APACHE-AF and SoSTART trials evaluated the resumption of apixaban post-ICH in patients with atrial fibrillation. The APACHE-AF was an open-label, randomized, phase 2 trial of patients with atrial fibrillation and ICH, assigned to either apixaban or avoidance of anticoagulation (though antiplatelets were allowed in the control group). Among 101 enrolled patients, the primary composite outcome of non-fatal stroke or vascular death occurred in 26% of patients randomized to apixaban versus 24% allocated to no anticoagulation over a median 1.9-year follow-up [78]. Over half of patients (51%) in the avoid apixaban group received antiplatelet agents. The SoSTART study was an open-label randomized trial of patients with ICH and atrial fibrillation allocating patients to start anticoagulation (either direct oral anticoagulant or warfarin) or avoid anticoagulants (antiplatelet agents were allowed). Starting oral anticoagulation (direct oral anticoagulant in 97%) was associated recurrent intracranial hemorrhage in 8% of patients with compared to 4% in the group that avoided anticoagulation (28% received an antiplatelet agent). Rates of symptomatic major vascular events was 12% in the start anticoagulation group compared to 24% in the avoid group ($P = 0.060$) and rates of stroke were also lower in the start group 11% compared to 22% ($P = 0.082$) [79]. Neither APACHE-AF nor SoSTART was powered to assess long-term efficacy of resuming anticoagulation versus not after ICH. To address this, an ongoing, large randomized, controlled, double-blinded trial evaluating apixaban versus aspirin in patients with atrial fibrillation and intracerebral hemorrhage [80] should provide more definitive data on appropriate antithrombotic strategies.

The ideal time to resume anticoagulation post intracranial hemorrhage (ICH) is unclear. Studies that assessed high-risk patients with mechanical valves found a benefit to resuming anticoagulation at approximately 3–10 days [81]. However, extensive retrospective cohort studies had found that the combined risk of recurrent ICH and ischemic stroke was lowest when anticoagulation was resumed 10–30 weeks post the index event [82]. Another observational study found resumption at 7–8 weeks optimized benefit and minimized risk [83]. Two meta-analyses found that resumption of anticoagulation after intracranial hemorrhage (including mixed populations of IPH, SAH and TBI) resulted in significantly fewer thromboembolic events (pooled RR 0.31, 96% CI 0.23–0.42) when resumed from 6–120 days [84] as well as 10–180 days (pooled RR, 0.34, 95% CI, 0.25–0.45) [77]. Data also demonstrate that the risk of recurrent ICH is higher earlier on. For example, one study found that restarting therapeutic anticoagulation less than 2 weeks post-ICH patients with mechanical heart valves demonstrated a higher risk of hemorrhagic complications (HR 7.06, 95% CI 2.33–21.37) [85]. Data also demonstrated that rebleeding risk may be higher than ischemic or thromboembolic event risk within the first few weeks after intracranial hemorrhage in LVAD patients [86]. This supports a more delayed timeframe for resumption. In practice, most resume anticoagulation at about 2–4 weeks post ICH [74]. Given that no randomized clinical trials are available that address this clinical question, the ideal time to resume anticoagulation remains unknown. Current literature suggests weighing patient risk and benefits on a case-by-case basis.

Alternatives to Resumption of Anticoagulants

Antiplatelets

The value of antiplatelet use to prevent thromboembolism in AF is unclear. Aspirin has been shown to reduce the risk of stroke by about 30% compared to placebo [87]. Additionally, lower hemorrhage rates have been found in patients on antiplatelet therapy compared to warfarin [88]. The AVERROES trial compared apixaban to aspirin for primary stroke prevention and found that apixaban reduced stroke without increasing the risk for hemorrhage compared to aspirin [54, 55]. The RESTART trial suggested that resuming antiplatelet agents after intracerebral hemorrhage is safe, but there was no difference in thromboembolic event rates between the aspirin and the no antiplatelet groups, so the efficacy remains unclear [89].

Left Atrial Appendage Closure

In patients with atrial fibrillation and contraindications to long-term anticoagulation, such as recurrent hemorrhage, closure of the left atrial appendage may be considered. The WATCHMAN is an FDA-approved implantable device that utilizes a self-expanding fabric-coated frame for atrial appendage closure [90]. Notable trials that evaluated the safety and efficacy of the WATCHMAN include the PREVAIL and the PROTECT AF trials. These trials compared the safety and efficacy of the WATCHMAN device versus warfarin therapy in patients with nonvalvular atrial fibrillation. In both trials, atrial appendage closure with WATCHMAN was non-inferior to warfarin to prevent vascular events [91, 92]. The Amplatzer Amulet Left Atrial Appendage Occluder (LAAO) is another atrial appendage closure device that utilizes a lobe with a covering disk for atrial appendage closure. One meta-analysis comparing WATCHMAN and Amplatzer found that the two devices were comparable in efficacy with low complication rates. Total bleeding rates were higher with Amplatzer use, while a higher percentage of little peri-device leakage was found among the WATCHMAN group [93]. More recently, the Amulet IDE randomized controlled trial found that the Amplatzer was non-inferior for safety and efficacy when compared to WATCHMAN but superior for left atrial appendage occlusion (98.9% for Amplatzer versus 96.8% for WATCHMAN, 95% CI, 0.41–3.66) [94]. Left atrial appendage closure devices require short-term anticoagulation after placement. For example, the PROTECT AF protocol required warfarin plus aspirin for 45 days after device placement, followed by clopidogrel plus aspirin for 6 months, followed by aspirin alone. The ASAP study required dual antiplatelet use for 6 months, with a minimum of 1–3 months of dual antiplatelet use for patients at very high risk of bleeding [95]. Left atrial appendage closure has not been directly compared to resumption of a direct oral anticoagulant, and the risks and benefits compared to these agents remain unknown.

References

1. Broos K, Feys HB, De Meyer SF, Vanhoorelbeke K, Deckmyn H. Platelets at work in primary hemostasis. Blood Rev. 2011;25:155–67.
2. Green D. Coagulation cascade. Hemodial Int. 2006;10(Suppl 2):S2–4.
3. Russeau AP, Vall H, Manna B. Bleeding time. In: StatPearls, Treasure Island, FL; 2022.
4. Chan MV, Armstrong PC, Papalia F, Kirkby NS, Warner TD. Optical multichannel (optimul) platelet aggregometry in 96-well plates as an additional method of platelet reactivity testing. Platelets. 2011;22:485–94.
5. Malinin A, Pokov A, Spergling M, Defranco A, Schwartz K, Schwartz D, Mahmud E, Atar D, Serebruany V. Monitoring platelet inhibition after clopidogrel with the VerifyNow-P2Y12(R) rapid analyzer: the VERIfy Thrombosis risk ASsessment (VERITAS) study. Thromb Res. 2007;119:277–84.
6. Othman M, Kaur H. Thromboelastography (TEG). Methods Mol Biol. 2017;1646:533–43.
7. Veigas PV, Callum J, Rizoli S, Nascimento B, da Luz LT. A systematic review on the rotational thrombelastometry (ROTEM(R)) values for the diagnosis of coagulopathy, prediction and guidance of blood transfusion and prediction of mortality in trauma patients. Scand J Trauma Resusc Emerg Med. 2016;24:114.
8. Lee EJ, Lee AI. Thrombocytopenia. Prim Care. 2016;43:543–57.
9. Schiffer CA, Bohlke K, Delaney M, Hume H, Magdalinski AJ, McCullough JJ, Omel JL, Rainey JM, Rebulla P, Rowley SD, Troner MB, Anderson KC. Platelet transfusion for patients with cancer: American Society of Clinical Oncology clinical practice guideline update. J Clin Oncol. 2018;36:283–99.
10. Kapila V, Wehrle CJ, Tuma F. Physiology, spleen. In: StatPearls. Treasure Island, FL; 2022.
11. Smock KJ, Perkins SL. Thrombocytopenia: an update. Int J Lab Hematol. 2014;36:269–78.
12. Ahmed I, Majeed A, Powell R. Heparin induced thrombocytopenia: diagnosis and management update. Postgrad Med J. 2007;83:575–82.
13. Nicolas D, Nicolas S, Hodgens A, Reed M. Heparin induced thrombocytopenia. In: StatPearls, Treasure Island, FL; 2022.
14. Napolitano LM, Warkentin TE, Almahameed A, Nasraway SA. Heparin-induced thrombocytopenia in the critical care setting: diagnosis and management. Crit Care Med. 2006;34:2898–911.
15. Lo GK, Juhl D, Warkentin TE, Sigouin CS, Eichler P, Greinacher A. Evaluation of pretest clinical score (4 T's) for the diagnosis of heparin-induced thrombocytopenia in two clinical settings. J Thromb Haemost. 2006;4:759–65.
16. Pishko AM, Fardin S, Lefler DS, Paydary K, Vega R, Arepally GM, Crowther M, Rice L, Cines DB, Cuker A. Prospective

comparison of the HEP score and 4Ts score for the diagnosis of heparin-induced thrombocytopenia. Blood Adv. 2018;2:3155–62.
17. Verma AK, Levine M, Shalansky SJ, Carter CJ, Kelton JG. Frequency of heparin-induced thrombocytopenia in critical care patients. Pharmacotherapy. 2003;23:745–53.
18. Crowther MA, Cook DJ, Meade MO, Griffith LE, Guyatt GH, Arnold DM, Rabbat CG, Geerts WH, Warkentin TE. Thrombocytopenia in medical-surgical critically ill patients: prevalence, incidence, and risk factors. J Crit Care. 2005;20:348–53.
19. Greinacher A, Selleng K, Palankar R, Wesche J, Handtke S, Wolff M, Aurich K, Lalk M, Methling K, Volker U, Hentschker C, Michalik S, Steil L, Reder A, Schonborn L, Beer M, Franzke K, Buttner A, Fehse B, Stavrou EX, Rangaswamy C, Mailer RK, Englert H, Frye M, Thiele T, Kochanek S, Krutzke L, Siegerist F, Endlich N, Warkentin TE, Renne T. Insights in ChAdOx1 nCoV-19 vaccine-induced immune thrombotic thrombocytopenia. Blood. 2021;138:2256–68.
20. Levi M, Sivapalaratnam S. Disseminated intravascular coagulation: an update on pathogenesis and diagnosis. Expert Rev Hematol. 2018;11:663–72.
21. Brohi K, Singh J, Heron M, Coats T. Acute traumatic coagulopathy. J Trauma. 2003;54:1127–30.
22. Chang R, Cardenas JC, Wade CE, Holcomb JB. Advances in the understanding of trauma-induced coagulopathy. Blood. 2016;128:1043–9.
23. Dadhwal US, Pathak N. Damage control philosophy in polytrauma. Med J Armed Forces India. 2010;66:347–9.
24. Kimmoun A, Novy E, Auchet T, Ducrocq N, Levy B. Hemodynamic consequences of severe lactic acidosis in shock states: from bench to bedside. Crit Care. 2015;19:175.
25. Hall K, Drobatz K. Volume resuscitation in the acutely hemorrhaging patient: historic use to current applications. Front Vet Sci. 2021;8:638104.
26. Kasotakis G, Sideris A, Yang Y, de Moya M, Alam H, King DR, Tompkins R, Velmahos G, Inflammation, and Investigators Host Response to Injury. Aggressive early crystalloid resuscitation adversely affects outcomes in adult blunt trauma patients: an analysis of the Glue Grant database. J Trauma Acute Care Surg. 2013;74:1215–21; discussion 21-2.
27. Finfer S, Bellomo R, Boyce N, French J, Myburgh J, Norton R, Safe Study Investigators. A comparison of albumin and saline for fluid resuscitation in the intensive care unit. N Engl J Med. 2004;350:2247–56.
28. Chatrath V, Khetarpal R, Ahuja J. Fluid management in patients with trauma: restrictive versus liberal approach. J Anaesthesiol Clin Pharmacol. 2015;31:308–16.
29. Maegele M, Schochl H, Menovsky T, Marechal H, Marklund N, Buki A, Stanworth S. Coagulopathy and haemorrhagic progression in traumatic brain injury: advances in mechanisms, diagnosis, and management. Lancet Neurol. 2017;16:630–47.
30. CRASH-3 Trial Collaborators. Effects of tranexamic acid on death, disability, vascular occlusive events and other morbidities in patients with acute traumatic brain injury (CRASH-3): a randomised, placebo-controlled trial. Lancet. 2019;394:1713–23.
31. Stein SC, Graham DI, Chen XH, Smith DH. Association between intravascular microthrombosis and cerebral ischemia in traumatic brain injury. Neurosurgery. 2004;54:687–91; discussion 91.
32. Mhatre M, Nguyen A, Kashani S, Pham T, Adesina A, Grammas P. Thrombin, a mediator of neurotoxicity and memory impairment. Neurobiol Aging. 2004;25:783–93
33. Zheng X, Majerus EM, Sadler JE. ADAMTS13 and TTP. Curr Opin Hematol. 2002;9:389–94.
34. Joly BS, Coppo P, Veyradier A. An update on pathogenesis and diagnosis of thrombotic thrombocytopenic purpura. Expert Rev Hematol. 2019;12:383–95.
35. Justiz Vaillant AA, Gupta N. ITP-immune thrombocytopenic purpura. In: StatPearls, Treasure Island, FL; 2022.
36. Lazzaro MA, Cochran EJ, Lopes DK, Prabhakaran S. Moyamoya syndrome in an adult with essential thrombocythemia. Neurol Int. 2011;3:e3.
37. Kim SY, Im K, Park SN, Kwon J, Kim JA, Lee DS. CALR, JAK2, and MPL mutation profiles in patients with four different subtypes of myeloproliferative neoplasms: primary myelofibrosis, essential thrombocythemia, polycythemia vera, and myeloproliferative neoplasm, unclassifiable. Am J Clin Pathol. 2015;143:635–44.
38. Schafer AI. Molecular basis of the diagnosis and treatment of polycythemia vera and essential thrombocythemia. Blood. 2006;107:4214–22.
39. Cervantes F. Management of essential thrombocythemia. Hematol Am Soc Hematol Educ Program. 2011;2011:215–21.
40. Grainger JD, Thachil J, Will AM. How we treat the platelet glycoprotein defects; Glanzmann thrombasthenia and Bernard Soulier syndrome in children and adults. Br J Haematol. 2018;182:621–32.
41. Escolar G, Cases A, Bastida E, Garrido M, Lopez J, Revert L, Castillo R, Ordinas A. Uremic platelets have a functional defect affecting the interaction of von Willebrand factor with glycoprotein IIb-IIIa. Blood. 1990;76:1336–40.
42. Gawaz MP, Dobos G, Spath M, Schollmeyer P, Gurland HJ, Mujais SK. Impaired function of platelet membrane glycoprotein IIb-IIIa in end-stage renal disease. J Am Soc Nephrol. 1994;5:36–46.
43. Steiner RW, Coggins C, Carvalho AC. Bleeding time in uremia: a useful test to assess clinical bleeding. Am J Hematol. 1979;7:107–17.
44. Hedges SJ, Dehoney SB, Hooper JS, Amanzadeh J, Busti AJ. Evidence-based treatment recommendations for uremic bleeding. Nat Clin Pract Nephrol. 2007;3:138–53.
45. Noris M, Remuzzi G. Uremic bleeding: closing the circle after 30 years of controversies? Blood. 1999;94:2569–74.
46. Afdhal N, McHutchison J, Brown R, Jacobson I, Manns M, Poordad F, Weksler B, Esteban R. Thrombocytopenia associated with chronic liver disease. J Hepatol. 2008;48:1000–7.
47. Bennani-Baiti N, Daw HA. Primary hyperfibrinolysis in liver disease: a critical review. Clin Adv Hematol Oncol. 2011;9:250–2.
48. Ferro D, Celestini A, Violi F. Hyperfibrinolysis in liver disease. Clin Liver Dis. 2009;13:21–31.
49. Blasi A, Calvo A, Prado V, Reverter E, Reverter JC, Hernandez-Tejero M, Aziz F, Amoros A, Cardenas A, Fernandez J. Coagulation failure in patients with acute-on-chronic liver failure and decompensated cirrhosis: beyond the international normalized ratio. Hepatology. 2018;68:2325–37.
50. Bedreli S, Sowa JP, Malek S, Blomeyer S, Katsounas A, Gerken G, Saner FH, Canbay A. Rotational thromboelastometry can detect factor XIII deficiency and bleeding diathesis in patients with cirrhosis. Liver Int. 2017;37:562–8.
51. Mehta P, Reddivari AKR. Hemophilia. In: StatPearls. Treasure Island, FL; 2022.
52. Young G, Liesner R, Chang T, Sidonio R, Oldenburg J, Jimenez-Yuste V, Mahlangu J, Kruse-Jarres R, Wang M, Uguen M, Doral MY, Wright LY, Schmitt C, Levy GG, Shima M, Mancuso ME. A multicenter, open-label phase 3 study of emicizumab prophylaxis in children with hemophilia A with inhibitors. Blood. 2019;134:2127–38.
53. Francis RB Jr. Clinical disorders of fibrinolysis: a critical review. Blut. 1989;59:1–14.
54. Connolly SJ, Eikelboom J, Joyner C, Diener HC, Hart R, Golitsyn S, Flaker G, Avezum A, Hohnloser SH, Diaz R, Talajic M, Zhu J, Pais P, Budaj A, Parkhomenko A, Jansky P, Commerford P, Tan RS, Sim KH, Lewis BS, Van Mieghem W, Lip GY, Kim JH, Lanas-Zanetti F, Gonzalez-Hermosillo A, Dans AL, Munawar M, O'Donnell M, Lawrence J, Lewis G, Afzal R, Yusuf S, Averroes

Steering Committee, and Investigators. Apixaban in patients with atrial fibrillation. N Engl J Med. 2011a;364:806–17.
55. Connolly SJ, Eikelboom JW, Ng J, Hirsh J, Yusuf S, Pogue J, de Caterina R, Hohnloser S, Hart RG, Active Steering Committee, and Investigators. Net clinical benefit of adding clopidogrel to aspirin therapy in patients with atrial fibrillation for whom vitamin K antagonists are unsuitable. Ann Intern Med. 2011b;155:579–86.
56. Connolly SJ, Ezekowitz MD, Yusuf S, Eikelboom J, Oldgren J, Parekh A, Pogue J, Reilly PA, Themeles E, Varrone J, Wang S, Alings M, Xavier D, Zhu J, Diaz R, Lewis BS, Darius H, Diener HC, Joyner CD, Wallentin L, Re-Ly Steering Committee, and Investigators. Dabigatran versus warfarin in patients with atrial fibrillation. N Engl J Med. 2009;361:1139–51.
57. Giugliano RP, Ruff CT, Braunwald E, Murphy SA, Wiviott SD, Halperin JL, Waldo AL, Ezekowitz MD, Weitz JI, Spinar J, Ruzyllo W, Ruda M, Koretsune Y, Betcher J, Shi M, Grip LT, Patel SP, Patel I, Hanyok JJ, Mercuri M, Antman EM, Engage Af-Timi Investigators. Edoxaban versus warfarin in patients with atrial fibrillation. N Engl J Med. 2013;369:2093–104.
58. Granger CB, Alexander JH, McMurray JJ, Lopes RD, Hylek EM, Hanna M, Al-Khalidi HR, Ansell J, Atar D, Avezum A, Bahit MC, Diaz R, Easton JD, Ezekowitz JA, Flaker G, Garcia D, Geraldes M, Gersh BJ, Golitsyn S, Goto S, Hermosillo AG, Hohnloser SH, Horowitz J, Mohan P, Jansky P, Lewis BS, Lopez-Sendon JL, Pais P, Parkhomenko A, Verheugt FW, Zhu J, Wallentin L, Aristotle Committees, and Investigators. Apixaban versus warfarin in patients with atrial fibrillation. N Engl J Med. 2011;365:981–92.
59. Patel MR, Mahaffey KW, Garg J, Pan G, Singer DE, Hacke W, Breithardt G, Halperin JL, Hankey GJ, Piccini JP, Becker RC, Nessel CC, Paolini JF, Berkowitz SD, Fox KA, Califf RM, Rocket Af Investigators. Rivaroxaban versus warfarin in nonvalvular atrial fibrillation. N Engl J Med. 2011;365:883–91.
60. Anderson CS, Heeley E, Huang Y, Wang J, Stapf C, Delcourt C, Lindley R, Robinson T, Lavados P, Neal B, Hata J, Arima H, Parsons M, Li Y, Wang J, Heritier S, Li Q, Woodward M, Simes RJ, Davis SM, Chalmers J, Interact Investigators. Rapid blood-pressure lowering in patients with acute intracerebral hemorrhage. N Engl J Med. 2013;368:2355–65.
61. Mayer SA, Brun NC, Begtrup K, Broderick J, Davis S, Diringer MN, Skolnick BE, Steiner T, Fast Trial Investigators. Efficacy and safety of recombinant activated factor VII for acute intracerebral hemorrhage. N Engl J Med. 2008;358:2127–37.
62. Qureshi AI, Palesch YY, Barsan WG, Hanley DF, Hsu CY, Martin RL, Moy CS, Silbergleit R, Steiner T, Suarez JI, Toyoda K, Wang Y, Yamamoto H, Yoon BW, Atach-Trial Investigators, and Network the Neurological Emergency Treatment Trials. Intensive blood-pressure lowering in patients with acute cerebral hemorrhage. N Engl J Med. 2016;375:1033–43.
63. Rosand J, Eckman MH, Knudsen KA, Singer DE, Greenberg SM. The effect of warfarin and intensity of anticoagulation on outcome of intracerebral hemorrhage. Arch Intern Med. 2004;164:880–4.
64. Huttner HB, Schellinger PD, Hartmann M, Kohrmann M, Juettler E, Wikner J, Mueller S, Meyding-Lamade U, Strobl R, Mansmann U, Schwab S, Steiner T. Hematoma growth and outcome in treated neurocritical care patients with intracerebral hemorrhage related to oral anticoagulant therapy: comparison of acute treatment strategies using vitamin K, fresh frozen plasma, and prothrombin complex concentrates. Stroke. 2006;37:1465–70.
65. Parry-Jones AR, Di Napoli M, Goldstein JN, Schreuder FH, Tetri S, Tatlisumak T, Yan B, van Nieuwenhuizen KM, Dequatre-Ponchelle N, Lee-Archer M, Horstmann S, Wilson D, Pomero F, Masotti L, Lerpiniere C, Godoy DA, Cohen AS, Houben R, Al-Shahi Salman R, Pennati P, Fenoglio L, Werring D, Veltkamp R, Wood E, Dewey HM, Cordonnier C, Klijn CJ, Meligeni F, Davis SM, Huhtakangas J, Staals J, Rosand J, Meretoja A. Reversal strategies for vitamin K antagonists in acute intracerebral hemorrhage. Ann Neurol. 2015;78:54–62.
66. Kuramatsu JB, Gerner ST, Schellinger PD, Glahn J, Endres M, Sobesky J, Flechsenhar J, Neugebauer H, Juttler E, Grau A, Palm F, Rother J, Michels P, Hamann GF, Huwel J, Hagemann G, Barber B, Terborg C, Trostdorf F, Bazner H, Roth A, Wohrle J, Keller M, Schwarz M, Reimann G, Volkmann J, Mullges W, Kraft P, Classen J, Hobohm C, Horn M, Milewski A, Reichmann H, Schneider H, Schimmel E, Fink GR, Dohmen C, Stetefeld H, Witte O, Gunther A, Neumann-Haefelin T, Racs AE, Nueckel M, Erbguth F, Kloska SP, Dorfler A, Kohrmann M, Schwab S, Huttner HB. Anticoagulant reversal, blood pressure levels, and anticoagulant resumption in patients with anticoagulation-related intracerebral hemorrhage. JAMA. 2015;313:824–36.
67. Frontera JA, Lewin JJ 3rd, Rabinstein AA, Aisiku IP, Alexandrov AW, Cook AM, del Zoppo GJ, Kumar MA, Peerschke EI, Stiefel MF, Teitelbaum JS, Wartenberg KE, Zerfoss CL. Guideline for reversal of antithrombotics in intracranial hemorrhage: a statement for healthcare professionals from the Neurocritical Care Society and Society of Critical Care Medicine. Neurocrit Care. 2016;24:6–46.
68. Kumar M, Ahmad J, Maiwall R, Choudhury A, Bajpai M, Mitra LG, Saluja V, Mohan Agarwal P, Bihari C, Shasthry SM, Jindal A, Bhardwaj A, Kumar G, Sarin SK. Thromboelastography-guided blood component use in patients with cirrhosis with non-variceal bleeding: a randomized controlled trial. Hepatology. 2020;71:235–46.
69. Pandit TN, Sarode R. Blood component support in acquired coagulopathic conditions: is there a method to the madness? Am J Hematol. 2012;87(Suppl 1):S56–62.
70. Shah NL, Intagliata NM, Northup PG, Argo CK, Caldwell SH. Procoagulant therapeutics in liver disease: a critique and clinical rationale. Nat Rev Gastroenterol Hepatol. 2014;11:675–82.
71. Zeigler ZR, Megaludis A, Fraley DS. Desmopressin (d-DAVP) effects on platelet rheology and von Willebrand factor activities in uremia. Am J Hematol. 1992;39:90–5.
72. Miller JB, Figueroa EJ, Haug RM, Shah NL. Thrombocytopenia in chronic liver disease and the role of thrombopoietin agonists. Gastroenterol Hepatol (N Y). 2019;15:326–32.
73. Gunther M, Witenko CJ, Prust M, Salerno D, Berger K. The safety and efficacy of desmopressin in patients with intracranial hemorrhage and a history of alcohol use. J Intensive Care Med. 2021:885066621103l494.
74. da Silva IRF, Frontera JA. Resumption of anticoagulation after intracranial hemorrhage. Curr Treat Options Neurol. 2017;19:39.
75. De Vleeschouwer S, Van Calenbergh F, van Loon J, Nuttin B, Goffin J, Plets C. Risk analysis of thrombo-embolic and recurrent bleeding events in the management of intracranial haemorrhage due to oral anticoagulation. Acta Chir Belg. 2005;105:268–74.
76. Nielsen PB, Larsen TB, Skjoth F, Gorst-Rasmussen A, Rasmussen LH, Lip GY. Restarting anticoagulant treatment after intracranial hemorrhage in patients with atrial fibrillation and the impact on recurrent stroke, mortality, and bleeding: a nationwide cohort study. Circulation. 2015;132:517–25.
77. Murthy SB, Gupta A, Merkler AE, Navi BB, Mandava P, Iadecola C, Sheth KN, Hanley DF, Ziai WC, Kamel H. Restarting anticoagulant therapy after intracranial hemorrhage: a systematic review and meta-analysis. Stroke. 2017;48:1594–600.
78. Schreuder FHBM, van Nieuwenhuizen KM, Hofmeijer J, Vermeer SE, Kerkhoff H, Zock E, Luijckx G-J, Messchendorp GP, van Tuijl J, Bienfait HP, Booij SJ, van den Wijngaard IR, Remmers MJM, Schreuder AHCML, Dippel DW, Staals J, Brouwers PJAM, Wermer MJH, Coutinho JM, Kwa VIH, van Gelder IC, Schutgens REG, Zweedijk B, Algra A, van Dalen JW, Kappelle LJ, Rinkel GJE, van der Worp HB, Klijn CJM, on behalf of the APACHE-AF Trial Investigators. Apixaban versus no antico-

agulation after anticoagulation-associated intracerebral haemorrhage in patients with atrial fibrillation in The Netherlands (APACHE-AF): a randomised, open-label, phase 2 trial. Lancet Neurol. 2021;20:907–16.
79. So, Start Collaboration. Effects of oral anticoagulation for atrial fibrillation after spontaneous intracranial haemorrhage in the UK: a randomised, open-label, assessor-masked, pilot-phase, non-inferiority trial. Lancet Neurol. 2021;20:842–53.
80. Yale University, National Institute of Neurological Disorders and Stroke. Anticoagulation in ICH survivors for stroke prevention and recovery; 2024.
81. Aguilar MI, Hart RG, Kase CS, Freeman WD, Hoeben BJ, Garcia RC, Ansell JE, Mayer SA, Norrving B, Rosand J, Steiner T, Wijdicks EF, Yamaguchi T, Yasaka M. Treatment of warfarin-associated intracerebral hemorrhage: literature review and expert opinion. Mayo Clin Proc. 2007;82:82–92.
82. Majeed A, Kim YK, Roberts RS, Holmstrom M, Schulman S. Optimal timing of resumption of warfarin after intracranial hemorrhage. Stroke. 2010;41:2860–6.
83. Pennlert J, Overholser R, Asplund K, Carlberg B, Van Rompaye B, Wiklund PG, Eriksson M. Optimal timing of anticoagulant treatment after intracerebral hemorrhage in patients with atrial fibrillation. Stroke. 2017;48:314–20.
84. Zhou Z, Yu J, Carcel C, Delcourt C, Shan J, Lindley RI, Neal B, Anderson CS, Hackett ML. Resuming anticoagulants after anticoagulation-associated intracranial haemorrhage: systematic review and meta-analysis. BMJ Open. 2018;8:e019672.
85. Kuramatsu JB, Sembill JA, Gerner ST, Sprugel MI, Hagen M, Roeder SS, Endres M, Haeusler KG, Sobesky J, Schurig J, Zweynert S, Bauer M, Vajkoczy P, Ringleb PA, Purrucker J, Rizos T, Volkmann J, Mullges W, Kraft P, Schubert AL, Erbguth F, Nueckel M, Schellinger PD, Glahn J, Knappe UJ, Fink GR, Dohmen C, Stetefeld H, Fisse AL, Minnerup J, Hagemann G, Rakers F, Reichmann H, Schneider H, Wopking S, Ludolph AC, Stosser S, Neugebauer H, Rother J, Michels P, Schwarz M, Reimann G, Bazner H, Schwert H, Classen J, Michalski D, Grau A, Palm F, Urbanek C, Wohrle JC, Alshammari F, Horn M, Bahner D, Witte OW, Gunther A, Hamann GF, Lucking H, Dorfler A, Achenbach S, Schwab S, Huttner HB. Management of therapeutic anticoagulation in patients with intracerebral haemorrhage and mechanical heart valves. Eur Heart J. 2018;39:1709–23.
86. Cho SM, Moazami N, Katz S, Starling R, Frontera JA. Reversal and resumption of antithrombotic therapy in LVAD-associated intracranial hemorrhage. Ann Thorac Surg. 2019;108:52–8.
87. Anonymous. Risk factors for stroke and efficacy of antithrombotic therapy in atrial fibrillation. Analysis of pooled data from five randomized controlled trials. Arch Intern Med. 1994;154:1449–57.
88. Melkonian M, Jarzebowski W, Pautas E, Siguret V, Belmin J, Lafuente-Lafuente C. Bleeding risk of antiplatelet drugs compared with oral anticoagulants in older patients with atrial fibrillation: a systematic review and meta-analysis. J Thromb Haemost. 2017;15:1500–10.
89. RESTART Collaboration. Effects of antiplatelet therapy after stroke due to intracerebral haemorrhage (RESTART): a randomised, open-label trial. Lancet. 2019;393:2613–23.
90. Reddy VY, Sievert H, Halperin J, Doshi SK, Buchbinder M, Neuzil P, Huber K, Whisenant B, Kar S, Swarup V, Gordon N, Holmes D, Protect Af Steering Committee, and Investigators. Percutaneous left atrial appendage closure vs warfarin for atrial fibrillation: a randomized clinical trial. JAMA. 2014;312:1988–98.
91. Holmes DR Jr, Kar S, Price MJ, Whisenant B, Sievert H, Doshi SK, Huber K, Reddy VY. Prospective randomized evaluation of the Watchman left atrial appendage closure device in patients with atrial fibrillation versus long-term warfarin therapy: the PREVAIL trial. J Am Coll Cardiol. 2014;64:1–12.
92. Holmes DR, Reddy VY, Turi ZG, Doshi SK, Sievert H, Buchbinder M, Mullin CM, Sick P, Investigators PA. Percutaneous closure of the left atrial appendage versus warfarin therapy for prevention of stroke in patients with atrial fibrillation: a randomised non-inferiority trial. Lancet. 2009;374:534–42.
93. Basu Ray I, Khanra D, Shah S, Char S, Jia X, Lam W, Mathuria N, Razavi M, Jain B, Lakkireddy D, Kar S, Natale A, Adeboye A, Jefferies JL, Bangalore S, Asirvatham S, Saeed M. Meta-analysis comparing Watchman(TM) and Amplatzer devices for stroke prevention in atrial fibrillation. Front Cardiovasc Med. 2020;7:89.
94. Lakkireddy D, Thaler D, Ellis CR, Swarup V, Sondergaard L, Carroll J, Gold MR, Hermiller J, Diener HC, Schmidt B, MacDonald L, Mansour M, Maini B, O'Brien L, Windecker S. Amplatzer amulet left atrial appendage occluder versus Watchman device for stroke prophylaxis (amulet IDE): a randomized, controlled trial. Circulation. 2021;144:1543–52.
95. Reddy VY, Mobius-Winkler S, Miller MA, Neuzil P, Schuler G, Wiebe J, Sick P, Sievert H. Left atrial appendage closure with the Watchman device in patients with a contraindication for oral anticoagulation: the ASAP study (ASA Plavix Feasibility Study With Watchman Left Atrial Appendage Closure Technology). J Am Coll Cardiol. 2013;61:2551–6.

Jaundice and Abnormal Liver Function Tests

17

Ramon O. Minjares, Paul Martin,
and Kalyan Ram Bhamidimarri

Contents

Abstract

Liver "function tests" include markers of liver injury, hepatobiliary abnormalitities, and synthetic function. Hepatic dysfunction is a marker of morbidity and mortality in critically ill patients. Hepatic dysfunction in the critical care patient may reflect a primary liver insult or more typically their underlying acute systemic dysregulation. Acute ischemic injury from circulatory shock, drug-induced liver injury, and intrahepatic cholestasis from sepsis or systemic inflammatory response syndrome (SIRS) are the most common causes of hepatic dysfunction in the intensive care unit. Unrecognized chronic liver disease can have an initial presentation as acute-on-chornic liver failure (ACLF) with index complications such as fluid overload, variceal hemorrhage, or hepatic encephalopathy. COVID-19 infection has been implicated in liver injury due to immune-mediated inflammation, sepsis, drug-induced injury, and/or viral replication in liver cells. Assessment of liver injury in the critical care setting can be challenging, but prompt recognition and identification of etiology can prevent unnecessary invasive testing and facilitate logical management.

R. O. Minjares (✉)
Department of Internal Medicine, University of Miami Miller School of Medicine, Miami, FL, USA
e-mail: rom25@miami.edu

P. Martin · K. R. Bhamidimarri
Division of Digestive Health and Liver Diseases, Department of Medicine, University of Miami Miller School of Medicine, Miami, FL, USA

E. Mahanna Gabrielli et al. (eds.), *Textbook of Neurointensive Care: Volume 1*, https://doi.org/10.1007/978-3-031-62220-5_17

Introduction

Hypoxic, toxic, and inflammatory insults are common in the intensive care unit (ICU) and can affect liver function potentially leading to systemic complications such as coagulopathy, increased risk of infection, hypoglycemia, encephalopathy, acute kidney injury, and multiorgan failure [1]. Liver chemistries (colloquially known as "liver function tests") include markers of hepatobiliary injury [2]. Liver injury in critical illness can be divided into two groups: (1) primary hepatic dysfunction, such as liver cirrhosis and subsequent acute-on-chronic liver failure (ACLF) or primary acute liver failure (ALF) and (2) secondary or acquired liver injury and failure (without underlying liver disease), such as hypoxic liver injury, cholestatic dysfunction in critical illness, sclerosing cholangitis in critically ill patients (SC-CIP), and drug-induced liver injury (DILI).

Multiple factors are involved in the pathogenesis of hepatic dysfunction in critical illness; cholestatic dysfunction mediated by alterations of intracellular bile acid (BA) transporters and impaired BA secretion leading to subsequent BA retention [3]. Hypoxic hepatitis caused by a disbalance in hepatic oxygen supply and expenditure eventually causing centrilobular liver cell necrosis. And finally, biliary strictures and cast formation (e.g., SC-CIP) that are a consequence of biliary epithelium destruction due to hypoxia and inflammation (cholangitis). It is estimated that up to 20% of patients in the ICU develop cholestasis [4]. However, cholestatic alterations are more frequently found in certain types of shock (33% in septic shock vs. 21% in cardiogenic shock) or following surgery (5%) [5]. Hypoxic hepatitis is by far the most common cause of massive elevation in aminotransferase levels in hospitalized patients. The prevalence of hypoxic hepatitis ranges between 1% and 12% in ICU and may be even higher in patients with cardiogenic shock, in whom the prevalence was reported to be greater than 20% [4, 6, 7]. Acute heart failure and cardiogenic shock are present in 50–70% of patients with hypoxic hepatitis, whereas sepsis is observed in 13–32% [4, 6–8].

Multiple studies have demonstrated that liver injury and failure in the critically ill patients are important predictors of overall worse clinical outcomes, prolonged hospitalization, increased morbidity, and mortality [2, 4, 9–12]. Decompensated cirrhosis/ACLF has a prevalence of 1.6–5.4% and a hospital mortality of 36–86%, whereas ALF has a prevalence of <10 cases per million persons/year with a hospital mortality of 23–53% [4]. Patients with serum bilirubin levels between 2 and 3 mg/dL had a 27% hospital mortality rate, and in those with bilirubin between 6 and 10 mg/dL and greater than 10 mg/dL, the hospital mortality was 38% and 47%, respectively [13]. Furthermore, critically ill patients with hypoxic liver injury have significantly decreased survival rates: 28-day mortality ranges between 40% and 60%, and 1-year mortality rate is about 75% [4, 6–8]. The highest mortality rates are observed in patients with septic shock, high severity of organ failure, and patients with preexistent chronic liver diseases. Hence, prompt diagnosis and multidisciplinary management of the liver injury and failure in the ICU is crucial.

Chapter Goals

- To provide a comprehensive overview and interpretation of liver chemistries
- To evaluate liver test abnormalities and distinguish the various patterns of liver injury
- To describe liver test abnormalities in critically ill patients
- To increase awareness regarding indirect or systemic insults to the liver and the concept of ACLF
- To review the management of liver-related complications in the ICU. Some key clinical questions that this chapter will answer are listed in Table 17.1.

Common Liver Biochemical and Function Tests

Serum aminotransferases such as aspartate aminotransferase (AST) and alanine aminotransferase (ALT) are intracellular enzymes involved in the transfer of amino groups of aspartate and alanine to ketoglutaric acid. They are released from injured hepatocytes and are useful markers of hepatocellular injury (inflammation or cell necrosis). AST is present in the liver and in other organs such as the skeletal muscle, cardiac muscle, kidney, and brain. ALT is a more specific marker of hepatocellular cell injury as its highest concentration is in the liver. An increase in AST without elevation in ALT is suggestive of cardiac or muscle injury [14]. In adults, normal ALT levels range from 29 to 33 units/L for males and 19 to 25 units/L for females [2]. Levels of ALT increase with body mass index (particularly trunk fat) and correlate with serum triglycerides, glucose, insulin, and leptin levels. Levels may rise acutely with a high caloric meal or ingestion of acetaminophen. Lactate dehydrogenase (LDH) is a cytoplasmic enzyme present in tissues throughout the body. LDH is not as sensitive as the serum aminotransferases and has poor sensitivity (even when using isoenzyme LDH5 analysis).

Table 17.1 Key clinical questions the chapter will answer

What are liver function tests?
How to interpret abnormal liver tests and pattern of liver injury?
What are the common etiologies of liver injury in the critically ill patient?
What is acute on chronic liver failure?
How to diagnose and treat liver injury in ICU?

However, the ALT/LDH ratio may help differentiate acute viral hepatitis (≥1.5) from ischemic hepatitis and acetaminophen toxicity (<1.5) [15].

Alkaline phosphatase (ALP) is part of a family of zinc metalloproteinase enzymes that catalyze the hydrolysis of phosphate esters at an alkaline pH. Serum ALP is derived predominantly from the liver (particularly in the hepatocytes on the canalicular membrane, and not from the bile duct cell), but it is also found in abundance in bone and in smaller quantities in the small intestine, kidney, and white blood cells. Levels are physiologically higher in childhood (bone growth) and in pregnancy (placental production) [16]. Pathologically increased levels occur mainly in bone disease (e.g., metastatic bone disease and fractures) and cholestatic liver disease—for example, primary biliary cholangitis (PBC), primary sclerosing cholangitis (PSC), common bile duct obstruction, intrahepatic duct obstruction, and drug-induced cholestasis (Table 17.2) [2]. Furthermore, hepatic congestion in right-sided heart failure can lead to a cholestatic pattern (elevated ALP levels and/or bilirubin).

Table 17.2 Causes of elevated serum alkaline phosphatase levels

Moderate elevation (<4 times ULN)
Hepatic
Hepatitis (viral, alcoholic, chronic)
Cirrhosis
Infiltrative disorders (sarcoidosis, amyloidosis, etc.)
Hypoperfusion (sepsis, shock, etc.)
Nonhepatic
Pregnancy (third trimester)
Physiologic (after eating a fatty meal in individuals with type O or B)
High bone turnover (healing fractures, osteomalacia, Paget disease of bone, hyperparathyroidism, hyperthyroidism, etc.)
Extrahepatic tumors (osteosarcoma, lung, gastric, head/neck, renal cell, ovarian, uterine, Hodgkin lymphoma)
Marked elevation (≥4 times ULN)
Extrahepatic biliary obstruction
Choledocholithiasis
Malignant obstruction (pancreas, ampulla, gallbladder, bile duct cancer, etc.)
Biliary strictures (PSC with extrahepatic duct stricture, complications after procedures, chronic pancreatitis, anastomotic stricture after LT)
Infections (AIDS cholangiopathy, *Ascaris lumbricoides*, liver fluke)
Intrahepatic cholestasis
Drugs associated with cholestasis (steroids, phenytoin, etc.)
Primary biliary cholangitis
Primary sclerosing cholangitis
Intrahepatic cholestasis of pregnancy
Infiltrative disorders (amyloidosis, lymphoma, sarcoidosis, tuberculosis, hepatic abscess)
Metastatic disease
Liver allograft rejection
Ischemic cholangiopathy
Sickle cell disease (hepatic crisis)

Abbreviations: ULN upper limit of normal, *LT* liver transplantation, *PSC* primary sclerosing cholangitis, *AIDS* acquired immunodeficiency syndrome

ALP is sensitive for detection of biliary tract obstruction; a normal value is highly unusual in significant biliary obstruction unless it is very recent. An increase in serum ALP results from increased hepatic synthesis of the enzyme, rather than leakage from bile duct cells or failure to clear circulating ALP [16]; because it is synthesized in response to biliary obstruction, the ALP level may be normal early during acute cholangitis when the serum aminotransferases are already elevated. Fractionated ALP level may help differentiate if it originates from the liver or other tissues (e.g., bones, kidney, placenta); however, in clinical practice a liver source is identified by confirming simultaneous elevation in other measures of cholestasis (e.g., GGT, 5′ nucleotidase). In children and the elderly (especially in females over 50 years of age), ALP levels increase in part due to bone turnover.

GGT is present in hepatocytes and biliary epithelial cells, as well as kidney, seminal versicles, pancreas, spleen, brain, and heart. GGT can be used to confirm the hepatic origin of an elevated ALP or to support a suspicion of alcohol abuse in a patient with alcoholic hepatitis (AST:ALT ratio > 2:1). An isolated elevation in GGT (with otherwise normal liver biochemical tests including ALP) should not lead to an exhaustive work-up for liver disease. Serum 5′ nucleotidase (5NT) is found in liver in association with canalicular and sinusoidal plasma membranes. 5NT is found in multiple organs (i.e., liver, intestine, brain, heart, vessels, pancreas) but only released into serum by the hepatobiliary tissue. Although the physiologic function of 5NT is unknown, it specifically catalyzes hydrolysis of nucleotides (i.e., adenosine 5′-phosphate and inosine 5′-phosphate). An elevated serum 5NT level in association with an elevated ALP level is specific for hepatobiliary dysfunction and is superior to GGT [15, 17].

Patterns of Liver Chemistry Test Elevations

Liver test abnormalities can often be grouped into one of the several patterns: the abnormalities may be acute, subacute, or chronic based on whether they have been present for less than 6 weeks, 6 weeks to 6 months, or more than 6 months, respectively. The most common classification is based on the pattern of elevation: (1) hepatocellular (disproportionate elevation in AST and ALT levels as compared with ALP or GGT levels), (2) cholestatic (disproportionate elevation in ALP and GGT level as compared with AST and ALT levels), (3) mixed (elevation of alkaline phosphatase and AST/ALT levels), and (4) isolated hyperbilirubinemia (elevated bilirubin with normal alkaline phosphatase and AST/ALT levels) [2]. These tests have been reported to be abnormal in as many as 61% of patients who are admitted to the ICU [1].

Hepatic dysfunction in the critical ill patient could be related to underlying liver disease or secondary to direct liver insults or systemic dysregulation. Acute ischemic injury from circulatory shock, drug-induced liver injury, intrahepatic cholestasis from sepsis or systemic inflammatory response syndrome (SIRS) are frequent etiologies for liver dysfunction and are commonly encountered in the critical care setting. However, the precise etiology—especially in mild elevations, may not always be elucidated [1, 18].

The R-value or R-factor is calculated by the formula $R = (ALT \div ULN\ ALT)/(ALP \div ULN\ ALP)$. It can be used to help determine the likely type of liver injury in patients with elevated aminotransferases and ALP. An R-value ≥5 is labeled as hepatocellular injury, whereas an R-value of ≤2 suggests cholestatic injury. An R-value between 2 and 5 is interpreted as a mixed pattern [19]. The serum bilirubin can be elevated in both hepatocellular and cholestatic conditions, hence it is not helpful in differentiating between the two patterns. Liver injury can be due to direct hepatotoxic insults or due to indirect insults resulting due to systemic derangements that are frequent in critically ill patients.

Table 17.3 Causes of elevated serum aminotransferase levels

Mild elevation (<5× ULN) [a]	Severe elevation (>15× ULN)
Hepatic (ALT>AST)	Acute viral hepatitis (A-E, HSV)
Chronic viral hepatitis	DILI, acetaminophen toxicity
Acute viral hepatitis (A-E, EBV, CMV, HSV)	Ischemic liver injury (LDH markedly elevated)
MAFLD (steatosis, NASH)	Autoimmune hepatitis
Hemochromatosis	Wilson disease
DILI	Acute bile duct obstruction
Autoimmune hepatitis	Acute Budd-Chiari syndrome
AAT deficiency	Hepatic artery ligation
Wilson disease	Toxin-related hepatitis
Celiac disease	HELLP
Glycogenic hepatology	Sinusoidal obstruction syndrome (veno-occlusive disease)
Hepatic (AST > ALT)	Malignant infiltration
Alcohol-related liver injury (AST/ALT >2:1)	
Cirrhosis	
Nonhepatic	
Strenuous exercise (rhabdomyolysis, muscular damage)	
Hemolysis	
Myopathy	
Thyroid disease	
Adrenal insufficiency	
Macro-AST	
Cardiac disease	

Abbreviations: ULN upper limit of normal, *ALT* alanine aminotransferase, *AST* aspartate aminotransferase, *CMV* cytomegalovirus, *DILI* drug-induced liver injury, *EBV* Epstein-Barr virus, *HSV* herpes simplex virus, *MAFLD* metabolic associated fatty liver disease, *A1AT* alpha-1 antitrypsin, *HELLP* hemolysis, elevated liver enzymes and low platelets

[a] Any liver disease may be associated with moderate elevation in ALT levels (5–15 times upper limit of normal)

Hepatocellular Injury

The magnitude of the liver chemistry abnormalities and the ratio of AST to ALT will help guide the evaluation. Most causes of hepatocellular injury are associated with a serum AST level that is lower than the ALT. Conversely, in alcoholic hepatitis the serum AST is usually no more than two to ten times the upper limit of normal (ULN), and the ALT is normal or nearly normal, with an AST:ALT ratio > 2:1, particularly with an elevated GGT. In metabolic fatty liver disease (MAFLD), ALT is typically higher than AST until cirrhosis develops [2, 20].

Mild elevations of AST and/or ALT (two to five times ULN) are seen in a variety of hepatic and nonhepatic conditions (Table 17.3). Moderate elevations of serum transaminases (5–15 times ULN) overlap with the mild and severe lists. Severe elevations of AST and/or ALT (>15 times ULN) can be caused by several disorders, including viral hepatitis, acute ischemic injury, septic shock, acute Budd–Chiari syndrome, acute hepatic artery occlusion, toxin or medication-induced liver injury, autoimmune hepatitis, acute biliary obstruction, diffuse infiltration of the liver with cancer, liver trauma/surgery, and Wilson's disease. Massive liver-related elevations in AST and/or ALT (>10,000 IU/L) are seen in acetaminophen toxicity, acute ischemic injury, and toxin-related liver injury (e.g., *Amanita phalloides*); and less commonly, in nonhepatic conditions such as rhabdomyolysis and heat stroke [21–23]. The diagnostic approach to elevations in serum transaminases is shown in Fig. 17.1.

Patients with moderate to massive elevations of ALT and/or AST require a prompt workup [2, 21]. Considerations include acute hepatitis (A–E), acute reactivation of chronic hepatitis B (HBV), and acute hepatitis from non-hepatotropic viruses including herpes simplex virus (HSV), Epstein–Barr virus (EBV), and/or cytomegalovirus (CMV). Acute autoimmune liver disease and idiosyncratic drug reactions are other possibilities. A history of hematologic malignancy with recent chemotherapy may suggest a diagnosis of sinusoidal obstruction syndrome (veno-occlusive disease). Finally, a history of a hypercoagulable state (i.e., polycythemia vera) in the setting of abnormal liver tests and ascites should suggest Budd–Chiari syndrome [22].

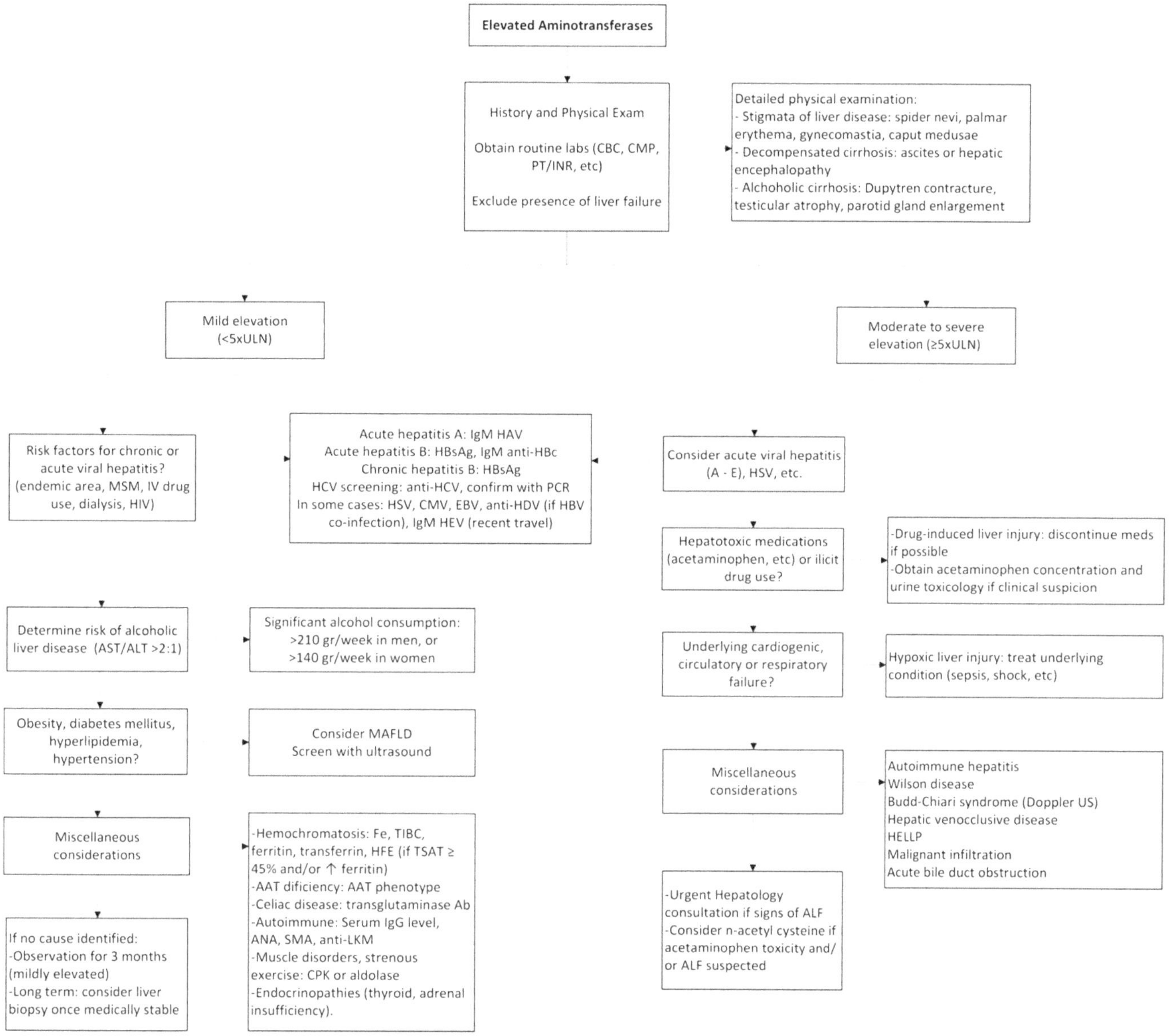

Fig. 17.1 Diagnostic approach to elevations in serum aminotransferases in the ICU. *Abbreviations: ALT* alanine aminotransferase, *ALF* acute liver failure, *AST* aspartate aminotransferase, *CBC* complete blood count, *CMP* comprehensive metabolic panel, *PT/INR* prothrombin time/international normalized ratio, *MAFLD* metabolic associated fatty liver disease, *MSM* men who have sex with men, *HIV* human immunodeficiency virus, *HSV* herpes simplex virus, *CMV* cytomegalovirus, *EBV* Epstein-Barr virus, *TSAT* transferrin saturation, *AAT* alpha-1 antitrypsin, *HELLP* hemolysis, elevated liver enzymes and low platelets

Cholestatic Injury

Cholestasis reflects altered bile production, secretion, or excretion. Consequently, laboratory abnormalities are related to the retention of substances in the blood that are normally excreted in bile (bile acids, conjugated bilirubin) and are associated with an increase in cholestatic enzymes such as ALP and GGT. There is no uniform laboratory definition of cholestasis. According to some authors, total bilirubin >2 mg/dL represents a reasonable cutoff in daily practice. Others use a two-fold to three-fold elevation in ALP and/or GGT to define cholestasis. Extrahepatic cholestasis is defined as the inability of a sufficient bile excretion due to bile duct obstruction, while intrahepatic cholestasis is a consequence of alterations in signaling and transport at the hepatocellular level. The magnitude of the serum ALP elevation does not distinguish extrahepatic from intrahepatic cholestasis. It is estimated that up to 20% of patients will develop cholestasis during their ICU stay [24].

The clinical association of cholestasis and systemic inflammation is well known. Alterations in hepatic transport and metabolism occur in the first hours of critical illness. Infections, hypoperfusion, retention of toxic molecules, and pathogen-associated molecular patterns (PAMPs) contribute to cholestasis in critical illness through inflammation-mediated repression of hepatobiliary transporters and reduced canalicular contractility, resulting in impaired bile flow and bile acids (BA) retention. BA have important signaling functions that regulate energy, lipid, and glucose homeostasis [25, 26].

Synthetic Function

The majority of circulating proteins are produced by the liver. Serum albumin and prothrombin time (PT) or internationalized normalized ratio (INR) are commonly used to test hepatic synthetic function. As reference range varies among laboratories, INR is used to standardize PT determinations performed in different laboratories; however, the results are less consistent in patients with liver disease than in those taking warfarin unless liver-disease controls are used [27]. Albumin is produced by the liver with a circulating half-life of 3 weeks and is a useful marker of the synthetic function of the liver. It has multiple biological actions, including maintenance of oncotic pressure, binding of other substances (fatty acids, bilirubin, thyroid hormone, drugs, etc.), metabolism of compounds, and antioxidant properties. Albumin concentrations may be reduced in many clinical situations, including sepsis, systemic inflammatory disorders, nephrotic syndrome, malabsorption, and gastrointestinal protein loss in addition to liver disease [28].

PT is a useful test to assess the severity and prognosis of acute liver disease as it may be prolonged in patients with severe liver disease of <24 h duration [29]. The one-stage PT measures the rate of conversion of prothrombin to thrombin after activation of the extrinsic coagulation pathway in the presence of a tissue extract (thromboplastin) and calcium ions. Deficiency of one or more of the liver-produced factors results in a prolonged PT. Apart from hepatocellular disease or vitamin K deficiency, PT may also be elevated in consumptive coagulopathies, inherited deficiencies of a coagulation factor, disseminated intravascular coagulation (DIC) or medications that antagonize the prothrombin complex. The PT and INR correlate with the severity of liver disease but not with the risk of bleeding because of counterbalancing decreases in levels of anticoagulant factors (e.g., proteins C and S, antithrombin) and enhanced fibrinolysis in patients with liver disease. Vitamin K deficiency as the cause of a prolonged PT can be excluded by oral administration of vitamin K. Correction or improvement of the PT by at least 30% within 24 h of administration of vitamin K implies that hepatic synthetic function is intact [15].

Most coagulation factors are synthesized by the liver, including factors I (fibrinogen), II (prothrombin), V, VII, IX, and X and have much shorter half-lives than that of albumin. Factor VII decreases first in liver disease because of its shortest half-life, followed by factors X and IX. Factor V is not vitamin K dependent, and its measurement can help distinguish vitamin K deficiency from hepatocellular dysfunction in a patient with prolonged PT. Measurement of factor II has also been used to assess liver function. Elevated levels are found in cirrhosis and hepatocellular carcinoma (HCC) and in patients taking warfarin (vitamin K antagonist). Administration of vitamin K results in normalization of factor II in patients taking warfarin but not in those with cirrhosis. Globulins are often increased nonspecifically in chronic liver disease. The pattern of elevation may suggest the cause of the underlying liver disease (i.e., elevated IgG in autoimmune hepatitis or elevated IgM in primary biliary cholangitis) [30, 31].

Bilirubin and Jaundice

Jaundice is clinically apparent when serum bilirubin exceeds 3 mg/dL, although patient may notice acholic stools and dark urine before the appearance of conjunctival icterus. Bilirubin is a breakdown product of hemoglobin, and to a lesser extent, heme-containing enzymes. After red blood cell breakdown in the reticuloendothelial system, heme is degraded by the enzyme heme oxygenase in the endoplasmic reticulum. Bilirubin tightly binds albumin after being released into the blood. Unconjugated bilirubin is taken up by the liver by a carrier-mediated process, attaches to intracellular storage proteins (ligands), and is conjugated by the enzyme uridine 5′-diphosphate (UDP)-glucuronyl transferase to form a diglucuronide and, to a lesser extent, a monoglucuronide. Conjugated bilirubin is water soluble and thus appears in urine. When serum levels of bilirubin glucuronides are elevated, some binding to albumin occurs (delta bilirubin), leading to absence of bilirubinuria despite conjugated hyperbilirubinemia; this phenomenon explains delayed resolution of jaundice during recovery from acute liver disease until albumin-bound bilirubin is catabolized [32, 33].

Laboratory analysis including reticulocyte count, serum haptoglobin, and peripheral smear should be obtained if hemolysis is suspected. Markedly elevated bilirubin levels usually represent hemolysis plus parenchymal liver disease or biliary obstruction. Bilirubin level > 60 mg/dL is typically seen in patients with hemoglobinopathies (e.g., sickle cell disease) in whom obstructive jaundice or acute hepatitis develops. The second group of disorders with unconjugated hyperbilirubinemia includes those with impaired hepatic uptake or conjugation of bilirubin. Certain medications, such as rifampin and probenecid, are commonly associated with diminished uptake of bilirubin, highlighting the importance of performing a detailed medication reconciliation, especially in the critical care setting. Conversely, conjugated hyperbilirubinemia is found in cholestasis (bile duct obstruction, PSC, PBC, biliary strictures, etc.). These conditions should be suspected in patients with mild hyperbilirubinemia in the absence of other abnormalities of routine liver biochemical.

Common Etiologies and Management of Liver Injury in Critically Ill Patients

Ischemic Hepatitis

Ischemic hepatitis is characterized by rapid and transient increases in either AST or ALT (>10 times ULN) in cardiac, circulatory, or respiratory failure. The typical histopathological pattern in ischemic hepatitis is centrilobular hepatocyte necrosis. It is characterized by a primary hepatocellular pattern of injury. Hepatic synthetic function usually remains normal or is only mildly impaired. Simultaneous onset of renal dysfunction and muscle necrosis (rapid rise in serum aminotransferase levels associated with rise in LDH level) may be noted. It represents the most common cause of massive elevation of serum transaminase in the critically ill patients [34]. This condition has been labeled with various terms over time (i.e., shock liver, hypoxic liver injury, acute ischemic injury, ischemic hepatopathy, and hypoxic hepatitis, etc.), which reflects the evolving pathophysiologic understanding of the contributing factors leading to liver cell necrosis. The term hepatitis is somewhat of a misnomer since the injury is not mediated by an inflammatory process.

The liver has dual blood supply, with the portal vein accounting for ~80% of the hepatic blood flow. Ischemic hepatitis may occur in a "two-hit" mechanism. A low-flow state, typically from right-sided heart failure leads to elevated hepatic pressures, placing the liver at risk for hypoxemic injury. The second hit occurs during acute cardiac, circulatory, or respiratory failure that provokes systemic hypotension and hepatic ischemia. Therefore, arterial hypotension by itself is rarely complicated by ischemic hepatitis. Ischemic injury can also be caused by focal interruption of blood supply, as it occurs in sickle cell crisis and hepatic artery thrombosis (post-transplanted patients with a preexisting portal vein thrombosis). The prevalence of ischemic hepatitis ranges between 1% and 12% in ICU and may be even higher in patients with cardiogenic shock (≥ 20%). The European Association of Studies of the Liver (EASL) has described ischemic hepatitis as an important cause of secondary ALF [4].

No specific therapeutic intervention has been described for ischemic hepatitis. Management should focus on reversing the underlying cause of hemodynamic instability. After hemodynamic stability, aminotransferase levels decline steadily usually returning to normal within a week. Although evidence shows that dopamine may lead to preservation of hepatic flow, no clinical benefit has been established for ischemic hepatitis. A study published by Drolz et al. included 851 patients who were prospectively screened for development of ischemic hepatitis within 48 h of admission to the ICU. Statin treatment prior to ICU admission was significantly associated with decreased incidence of ischemic hepatitis (OR = 0.42, 95% CI 0.19–0.95; $p < 0.05$). Overall survival benefit of statins was not identified [35].

Acute Liver Failure

Acute liver failure (previously known as fulminant hepatic failure or necrosis, fulminant hepatitis, and acute hepatic necrosis) is defined as the development of hepatocellular dysfunction manifesting with coagulopathy (INR ≥ 1.5, or prolonged PT) and altered level of consciousness due to hepatic encephalopathy (HE) in patients without an underlying liver disease [36]. Disease duration of greater than 28 weeks before the onset of encephalopathy suggests chronic liver disease. Other findings include jaundice, RUQ tenderness, fever, ascites, signs of intravascular depletion and vesicular skin lesions (ALF due to HSV). Serum aminotransferases and bilirubin are often also elevated. Other laboratory findings include hemolytic anemia, elevated serum creatinine, hypoglycemia and electrolyte and acid–base disturbances.

ALF presents a unique set of complications and management strategies with liver transplantation (LT) as the common end point in most cases. DILI and viral hepatitis represent the most common causes of ALF in the United States (Table 17.4), with acetaminophen toxicity being the

Table 17.4 Common etiologies of acute liver failure

Most common causes	Less frequent causes
Acetaminophen toxicity	Autoimmune hepatitis
Hepatitis (HAV, HBV)	Genetic (Wilson)
Medications Antimicrobials Antiepileptic agents (carbamazepine, phenytoin) Statins Chemotherapy NSAIDs	Metabolic disease
	Vascular Budd Chiari Ischemic hepatopathy
	Pregnancy HELLP Fatty liver disease of pregnancy Pre-eclamptic liver rupture
Toxic agents Herbal supplements Cocaine Ecstasy	Malignancy, lymphoma, HLH
	Mushroom poisoning (*Amanita phalloides*)

Abbreviations: NSAID non-steroidal anti-inflammatory drugs, *HELLP* hemolysis, elevated liver enzymes and low platelets, *HLH* hemophagocytic lymphohistiocytosis most common reason for liver transplantation. ALF can be further classified as hyperacute (<7 days), acute (7–21 days), or subacute (>21 days and < 26 weeks). In patients with hyperacute or ALF, cerebral edema is common, whereas renal failure and portal hypertension are more frequently observed in patients with subacute liver failure. The diagnostic approach of ALF is described in Fig. 17.2. Imaging with abdominal Doppler ultrasonography should be obtained to exclude Budd–Chiari syndrome and evaluate for portal hypertension, hepatic steatosis, hepatic congestion, and underlying cirrhosis. Computed tomography (CT), magnetic resonance imaging (MRI), and venography (MRV) are typically reserved for patients with a negative ultrasound in whom the suspicion for Budd–Chiari syndrome or malignancy remains high. Patients with ALF may also develop renal dysfunction; therefore, the risk of further renal injury associated with contrast agents (e.g., nephrogenic systemic fibrosis with gadolinium) should be weighed against the need for the examination. Contrast-enhanced, cross-sectional imaging with either a CT scan or an MRI of the liver are recommended for patients who are being considered for LT to assess for thrombosis or malignancy.

Early recognition of ALF with serial neurologic examinations is the key to initiating appropriate management of HE and cerebral edema. The pathophysiology that leads to the development of HE is mediated by elevation in ammonia levels, inflammation, and increased cerebral blood flow. An acute rise in ammonia levels triggers osmotic shifts, which subsequently lead to astrocyte swelling and cerebral edema. Hence, HE is considered a precursor to the development of cerebral edema and intracranial hypertension. Though the incidence of intracranial hypertension has decreased recently, it may still develop in up to a third of patients with ALF who progress to grade 3–4 HE and can lead to transtentorial herniation and death [36, 37]. Clinical features of intracranial hypertension include pupillary changes, Cushing's triad (systemic hypertension, bradycardia, respiratory depression), seizures, and abnormal brain stem reflexes.

Whenever possible, patients with acute liver failure should be managed in an ICU preferably located in a liver transplantation center. Patients with HE should undergo non-contrasted CT scan of the head to rule out other causes of altered mental status or complication of ALF (e.g., space-occupying lesion, intracranial hypertension). HE is graded from 1 to 4 and ranges from changes in behavior to coma. The grade of HE correlates with development of cerebral edema and prognosis. While lactulose and rifaximin are commonly used in patients with HE and chronic liver disease, their role in patients with ALF is unclear. Progression to grade 3–4 HE may warrant intubation and mechanical ventilation for airway protection. Ventilation strategies should target prevention of hypercapnia in the setting of cerebral edema and intracranial hypertension. Neurotherapeutic interventions should be initiated for the management of cerebral edema and intracranial hypertension with the primary goal of limiting increased intracranial pressure (ICP) while maintaining adequate cerebral perfusion pressure. Although the placement of invasive ICP monitoring devices remains a matter of intense debate, some LT programs routinely use these invasive techniques in patients who are at greater risk for cerebral edema (e.g., grade 4 HE, or rapidly progressive grade 3 HE) [36, 38]. Major complications from ICP monitoring are infections and bleeding. Once established, the medical treatment of intracranial hypertension must bridge patients to LT because no treatment permanently reverses cerebral edema [21], although uncontrolled ICP elevation is a contraindication to LT.

The hepatocellular injury present in ALF leads to a significant reduction in the production of procoagulation and anticoagulation factors that are normally synthesized by the liver. Factors II, V, VII, and X are significantly decreased, while factor XIII is increased. This has been attributed to acute inflammation and increased consumption. Thrombocytopenia is variable and associated with portal hypertension. There is a higher incidence of deep vein thrombosis in the setting of a hypercoagulable state despite elevated INR and thrombocytopenia. Since conventional coagulation tests such as INR are not helpful in determining a patient's risk of bleeding, those who require an invasive procedure or who develop bleeding may need additional testing. (i.e., fibrinogen, thromboelastography) to guide management. There is no clear role for administration of blood products such as fresh frozen plasma (FFP) to correct coagulation abnormalities in the absence of active bleeding, since it has not been shown to influence mortality [39]. There has been much debate regarding the use of recombinant factor VIIa to aid in reversal of coagulopathy; however, its use has been limited by the increased risk of thrombosis.

Early identification of the etiology of ALF is crucial to guide potential specific management and predict its outcome. The leading causes of mortality in ALF are intracranial hypertension and infections; however, patients can also develop other complications with varying degrees of hemodynamic derangements and renal dysfunction. The transplant-free survival of patients with ALF related to acetaminophen, HAV, hypoxic hepatitis or pregnancy is >50%. Conversely, when ALF is associated with HBV, drugs other than acetaminophen, autoimmune hepatitis (AIH), Wilson's disease, or Budd–Chiari syndrome, the transplant-free survival rate is lower than 25% [40]. Predicting which ALF patients will ultimately require transplantation may be challenging. The King's College Hospital (KCH) criteria is the most clinically useful model to guide referral to specialized units for LT (Table 17.5). It has a sensitivity of 68–69% and a specificity of 82–92% [41, 42]. Newer models, including the model for

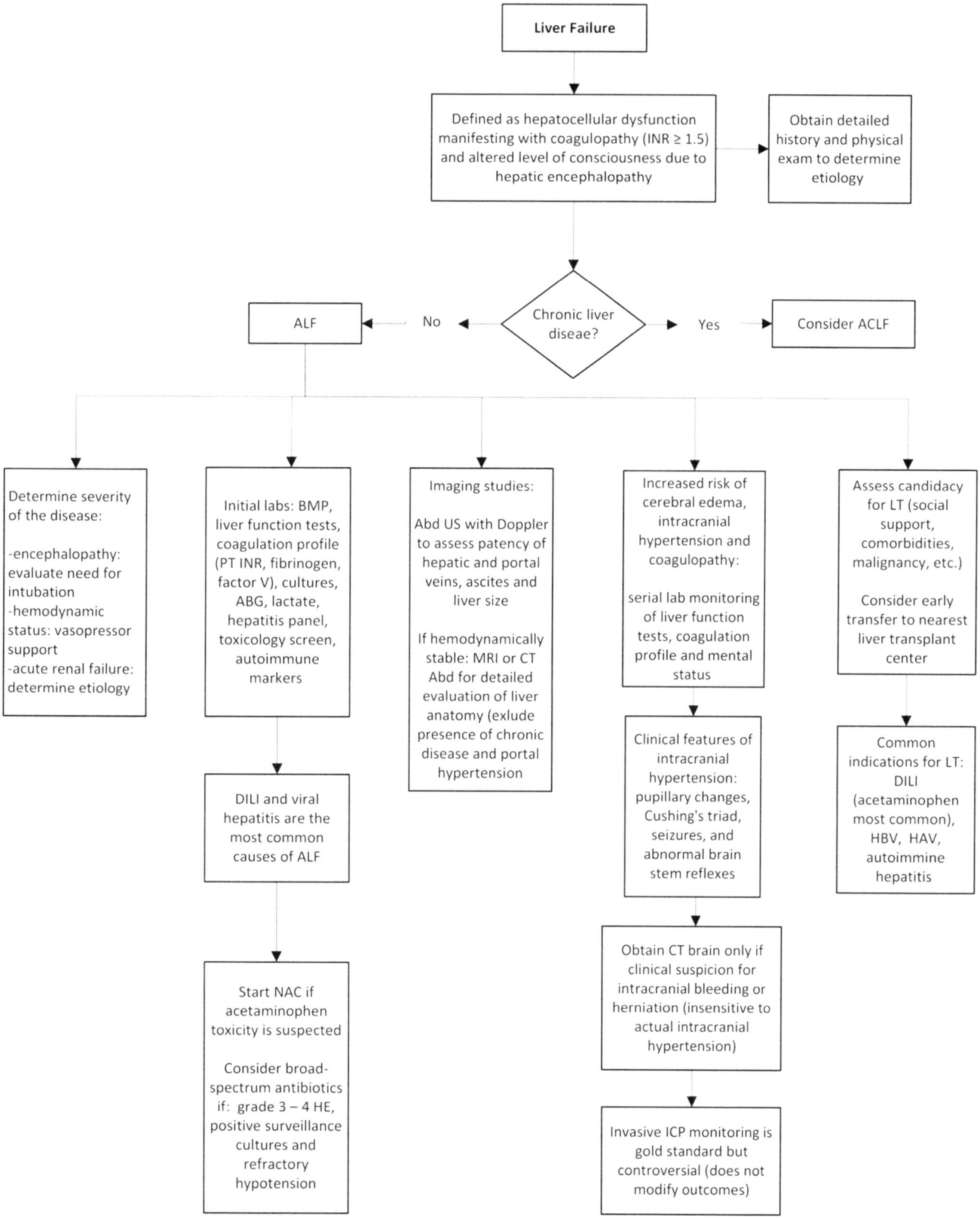

Fig. 17.2 Management of acute liver failure. *Abbreviations: ALF* acute liver failure, *ACLF* acute-on-chronic liver failure, *BMP* basic metabolic panel, *PT* prothrombin time, *INR* international normalized ratio, *ABG* arterial blood gas, *HE* hepatic encephalopathy, *NAC* N-acetylcysteine, *CT* computed tomography, *MRI* magnetic resonance imaging, *US* ultrasound, *LT* liver transplant, *DILI* drug-induced liver injury

Table 17.5 King's college criteria for liver transplantation[a]

ALF due to acetaminophen	ALF not due to acetaminophen
Arterial pH <7.3	Prothrombin time > 100 s (INR >6.5)
All of the following three criteria: • Hepatic encephalopathy grade 3–4 • Serum creatinine >3.4 mg/dL (>300 μmol/L) • Prothrombin time > 100 s (INR >6.5)	*Any* of the following criteria • Non-A, non-B viral hepatitis, drug-induced or indeterminate etiology of ALF • Time from jaundice to encephalopathy >7 days • Age < 10 years or > 40 years • Prothrombin time > 50 s (INR >3.5) • Serum Bilirubin >17.4 mg/dL (>300 μmol/L)

Abbreviations: ALF acute liver failure, *INR* international normalized ratio
[a]Adapted from O'Grady JG et al. [42]

end-stage liver disease (MELD) score, have not improved accuracy. In fact, the discriminative power of the MELD was not found to be superior to that of the INR or the KCH criteria [21, 43].

N-acetylcysteine (NAC) is used for the treatment of acetaminophen toxicity as it can dramatically improve prognosis. NAC should be given to any patient with a history suggestive of acetaminophen toxicity. Although additional studies are needed before NAC can be routinely recommended for ALF from causes other than acetaminophen toxicity, it is sometimes administered in patients who are not candidates for LT, patients taking medications that induce cytochrome P450 activity, patients with chronic liver disease, and patients with an indeterminate cause for the ALF. A placebo-controlled trial involving 173 patients and conducted by Lee et al. reported improved transplant-free survival in patients with non-acetaminophen-related ALF toxicity who were treated with NAC (40% vs. 27% in placebo group; $P = 0.043$). The benefit appeared to be confined to patients with early-stage HE [44].

The features of coagulopathy, increased serum transaminases, abnormal bilirubin, and altered levels of consciousness may be seen in patients with a variety of systemic disease processes. Therefore, if there is no primary liver insult, these patients should be considered to have a secondary liver injury and not ALF; management should focus on the treatment of any underlying disease processes. Secondary forms of liver injury can also fulfill diagnostic criteria of ALF and are consequently incorporated into the recent European guidelines on ALF. In contrast to primary ALF, LT is usually contraindicated in patients with secondary ALF.

Finally, patients with ALF are at increased risk for infection and sepsis. Common offenders include gram-positive cocci, enteric gram-negative bacilli, and Candida species. However, prophylactic use of antimicrobials in patients with ALF is not associated with increased survival. The EASL and the American Association for the Study of Liver Diseases (AASLD) recommend that all patients should have routine urine, sputum, and blood cultures, as well as chest radiographs to detect bacterial or fungal infections (including those without signs of infection) [36]. Based on current guidelines, broad-spectrum antibiotics should be administered in patients with ALF who have evidence of systemic inflammatory response syndrome (SIRS), unexplained progression to higher grades of HE, and refractory hypotension without an identified source of infection [36]. The initial antibiotic regimen should target enteric gram-negatives and anaerobes with addition of vancomycin in patients with increased risk of MRSA infection (i.e., catheter-related blood stream infections or known colonization). Fungal infections are frequently encountered but diagnosis and management are often delayed [45]; hence, a low threshold for initiating antifungal coverage for patients who are at increased risk for fungal infection is advised.

Acute-on-Chronic Liver Failure

ACLF is a recently recognized and defined clinical syndrome encompassing an acute deterioration of liver function in patients with chronic liver disease, which is usually associated with a precipitating event and results in the failure of one or more extrahepatic organs and high short-term mortality [46, 47]. Alcohol and chronic viral hepatitis are the most common underlying causes of chronic liver disease. Although up to 50% of the cases of ACLF have no identifiable trigger; in the remaining patients, sepsis, active alcoholism, and relapse of chronic viral hepatitis are the most common reported precipitating factors. Table 17.6 describes the ACLF-grading system.

An excessive systemic inflammatory response seems to play a crucial role in the development of ACLF. Elevated levels of multiple pro- and anti-inflammatory cytokines (TNF-α, sTNF-αR1, sTNF-αR2, IL-2, IL-2R, IL-6, IL-8, IL-10, and IFN-ϒ) have been described in ACLF [47]. Infection is a common feature of ACLF, which complicates the natural history and is associated with significant morbidity and mortality. Genetic predisposition may underlie the risk of infection in cirrhotic patients. A recent study focused on Toll-like receptor (TLR) 2 and nucleotide-binding oligomerization domain (NOD) 2 which recognize pathogen-associated molecular patterns. Investigators confirmed that TLR2 GT microsatellite polymorphism and NOD2 variants were independent predictors of spontaneous bacterial peritonitis (SBP) when both risk factors were present the risk of SBP was dramatically increased (OR: 11.3; $p = 0.00002$) [48].

Using a liver-adapted sequential organ assessment failure score, it is possible to triage and prognosticate the outcome of patients with ACLF. The course of ACLF is dynamic and changes over the course of hospital admission. Most of the patients will have a clear prognosis between day 3 and 7 of hospital admission and clinical decisions such as evaluation for LT or discussion over goals of care could be tailored using clinical scores. Bioartificial liver support systems, granulocyte-colony stimulating factors (G-CSF), or stem-cell transplant are in the horizon of medical care of this patient population; however, data are too premature to implement them as standard of care.

A large prospective observational European study, called the "European Association for the Study of the Liver (EASL)—Chronic Liver Failure (CLIF) Consortium Acute-on-Chronic Liver Failure in Cirrhosis (CANONIC)" study is the most comprehensive registry to understand outcomes on hospitalized patients with cirrhosis [49]. Jalan et al. developed and independently validated a scoring system based on the CANONIC study population that showed significantly higher prognostic accuracy than conventional measures (MELD, MELD-Na and Child-Pugh-Turcotte scores) after ACLF diagnosis [50]. This is the so-called CLIF-C ACLF score (Table 17.7).

There is no specific effective treatment available for ACLF, and therefore treatment is based on organ support and treatment of associated complications. When ACLF is associated with a precipitating factor (i.e., bacterial infections, GI bleeding, alcoholism, drug toxicity), early identification and treatment of the precipitating factor are essential. Ideally, patients with ACLF should be admitted to the ICU and preferably managed in a transplant center. General management should be based on current guidelines on the management of critically ill patients with cirrhosis. LT represents the definitive treatment for patients with ACLF [46].

Innovative therapies based on immunomodulatory or liver regenerative effects (including administration of G-CSF and stem cell transplantation) have been proposed as therapeutic approaches in ACLF. A randomized control trial (RCT) conducted by Garg et al. included 47 patients with ACLF (defined by the APASL criteria); 23 patients were treated with G-CSF and 24 were treated with placebo. The investigators reported improvement in 60-day survival in the G-CSF group vs. placebo (66% vs. 26%, respectively; $p = 0.001$) along with a reduction in Child-Pugh, SOFA, and MELD scores and a decrease in the occurrence of hepatorenal syndrome, HE, and sepsis in G-CSF treated patients. Although these results are promising, the evidence is still very preliminary, and no recommendations can be made regarding their potential use in clinical practice [51].

Extracorporeal liver support systems, particularly albumin dialysis and/or plasma exchange, have been proposed as new therapeutic options that could be used as a bridge to LT in patients with ACLF. The most studied liver support devices include molecular adsorbent recirculating system (MARS) and fractionated plasma separation and absorption (FPSA) system, which are based on the principles of albumin dialysis. These systems remove albumin-bound substances and other substances that accumulate in the context of ACLF and may have deleterious effects on the function of different organs. A multicenter European RCT known as the RELIEF trial, failed to demonstrate differences in 28- and 90-day transplant-free survival between MARS and standard medical therapy in patients with ACLF [52]. Another European RCT showed that the use of FPSA in patients with ACLF

Table 17.6 Acute-on-chronic liver failure (ACLF) grading system

ACLF Grade	Characteristics Acute liver failure associated with:
Grade I	Single organ failure (kidney, liver, circulatory, respiratory) in patients with serum creatinine 1.5–1.9 mg/dL and/or HE grade 1–2 OR Brain failure with serum creatinine 1.5–1.9 mg/dL
Grade II	Two organ failures
Grade III	Three or more organ failures

Abbreviations: ACLF acute-on-chronic liver failure, *HE* hepatic encephalopathy

Table 17.7 CLIF consortium organ failure score and the CLIF-C ACLF Score

Organ system	Variable	Score = 1	Score = 2	Score = 3
CLIF Consortium Organ Failure Score (CLIF-C OF)				
Liver	Bilirubin (mg/dL)	<6	6 to <12	≥12
Kidney	Creatinine (md/dL)	<2	2 to <3.5	≥3.5 or RRT
Brain	Encephalopathy grade (west-haven)	0	1–2	3–4
Coagulation	INR	<2	2 to <2.5	≥2.5
Circulation	MAP (mmHg)	≥70	<70	Vasopressors
Respiratory	PaO_2/FiO_2 or SpO_2/FiO_2	>300 >357	≤300 and > 200 >200 and ≤ 357	≤ 200 ≤ 214

CLIF-C ACLF score
CLIF-C ACLF score = 10 × [0.33 × CLIF organ failure score + 0.04 × age, years + 0.63 × ln(WBC count, 10^9 cells/L) − 2]

Abbreviations: CLIF chronic liver failure, *ACLF* acute-on-chronic liver failure, *FiO_2* fraction of inspired oxygen, *INR* international normalized ratio, *MAP* mean arterial pressure, *PaO_2* partial pressure of arterial oxygen, *RRT* renal replacement therapy, *SOFA* sequential organ failure assessment, *SpO_2* pulse oximetry saturation was safe and well tolerated but did not increase the probability of survival at 28 days [53]. The usefulness of these devices, particularly in patients with ACLF, is difficult to assess due to the heterogeneity of patient populations, definitions, and modalities. Therefore, further studies with a homogenous definition of the syndrome are needed to reach a level sufficient to gain approval for widespread use.

Decompensated Cirrhosis

Cirrhosis is a pathological diagnosis characterized by diffuse fibrosis, severe disruption of the intrahepatic arterial and venous flow, portal hypertension and, ultimately, liver failure. These architectural changes are associated with life-threatening complications related to portal hypertension and/or hepatic dysfunction that may require ICU hospitalization. Historically, it has been subdivided into compensated and decompensated disease. The transition to decompensated cirrhosis happens when any of the following hallmarks are present: ascites, variceal hemorrhage, HE, and/or hepatocellular carcinoma. Once decompensation has occurred, cirrhosis becomes a systemic disease, with multi-organ/system dysfunction. The clinical manifestations of decompensated cirrhosis are a consequence of hemodynamic disturbances with splanchnic vasoconstriction, as well as cirrhosis-associated immune dysfunction, which often lead to renal dysfunction and bacterial infections. In addition, given the prevalence of this disease, it is frequent that the reason for initial ICU admission is not a complication of cirrhosis but rather another condition likely to lead to organ failure such as pneumonia-related septic shock, community-acquired peritonitis, stroke, trauma, etc. [51].

Patient with cirrhosis have increased levels of pro-inflammatory cytokines and chemokines, likely caused by systemic spread of bacteria and bacterial products (e.g., PAMPs) after abnormal bacterial translocation. Danger associated molecular patterns (DAMPs) are released by the diseased liver because of local inflammation and cell apoptosis and necrosis. Both, PAMPs and DAMPs lead to release of pro-inflammatory molecules, reactive oxygen and nitrogen species that contribute to the development of circulatory dysfunction and failure [54]. As described previously, the ratio of AST to ALT may be useful in determining the etiology of abnormal liver chemistries. ALT levels are higher than AST levels in most liver conditions including chronic viral hepatitis and MAFLD. While most patients with alcoholic liver disease have AST > ALT, this pattern can also be seen in patients with cirrhosis of any etiology, although the AST:ALT ratio is typically not >2:1. In one study examining HCV patients, non-cirrhotics had an AST/ALT ratio of 0.60, while the mean ratio in cirrhotics was 1.05 [55].

The in-hospital mortality rate in cirrhotic patients requiring ICU hospitalization is typically high (ranging from 30% to 50%). The severity of cirrhosis was initially established by the Child–Turcotte score and subsequently modified by Pugh. ACLF can occur in patients with or without a prior history of acute decompensation. The diagnosis of ACLF and its classification (four grades of severity based on the number of organs failing) was made using the CLIF SOFA score. It is important to highlight that an ACLF grading system based on organ failure has been shown to better predict the outcomes of ICU cirrhotic patients than the standard prognostic methods (i.e., MELD or Child–Pugh scores) [56].

The major goals of managing patients with cirrhosis include slowing or reversing the progression of liver disease, preventing superimposed insults to the liver, as well as preventing, identifying, and treating the complications of cirrhosis [57]. HE is a brain dysfunction caused by liver insufficiency and/or portosystemic shunting that describes a wide spectrum of potentially reversible neuropsychiatric abnormalities ranging from subclinical alterations and coma. HE is a frequent complication and one of the most debilitating manifestations or liver disease. The prevalence of overt HE is 16–21% in patients with decompensated cirrhosis [58, 59]. Diagnosis of overt HE is based on a clinical examination and a clinical decision. The West Haven Criteria is the gold standard clinical scale to analyze the severity of HE. Patients with Grade 1 HE typically will exhibit inattention, euphoria, anxiety, altered sleep pattern, and decreased attention span. Those with Grade 2 HE have lethargy, behavior and/or personality changes, disorientation, asterixis, and hypoactive deep tendon reflexes (DTRs). Grade 3 HE is characterized by varying degrees of somnolence to semistupor (but responsive to stimuli), asterixis, disorientation, and hyperactive DTRs. And finally, coma in Grade 4 HE [57].

Management of HE includes addressing any predisposing conditions (e.g., infection or gastrointestinal bleeding). Most drugs have not been tested by rigorous RCTs and are utilized based on circumstantial observations. These agents include nonabsorbable disaccharides (e.g., lactulose) and antibiotics such as rifaximin. Lactulose should be titrated to maintain two to three bowel movements per day. Overuse of lactulose leads to several complications, such as aspiration, dehydration, hypernatremia, and may also precipitate HE. Rifaximin has been shown to be equivalent or superior to placebo, other antibiotics, and disaccharides for the management of HE [60].

A diagnostic paracentesis is recommended in all patients with new onset of clinically evident ascites, or in hospitalized patients with any complication of cirrhosis [51]. A neutrophil count above 250 cells/μl is required to diagnose SBP. Third generation cephalosporins are recommended as first-line antibiotic treatment for community-acquired SBP. The serum-ascites albumin gradient (SAAG) should be calculated when the cause of ascites is not immediately evident, and/or when conditions other than cirrhosis are suspected, as a SAAG ≥1.1 g/dL indicates that portal hypertension is involved in ascites formation with an accuracy of 97%. Cytology should also be performed to differentiate from malignancy-related ascites. Large volume paracentesis (> 5 L) should be followed by plasma volume expansion with albumin to decrease risk of circulatory dysfunction. An anti-mineralocorticoid drug alone should be started in patients with the first episode of moderate grade ascites. Furosemide should be added in patients who do not respond to anti-mineralocorticoids, or in those who develop hyperkalemia. Patients with long-standing or recurrent ascites should be treated with a combination of furosemide and anti-mineralocorticoids. Once ascites has largely resolved, the dose of diuretics should be reduced to the lowest effective dose. Transjugular intrahepatic portosystemic shunt (TIPS) insertion is recommended in patients with recurrent ascites as it improves survival [51].

Upper gastrointestinal (GI) bleeding events in patients with portal hypertension remains one of the most severe and immediate life-threatening complications in patients with cirrhosis and constitutes the second most frequent event that leads to decompensated disease [61, 62]. In acute GI bleeding, volume replacement should be initiated promptly to restore and maintain hemodynamic stability. A restrictive transfusion strategy is recommended in most patients with a hemoglobin threshold for transfusion of 7 g/dL and a target range of 7–9 g/dL [63]. Antibiotic prophylaxis is recommended in cirrhotic patients with acute GI bleeding because it reduces the incidence of infections and improves control of bleeding and survival. Treatment should be initiated on presentation of bleeding and continued for up to 7 days. Ceftriaxone is the first choice in patients with decompensated cirrhosis. Vasoactive drug therapy (terlipressin or octreotide) should be initiated as soon as acute variceal bleeding is suspected, and before endoscopy. Gastroscopy should be performed within the first 12 h after admission once hemodynamic stability has been achieved, to ascertain the cause of hemorrhage and to provide endoscopic therapy. Balloon tamponade should be placed by a specialist in case of uncontrolled bleeding, as a temporary "bridge" until definitive treatment can be instituted and for a maximum of 24 h [64].

Patients with decompensated cirrhosis should have esophagogastroduodenoscopy (EGD) performed to screen for gastroesophageal varices if hemodynamically stable, unless previously diagnosed and treated. If the state of decompensation continues, screening EGD should be repeated every year. The AASLD guidelines primarily recommend nonselective betablockers (NSBBs) for primary prophylaxis of variceal hemorrhage (VH) in patients with cirrhosis who have high-risk varices and combined with endoscopic band ligation (EBL), for secondary prophylaxis of VH. However, beta-blockers and vasodilators should be avoided during the acute bleeding episode [51, 64].

Drug-Induced Liver Injury

DILI can occur due to direct hepatotoxicity or due to idiosyncratic or immune-mediated toxicity. The risk of DILI in critically ill patients is significantly increased because of polypharmacy, and due to potential drug–drug interactions. DILI can present with mild asymptomatic elevation in liver chemistries to profound hepatocellular or cholestatic pattern of injury resulting in jaundice and/or liver failure [65]. Nearly all medications are associated with at least a small risk of elevation of transaminases, ALP, or bilirubin with or without hepatotoxicity. Two primary mechanisms are responsible for DILI: 1) intrinsic, which refers to drugs that can cause liver injury when given in sufficiently high doses (reaction stereotypic and dose-dependent) and 2) idiosyncratic reactions, which affects only susceptible individuals, is less consistently related to dose and is more varied in its presentation.

Acetaminophen is the best-known drug to cause intrinsic DILI. Chronic DILI occurs when liver enzymes or bilirubin fail to return to a pre-DILI baseline after 6–9 months of DILI onset, and/or there are signs and symptoms of ongoing liver disease. Several mechanisms may initiate or contribute to drug-induced hepatotoxicity: phase one reactions (cytochrome p450) result in the production of highly reactive oxygen species (ROS) that often are more cytotoxic to liver than the pre-metabolized drug. In phase two reactions, depletion of glucuronide, sulfate, and glutathione can result in hepatocyte necrosis [18]. Other cellular mechanisms of drug-induced hepatotoxicity include 1) disruption of cell membranes, 2) inhibition of cellular pathways of drug metabolism, 3) abnormal bile flow resulting from disruption of subcellular actin filaments or interruption of transport pumps leading to cholestasis or jaundice, and 4) inhibition of mitochondrial function with accumulation of ROS and lipid peroxidation, fat accumulation, and cell death [66].

Common drug classes that may cause DILI are antibiotics and antiepileptics, accounting for more than half of all DILI. Other medications include nonsteroidal anti-inflammatory agents (NSAIDs), anti-retroviral treatment for HIV, biologic agents (e.g., anti-tumor necrosis factor drugs), and chemotherapeutic agents. Although statins have been associated with elevated liver chemistries, there is an extensive literature on the safety in those with chronic liver disease with only rare cases of hepatotoxicity reported. DILI remains a diagnosis of exclusion based primarily on a detailed history and use of laboratory tests, imaging, and liver biopsy. Physicians should also consider non-prescribed complimentary alternative medicines (CAM's) or herbal supplements (e.g., chaparral, ephedra, germander, green tea extract, and shark cartilage) as potential etiologies of hepatotoxicity. Illicit drugs such as methylenedioxymethamphetamine have been linked to liver injury, and in some instances ALF [67]. Readers may also refer to *LiverTox*, a free online resource produced by the National Institute of Diabetes and Digestive and Kidney Diseases and the National Library of Medicine consisting of helpful detailed information on more than 1200 agents (http://livertox.nih.gov).

Frequently prescribed medications in the ICU that may potentially lead to DILI are described in Table 17.8. Based on the R-value at presentation, DILI may be categorized into hepatocellular, cholestatic, or mixed types. Antibiotics such as macrolides, isoniazid, minocycline, nitrofurantoin, and rifampicin may lead to liver injury evidenced in a hepatocellular pattern. Some antivirals like acyclovir and valacyclovir, or antifungals (e.g., ketoconazole) are also associated with this pattern of injury. Amoxicillin and trimethoprim/sulfamethoxazole usually cause cholestatic injury but can also present with a hepatocellular pattern. Common antiepileptics like valproate and lamotrigine cause hepatocellular injury, whereas phenytoin and carbamazepine have variable patterns (i.e., hepatocellular, mixed or cholestatic). Acetaminophen and NSAIDs (e.g., diclofenac) are associated with a hepatocellular pattern. Azathioprine can cause cholestatic or hepatocellular injury but can present with portal hypertension (veno-occlusive disease and nodular regenerative hyperplasia).

Table 17.8 Frequently prescribed medications in the ICU that may potentially cause DILI[a]

Drugs	Pattern
Antiinfectious agents	
Ketoconazole	Hepatocellular
Isoniazid	Hepatocellular
Minocycline	Hepatocellular
Nitrofurantoin	Hepatocellular
Rifampicin	Hepatocellular
Acyclovir/Valacyclovir	Hepatocellular
Amoxicillin or clavulanate	Cholestasis > hepatocellular
Trimethoprim/	Cholestasis > hepatocellular
sulfamethoxazole	Cholestasis
Ceftriaxone	Hepatocellular > cholestasis
Macrolides	Mixed
Clindamycin	Hepatocellular, mixed or
Fluoroquinolones	Cholestatic
Antiepileptics	
Valproic acid	Hepatocellular
Lamotrigine	Hepatocellular
Phenytoin	Hepatocellular, mixed or
Carbamazepine	Cholestatic
Phenobarbital	Hepatocellular, mixed or
	Cholestatic
	Mixed
Analgesics	
Acetaminophen	Hepatocellular
Diclofenac	Hepatocellular
Immune modulators	
Interferon-beta	Hepatocellular
Interferon-alpha	Hepatocellular
Anti-TNF agents	Hepatocellular
Azathioprine	Cholestatic or hepatocellular
Others	
Amiodarone	Hepatocellular, mixed or
Statins	Cholestatic
Propofol	Hepatocellular
Proton pump inhibitors	Hepatocellular
Heparins	Hepatocellular
Rivaroxaban	Hepatocellular
Allopurinol	Mixed
Androgen-containing	Hepatocellular or mixed
steroids	Cholestatic

Abbreviations: ICU intensive care unit, *DILI* drug-induced liver injury

[a] Adapted from Lescot T, et al. [18], Horvatits T. et al. [4], and Chalasani et al. [65]

In those patients with high ALT levels (>1000 IU/l), an accurate history of acetaminophen use (single or in combination with analgesic-narcotics) is essential. Individuals with suspected hepatocellular or mixed DILI should undergo serologic testing to exclude viral hepatitis (A, B, and C) and AIH. Anti-HEV may be considered in selected patients with risk factors (recent travel, etc.). If classical viral hepatitis has been excluded or clinical features (i.e., atypical lymphocytosis or lymphadenopathy) suggest other causes, patients should also be tested for EBV, CMV, and HSV. In those individuals with cholestatic DILI, abdominal imaging (ultrasound, CT scan, MRI) should be performed to exclude biliary tract pathology or infiltrative processes. Endoscopic retrograde cholangiography (ERCP) should be limited to instances where routine imaging or endoscopic ultrasound is unable to exclude impacted common bile duct stones, PSC, or pancreaticobiliary malignancy. Liver biopsy should be considered if: (1) AIH is suspected and immunosuppressive therapy is being contemplated, (2) unrelenting rise in liver chemistries or worsening liver function despite stopping the offending drug, (3) peak ALT has not fallen >50% in 30–60 days after DILI onset or peak ALP has not fallen by >50% at 180 days despite stopping the offending drug, (4) re-exposure to the implicated agent is contemplated, or (5) liver chemistries abnormalities persist beyond 180 days [65]. Table 17.9 describes other common indications for liver biopsy [68, 69].

Attributing liver injury to a specific agent is complicated and frequently requires empiric trials of drug discontinuation to observe full recovery of liver chemistries. In cases in which the suspected agent is medically required, efforts should be made to identify potential drug alternatives and to establish a surveillance plan to monitor for progressive liver injury or failure. Currently, there is no approved antidote for ALF due to idiosyncratic DILI. Antihistamines (e.g., diphenhydramine and hydroxyzine) may be used for symptomatic pruritus.

Table 17.9 Indications and contraindications to liver biopsy[a]

Indications for liver biopsy	
Abnormal liver chemistries and hepatomegaly of unknown etiology	
Evaluation and staging of chronic hepatitis	
Identification and staging of alcoholic liver disease	
Recognition of systemic inflammatory or granulomatous disorders	
Evaluation of the pattern and extent of DILI	
Focal or diffuse abnormalities on imaging studies	
Diagnosis of multisystemic infiltrative disorders	
Evaluation and staging of cholestatic liver disease (PBC, PSC)	
Screening of relatives of patients with familial diseases	
Obtaining tissue to culture infectious agents (e.g., mycobacteria)	
Evaluation of effectiveness of therapies for liver diseases (e.g., Wilson disease, hemochromatosis, autoimmune hepatitis, chronic viral hepatitis	
Evaluation of liver biochemical test abnormalities following transplantation	
Contraindications to liver biopsy	
Absolute	*Relative*
History of unexplained bleeding	Ascites
Severe coagulopathy	Infection in right pleural cavity
Platelets <60,000/mm^3	Hydatid disease
Unavailability of blood transfusion support	Morbid obesity
Infection of hepatic bed	Possible vascular lesions
Suspected hemangioma	Amyloidosis
Uncooperative patient	
Extrahepatic biliary obstruction	

Abbreviations: DILI drug-induced liver injury, *PBC* primary biliary cirrhosis, *PSC* primary sclerosing cholangitis, *PT* prothrombin time
[a] Adapted from Friedman LS and Rockey DC [68, 69]

Although no definitive therapies are available either for idiosyncratic DILI with or without ALF, the American College of Gastroenterology recent guidelines suggest consideration of NAC treatment in adults with early stage ALF, given its good safety profile and some evidence for efficacy in early coma stage patients. While a limited number of retrospective studies have suggested that steroid therapy may be associated with improvement, there have been no randomized controlled trials to evaluate their efficacy and safety. Steroids should only be considered in a subset of patients with DILI exhibiting AIH-like features [65].

Prognosis is generally dependent on the type of DILI with most patients experiencing complete recovery once the offending medication is discontinued or the dosage is decreased. Acute liver failure may occur in ~10% of patients with idiosyncratic DILI and fewer than 20% will develop chronic liver injury [70, 71]. However, DILI that results in ALF carries a poor prognosis with 40% of patients requiring LT. Prognostic scores may identify individuals at risk of death from DILI by incorporating clinical and laboratory data, including the one developed and validated by Ghabril et al. [72]. This model accurately predicts six-month mortality in individuals presenting with suspected DILI by incorporating MELD, Charlson comorbidity index, and serum albumin.

Secondary Sclerosing Cholangitis in Critically Ill Patients

Secondary sclerosing cholangitis in critically ill patients (SC-CIP) is a recently identified cholestatic liver disease occurring in patients with no previous history of hepatobiliary disease. It is a rare entity that was first described by Scheppach et al. in 2001 [73] with an estimated frequency of 1 in 2000 ICU admissions [74]. However, the prognosis is dire with a high mortality in the ICU and many surviving patients eventually requiring LT [74]. The pathogenesis of SC-CIP is not fully understood, but the main pathogenic mechanisms seem to be ischemic cholangiopathy, changes in bile composition, and biliary infection. Several drugs commonly used in the ICU setting have been implicated in drug-induced secondary sclerosing cholangitis, including antibiotics and anesthetics such as ketamine [75, 76].

The differential diagnosis for SC-CIP is extensive, most notably sepsis-induced cholestasis, total parenteral nutrition-associated cholestasis, hypoxic hepatitis, choledocholithiasis, and DILI [77]. SC-CIP manifests with a pattern of cholestasis. GGT increases first (7–9 days after the initial insult) and is followed by elevation in ALP a few days later. Bilirubin is the last to rise, taking ~20 days. GGT elevation is more pronounced, peaking at around 20–50 times the ULN, while ALP and bilirubin elevation reach a maximum of 15 times the ULN. Conversely, ALT and AST show only a mild increase of up to three times the ULN. Bilirubin levels may spontaneously decrease after 2–6 months while SC-CIP keeps progressing [77].

Diagnosis is established with magnetic resonance cholangiopancreatography (MRCP) or ERCP, revealing dilatations and PSC-like diffuse strictures of the intrahepatic bile ducts as well as biliary casts. No treatment has been shown to slow the rapid progression of the disease, and patients can develop liver cirrhosis over weeks to months. Endoscopic removal of biliary casts and sphincterotomy improve biliary drainage, resulting in transient clinical and biochemical improvement even when biliary cirrhosis has already occurred. Recurrent episodes of cholangitis are treated with antimicrobials and endoscopic therapy to alleviate obstruction. Liver transplant referral should be considered early after the diagnosis of SC-CIP [78].

Acute Acalculous Cholecystitis

Acute acalculous cholecystitis (AAC) is defined as an acute necroinflammatory disease of the gallbladder in the absence of gallstones. It accounts for approximately 10% of all cases of acute cholecystitis and has an incidence of ~0.4% in critically ill patients [79]. The proposed common pathophysiology among ICU patients is gallbladder ischemia from hypoperfusion and bile stasis. Hypoperfusion is often multifactorial, due to splanchnic vasoconstriction from hypotension or vasopressors, atherosclerotic vascular disease, or increased gallbladder pressure from biliary stasis. Known risk factors for AAC in the critically ill patients include shock of any kind, trauma, infections, TPN, prolonged fasting, mechanical ventilation, and opioid-induced ileus. AAC is nearly clinically indistinguishable from calculous cholecystitis. The most common findings include right upper quadrant pain, fever, leukocytosis, and abnormal liver chemistries (mild elevation in aminotransferases and alkaline phosphatase, conjugated hyperbilirubinemia). In critically ill and sedated patients the diagnosis can be challenging, and the appearance of unexplained fever may be the only sign of AAC. Because the presentation may be insidious, patients may develop sepsis, shock, and peritonitis due to complications (e.g., gangrene, perforation, and empyema) [80, 81].

Radiologic criteria for the diagnosis of AAC have been developed for the use of ultrasound (US), computerized tomography (CT), and hepatobiliary iminodiacetic acid scan (HIDA). CT scan has little benefit over US in the evaluation for AAC, however it can be employed to investigate alternative intraabdominal processes. Considerations in the critically ill patient are the difficulties in transportation and hemodynamic status, thus a bedside study like ultrasound (sensitivity ranging 30–92% and specificity 89–100%) is preferred. Accepted US criteria for AAC include gallbladder wall thickness > 3.5 mm, pericholecystic fluid, intramural gas, sloughed mucosal membrane, biliary sludge, and gallbladder hydrops (gallbladder distention >5 cm transversely or > 8 cm longitudinally). In the critical care setting, these criteria are sensitive but not specific as ICU patients without AAC may also manifest several of these findings. HIDA is a procedure that lasts from 1 to 6 h and involves the transportation of a patient to the nuclear medicine suite, hence it should only be considered in stable patients. Sensitivity of HIDA ranges from 67% to 100% and the specificity ranges from 38% to 100% [79].

Initial management includes fluid resuscitation and systemic IV antibiotics (gram-negative coverage). The two mainstays of treatment for AAC are cholecystostomy (drainage of gallbladder) and cholecystectomy. Cholecystostomy is generally plausible, rapid, and safe. It can be performed under US or CT guidance by surgeons or by interventional radiology. For uncomplicated cases of AAC with no evidence of gallbladder necrosis, emphysematous gallbladder, perforation, or empyema, percutaneous cholecystostomy is preferred for decompression and drainage. For more critically ill patients, if there is evidence of significant gallbladder ischemia or necrosis, or persistent symptoms beyond 1–2 days, surgery is needed. When neither cholecystostomy nor cholecystectomy can be performed, direct gallbladder drainage via ERCP can be attempted to assist decompression. This generally is believed to be inferior therapy and seldom performed [79, 82, 83].

COVID-19 Infection

Abnormal liver chemistries have been reported in up to one-half of patients with COVID-19, and the occurrence of liver injury is associated with a nine-fold greater risk of severe infection [84]. Several mechanisms have been proposed to explain hepatic injury during COVID-19. High levels of positive end expiratory pressure (PEEP) during mechanical ventilation can contribute to hepatic congestion by increasing right atrial pressure and impeding venous return. Hypoxia and shock in the critically affected COVID-19 patients can predispose them to hypoxic hepatitis—although the pattern of aminotransferase rise in this set of patients is not consistent with that of hypoxic hepatitis. Finally, liver damage in patients with coronavirus infections might also be caused by direct viral replication in liver cells (viral hepatitis), immune-mediated inflammation (i.e., cytokine storm, pneumonia-associated inflammation) and DILI [84–86].

Liver chemistry abnormalities induced by COVID-19 are mainly manifested as an elevation of serum aminotransferases (AST and ALT) and LDH in ~20% of mild to moderate cases and in greater than 60% of critically ill patients. Elevation in bilirubin is less commonly reported (<3%). Although ALP is normal in almost all cases, GGT levels were increased by up to 72% in severe cases of COVID-19 [86–88]. While synthetic function can be largely preserved, late cholestasis is frequently observed and may be related to the critical illness itself (i.e., inflammation), TPN, or drug toxicity [89].

Liver involvement in mild COVID-19 cases is usually transient and does not require specific treatment [87]. The AASLD recommends that all COVID-19 patients with abnormal liver functions should be screened for HCV and HBV and encourages clinicians to avoid unnecessary imaging studies. Moreover, the presence of abnormal liver biochemistries should not be a contraindication to using investigational or off-label therapeutics for COVID-19 (e.g., remdesivir, tocilizumab), although AST or ALT levels >5 times ULN may exclude patients from consideration of some investigational agents [90]. Overall, attention to modifiable factors, such as control of inflammation, timing of TPN, and avoiding drugs with worse liver toxicity profile, may be important to prevent cholestasis progression in these patients.

Conclusion

Clinicians often encounter elevated liver chemistries in the critical ill patient, and the presence of jaundice or liver failure poses additional challenge. The assessment of elevated liver chemistries is guided by the clinical presentation and the degree of elevation. A thorough history dating back to 3–6 months prior to the presentation is necessary to identify the etiology of the liver injury. History that is not usually forthcoming or forgotten or unclear from patients like short courses of antibiotics, use of herbals, CAM's/ OTC medication use, alcohol consumption, travel history, sick contacts, and other high-risk behaviors need to be elicited with specifically directed questionnaire to the patient or patient's family/ close contacts. Minimal elevation of liver enzymes can be managed conservatively without many interventions. However, higher degrees of elevation in serum transaminases should be approached with a systematic evaluation of direct and indirect liver insults. Cholestatic injury typically results in a protracted recovery compared to hepatocellular injury. If there are signs of acute liver failure, urgent hepatology consultation and referral to a liver transplant center should be undertaken. Early referral to a transplant center is paramount so as to allow time for a thorough workup and also to monitor the prognosis. Patients for LT in the acute setting can eventually be delisted if they improve significantly with prompt diagnosis and early treatment. In summary, liver dysfunction is common in critically ill patients and the management can be challenging due to the dynamic pathophysiologic alterations. The prognosis generally depends on the underlying hepatic reserve of the patient and expert management in concert with different disciplines.

References

1. Thomson SJ, Cowan ML, Johnston I, Musa S, Grounds M, Rahman TM. 'Liver function tests' on the intensive care unit: a prospective, observational study. Intensive Care Med. 2009;35(8):1406–11. https://doi.org/10.1007/s00134-009-1511-7.
2. Kwo PY, Cohen SM, Lim JK. ACG clinical guideline: evaluation of abnormal liver chemistries. Am J Gastroenterol. 2017;112(1):18–35. https://doi.org/10.1038/ajg.2016.517.
3. Trauner M, Meier PJ, Boyer JL. Molecular pathogenesis of cholestasis. N Engl J Med. 1998;339(17):1217–27. https://doi.org/10.1056/NEJM199810223391707.
4. Horvatits T, Drolz A, Trauner M, Fuhrmann V. Liver injury and failure in critical illness. Hepatology. 2019;70(6):2204–15. https://doi.org/10.1002/hep.30824.
5. Horvatits T, Drolz A, Rutter K, Roedl K, Langouche L, Van den Berghe G, et al. Circulating bile acids predict outcome in critically ill patients. Ann Intensive Care. 2017;7(1):48. https://doi.org/10.1186/s13613-017-0272-7.
6. Van den Broecke A, Van Coile L, Decruyenaere A, Colpaert K, Benoit D, Van Vlierberghe H, et al. Epidemiology, causes, evolution and outcome in a single-center cohort of 1116 critically ill patients with hypoxic hepatitis. Ann Intensive Care. 2018;8(1):15. https://doi.org/10.1186/s13613-018-0356-z.
7. Henrion J, Descamps O, Luwaert R, Schapira M, Parfonry A, Heller F. Hypoxic hepatitis in patients with cardiac failure: incidence in a coronary care unit and measurement of hepatic blood flow. J Hepatol. 1994;21(5):696–703. https://doi.org/10.1016/s0168-8278(94)80226-2.
8. Raurich JM, Perez O, Llompart-Pou JA, Ibanez J, Ayestaran I, Perez-Barcena J. Incidence and outcome of ischemic hepatitis complicating septic shock. Hepatol Res. 2009;39(7):700–5. https://doi.org/10.1111/j.1872-034X.2009.00501.x.
9. Ruhl CE, Everhart JE. Elevated serum alanine aminotransferase and gamma-glutamyltransferase and mortality in the United States population. Gastroenterology. 2009;136(2):477–85 e11. https://doi.org/10.1053/j.gastro.2008.10.052.
10. Jager B, Drolz A, Michl B, Schellongowski P, Bojic A, Nikfardjam M, et al. Jaundice increases the rate of complications and one-year mortality in patients with hypoxic hepatitis. Hepatology. 2012;56(6):2297–304. https://doi.org/10.1002/hep.25896.
11. Fuhrmann V, Kneidinger N, Herkner H, Heinz G, Nikfardjam M, Bojic A, et al. Impact of hypoxic hepatitis on mortality in the intensive care unit. Intensive Care Med. 2011;37(8):1302–10. https://doi.org/10.1007/s00134-011-2248-7.
12. Vincent JL, Lefrant JY, Kotfis K, Nanchal R, Martin-Loeches I, Wittebole X, et al. Comparison of European ICU patients in 2012 (ICON) versus 2002 (SOAP). Intensive Care Med. 2018;44(3):337–44. https://doi.org/10.1007/s00134-017-5043-2.
13. Kramer L, Jordan B, Druml W, Bauer P, Metnitz PG, Austrian Epidemiologic Study on Intensive Care ASG. Incidence and prognosis of early hepatic dysfunction in critically ill patients--a prospective multicenter study. Crit Care Med. 2007;35(4):1099–104. https://doi.org/10.1097/01.CCM.0000259462.97164.A0.
14. Karmen A, Wroblewski F, Ladue JS. Transaminase activity in human blood. J Clin Invest. 1955;34(1):126–31. https://doi.org/10.1172/JCI103055.
15. Friedman LS, Martin P. Assessment of liver function and diagnostic studies. In: Handbook of liver disease. 4th ed. Philadelphia, PA: Elsevier; 2018. p. 1–17.
16. Vroon DH, Israili Z. Alkaline phosphatase and gamma Glutamyltransferase. In: Rd WHK, Hall WD, Hurst JW, editors. Clinical methods: the history, physical, and laboratory examinations. Boston; 1990.
17. O'Shea RS, Dasarathy S, McCullough AJ. Alcoholic liver disease. Am J Gastroenterol. 2010;105(1):14–32.; quiz 3. https://doi.org/10.1038/ajg.2009.593.
18. Lescot T, Karvellas C, Beaussier M, Magder S. Acquired liver injury in the intensive care unit. Anesthesiology. 2012;117(4):898–904. https://doi.org/10.1097/ALN.0b013e318266c6df.
19. Benichou C. Criteria of drug-induced liver disorders. Report of an international consensus meeting. J Hepatol. 1990;11(2):272–6. https://doi.org/10.1016/0168-8278(90)90124-a.
20. Cohen JA, Kaplan MM. The SGOT/SGPT ratio--an indicator of alcoholic liver disease. Dig Dis Sci. 1979;24(11):835–8. https://doi.org/10.1007/BF01324898.
21. Lee WM, Stravitz RT, Larson AM. Introduction to the revised American Association for the Study of Liver Diseases position paper on acute liver failure 2011. Hepatology. 2012;55(3):965–7. https://doi.org/10.1002/hep.25551.
22. Green RM, Flamm S. AGA technical review on the evaluation of liver chemistry tests. Gastroenterology. 2002;123(4):1367–84. https://doi.org/10.1053/gast.2002.36061.

23. Kim WR, Flamm SL, Di Bisceglie AM, Bodenheimer HC. Public policy Committee of the American Association for the study of liver D. Serum activity of alanine aminotransferase (ALT) as an indicator of health and disease. Hepatology. 2008;47(4):1363–70. https://doi.org/10.1002/hep.22109.
24. Mesotten D, Wauters J, Van den Berghe G, Wouters PJ, Milants I, Wilmer A. The effect of strict blood glucose control on biliary sludge and cholestasis in critically ill patients. J Clin Endocrinol Metab. 2009;94(7):2345–52. https://doi.org/10.1210/jc.2008-2579.
25. Sun J, Zhang J, Wang X, Ji F, Ronco C, Tian J, et al. Gut-liver crosstalk in sepsis-induced liver injury. Crit Care. 2020;24(1):614. https://doi.org/10.1186/s13054-020-03327-1.
26. Keitel V, Kubitz R, Haussinger D. Endocrine and paracrine role of bile acids. World J Gastroenterol. 2008;14(37):5620–9. https://doi.org/10.3748/wjg.14.5620.
27. Deitcher SR. Interpretation of the international normalised ratio in patients with liver disease. Lancet. 2002;359(9300):47–8. https://doi.org/10.1016/S0140-6736(02)07282-3.
28. Rothschild MA, Oratz M, Schreiber SS. Serum albumin. Hepatology. 1988;8(2):385–401. https://doi.org/10.1002/hep.1840080234.
29. Dufour DR, Lott JA, Nolte FS, Gretch DR, Koff RS, Seeff LB. Diagnosis and monitoring of hepatic injury. II. Recommendations for use of laboratory tests in screening, diagnosis, and monitoring. Clin Chem. 2000;46(12):2050–68.
30. Gatselis NK, Zachou K, Koukoulis GK, Dalekos GN. Autoimmune hepatitis, one disease with many faces: etiopathogenetic, clinico-laboratory and histological characteristics. World J Gastroenterol. 2015;21(1):60–83. https://doi.org/10.3748/wjg.v21.i1.60.
31. Senzolo M, Burra P, Cholongitas E, Burroughs AK. New insights into the coagulopathy of liver disease and liver transplantation. World J Gastroenterol. 2006;12(48):7725–36. https://doi.org/10.3748/wjg.v12.i48.7725.
32. Dufour DR, Lott JA, Nolte FS, Gretch DR, Koff RS, Seeff LB. Diagnosis and monitoring of hepatic injury. I. Performance characteristics of laboratory tests. Clin Chem. 2000;46(12):2027–49.
33. Scharschmidt BF, Blanckaert N, Farina FA, Kabra PM, Stafford BE, Weisiger RA. Measurement of serum bilirubin and its mono- and diconjugates: application to patients with hepatobiliary disease. Gut. 1982;23(8):643–9. https://doi.org/10.1136/gut.23.8.643.
34. Tapper EB, Sengupta N, Bonder A. The incidence and outcomes of ischemic hepatitis: a systematic review with meta-analysis. Am J Med. 2015;128(12):1314–21. https://doi.org/10.1016/j.amjmed.2015.07.033.
35. Drolz A, Horvatits T, Michl B, Roedl K, Schellongowski P, Holzinger U, et al. Statin therapy is associated with reduced incidence of hypoxic hepatitis in critically ill patients. J Hepatol. 2014;60(6):1187–93. https://doi.org/10.1016/j.jhep.2014.01.019.
36. European Association for the Study of the Liver. Electronic address eee, Clinical practice guidelines p, Wendon J, Panel M, Cordoba J, Dhawan A, et al. EASL clinical practical guidelines on the management of acute (fulminant) liver failure. J Hepatol. 2017;66(5):1047–81. https://doi.org/10.1016/j.jhep.2016.12.003.
37. Bernal W, Hyyrylainen A, Gera A, Audimoolam VK, McPhail MJ, Auzinger G, et al. Lessons from look-back in acute liver failure? A single Centre experience of 3300 patients. J Hepatol. 2013;59(1):74–80. https://doi.org/10.1016/j.jhep.2013.02.010.
38. Bernuau J, Durand F. Intracranial pressure monitoring in patients with acute liver failure: a questionable invasive surveillance. Hepatology. 2006;44(2):502–4. https://doi.org/10.1002/hep.21243.
39. Gazzard BG, Henderson JM, Williams R. Early changes in coagulation following a paracetamol overdose and a controlled trial of fresh frozen plasma therapy. Gut. 1975;16(8):617–20. https://doi.org/10.1136/gut.16.8.617.
40. Ostapowicz G, Fontana RJ, Schiodt FV, Larson A, Davern TJ, Han SH, et al. Results of a prospective study of acute liver failure at 17 tertiary care centers in the United States. Ann Intern Med. 2002;137(12):947–54. https://doi.org/10.7326/0003-4819-137-12-200212170-00007.
41. McPhail MJ, Wendon JA, Bernal W. Meta-analysis of performance of Kings's college hospital criteria in prediction of outcome in non-paracetamol-induced acute liver failure. J Hepatol. 2010;53(3):492–9. https://doi.org/10.1016/j.jhep.2010.03.023.
42. O'Grady JG, Alexander GJ, Hayllar KM, Williams R. Early indicators of prognosis in fulminant hepatic failure. Gastroenterology. 1989;97(2):439–45. https://doi.org/10.1016/0016-5085(89)90081-4.
43. Schmidt LE, Larsen FS. MELD score as a predictor of liver failure and death in patients with acetaminophen-induced liver injury. Hepatology. 2007;45(3):789–96. https://doi.org/10.1002/hep.21503.
44. Lee WM, Hynan LS, Rossaro L, Fontana RJ, Stravitz RT, Larson AM, et al. Intravenous N-acetylcysteine improves transplant-free survival in early stage non-acetaminophen acute liver failure. Gastroenterology. 2009;137(3):856–64. ; 64 e1. https://doi.org/10.1053/j.gastro.2009.06.006.
45. Rolando N, Harvey F, Brahm J, Philpott-Howard J, Alexander G, Casewell M, et al. Fungal infection: a common, unrecognised complication of acute liver failure. J Hepatol. 1991;12(1):1–9. https://doi.org/10.1016/0168-8278(91)90900-v.
46. Hernaez R, Sola E, Moreau R, Gines P. Acute-on-chronic liver failure: an update. Gut. 2017;66(3):541–53. https://doi.org/10.1136/gutjnl-2016-312670.
47. Jalan R, Gines P, Olson JC, Mookerjee RP, Moreau R, Garcia-Tsao G, et al. Acute-on chronic liver failure. J Hepatol. 2012;57(6):1336–48. https://doi.org/10.1016/j.jhep.2012.06.026.
48. Nischalke HD, Berger C, Aldenhoff K, Thyssen L, Gentemann M, Grunhage F, et al. Toll-like receptor (TLR) 2 promoter and intron 2 polymorphisms are associated with increased risk for spontaneous bacterial peritonitis in liver cirrhosis. J Hepatol. 2011;55(5):1010–6. https://doi.org/10.1016/j.jhep.2011.02.022.
49. Moreau R, Jalan R, Gines P, Pavesi M, Angeli P, Cordoba J, et al. Acute-on-chronic liver failure is a distinct syndrome that develops in patients with acute decompensation of cirrhosis. Gastroenterology. 2013;144(7):1426–37; 37 e1–9. https://doi.org/10.1053/j.gastro.2013.02.042.
50. Jalan R, Saliba F, Pavesi M, Amoros A, Moreau R, Gines P, et al. Development and validation of a prognostic score to predict mortality in patients with acute-on-chronic liver failure. J Hepatol. 2014;61(5):1038–47. https://doi.org/10.1016/j.jhep.2014.06.012.
51. European Association for the Study of the liver. Electronic address eee, European Association for the Study of the L. EASL clinical practice guidelines for the management of patients with decompensated cirrhosis. J Hepatol. 2018;69(2):406–60. https://doi.org/10.1016/j.jhep.2018.03.024.
52. Banares R, Nevens F, Larsen FS, Jalan R, Albillos A, Dollinger M, et al. Extracorporeal albumin dialysis with the molecular adsorbent recirculating system in acute-on-chronic liver failure: the RELIEF trial. Hepatology. 2013;57(3):1153–62. https://doi.org/10.1002/hep.26185.
53. Kribben A, Gerken G, Haag S, Herget-Rosenthal S, Treichel U, Betz C, et al. Effects of fractionated plasma separation and adsorption on survival in patients with acute-on-chronic liver failure. Gastroenterology. 2012;142(4):782–9 e3. https://doi.org/10.1053/j.gastro.2011.12.056.
54. Bernardi M, Moreau R, Angeli P, Schnabl B, Arroyo V. Mechanisms of decompensation and organ failure in cirrhosis: from peripheral arterial vasodilation to systemic inflammation hypothesis. J Hepatol. 2015;63(5):1272–84. https://doi.org/10.1016/j.jhep.2015.07.004.
55. Sheth SG, Flamm SL, Gordon FD, Chopra S. AST/ALT ratio predicts cirrhosis in patients with chronic hepatitis C virus infection. Am J Gastroenterol. 1998;93(1):44–8. https://doi.org/10.1111/j.1572-0241.1998.044_c.x.

56. Paugam-Burtz C, Levesque E, Louvet A, Thabut D, Amathieu R, Bureau C, et al. Management of liver failure in general intensive care unit. Anaesth Crit Care Pain Med. 2020;39(1):143–61. https://doi.org/10.1016/j.accpm.2019.06.014.
57. Vilstrup H, Amodio P, Bajaj J, Cordoba J, Ferenci P, Mullen KD, et al. Hepatic encephalopathy in chronic liver disease: 2014 practice guideline by the American Association for the Study of Liver Diseases and the European Association for the Study of the liver. Hepatology. 2014;60(2):715–35. https://doi.org/10.1002/hep.27210.
58. D'Amico G, Morabito A, Pagliaro L, Marubini E. Survival and prognostic indicators in compensated and decompensated cirrhosis. Dig Dis Sci. 1986;31(5):468–75. https://doi.org/10.1007/BF01320309.
59. Coltorti M, Del Vecchio-Blanco C, Caporaso N, Gallo C, Castellano L. Liver cirrhosis in Italy. A multicentre study on presenting modalities and the impact on health care resources. National Project on liver cirrhosis group. Ital J Gastroenterol. 1991;23(1):42–8.
60. Lawrence KR, Klee JA. Rifaximin for the treatment of hepatic encephalopathy. Pharmacotherapy. 2008;28(8):1019–32. https://doi.org/10.1592/phco.28.8.1019.
61. D'Amico G, De Franchis R, Cooperative Study G. Upper digestive bleeding in cirrhosis. Post-therapeutic outcome and prognostic indicators. Hepatology. 2003;38(3):599–612. https://doi.org/10.1053/jhep.2003.50385.
62. Jepsen P, Ott P, Andersen PK, Sorensen HT, Vilstrup H. Clinical course of alcoholic liver cirrhosis: a Danish population-based cohort study. Hepatology. 2010;51(5):1675–82. https://doi.org/10.1002/hep.23500.
63. Villanueva C, Colomo A, Bosch A, Concepcion M, Hernandez-Gea V, Aracil C, et al. Transfusion strategies for acute upper gastrointestinal bleeding. N Engl J Med. 2013;368(1):11–21. https://doi.org/10.1056/NEJMoa1211801.
64. Garcia-Tsao G, Sanyal AJ, Grace ND, Carey W. Practice guidelines Committee of the American Association for the study of liver D, practice parameters Committee of the American College of G. Prevention and management of gastroesophageal varices and variceal hemorrhage in cirrhosis. Hepatology. 2007;46(3):922–38. https://doi.org/10.1002/hep.21907.
65. Chalasani NP, Maddur H, Russo MW, Wong RJ, Reddy KR. Practice parameters Committee of the American College of G. ACG clinical guideline: diagnosis and Management of Idiosyncratic Drug-Induced Liver Injury. Am J Gastroenterol. 2021;116(5):878–98. https://doi.org/10.14309/ajg.0000000000001259.
66. Navarro VJ, Senior JR. Drug-related hepatotoxicity. N Engl J Med. 2006;354(7):731–9. https://doi.org/10.1056/NEJMra052270.
67. Cajanding RJM. MDMA-associated liver toxicity: pathophysiology, management, and current state of knowledge. AACN Adv Crit Care. 2019;30(3):232–48. https://doi.org/10.4037/aacnacc2019852.
68. Friedman LS. Controversies in liver biopsy: who, where, when, how, why? Curr Gastroenterol Rep. 2004;6(1):30–6. https://doi.org/10.1007/s11894-004-0023-4.
69. Rockey DC, Caldwell SH, Goodman ZD, Nelson RC, Smith AD. American Association for the Study of liver D. Liver biopsy Hepatology. 2009;49(3):1017–44. https://doi.org/10.1002/hep.22742.
70. Temple R. Hy's law: predicting serious hepatotoxicity. Pharmacoepidemiol Drug Saf. 2006;15(4):241–3. https://doi.org/10.1002/pds.1211.
71. Chalasani N, Bonkovsky HL, Fontana R, Lee W, Stolz A, Talwalkar J, et al. Features and outcomes of 899 patients with drug-induced liver injury: the DILIN prospective study. Gastroenterology. 2015;148(7):1340–52 e7. https://doi.org/10.1053/j.gastro.2015.03.006.
72. Ghabril M, Gu J, Yoder L, Corbito L, Ringel A, Beyer CD, et al. Development and validation of a model consisting of comorbidity burden to calculate risk of death within 6 months for patients with suspected drug-induced liver injury. Gastroenterology. 2019;157(5):1245–52 e3. https://doi.org/10.1053/j.gastro.2019.07.006.
73. Scheppach W, Druge G, Wittenberg G, Mueller JG, Gassel AM, Gassel HJ, et al. Sclerosing cholangitis and liver cirrhosis after extrabiliary infections: report on three cases. Crit Care Med. 2001;29(2):438–41. https://doi.org/10.1097/00003246-200102000-00042.
74. Leonhardt S, Veltzke-Schlieker W, Adler A, Schott E, Hetzer R, Schaffartzik W, et al. Trigger mechanisms of secondary sclerosing cholangitis in critically ill patients. Crit Care. 2015;19:131. https://doi.org/10.1186/s13054-015-0861-5.
75. Turkish A, Luo JJ, Lefkowitch JH. Ketamine abuse, biliary tract disease, and secondary sclerosing cholangitis. Hepatology. 2013;58(2):825–7. https://doi.org/10.1002/hep.26459.
76. Gudnason HO, Bjornsson HK, Gardarsdottir M, Thorisson HM, Olafsson S, Bergmann OM, et al. Secondary sclerosing cholangitis in patients with drug-induced liver injury. Dig Liver Dis. 2015;47(6):502–7. https://doi.org/10.1016/j.dld.2015.03.002.
77. Martins P, Verdelho MM. Secondary Sclerosing cholangitis in critically ill patients: an underdiagnosed entity. GE Port J Gastroenterol. 2020;27(2):103–14. https://doi.org/10.1159/000501405.
78. Voigtlander T, Jaeckel E, Lehner F, Manns MP, Lankisch TO. Liver transplantation for critically ill patients with secondary sclerosing cholangitis: outcome and complications. Liver Transpl. 2015;21(10):1295–9. https://doi.org/10.1002/lt.24192.
79. Huffman JL, Schenker S. Acute acalculous cholecystitis: a review. Clin Gastroenterol Hepatol. 2010;8(1):15–22. https://doi.org/10.1016/j.cgh.2009.08.034.
80. Barie PS, Eachempati SR. Acute acalculous cholecystitis. Curr Gastroenterol Rep. 2003;5(4):302–9. https://doi.org/10.1007/s11894-003-0067-x.
81. McChesney JA, Northup PG, Bickston SJ. Acute acalculous cholecystitis associated with systemic sepsis and visceral arterial hypoperfusion: a case series and review of pathophysiology. Dig Dis Sci. 2003;48(10):1960–7. https://doi.org/10.1023/a:1026118320460.
82. Kjaer DW, Kruse A, Funch-Jensen P. Endoscopic gallbladder drainage of patients with acute cholecystitis. Endoscopy. 2007;39(4):304–8. https://doi.org/10.1055/s-2007-966335.
83. Owen CC, Jain R. Acute Acalculous Cholecystitis. Curr Treat Options Gastroenterol. 2005;8(2):99–104. https://doi.org/10.1007/s11938-005-0001-4.
84. Cai Q, Huang D, Yu H, Zhu Z, Xia Z, Su Y, et al. COVID-19: abnormal liver function tests. J Hepatol. 2020;73(3):566–74. https://doi.org/10.1016/j.jhep.2020.04.006.
85. Chau TN, Lee KC, Yao H, Tsang TY, Chow TC, Yeung YC, et al. SARS-associated viral hepatitis caused by a novel coronavirus: report of three cases. Hepatology. 2004;39(2):302–10. https://doi.org/10.1002/hep.20111.
86. Metawea MI, Yousif WI, Moheb I. COVID 19 and liver: an A-Z literature review. Dig Liver Dis. 2021;53(2):146–52. https://doi.org/10.1016/j.dld.2020.09.010.
87. Zhang C, Shi L, Wang FS. Liver injury in COVID-19: management and challenges. Lancet Gastroenterol Hepatol. 2020;5(5):428–30. https://doi.org/10.1016/S2468-1253(20)30057-1.
88. Huang C, Wang Y, Li X, Ren L, Zhao J, Hu Y, et al. Clinical features of patients infected with 2019 novel coronavirus in Wuhan, China. Lancet. 2020;395(10223):497–506. https://doi.org/10.1016/S0140-6736(20)30183-5.
89. Cardoso FS, Pereira R, Germano N. Liver injury in critically ill patients with COVID-19: a case series. Crit Care. 2020;24(1):190. https://doi.org/10.1186/s13054-020-02924-4.
90. Fix OK, Hameed B, Fontana RJ, Kwok RM, McGuire BM, Mulligan DC, et al. Clinical best practice advice for Hepatology and liver transplant providers during the COVID-19 pandemic: AASLD expert panel consensus statement. Hepatology. 2020;72(1):287–304. https://doi.org/10.1002/hep.31281.

Gastrointestinal Emergencies

18

Andreas Zori, Brett Styskel, and Nanlong Liu

Contents

Abstract

Patients with critical neurologic injuries are at increased risk for potentially life-threatening gastrointestinal and hepatobiliary conditions. Neurointensivists must recognize and be familiar with these conditions to ensure early and proper interventions in order to reduce complications. The most common and most severe of these conditions including gastrointestinal hemorrhage, intestinal ischemia, acute ascending cholangitis, and acute liver failure are discussed in this chapter.

A. Zori (✉) · B. Styskel · N. Liu
University of Florida College of Medicine, Gastroenterology, Hepatology, and Nutrition, Gainesville, FL, USA

University of Florida, Gastroenterology, Hepatology, and Nutrition, Gainesville, FL, USA

University of Louisville, Gastroenterology, Hepatology, and Nutrition, Louisville, KY, USA
e-mail: andreas.zori@medicine.ufl.edu; brett.styskel@medicine.ufl.edu; nanlong.liu@medicine.ufl.edu

E. Mahanna Gabrielli et al. (eds.), *Textbook of Neurointensive Care: Volume 1*, https://doi.org/10.1007/978-3-031-62220-5_18

Introduction

The field of gastroenterology (GI) has evolved tremendously over the past few decades with procedural interventions such as Endoscopic Retrograde Cholangiopancreatography (ERCP) to device breakthroughs such as endoscopic clips utilized for treating gastrointestinal bleeds and perforations. The role of gastroenterologist consultants in the management of neuro-intensive care unit (ICU) patients is integral to patient care. Breakthroughs in nutrition and management of GI complications have continued to grow. The GI armamentarium continues to evolve. Even with these advancements in endoscopy, the first line in managing GI complications and emergencies is medical management and resuscitation of the patient before intervention can safely be performed. While not all GI emergencies are covered in this chapter, the pertinent GI issues encountered in the Neuro ICU are highlighted. Acute liver failure was included in this chapter because of the close association between the fields of Gastroenterology and Hepatology.

Gastrointestinal Hemorrhage

Gastrointestinal bleeding (GIB) is common in the neurocritical intensive critical care unit (ICU) and may negatively affect prognosis. The risk factors most strongly associated with GIB in critically ill patients are respiratory failure (OR = 15.6) and coagulopathy (OR = 4.3) [1]. Risk factors for GIB in patients after acute cerebral infarction found that risk factors include advanced age, low Glasgow Coma Scale (GCS) score, high NIHSS score, infection, and posterior circulation infarction [2]. Patients with a GIB had a higher rate of mortality and disability, which is an independent risk factor for death within 1 year after stroke [2].

Presentation

GIB can be divided into upper gastrointestinal bleed (UGIB) and lower gastrointestinal bleed (LGIB) based on its location concerning the ligament of Treitz at the junction of the duodenum and jejunum. Overt GI bleeding can include hematemesis, melena, and hematochezia. Hematemesis suggests a UGIB. Melena, a product of blood degradation within the GI tract, arises from an upper GI source about 90% of the time, while 10% of cases may arise from the small bowel distal to the ligament of Treitz or right colon [3]. Hematochezia is usually due to bleeding from a lower gastrointestinal source, though it can occasionally arise from a massive UGIB. However, UGIB causing hematochezia is generally accompanied by signs of hypovolemia and hypoperfusion manifesting as hypotension [3]. When there is clinical suspicion of an acute GI bleed, the recommended strategy for diagnosis is a thorough history and physical, including visual inspection of gastric output, if concern for hematemesis, and the stool by the clinician to assess for hematochezia or melena. Patients with upper GI bleeds should be evaluated for the possibility of chronic liver disease or portal hypertension, which would raise concern for esophageal variceal hemorrhage [3]. Determining the severity and likely location of the bleed is critical to determine which diagnostic and treatment modality is indicated if any, and the urgency of the procedure.

GIB occurs in 1–8% of patients with an acute ischemic stroke [4, 5]. Risk factors for GIB in this setting appear to be increasing age, Asian descent, history of peptic ulcer disease, liver disease, cancer, coagulopathy, and alcohol use [4]. GIB in this setting is associated with prolonged length of stay (LOS), increased hospital costs, in-hospital mortality, and 3-year mortality [4, 6]. Antiplatelet drugs are widely used in the secondary prevention of cardiovascular disease, specifically when pertinent to the neurological ICU in treating TIA or ischemic stroke. The risk for major GIB resulting in death or hospitalization is more significant in patients on dual antiplatelet therapy (DAPT) than single antiplatelet therapy, and this risk appears to decline after the first month of DAPT [7]. A study assessing the etiology of GIB in an ICU setting found that out of 4439 patients who entered the medical ICU without pre-existing GIB, 58 (1.3%) developed GIB; of these, 69% of bleeds were from a UGIB, while 10% were from a LGIB (Table 18.1) [8].

Table 18.1 Causes of GI bleeding in an intensive care unit setting (adapted from Kumar S, Ramos C, Garcia-Carrasquillo RJ, et al. Frontline Gastroenterology 2017;8:167–173)

Source of bleeding	% of patients
Upper GI bleeding	**69**
Gastric or duodenal ulcer	12
Gastropathy	10
Erosions	10
Variceal hemorrhage	7
Esophagitis	5
Vascular (angioectasia, Dieulafoy's)	5
Mallory Weiss or other esophageal tear	3
Tumor	2
No source identified but upper GI source suspected	14
Lower GI bleeding	**10**
Colonic ulcers	3
Diverticular bleeding	2
Colitis	2
Rectal artery	2
Friable mucosa	2
GI bleeding, source not identified after endoscopy	**19**
GI bleeding, no endoscopic workup performed	**2**

Upper GI Bleeding

The use of proton pump inhibitors (PPIs) and histamine-2 receptor antagonists (H2RAs) as prophylaxis against gastrointestinal stress ulceration in an ICU has been included in major international critical care guidelines [9, 10]. A recent large meta-analysis involving 72 trials, including 12,660 patients, aimed to determine the relative impact of PPIs, H2RAs, sucralfate, and placebo or no prophylaxis on GIB in the ICU [11]. This study grouped patients by risk to assess treatment outcomes with each medication (Table 18.2). This study found that in critically ill patients at high risk for GIB, PPIs and H2RAs likely reduced GIB compared to no prophylaxis (PPIs with more significant benefit than H2RAs) and are recommended for these groups [10, 11]. For patients at moderate or low risk, the reduction was modest and was not recommended [10, 11]. Sucralfate did not significantly affect the patient for any level of risk [11]. PPIs and H2RAs for prophylaxis may increase the risk for pneumonia and do not seem to affect mortality compared with no prophylaxis [11, 12].

Intravascular volume resuscitation should be initiated for all patients with an acute upper GI bleed and hemodynamic instability as early intensive resuscitation significantly decreases mortality [13, 14]. There is debate regarding the type of fluid (colloid vs. crystalloid). A recent large randomized control trial of critically ill patients found a small reduction in acute kidney injury and a possible reduction in in-hospital mortality with balanced crystalloids such as lactated Ringer's solution versus normal saline [15]. The target endpoint for resuscitation is unclear. However, an increase in blood urine nitrogen at 24 h (which likely reflects under resuscitation) is a predictor of worse outcomes in patients with acute nonvariceal UGIB [16]. Clinicians should obtain large-bore (14–16 gauge) IV access and keep an active type and screen. A restrictive transfusion goal (transfuse for hemoglobin <7 g/dL for a goal of 7–9 g/dL) is associated with higher survival at 6 weeks than a liberal transfusion goal (transfuse for hemoglobin <9 g/dL for goal 9–11 g/dL) [17]. For patients with an acute UGIB and underlying cardiovascular disease, a transfusion threshold of 8 g/dL has been recommended [13, 18]. An upper endoscopy will be indicated in many cases of UGIB. For coagulopathy, a goal international normalized ratio (INR) < 1.8 and goal platelets above 50,000 is generally advised ahead of endoscopy, though if the patient has active bleeding and needs urgent endoscopy, the safety of upper endoscopy has been demonstrated with a goal INR < 2.5 and a platelet goal of above 20,000 [19, 20]. In patients with coagulopathy due to cirrhosis, correction of coagulopathy based on thromboelastography has been associated with lower use of blood components without an increase in failure to control bleeding, rebleeding, or mortality [21]. Worse outcomes are associated with urgent endoscopy (<12 h) for non-variceal bleeding compared to urgent (<24 h) possibly due to inadequate resuscitation [22].

Table 18.2 Baseline risk level of clinically important gastrointestinal bleeding for each group

Risk level	Risk factors	Percent risk of clinically important gastrointestinal bleeding
Low risk	Critical illness, acute liver failure, use of immunosuppression including steroids, use of anticoagulants, cancer, male gender	1–2
Moderate risk	Mechanical ventilation with enteral nutrition, sepsis, shock, acute kidney injury	2.1–4
High risk	Coagulopathy	4.1–8
Highest risk	Mechanical ventilation without enteral nutrition, chronic liver disease	8.1–10

Intravenous administration of PPIs is recommended as part of pre-endoscopy treatment [13]. Intravenous PPI use before endoscopy reduces the proportion of patients with high-risk stigmata and the need for endoscopic therapy. However, it does not significantly decrease mortality, rebleeding, or need for surgery [23, 24]. The optimal PPI dose for this effect is unclear. Many of the large randomized control trials use a high dose (pantoprazole 80 mg bolus IV followed by continuous drip at 8 mg per hour), and this may be more effective at reducing the chance of high-risk peptic ulcer bleeding compared to the standard dose (pantoprazole 40 mg IV twice daily) [23, 25].

Patients with a history of liver cirrhosis or portal hypertension with UGIB should raise suspicion for acute esophageal or gastric variceal hemorrhage, which demands specific management considerations. Patients with cirrhosis who have gastrointestinal bleeding of any etiology should be given a short course (2–5 days) of antibiotics, as antibiotic prophylaxis in such patients significantly reduces bacterial infections, all-cause mortality, bacterial infection mortality, and rebleeding events [26, 27]. Ceftriaxone 1 g every 24 h is the preferred antibiotic [26]. When variceal hemorrhage is suspected, vasoactive drugs such as octreotide, vasopressin, or terlipressin should be initiated immediately, as these medications improve outcomes, including reducing mortality [28]. In suspected variceal hemorrhage, endoscopy should be performed within 12 h when the patient is hemodynamically stable. If esophageal varices are the likely source of bleeding, endoscopic variceal ligation should be performed, and vasoactive drugs continued for 2–5 days afterward [26]. If gastric varices are found during endoscopy, the management may depend on the local availability of treatment options and is often done through a multidisciplinary approach, including gastroenterologists, hepatologists, interventional radiologists, and interventional endoscopists [29]. Potential endoscopic treatment options include endoscopic cyanoacrylate injection (not available in the United States), alcohol-based agents, and band ligation. Balloon tamponade and endoscopically placed stents (if available) are potential temporizing measures, until more definitive therapy can be pursued. Endovascular management to reduce portal hypertension may include transjugular intrahepatic portosystemic shunt TIPS, and balloon retrograde transvenous obliteration (BRTO) [29]. TIPS is the recommended intervention for variceal bleeding in patients with Child-Pugh class B cirrhosis and active bleeding on endoscopy and patients who have Child-Pugh C cirrhosis with a Child-Pugh score < 14. TIPS is also recommended for patients with two or more episodes of variceal bleeding [26, 30].

Lower GI Bleeding

Similar to upper GI bleeding, patients with lower GI bleed (LGIB) with hemodynamic instability or active bleeding should receive prompt intravenous fluid resuscitation and transfusion of blood products as required to maintain desired hematologic parameters [31–33]. The hemoglobin and platelet goals in patients with LGIB are similar to those with UGIB [31–33]. In patients with a brisk bleed who are hemodynamically unstable or in whom active bleeding is suspected, CT angiography (CTA) may provide a fast and less invasive means to identify the location of bleeding, which may aid in planning for endoscopic or endovascular therapy [33]. CTA is highly sensitive and specific for detecting the bleeding site if the velocity of blood loss into the lumen is 0.3–1.0 mL/min [34]. Vitamin K antagonists and direct oral anticoagulants should be stopped in patients with lower GI bleeding. The decision to stop DAPT may be more difficult, particularly in patients with prior coronary stents. Therefore, risks and benefits may need to be weighed with specialists familiar with the risks associated with DAPT [32]. When patients are hemodynamically stable, colonoscopy should be performed after adequate colon preparation [31]. A rapid prep, which is four to six liters of polyethylene glycol-based solution administered over 3–4 h, maybe considered if the patient is hemodynamically stable. A nasogastric tube may be needed for patients to tolerate rapid ingestion of this large volume. Unprepped colonoscopy or sigmoidoscopy is not recommended [31]. The optimal timing of colonoscopy for acute LGIB is unclear. Urgent (<24 h) colonoscopy may increase diagnostic and therapeutic yield and decrease the length of stay but has not been shown to reduce mortality [33].

While bleeding in the small intestine distal to the ligament of Treitz is considered an LGIB, its management is distinct from bleeding involving the colon or rectum. Bleeding in the small intestine only accounts for about 5–10% of patients presenting with gastrointestinal bleeding [35]. While assessing the small intestine can be difficult, endoscopic visualization of the small intestine may be achieved through video capsule endoscopy, deep enteroscopy, and intraoperative enteroscopy.

Intestinal Ischemia

Intestinal ischemia is classified based on chronicity and the area of bowel affected. Ischemia of the small bowel is mesenteric ischemia, while ischemia involving the large bowel is referred to as colonic ischemia. For this chapter, the focus will be on acute small and large bowel ischemia.

Acute Mesenteric Ischemia

Causes of acute mesenteric ischemia (AMI) include acute mesenteric arterial embolism, acute mesenteric arterial thrombosis, and acute non-occlusive mesenteric ischemia (low splanchnic blood flow states), and mesenteric venous thrombosis [36]. The classically described presentation is severe abdominal pain out of proportion to the abdominal exam findings. It should be suspected in critically ill patients with abdominal pain or distention, and multi-organ dysfunction requiring vasopressor support [36, 37]. Risk factors associated with acute mesenteric ischemia overlap with risk factors for CVA, including atherosclerotic disease and conditions predisposing patients to embolism including atrial fibrillation and recent myocardial infarction [38]. As mortality rates are high (60–80%), diagnostic workup with a CTA should be performed as soon as possible when AMI is suspected [36, 38]. CTA has a 95–100% accuracy for diagnosing visceral ischemic syndromes [39]. Endoscopic examination is not often helpful in ruling in mesenteric ischemia as often endoscopic examination does not reach the majority of sections of the small bowel that are most frequently involved in AMI [38].

Fluid resuscitation and broad-spectrum antibiotic treatment should be initiated promptly, and surgical consultation should be obtained when AMI is diagnosed [36]. Additionally, oral intake should be avoided in patients with AMI since it can exacerbate intestinal ischemia [40]. Treatment options include endovascular repair and open repair, and surgical consultants should assist in this decision [38]. If massive gut necrosis is found, careful assessment of patients' co-morbidities and goals of care should be considered to determine if comfort care may be the best treatment option [36].

Acute Colonic Ischemia

Acute colonic ischemia (CI) is caused by local hypoperfusion and reperfusion injury from low blood flow states, embolic and thrombotic arterial occlusion, and mesenteric vein thrombosis [41]. Non-occlusive CI due to hypoperfusion of the mesenteric microvasculature accounts for 95% of cases [41]. Symptoms of acute colonic ischemia include sudden crampy abdominal pain, bright red or maroon blood per rectum, vomiting, and diarrhea [42, 43]. There is overlap among risk factors for CI and CVA, including atherosclerotic disease, diabetes, coronary artery disease, and peripheral vascular disease [41, 44]. Additional risk factors for CI include irritable bowel syndrome, surgical procedures such as abdominal aortic aneurysm repair, hypotension, and shock [43]. The "watershed" areas of the colon are most susceptible to ischemia due to their location between separate vascular supplies and include the splenic flexure and the rectosigmoid junction. However, any area of the colon may be affected [41, 43]. CT with IV and oral contrast is the imaging modality of choice for patients with suspected CI [41, 43]. Performing a colonoscopy early (within 48 h of presentation) is recommended to confirm the diagnosis unless the patient has peritonitis or irreversible ischemic damage such as gangrene or pneumatosis [43].

According to recent guidelines, patients can present with variable disease severity. If known, their risk-stratified before admission to the ICU will help guide management [43]. Patients with mild disease have typical symptoms of CI with segmental colitis not isolated to the right colon and none of the commonly associated risk factors for worse outcomes seen in more advanced disease. Patients with moderate disease include patients with CI and three of the following factors: Male gender, hypotension, tachycardia, abdominal pain without rectal bleeding, BUN >20 mg/dL, Hgb < 12 g/dL, LDH > 350 U/L, serum sodium <136 mEq/L, WBC > 15 × 10 [9]/L, or mucosal ulcerations on colonoscopy. Unfortunately, many of these symptoms are generic and easily confounded with other neurological co-morbidities. Severe diseases are easier to recognize in critical neurological patients. Signs of severe CI can include patients with CI and more than three of the criteria for moderate disease and peritoneal signs on physical examination, pneumatosis or portal venous gas on radiologic imaging, gangrene on colonoscopy or pancolonic distribution or isolated right-colon ischemia on imaging or colonoscopy. Mild disease is often unrecognized in the ICU or interpreted as a sign of malabsorption or dynamic ileus. In patients with known severe disease, worsening hemodynamics and increased requirement of vasopressors requires emergent surgical consultation. Correction of cardiovascular abnormalities and broad-spectrum antibiotic therapy is recommended while consideration for abdominal surgical exploration may be necessary. The presence of an unexplained lactic acidosis, especially if not cleared with more aggressive resuscitation, can often unmask severe CI in the ICU [43].

Diagnosis and Management of Cholangitis for Intensive Care Unit Patients

Introduction to Cholangitis

Ascending cholangitis, also known as acute bacterial cholangitis, is a gastrointestinal (GI) emergency defined as an infection of the biliary tract. This infection is typically caused by an obstruction in the bile duct, usually gallstones, neoplastic tissue, or retained stents. Uncommon causes include parasitic infections, autoimmune-related strictures, and altered anatomy such as biliary-enteric anastomotic strictures. This condition should not be confused with Primary Biliary Cholangitis or Primary Sclerosing Cholangitis, which are different chronic auto-immune conditions. Acute cholangitis causes a severe systemic response that leads to septic shock if not treated with resuscitation, antibiotics, and biliary decompression. In addition, cholangitis causes altered mental status changes that can be confused with a primary neurological condition if not carefully differentiated. Patients diagnosed with cholangitis have a high mortality rate. In a study cohort of 256 patients with cholangitis secondary to choledocholithiasis, the in-hospital overall mortality rate was 3.5% [45]. The 3-month mortality for this group was 8.2% [45]. Prompt diagnosis and treatment are essential since the infection can quickly progress and is a treatable condition. A delay in treatment is associated with prolonged hospitalization and worse outcomes [46].

Etiology

Acute cholangitis usually involves an obstruction or previous instrumentation that allows gut bacteria to migrate into the bile duct, hence the term ascending cholangitis. The most common cause of obstructive cholangitis is common bile duct stones called choledocholithiasis. About 48 malignant lesions can also obstruct the bile duct, the most common of which are pancreatic head tumors and ampullary neoplasms, cholangiocarcinoma, and gallbladder cancer. Previous instrumentation with ERCP and placement of stents can also cause cholangitis [47]. Plastic and fully covered metal stents are temporary. They should be removed in a timely fashion as dictated in the post-procedure note at the time of placement as standard practice. These stents can occlude and precipitate a nidus for infection leading to cholangitis. In general, plastic stents can stay patent for up to 3–4 months, with covered metal stent patency around 6–8 months [48]. This time frame can be variable depending on the size of the stents and the initial indication for placement. Narrowing of the bile duct caused by strictures can also lead to obstruction. These strictures can be benign, such as biliary-enteric anastomotic strictures, or malignant such as in cholangiocarcinoma. Other less common causes are round or tapeworm infections of the bile duct. The most common bacterial organisms that cause cholangitis are Escherichia coli, Enterococcus, and Klebsiella [49].

Diagnosis

Traditionally, the clinical diagnosis of cholangitis was described as Charcot's "Triad," which consisted of abdominal pain, fever, and jaundice and was first described in the 1800s [50]. In addition to the triad, patients with severe disease can present with shock requiring pressor support and mental confusion known as Reynold's Pentad when all five are present. However, patients with cholangitis often do not present with all three diagnostic criteria of Charcot's Triad; therefore, a high index of suspicion is needed to make the diagnosis. One systematic review found that the sensitivity of Charcot's Triad was only 36.2% compared to the specificity, which was high at 93.2% [51]. Given the low ability to rule out cholangitis, additional diagnostic criteria have recently evolved to identify a broader range of patients presenting with cholangitis that present without all three classic symptoms. To add to the complexity, differentials such as cholecystitis and pancreatitis can present with similar clinical symptoms, so it is essential to consider these conditions with labs and imaging.

Given this clinical issue and the importance of recognizing cholangitis, various consensus criteria and guidelines have been published to help clinicians with earlier and widespread detection. The Tokyo Guidelines helped address this clinical conundrum by defining the diagnosis and grading the severity of cholangitis first published in 2007 [52]. These guidelines were then updated in 2013 and 2018 [53, 54]. As described in Table 18.3, if the patient meets criteria from row A plus either row B or C, then there should be a clinical suspicion for cholangitis. If the patient meets the criteria for all three rows, then the patient is diagnosed as having definite cholangitis. The numerical criteria that correspond with Table 18.3 are listed in Table 18.4 below, adapted from the 2018 guidelines [54].

The diagnosis of cholangitis can be aided by blood chemistry and imaging in addition to the clinical presentation of abdominal pain and fever that Charcot first described in the 1800s. A few studies show improvement with a sensitivity of the Tokyo 2013/2018 guidelines and identification of cholangitis to 90–92% [55]. The main limitations are patients with only mild or moderate cholangitis who may not present with prominent imaging findings or systemic inflammatory response. Given an initial negative workup, as the patient worsens during their hospitalization, cholangitis may become overlooked, especially if liver function tests are no longer ordered. The patient may develop neurological and cognitive changes due to sepsis inflammatory status or shock, which can be occasionally confused with a primary neurological manifestation. The presence of septic shock in severe acute cholangitis requires emergent biliary decompression. Any other signs of organ dysfunction in the recent Tokyo 2018 Guidelines indicate severe cholangitis, including respiratory failure, renal dysfunction, and hypotension [54].

Table 18.3 Tokyo Guidelines 2018 Diagnosis of Cholangitis

Definite diagnosis of cholangitis: One criterion each from A, B, and C	
Suspicious diagnosis of cholangitis: One criterion from A with a criteria from either B or C	
A. Systemic inflammation	A-1 fever and/or chills
	A-2 abnormal inflammatory response markers
B. Cholestasis	B-1 jaundice
	B-2 abnormal liver function tests
C. Imaging	C-1 biliary dilation
	C-2 evidence of etiology on imaging such as stones and occluded stents

Table 18.4 Abnormal values for diagnostic criteria of cholangitis

A-1 fever	Temperature > 38 °C
A-2 abnormal inflammatory response markers	WBC < 4000 or > 10,000/μL or CRP (mg/dL) >1
B-1 jaundice	Total bilirubin >2 mg/dL
B-2 abnormal liver function tests	Alkaline phosphatase/AST/ALT/GGT values >1.5 upper limit normal

Non-invasive Imaging Modalities

In addition to clinical symptoms and laboratory investigations, imaging is paramount in helping to assess for cholangitis. Non-invasive imaging modalities include Trans-abdominal Ultrasound (US), Computed Tomography (CT), Magnetic Resonance Cholangiopancreatography (MRCP), and Endoscopic Ultrasound (EUS). US has low sensitivity (73%) in detecting stones but is more reliable in detecting ductal dilation [56]. A CT with contrast appears to have a higher sensitivity for detecting CBD stones (88%) and is also valuable for further helping identify a cause of obstruction, such as a pancreatic head mass compressing the distal bile duct [57]. MRCP seems to carry a similar sensitivity of 88% but does not require IV contrast. If there is a concern for a pancreatic mass causing compression, an MRI abdomen with contrast would be recommended. When interpreting these radiological studies, the primary consideration is evaluating for biliary dilation, strictures, and stones. Findings of air in the biliary tree, also termed pneumobilia, can signify an infection; however, patients that have had previous sphincterotomy or biliary stent placement will frequently have these findings. EUS carries a higher sensitivity than CT or MRCP [57]. In addition, if the EUS is positive for a finding, ERCP can often be performed immediately after to EUS in the same endoscopic session.

Treatment

The initial management phase of cholangitis is fluid resuscitation and antibiotics. Lab studies, imaging, and blood cultures should also be obtained. Hypotension and lactic acidosis should be aggressively treated and monitored. Depending on the patient's allergies, broad-spectrum antibiotics should cover gram negatives and anaerobes such as piperacillin/tazobactam, cefepime, and ciprofloxacin/metronidazole [49]. After cultures return, antibiotic coverage should be narrowed and continued for at least 7 days. Duration should be extended to 14 days if bacteremia is confirmed by blood culture [49]. If the patient is coagulopathic due to liver dysfunction from biliary obstruction, the patient should be given vitamin K and fresh frozen plasma and monitored for bleeding.

After initial stabilization and medical management, biliary drainage is required. In most situations, ERCP will be the primary therapeutic intervention in cases of confirmed cholangitis. The procedure can be performed with deep or general sedation, a logistic that needs to be carefully planned not to interfere with the underlying neurological dysfunction. The procedure does require fluoroscopy. However, transport to a specialized endoscopy unit should be carefully arranged only if continuous neurological monitoring is feasible and can be done safely. Typically, when an ERCP is performed, an incision into the biliary orifice, also called a biliary sphincterotomy, will allow for biliary drainage. A temporary stent is placed to allow for further processing of biliary decompression. In cholangitis, if severe coagulopathy or the patient is taking an anti-platelet or is on anticoagulation, then not performing a sphincterotomy is advised, and a plastic biliary stent can be placed for decompression. Large stones in the bile duct can be extracted later on follow-up ERCP since a stent allows biliary decompression. Fig. 18.1 depicts an extraction of a large stone removed during ERCP that caused cholangitis. In the setting of ascending cholangitis, a systematic review found that ERCP performed <48 h led to a decrease in inpatient mortality as compared to >48 h [46]. Unsuccessful ERCP and delayed biliary decompression >72 h have been shown to carry increased mortality for the patient [58]. It is crucial that a stent is placed to allow for continued drainage, and a follow-up ERCP is performed in a timely fashion to prevent the stent from occlusion, precipitating repeat cholangitis.

When ERCP cannot be performed safely, Interventional Radiology should be consulted for Percutaneous Transhepatic Biliary Drainage (PTBD), where a catheter is left to provide continuous external drainage of the biliary system. PTBD can be performed rapidly using a local anesthetic, in general, better tolerated without interfering with the neurological exam. Complications from PTBD include biliary peritonitis and bleeding.

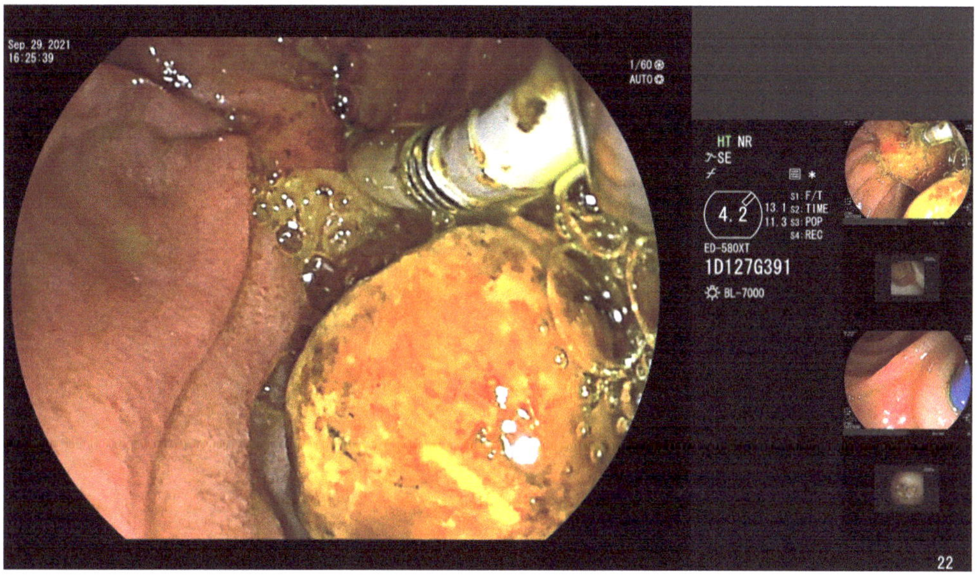

Fig. 18.1 A large biliary stone is being removed from the biliary tree into the duodenum during an ERCP

Conclusion

Ascending cholangitis is a medical emergency that requires prompt recognition. The limitations of a low sensitivity using Charcot's triad led to further expansion of guidelines involving imaging and labs to help clinicians detect this infection earlier. Delayed or late presentations of this condition can deteriorate to septic shock, associated with higher mortality. Initial management with antibiotics and fluid resuscitation followed by biliary drainage within 48 h is critical for control. ERCP is typically the first-line therapy for biliary decompression, but PTBD may be needed in selected situations.

Acute Liver Failure

Acute liver failure (ALF) is a sudden, severe deterioration of liver function due to an acute insult. The diagnosis is made clinically and is defined as acute onset coagulopathy with an INR >1.5 and altered mentation in patients without preexisting liver disease. The duration of symptoms varies considerably depending on etiology. The symptom duration of hyperacute failure, commonly seen after acetaminophen toxicity, is a week or less compared to subacute failure, where the time can be up to 26 weeks [59]. Direct hyperbilirubinemia is not always included in the clinical definition but is almost universally present. The degree of elevation in transaminases varies by etiology, with marked elevation, often more significant than 1000 U/L, seen commonly if symptom duration is short or if ALF is due to ischemia, viral hepatitis, or acetaminophen toxicity. Severe transaminase elevation may not be apparent at the time of presentation in subacute ALF or later in the course of acute ALF due to severe hepatic necrosis causing depletion of transaminases. Therefore, transaminase improvement is not necessarily a sign of clinical improvement and should be viewed in the clinical context. Improvement in encephalopathy and markers of synthetic liver function such as INR and bilirubin are more reliable indicators of improvement in ALF. However, the peak in bilirubin usually lags several days behind the peak in transaminases.

Encephalopathy is the distinguishing clinical feature of ALF and is similar in presentation to hepatic encephalopathy caused by chronic liver disease. It is characterized by disorientation, mild confusion, slurred speech, and somnolence which progresses to a stuporous state and eventually to a coma. Physical exam may demonstrate asterixis, an inability to maintain sustained muscle contraction where a compensatory jerk follows a brief loss of tone. This is shown classically by asking the patient to support wrist extension, resulting in the patient's hands "flapping." Alternatively, this can be shown by having the patient keep a firm hand grip where irregular loosening followed by tightening is indicative of asterixis. Progression of encephalopathy is one of the most concerning clinical features in ALF and warrants aggressive intervention, transfer to a liver transplant center, and monitoring of serum ammonia, which will be discussed in detail later in this section. Because of altered mentation and risk of increased intracranial pressure (ICP), patients with ALF are often evaluated by or in conjunction with neurocritical care providers.

Acute onset worsening of liver function in a patient with underlying cirrhosis, commonly referred to as acute on chronic liver failure (ACLF), is considered a separate entity and will not be discussed in this section. Although ALF is rare, with about 2000–2800 cases yearly in the United States, it is associated with death or multi-organ failure in about half of cases [60–62]. Early recognition and aggressive ICU management in ALF management are crucial to recovery or stabilization until liver transplantation can be performed.

Causes/Evaluation

The cause of ALF varies considerably across the world. In the developing world, viral infections, especially Hepatitis A, B, and E, are the most common causes. In the United States and most Western Europe, acetaminophen and other drugs are the most common cause, although the cause is indeterminate in 17–43% of cases [61, 63].

Obtaining a detailed clinical history is often critical to determining the cause of ALF and determining their transplant candidacy should their disease progress. Because encephalopathy often progresses rapidly, it is essential to take a detailed history immediately on presentation if the patient is coherent, including drug exposures, travel, sick contacts, history of auto-immune disorders, psycho-social history (including a history of past suicide attempts), history of malignancy, and history of thrombosis. A detailed drug history (alcohol, illicit drugs, over-the-counter medications, and supplements/herbals) is essential since non-acetaminophen drug toxicity accounts for about 9% of ALF in the United States [64]. Although antibiotics account for nearly 50% of non-acetaminophen drug-induced ALF, this is primarily due to their prescription frequency, and risk of ALF from antibiotics is low. Other drugs have a higher likelihood causing ALF, including halothane, isoniazid/rifampin, NSAIDs, sulfonamides, flutamide, sodium valproate, carbamazepine, ecstasy (MDMA) [62, 65].

Radiologic evaluation is important to evaluate for causes of ALF including Budd–Chiari syndrome and malignant liver infiltration. In addition, it is essential to exclude the presence of cirrhosis. The nodular contour to the liver in patients with cirrhosis can be masked by severe hepatic swelling, often present in ALF. However, patients with underlying cirrhosis will typically display signs of chronic portal hypertension, including splenomegaly, recanalized umbilical vein, ascites, and varices on imaging. Laboratory evaluation should include a metabolic panel, liver function panel, arterial blood gas, serum ammonia, complete blood count, acetaminophen level, toxicology screen, viral hepatitis serology, autoimmune markers (ANA, anti-smooth muscle, immunoglobulins, and in children anti-liver kidney microsomal antibody), pregnancy test in females, and HIV testing [59]. In specific clinical scenarios, additional testing for Wilson's disease and other viral infections should be considered (Table 18.5). Liver biopsy may be helpful in some situations, especially if autoimmune hepatitis or infiltrative malignancy is likely etiologies of ALF. The transjugular route is preferred due to a lower bleeding risk than percutaneous liver biopsies.

Table 18.5 Acute liver failure etiology-specific epidemiology and management

Cause of ALF	Relative frequency in USA	Transplant free survival	Common clinical scenario	Specific evaluation	Specific intervention
Acetaminophen	39%	65–75%	Suicide attempt Accidental, polypharmacy	Acetaminophen level	Acetylcysteine
Other drugs	13%	70% If encephalopathy occurs <25%	Exposure to a drug known to cause ALF	Urine tox screen	Consider Acetylcysteine
Hepatitis B	7%	20–30%	New infection—IV drug use, multiple sexual partners Reactivation—Untreated HBV	HBsAg, anti-HBc total and IgM, HBV DNA, HDV IgM	Nucleos(t)ide inhibitors—Tenofovir, entecavir
Ischemic Hepatopathy	6%	60%	Severe shock, multiorgan failure Marked, rapid rise in transaminases	Evaluate for underlying cause of hypoprofusion	Treat underlying cause of hypoprofusion
Other viral hepatitis (HAV, HEV, VZV, HSV)	4% (primarily HAV)	HAV—60-70%	HEV—Travel to endemic country, pregnant females	Anti-HAV, HSV1 IgM, VZV IgM, HEV IgM[a]	HSV/VZV—Acyclovir
Autoimmune	4%	10–20%	Often young Female: Male 4:1 Acute or subacute	ANA, anti-smooth muscle antibody, immunoglobulins, anti-liver kidney antigen (children)	Consider corticosteroids in early stages, without infection
Wilson's	3%	<1%	Age < 40 Low alkaline phosphatase or uric acid Bilirubin to alkaline phosphatase ratio > 2 Coombs negative hemolytic anemia	Ceruloplasmin, serum copper, 24 h urine copper, uric acid	Early liver transplant evaluation
Budd-Chiari syndrome	2%	20%	History of malignancy or thrombosis	Cross-sectional imaging Pregnancy test Evaluation for malignancy	Thrombolysis, endovascular intervention/TIPS, early liver transplant evaluation
Pregnancy associated	2%	78%	AFLP—Third trimester, 20% post-natal HELLP syndrome after 20th week Eclampsia	Abdominal imaging -HELLP associated with hemorrhage in 45%	Delivery of fetus when possible
Mushroom poisoning *(amanita phalloides)*	<1%	Unknown, likely similar to non-acetaminophen drugs	Severe gastrointestinal symptoms within hours of ingestion	No serologic testing available	Penicillin G, Silibinin[b] NG lavage and activated charcoal if present within 4 h of ingestion

[a] Testing for hepatitis E is indicated if there is history of recent travel to endemic area
[b] Not available in the US

Management

Management of ALF is complex with often rapid and unpredictable disease progression (Table 18.6). Transfer to a tertiary care center with liver transplant capability should be sought after initial stabilization if the patient develops even mild encephalopathy [59]. On initial presentation shock and multiorgan failure are common due release of pro-inflammatory cytokines and cell damage-associated molecular patterns [65]. Resuscitation with either crystalloid or albumin can be used, but neither has demonstrated a clear advantage [59, 66]. Care should be taken to avoid volume overload, which is associated with higher mortality [63]. Norepinephrine is the initial vasopressor of choice if hypotension persists after initial volume resuscitation. Ideal MAP targets have not been established, but some favor targeting MAPs greater than 75 prior to developing renal failure and in patients with chronic hypertension. This MAP target is of little benefit after the initiation of renal replacement therapy and should be reconsidered to a lower level [63]. Aggressive management of shock and the metabolic disturbances associated with ALF are essential to allow the patient to either recover from the hepatic insult or to allow enough time for liver transplant evaluation, listing, and organ allocation.

One of the most severe consequences of ALF is cerebral edema and herniation, which occurs primarily due to hyperammonemia. Patients should be monitored closely with regular neuro checks before the development of encephalopathy. Once encephalopathy develops, patients should be monitored in the ICU with a neurologist consultant and have general measures to prevent elevated intracranial pressure instituted. In addition to clinical monitoring, monitoring serum ammonia is essential. When drawing serum ammonia, the sample should be taken promptly to the lab on ice and, if possible, drawn from an arterial line as this reduces falsely elevated results. Serum ammonia above 150–200 μmol/L increases the risk of intracranial hypertension, therefore it should be treated aggressively [67].

Hyperammonemia in the setting of ALF can progress rapidly due to the liver's central role in ammonia metabolism and requires an aggressive multimodal approach rather than a stepwise response. Although lactulose and rifaximin are the standard of care for managing hepatic encephalopathy in cirrhosis, limited evidence supports their use in ALF [63]. However, many practitioners utilize lactulose and rifaximin as they are associated with lowering ammonia and there is little potential harm. Ammonia scavengers such as sodium benzoate and sodium phenylacetate conjugate with ammonia to form water-soluble compounds excretable in the urine and can lower serum ammonia but have not been specifically studied in ALF [68]. However, to be useful, the patient must be producing urine which is often not the case in patients with severe ALF. Often the most effective strategy for decreasing serum ammonia in ALF is the early and aggressive use of hemodialysis. Continuous venovenous hemodialysis (CVVHD) is preferred as it is associated with fewer hemodynamic disturbances [59]. Various external liver support devices have been evaluated in ALF, but none have improved mortality or reduced need for liver transplantation [69].

Table 18.6 General management in acute liver failure

General management	Evaluate for cause of ALF Avoid sedatives Head of the bed elevation at 30° Neck in a neutral position Avoiding excessive stimulus and suctioning Stress ulcer prophylaxis
General monitoring	Every 1–2 h neuro checks Close monitoring of urine output
Hemodynamics	Invasive hemodynamic monitoring early Norepinephrine preferred vasopressor
Anti-infection	Close surveillance for infection (cultures, imaging) Low threshold to initiate antibiotics Prophylaxis not established may be helpful in severe cases
Ventilator management	Low tidal volume and low PEEP strategy in patients with ARDS Hyperventilation ($PaCO_2$ 25–30)
Encephalopathy/ Hyperammonemia	Grade 1–2 Transfer to liver transplant center Lactulose and Rifaximin Grade 3–4 Intubate, monitor for signs of increased ICP, CT head, monitor serum ammonia If patients make urine, consider ammonia scavengers Early CVVHD Target Na 145–155 meq/L
Coagulation	Hemoglobin transfusion threshold 7 g/dL Restrict clotting factor and platelet transfusion unless bleeding Use Thromboelastography for correction of coagulopathy
Other considerations	N-acetyl cystine—Consider in patients with both acetaminophen induced and ALF of unclear etiology

ALF acute liver failure, *PEEP* positive end expiratory pressure, *CVVHD* continuous venovenous hemodialysis

The management of patients who develop signs of increased ICP is similar to other causes of increased ICP, including mannitol, hypertonic saline, and head elevated but will not be covered in detail in this section [59]. Even in patients without elevated ICP, hypertonic saline can be utilized to target serum sodium levels of 145–155 meq/L as it has been associated with a decreased vasopressor requirement in patients with ALF [70]. Invasive intracranial pressure (ICP) monitoring in ALF has been used in the past but is not associated with improved outcomes [71].

Increased INR and thrombocytopenia are common but do not always reflect true coagulopathy or bleeding risk since ALF is often associated with balanced disturbance in endogenous pro and anticoagulation factors. Therefore, the decision to correct coagulopathy should be based on clinical bleeding or thromboelastography, as this is a more physiologic assessment of bleeding propensity [72].

In patients with acetaminophen-induced ALF, N-acetylcysteine (NAC) administration is recommended as early as possible, and it is occasionally helpful even >48 h after ingestion [59, 73]. In patients with non-acetaminophen drug-induced ALF, NAC has also been associated with improved transplant-free survival and should be considered as well [74].

Conclusions

Despite continuous improvement in the quality, safety, diagnostic, and treatment management of critically ill patients, gastrointestinal dysfunction is often present and associated with severe neurological impairment. Gastrointestinal dysfunction is also common when the primary reason for ICU admission is neurological or neurosurgical. While the etiology is often multifactorial, it largely relates to severe physiologic stress, causing reduced splanchnic blood flow, mucosal ischemia, and reperfusion injury. Mechanical ventilation and comorbidities (e.g., shock, coagulopathy, liver disease) contribute to worse clinical outcomes. New diagnostic tools have facilitated early recognition of life-threatening GI complications in the ICU. However, the key strategies to manage GI dysfunction are multidisciplinary and based on scientific evidence approach to prophylaxis of known complications, diagnostic, and therapeutic algorithms.

References

1. Cook DJ, Fuller HD, Guyatt GH, et al. Risk factors for gastrointestinal bleeding in critically ill patients. Canadian critical care trials group. N Engl J Med. 1994;330(6):377. https://doi.org/10.1056/NEJM199402103300601.
2. Fu J. Factors affecting the occurrence of gastrointestinal bleeding in acute ischemic stroke patients. Medicine (United States). 2019;98(28):e16312. https://doi.org/10.1097/MD.0000000000016312.
3. Cappell MS, Friedel D. Initial Management of Acute Upper Gastrointestinal Bleeding: from initial evaluation up to gastrointestinal endoscopy. Med Clin North Am. 2008;92(3):491–509. https://doi.org/10.1016/j.mcna.2008.01.005.
4. Rumalla K, Mittal MK. Gastrointestinal bleeding in acute ischemic stroke: a population-based analysis of hospitalizations in the United States. J Stroke Cerebrovasc Dis. 2016;25(7):1728–35. https://doi.org/10.1016/j.jstrokecerebrovasdis.2016.03.044.
5. Siddiqui MT, Bilal M, Gollapudi LA, et al. Endoscopy is relatively safe in patients with acute ischemic stroke and gastrointestinal hemorrhage. Dig Dis Sci. 2019;64(6):1588–98. https://doi.org/10.1007/s10620-018-5399-3.
6. Chou YF, Weng WC, Huang WY. Association between gastrointestinal bleeding and 3-year mortality in patients with acute, first-ever ischemic stroke. J Clin Neurosci. 2017;44:289–93. https://doi.org/10.1016/j.jocn.2017.06.068.
7. Hilkens NA, Algra A, Kappelle LJ, et al. Early time course of major bleeding on antiplatelet therapy after TIA or ischemic stroke. Neurology. 2018;90(8):e683–9. https://doi.org/10.1212/WNL.0000000000004997.
8. Kumar S, Ramos C, Garcia-Carrasquillo RJ, Green PH, Lebwohl B. Incidence and risk factors for gastrointestinal bleeding among patients admitted to medical intensive care units. *Frontline*. Gastroenterology. 2017;8(3):167. https://doi.org/10.1136/flgastro-2016-100722.
9. Rhodes A, Evans LE, Alhazzani W, et al. Surviving sepsis campaign: international guidelines for Management of Sepsis and Septic Shock: 2016. Intensive Care Med. 2017;43(3):304–77. https://doi.org/10.1007/s00134-017-4683-6.
10. Ye Z, Reintam Blaser A, Lytvyn L, et al. Gastrointestinal bleeding prophylaxis for critically ill patients: a clinical practice guideline. BMJ. 2020;368:l6722. https://doi.org/10.1136/bmj.l6722.
11. Wang Y, Ye Z, Ge L, et al. Efficacy and safety of gastrointestinal bleeding prophylaxis in critically ill patients: systematic review and network meta-analysis. BMJ. 2020;368:l6744. https://doi.org/10.1136/bmj.l6744.
12. Krag M, Marker S, Perner A, et al. Pantoprazole in patients at risk for gastrointestinal bleeding in the ICU. N Engl J Med. 2018;379(23):2199–208. https://doi.org/10.1056/nejmoa1714919.
13. Barkun AN, Almadi M, Kuipers EJ, et al. Management of non-variceal upper gastrointestinal bleeding: guideline recommendations from the international consensus group. Ann Intern Med. 2019;171(11):805–22. https://doi.org/10.7326/M19-1795.
14. Baradarian R, Ramdhaney S, Chapalamadugu R, et al. Early intensive resuscitation of patients with upper gastrointestinal bleeding decreases mortality. Am J Gastroenterol. 2004;99(4):619. https://doi.org/10.1111/j.1572-0241.2004.04073.x.
15. Semler MW, Self WH, Wanderer JP, et al. Balanced crystalloids versus saline in critically ill adults. N Engl J Med. 2018;378(9):829–39. https://doi.org/10.1056/nejmoa1711584.
16. Kumar NL, Claggett BL, Cohen AJ, Nayor J, Saltzman JR. Association between an increase in blood urea nitrogen at 24 hours and worse outcomes in acute nonvariceal upper GI bleeding. Gastrointest Endosc. 2017;86(6):1022. https://doi.org/10.1016/j.gie.2017.03.1533.
17. Villanueva C, Colomo A, Bosch A, et al. Transfusion strategies for acute upper gastrointestinal bleeding. N Engl J Med. 2013;368(1):11–21. https://doi.org/10.1056/nejmoa1211801.
18. Carson JL, Guyatt G, Heddle NM, et al. Clinical practice guidelines from the AABB: red blood cell transfusion thresholds and storage. JAMA. 2016;316(19):2025–35. https://doi.org/10.1001/jama.2016.9185.
19. Acosta RD, Abraham NS, Chandrasekhara V, et al. The management of antithrombotic agents for patients undergoing GI endoscopy. Gastrointest Endosc. 2016;83(1):3–16. https://doi.org/10.1016/j.gie.2015.09.035.
20. Ramos GP, Binder M, Hampel P, et al. Outcomes of endoscopic intervention for overt GI bleeding in severe thrombocytopenia. Gastrointest Endosc. 2018;88(1):55–61. https://doi.org/10.1016/j.gie.2018.01.028.
21. Kumar M, Ahmad J, Maiwall R, et al. Thromboelastography-guided blood component use in patients with cirrhosis with Nonvariceal bleeding: a randomized controlled trial. Hepatology. 2020;71(1):235. https://doi.org/10.1002/hep.30794.
22. Kumar NL, Cohen AJ, Nayor J, Claggett BL, Saltzman JR. Timing of upper endoscopy influences outcomes in patients with acute non-variceal upper GI bleeding. Gastrointest Endosc. 2017;85(5):945. https://doi.org/10.1016/j.gie.2016.09.029.

23. Lau JY, Leung WK, Wu JCY, et al. Omeprazole before endoscopy in patients with gastrointestinal bleeding. N Engl J Med. 2007;356(16):1631. https://doi.org/10.1056/NEJMoa065703.
24. Dorward S, Sreedharan A, Leontiadis GI, Howden CW, Moayyedi P, Forman D. Proton pump inhibitor treatment initiated prior to endoscopic diagnosis in upper gastrointestinal bleeding. Cochrane Database Syst Rev. 2006;4:CD005415. https://doi.org/10.1002/14651858.CD005415.pub2.
25. Rattanasupar A, Sengmanee S. Comparison of high dose and standard dose proton pump inhibitor before endoscopy in patients with non-portal hypertension bleeding. J Med Assoc Thai. 2016;99(9):988.
26. Garcia-Tsao G, Abraldes JG, Berzigotti A, Bosch J. Portal hypertensive bleeding in cirrhosis: risk stratification, diagnosis, and management: 2016 practice guidance by the American association for the study of liver diseases. Hepatology. 2017;65(1):310–35. https://doi.org/10.1002/hep.28906.
27. Chavez-Tapia NC, Barrientos-Gutierrez T, Tellez-Avila F, et al. Meta-analysis: antibiotic prophylaxis for cirrhotic patients with upper gastrointestinal bleeding - an updated Cochrane review. Aliment Pharmacol Ther. 2011;34(5):509. https://doi.org/10.1111/j.1365-2036.2011.04746.x.
28. Wells M, Chande N, Adams P, et al. Meta-analysis: vasoactive medications for the management of acute variceal bleeds. Aliment Pharmacol Ther. 2012;35(11):1267. https://doi.org/10.1111/j.1365-2036.2012.05088.x.
29. Henry Z, Patel K, Patton H, Saad W. AGA clinical practice update on Management of Bleeding Gastric Varices: expert review. Clin Gastroenterol Hepatol. 2021;19(6):1098. https://doi.org/10.1016/j.cgh.2021.01.027.
30. de Franchis R. Expanding consensus in portal hypertension. J Hepatol. 2015;63(3):743. https://doi.org/10.1016/j.jhep.2015.05.022.
31. Strate LL, Gralnek IM. ACG clinical guideline: Management of Patients with Acute Lower Gastrointestinal Bleeding. Am J Gastroenterol. 2016;111(4):459. https://doi.org/10.1038/ajg.2016.41.
32. Triantafyllou K, Gkolfakis P, Gralnek IM, et al. Diagnosis and management of acute lower gastrointestinal bleeding: European Society of Gastrointestinal Endoscopy (ESGE) guideline. Endoscopy. 2021;53(08):850. https://doi.org/10.1055/a-1496-8969.
33. Oakland K, Chadwick G, East JE, et al. Diagnosis and management of acute lower gastrointestinal bleeding: guidelines from the British Society of Gastroenterology. Gut. 2019;68(5):776. https://doi.org/10.1136/gutjnl-2018-317807.
34. Dobritz M, Engels HP, Schneider A, et al. Evaluation of dual-phase multi-detector-row CT for detection of intestinal bleeding using an experimental bowel model. Eur Radiol. 2009;19(4):875. https://doi.org/10.1007/s00330-008-1205-5.
35. Gerson LB, Fidler JL, Cave DR, Leighton JA. ACG clinical guideline: diagnosis and Management of Small Bowel Bleeding. Am J Gastroenterol. 2015;110(9):1265. https://doi.org/10.1038/ajg.2015.246.
36. Bala M, Kashuk J, Moore EE, et al. Acute mesenteric ischemia: guidelines of the world Society of Emergency Surgery. World J Emerg Surgery. 2017;12(1):38. https://doi.org/10.1186/s13017-017-0150-5.
37. Carver TW, Vora RS, Taneja A. Mesenteric ischemia. Crit Care Clin. 2016;32(2):155. https://doi.org/10.1016/j.ccc.2015.11.001.
38. Clair DG, Beach JM. Mesenteric Ischemia. N Engl J Med. 2016;374(10):959. https://doi.org/10.1056/NEJMra1503884.
39. Hagspiel KD, Flors L, Hanley M, Norton PT. Computed tomography angiography and magnetic resonance angiography imaging of the mesenteric vasculature. Tech Vasc Interv Radiol. 2015;18(1):2–13. https://doi.org/10.1053/j.tvir.2014.12.002.
40. Kles KA, Wallig MA, Tappenden KA. Luminal nutrients exacerbate intestinal hypoxia in the Hypoperfused jejunum. J Parenter Enter Nutr. 2001;25(5):246. https://doi.org/10.1177/0148607101025005246.
41. Cotter TG, Bledsoe AC, Sweetser S. Colon ischemia. Mayo Clin Proc. 2016;91(5):671. https://doi.org/10.1016/j.mayocp.2016.02.006.
42. Longstreth GF, Yao JF. Epidemiology, clinical features, high-risk factors, and outcome of acute large bowel ischemia. Clin Gastroenterol Hepatol. 2009;7(10):1075. https://doi.org/10.1016/j.cgh.2009.05.026.
43. Brandt LJ, Feuerstadt P, Longstreth GF, Boley SJ. ACG clinical guideline: epidemiology, risk factors, patterns of presentation, diagnosis, and Management of Colon Ischemia (CI). Am J Gastroenterol. 2015;110(1):18. https://doi.org/10.1038/ajg.2014.395.
44. Yadav S, Dave M, Edakkanambeth Varayil J, et al. A population-based study of incidence, risk factors, clinical Spectrum, and outcomes of ischemic colitis. Clin Gastroenterol Hepatol. 2015;13(4):731. https://doi.org/10.1016/j.cgh.2014.07.061.
45. Thuluvath AJ, Ahn JC, Rattan P, et al. Evaluation of Charcot triad, Reynolds pentad, and Tokyo guidelines for diagnosis of cholangitis secondary to Choledocholithiasis across patient age groups. Mayo Clin Proc Innov Qual Outcomes. 2021;5(2):377. https://doi.org/10.1016/j.mayocpiqo.2021.01.008.
46. Buxbaum JL, Buitrago C, Lee A, et al. ASGE guideline on the management of cholangitis. Gastrointest Endosc. 2021;94(2):207. https://doi.org/10.1016/j.gie.2020.12.032.
47. Gigot JF, Leese T, Dereme T, Coutinho J, Castaing D, Bismuth H. Acute cholangitis. Multivariate analysis of risk factors. Ann Surg. 1989;209(4):435. https://doi.org/10.1097/00000658-198904000-00008.
48. Soderlund C, Linder S. Covered metal versus plastic stents for malignant common bile duct stenosis: a prospective, randomized, controlled trial. Gastrointest Endosc. 2006;63(7):986. https://doi.org/10.1016/j.gie.2005.11.052.
49. Gomi H, Solomkin JS, Schlossberg D, et al. Tokyo guidelines 2018: antimicrobial therapy for acute cholangitis and cholecystitis. J Hepatobiliary Pancreat Sci. 2018;25(1):15. https://doi.org/10.1002/jhbp.518.
50. Kimura Y, Takada T, Kawarada Y, et al. Definitions, pathophysiology, and epidemiology of acute cholangitis and cholecystitis: Tokyo guidelines. J Hepato-Biliary-Pancreat Surg. 2007;14(1):15. https://doi.org/10.1007/s00534-006-1152-y.
51. Rumsey S, Winders J, MacCormick AD. Diagnostic accuracy of Charcot's triad: a systematic review. ANZ J Surg. 2017;87(4):232. https://doi.org/10.1111/ans.13907.
52. Wada K, Takada T, Kawarada Y, et al. Diagnostic criteria and severity assessment of acute cholangitis: Tokyo guidelines. J Hepato-Biliary-Pancreat Surg. 2007;14(1):52. https://doi.org/10.1007/s00534-006-1156-7.
53. Takada T, Strasberg SM, Solomkin JS, et al. TG13: updated Tokyo guidelines for the management of acute cholangitis and cholecystitis. J Hepatobiliary Pancreat Sci. 2013;20(1):1–7. https://doi.org/10.1007/s00534-012-0566-y.
54. Kiriyama S, Kozaka K, Takada T, et al. Tokyo guidelines 2018: diagnostic criteria and severity grading of acute cholangitis (with videos). J Hepatobiliary Pancreat Sci. 2018;25(1):17. https://doi.org/10.1002/jhbp.512.
55. Gravito-Soares E, Gravito-Soares M, Gomes D, Almeida N, Tomé L. Clinical applicability of Tokyo guidelines 2018/2013 in diagnosis and severity evaluation of acute cholangitis and determination of a new severity model. Scand J Gastroenterol. 2018;53(3):329. https://doi.org/10.1080/00365521.2018.1430255.
56. Gurusamy KS, Giljaca V, Takwoingi Y, et al. Ultrasound versus liver function tests for diagnosis of common bile duct stones.

Cochrane Database Syst Rev. 2015;26:CD011548. https://doi.org/10.1002/14651858.CD011548.
57. Kondo S, Isayama H, Akahane M, et al. Detection of common bile duct stones: comparison between endoscopic ultrasonography, magnetic resonance cholangiography, and helical-computed-tomographic cholangiography. Eur J Radiol. 2005;54(2):271. https://doi.org/10.1016/j.ejrad.2004.07.007.
58. Khashab MA, Tariq A, Tariq U, et al. Delayed and unsuccessful endoscopic retrograde Cholangiopancreatography are associated with worse outcomes in patients with acute cholangitis. Clin Gastroenterol Hepatol. 2012;10(10):1157. https://doi.org/10.1016/j.cgh.2012.03.029.
59. Polson J, Lee WM. AASLD position paper: the management of acute liver failure. Hepatology. 2005;41(5):1179. https://doi.org/10.1002/hep.20703.
60. Kwong AJ, Kim WR, Lake JR, et al. OPTN/SRTR 2019 annual data report: liver. Am J Transplant. 2021;21(Suppl 2):208. https://doi.org/10.1111/ajt.16494.
61. Bernal W, Wendon J. Acute Liver Failure. N Engl J Med. 2013;369(26):2525. https://doi.org/10.1056/NEJMra1208937.
62. Khashab M, Tector AJ, Kwo PY. Epidemiology of acute liver failure. Curr Gastroenterol Rep. 2007;9(1):66. https://doi.org/10.1007/s11894-008-0023-x.
63. European Association for the Study of the Liver. Electronic address: easloffice@easloffice.eu, Clinical practice guidelines panel, Wendon J, et al. EASL clinical practical guidelines on the management of acute (fulminant) liver failure. J Hepatol. 2017;66(5):1047. https://doi.org/10.1016/j.jhep.2016.12.003.
64. Fontana RJ. Acute liver failure due to drugs. Semin Liver Dis. 2008;28(2):175. https://doi.org/10.1055/s-2008-1073117.
65. Stravitz RT, Lee WM. Acute liver failure. Lancet. 2019;394(10201):869. https://doi.org/10.1016/S0140-6736(19)31894-X.
66. Nanchal R, Subramanian R, Karvellas CJ, et al. Guidelines for the Management of Adult Acute and Acute-on-Chronic Liver Failure in the ICU. Crit Care Med. 2020;48(3):e173–91. https://doi.org/10.1097/CCM.0000000000004192.
67. Bernal W, Hall C, Karvellas CJ, Auzinger G, Sizer E, Wendon J. Arterial ammonia and clinical risk factors for encephalopathy and intracranial hypertension in acute liver failure. Hepatology. 2007;46(6):1844. https://doi.org/10.1002/hep.21838.
68. de Las HJ, Aldámiz-Echevarría L, Martínez-Chantar ML, Delgado TC. An update on the use of benzoate, phenylacetate and phenylbutyrate ammonia scavengers for interrogating and modifying liver nitrogen metabolism and its implications in urea cycle disorders and liver disease. Expert Opin Drug Metab Toxicol. 2017;13(4):439. https://doi.org/10.1080/17425255.2017.1262843.
69. Kanjo A, Ocskay K, Gede N, et al. Efficacy and safety of liver support devices in acute and hyperacute liver failure: a systematic review and network meta-analysis. Sci Rep. 2021;11(1):4189. https://doi.org/10.1038/s41598-021-83292-z.
70. Murphy N, Auzinger G, Bernel W, Wendon J. The effect of hypertonic sodium chloride on intracranial pressure in patients with acute liver failure. Hepatology (Baltimore, MD). 2004;39(2):464. https://doi.org/10.1002/hep.20056.
71. Vaquero J, Fontana RJ, Larson AM, et al. Complications and use of intracranial pressure monitoring in patients with acute liver failure and severe encephalopathy. Liver Transpl. 2005;11(12):1581. https://doi.org/10.1002/lt.20625.
72. Lisman T, Caldwell SH, Burroughs AK, et al. Hemostasis and thrombosis in patients with liver disease: the ups and downs. J Hepatol. 2010;53(2):362. https://doi.org/10.1016/j.jhep.2010.01.042.
73. Harrison PM, Keays R, Bray GP, Alexander GJ, Williams R. Improved outcome of paracetamol-induced fulminant hepatic failure by late administration of acetylcysteine. Lancet (London, England). 1990;335(8705):1572. https://doi.org/10.1016/0140-6736(90)91388-q.
74. Lee WM, Hynan LS, Rossaro L, et al. Intravenous N-acetylcysteine improves transplant-free survival in early-stage non-acetaminophen acute liver failure. Gastroenterology. 2009;137(3):856. https://doi.org/10.1053/j.gastro.2009.06.006.

Fever and Therapeutic Hypothermia

19

Thanujaa Subramaniam, Melvin Parasram, Erin C. Barnes, John M. Picard, and Kevin N. Sheth

Contents

Abstract

Fever is a common phenomenon in the critical care setting but damaging to the injured brain. Therapeutic hypothermia (TH) is the intentional cooling of a patient by artificial means for a therapeutic purpose. Targeted Temperature Management (TTM) is the practice of setting a specified goal core temperature for the management of fever, maintaining normothermia, and induction of hypothermia. This chapter discusses fever and the use of TTM and TH in the neurocritical care unit for various neurological diseases. TTM in the context of post-cardiac arrest is addressed separately in another chapter. Basic definitions and methods for cooling are described and side effects of the use of TH are also presented. While this is an intriguing therapy with enormous potential, its efficacy for various neurologic diseases remains highly debated. In summary, this chapter will provide a review of the current literature and provide context for the use of TH and TTM in neurologically injured patients.

Introduction

Fever

Fever is a relatively common occurrence among critically ill patients, with one study noting fevers in up to 70% of patients during their hospital course [1]. While there is no universal threshold temperature for fever, a temperature greater than or equal to 38.3 °C is usually considered a fever in most intensive care units (ICUs) [2]. Fever is a physiologic response to stressors from infectious and noninfectious etiologies, which activate pyogenic and anti-pyretic pathways to increase the temperature set point in the hypothalamus [3]. The incidence

T. Subramaniam · M. Parasram · E. C. Barnes · J. M. Picard · K. N. Sheth (✉)
Division of Neurocritical Care and Emergency Neurology, Yale School of Medicine, New Haven, CT, USA
e-mail: thanujaa_subramaniam@brown.edu; Melvin.parasram@yale.edu; erin.barnes@yale.edu; kevin.sheth@yale.edu

E. Mahanna Gabrielli et al. (eds.), *Textbook of Neurointensive Care: Volume 1*, https://doi.org/10.1007/978-3-031-62220-5_19

of fevers in critically ill patients with acute neurological injury is 23–51% [4–6]. In a retrospective matched cohort study by Rincon et al. [4], critically ill neurological patients admitted to the ICU experienced more fevers when compared to non-neurological patients. Another study demonstrated that patients with traumatic brain injury (TBI) and aneurysmal subarachnoid hemorrhage (SAH) have higher rates of fevers compared to other acute neurological diagnoses [5].

In a subset of critically ill patients with central nervous system (CNS) injury, fever may be of central origin, also known as neurogenic fever. The concept of a neurogenic fever has been described for many years. It was first reported as a syndrome seen after brain surgery in 1939 by Ericson [7]. Neurogenic fever affects patients with severe CNS injuries, and is often associated with SAH, intraventricular hemorrhage (IVH), TBI, intracerebral hemorrhage (ICH), acute ischemic stroke (AIS), CNS proliferative processes, and acute spinal cord injury (SCI) [8]. Major characteristics of central fever include exclusion of other causes of fever, existing injury to thermoregulatory centers, higher body temperatures than those associated with infection, resistance to antipyretics, and lasting for several days to weeks [8]. The pathophysiology of neurogenic fever is not entirely understood, but lesions to the hypothalamus and thermoregulatory centers with corresponding elevations in prostaglandin E have been implicated.

Fever causes deleterious effects in the brain by promoting the release of excitotoxic neurotransmitters, inducing blood–brain barrier breakdown, increasing metabolic demand, and cerebral blood flow, which results in neuronal damage, elevated intracranial pressure (ICP), and brain ischemia [9]. Core body temperatures have been shown to correlate with brain temperatures that are, at times, 1–2 °C higher, and in the already injured brain, this temperature fluctuation can contribute to greater degrees of damage and ischemia [10]. In neurological patients, fever was independently associated with longer ICU stays, worse functional outcomes, and higher mortality rates [4, 11]. Thus, temperature management in the acutely ill neurological patient is an important consideration. However, whether there is a causal relationship between temperature elevations and mechanisms of injury is not clear, nor is the direction of causality if one exists. Preclinical and clinical observations are inconclusive to date.

Therapeutic Hypothermia and Targeted Temperature Management

Primary neurological injury in the critically ill patient may occur by trauma, hemorrhage, and/or ischemia, and is then followed by a cascade of events that contribute to secondary brain injury. When secondary brain injury is unmitigated, the initial injury can worsen and, in some cases, leads to further neurological deterioration. Secondary brain injury is thought to be caused by a combination of all or some of the following: blood brain barrier disruption, microthrombi, cerebral vasoconstriction, impaired cerebral autoregulation, development of cerebral edema, increased oxidized free radicals, induction of apoptosis, and decreased seizure threshold [12]. These processes are similar in most causes of neurological injury and have been shown to be temperature dependent—strikingly increased by hyperthermia and inhibited by mild hypothermia [13, 14]. In animal models, hypothermia reduces secondary cerebral injury by decreasing metabolic demand, reducing excitatory neurotransmitters, preventing formation of reactive oxygen species, decreasing inflammation, and maintaining integrity of the blood–brain barrier [15]. Table 19.1 provides a summary of the neuroprotective effects of hypothermia. The basis for the use of hypothermia for neuroprotection in humans is extrapolated from this data.

Therapeutic hypothermia (TH) is the intentional cooling of a patient for a specific therapeutic purpose. Hypothermia can be defined as body temperature less than 36 °C and can be further subdivided into mild TH (34–35.9 °C), moderate TH (32–33.9 °C), moderate/deep TH (30–31.9 °C) and deep TH (<30 °C) [14]. Targeted temperature management (TTM) is the more general term describing the practice of setting a specified goal temperature and actively treating a patient to achieve and maintain that set temperature with the aid of protocols and devices. TTM has been used prophylactically, immediately after the occurrence of brain injury, or therapeutically, as an intervention to treat fevers or various pathological state due to secondary brain injury.

The earliest observations of the neuroprotective effects of TH were made by Fay in 1943 [16]. He noted improved outcomes in patients with brain injury when they were cooled to 28–32 °C [16, 17]. In the 1950s, detailed experiments by Bigelow et al. [18] and Rosomoff et al. [19] showed neuroprotective effects of TH in surgical animal models. By the 1960s, several case reports of clinical use of TH during neurosurgical procedures were published highlighting its benefits [20–23]. Spencer et al. [24] used TH at 30–34 °C in 4 comatose survivors after cardiac arrest and reported complete recovery in 3 of these patients. Subsequently, interest in TH waned due to difficulty in managing the adverse effects of hypothermia, such as coagulopathy, electrolyte abnormalities, cardiac arrythmias, and infection [17].

Renewed interest in clinical use of TH occurred in the 1990s after publication of a randomized controlled trial (RCT) comparing TH and normothermia after TBI, which showed a trend towards improved outcomes in the moderate hypothermia group [25]. In 2002, two landmark randomized controlled trials using TH (32–34 °C for 12–24 h) in out-of-hospital comatose cardiac arrest survivors with

Table 19.1 Neuroprotective effects of hypothermia

Factor	Pathophysiology after injury	Neuroprotection with hypothermia
Early mechanisms: Minutes to hours after injury		
Mitochondrial function	Cerebral injury leads to mitochondrial dysfunction and dysregulated energy homeostasis	Hypothermia reduces mitochondrial injury and improves energy homoeostasis
Cerebral metabolism	Increased cerebral blood flow and increased glucose and oxygen consumption which leads to anaerobic glycolysis and increased lactate	Cellular oxygen and glucose requirements decrease by 6–10% per 1 °C below 37 °C
ATPase pump and calcium ion homeostasis	Cerebral hypoxia leads to loss of ATP and results in dysfunction in the ATP-dependent Na-K pumps in the cell membrane. This dysfunction increases calcium influx leading to release of glutamate and subsequent excitotoxic injury	Hypothermia prevents depletion of ATP and decreases ATPase pump dysfunction which reduces calcium influx and prevents excitotoxic injury
Cytotoxic edema	ATPase pump dysfunction and cellular membrane damage leads to cytotoxic edema	Hypothermia decreases cell membrane leakage and formation of cytotoxic edema
Free radical formation	After injury, there is an increased production of superoxide (O_2^-), peroxynitrite (NO_2^-), hydrogen peroxide (H_2O_2), and hydroxyl radicals (OH^-), which oxidize and damage numerous cellular components	Core body temperatures of 30–35 °C prevents free radical formation that is common after ischemic injury
Late mechanisms: Hours to days/weeks after injury		
Apoptosis	Caspases, cysteine proteases which execute apoptosis, are upregulated after cerebral injury and ischemia	Caspases are reduced up to 1 week after induced hypothermia in animal studies
Blood brain barrier permeability	Disruption of BBB and increased vascular permeability occurs after injury leading to increased cerebral edema	Hypothermia stabilizes BBB integrity and decreases vascular permeability which results in reduced cerebral edema
Neuroinflammation	Cerebral injury activates an inflammatory cascade which involves the production of proinflammatory cytokines (IL-1, MMP, TNFa). This inflammatory state results in secondary brain injury	Hypothermia reduces inflammatory reactions and decreases release of proinflammatory cytokines, preventing further injury
Epileptic activity	Seizures are common after primary brain injury and cause secondary injury	Numerous animal and clinical studies have shown cessation and reduction of seizures with hypothermia
Reperfusion injury	Reperfusion after initial brain injury leads to secondary injury	Hypothermia mitigates reperfusion injury by improving brain tolerance for ischemia
Coagulation	Microthrombus formation commonly occurs after cardiopulmonary resuscitation, which may play a role in secondary injury	Hypothermia induces anticoagulation effects
Cerebral Thermo-pooling	Normally, brain temperature is 1–2 °C higher than core temperature. Brain injury results in higher gradient of temperature difference, up to 2–4 °C. Higher brain temperature prompts secondary injury	Hypothermia reduces cerebral thermo-pooling, resulting in reduced secondary injury
Gene expression	Heat shock proteins are upregulated in hyperthermic states after ischemic injury, which expands ischemic core	Hypothermia increases the expression of genes which upregulate cold shock proteins that protects cells from further ischemic and traumatic injury
Cortical spreading depression-like depolarization	Cortical spreading depression-like depolarization increases neuronal damage after primary brain injury	Hypothermia reduces spreading depolarizations which protect neurons from further injury

initial shockable rhythms showed significant survival and functional outcomes benefit in the TH group compared with the normothermia group [26, 27]. The positive impact of these two trials resulted in the standardization of care for the use of TH for neuroprotection in out-of-hospital comatose cardiac arrest survivors from shockable rhythms by the Task Force of the International Liaison Committee on Resuscitation (ILCOR) [28] and the American Heart Association (AHA) [29].

The therapeutic neuroprotective benefits of TH in survivors of cardiac arrest have led to the evaluation of TH in other acute neurological disease states. This chapter will comprehensively review the pathophysiology and the management of fever in the critically ill neurological patient, the neuroprotective effects of TH, and the use of TH in various acute neurological disease states.

Disease States (See Table 19.2)

Acute Ischemic Stroke

Prior research has suggested that fever adversely influences outcomes in AIS patients, likely in part due to oxidative stress and increased metabolic demand in penumbral tissue. In a large retrospective cohort study of fever in brain injury patients, a subgroup analysis revealed AIS patients with fever had the highest risk of death when compared with patients with ICH, TBI, and SAH [5]. Similarly, in a meta-analysis by Greer et al., of 39 studies reviewed, those focusing exclusively on AIS more consistently demonstrated a relationship between fever and outcome measures, including both higher mortality and lower Glasgow Outcome Scale (GOS) scores [11]. A more recent retrospective cohort study examined the body temperature trends of AIS patients in the first 24 h after endovascular therapy [30]. Investigators concluded that peak body temperature ≥ 37.5 °C led to a reduction in functional independence while peak body temperature ≥ 38 °C was significantly associated with poor 3-month outcomes.

Table 19.2 Summary of Guideline Statements and Recommendations for Each Disease State

Disease States	Summary of Guideline Statements and Recommendations
Acute ischemic stroke	NCS: Strong recommendation for controlled normothermia to "reduce fever burden in patients with fever refractory to conventional therapy." no recommendation regarding therapeutic hypothermia AHA/ASA: Prompt identification of hyperthermia and its potential sources and the use of antipyretic medications. Benefit of treatment with therapeutic hypothermia is uncertain
Intracerebral hemorrhage	AHA/ASA: Treatment of fever may be reasonable. Benefit of treatment with therapeutic hypothermia is uncertain
Subarachnoid Hemorrhage	NCS: Strong recommendation for fever control during the period of high delayed cerebral ischemia risk. No recommendation regarding therapeutic hypothermia AHA/ASA: Aggressive control of fever to a target of normothermia is reasonable in the acute phase. No recommendation regarding therapeutic hypothermia
Traumatic brain injury	NCS: Conditional recommendation for the use of longer duration TTM for ICP control in severe TBI. No recommendation for prophylactic application of therapeutic hypothermia BTF: Level IIB recommendation that early (within 2.5 h), short-term (48 h post-injury) prophylactic hypothermia is not recommended to improve outcomes
Status epilepticus	No guideline recommendations: Limited clinical data to support the use of controlled normothermia or hypothermia
Spinal cord injury	No guideline recommendations: Limited clinical data to support the use of controlled normothermia or hypothermia

Regarding temperature management in ischemic stroke, most studies to date have focused on the role of TH as opposed to controlled normothermia. Schwab et al. conducted an early study on TH in patients with severe middle cerebral artery (MCA) territory infarction by inducing hypothermia to 33 °C and maintaining this temperature for 72 h [31]. Mortality was 44% and survivors had a favorable outcome by Barthel index assessment. Of note, investigators identified risk for a secondary rise in ICP during rewarming which required additional treatment with osmotherapy. Similar results were reported in a multicenter, prospective observational study involving 50 patients with at least complete MCA territory infarction and the initiation of TH to 33 °C [32]. Mortality was 38% with 30% of patients dying during the rewarming phase secondary to ICP crisis. In the Cooling for Acute Ischemic Brain Damage (COOL AID) 1 study [33], patients were randomized to hypothermia (32 ± 1 °C) or standard of care with duration of TH determined by assessment of culprit vessel patency by posttreatment angiogram or transcranial doppler sonography. Of note, all patients undergoing TH were endotracheally intubated and mechanically ventilated to allow for aggressive management of shivering. Results showed no significant difference in Modified Rankin Scale (mRS) at 3 months between the two groups, and mortality rate was comparable. In a follow-up study, De Georgia et al. [34] demonstrated the feasibility and safety of endovascular cooling to 33 °C; however, similarly, there was no significant difference between the hypothermia and control groups in diffusion weighted imaging (DWI) lesion growth or mRS scores at 1 month.

For patients with large hemispheric infarction (LHI), defined as infarct involving at least 2/3 MCA territory, several studies have explored whether TH could be an adjunct or even an alternative to decompressive hemicraniectomy. In one study, a total of 36 patients with LHI were treated with hemicraniectomy or moderate hypothermia [35]. Mortality was 12% for hemicraniectomy and 47% for moderate hypothermia. Of those receiving TH, one died of septic shock and three due to ICP crisis during rewarming. Els et al. [36] randomized 25 patients with LHI to hemicraniectomy alone or to the combination of hemicraniectomy and TH to 35 °C for 48 h. The investigators observed a tendency to lower mortality at 6 months in the combination group and concluded that TH may be useful in this population. Similarly, Su et al. [37] randomized patients with LHI to either endovascular cooling (goal 33–34 °C) or normothermia. Mortality was similar in both groups, but survivors treated with hypothermia achieved better neurologic outcomes at 6 months. Of note, there were significantly more complications in the hypothermia group including electrolyte disorders, gastrointestinal bleeding, gastric retention, and stress hyperglycemia. In contrast, the more recently published Decompressive Surgery Plus Hypothermia for Space-Occupying Stroke (DEPTH-SOS), a multicenter RCT found that moderate hypothermia early after hemicraniectomy did not improve mortality or functional outcome when compared to standard of care. In fact, it was concluded that TH may cause harm as rates of serious adverse events were 80% in the hypothermia group and 43% in the standard care (hemicraniectomy alone) group [38, 39].

Additional studies on TH in AIS have had mixed results. Some have identified a trend toward better outcomes in patients managed with TH. Hong et al. [40] randomized patients after successful endovascular recanalization (TICI ≥2b) within 6 h of symptom onset to cooling (34.5–35 °C) for 48 h or normothermia. Investigators reported improved outcomes (mRS 0–2) in the hypothermia group at 3 months, as well as less hemorrhagic transformation and less cerebral edema. Other studies, however, have revealed higher rates of adverse events (most notably pneumonia) and little evidence to suggest an outcome benefit to TH. Studies by Geurts et al. [41], Lyden et al. [42], and Piironen et al. [43] revealed an increased risk of pneumonia with TH. Ovesen et al. [44] and Hemmen et al. [45] utilized endovascular cooling and concluded no clear benefit of TH with regards to mRS and mortality.

The 2017 Neurocritical Care Society (NCS) guideline on TTM [46] recommends the use of controlled normothermia to "reduce fever burden in patients with fever refractory to conventional therapy." Similarly, American Heart Association/American Stroke Association (AHA/ASA) guidelines [47] recommend prompt identification of fever (>38 °C) and its potential sources and the use of antipyretic medications for treatment. It is worth noting that no definitive studies to date have shown improved post-discharge outcome in a clinical trial which treats fever. A recently completed study, Impact of Fever Prevention in Brain Injured Patients (INTREPID) may help shed some light. The trial aimed to assess neurologic outcomes in patients who underwent fever prevention with an advanced temperature management device. Patients were assigned to either prophylactic TTM or reactive treatment of fever following a stepwise algorithm (*ClinicalTrials.gov Identifier: NCT02996266*) [48]. Results from this study are greatly anticipated.

Current guidelines from NCS and AHA/ASA reflect the uncertainty surrounding the use of TH in the management of AIS with NCS providing no recommendation and AHA/ASA stating uncertain benefits for TH in AIS.

Intracerebral Hemorrhage

As in AIS, fever in primary ICH has been associated with suboptimal outcomes. In a study by Schwarz et al. [49], of 251 patients with spontaneous supratentorial ICH, fever occurred in almost all (91%) patients during the first 72 h after hospitalization. Moreover, duration of fever in the first 72 h was found to be an independent prognostic factor. Similarly, Leira et al. [50] reported that body temperature > 37.5 °C was an independent predictor of early neurologic deterioration, with worsening of stroke scale assessments between admission and 48 h.

When ictus of ICH has resolved and hematoma growth stabilized, secondary injury remains a concern due to perihematomal edema (PHE) formation and progression with increased ICP [51, 52]. It is unclear to what extent TTM can mitigate secondary injury due to PHE. In animal models of ICH, there has been a suggested benefit of TH at a molecular level, but an observed lack of effect when considering measures of clinical improvement.

Several clinical trials have explored the use of both controlled normothermia and TH in the management of primary ICH. In a prospective, randomized controlled trial by Broessner et al. [53], 102 patients (40% of whom had spontaneous ICH) were randomized to either conventional fever management or prophylactic TTM with a goal of normothermia (36.5 °C). Investigators successfully and safely achieved normothermia in the treatment group with a significant reduction in fever burden; however, there was no clear difference in neurologic outcome at 6-month follow-up. Lord et al. [54] concluded in a retrospective case-control study that while the mean daily maximum temperature was significantly higher in a control group versus a matched controlled normothermia group, there was no difference in discharge outcomes. Additionally, the controlled normothermia group had more days of intravenous sedation, mechanical ventilation, and more frequently underwent tracheostomy.

With regard to TH in ICH, Kollmar et al. [55] found that PHE remained stable over 14 days in patients treated with TH to 35 °C but increased significantly in a matched control group. Staykov et al. [56] controlled 25 patients at 35 °C for 8–10 days following presentation with large supratentorial ICH via endovascular cooling catheters. Compared to historical controls, a significant difference was found in the extent of PHE between the two groups with largely stable PHE during hospitalization for those undergoing TH. Volbers et al. [57] found in a retrospective case-control study that while early TH to 35 °C led to a relative decrease in PHE between admission and day 3 compared to control and late TH groups, PHE increased in all groups after day 3. Moreover, there was no clear difference in functional outcomes between groups.

Current guidelines on spontaneous ICH from AHA/ASA [58] state that "treatment of fever may be reasonable." Similar to ischemic stroke, no clinical trials have yet to show improved post-discharge outcomes from fever treatment. This may be in part because we have yet to identify the appropriate outcomes of interest to measure, or we have yet to identify the subgroup of patients who might benefit the most. TH for ICH is still considered largely investigational.

Subarachnoid Hemorrhage

Fever is associated with poor outcomes in aneurysmal SAH [11, 59–62], and TTM may play a role in mitigating secondary brain injury. Douds et al. [63] demonstrated that aneurysmal SAH patients with just 1–2 days of fever were less likely to have a favorable outcome when compared to patients who remained afebrile throughout the hospital course. It remains unclear if fever is a marker of injury severity or an independent factor influencing outcome. More recently, a case-control study by Badjatia et al. [64] compared the outcomes of febrile patients with nontraumatic SAH who underwent either conventional fever control (acetaminophen ± cooling blanket) or TTM with surface cooling and goal normothermia (37 °C) for 7 days. The investigators found that the average daily fever burden was significantly lower for those patients undergoing controlled normothermia. In outcomes assessment, TTM was associated with a significantly reduced risk for poor outcome at 12 months, but not at 14 days or 3 months. The lack of improved outcome at 14 days and 3 months was felt to be reflective of longer ICU length of stay due to the need for prolonged sedation for control of shivering and higher rates of tracheostomy in the TTM group.

Studies investigating TH in SAH are few. Gasser et al. [65] performed a feasibility study and treated 21 patients with poor-grade SAH (Hunt & Hess grade 4 or 5) with TH to goal 33–34 °C combined with barbiturate coma given severe brain edema and elevated ICP after early aneurysm clipping. A GOS of 4–5 was achieved in 48% of patients at 3 months. Todd et al. [66] assigned low-grade SAH patients to intraoperative hypothermia (33 °C) or normothermia (36.5 °C) during aneurysm clipping. There was no difference in the GOS between the two groups at 90 days post-surgery but there was a higher rate of bacteremia in the hypothermia group than in the normothermia group.

The 2011 NCS guideline on SAH management [67] strongly recommends fever control during the period of high delayed cerebral ischemia (DCI) risk. TH is not discussed as a treatment modality to improve outcomes. Similarly, the AHA/ASA [68] states that aggressive control of fever to a target of normothermia is reasonable in the acute phase of SAH. There seem to be a paucity of good quality studies examining the benefit of prophylactic fever prevention or TH in the SAH patient population.

Traumatic Brain Injury

Fever after TBI is associated with prolonged intensive care unit stays and higher patient mortality rates, although a causal link has yet to be established [69, 70]. It is worth noting that aside from cardiac arrest, TBI is the most studied clinical condition in relation to the therapeutic effects of hypothermia. Hypothermia in TBI has been investigated as a prophylactic application, i.e., immediately post-injury and as a treatment applied therapeutically to address various pathological states following TBI such as ICP. Historically, a large body of laboratory research involving multiple models and species have demonstrated compelling results for neuroprotection, particularly when delivered early [71]. Unfortunately, these highly encouraging results have not borne out in a similar fashion in the clinical world.

Over the last two decades, several large multicenter trials failed to show an effect on mortality or functional outcome with TH in TBI [72]. A recent meta-analysis by Chen et al. [73] involving 23 major trials concluded that induced hypothermia did not reduce but may increase mortality rate of patients with TBI, with the caveat that the population of TBI patients with elevated ICP could benefit from hypothermia when used therapeutically. The Brain Trauma Foundation (BTF) 2016 guideline [74] provides a level IIB recommendation that early (within 2.5 h), short-term (48 h post-injury) prophylactic hypothermia is not recommended to improve outcomes in patients with diffuse injury, while acknowledging that there is insufficient data to guide level I or IIA recommendations. The 2017 NCS guideline [46] provides a conditional recommendation for the use of longer duration TTM for ICP control in severe TBI patients but has no recommendation for prophylactic hypothermia.

One key criticism of these previously conducted clinical trials was the lack of early application of hypothermia. Prophylactic Hypothermia Trial to Lessen Traumatic Brain Injury—Randomized Clinical Trial (POLAR-RCT) [75] was a well-designed, international, multi-center study in 2018 involving 511 patients that attempted to address the issue of early hypothermic application. Patients were randomized to receive either hypothermia or normothermia. In the intervention group, hypothermia was induced and maintained for 72 h at 33 °C (or 35 °C if there were concerns for bleeding) and initiated either in the out-of-hospital setting before arrival or in the emergency department. A key point in this study was the initiation of intervention as early as possible regardless of intracranial pressure. Results from this trial did not show a difference in long-term favorable functional outcomes between treatment and control group in patients with moderate and severe TBI. Additionally, there were no significant differences in the secondary outcomes and there was an increased risk of pneumonia among those who received hypothermia. Another critique was TH was generally applied for less than 72 h in most trials which may be an interval too short to cover the entirety of secondary brain injury following TBI. A recent RCT by Hui et al. [76] examined the safety and efficacy of long-term mild hypothermia (5 days) and did not find improvements in neurological outcomes at 6 months for the hypothermic group when compared to the normothermic group. However, patients with ICP > 30 mmHg did have significantly increased favorable outcomes compared to the normothermia group.

It is unclear why hypothermia has failed in translation from the bench to the bedside. Differences in animal versus human brain, imbalances in co-interventions between the groups, time taken to achieve hypothermia in humans are some of the proposed theories for this observed discrepancy [77]. In summary, fever should be avoided in TBI patients and extensive efforts should be made to maintain normothermia. Further, there is no clinical evidence currently to support the broad application of induced hypothermia for TBI patients, particularly when it is applied prophylactically. However, hypothermia can be considered on a case-by-case basis to treat manifestations of secondary brain injury following TBI such as refractory ICP issues or evidence of brain metabolic crisis via invasive multimodal monitoring, while taking into consideration other medical and surgical issues inherent to trauma patients.

Status Epilepticus

Status epilepticus (SE) carries a high mortality rate and frequently fails to respond to conventional treatments. In refractory SE, treatment often involves a combination of several antiseizure drugs, benzodiazepines and anesthetics infusions, which can cause substantial side effects. Additionally, 8–21% of SE patients develop super refractory SE, requiring alternate and high-risk treatments such as induced pentobarbital coma, electroconvulsive therapy, or inhaled anesthetic agents [78].

While the aggravating effect of hyperthermia on seizure activity is well known, there has been growing interest in hypothermia as an alternative therapy to treat refractory seizures. Animal studies have provided strong experimental evidence supporting the anticonvulsant and neuroprotective effects of hypothermia in SE [79]. These experimental models used a wide variety of temperatures and applied hypothermia prophylactically or during the ictal phase [79].

Clinical research on TH in SE has been limited to case reports/series and one RCT. Reports describing successful use of TH involved pediatric and adult population with hypothermia applied to patients with highly refractory epileptic activity that remained uncontrolled despite extensive pharmacological treatment [79]. The one RCT was designed to investigate the potential neuroprotective effects of therapeutic hypothermia in adults with convulsive SE. Patients were randomized to treatment with or without hypothermia (32 and 34 °C) for 24 h. Functional outcomes assessed at 90 days did not differ between groups, but TH was significantly associated with less progression to SE in patients with coma [80].

The available clinical research suggests that the temperatures needed to achieve burst suppression vary from patient to patient but generally tend to be colder than mild hypothermia. If a patient cannot tolerate induction of burst suppression with pentobarbital or all other treatments have failed, the use of TH can be considered to control brain activity. However, the use of TH must be tempered with the caveat that the deeper a patient is cooled, the greater the potential for side effects. Overall, refractory SE is associated with high mortality, and the limited available literature suggests that TH can be effective in controlling seizures but is not without the potential for harm in this patient population.

Spinal Cord Injury

Animal studies for SCI are largely focused on TH, with mixed evidence supporting its beneficial effect. Overall, animal studies of hypothermia after SCI encompass various animal models, mechanisms, and severity of cord injury, with variations in the timing, duration, and depth of hypothermia, complicating its interpretation [81].

From a clinical standpoint, Levi et al. [82] reported a series of 14 patients with acute, complete cervical SCI who underwent TH to 33 °C via an intravascular cooling catheter. The investigators determined that the approach was safe and found that six of the 14 patients (42.8%) improved to incomplete cord injury by follow-up. Moreover, Dididze et al. [83] performed a case-control study of 35 patients with acute cervical SCI with International Standards for Neurological Classification of Spinal Cord Injury (ISNCSCI) grade A who underwent TH to goal 33 °C via intravascular cooling. They found that 35% of cervical ISNCSCI A patients improved by at least one grade with a low risk of systemic complications. Finally, local hypothermia was explored by Hansebout et al. [84] using an intraoperative extradural saddle with localized cord cooling to a dural temperature of 6 °C for 4 h. The investigators reported that 80% of the 20 enrolled patients (12 cervical and 4 thoracic) with an initially complete cord injury (ASIA A) had some recovery of sensory or motor function.

Overall, guidelines at this time have indicated that there is little available clinical data to support the use of either systemic or local hypothermia in the management of acute SCI [81].

Management

Given the impact of fever, a thorough evaluation for underlying causes should be pursued. An infectious workup, a review of medications to assess for the possibility of drug fever, as well as consideration of studies to assess for other causes of fevers such as deep vein thrombosis, pulmonary embolism, and/or acalculous cholecystitis should be done. While pursuing fever etiology, efforts to defervesce the patient should occur in tandem. First line treatments include antipyretics (acetaminophen, non-steroidal anti-inflammatory drugs) and nonpharmacological methods. Should the fever prove difficult to control with these standard methods, normothermia can be enforced with more advanced TTM techniques.

The means by which body temperature can be lowered range from conventional cooling blankets, ice packs, and chilled intravenous fluids to more active methods that allow for automated feedback and adjustments to achieve their temperature goals. Ice packs and cooling blankets are easily applied and entail lower costs, however, a survey of ICU nursing found that ice packs and cooling blankets are generally less efficacious for temperature maintenance and more labor intensive to maintain than modern methods for temperature management [85]. More technologically advanced methods of temperature management modern devices were found to be more effective in temperature maintenance with less workload on ICU nursing [85]. Modern devices target and control core temperature by means of a feedback loop, i.e. when the core body temperature is not equal to the target temperature, the device adjusts its settings accordingly, either providing warmth or cool to get the body to the desired temperature.

There are a variety methods by which temperature management devices operate; more popular methods use surface gel pads and intravascular catheters. There are also less frequently used devices, such as intranasal and esophageal devices, with many more in development [86]. In general, these devices allow for faster time to target temperature and offer a higher likelihood of success in achieving target temperature when compared to standard methods. Investigators have tried to determine the best advanced cooling method to use for TTM, but while some studies trend toward favoring the intravascular cooling catheter devices for cardiac arrest patients, there does not yet exist robust data to support one of these methods over another as superior in terms of clinical outcomes [46, 86, 87]. Additionally, there is a low, but non-zero, risk of catheter associated deep vein thrombosis as well as catheter associated line infection with intravascular cooling devices [88].

Special consideration should be given to patients with suspected fever of central origin. Various case studies have invoked the use of bromocriptine, propranolol, baclofen, and other agents to control this entity. However, there is no robust evidence to suggest the superiority of any single agent [89].

Shivering

In the human body, there exists a thermoregulatory set-point within the pre-optic and anterior hypothalamic region that works to maintain the body at a set temperature window [10]. Chemicals released in the inflammatory cascade as a response to infection or stressors, or injury to the thermoregulatory regions of the brain themselves can cause an increase in this "set-point" causing fever [10]. Core body temperatures lower than the normal "set-point" of 36.5–37.5 °C trigger a shivering response, which in TTM actively works against the device to try to raise the body temperature, increasing metabolic demand of the brain and body, and negating the benefits of TTM [90].

The Bedside Shivering Assessment Scale (BSAS) is a simple 4-point bedside scale widely used for the evaluation shivering with high interobserver reliability and validity [91]. The BSAS assesses for shivering in muscles, which allows for quantification of the metabolic impact of shivering (Table 19.3) [91]. Given the deleterious effects of shivering, which works against TTM, therapeutics are used to counteract it. For all patients undergoing TTM, a stepwise, protocoled approach based on an objective measurement of shivering (BSAS score) is recommended to combat shivering [46]. Firstly, skin counter-warming is recommended in all patients undergoing TTM. This measure is exceptionally beneficial as a first step as it helps to decrease the shivering threshold by as much as 1 °C [92]. Other baseline interventions with little risk to the patient include around the clock acetaminophen as well as administration of magnesium sulfate to target a serum range between 3 and 4 mg/dL which acts by reducing smooth muscle tone and incidence of shivering [92]. Figure 19.1 includes a flow chart for shivering management based on the Columbia anti-shivering protocol.

Table 19.3 The Bedside Shivering Assessment Scale (BSAS)

Score	Severity of shivering	Location
None	0	No shivering is detected
Mild	1	Shivering localized to the neck and thorax
Moderate	2	Shivering involves gross movements of the upper extremities, including neck and thorax
Severe	3	Shivering involves gross movements of the trunk, upper and lower extremities

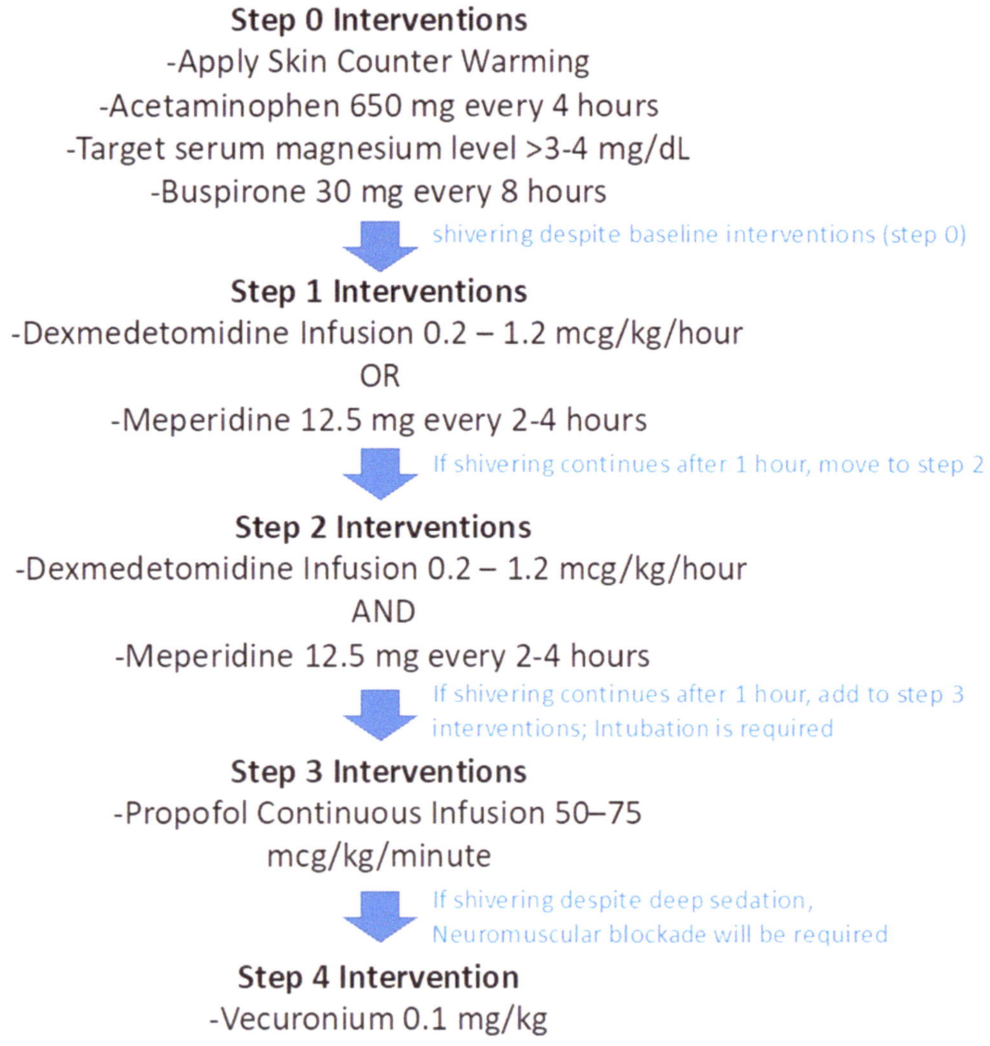

Fig. 19.1 Shivering Management based on the Columbia Anti Shivering Protocol

Other commonly used pharmacological agents to prevent shivering include buspirone and meperidine. Buspirone alone has a modest effect on lowering the shivering threshold, but in low doses and in conjunction with low dose meperidine, a synergistic effect is seen, and the shivering threshold can be lowered by as much as 2 °C [93]. A similar effect is seen with dexmedetomidine and meperidine, as well as dexmedetomidine and buspirone [94]. When these agents are ineffective, intermittent dosing or infusions of opioids or intravenous anesthetics, are next line [92]. In general, when choosing an opioid or sedative drip for shivering management in TTM, it is advisable to choose a drug with a short half-life, as longer-acting drugs have been associated with delayed reawakening and more days on ventilator. Lastly, neuromuscular blockade can be considered as an additional method to stop shivering in patients undergoing TTM. While highly effective at stopping shivering, the associated risks of neuromuscular blockade, including the risk for critical illness neuromyopathy should be considered [92].

Stöckl et al. randomized all patients presenting within 6 h of cardiac arrest and starting on TTM to on-demand rocuronium by bolus vs. continuous infusion of rocuronium, in addition to baseline infusions of midazolam and fentanyl [95]. This study found that the group that was placed on continuously infused rocuronium received increased total doses of neuromuscular blockade but experienced decreased shivering events, decreased time in the ICU, decreased exposure to fentanyl and midazolam, and decreased time to awakening without clear harm [95]. This study challenges the presumption that neuromuscular blockade should be avoided until other agents have failed, and while this one study should be taken into consideration against existing consensus, it is intriguing and worth investigating early neuromuscular blockade with future studies.

Other Management Considerations

When artificially changing body temperatures, there should be careful monitoring for potassium shifts, as hypothermia induces hypokalemia and rewarming can cause rebound hyperkalemia, putting the patient at risk for dysrhythmias [46, 96]. As such, NCS recommends that during induction and maintenance phases of TTM, potassium levels are maintained between 3.0 and 3.5 mmol/L [46].

Bleeding and coagulopathies are of concern during induced hypothermia; temperatures below 35 °C are known to influence platelet function and the coagulation pathway. Despite higher rates of thrombocytopenia, two meta-analyses in cardiac arrest populations treated with TTM found no difference in bleeding rates [97, 98]. Similarly, in patient populations undergoing therapeutic hypothermia for AIS and TBI, there was no demonstrable increased risk of bleeding or hemorrhagic complications in these populations while undergoing therapeutic hypothermia [42].

Providers should maintain vigilance for underlying infectious processes with patients undergoing TTM. While there is no significant difference in the rates of infection between critically ill patients on TTM and those not on TTM, with advanced cooling devices it may not always be readily evident when a patient is trying to mount a fever. Some institutions practice monitoring water temperatures on certain TTM devices; water temperatures below a certain threshold suggest a mounting fever (or shivering) and this can serve as a method to trigger infectious workup, though this is not a practice that has been broadly investigated [46]. Lastly, patients undergoing TTM may be at increased risk of skin complications due to immobility and the contact of cooling devices with the skin.

Conclusions

Fever is independently associated with worsened morbidity and mortality in patients with acute neurologic injury. Accordingly, fever treatment and emphasis on maintaining normothermia is an important aspect in the management of neurocritical care patients. This can be achieved with various pharmacologic and non-pharmacologic interventions. When applying interventions to lower body temperatures, special consideration should be given to potential side effects and management of shivering.

TH as a treatment modality for neurocritical care disease has garnered much interest for almost 60 years, stemming from early laboratory research showing its tremendous potential for neuroprotection and prevention of secondary brain injury. Given its pleiotropic effects, TH has the potential to treat a wide variety of neurological conditions; however, measuring its true clinical impact can be a challenging task. Extensive laboratory and animal studies have shown that fever prevention and TH in acute neurological injury may provide neuroprotective effects by mitigating secondary brain injury. However, the clinical data describing the use of induced hypothermia in various neurologic diseases described in this chapter have shown equivocal, if not contradictory, results. It is possible that these neurological conditions may respond differently to timing of hypothermia induction and maintenance, varying temperature set-point targets, and different rewarming strategies. Additionally, strict management of complications of cooling and rewarming is necessary to limit adverse effects, which, if not well controlled, may play a role in negative outcomes.

In summary, most guidelines recommend prompt treatment of fever in acute neurological disease and various clinical reports have suggested possible prevention of neurological deterioration with fever control. However, it is worth noting that aggressive fever treatment has not yet been conclusively shown to have a durable effect on clinical outcomes. It is likely that we have yet to identify the subgroup of patients who might benefit the most from this intervention or the appropriate outcomes of interest to measure.

With regards to therapeutic hypothermia, most guidelines cannot provide recommendations or advise against induced hypothermia for acute neurological injuries other than in the post-cardiac arrest setting. However, there are certain circumstances that TH may be beneficial, such as treating refractory ICP in TBI patients. For several neurological diseases described in this chapter, more well-designed trials are needed to assess the clinical impact of therapeutic hypothermia. Further research should aim to refine understanding of which pathophysiological state could benefit most from TH or strict normothermia, perhaps with the aid of invasive multimodal monitoring tools.

References

1. Circiumaru B, Baldock G, Cohen J. A prospective study of fever in the intensive care unit. Intensive Care Med. 1999;25(7):668–73. https://doi.org/10.1007/s001340050928.
2. O'Grady NP, Barie PS, Bartlett JG, Bleck T, Carroll K, Kalil AC, et al. Guidelines for evaluation of new fever in critically ill adult patients: 2008 update from the American College of Critical Care Medicine and the Infectious Diseases Society of America. Crit Care Med. 2008;36(4):1330–49. https://doi.org/10.1097/CCM.0b013e318169eda9.
3. Niven DJ, Laupland KB. Pyrexia: aetiology in the ICU. Crit Care. 2016;20(1):247. https://doi.org/10.1186/s13054-016-1406-2.
4. Rincon F, Patel U, Schorr C, Lee E, Ross S, Dellinger RP, et al. Brain injury as a risk factor for fever upon admission to the intensive care unit and association with in-hospital case fatality: a matched cohort study. J Intensive Care Med. 2015;30(2):107–14. https://doi.org/10.1177/0885066613508266.
5. Rincon F, Hunter K, Schorr C, Dellinger RP, Zanotti-Cavazzoni S. The epidemiology of spontaneous fever and hypothermia on admission of brain injury patients to intensive care units: a multicenter cohort study. J Neurosurg. 2014;121(4):950–60. https://doi.org/10.3171/2014.7.Jns132470.

6. Commichau C, Scarmeas N, Mayer SA. Risk factors for fever in the neurologic intensive care unit. Neurology. 2003;60(5):837–41. https://doi.org/10.1212/01.wnl.0000047344.28843.eb.
7. Erickson TC. Neurogenic hyperthermia (a clinical syndrome and its treatment). Brain. 1939;62(2):172–90.
8. Zawadzka M, Szmuda M, Mazurkiewicz-Bełdzińska M. Thermoregulation disorders of central origin - how to diagnose and treat. Anaesthesiol Intensive Ther. 2017;49(3):227–34. https://doi.org/10.5603/ait.2017.0042.
9. Chavali S, Tripathi M, Rajagopalan V. Fever in the Neurointensive care unit. J Neuroanaesth Crit Care. 2019;6:275. https://doi.org/10.1055/s-0039-3399399.
10. Childs C. Human brain temperature: regulation, measurement and relationship with cerebral trauma: part 1. Br J Neurosurg. 2008;22(4):486–96. https://doi.org/10.1080/02688690802245541.
11. Greer DM, Funk SE, Reaven NL, Ouzounelli M, Uman GC. Impact of fever on outcome in patients with stroke and neurologic injury: a comprehensive meta-analysis. Stroke. 2008;39(11):3029–35. https://doi.org/10.1161/strokeaha.108.521583.
12. Sekhon MS, Ainslie PN, Griesdale DE. Clinical pathophysiology of hypoxic ischemic brain injury after cardiac arrest: a "two-hit" model. Crit Care. 2017;21(1):90. https://doi.org/10.1186/s13054-017-1670-9.
13. Polderman KH. Induced hypothermia and fever control for prevention and treatment of neurological injuries. Lancet. 2008;371(9628):1955–69. https://doi.org/10.1016/s0140-6736(08)60837-5.
14. Polderman KH. Mechanisms of action, physiological effects, and complications of hypothermia. Crit Care Med. 2009;37(7 Suppl):S186–202. https://doi.org/10.1097/CCM.0b013e3181aa5241.
15. Liu L, Yenari MA. Therapeutic hypothermia: neuroprotective mechanisms. Front Biosci. 2007;12:816–25. https://doi.org/10.2741/2104.
16. Fay T. Observations on generalized refrigeration in cases of severe cerebral trauma. Assoc Res Nerv Ment Dis Proc. 1943;24:611–9.
17. Karnatovskaia LV, Wartenberg KE, Freeman WD. Therapeutic hypothermia for neuroprotection: history, mechanisms, risks, and clinical applications. Neurohospitalist. 2014;4(3):153–63. https://doi.org/10.1177/1941874413519802.
18. Bigelow WG, McBirnie JE. Further experiences with hypothermia for intracardiac surgery in monkeys and groundhogs. Ann Surg. 1953;137(3):361–5. https://doi.org/10.1097/00000658-195303000-00010.
19. Rosomoff HL, Holaday DA. Cerebral blood flow and cerebral oxygen consumption during hypothermia. Am J Phys. 1954;179(1):85–8. https://doi.org/10.1152/ajplegacy.1954.179.1.85.
20. Botterell EH, Lougheed WM, Scott JW, Vandewater SL. Hypothermia, and interruption of carotid, or carotid and vertebral circulation, in the surgical management of intracranial aneurysms. J Neurosurg. 1956;13(1):1–42. https://doi.org/10.3171/jns.1956.13.1.0001.
21. Lazorthes G, Campan L. Hypothermia in the treatment of Craniocerebral traumatism. J Neurosurg. 1958;15(2):162–7. https://doi.org/10.3171/jns.1958.15.2.0162.
22. Drake CG, Barr HWK, Coles JC, Gergely NF. The use of extracorporeal circulation and profound hypothermia in the treatment of ruptured intracranial aneurysm. J Neurosurg. 1964;21(7):575–81. https://doi.org/10.3171/jns.1964.21.7.0575.
23. Lundberg N, Nielsen KC, Nilsson E. Deep hypothermia in intracranial surgery. J Neurosurg. 1956;13(3):235–47. https://doi.org/10.3171/jns.1956.13.3.0235.
24. Williams GR Jr, Spencer FC. The clinical use of hypothermia following cardiac arrest. Ann Surg. 1958;148(3):462–8. https://doi.org/10.1097/00000658-195809000-00014.
25. Marion DW, Penrod LE, Kelsey SF, Obrist WD, Kochanek PM, Palmer AM, et al. Treatment of traumatic brain injury with moderate hypothermia. N Engl J Med. 1997;336(8):540–6. https://doi.org/10.1056/nejm199702203360803.
26. Bernard SA, Gray TW, Buist MD, Jones BM, Silvester W, Gutteridge G, et al. Treatment of comatose survivors of out-of-hospital cardiac arrest with induced hypothermia. N Engl J Med. 2002;346(8):557–63. https://doi.org/10.1056/NEJMoa003289.
27. The Hypothermia after Cardiac Arrest Study Group. Mild therapeutic hypothermia to improve the neurologic outcome after cardiac arrest. N Engl J Med. 2002;346(8):549–56. https://doi.org/10.1056/NEJMoa012689.
28. Wyckoff MH, Singletary EM, Soar J, Olasveengen TM, Greif R, Liley HG, et al. International consensus on cardiopulmonary resuscitation and emergency cardiovascular care science with treatment recommendations: summary from the basic life support; advanced life support; neonatal life support; education, implementation, and teams; first aid task forces; and the COVID-19 working group. Circulation. 2021;145:e645. https://doi.org/10.1161/CIR.0000000000001017.
29. Panchal AR, Bartos JA, Cabañas JG, Donnino MW, Drennan IR, Hirsch KG, et al. Part 3: adult basic and advanced life support: 2020 American Heart Association guidelines for cardiopulmonary resuscitation and emergency cardiovascular care. Circulation. 2020;142(16_suppl_2):S366–468. https://doi.org/10.1161/CIR.0000000000000916.
30. Chen M, Fang J, Wu X, Liu Q, Feng L, He L. Association between hyperpyrexia and poststroke outcomes in patients with recanalization after mechanical thrombectomy: a retrospective cohort study. BMC Neurol. 2021;21(1):365. https://doi.org/10.1186/s12883-021-02400-8.
31. Schwab S, Schwarz S, Spranger M, Keller E, Bertram M, Hacke W. Moderate hypothermia in the treatment of patients with severe middle cerebral artery infarction. Stroke. 1998;29(12):2461–6. https://doi.org/10.1161/01.str.29.12.2461.
32. Schwab S, Georgiadis D, Berrouschot J, Schellinger PD, Graffagnino C, Mayer SA. Feasibility and safety of moderate hypothermia after massive hemispheric infarction. Stroke. 2001;32(9):2033–5. https://doi.org/10.1161/hs0901.095394.
33. Krieger DW, Georgia MAD, Abou-Chebl A, Andrefsky JC, Sila CA, Katzan IL, et al. Cooling for acute ischemic brain damage (COOL AID). Stroke. 2001;32(8):1847–54. https://doi.org/10.1161/01.STR.32.8.1847.
34. De Georgia MA, Krieger DW, Abou-Chebl A, Devlin TG, Jauss M, Davis SM, et al. Cooling for acute ischemic brain damage (COOL AID): a feasibility trial of endovascular cooling. Neurology. 2004;63(2):312–7. https://doi.org/10.1212/01.wnl.0000129840.66938.75.
35. Georgiadis D, Schwarz S, Aschoff A, Schwab S. Hemicraniectomy and moderate hypothermia in patients with severe ischemic stroke. Stroke. 2002;33(6):1584–8. https://doi.org/10.1161/01.str.0000016970.51004.d9.
36. Els T, Oehm E, Voigt S, Klisch J, Hetzel A, Kassubek J. Safety and therapeutical benefit of hemicraniectomy combined with mild hypothermia in comparison with hemicraniectomy alone in patients with malignant ischemic stroke. Cerebrovasc Dis. 2006;21(1–2):79–85. https://doi.org/10.1159/000090007.
37. Su Y, Fan L, Zhang Y, Zhang Y, Ye H, Gao D, et al. Improved neurological outcome with mild hypothermia in surviving patients with massive cerebral hemispheric infarction. Stroke. 2016;47(2):457–63. https://doi.org/10.1161/strokeaha.115.009789.
38. Neugebauer H, Kollmar R, Niesen W D, Bösel J, Schneider H, Hobohm C, et al. DEcompressive surgery plus hypoTHermia for space-occupying stroke (DEPTH-SOS): a protocol of a multicenter randomized controlled clinical trial and a literature review. Int J Stroke. 2013;8(5):383–7. https://doi.org/10.1111/ijs.12086.
39. Neugebauer H, Schneider H, Bösel J, Hobohm C, Poli S, Kollmar R, et al. Outcomes of hypothermia in addition to Decompressive

Hemicraniectomy in treatment of malignant middle cerebral artery stroke: a randomized clinical trial. JAMA Neurol. 2019;76(5):571–9. https://doi.org/10.1001/jamaneurol.2018.4822.
40. Hong JM, Lee JS, Song HJ, Jeong HS, Choi HA, Lee K. Therapeutic hypothermia after recanalization in patients with acute ischemic stroke. Stroke. 2014;45(1):134–40. https://doi.org/10.1161/strokeaha.113.003143.
41. Geurts M, Petersson J, Brizzi M, Olsson-Hau S, Luijckx GJ, Algra A, et al. COOLIST (cooling for ischemic stroke trial): a multicenter, open, randomized, phase II. Clinical Trial Stroke. 2017;48(1):219–21. https://doi.org/10.1161/strokeaha.116.014757.
42. Lyden P, Hemmen T, Grotta J, Rapp K, Ernstrom K, Rzesiewicz T, et al. Results of the ICTuS 2 trial (intravascular cooling in the treatment of stroke 2). Stroke. 2016;47(12):2888–95. https://doi.org/10.1161/strokeaha.116.014200.
43. Piironen K, Tiainen M, Mustanoja S, Kaukonen KM, Meretoja A, Tatlisumak T, et al. Mild hypothermia after intravenous thrombolysis in patients with acute stroke: a randomized controlled trial. Stroke. 2014;45(2):486–91. https://doi.org/10.1161/strokeaha.113.003180.
44. Ovesen C, Brizzi M, Pott FC, Thorsen-Meyer HC, Karlsson T, Ersson A, et al. Feasibility of endovascular and surface cooling strategies in acute stroke. Acta Neurol Scand. 2013;127(6):399–405. https://doi.org/10.1111/ane.12059.
45. Hemmen TM, Raman R, Guluma KZ, Meyer BC, Gomes JA, Cruz-Flores S, et al. Intravenous thrombolysis plus hypothermia for acute treatment of ischemic stroke (ICTuS-L): final results. Stroke. 2010;41(10):2265–70. https://doi.org/10.1161/strokeaha.110.592295.
46. Madden LK, Hill M, May TL, Human T, Guanci MM, Jacobi J, et al. The implementation of targeted temperature management: an evidence-based guideline from the Neurocritical care society. Neurocrit Care. 2017;27(3):468–87. https://doi.org/10.1007/s12028-017-0469-5.
47. Powers WJ, Rabinstein AA, Ackerson T, Adeoye OM, Bambakidis NC, Becker K, et al. 2018 guidelines for the early Management of Patients with Acute Ischemic Stroke: a guideline for healthcare professionals from the American Heart Association/American Stroke Association. Stroke. 2018;49(3):e46–99. https://doi.org/10.1161/STR.0000000000000158.
48. Greer DM, Ritter J, Helbok R, Badjatia N, Ko SB, Guanci M, et al. Impact of fever prevention in brain-injured patients (INTREPID): study protocol for a randomized controlled trial. Neurocrit Care. 2021;35(2):577–89. https://doi.org/10.1007/s12028-021-01208-1.
49. Schwarz S, Häfner K, Aschoff A, Schwab S. Incidence and prognostic significance of fever following intracerebral hemorrhage. Neurology. 2000;54(2):354–61. https://doi.org/10.1212/wnl.54.2.354.
50. Leira R, Dávalos A, Silva Y, Gil-Peralta A, Tejada J, Garcia M, et al. Early neurologic deterioration in intracerebral hemorrhage: predictors and associated factors. Neurology. 2004;63(3):461–7. https://doi.org/10.1212/01.wnl.0000133204.81153.ac.
51. Gebel JM Jr, Jauch EC, Brott TG, Khoury J, Sauerbeck L, Salisbury S, et al. Natural history of perihematomal edema in patients with hyperacute spontaneous intracerebral hemorrhage. Stroke. 2002;33(11):2631–5. https://doi.org/10.1161/01.str.0000035284.12699.84.
52. Fernandes HM, Siddique S, Banister K, Chambers I, Wooldridge T, Gregson B, et al. Continuous monitoring of ICP and CPP following ICH and its relationship to clinical, radiological and surgical parameters. Acta Neurochir Suppl. 2000;76:463–6. https://doi.org/10.1007/978-3-7091-6346-7_96.
53. Broessner G, Beer R, Lackner P, Helbok R, Fischer M, Pfausler B, et al. Prophylactic, endovascularly based, long-term normothermia in ICU patients with severe cerebrovascular disease: bicenter prospective, randomized trial. Stroke. 2009;40(12):e657–65. https://doi.org/10.1161/strokeaha.109.557652.
54. Lord AS, Karinja S, Lantigua H, Carpenter A, Schmidt JM, Claassen J, et al. Therapeutic temperature modulation for fever after intracerebral hemorrhage. Neurocrit Care. 2014;21(2):200–6. https://doi.org/10.1007/s12028-013-9948-5.
55. Kollmar R, Staykov D, Dörfler A, Schellinger PD, Schwab S, Bardutzky J. Hypothermia reduces Perihemorrhagic edema after intracerebral hemorrhage. Stroke. 2010;41(8):1684–9. https://doi.org/10.1161/STROKEAHA.110.587758.
56. Staykov D, Wagner I, Volbers B, Doerfler A, Schwab S, Kollmar R. Mild prolonged hypothermia for large intracerebral hemorrhage. Neurocrit Care. 2013;18(2):178–83. https://doi.org/10.1007/s12028-012-9762-5.
57. Volbers B, Herrmann S, Willfarth W, Lücking H, Kloska SP, Doerfler A, et al. Impact of hypothermia initiation and duration on Perihemorrhagic edema evolution after intracerebral hemorrhage. Stroke. 2016;47(9):2249–55. https://doi.org/10.1161/strokeaha.116.013486.
58. Hemphill JC 3rd, Greenberg SM, Anderson CS, Becker K, Bendok BR, Cushman M, et al. Guidelines for the Management of Spontaneous Intracerebral Hemorrhage: a guideline for healthcare professionals from the American Heart Association/American Stroke Association. Stroke. 2015;46(7):2032–60. https://doi.org/10.1161/str.0000000000000069.
59. Kramer CL, Pegoli M, Mandrekar J, Lanzino G, Rabinstein AA. Refining the Association of Fever with functional outcome in aneurysmal subarachnoid hemorrhage. Neurocrit Care. 2017;26(1):41–7. https://doi.org/10.1007/s12028-016-0281-7.
60. Fernandez A, Schmidt JM, Claassen J, Pavlicova M, Huddleston D, Kreiter KT, et al. Fever after subarachnoid hemorrhage: risk factors and impact on outcome. Neurology. 2007;68(13):1013–9. https://doi.org/10.1212/01.wnl.0000258543.45879.f5.
61. Naidech AM, Bendok BR, Bernstein RA, Alberts MJ, Batjer HH, Watts CM, et al. Fever burden and functional recovery after subarachnoid hemorrhage. Neurosurgery. 2008;63(2):212–7; discussion 7–8. https://doi.org/10.1227/01.Neu.0000320453.61270.0f.
62. Springer MV, Schmidt JM, Wartenberg KE, Frontera JA, Badjatia N, Mayer SA. Predictors of global cognitive impairment 1 year after subarachnoid hemorrhage. Neurosurgery. 2009;65(6):1043–50.; discussion 50-1. https://doi.org/10.1227/01.Neu.0000359317.15269.20.
63. Douds GL, Tadzong B, Agarwal AD, Krishnamurthy S, Lehman EB, Cockroft KM. Influence of fever and hospital-acquired infection on the incidence of delayed neurological deficit and poor outcome after aneurysmal subarachnoid hemorrhage. Neurol Res Int. 2012;2012:479865. https://doi.org/10.1155/2012/479865.
64. Badjatia N, Fernandez L, Schmidt JM, Lee K, Claassen J, Connolly ES, et al. Impact of induced normothermia on outcome after subarachnoid hemorrhage: a case-control study. Neurosurgery. 2010;66(4):696–700; discussion −1. https://doi.org/10.1227/01.Neu.0000367618.42794.Aa.
65. Gasser S, Khan N, Yonekawa Y, Imhof HG, Keller E. Long-term hypothermia in patients with severe brain edema after poor-grade subarachnoid hemorrhage: feasibility and intensive care complications. J Neurosurg Anesthesiol. 2003;15(3):240–8. https://doi.org/10.1097/00008506-200307000-00012.
66. Todd MM, Hindman BJ, Clarke WR, Torner JC. Mild intraoperative hypothermia during surgery for intracranial aneurysm. N Engl J Med. 2005;352(2):135–45. https://doi.org/10.1056/NEJMoa040975.
67. Diringer MN, Bleck TP, Claude Hemphill J 3rd, Menon D, Shutter L, Vespa P, et al. Critical care management of patients following aneurysmal subarachnoid hemorrhage: recommendations from the Neurocritical care Society's multidisciplinary consensus conference. Neurocrit Care. 2011;15(2):211–40. https://doi.org/10.1007/s12028-011-9605-9.

68. Connolly ES, Rabinstein AA, Carhuapoma JR, Derdeyn CP, Dion J, Higashida RT, et al. Guidelines for the Management of Aneurysmal Subarachnoid Hemorrhage. Stroke. 2012;43(6):1711–37. https://doi.org/10.1161/STR.0b013e3182587839.
69. Bao L, Chen D, Ding L, Ling W, Xu F. Fever burden is an independent predictor for prognosis of traumatic brain injury. PLoS One. 2014;9(3):e90956. https://doi.org/10.1371/journal.pone.0090956.
70. Birg T, Ortolano F, Wiegers EJA, Smielewski P, Savchenko Y, Ianosi BA, et al. Brain temperature influences intracranial pressure and cerebral perfusion pressure after traumatic brain injury: a CENTER-TBI study. Neurocrit Care. 2021;35(3):651–61. https://doi.org/10.1007/s12028-021-01294-1.
71. Hirst TC, Klasen MG, Rhodes JK, Macleod MR, Andrews PJD. A systematic review and meta-analysis of hypothermia in experimental traumatic brain injury: why have promising animal studies not been replicated in pragmatic clinical trials? J Neurotrauma. 2020;37(19):2057–68. https://doi.org/10.1089/neu.2019.6923.
72. Watson HI, Shepherd AA, Rhodes JKJ, Andrews PJD. Revisited: a systematic review of therapeutic hypothermia for adult patients following traumatic brain injury. Crit Care Med. 2018;46(6):972–9. https://doi.org/10.1097/ccm.0000000000003125.
73. Chen H, Wu F, Yang P, Shao J, Chen Q, Zheng R. A meta-analysis of the effects of therapeutic hypothermia in adult patients with traumatic brain injury. Crit Care. 2019;23(1):396. https://doi.org/10.1186/s13054-019-2667-3.
74. Carney N, Totten AM, O'Reilly C, Ullman JS, Hawryluk GW, Bell MJ, et al. Guidelines for the Management of Severe Traumatic Brain Injury. Fourth Edition Neurosurgery. 2017;80(1):6–15. https://doi.org/10.1227/neu.0000000000001432.
75. Cooper DJ, Nichol AD, Bailey M, Bernard S, Cameron PA, Pili-Floury S, et al. Effect of early sustained prophylactic hypothermia on neurologic outcomes among patients with severe traumatic brain injury: the POLAR randomized clinical trial. JAMA. 2018;320(21):2211–20. https://doi.org/10.1001/jama.2018.17075.
76. Hui J, Feng J, Tu Y, Zhang W, Zhong C, Liu M, et al. Safety and efficacy of long-term mild hypothermia for severe traumatic brain injury with refractory intracranial hypertension (LTH-1): a multicenter randomized controlled trial. EClinicalMedicine. 2021;32:100732. https://doi.org/10.1016/j.eclinm.2021.100732.
77. Elstrott B, Hinson HE. Commentary on "brain temperature influences intracranial pressure and cerebral perfusion pressure after traumatic brain injury". Neurocrit Care. 2021;35(3):615–6. https://doi.org/10.1007/s12028-021-01295-0.
78. Rossetti AO, Logroscino G, Bromfield EB. Refractory status epilepticus: effect of treatment aggressiveness on prognosis. Arch Neurol. 2005;62(11):1698–702. https://doi.org/10.1001/archneur.62.11.1698.
79. Legriel S. Hypothermia as a treatment in status epilepticus: a narrative review. Epilepsy Behav. 2019;101(Pt B):106298. https://doi.org/10.1016/j.yebeh.2019.04.051.
80. Legriel S, Lemiale V, Schenck M, Chelly J, Laurent V, Daviaud F, et al. Hypothermia for neuroprotection in convulsive status epilepticus. N Engl J Med. 2016;375(25):2457–67. https://doi.org/10.1056/NEJMoa1608193.
81. Kwon BK, Mann C, Sohn HM, Hilibrand AS, Phillips FM, Wang JC, et al. Hypothermia for spinal cord injury. Spine J. 2008;8(6):859–74. https://doi.org/10.1016/j.spinee.2007.12.006.
82. Levi AD, Casella G, Green BA, Dietrich WD, Vanni S, Jagid J, et al. Clinical outcomes using modest intravascular hypothermia after acute cervical spinal cord injury. Neurosurgery. 2010;66(4):670–7, https://doi.org/10.1227/01.Neu.0000367557.77973.5f.
83. Dididze M, Green BA, Dietrich WD, Vanni S, Wang MY, Levi AD. Systemic hypothermia in acute cervical spinal cord injury: a case-controlled study. Spinal Cord. 2013;51(5):395–400. https://doi.org/10.1038/sc.2012.161.
84. Hansebout RR, Hansebout CR. Local cooling for traumatic spinal cord injury: outcomes in 20 patients and review of the literature. J Neurosurg Spine. 2014;20(5):550–61. https://doi.org/10.3171/2014.2.Spine13318.
85. Papageorgiou DE, Tsikritsaki K, Javed F, Stathopoulos T, Ntinou E, Mavrogenis AF, et al. Therapeutic hypothermia in the ICU: the nursing aspect. J Long-Term Eff Med Implants. 2017;27(1):21–4. https://doi.org/10.1615/JLongTermEffMedImplants.2017019969.
86. Sonder P, Janssens GN, Beishuizen A, Henry CL, Rittenberger JC, Callaway CW, et al. Efficacy of different cooling technologies for therapeutic temperature management: a prospective intervention study. Resuscitation. 2018;124:14–20. https://doi.org/10.1016/j.resuscitation.2017.12.026.
87. Calabró L, Bougouin W, Cariou A, De Fazio C, Skrifvars M, Soreide E, et al. Effect of different methods of cooling for targeted temperature management on outcome after cardiac arrest: a systematic review and meta-analysis. Crit Care. 2019;23(1):285. https://doi.org/10.1186/s13054-019-2567-6.
88. Andremont O, du Cheyron D, Terzi N, Daubin C, Seguin A, Valette X, et al. Endovascular cooling versus standard femoral catheters and intravascular complications: a propensity-matched cohort study. Resuscitation. 2018;124:1–6. https://doi.org/10.1016/j.resuscitation.2017.12.014.
89. Meier K, Lee K. Neurogenic Fever. J Intensive Care Med. 2017;32(2):124–9. https://doi.org/10.1177/0885066615625194.
90. Badjatia N. Hyperthermia and fever control in brain injury. Crit Care Med. 2009;37(7 Suppl):S250–7. https://doi.org/10.1097/CCM.0b013e3181aa5e8d.
91. Badjatia N, Strongilis E, Gordon E, Prescutti M, Fernandez L, Fernandez A, et al. Metabolic impact of shivering during therapeutic temperature modulation. Stroke. 2008;39(12):3242–7. https://doi.org/10.1161/STROKEAHA.108.523654.
92. Choi HA, Ko S-B, Presciutti M, Fernandez L, Carpenter AM, Lesch C, et al. Prevention of shivering during therapeutic temperature modulation: the Columbia anti-shivering protocol. Neurocrit Care. 2011;14(3):389–94. https://doi.org/10.1007/s12028-010-9474-7.
93. Mokhtarani M, Mahgoub AN, Morioka N, Doufas AG, Dae M, Shaughnessy TE, et al. Buspirone and meperidine synergistically reduce the shivering threshold. Anesth Analg. 2001;93(5):1233–9. https://doi.org/10.1097/00000539-200111000-00038.
94. Doufas AG, Lin CM, Suleman MI, Liem EB, Lenhardt R, Morioka N, et al. Dexmedetomidine and meperidine additively reduce the shivering threshold in humans. Stroke. 2003;34(5):1218–23. https://doi.org/10.1161/01.Str.0000068787.76670.A4.
95. Stöckl M, Testori C, Sterz F, Holzer M, Weiser C, Schober A, et al. Continuous versus intermittent neuromuscular blockade in patients during targeted temperature management after resuscitation from cardiac arrest-a randomized, double blinded, double dummy, clinical trial. Resuscitation. 2017;120:14–9. https://doi.org/10.1016/j.resuscitation.2017.08.238.
96. Mirzoyev SA, McLeod CJ, Bunch TJ, Bell MR, White RD. Hypokalemia during the cooling phase of therapeutic hypothermia and its impact on arrhythmogenesis. Resuscitation. 2010;81(12):1632–6. https://doi.org/10.1016/j.resuscitation.2010.08.007.
97. Stockmann H, Krannich A, Schroeder T, Storm C. Therapeutic temperature management after cardiac arrest and the risk of bleeding: systematic review and meta-analysis. Resuscitation. 2014;85(11):1494–503. https://doi.org/10.1016/j.resuscitation.2014.07.018.
98. Wang CH, Chen NC, Tsai MS, Yu PH, Wang AY, Chang WT, et al. Therapeutic hypothermia and the risk of hemorrhage: a systematic review and meta-analysis of randomized controlled trials. Medicine (Baltimore). 2015;94(47):e2152. https://doi.org/10.1097/md.0000000000002152.

Part III

Specific Diagnosis, Diseases and Management

Subarachnoid Hemorrhage: Overview of Management

20

Brandon P. Lucke-Wold and Brian L. Hoh

Contents

Abstract

Aneurysmal subarachnoid hemorrhage (aSAH) continues to be a challenging disease for treatment. Patients have high morbidity and mortality. Hospital courses can be complicated by hydrocephalus, cerebral salt wasting, vasospasm, and delayed cerebral ischemia. Over the past several decades high quality studies have been conducted to determine the optimal management of this patient population. Although much work is still needed, some evidence-based standards have emerged. In this chapter, we present the epidemiology of SAH, highlight the supported evidence, and present emerging areas requiring further investigation.

B. P. Lucke-Wold · B. L. Hoh (✉)
Department of Neurosurgery, University of Florida, Gainesville, FL, USA
e-mail: Brandon.Lucke-Wold@neurosurgery.ufl.edu; Brian.Hoh@neurosurgery.ufl.edu

Chapter Goals

- Understand the epidemiology and pathophysiology of subarachnoid hemorrhage.
- Appreciate how to diagnose subarachnoid hemorrhage and what imaging modalities are utilized.

E. Mahanna Gabrielli et al. (eds.), *Textbook of Neurointensive Care: Volume 1*, https://doi.org/10.1007/978-3-031-62220-5_20

- Gain an understanding of the medial management of subarachnoid hemorrhage patients.
- Become familiar with common treatment modalities for brain aneurysms.
- Allow a greater appreciation for determining symptomatic vasospasm and delayed cerebral ischemia.

Background

Aneurysmal subarachnoid hemorrhage (aSAH) is associated with high levels of morbidity and mortality [1]. It accounts for 5% of all strokes and affects 30,000–40,000 patients annually in the United States [2]. An estimated 12–15% of patients don't make it to the hospital for treatment [3]. For patients that make it to the hospital, hydrocephalus, vasospasm, cerebral salt wasting, and delayed cerebral ischemia (DCI) are well-known complications [4]. Overall mortality ranges from 32% to 50% [5]. Over the past several years several high-quality studies have been conducted to look at optimal treatment regimens for this patient population. These studies have investigated a variety of factors ranging from optimal timing of treatment, control of blood pressure, use of antiepileptic medications, and supportive management of fluid balance [6]. A wide variance in genetic predisposition to aneurysm formation and rupture has been shown. Age; however, is the biggest risk factor with the majority of aSAH presenting in adults from the fifth to seventh decades [7]. This chapter will highlight the epidemiology of aSAH, address initial diagnosis and management, discuss the evidence, and present emerging areas that warrant further investigation.

Epidemiology

The incidence for aSAH based on different population demographics has ranged from 2 to 22.5 per 100,000 [8]. The highest reported incidence is for patients of Scandinavian descent compared to lowest incidence amongst patients of central Asian descent [9]. The incidence has remained overall stable for the past 4 decades, with increased survival as care has become standardized. Patients with a family history of intracranial aneurysms are more likely to have aneurysms themselves [10]. Furthermore, certain conditions such as Ehlers-Danlos and polycystic kidney disease have a higher risk of aneurysm formation [11, 12]. Within the United States, the average is 9.7 per 100,000 [13]. However, differences in aSAH incidence have been documented based on socioeconomic status, race, and ethnicity. Black and Hispanics have a higher incidence than white Americans [14]. Sex also plays an important role. aSAH is 1.24 to 1.6 times higher in women depending on the study and peaks around age 55 [15]. Women who are post-menopausal have a slightly higher risk for aneurysm rupture than pre-menopausal women [16]. Incidence increases with age, especially in the >50-year-old population [17].

Several modifiable risk factors have also been linked to aSAH including smoking, alcohol abuse, and use of sympathomimetic drugs [18]. The extent of contribution to rupture and clinical course is debated in the literature. Besides drugs of abuse, other medical comorbidities have been linked to aneurysm formation and rupture rate including hypertension, atrial fibrillation, congestive heart failure, renal disease, and coronary artery disease [19]. The combination of smoking and hypertension has been shown to have a synergistic effect on increasing the risk for aneurysm rupture and has the most well-supported data [20]. Understanding the underlying patient comorbidities can help guide appropriate treatment after aneurysm rupture and help tailor further preventative strategies [21].However, initial presentation is more important than pre-existing comorbidities for predicting outcome [22].

A total of 12–15% of patients fail to reach the hospital after aSAH. In recent years, 8% of those who make it to the hospital die from progressive deterioration or family withdrawal of care. This represents improved survival compared to prior decades [23]. Patients who have lower Hunt and Hess (HH) scores and World Federation of Neurologic Surgeons (WFNS) grades upon arrival compared to those who survive. Hunt and Hess score descriptions with associated mortality are listed in Table 20.1 [24]. WFNS grade is documented in Table 20.2 [25]. The majority of those who die deteriorate quickly within the first 7 days of hospital stay [26]. Rebleeding was the primary cause of further deterioration [27]. There is a 4.1% risk of rebleed in the first 24 h followed by 1% per day for the next 2 weeks [28]. Of those

Table 20.1 Hunt and Hess Scores with associated mortality

Grade	Characteristic	Mortality (%)
0	Unruptured/without symptoms	0
1	Minimal headache/slight nuchal rigidity	1
2	Moderate/severe headache, nuchal rigidity, possible cranial nerve palsy	5
3	Drowsy, confused, focal deficit	19
4	Stupor, potential hemiparesis, early decerebrate rigidity	42
5	Coma, decerebrate rigidity, moribund	77

Table 20.2 World Federation of Neurologic Surgeons Grade

WFNS grade	Glasgow coma score	Major focal deficit
1	15	No
2	13–14	No
3	13–14	Yes
4	7–12	Yes or no
5	3–6	Yes or no

that survive, vasospasm and DCI are the primary contributors to neurologic morbidity [29].

It is estimated that 20–30% of aSAH patients develop hydrocephalus and need permanent cerebral spinal fluid (CSF) drainage [30]. Ventriculoperitoneal shunt (VPS) is the most commonly performed definitive treatment [31]. Cerebral vasospasm is also common with 70% of SAH patients showing evidence on imaging and 30% becoming symptomatic [32]. The peak is day 7 with a window for vasospasm between the fourth and twenty-first days [33]. Not surprisingly, severity of SAH is directly linked to symptomatic vasospasm, but other factors such as smoking, hypertension, and left ventricular heart strain have also been correlated [34]. Similar to vasospasm, the peak for DCI is 6 to 8 days after injury [35]. Although no definitive treatment yet exists for delayed cerebral edema, continuous electroencephalography (EEG) can help detect DCI early in order to guide management stratregies [36].

Standard Case Presentation

A 55-year-old-female who was driving to work and experienced sudden onset thunderclap headache. Had associated seizure and loss of consciousness. Bystanders found her unresponsive. Emergency medical services were notified, and she was brought to the nearby hospital via ambulance. Upon arrival, she was intubated. Computed tomography (CT) scan was obtained showing diffuse SAH, with the greatest clot burden around the left side of Circle of Willis and Sylvian Fissure. She was subsequently flown to the larger tertiary care center for further management. Upon arrival at the hospital, CT angiography (CTA) was obtained showing a ruptured left superior cerebellar artery (SCA) aneurysm (Fig. 20.1).

Imaging characteristics were consistent with Fisher Grade 3/4 subarachnoid hemorrhage and upon clinical evaluation, patient was Hunt Hess 4. Fisher Grade scores and modified Fisher Grade scores are described with the associated risk of vasospasm in Table 20.3 [37]. She was admitted to the neurosurgical service with the following aSAH protocol: goal SBP < 140 mmHg for unsecured aneurysm including intravenous antihypertensives to maintain goal, arterial line placement left radial artery to spare right side for potential angiography, every hour vital signs and neuro exam assessment, sequential compression device placement, nimodipine 60 mg every 4 h, levetiracetam 500 mg every 12 h for 3 days, aminocaproic acid to be stopped 3 h before angiography, and daily transcranial dopplers (TCD). An external ventricular drain (EVD) was placed via the right frontal approach. She was subsequently taken to the interventional suite where a cerebral angiogram was performed via right femoral access followed by successful coiling (Fig. 20.2). She was transferred back to the neurocritical care unit for continued monitoring. Attempts to wean the EVD failed and a VPS was placed on post-bleed day 11. The patient was monitored for symptomatic vasospasm and did not require further intervention. After the patient was outside the vasospasm window,

Table 20.3 Associated symptomatic vasospasm with Fisher Scale or Modified Fisher Scale scores

Grade	Fisher scale	% Symptomatic vasospasm	Modified fisher scale	% Symptomatic vasospasm
1	Focal/thin	21	Focal or diffuse thin SAH with no IVH	24
2	Diffuse thin SAH	25	Focal or diffuse thin SAH with IVH	33
3	Thick SAH	37	Thick SAH with no IVH	33
4	Focal or diffuse SAH with significant ICH or IVH	31	Thick SAH with IVH	40

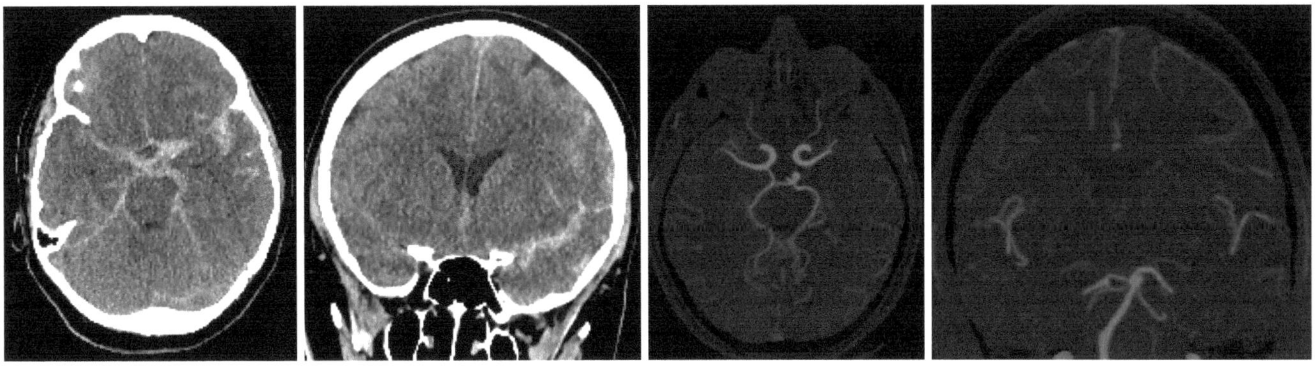

Fig. 20.1 ruptured left SCA aneurysm with extensive clot burden along Circle of Willis and left Sylvian Fissure

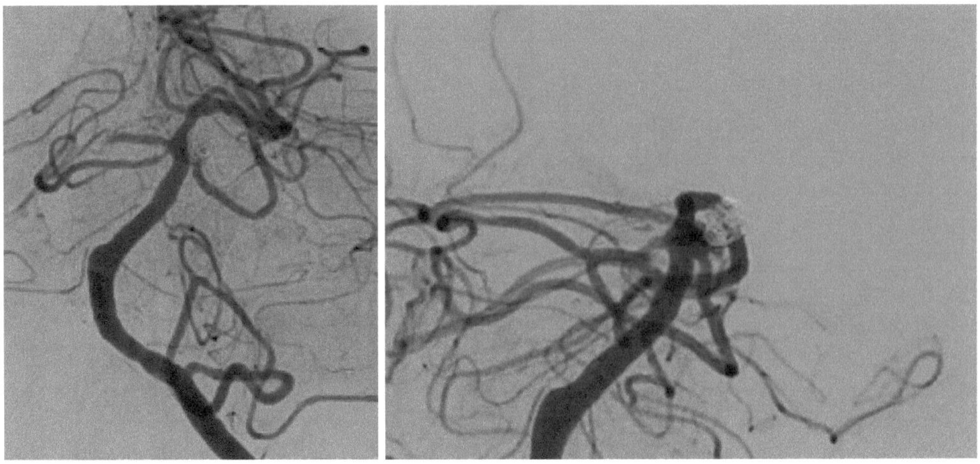

Fig. 20.2 Coiling of left SCA aneurysm with successful obliteration

she was discharged to a rehabilitation center to continue her neurologic recovery.

Imaging Diagnostics

CTA can be used for the initial evaluation of aSAH. It can be obtained quickly, provides good three-dimensional reconstructions, and aids appreciation for the relationship of aneurysms to bony landmarks. For aneurysms >5 mm, the sensitivity is 95% but drops to 83% for aneurysms <5 mm [38]. The average specificity is 98.9% and positive likelihood ratio ranges from 3.9 to 56 depending on aneurysm size [39]. CTA is 90% accurate in determining correct aneurysm neck diameter compared to the gold standard diagnostic cerebral angiography (DSA) [40]. The diagnostic challenge is when subarachnoid blood cannot be detected on CT Head. Historically, lumbar puncture has been the preferred next step in this scenario. It is important for the clinician to perform a nontraumatic lumbar puncture and collect 4 tubes of cerebrospinal fluid to assess xanthochromia and RBC clearing. Xanthochromia does not appear until 2–4 h after aneurysmal hemorrhage but is present in 100% of patients by 12 h and remains present for 3 weeks after initial bleeding. Comparison of RBC count from the first and fourth tubes as well as examination of the supernatant fluid for xanthochromia helps distinguish aSAH from a traumatic lumbar puncture. Determination of SAH verse traumatic tap is documented in Table 20.4 [41].

Table 20.4 CSF results to differentiate between SAH and traumatic tap

CSF features	SAH	Traumatic tap
Opening pressure	Often elevated	Normal
Fluid appearance	Xanthochromia (yellow/pink)	Bloody
Supernatant appearance	Xanthochromia	Clear
Clotting	Does not clot	Clots
Red blood cell count	>100,000 RBC/mm^3 with persistence between first and fourth tubes	Elevated count in first tube with decrease by fourth tube
WBC/RBC ratio	Slight leukocytosis	Same as peripheral blood
Protein	Elevated	Slightly elevated

MRI was until recently of little diagnostic value for SAH due to the inability to detect methemoglobin in the first 24–48 h. It also is more expensive and takes longer to obtain. MRA has decreased sensitivity for detecting small aneurysms compared to CTA and therefore is only used in patients unable to get CTAs (pregnant, renal failure, renal insufficiency). New MRI modalities have emerged in recent years however, including the basiparallel anatomic scanning and volumetric isotropic TSE acquisition (black blood imaging) that can detect subarachnoid blood not caught on traditional CT. FLAIR sequencing has also been useful to identify occult SAH [42]. Initial studies for detection of small aneurysms and early subarachnoid blood on MRI are promising and can aid in diagnosis [43]. This modality is now considered as a potential alternative to lumbar puncture when CT is non-diagnostic [44]. Lumbar puncture should still be obtained if black blood imaging is negative.

Cerebral DSA is another diagnostic modality when aneurysmal SAH is suspected and is often employed for confirmation after the above modalities are utilized for initial diagnosis. The sequential evaluation of each major intracranial vessel offers real-time assessment with PA and lateral projections. The ability to adjust projections allows for ideal visualization of surrounding cerebral vasculature when an aneurysm is suspected. Contrast load can also be carefully monitored. In CTA-negative SAH, cerebral angiography also fails to detect aneurysmal cause in 20–25% of cases. Repeat angiography performed 1 week later however, may identify an aneurysm in 1–2% of patients and they may be treated accordingly [45]. Therefore, repeat angiography is indicated if initial imaging is negative but suspicion remains high.

Table 20.5 Contrast allergy prophylaxis protocol

Elective (13 h protocol)	Accelerated (4 h protocol)	Emergent (1 h protocol)
Prednisone 50 mg PO given 13, 7, and 1 h prior	Methylprednisolone 40 mg IV given now and 1 h prior	Methylprednisolone 40 mg IV given 1 h prior
Diphenhydramine 50 mg PO given 1 h prior	Diphenhydramine 50 mg IV given 1 h prior	Diphenhydramine 50 mg IV given 1 h prior

Another key benefit of angiography is that intervention can be initiated at the time of diagnosis thereby limiting unnecessary subsequent procedures and increasing the efficiency of management.

As endovascular intervention options have improved, more and more patients are undergoing endovascular procedures. The current contrast agents are low-osmolality and help reduce pain and adverse events such as rash, flushing, angioedema, or vasomotor collapse. The current risk for reaction or kidney damage is 4% [46]. Associated risk factors for kidney injury include age > 70, increased contrast volume, pre-existing renal disease, and poorly controlled hypertension [47]. Risk for adverse reactions is increased in patients with asthma, heart disease, diabetes mellitus, myeloma, sickle cell disease, and polycythemia [48]. The risk for a subsequent reaction in a patient who has had prior reaction is 17–35% [49]. Routine premedication is not recommended, but some approved protocols have been supported by American College of Radiology for those with documented contrast allergies. These are documented in Table 20.5.

Data Supported Guidelines

The following guidelines are based on the AHA consortium with level of evidence summarized by Class and Level as outlined in Table 20.6 [6].

Recommendations for Diagnosis

As previously mentioned, aneurysmal SAH can be misdiagnosed when CT head is negative. Therefore, there is Class I, Level B data to support a high clinical suspicion for aneurysmal SAH if a patient presents with acute onset of severe headache. As emergency physicians and first responders often are the initial gateway, cross-disciplinary education is critical for early recognition and funneling towards early treatment. Non-contrast CT and CTA head is often performed, but if non diagnostic there is AHA Class I, Level B data to support lumbar puncture to rule out SAH as previously described. If CTA head is non-diagnostic, there is AHA Class IIb, Level C evidence to proceed with an angiogram. Black blood sequence MRIs have AHA Class IIB, Level C evidence but should not negate the need for lumbar puncture if negative as previously mentioned. If the above modalities confirm SAH, cerebral angiography is indicated for treatment planning as well as early intervention (AHA Class I, Level B evidence).

Stabilization and Preventing Rebleed

Attention to the airway, breathing, and ensuring hemodynamic stability should be the first priority for all patients. If a patient requires intubation, efforts should be made to control blood pressure, avoid pharmacologic agents that can cause dysrhythmias, and limit hemodynamic instability and hypertension to prevent potential for rebleeding. Preoxygenation should be performed prior to endotracheal intubation as well as initiation of antihypertensives [50]. Target SBP has been proposed as <160 mmHg in most studies of aSAH [51]. Beta-blockers, hydralazine, and nicardipine infusion can all be utilized but sodium nitroprusside should be avoided as venodilation may raise intracranial pressure and side effects include cyanide toxicity.

The risk of rebleeding is maximal between 2 h and 12 h [52] and 1/3 of rebleeds occur within the first 3 h [53]. Larger aneurysms, worse neurologic status upon admission, and sustained SBP > 160 mm Hg have all been associated with increased rebleeding rates [54]. Interestingly, aneurysms associated with genetic syndromes do not have increased rates of rupture compared to those not associated with genetic syndromes and should be managed similarly [55]. Of the above-mentioned antihypertensives, nicardipine has been shown to be most useful in preventing BP swings prior to securing the aneurysm [56]. Early treatment with microsurgical clip obliteration or endovascular occlusion greatly reduces rebleeding potential [57]. The summarized recommendations include: utilizing a titratable antihypertensive to control BP, which has been shown to reduce rebleeding rate until the aneurysm is secured (AHA Class I, Level B). SBP should be maintained <160 mm Hg until aneurysm is secured (AHA Class IIa; Level C).

Antifibrinolytic Therapy

Antifibrinolytics have been studied for SAH since the late 1960s. Early studies of antifibrinolytics showed promise to reduce the rates of early rebleeding. Subsequent studies, however, found an increased risk of cerebral infarction or deep venous thrombosis (DVT). The two major medications

Table 20.6 Level of evidence recommendations

	Level A: Multiple Clinical Trials	Level B: Single Clinical Trial or Nonrandomized Studies	Level C: Limited Evaluation with Case Studies or Expert Opinion Dictating Recommendations
Type 1: Risk/benefit ratio favors intervention	Strong support for intervention	Support for intervention	Support for intervention
Type 2a: Risk/benefit ratio favors intervention although further studies warranted	Support for intervention	Weak support for intervention	Weak support for intervention
Type 2b: Risk/benefit ratio favors intervention based on majority but conflicting studies reported	Interpret available literature; some support for intervention	Further studies warranted: Some support for intervention	Further studies warranted: No strong evidence to support intervention
Type 3: Risk/benefit ratio favors no benefit or harm	Intervention not supported	Intervention not supported	Intervention not supported

utilized are tranexamic acid and epsilon-aminocaproic acid. A 40–60% reduction in rebleeding has been reported in aSAH patients treated with tranexamic acid [58].However, some studies report up to 43% risk of neurologic deficits [59]. aSAH patients treated with epsilon-aminocaproic acid had a reduction in rebleed rate but an eight-fold increase in DVTs [60, 61]. Several groups have therefore argued for short-duration antifibrinolytics to reduce rebleeding rates acutely but also rapid discontinuation within the first 72 h to prevent complication risk [62]. Current evidence to support the use of short-term antifibrinolytic is AHA Class IIa, Level B.

Seizures

The true incidence of seizures following aSAH is still debated. Large studies have found that 21% of patients will experience seizures during their hospital stay but only 3.8% go on to develop epilepsy [63]. The majority of seizures that do occur, happen during the first 72 h. Therefore, the use of anti-epileptic drugs has been limited to this time window to avoid long-term consequences of these medications. When antiepileptic medications are not discontinued by 3 days, up to 23% of patients may have associated complications [64]. Historically, phenytoin was the agent of choice, but due to the side effect profile and need for laboratory monitoring, it has fallen out of favor [65]. Levetiracetam has now emerged as the agent of choice due to its more favorable side effect profile and ability to be titrated without extensive monitoring [66]. Perioperative seizures were slightly more common in patients undergoing clipping, but not significant enough to dictate change in practice pattern [67]. There is AHA Class IIb; Level B evidence to support the use of antiepileptics for the first 72 h. AHA Class III, Level B evidence is available that recommends against long-term anticonvulsant use in aSAH patients.

Hydrocephalus

Depending on the study, 15–87% of patients with aSAH have ventriculomegaly. When associated with neurologic deficit, EVD or lumbar drain (LD) placement provides symptomatic relief [68]. EVD placement has not been associated with increased rebleed rates [69]. Early EVD weaning has had some success in preventing the need for subsequent surgical shunt placement [70]. A fast wean <24 h, has proven most effective and patients that are successfully weaned have decreased length of stay in the intensive care unit [71]. Despite weaning attempts, 8.9–48% go on to require shunt placement for permanent cerebral spinal fluid diversion [72]. AHA Class I, level C evidence supports the use of a shunt for permanent CSF diversion if EVD cannot be weaned. Treatment modality (coiling verse clipping) does not have a significant effect on the need for subsequent shunt placement [73]. The type of shunt placed is usually decided at discretion of neurosurgeon without significant evidence to support one type over another. Insufficient evidence is available to support the use of lamina terminalis fenestration (AHA Class III, Level B) [74]. AHA Class I, level B evidence supports early treatment of hydrocephalus with external drain. Early EVD weaning is preferred (AHA Class III, level B).

Medical Complications

Complications associated with SAH are common and can increase morbidity and mortality. Forty Percent of SAH patients experience complications while admitted [75]. One of the most common complications is disturbance of sodium homeostasis. Hyponatremia (Na < 135) is most commonly associated with cerebral salt wasting, which has been linked to cerebral vasospasm [76]. Patients who experience cerebral salt wasting often have worse HH grade, hydrocephalus, and anterior circulation aneurysms [77]. In its most severe state cerebral salt wasting can cause Na to drop below 125 and induce seizures. The use of hypertonic saline infusion (3%) has been shown to be effective in treating hyponatremia, increasing cerebral blood flow, and improving brain tissue oxygenation [78]. The mineralocorticoid fludrocortisone can also be used as it promotes sodium reabsorption from the kidneys while not significantly altering pulmonary or cardiovascular functioning [79]. Occasionally hyponatremia can be

Table 20.7 Differentiating cause of hyponatremia

Biomarker	SIADH	CSW
Blood BUN/creatinine	Low	High
Brain natriuretic peptide level	Normal	High
Serum potassium level	Normal	Normal to high
Serum uric acid level	Low	Low
Serum osmolality	Low	Low
Urinary sodium level	>40 mEq/L	>40 mEq/L
Initial fractional excretion of urate	High	High
Fractional excretion of urate after correction	Normal	High
Urinary osmolality	High	High
Pulmonary capillary wedge pressure	Normal to high	Low
Central venous pressure	Normal to high	Low
Extracellular fluid volume	Normal to high	Low

caused by the syndrome of inappropriate antidiuretic hormone secretion (SIADH). Standard treatment for SIADH in other clinical scenarios is volume restriction, but due to the increased risk for ischemia due to vasospasm with aSAH, hypertonic saline is also the preferred method for treating SIADH in this population [80]. Interpretation of laboratory values to differentiate between cerebral salt wasting and SIADH is shown in Table 20.7. Current evidenced based recommendations discourage the use of volume contraction or administration of hypotonic fluids (AHA Class III, Level B). Monitoring fluid balance to determine when to give hypertonic crystalloids (AHA Class IIa, Level B). The use of fludrocortisone and hypertonic saline to correct hyponatremia is indicated (AHA Class IIa, Level B).

Cardiac complications are also prominent after SAH. Myocardial injury and dysfunction have been postulated to be due to hypothalamic dysregulation and an elevated catecholamine surge [81]. In severe cases, the catecholamine surge can induce myocardial necrosis [82]. Early detection is critical with troponin elevations indicating cardiac strain [83]. These patients warrant electrocardiogram (ECG) and echocardiography for further assessment. T-wave inversion and QT prolongation are common for SAH patients [75]. Therefore, careful monitoring of magnesium and potassium is critical to ensure electrolyte optimization in order to reduce arrhythmias. On echocardiography, left ventricular dysfunction is most often seen in SAH patients [84]. Eighteen percent of SAH patients have regional wall motion abnormalities, and this is increased to 35% for the HH 3–5 cohort [85]. Another unique cardiovascular complication associated with SAH is takotsubo cardiomyopathy. The akinesia is predominantly at the apex with relative sparing of the basal segment thereby inducing apical ballooning [86]. This produces the classic Japanese crab cage imaging characteristics. With supportive care and medications that target sympathetic dysregulation, takotsubo cardiomyopathy can be successfully reversed with restoration of normal ejection fraction [87].

Pulmonary complications are also common after aSAH. 27% of SAH patients have pulmonary-related abnormalities [88]. The best-accepted metric is a pulmonary arterial O_2 over fraction of inspired O_2 (P/F) ratio of <300 [89]. This has been correlated with pulmonary infiltrates and edema on chest x-rays. The pulmonary edema is often neurogenic in origin, which is distinct from cardiac-induced pulmonary edema. Euvolemic volume targets have had some benefit in decreasing pulmonary edema [90]. Another common complication that affects 15% of SAH patients is pneumonia [91]. One of the postulated mechanisms is that acute lung injury commonly associated with SAH prevents adequate clearance of hospital-acquired pathogens [92]. Early recognition of infection including rising white blood cell count, increased ventilator requirements, and fever should be carefully managed. An elevated neutrophil/lymphocyte ratio is an early indicator of pneumonia in the SAH population [93]. Empiric antibiotics should be started early when suspicion is high. There is AHA Class IIa, Level B evidence to support maintaining normothermia and treating fever aggressively. When feasible, early mobilization and initiation of physical therapy have shown benefit in preventing pneumonia following SAH [94]. Careful glucose management to decrease the risk of infection is indicated by both avoiding hyper and hypoglycemia (AHA Class IIb, Level B evidence).

Another common issue for SAH patients is anemia. More severe SAH is associated with worse anemia and a poor outcome. Restricted transfusion strategies that maintain Hgb > 7 g/dL have been shown to be superior to maintaining Hgb > 10 g/dL with fewer transfusion reactions and no change in mortality between groups [95]. Repetitive transfusions are associated with worse outcomes [96]. Maintaining Hgb is critical for cerebral oxygen delivery and transfusions to maintain goal Hg targets are supported by Class IIb, Level B evidence [97].. With the impaired cerebrovascular response following SAH, adequate circulating volume and tissue oxygen delivery must be maintained with crystalloid administration.

Thromboembolic complications are common after aSAH. aSAH patients are often bedbound with extended intensive care unit stays that predispose them to DVT development. 7.9% of aSAH patients will develop a DVT during admission [98]. Some of these patients go on to develop life-threatening pulmonary embolus [99]. These patients then require systemic anticoagulation, which is complicated in SAH patients, due to the increased bleeding risk [100]. Subcutaneous heparin prophylaxis and sequential compression devices are recommended and supported by AHA Class I, Level B evidence. Heparin-induced thrombocytopenia is rare and can be managed quickly when recognized early [101]. Although it increases the risk for vasospasm and death when not recognized and treated, heparin-induced thrombocytopenia occurs in <5% of patients and should not be a contraindication to starting DVT prophylaxis.

Systems of Care

Although academic centers are often treating more complex aSAH patients urban teaching hospitals have a 1.62 odds ratio of definitive treatment of aneurysms compared to rural or non-teaching hospitals [4] [102]. Patients have better outcomes after both clipping and coiling at the larger academic hospitals [103]. An added gain of 1.6 quality-adjusted life-years is provided if the patient is treated at a large academic center [104]. It is suggested that aneurysms be treated at hospitals that treat >35 SAH patients per year [105]. All providers should have completed an appropriate Endovascular CAST or ACGME accredited program, with options for open fellowships also available [106]. For neurosurgeons this provides sufficient volume to obtain proficiency at both endovascular and clipping techniques [107]. Neurology and radiology teams obtain sufficient volume during their endovascular training. Furthermore, large academic centers have 24/7 intensive care unit staffing to support consistent management and implementation of evidence-based guidelines [108].

Treatment

Ruptured aneurysms should be treated in a timely manner, ideally within the first 24 h post rupture. Aneurysm size and morphology dictate treatment options, which can vary from coiling, clipping, synthetic wrapping, or in extreme circumstances vessel sacrifice. Historically, carotid ligation was a commonly performed procedure with high morbidity and mortality, then advances in clip design and application provided better alternatives and became standard of care up until 1991 when coiling became available [109]. Endovascular techniques have continued to evolve allowing for a broader spectrum of aneurysms that can be successfully treated. The ISAT trial showed that both clipping and coiling offered no difference in patient mortality but that morbidity was higher in the clipping group at 1 year [110]. This was especially true with regard to verbal memory [111]. This needs to be taken into context of the potential necessity of repeat procedures for endovascular treatment and a higher rebleeding rate (ref).

Clipping

Surgical clipping is highly effective in treating ruptured aneurysms and has low recanalization and re-hemorrhage rates. The reported re-hemorrhage rate post clipping is 1.2–2% [112]. Furthermore, complete obliteration rate on follow-up angiography is high (91.8%) with late recurrence minimal (0.5%) [113]. AHA Class I, level B evidence supports coiling over clipping when coiling is feasible. Clipping is ideal however for aneurysms that are difficult to treat endovascularly. Middle cerebral artery bifurcation aneurysms are amenable to clipping with favorable outcomes and are often difficult to treat via coiling due to their distal nature [114]. Aneurysms with neck morphology not amenable to coiling or other endovascular device treatment should be treated by clipping. Patients presenting with large intraparenchymal hematomas from ruptured aneurysms may benefit from surgical clipping as clot evacuation can be performed at the same time [115]. Clipping can also be performed as salvage treatment in patients with coil compaction or intraoperative rupture during coil embolization [116]. An example of a patient that had a right PCOM aneurysm clipped after attempted pipeline-assisted coiling is shown in Fig. 20.3.

Coiling

Aneurysm embolization has continued to evolve over the last three decades and is appealing for older patients with multiple co-morbidities [117]. Traditional platinum-based coils are still used, but new modalities are being developed and tested as well as new coil designs. Standard coiling has a rebleeding rate of 0.9–2.9% [21]. Clinical superiority for coiling posterior circulation aneurysms has been shown due to the inherent risks of complications from surgical clipping in this region [118]. Recurrence is a concern with coiling and is related to compaction over time and insufficient packing density based on aneurysm characteristics. Large aneurysms and those with wide necks are less likely to have the coiling packing density necessary to achieve complete obliteration. Stent-assisted and balloon-assisted coiling offer new opportunities for treating some of these complex aneurysms. Stenting also is valuable to treat dissecting aneurysms where traditional methods are not feasible. Stent -assisted treatment requires the use of post-operative antiplatelets and this can be problematic due to increased bleeding risk if invasive procedures such as ventriculostomy placement become necessary. Class III, Level C evidence supports only using stenting when lower risk options have been excluded. Some groups have been investigating coated bioactive coils to enhance aneurysm obliteration at faster rates than standard platinum coils, which may provide a tangible solution [114]. Large clinical trials to determine efficacy are still lacking. Due to the risk of recurrence, patients should be screened with follow-up angiography and retreated if indicated (AHA Class I, Level B evidence). The

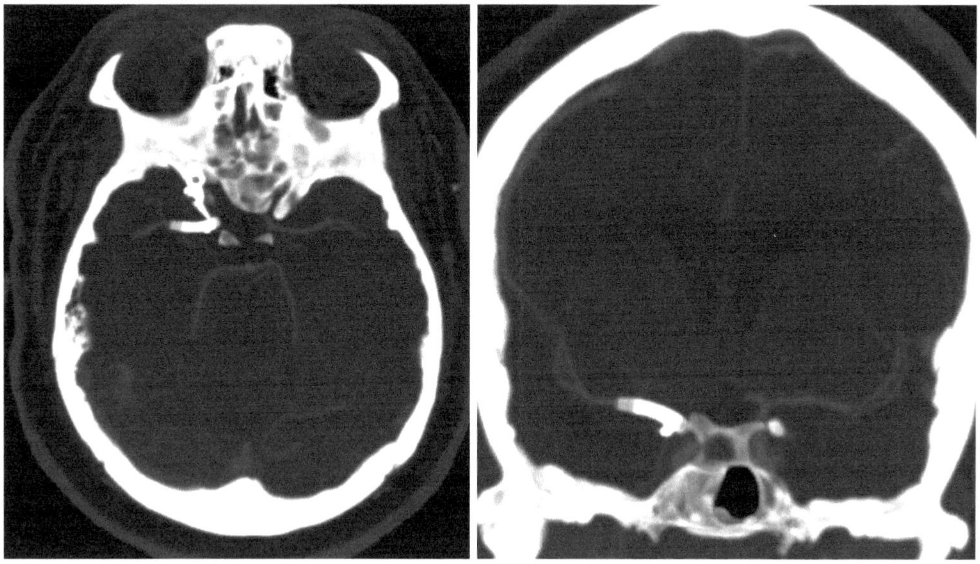

Fig. 20.3 A 37 year-old with ruptured right PCOM aneurysm had pipeline-assisted coiling performed. Repeat angiography had demonstrated residual aneurysm filling and the patient elected to proceed with clip placement at that time

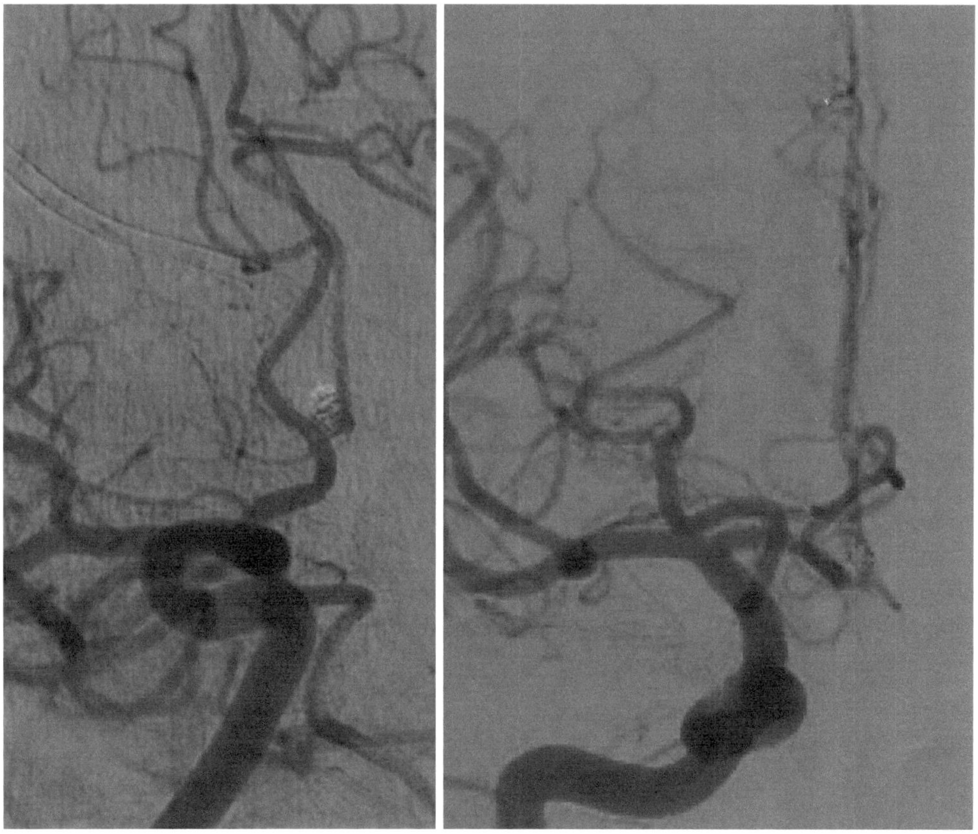

Fig. 20.4 A 55-year-old female at 5 years follow up from ruptured Acom aneurysm. Patient underwent stent-assisted coiling with 100% obliteration with no recurrence out to 5 years

standard duration of follow-up has not been clearly defined based on evidence-based guidelines and is at the discretion of the provider. Most providers will continue to follow for several years after aSAH. The successful stent coiling of an anterior communicating (Acom) aneurysm is shown in Fig. 20.4.

Alternatives

AHA Class I, Level B data exists to support early coiling/clipping with the goal of complete obliteration. Rarely, due to aneurysm characteristics, endovascular or clipping options are not feasible. Formulation of a treatment plan should be multidisciplinary to consider viable alternatives. Clip-wrapping has been studied, but results in high re-hemorrhage rates and rates of recurrence, and large clinical trials are lacking. Blister aneurysms offer a unique challenge. Gore-Tex clip-wrapping has been performed in case series with evidence of good long-term outcomes for these patients [119]. For very large ruptured aneurysms, vessel sacrifice with or without bypass might be the only feasible option [120]. This should be reserved as an end-stage option when no other viable alternatives exist due to the very high associated morbidity and mortality (ref) [121–126].

Cerebral Vasospasm

Vasospasm can lead to delayed cerebral ischemia and neurologic deficits. Vessel narrowing is first induced by oxyhemoglobin contacting the vessel wall [127]. The downstream mechanisms responsible for sustained vasoconstriction are still being investigated but are thought to be due to an inflammatory surge of cytokines and dysregulation of vasoregulatory endothelins and disturbance of the nitric oxide pathway [128, 129]. Vasospasm is the major cause of morbidity for SAH patients and occurs between 4 and 21 days with a peak on day 7 [29]. 4–23% of aSAH patients have ischemic infarcts on follow-up head CTs with associated worse modified Rankin Scores compared to those without infarcts [130]. These patients are often those with documented clinically symptomatic vasospasm during the intensive care unit stay.

Table 20.8 standard transcranial doppler cut-off interpretations for vasospasm (ref)

Artery	Normal MFV (cm/s)	Cut off for vasospasm
MCA	<80	>100
ACA	<80	>90
ICA	<70	>90
PCA	<50	>70
VA	<60	>70
BA	<50	>70
Lindegaard ratio; MCA/ICA	<3	>3

Diagnosis

Transcranial Doppler (TCD) is recommended daily during the intensive care unit stay. Age, hematocrit, mean arterial blood pressure, and individual anatomic differences may impact readings [131]. Normal flow velocity and vasospasm cut-offs are reported in Table 20.8. Mean Flow Velocity trends should be monitored closely and specific interventions implemented based on symptomatology.

For patients who experience neurologic decline in the vasospasm window, CTA should be performed to assess for marked narrowing in large vessels. Although clip/coil artifacts can sometimes limit interpretation, perfusion imaging can be considered to identify areas of ischemia [132]. If CTA is negative, but small vessel vasospasm is suspected then DSA should be performed [133]. DSA showing diffuse vasospasm is shown in Fig. 20.5.

Treatment

Several experimental treatments such as papaverine, tissue plasminogen activators, and rho-kinase inhibitors have been trialed in case studies, but efficacy with large clinical trials

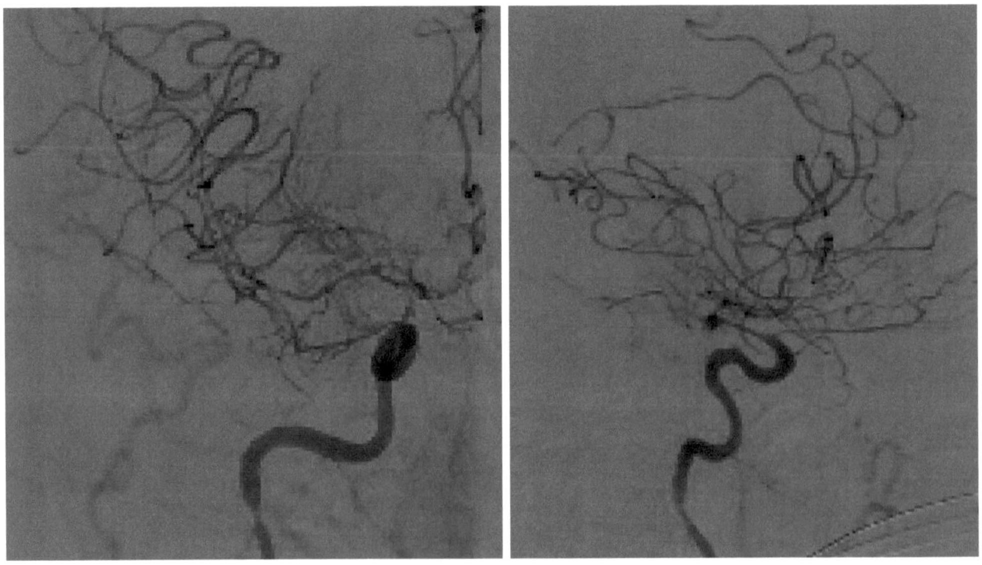

Fig. 20.5 A 38-year-old female who had neurologic decline with diffuse vasospasm in right ACA/MCA territories

are lacking [134–136]. Mixed data are available with some studies showing benefit and others with no benefit or harm. A key difficulty in designing clinical trials for vasospasm treatment is incomplete understanding of pathophysiology. Vasospasms can occur both in large arteries as well as smaller arterioles. The exact mechanisms are still being investigated. Cross talk with the glymphatic system is a topic of growing interest [137]. Furthermore, DCI can manifest in sites remote from documented vasospasm indicating that other factors are likely at play [138]. Nimodipine and maintenance of euvolemia have shown benefit, but exact mechanisms are still under investigation [139]. Statins have been trialed to target oxidative stress, endothelin-1 antagonists have been used for endothelial dysfunction, and magnesium infusion has been investigated for delaying DCI [140–142]. None of these clinical trials have demonstrated consistent clinical benefit.

Intra-arterial treatment of vasospasm with calcium channel blockers with or without balloon angioplasty has been the mainstay of treatment [143]. Small case series have also investigated intra-arterial nitric oxide pathway modulators [144]. For symptomatic patients, this often involves multiple endovascular interventions until vasospasm improves [145]. Early interventions for symptomatic patients have proven beneficial in improving long-term outcomes [146]. More recently, stent retrievers have been utilized and studies show similar efficacy to balloon angioplasty with decreased risk of vessel rupture [147]. An added benefit of stent retrievers is the ability to administer intra-arterial verapamil simultaneously [148].

Conclusion

aSAH continues to be a devastating neurologic injury that requires multidisciplinary care to optimize management. Over the past several decades, clinical-based guidelines have emerged and are supported by the AHA. Institution of these guidelines has improved morbidity and mortality through early recognition and implementation of treatment goals. Ongoing investigations into the best treatment options for vasospasm and DCI are underway. As understanding of the pathophysiology improves, new modalities may offer improved outcomes for this patient population.

References

1. Lucke-Wold BP, Logsdon AF, Manoranjan B, Turner RC, McConnell E, Vates GE, Huber JD, Rosen CL, Simard JM. Aneurysmal subarachnoid hemorrhage and Neuroinflammation: a comprehensive review. Int J Mol Sci. 2016;17(4):497.
2. King JT Jr. Epidemiology of aneurysmal subarachnoid hemorrhage. Neuroimaging Clin N Am. 1997;7(4):659–68.
3. Schievink WI, Wijdicks EF, Parisi JE, Piepgras DG, Whisnant JP. Sudden death from aneurysmal subarachnoid hemorrhage. Neurology. 1995;45(5):871–4.
4. Shea AM, Reed SD, Curtis LH, Alexander MJ, Villani JJ, Schulman KA. Characteristics of nontraumatic subarachnoid hemorrhage in the United States in 2003. Neurosurgery. 2007;61(6):1131–7; discussion 1137–8.
5. Hop JW, Rinkel GJ, Algra A, van Gijn J. Case-fatality rates and functional outcome after subarachnoid hemorrhage: a systematic review. Stroke. 1997;28(3):660–4.
6. Connolly ES Jr, Rabinstein AA, Carhuapoma JR, Derdeyn CP, Dion J, Higashida RT, Hoh BL, Kirkness CJ, Naidech AM, Ogilvy CS, et al. Guidelines for the management of aneurysmal subarachnoid hemorrhage: a guideline for healthcare professionals from the American Heart Association/american Stroke Association. Stroke. 2012;43(6):1711–37.
7. Ruigrok YM, Buskens E, Rinkel GJ. Attributable risk of common and rare determinants of subarachnoid hemorrhage. Stroke. 2001;32(5):1173–5.
8. Feigin VL, Lawes CM, Bennett DA, Barker-Collo SL, Parag V. Worldwide stroke incidence and early case fatality reported in 56 population-based studies: a systematic review. Lancet Neurol. 2009;8(4):355–69.
9. Ingall T, Asplund K, Mahonen M, Bonita R. A multinational comparison of subarachnoid hemorrhage epidemiology in the WHO MONICA stroke study. Stroke. 2000;31(5):1054–61.
10. Bor AS, Koffijberg H, Wermer MJ, Rinkel GJ. Optimal screening strategy for familial intracranial aneurysms: a cost-effectiveness analysis. Neurology. 2010;74(21):1671–9.
11. Lozano AM, Leblanc R. Cerebral aneurysms and polycystic kidney disease: a critical review. Can J Neurol Sci. 1992;19(2):222–7.
12. Kato T, Hattori H, Yorifuji T, Tashiro Y, Nakahata T. Intracranial aneurysms in Ehlers-Danlos syndrome type IV in early childhood. Pediatr Neurol. 2001;25(4):336–9.
13. Labovitz DL, Halim AX, Brent B, Boden-Albala B, Hauser WA, Sacco RL. Subarachnoid hemorrhage incidence among whites, blacks and Caribbean Hispanics: the northern Manhattan study. Neuroepidemiology. 2006;26(3):147–50.
14. Broderick JP, Brott T, Tomsick T, Huster G, Miller R. The risk of subarachnoid and intracerebral hemorrhages in blacks as compared with whites. N Engl J Med. 1992;326(11):733–6.
15. de Rooij NK, Linn FH, van der Plas JA, Algra A, Rinkel GJ. Incidence of subarachnoid haemorrhage: a systematic review with emphasis on region, age, gender and time trends. J Neurol Neurosurg Psychiatry. 2007;78(12):1365–72.
16. Algra AM, Klijn CJ, Helmerhorst FM, Algra A, Rinkel GJ. Female risk factors for subarachnoid hemorrhage: a systematic review. Neurology. 2012;79(12):1230–6.
17. Mahindu A, Koivisto T, Ronkainen A, Rinne J, Assaad N, Morgan MK. Similarities and differences in aneurysmal subarachnoid haemorrhage between eastern Finland and northern Sydney. J Clin Neurosci. 2008;15(6):617–21.
18. Andreasen TH, Bartek J Jr, Andresen M, Springborg JB, Romner B. Modifiable risk factors for aneurysmal subarachnoid hemorrhage. Stroke. 2013;44(12):3607–12.
19. Broderick JP, Viscoli CM, Brott T, Kernan WN, Brass LM, Feldmann E, Morgenstern LB, Wilterdink JL, Horwitz RI, Hemorrhagic Stroke Project I. Major risk factors for aneurysmal subarachnoid hemorrhage in the young are modifiable. Stroke. 2003;34(6):1375–81.
20. Lindekleiv H, Sandvei MS, Romundstad PR, Wilsgaard T, Njolstad I, Ingebrigtsen T, Vik A, Mathiesen EB. Joint effect of modifiable risk factors on the risk of aneurysmal subarachnoid hemorrhage: a cohort study. Stroke. 2012;43(7):1885–9.

21. Bederson JB, Connolly ES Jr, Batjer HH, Dacey RG, Dion JE, Diringer MN, Duldner JE Jr, Harbaugh RE, Patel AB, Rosenwasser RH, et al. Guidelines for the management of aneurysmal subarachnoid hemorrhage: a statement for healthcare professionals from a special writing group of the stroke council, American Heart Association. Stroke. 2009;40(3):994–1025.
22. Rahmanian A, Derakhshan N, Mohsenian Sisakht A, Karamzade Ziarati N, Raeisi Shahraki H, Motamed S. Risk factors for unfavorable outcome in aneurysmal subarachnoid hemorrhage revisited. Odds and Ends Bull Emerg Trauma. 2018;6(2):133–40.
23. Adams HP Jr, Kassell NF, Torner JC, Nibbelink DW, Sahs AL. Early management of aneurysmal subarachnoid hemorrhage. A report of the cooperative aneurysm study. J Neurosurg. 1981;54(2):141–5.
24. Hacein-Bey L, Provenzale JM. Current imaging assessment and treatment of intracranial aneurysms. AJR Am J Roentgenol. 2011;196(1):32–44.
25. Teasdale GM, Drake CG, Hunt W, Kassell N, Sano K, Pertuiset B, De Villiers JC. A universal subarachnoid hemorrhage scale: report of a committee of the world federation of neurosurgical societies. J Neurol Neurosurg Psychiatry. 1988;51(11):1457.
26. Broderick JP, Brott TG, Duldner JE, Tomsick T, Leach A. Initial and recurrent bleeding are the major causes of death following subarachnoid hemorrhage. Stroke. 1994;25(7):1342–7.
27. Sarti C, Tuomilehto J, Salomaa V, Sivenius J, Kaarsalo E, Narva EV, Salmi K, Torppa J. Epidemiology of subarachnoid hemorrhage in Finland from 1983 to 1985. Stroke. 1991;22(7):848–53.
28. Laidlaw JD, Siu KH. Poor-grade aneurysmal subarachnoid hemorrhage: outcome after treatment with urgent surgery. Neurosurgery. 2003;53(6):1275–80; discussion 1280–2.
29. Fisher CM, Roberson GH, Ojemann RG. Cerebral vasospasm with ruptured saccular aneurysm--the clinical manifestations. Neurosurgery. 1977;1(3):245–8.
30. Chen S, Luo J, Reis C, Manaenko A, Zhang J. Hydrocephalus after subarachnoid hemorrhage: pathophysiology, diagnosis, and treatment. Biomed Res Int. 2017;2017:8584753.
31. Chen Q, Feng Z, Tan Q, Guo J, Tang J, Tan L, Feng H, Chen Z. Post-hemorrhagic hydrocephalus: recent advances and new therapeutic insights. J Neurol Sci. 2017;375:220–30.
32. Findlay JM, Nisar J, Darsaut T. Cerebral Vasospasm: A Review. Can J Neurol Sci. 2016;43(1):15–32.
33. Heros RC, Zervas NT, Varsos V. Cerebral vasospasm after subarachnoid hemorrhage: an update. Ann Neurol. 1983;14(6):599–608.
34. Inagawa T. Risk factors for cerebral vasospasm following aneurysmal subarachnoid hemorrhage: a review of the literature. World Neurosurg. 2016;85:56–76.
35. Hijdra A, Van Gijn J, Stefanko S, Van Dongen KJ, Vermeulen M, Van Crevel H. Delayed cerebral ischemia after aneurysmal subarachnoid hemorrhage: clinicoanatomic correlations. Neurology. 1986;36(3):329–33.
36. Guo Y, Fang S, Wang J, Wang C, Zhao J, Gai Y. Continuous EEG detection of DCI and seizures following aSAH: a systematic review. Br J Neurosurg. 2020;34(5):543–8.
37. Claassen J, Bernardini GL, Kreiter K, Bates J, Du YE, Copeland D, Connolly ES, Mayer SA. Effect of cisternal and ventricular blood on risk of delayed cerebral ischemia after subarachnoid hemorrhage: the Fisher scale revisited. Stroke. 2001;32(9):2012–20.
38. Hope JK, Wilson JL, Thomson FJ. Three-dimensional CT angiography in the detection and characterization of intracranial berry aneurysms. AJNR Am J Neuroradiol. 1996;17(3):439–45.
39. van Gelder JM. Computed tomographic angiography for detecting cerebral aneurysms: implications of aneurysm size distribution for the sensitivity, specificity, and likelihood ratios. Neurosurgery. 2003;53(3):597–605; discussion 605–6.
40. McCormack RF, Hutson A. Can computed tomography angiography of the brain replace lumbar puncture in the evaluation of acute-onset headache after a negative noncontrast cranial computed tomography scan? Acad Emerg Med. 2010;17(4):444–51.
41. Shah KH, Richard KM, Nicholas S, Edlow JA. Incidence of traumatic lumbar puncture. Acad Emerg Med. 2003;10(2):151–4.
42. Takemoto K, Takano K, Abe H, Okawa M, Iwaasa M, Higashi T, Inoue T. The new MRI modalities "BPAS and VISTA" for the diagnosis of VA dissection. Acta Neurochir Suppl. 2011;112:59–65.
43. Obusez EC, Jones SE, Mandell D, Bullen J, Gonzalez F, Hui FK. Feasibility of vessel wall imaging in assessing unruptured paraclinoid aneurysms: clinical observations and preliminary experience. J Clin Neurosci. 2019;61:59–65.
44. Endo H, Niizuma K, Fujimura M, Sato K, Inoue T, Osawa S, Tominaga T. Ruptured cerebral microaneurysm diagnosed by 3-dimensional fast spin-Echo T1 imaging with variable Flip angles. J Stroke Cerebrovasc Dis. 2015;24(8):e231–5.
45. Yeole U, Nagesh M, Shukla D, R AH, R PA. The yield of repeat angiography in angiography-negative spontaneous subarachnoid hemorrhage. J Neurosci Rural Pract. 2020;11(4):565–72.
46. Canter LM. Anaphylactoid reactions to radiocontrast media. Allergy Asthma Proc. 2005;26(3):199–203.
47. Zaraca F, Wiedermann CJ, Ebner H. Contrast media-induced nephropathy in patients undergoing angiography prior to or during vascular surgery: a systematic review. Minerva Chir. 2011;66(6):553–60.
48. Morcos SK, Thomsen HS. Adverse reactions to iodinated contrast media. Eur Radiol. 2001;11(7):1267–75.
49. Bush WH, Swanson DP. Acute reactions to intravascular contrast media: types, risk factors, recognition, and specific treatment. AJR Am J Roentgenol. 1991;157(6):1153–61.
50. Wijdicks EF, Vermeulen M, Murray GD, Hijdra A, van Gijn J. The effects of treating hypertension following aneurysmal subarachnoid hemorrhage. Clin Neurol Neurosurg. 1990;92(2):111–7.
51. Stornelli SA, French JD. Subarachnoid hemorrhage--factors in prognosis and management. J Neurosurg. 1964;21:769–80.
52. Hillman J, Fridriksson S, Nilsson O, Yu Z, Saveland H, Jakobsson KE. Immediate administration of tranexamic acid and reduced incidence of early rebleeding after aneurysmal subarachnoid hemorrhage: a prospective randomized study. J Neurosurg. 2002;97(4):771–8.
53. Tanno Y, Homma M, Oinuma M, Kodama N, Ymamoto T. Rebleeding from ruptured intracranial aneurysms in north Eastern Province of Japan. A cooperative study J Neurol Sci. 2007;258(1–2):11–6.
54. Naidech AM, Janjua N, Kreiter KT, Ostapkovich ND, Fitzsimmons BF, Parra A, Commichau C, Connolly ES, Mayer SA. Predictors and impact of aneurysm rebleeding after subarachnoid hemorrhage. Arch Neurol. 2005;62(3):410–6.
55. Kassell NF, Torner JC, Jane JA, Haley EC Jr, Adams HP. The international cooperative study on the timing of aneurysm surgery. Part 2: surgical results. J Neurosurg. 1990;73(1):37–47.
56. Liu-Deryke X, Janisse J, Coplin WM, Parker D Jr, Norris G, Rhoney DH. A comparison of nicardipine and labetalol for acute hypertension management following stroke. Neurocrit Care. 2008;9(2):167–76.
57. Ruigrok YM, Slooter AJ, Rinkel GJ, Wijmenga C, Rosendaal FR. Genes influencing coagulation and the risk of aneurysmal subarachnoid hemorrhage, and subsequent complications of secondary cerebral ischemia and rebleeding. Acta Neurochir. 2010;152(2):257–62.
58. Torner JC, Kassell NF, Wallace RB, Adams HP Jr. Preoperative prognostic factors for rebleeding and survival in aneurysm patients receiving antifibrinolytic therapy: report of the cooperative aneurysm study. Neurosurgery. 1981;9(5):506–13.
59. Kassell NF, Torner JC, Adams HP Jr. Antifibrinolytic therapy in the acute period following aneurysmal subarachnoid hemorrhage.

Preliminary observations from the cooperative aneurysm study. J Neurosurg. 1984;61(2):225–30.
60. Starke RM, Kim GH, Fernandez A, Komotar RJ, Hickman ZL, Otten ML, Ducruet AF, Kellner CP, Hahn DK, Chwajol M, et al. Impact of a protocol for acute antifibrinolytic therapy on aneurysm rebleeding after subarachnoid hemorrhage. Stroke. 2008;39(9):2617–21.
61. Park J, Woo H, Kang DH, Kim YS, Kim MY, Shin IH, Kwak SG. Formal protocol for emergency treatment of ruptured intracranial aneurysms to reduce in-hospital rebleeding and improve clinical outcomes. J Neurosurg. 2015;122(2):383–91.
62. Harrigan MR, Rajneesh KF, Ardelt AA, Fisher WS 3rd. Short-term antifibrinolytic therapy before early aneurysm treatment in subarachnoid hemorrhage: effects on rehemorrhage, cerebral ischemia, and hydrocephalus. Neurosurgery. 2010;67(4):935–9. discussion 939-40
63. Lin CL, Dumont AS, Lieu AS, Yen CP, Hwang SL, Kwan AL, Kassell NF, Howng SL. Characterization of perioperative seizures and epilepsy following aneurysmal subarachnoid hemorrhage. J Neurosurg. 2003;99(6):978–85.
64. Choi KS, Chun HJ, Yi HJ, Ko Y, Kim YS, Kim JM. Seizures and epilepsy following aneurysmal subarachnoid hemorrhage : incidence and risk factors. J Korean Neurosurg Soc. 2009;46(2):93–8.
65. Chumnanvej S, Dunn IF, Kim DH. Three-day phenytoin prophylaxis is adequate after subarachnoid hemorrhage. Neurosurgery. 2007;60(1):99–102; discussion 102–3.
66. Mahmoud SH, Buxton J. Seizures and choice of antiepileptic drugs following subarachnoid hemorrhage: a review. Can J Neurol Sci. 2017;44(6):643–53.
67. Butzkueven H, Evans AH, Pitman A, Leopold C, Jolley DJ, Kaye AH, Kilpatrick CJ, Davis SM. Onset seizures independently predict poor outcome after subarachnoid hemorrhage. Neurology. 2000;55(9):1315–20.
68. Hasan D, Vermeulen M, Wijdicks EF, Hijdra A, van Gijn J. Management problems in acute hydrocephalus after subarachnoid hemorrhage. Stroke. 1989;20(6):747–53.
69. McIver JI, Friedman JA, Wijdicks EF, Piepgras DG, Pichelmann MA, Toussaint LG 3rd, McClelland RL, Nichols DA, Atkinson JL. Preoperative ventriculostomy and rebleeding after aneurysmal subarachnoid hemorrhage. J Neurosurg. 2002;97(5):1042–4.
70. Chung DY, Mayer SA, Rordorf GA. External ventricular drains after subarachnoid hemorrhage: is less more? Neurocrit Care. 2018;28(2):157–61.
71. Klopfenstein JD, Kim LJ, Feiz-Erfan I, Hott JS, Goslar P, Zabramski JM, Spetzler RF. Comparison of rapid and gradual weaning from external ventricular drainage in patients with aneurysmal subarachnoid hemorrhage: a prospective randomized trial. J Neurosurg. 2004;100(2):225–9.
72. Kwon JH, Sung SK, Song YJ, Choi HJ, Huh JT, Kim HD. Predisposing factors related to shunt-dependent chronic hydrocephalus after aneurysmal subarachnoid hemorrhage. J Korean Neurosurg Soc. 2008;43(4):177–81.
73. de Oliveira JG, Beck J, Setzer M, Gerlach R, Vatter H, Seifert V, Raabe A. Risk of shunt-dependent hydrocephalus after occlusion of ruptured intracranial aneurysms by surgical clipping or endovascular coiling: a single-institution series and meta-analysis. Neurosurgery. 2007;61(5):924–33; discussion 933–4.
74. Komotar RJ, Hahn DK, Kim GH, Starke RM, Garrett MC, Merkow MB, Otten ML, Sciacca RR, Connolly ES Jr. Efficacy of lamina terminalis fenestration in reducing shunt-dependent hydrocephalus following aneurysmal subarachnoid hemorrhage: a systematic review. Clinical article. J Neurosurg. 2009;111(1):147–54.
75. Solenski NJ, Haley EC Jr, Kassell NF, Kongable G, Germanson T, Truskowski L, Torner JC. Medical complications of aneurysmal subarachnoid hemorrhage: a report of the multicenter, cooperative aneurysm study. Participants of the multicenter cooperative aneurysm study. Crit Care Med. 1995;23(6):1007–17.
76. Rahman M, Friedman WA. Hyponatremia in neurosurgical patients: clinical guidelines development. Neurosurgery. 2009;65(5):925–35; discussion 935–6.
77. Qureshi AI, Suri MF, Sung GY, Straw RN, Yahia AM, Saad M, Guterman LR, Hopkins LN. Prognostic significance of hypernatremia and hyponatremia among patients with aneurysmal subarachnoid hemorrhage. Neurosurgery. 2002;50(4):749–55; discussion 755–6.
78. Suarez JI, Qureshi AI, Parekh PD, Razumovsky A, Tamargo RJ, Bhardwaj A, Ulatowski JA. Administration of hypertonic (3%) sodium chloride/acetate in hyponatremic patients with symptomatic vasospasm following subarachnoid hemorrhage. J Neurosurg Anesthesiol. 1999;11(3):178–84.
79. Mori T, Katayama Y, Kawamata T, Hirayama T. Improved efficiency of hypervolemic therapy with inhibition of natriuresis by fludrocortisone in patients with aneurysmal subarachnoid hemorrhage. J Neurosurg. 1999;91(6):947–52.
80. Wijdicks EF, Vermeulen M, Hijdra A, van Gijn J. Hyponatremia and cerebral infarction in patients with ruptured intracranial aneurysms: is fluid restriction harmful? Ann Neurol. 1985;17(2):137–40.
81. Naredi S, Lambert G, Eden E, Zall S, Runnerstam M, Rydenhag B, Friberg P. Increased sympathetic nervous activity in patients with nontraumatic subarachnoid hemorrhage. Stroke. 2000;31(4):901–6.
82. Todd GL, Baroldi G, Pieper GM, Clayton FC, Eliot RS. Experimental catecholamine-induced myocardial necrosis. II. Temporal development of isoproterenol-induced contraction band lesions correlated with ECG, hemodynamic and biochemical changes. J Mol Cell Cardiol. 1985;17(7):647–56.
83. van der Bilt IA, Hasan D, Vandertop WP, Wilde AA, Algra A, Visser FC, Rinkel GJ. Impact of cardiac complications on outcome after aneurysmal subarachnoid hemorrhage: a meta-analysis. Neurology. 2009;72(7):635–42.
84. Kothavale A, Banki NM, Kopelnik A, Yarlagadda S, Lawton MT, Ko N, Smith WS, Drew B, Foster E, Zaroff JG. Predictors of left ventricular regional wall motion abnormalities after subarachnoid hemorrhage. Neurocrit Care. 2006;4(3):199–205.
85. Sugimoto K, Watanabe E, Yamada A, Iwase M, Sano H, Hishida H, Ozaki Y. Prognostic implications of left ventricular wall motion abnormalities associated with subarachnoid hemorrhage. Int Heart J. 2008;49(1):75–85.
86. Amin HZ, Amin LZ, Pradipta A. Takotsubo cardiomyopathy: a brief review. J Med Life. 2020;13(1):3–7.
87. Lee VH, Connolly HM, Fulgham JR, Manno EM, Brown RD Jr, Wijdicks EF. Tako-tsubo cardiomyopathy in aneurysmal subarachnoid hemorrhage: an underappreciated ventricular dysfunction. J Neurosurg. 2006;105(2):264–70.
88. Kahn JM, Caldwell EC, Deem S, Newell DW, Heckbert SR, Rubenfeld GD. Acute lung injury in patients with subarachnoid hemorrhage: incidence, risk factors, and outcome. Crit Care Med. 2006;34(1):196–202.
89. Kramer AH, Bleck TP, Dumont AS, Kassell NF, Olson C, Nathan B. Implications of early versus late bilateral pulmonary infiltrates in patients with aneurysmal subarachnoid hemorrhage. Neurocrit Care. 2009;10(1):20–7.
90. Sharma D. Perioperative Management of Aneurysmal Subarachnoid Hemorrhage. Anesthesiology. 2020;133(6):1283–305.
91. Friedman JA, Pichelmann MA, Piepgras DG, McIver JI, Toussaint LG 3rd, McClelland RL, Nichols DA, Meyer FB, Atkinson JL, Wijdicks EF. Pulmonary complications of aneurysmal subarachnoid hemorrhage. Neurosurgery. 2003;52(5):1025–31; discussion 1031–2.

92. Peterson E, Heros RC. Don't lose the lungs for the brain: pulmonary complications after subarachnoid hemorrhage. World Neurosurg. 2014;82(1–2):e167–8.
93. Jamali SA, Turnbull MT, Kanekiyo T, Vishnu P, Zubair AC, Raper CC, Tawk RG, Freeman WD. Elevated neutrophil-lymphocyte ratio is predictive of poor outcomes following aneurysmal subarachnoid hemorrhage. J Stroke Cerebrovasc Dis. 2020;29(4):104631.
94. Karic T, Roe C, Nordenmark TH, Becker F, Sorteberg W, Sorteberg A. Effect of early mobilization and rehabilitation on complications in aneurysmal subarachnoid hemorrhage. J Neurosurg. 2017;126(2):518–26.
95. McIntyre LA, Fergusson DA, Hutchison JS, Pagliarello G, Marshall JC, Yetisir E, Hare GM, Hebert PC. Effect of a liberal versus restrictive transfusion strategy on mortality in patients with moderate to severe head injury. Neurocrit Care. 2006;5(1):4–9.
96. Smith MJ, Le Roux PD, Elliott JP, Winn HR. Blood transfusion and increased risk for vasospasm and poor outcome after subarachnoid hemorrhage. J Neurosurg. 2004;101(1):1–7.
97. Dhar R, Zazulia AR, Videen TO, Zipfel GJ, Derdeyn CP, Diringer MN. Red blood cell transfusion increases cerebral oxygen delivery in anemic patients with subarachnoid hemorrhage. Stroke. 2009;40(9):3039–44.
98. Ji R, Li G, Zhang R, Hou H, Zhao X, Wang Y. Higher risk of deep vein thrombosis after hemorrhagic stroke than after acute ischemic stroke. J Vasc Nurs. 2019;37(1):18–27.
99. Stecker M, Michel K, Antaky K, Cherian S, Koyfmann F. Risk factors for DVT/PE in patients with stroke and intracranial hemorrhage. Open Neurol J. 2014;8:1–6.
100. Guo JD, Rajpura J, Hlavacek P, Keshishian A, Sah J, Delinger R, Mu Q, Mardekian J, Russ C, Okano GJ, et al. Comparative clinical and economic outcomes associated with warfarin versus Apixaban in the treatment of patients with venous thromboembolism in a large U.S. Commercial Claims Database. J Manag Care Spec Pharm. 2020;26(8):1017–26.
101. Alaraj A, Wallace A, Mander N, Aletich V, Charbel FT, Amin-Hanjani S. Risk factors for heparin-induced thrombocytopenia type II in aneurysmal subarachnoid hemorrhage. Neurosurgery. 2011;69(5):1030–6.
102. Adamczak S, Fritz R, Patel D, Geh N, Laurent D, Polifka A, Hoh BL, Fox WC. Trends in hospital-to-hospital transfers for aneurysmal subarachnoid hemorrhage: a single-institution experience from 2006 to 2017. World Neurosurg. 2021;148:e17–26.
103. Andaluz N, Zuccarello M. Recent trends in the treatment of cerebral aneurysms: analysis of a nationwide inpatient database. J Neurosurg. 2008;108(6):1163–9.
104. Bardach NS, Zhao S, Gress DR, Lawton MT, Johnston SC. Association between subarachnoid hemorrhage outcomes and number of cases treated at California hospitals. Stroke. 2002;33(7):1851–6.
105. Cross DT 3rd, Tirschwell DL, Clark MA, Tuden D, Derdeyn CP, Moran CJ, Dacey RG Jr. Mortality rates after subarachnoid hemorrhage: variations according to hospital case volume in 18 states. J Neurosurg. 2003;99(5):810–7.
106. Alberts MJ, Latchaw RE, Selman WR, Shephard T, Hadley MN, Brass LM, Koroshetz W, Marler JR, Booss J, Zorowitz RD, et al. Recommendations for comprehensive stroke centers: a consensus statement from the brain attack coalition. Stroke. 2005;36(7):1597–616.
107. Johnston SC. Effect of endovascular services and hospital volume on cerebral aneurysm treatment outcomes. Stroke. 2000;31(1):111–7.
108. Stevens RD, Naval NS, Mirski MA, Citerio G, Andrews PJ. Intensive care of aneurysmal subarachnoid hemorrhage: an international survey. Intensive Care Med. 2009;35(9):1556–66.
109. Murayama Y, Nien YL, Duckwiler G, Gobin YP, Jahan R, Frazee J, Martin N, Vinuela F. Guglielmi detachable coil embolization of cerebral aneurysms: 11 years' experience. J Neurosurg. 2003;98(5):959–66.
110. Molyneux AJ, Kerr RS, Yu LM, Clarke M, Sneade M, Yarnold JA, Sandercock P, International Subarachnoid Aneurysm Trial Collaborative G. International subarachnoid aneurysm trial (ISAT) of neurosurgical clipping versus endovascular coiling in 2143 patients with ruptured intracranial aneurysms: a randomised comparison of effects on survival, dependency, seizures, rebleeding, subgroups, and aneurysm occlusion. Lancet. 2005;366(9488):809–17.
111. Proust F, Martinaud O, Gerardin E, Derrey S, Leveque S, Bioux S, Tollard E, Clavier E, Langlois O, Godefroy O, et al. Quality of life and brain damage after microsurgical clip occlusion or endovascular coil embolization for ruptured anterior communicating artery aneurysms: neuropsychological assessment. J Neurosurg. 2009;110(1):19–29.
112. Sahs AL. Report on the cooperative study of intracranial aneurysms and subarachnoid hemorrhage. Section VII. 2. Hypotension and hypothermia in the treatment of intracranial aneurysms. J Neurosurg. 1966;25(5):593–600.
113. David CA, Vishteh AG, Spetzler RF, Lemole M, Lawton MT, Partovi S. Late angiographic follow-up review of surgically treated aneurysms. J Neurosurg. 1999;91(3):396–401.
114. Deng J, Zhao Z, Gao G. Periprocedural complications associated with endovascular embolisation of intracranial ruptured aneurysms with matrix coils. Singapore Med J. 2007;48(5):429–33.
115. Rinne J, Hernesniemi J, Niskanen M, Vapalahti M. Analysis of 561 patients with 690 middle cerebral artery aneurysms: anatomic and clinical features as correlated to management outcome. Neurosurgery. 1996;38(1):2–11.
116. Short JG, Marx WF, Lanzino G, Ellegala DB, Kassell NF. Surgical salvage of microcatheter-induced aneurysm perforation during coil embolization. AJNR Am J Neuroradiol. 2002;23(4):682–5.
117. Karamanakos PN, Koivisto T, Vanninen R, Khallaf M, Ronkainen A, Parviainen I, Manninen H, von und zu Fraunberg M, Morgan MK, Jaaskelainen JE and others. The impact of endovascular management on the outcome of aneurysmal subarachnoid hemorrhage in the elderly in eastern Finland. Acta Neurochir. 2010;152(9):1493–502.
118. Lusseveld E, Brilstra EH, Nijssen PC, van Rooij WJ, Sluzewski M, Tulleken CA, Wijnalda D, Schellens RL, van der Graaf Y, Rinkel GJ. Endovascular coiling versus neurosurgical clipping in patients with a ruptured basilar tip aneurysm. J Neurol Neurosurg Psychiatry. 2002;73(5):591–3.
119. Meling TR, Patet G. Clip-wrapping of ruptured blood blister-like aneurysms of the internal carotid artery. Neurosurg Rev. 2020;43(5):1365–71.
120. Gross BA, Du R. STA-MCA bypass. Acta Neurochir. 2012;154(8):1463–7.
121. Farrar JK, Gamache FW Jr, Ferguson GG, Barker J, Varkey GP, Drake CG. Effects of profound hypotension on cerebral blood flow during surgery for intracranial aneurysms. J Neurosurg. 1981;55(6):857–64.
122. Pasternak JJ, McGregor DG, Schroeder DR, Lanier WL, Shi Q, Hindman BJ, Clarke WR, Torner JC, Weeks JB, Todd MM, et al. Hyperglycemia in patients undergoing cerebral aneurysm surgery: its association with long-term gross neurologic and neuropsychological function. Mayo Clin Proc. 2008;83(4):406–17.
123. Todd MM, Hindman BJ, Clarke WR, Torner JC. Intraoperative hypothermia for aneurysm surgery trial I. Mild intraoperative hypothermia during surgery for intracranial aneurysm. N Engl J Med. 2005;352(2):135–45.
124. Sorar M, Altay O. Subarachnoid hemorrhage and Sevoflurane. Turk Neurosurg. 2020;30(3):354–60.
125. Park SD, Kim JH, Chang CH, Jung YJ. Procedure-related complication rate for the endovascular treatment of aneurysmal sub-

arachnoid hemorrhage under local anesthesia. J Cerebrovasc Endovasc Neurosurg. 2016;18(3):215–22.
126. Kundra S, Mahendru V, Gupta V, Choudhary AK. Principles of neuroanesthesia in aneurysmal subarachnoid hemorrhage. J Anaesthesiol Clin Pharmacol. 2014;30(3):328–37.
127. Weir BK, Kongable GL, Kassell NF, Schultz JR, Truskowski LL, Sigrest A. Cigarette smoking as a cause of aneurysmal subarachnoid hemorrhage and risk for vasospasm: a report of the cooperative aneurysm study. J Neurosurg. 1998;89(3):405–11.
128. Lucke-Wold B, Hosaka K, Dodd W, Motwani K, Laurent D, Martinez M, Hoh B. Interleukin-6: important mediator of vasospasm following subarachnoid hemorrhage. Curr Neurovasc Res. 2021;18(3):364–9.
129. Dodd WS, Patel D, Lucke-Wold B, Hosaka K, Chalouhi N, Hoh BL. Adropin decreases endothelial monolayer permeability after cell-free hemoglobin exposure and reduces MCP-1-induced macrophage transmigration. Biochem Biophys Res Commun. 2021;582:105–10.
130. Schmidt JM, Wartenberg KE, Fernandez A, Claassen J, Rincon F, Ostapkovich ND, Badjatia N, Parra A, Connolly ES, Mayer SA. Frequency and clinical impact of asymptomatic cerebral infarction due to vasospasm after subarachnoid hemorrhage. J Neurosurg. 2008;109(6):1052–9.
131. Sloan MA, Alexandrov AV, Tegeler CH, Spencer MP, Caplan LR, Feldmann E, Wechsler LR, Newell DW, Gomez CR, Babikian VL, et al. Assessment: transcranial Doppler ultrasonography: report of the therapeutics and technology assessment Subcommittee of the American Academy of neurology. Neurology. 2004;62(9):1468–81.
132. van der Schaaf I, Wermer MJ, van der Graaf Y, Velthuis BK, van de Kraats CI, Rinkel GJ. Prognostic value of cerebral perfusion-computed tomography in the acute stage after subarachnoid hemorrhage for the development of delayed cerebral ischemia. Stroke. 2006;37(2):409–13.
133. Anderson GB, Ashforth R, Steinke DE, Findlay JM. CT angiography for the detection of cerebral vasospasm in patients with acute subarachnoid hemorrhage. AJNR Am J Neuroradiol. 2000;21(6):1011–5.
134. Shibuya M, Suzuki Y, Sugita K, Saito I, Sasaki T, Takakura K, Nagata I, Kikuchi H, Takemae T, Hidaka H, et al. Effect of AT877 on cerebral vasospasm after aneurysmal subarachnoid hemorrhage. Results of a prospective placebo-controlled double-blind trial. J Neurosurg. 1992;76(4):571–7.
135. Hamada J, Kai Y, Morioka M, Yano S, Mizuno T, Hirano T, Kazekawa K, Ushio Y. Effect on cerebral vasospasm of coil embolization followed by microcatheter intrathecal urokinase infusion into the cisterna magna: a prospective randomized study. Stroke. 2003;34(11):2549–54.
136. Kassell NF, Helm G, Simmons N, Phillips CD, Cail WS. Treatment of cerebral vasospasm with intra-arterial papaverine. J Neurosurg. 1992;77(6):848–52.
137. Luo C, Yao X, Li J, He B, Liu Q, Ren H, Liang F, Li M, Lin H, Peng J, et al. Paravascular pathways contribute to vasculitis and neuroinflammation after subarachnoid hemorrhage independently of glymphatic control. Cell Death Dis. 2016;7:e2160.
138. Yundt KD, Grubb RL Jr, Diringer MN, Powers WJ. Autoregulatory vasodilation of parenchymal vessels is impaired during cerebral vasospasm. J Cereb Blood Flow Metab. 1998;18(4):419–24.
139. Allen GS, Ahn HS, Preziosi TJ, Battye R, Boone SC, Boone SC, Chou SN, Kelly DL, Weir BK, Crabbe RA, et al. Cerebral arterial spasm--a controlled trial of nimodipine in patients with subarachnoid hemorrhage. N Engl J Med. 1983;308(11):619–24.
140. Vergouwen MD. Effect of endothelin-receptor antagonists on delayed cerebral ischemia after aneurysmal subarachnoid hemorrhage remains unclear. Stroke. 2009;40(12):e714:author reply e715-6.
141. Vergouwen MD, Meijers JC, Geskus RB, Coert BA, Horn J, Stroes ES, van der Poll T, Vermeulen M, Roos YB. Biologic effects of simvastatin in patients with aneurysmal subarachnoid hemorrhage: a double-blind, placebo-controlled randomized trial. J Cereb Blood Flow Metab. 2009;29(8):1444–53.
142. Wong GK, Poon WS, Chan MT, Boet R, Gin T, Ng SC, Zee BC. Plasma magnesium concentrations and clinical outcomes in aneurysmal subarachnoid hemorrhage patients: post hoc analysis of intravenous magnesium sulphate for aneurysmal subarachnoid hemorrhage trial. Stroke. 2010;41(8):1841–4.
143. Jun P, Ko NU, English JD, Dowd CF, Halbach VV, Higashida RT, Lawton MT, Hetts SW. Endovascular treatment of medically refractory cerebral vasospasm following aneurysmal subarachnoid hemorrhage. AJNR Am J Neuroradiol. 2010;31(10):1911–6.
144. Shankar JJ, dos Santos MP, Deus-Silva L, Lum C. Angiographic evaluation of the effect of intra-arterial milrinone therapy in patients with vasospasm from aneurysmal subarachnoid hemorrhage. Neuroradiology. 2011;53(2):123–8.
145. Jabbarli R, Pierscianek D, Rolz R, Darkwah Oppong M, Kaier K, Shah M, Taschner C, Monninghoff C, Urbach H, Beck J, et al. Endovascular treatment of cerebral vasospasm after subarachnoid hemorrhage: more is more. Neurology. 2019;93(5):e458–66.
146. Boulouis G, Labeyrie MA, Raymond J, Rodriguez-Regent C, Lukaszewicz AC, Bresson D, Ben Hassen W, Trystram D, Meder JF, Oppenheim C, et al. Treatment of cerebral vasospasm following aneurysmal subarachnoid haemorrhage: a systematic review and meta-analysis. Eur Radiol. 2017;27(8):3333–42.
147. Kwon HJ, Lim JW, Koh HS, Park B, Choi SW, Kim SH, Youm JY, Song SH. Stent-retriever angioplasty for recurrent post-subarachnoid hemorrhagic vasospasm - a single center experience with long-term follow-up. Clin Neuroradiol. 2019;29(4):751–61.
148. Su YS, Ali MS, Pukenas BA, Favilla CG, Zanaty M, Hasan DM, Kung DK. Novel treatment of cerebral vasospasm using solitaire stent retriever-assisted angioplasty: case series. World Neurosurg. 2020;135:e657–63.

Intracerebral Hemorrhage

21

Trevor Hardigan, Colton J. Smith, Alexandra S. Reynolds, and Christopher P. Kellner

Contents

Abstract

Primary spontaneous intracerebral hemorrhage (ICH), or extravasation of blood into the brain parenchyma, typically results from either hypertension or cerebral amyloid angiopathy (CAA). This is in contrast to secondary ICH that results from underlying vascular lesions including aneurysms or malformations as well as pathologies like venous thrombosis, neoplasms, coagulopathies, or antithrombotic use. The management of primary ICH for many years has emphasized medical management as opposed to surgical intervention based on the failure of several large, randomized trials to show a benefit of open craniotomy with hematoma evacuation [1]. The treatment of ICH is a multidisciplinary effort, with neurologists, neurosurgeons, neurointensivists, internists, and rehabilitation specialists all playing critical roles in the care of these patients. The most recent guidelines from the American Heart Association/American Stroke Association in 2022 served as an update to the previous 2015 guidelines [2]. Even with recent advances in medical care and technology, the short-term case fatality still approaches 50%, indicating a continued treatment gap that further trials with novel therapies must seek to overcome [3]. This chapter will focus on the diagnosis and management of primary ICH, with particular attention to recent advances in surgical management including minimally invasive evacuation.

T. Hardigan · C. J. Smith · A. S. Reynolds · C. P. Kellner (✉)
Department of Neurosurgery, Icahn School of Medicine at Mount Sinai, New York, NY, USA
e-mail: trevor.hardigan@mountsinai.org; colton.smith@mountsinai.org

E. Mahanna Gabrielli et al. (eds.), *Textbook of Neurointensive Care: Volume 1*, https://doi.org/10.1007/978-3-031-62220-5_21

Introduction

Primary spontaneous intracerebral hemorrhage (ICH), or extravasation of blood into the brain parenchyma, typically results from either hypertension or cerebral amyloid angiopathy (CAA). This is in contrast to secondary ICH that results from underlying vascular lesions including aneurysms or malformations as well as pathologies like venous thrombosis, neoplasms, coagulopathies, or antithrombotic use. The management of primary ICH for many years has emphasized medical management as opposed to surgical intervention based on the failure of several large, randomized trials to show a benefit of open craniotomy with hematoma evacuation [1]. The treatment of ICH is a multidisciplinary effort, with neurologists, neurosurgeons, neurointensivists, internists, and rehabilitation specialists all playing critical roles in the care of these patients. The most recent guidelines from the American Heart Association/American Stroke Association in 2022 served as an update to the previous 2015 guidelines [2]. Even with recent advances in medical care and technology, the short-term case fatality still approaches 50%, indicating a continued treatment gap that further trials with novel therapies must seek to overcome [3]. This chapter will focus on the diagnosis and management of primary ICH, with particular attention to recent advances in surgical management including minimally invasive evacuation.

Epidemiology

Approximately 10–20% of all strokes are hemorrhagic [4, 5], with only 20% of patients regaining functional independence at 6 months. Of these cases, approximately 78–88% of them are primary ICH [6–8]. The incidence of ICH hospital admission rates increased over a 30-year period from 1979 to 2008, from an average of 24,000 cases (12.9 per 100,000 persons per year) to an average of 63,000 cases (21 per 100,000 per year) [9]. Over that time, in-hospital mortality fell significantly, from approximately 45% to 34%, which demonstrates the ongoing need for improvement in care of this patient population. The majority of these changes occurred during the first 10 years of the study, with the previous 20 years being relatively stable in regard to incidence and mortality. Multiple other studies confirm this concerning lack of improvement in decreasing the incidence of ICH over the last 30 years [5, 10, 11]

Risk Factors

The risk factors for spontaneous ICH are grouped into either non-modifiable risk factors including age, ethnicity, genetic predisposition, and cerebral amyloid angiopathy (CAA), or modifiable risk factors including hypertension (HTN), hypercholesterolemia, smoking, heavy alcohol consumption, drug use, and diet. In the INTERSTROKE study, an international case-control study on risk factors for stroke with 3059 ICH patients, HTN, physical activity, diet, alcohol consumption, and cardiac disease was associated with ICH [12]. A prospective cohort study of 15,792 patients determined that African American ethnicity and HTN were positively associated with the incidence of ICH, while smoking, diabetes, alcohol, and body mass index had no association [13]. Hypertension is perhaps the greatest risk factor for primary ICH [14, 15]. The odds ratio for ICH in the presence of HTN is approximately 2.5–5.5 [16–18]. Hypertension has been shown to be up to twice as common in patients with deep cerebral ICH compared with lobar ICH [19–21]. In a recent systematic review and metaanalysis, 26,174 patients from 42 studies were examined, with 9141 lobar and 17,033 non-lobar hemorrhage observed. Risk factors for non-lobar ICH were HTN (relative risk (RR) 4.25, 95% confidence interval (CI) 3.05–5.91), diabetes (RR 1.35, 95% CI 1.11–1.64), male sex (RR1.63, 95% CI 1.25–2.14), alcohol abuse (RR 1.48, 95% CI 1.21–1.81), underweight status (RR 2.12, 95% CI 1.12–4.01), and Black race/Hispanic ethinicity (RR 2.83 95% CI 1.02–7.84 and RR 2.95, 95% CI 1.69 = 5.14, respectively vs. Caucasian race) [22]. For lobar ICH, only HTN was a risk factor (RR 1.83, 95% CI 1.39–2.42). In this meta-analysis, neither smoking nor hypercholesterolemia were associated. This large study highlights the importance of referring to ICH located in the deep cerebral area by location-specific terminology, as opposed to labeling them as "hypertensive ICH". Despite the common association of lobar hemorrhages with CAA, HTN increases the risk of ICH significantly in this location as well, even if the risk is comparatively lower than with deep cerebral ICH.

CAA is the deposition of beta-amyloid in the media of cortical and leptomeningeal arteries, arterioles, and capillaries [23]. It is often presumed to be the cause of ICH in lobar hemorrhages, particularly in elderly patients or in the setting of recurrent bleeds [24]. The greatest risk factor for the development of CAA is advancing age, with approximately 30% of people over the age of 60 demonstrating evidence of this pathology [25]. There are certain genetic predispositions to the development of CAA as well, with an increased risk of lobar ICH in carriers of the APOE-ε2 or APOE-ε4 allele [18]. These genetic mutations are also linked to the familial forms of Alzheimer's disease, with accelerated formation of deposition of the amyloid-beta into the blood vessels [26].. In carriers of both of these two alleles (APOE-ε2/APOE-ε4) there is an association with increased CAA and recurrent lobar hemorrhages [27]. Further research into the genetic and familial causes of CAA and their association with lobar ICH are ongoing.

Age is the most significant non-modifiable risk factor for ICH [3]. There is an exponential incidence of ICH as patients age, from approximately 1.9 per 100,000 below age 44 up to 196 per 100,000 over the age of 85 [3]. Age greater than 80 was associated with a significant increase in 30-day mortality [24]. Importantly, the association with age on outcomes in ICH is difficult to assess, with multiple studies suggesting disparate results

[28–30]. This may be due to confounding issues related to goals of care and other medical comorbidities affecting prognosis in this age group compared to younger cohorts. Nevertheless, age remains a clear risk factor for the occurrence of ICH.

Clinical Presentation

The clinical presentation of patients with spontaneous ICH can vary greatly based on factors such as the size and location of the hemorrhage. Patients present commonly with headache and altered mental status [10, 31]. Additional symptoms commonly include vomiting, hypertension, and seizures, although these can be nonspecific for other intracranial pathologies, thus necessitating imaging for diagnosis [2]. The most common site of primary ICH is deep cerebral (basal ganglia/thalamic) bleeds, with an incidence of up to 69%, followed by lobar ICH with an incidence of up to 52% [32]. Primary ICH in the cerebellum and brainstem are less common, with incidences of 9% and 11% respectively. The neurological symptoms presentation are related to the anatomical location of the bleed: for instance, thalamic/basal ganglia ICH can present with hemiparesis, sensory deficits, and decreased consciousness, while dominant temporal ICH often present with aphasia and hemianopsia [10, 31]. The disparity of neurological presentations leads to inconsistency in the clinical assessment of these patients, with no accepted standardized model or grading scale. Hemphill et al. proposed the ICH Score in 2001, identifying factors independently associated with 30-day mortality [33]. These factors included GCS, age ≥ 80 years, infratentorial location, ICH volume ≥ 30 cm [3], and the presence of IVH. These factors were tabulated to a score on a scale of 0–6, with the overall score accurately predicting worsening outcomes of 30-day mortality rates as more risk factors were present (Table 21.1). The authors cautioned then [33] and now [34] against over-reliance on the ICH score and the potential for self-fulfilling poor outcomes, where the prognostication of mortality from this score is viewed within the overall framework of patient evaluation and management decisions. Several modifications to the original ICH score have been proposed which include factors such as the National Institutes of Health Stroke Severity Scale (NIHSS) and differences in hematoma volume between infratentorial and supratentorial locations have been shown to improve the prediction of good function outcomes [35–37]

Table 21.1 ICH score

Criterion		Points
GCS	3 to 4	2
	5 to 12	1
	13 to 15	0
Age ≥ 80	Yes	1
	No	0
Infratentorial origin	Yes	1
	No	0
ICH volume	30 cm^3 or greater	1
	Less than 30 cm^3	0

Essential Management Priorities

Early: Immediate/First 24 h

Airway

Patients with ICH may require intubation for several reasons: recurrent vomiting with concern for aspiration, depressed level of consciousness, and hypoventilation contributing to vasodilation and worsening intracranial pressure (ICP). Early securing of the airway is reasonable in ICH patients given the risk of early decompensation and hematoma expansion. The airway should be secured with ICP precautions when necessary, including minimizing flat time, minimizing apnea time, and consideration of use of fentanyl or lidocaine to blunt the sympathetic response. Patients should be well-sedated after intubation.

Blood Pressure

Initial hypertension has not consistently been shown to contribute to hematoma expansion [38–41]. However, initial hypertension on presentation has been associated with neurologic deterioration, death, and dependency [2]. Early intensive reduction of blood pressure (BP) to a systolic BP <140 mmHg has not been shown to improve outcomes [39, 42] and may be associated with increased incidence of renal adverse events [42]. That said, acutely decreasing BP has not been shown to result in worsened perihematomal edema [39] or ischemia [39, 43].

Current guidelines state that for ICH patients presenting with SBP between 150 and 220 mmHg and without contraindication to acute BP treatment, acute lowering of SBP to 140 mmHg is safe and that for ICH patients presenting with SBP >220 mmHg to consider aggressive reduction with continuous infusion of antihypertensive medication [2]. This recommendation comes in large part due to the improvements in functional recovery seen with a targeted reduction to SBP level < 140 mmHg that was demonstrated in the INTERACT2 trial, a phase 3 trial with 2839 patients examining intensive SBP reduction vs. standard management [40]. In general, shorter acting agents should be used to reduce BP. Nitrates should be avoided due to the risk of vasodilation that can increase ICP. In patients with elevated ICP, attention should be paid to cerebral perfusion pressure (CPP) when acutely lowering systemic BP (see below).

Intracranial Pressure

Patients with large ICH or with significant IVH and hydrocephalus may acutely present with elevated ICP. Patients with hydrocephalus may need an external ventricular drain for therapeutic

Table 21.2 Management of anti-coagulant related hemorrhage

Anticoagulant	Subgroup	First step	Reversal
Vitamin K antagonists	INR 1.3–1.9	Stop anticoagulant	4-factor PCC 10–20 IU/kg + IV vitamin K
	INR ≥ 2.0	Stop anticoagulant	4-factor PCC 25–50 IU/kg + IV vitamin K
Dabigatran		Stop anticoagulant activated charcoal if last dose <8 h ago	Idarucizumab if available, or PCC (37.5–50 IU/kg) +/– RRT
Factor Xa inhibitor		Stop anticoagulant activated charcoal if last dose <8 h ago	Andexanet alfa if available, or 4-factor PCC (37.5–50 IU/kg)
Heparins	Unfractionated	Stop anticoagulant	Protamine
	Low molecular weight heparin	Stop anticoagulant	Protamine (may need redosing)

INR international normalized ratio, *PCC* prothrombin concentrate, *RRT* renal replacement therapy

drainage of cerebrospinal fluid. In patients suspected of having elevated ICP and impending herniation, empiric treatment with hypertonic saline or hyperosmolar therapy can be pursued until ventricular drain placement, surgical evacuation or decompressive craniectomy can be performed [2]. Continuous hyperosmolar therapy has not been shown to be beneficial [2]. Corticosteroids should not be used to reduce ICP [2].

Patients who present in a coma (GCS ≤ 8) and have evidence of cerebral edema may benefit from ICP monitoring [2]. In those with significant IVH and hydrocephalus, a ventricular drain should be placed for therapeutic benefit. In cases where hydrocephalus is not present, an intraparenchymal ICP monitor can be considered.

Coagulopathy Reversal

Patients on antiplatelets and anticoagulation should have their medications held. Anticoagulation should be immediately reversed (Table 21.2). Warfarin can be most efficiently reversed with prothrombin complex concentrate (PCC) (25–50 U/kg) and intravenous vitamin K (10 mg). A study comparing the use of 20 mL/kg FFP versus 30 U/kg of 4-factor PCC found no difference in death and functional outcome at 90 days, although there was more hematoma expansion and correction of INR took longer in the FFP group [44], so 4 factor PCC is recommended in formal guidelines [45]. Dabigatran can be reversed with idarucizumab, a specific humanized antibody against dabigatran, given as an intravenous bolus (5 g) [45, 46]. Factor Xa inhibitors can be reversed with either PCC (25–50 U/kg) or bolus followed by 2-h infusion of andexanet alfa (dose depending on the timing of last intake), a recombinant factor Xa that competitively binds to Xa inhibitors [47]. Any patient who has ingested a direct oral anticoagulant (DOAC) within 2 h can be given activated charcoal 25 to 50 g to prevent absorption [45, 48]. Reversal of unfractionated heparin or low molecular weight heparin can be achieved with protamine [45].

Platelet transfusion has not been shown to confer benefit in spontaneous hemorrhages <30 mL as shown in the PATCH trial and was associated with a higher risk of adverse events and death [49]. However, if patients are undergoing a neurosurgical procedure, then platelet transfusion and administration of desmopressin 0.4 mcg/kg IV is reasonable [45]. Transfusion to a platelet goal >100,000/uL and fibrinogen >100 mg/dL is reasonable in patients with underlying thrombocytopenia or cirrhosis.

Seizure Management

Anywhere from 5% to 15% of patients with ICH will have seizures in their index hospitalization [50]. Patients who present with seizures after ICH should be loaded with an antiepileptic drug, as seizures may increase both systemic blood pressure and ICP. Patients should be maintained on antiepileptic drugs throughout their hospitalization. Continuous electroencephalography (EEG) should be considered in patients with persistently poor exams out of proportion to their imaging, as this may be indicative of nonconvulsive seizures [51]. It has been shown that in ICU patients with ICH-related seizures, between 53% and 76% of these were nonconvulsive and clinically not recognized [51, 52].

Routine use of seizure prophylaxis has not been shown to improve functional outcome or mortality and may even be associated with worse outcomes [53, 54]. However, in patients at high risk of decompensation due to elevated ICP or impending herniation, it may be reasonable to administer seizure prophylaxis until definitive treatment can be undertaken. Patients may be at higher risk of late development of seizures if ICH involves the cerebral cortex if the patient is <65 years old, if the hemorrhage is >10 mL, and if the patient had early seizures within the first 7 days [55]. Therefore, some studies advocate the use of anti-seizure medication with large bleeds and bleed involving the cortical surface, typically for up to 1-week post-hemorrhage [56].

Neuroimaging

Noncontrast head computed tomography (CT) is the gold-standard neuroimaging technique for evaluation of ICH, providing fast, and accurate evaluation of the hemorrhage size, location, age, and effects on the surrounding parenchyma (Fig. 21.1) [57, 58]. The volume of ICH is typically calculated using the easily accessible equation of (A×B×)/2, with A, B, and C equaling the largest cross-sectional diameter, the perpendicular diameter, and the number of CT slices with hemorrhage multiplied by the thickness of the CT slice, respectively [59]. Following identification of ICH on CT, CT angiography (CTA) is typically performed to evaluate for any underlying vascular pathologies like aneurysms or arteriovenous malformations. Besides its use in identifying vascular lesions, CTA is used to identify likely sites of active bleeding by visualizing the imaging biomarker known as the "spot sign" (Fig. 21.2) [60]. The spot sign is a tiny enhancing focus within the hematoma caused by contrast extravasation and indicates likely hematoma expansion. Up to 33% of hemorrhages in a study by Wada et al. [60] demonstrated this spot sign and it has been shown that the presence of a spot sign is associated with increased mortality [61]. Additionally, multiple spot signs further increase the risk of ICH expansion [62]. Other imaging signs in ICH that have been studied include the satellite sign [63], island sign [63, 64], swirl sign [65], black hole sign [66], and blend sign [67], all of which are visualized on noncontrast CT head scans Table 21.3. MRI imaging in ICH is more sensitive for the presence of hemorrhage but less commonly utilized as an initial/emergent study due to less availability, increased acquisition time, and increased costs [68]. MRI also more specifically indicates the age of ICH

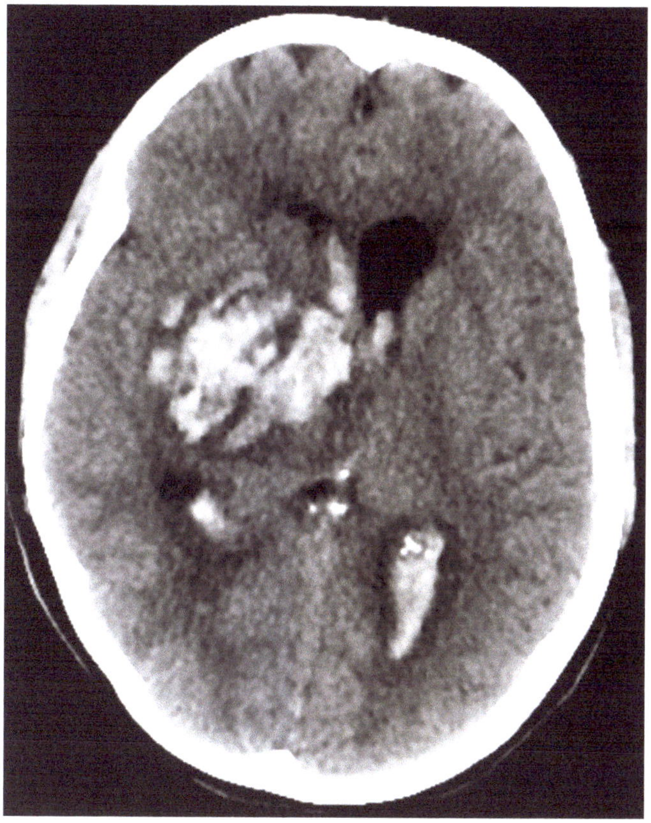

Fig. 21.1 Large Right thalamic ICH with intraventricular extension

Table 21.3 Imaging biomarker incidence and sensitivity/specificity for hematoma expansion

Imaging sign	Incidence (%)	Sensitivity/specificity for expansion
Spot sign [60]	33	91% sensitivity/89%specificity
Island sign [63, 64]	15	45% sensitivity/98%specificity
Satellite sign [63]	49.2	50% sensitivity/71% specificity
Black hole sign [66]	14.6	31.9% sensitivity/94.1% specificity
Swirl sign [65]	35	46.5% sensitivity/71.3% specificity
Blend sign [67]	16.90	39.3% sensitivity/95.5% specificity

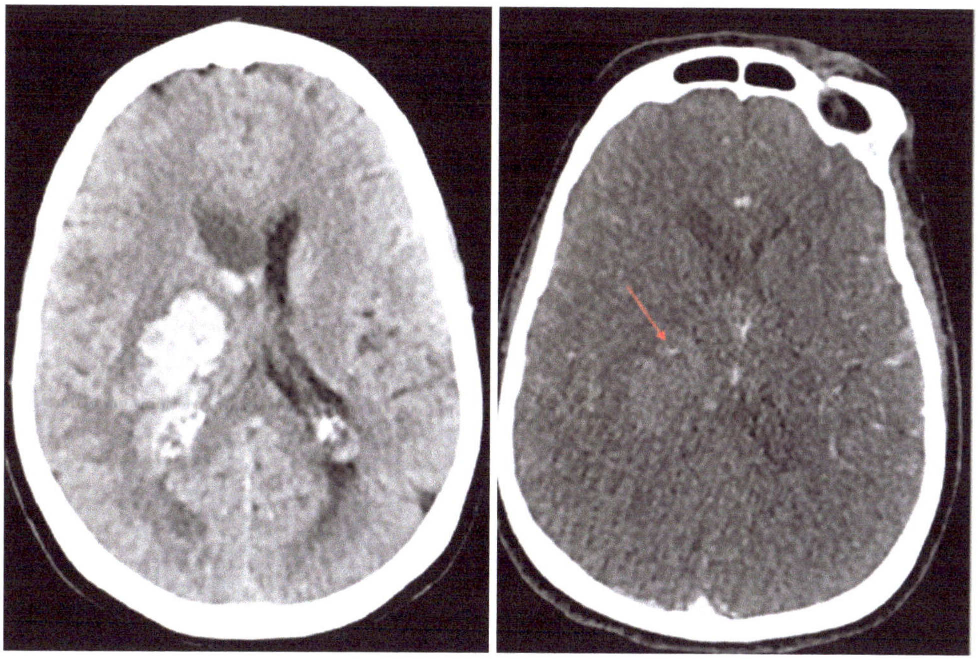

Fig. 21.2 ICH demonstrating classic "Spot sign" indicating likely active bleeding and risk for expansion. Left: Right thalamic ICH. Right: Spot sign within hemorrhage indicated by arrow

[69]. The use of gradient echo sequences in MRI is particularly useful in the evaluation of ICH due to CAA-related microhemorrhages Fig. 21.3. Key findings of amyloid angiopathy on MRI include lobar microbleeds, cortical superficial siderosis, and cortical microinfarcts [70]. Knudsen et al. [24] developed the Boston criteria to assist in the diagnosis of CAA, with 100% of patients meeting the criteria for probable CAA found to have histopathological confirmation of the disease. Further modifications to the Boston criteria occurred in 2010 and 2022 (Table 21.4 Boston Criteria 2.0) [71, 72]

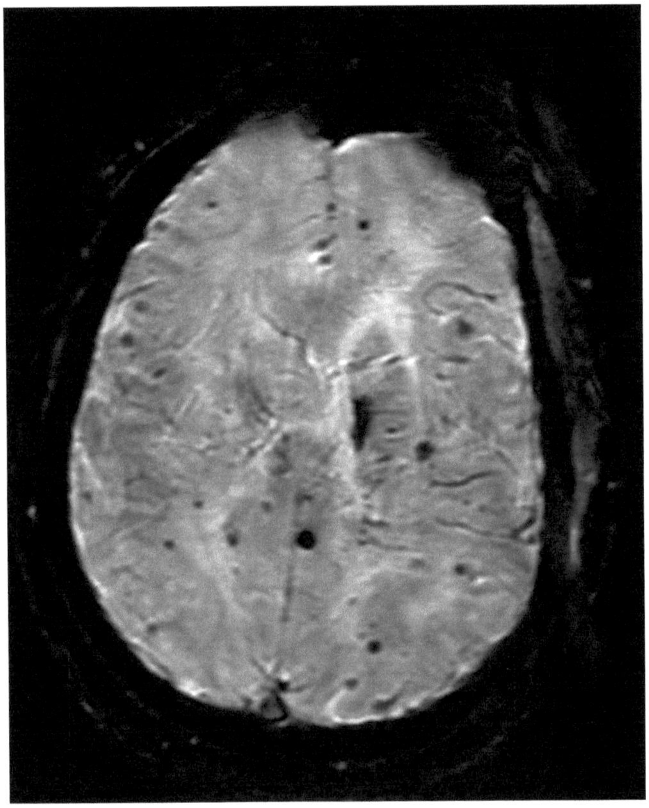

Fig. 21.3 Characteristic microhemorrhages indicative of CAA see on Gradient Echo MRI

While CTA and MRI are highly sensitive for detecting underlying vascular lesions in ICH, they are not always definitive. The Secondary Intracerebral Hemorrhage Score (SICH) was developed to stratify patients with ICH according to their risk of a causative vascular etiology [73]. Utilizing CTA imaging in the formulation of the scoring system, baseline clinical characteristics, sex, neither known HTN nor impaired coagulation, and noncontast CT categorization were used to predict the risk of a vascular lesion. Patients with SICH scores >2 was found to have higher incidences of vascular ICH etiologies (Tables 21.5 and 21.6). The use of the SICH assists with determination of the need for further investigation with a diagnostic cerebral angiogram. Digital subtraction angiography (DSA) is the gold standard for the evaluation of cerebral vasculature, and in young patients without hypertension (age < 45) it has been shown to reveal underlying vascular lesions approximately 48% of the time in deep cerebral/cerebellar ICH and 65% of the time in lobar ICH [74] In older patients with hypertension, the yield of performing a DSA is significantly lower and not typically recommended unless concerning findings are seen on CT/CTA or MRI.

More recent advances in neuroimaging such as diffusion tensor imaging also hold promise for aiding with outcome prediction in ICH [75]. While there are no large, prospective, randomized trials to date, smaller studies have found that fractional anisotropy and mean diffusivity of the pyramidal tracts were correlated with changes in functional outcome [76, 77]. DTI was examined at 3 days post hemorrhage and 2 weeks post hemorrhage, with more accurate predictions of motor outcomes and ability to conduct daily living activities coming from the 2-week post-hemorrhage imaging analysis [76]. Further work will be necessary to establish DTI as a powerful predictive tool to assess prognosis in ICH patients and identify potential therapeutic targets to promote motor recovery and outcomes (Table 21.7).

Table 21.4 Boston criteria 2.0 for diagnosis of cerebral amyloid angiopathy

Confidence of CAA diagnosis	Data source	Data findings
Definitive CAA	Full post-mortum examination	Presentation with spontaneous ICH, transient focal neurological episodes, convexity SAH, or cognitive impairment/dementia
		Severe CAA with vasculopathy
		Absence of another diagnostic lesion
Probable CAA with supporting pathology	Clinical data and pathologic tissue	Presentation with spontaneous ICH, transient focal neurological episodes, convexity SAH, or cognitive impairment/dementia
		Some degree of CAA in specimen
		Absence of another diagnostic lesion
Probable CAA	Clinical data and MRI	Age 50 years and older
		Presentation with spontaneous ICH, transient focal neurological episodes, convexity SAH, or cognitive impairment/dementia
		Two or more of the following strictly lobar hemorrhagic lesions on T2*weighted MRI in any combination: ICH, cerebral microbleeds, cortical superficial siderosis/convexity SAH foci
		OR
		One lobar hemorrhagic lesion with one white matter feature (severe perivascular spaces in the centrum semiovale [>20 visible in one hemisphere] or white matter hyperintensities in a multispot pattern)

Table 21.4 (continued)

Confidence of CAA diagnosis	Data source	Data findings
		Absence of any deep hemorrhagic lesions (ICH, cerebral microbleeds) on T2*weighted MRI
		Absence of another cause of hemorrhagic lesions
		Hemorrhagic lesion in cerebellum not counted as either lobar or deep hemorrhagic lesion
Possible CAA	Clinical data and MRI	Age 50 years and older
		Presentation with spontaneous ICH, transient focal neurological episodes, convexity SAH, or cognitive impairment/dementia
		Absence of another cause of hemorrhagic lesions
		One strictly lobar hemorrhagic lesion on T2*weighted MRI: ICH, cerebral microbleeds, cortical superficial siderosis/convexity SAH foci
		OR
		One white matter feature (severe perivascular spaces in the centrum semiovale [>20 visible in one hemisphere] or white matter hyperintensities in a multispot pattern)
		Absence of any deep hemorrhagic lesions (ICH, cerebral microbleeds) on T2*weighted MRI
		Absence of another cause of hemorrhagic lesion
		Hemorrhagic lesion in cerebellum not counted as either lobar or deep hemorrhagic lesion

CAA cerebral amyloid angiopathy, *ICH* intracranial hemorrhage, *MRI* magnetic resonance imaging, *SAH* subarachnoid hemorrhage

Table 21.5 Secondary hemorrhage score for likelihood of underlying vascular lesion

Parameter		Points
Noncontrast head CT	High probability: Enlarged vessels, calcifications along margins or hyperattenuation within a dural venous sinus or cortical vein	2
	Indeterminate	1
	Low probability: No high probability signs are present, and ICH is in the basal ganglia, thalamus, or brainstem	0
Age group	18–45 years	2
	46–70 years	1
	71 years and older	0
Sex	Female	1
	Male	0
Neither known hypertension nor coagulopathy	Yes	1
	No	0

CT computed tomography

Table 21.6 SICH score and percentage of CTAs positive for vascular lesion [67]

SICH Score	% Positive CTA
0	0
1	1.4
2	5.1
3	18.5
4	39
5	84.2
6	100

Table 21.7 Early priorities checklist

Imaging:	• STAT head CT at time of presentation • Repeat head CT 4–6 h
Neurological exam:	• Frequent neuromonitoring (q1h) to assess for neurodeterioration
Monitoring:	• Telemetry • Frequent blood pressure (arterial line or q1h BP) • Continuous pulse oximetry and respiratory rate
Airway:	• Intubate if inability to protect airway or inadequate oxygenation or ventilation
Blood pressure:	• For SBP 150–220 mmHg, lower to SBP 130–150 mmHg • For SBP >220 mmHg, aggressive lower to 150 mmHg • Limit variability in BP • Consider continuous infusions
Anticoagulants:	• Determine if the patient was taking any anticoagulants and stop them • Prompt reversal of anticoagulants within first 3–4 h of presentation
ICP monitoring:	• Consider in patients with evidence of high ICP clinically or radiograph or GCS <8 • EVD in patients with hydrocephalus • CPP goal 60–70 in patients with large ICH (>30 mL)
Surgical evacuation:	• Posterior fossa ICH >15 mL, declining exam, increased ICP • Supratentorial ICH > 20 30 mL, GCS 5–12 consider surgical evacuation

BP Blood pressure, *CT* computed tomography, *GCS* Glasgow coma scale, *h* hour, *q* every, *SBP* systolic blood pressure

Medical Management After Stabilization

Hematoma Expansion

ICH expansion most commonly occurs within the first 3–6 h [78, 79] and is generally defined in the literature as a 33% increase in volume from baseline CT [41, 80, 81], though other definitions have also been used including an absolute change of ≥12.5 mL [41, 80]. The major risk factor for hematoma expansion is coagulopathy, whether due to organ dysfunction, thrombocytopenia, or use of anticoagulant medications [79, 81, 82]. Radiographic predictors of hematoma expansion include irregular shape and density of hematoma [79, 83], presence of IVH [81], and spot sign on CTA [60, 84–86]. In regards to the relationship of the spot sign to hematoma expansion, the positive predictive value of the spot sign is inversely associated with hemorrhage onset to CTA time, suggesting that it is a dynamic and time-sensitive biomarker [87]. Meta-analysis of the predictive accuracy of the spot sign for hematoma expansion revealed a 62% sensitivity and 88% specificity, with an odds ratio of 8.49 [88], Presence of an area of hypoattenuation adjacent to a hyperintense area on a non-contrast CT, also called the "black hole" sign, has also been shown to predict hematoma expansion [66].

A recent meta-analysis of 36 cohorts included 5435 ICH patients [89]. It was shown that in ICH patients not on anticoagulant therapy that the probability of hematoma expansion declined with increasing time from symptom onset, with the greatest decrease in rate of decline at the 0.5–3 h post hemorrhage timepoint. The probability of ICH expansion increased with increasing ICH volume on baseline imaging, peaking at about 75 cm^3. The incidence of hematoma expansion varies widely in reports, from approximately 13–38% at 6 h post hemorrhage to 20% at 48 h [90, 91]. One study of 419 cases of ICH demonstrated a 24-h incidence of hematoma expansion of 14.3%, with a significant risk of expansion in those with irregularly shaped ICH and coagulation abnormalities [78]. Overall, the incidence and effects of hematoma expansion are variable but often portend poor functional outcomes [92]. Further clinical studies aimed at therapies reducing the incidence and associated risk factors of hematoma expansion are ongoing.

Cerebral Edema

Perihematomal edema develops within several hours of onset of ICH, rapidly progressing within the first 48 h and reaching a maximum volume on average 12 days after onset [31, 93]. Perihematomal edema growth positively correlates to ICH volume [94, 95], with the edema volume typically exceeding the hematoma volume by 100–600% [93, 96, 97].

Expert guidelines suggest preferentially using hypertonic saline rather than mannitol for patients with ICH, [98] though there is no strong evidence supporting this. There is no evidence to suggest that symptom-based bolus dosing of hypertonics is any different than employing a target sodium strategy and either strategy may be acceptable [98]. Patients should be closely monitored over the first week after their hemorrhage given the potential for decompensation related to worsening edema.

Intracranial Pressure Monitoring

ICP monitoring is indicated in any patient with evidence of elevated ICP either radiographically or clinically, and in comatose patients (GCS ≤8) with evidence of cerebral edema [2, 55]. Elevated ICP should be treated aggressively. Elevated ICP has not been shown to be independently associated with mRS scores and should not, in isolation, be assumed to portend a poor prognosis [99].

There is currently no high-quality evidence to guide use of more advanced neuromonitoring such as brain tissue oxygen, jugular bulb venous oximetry, or cerebral blood flow monitoring in ICH [100]. Small case series have been done using multimodal monitoring to identify optimal CPP and SBP which notably, have been higher than the most recent expert guidelines [101–103]. The optimal location of probe placement has not yet been established though most studies have placed probes in the perihematomal region. One center has described the identification of spreading depolarizations and focal brain fever in ICH patients using multimodal electrocorticography in the perihematomal area, which may be associated with progression of perihematomal edema [104–106].

There is no well-studied CPP goal in ICH, but guidelines suggest a CPP of 50–70 may be appropriate, depending on the integrity of cerebral autoregulation [2]. Despite this general guide, one retrospective study using a brain tissue oxygen monitor showed a CPP <70–80 mmHg was associated with brain tissue hypoxia and poor outcome [102]. It does appear that low CPP events (and high ICP events) are less frequent in patients that undergo reduction of ICH volume by surgery [107, 108]. Increased mortality and worse functional outcome have been associated with large ICH (>30 mL) requiring ICP monitoring with CPP of <60–70 mmHg, and recent guidelines suggest that blood pressure reduction is performed with a CPP target of >60–70 mmHg in patients with large ICH, ICP elevation, or decreased CPP [2].

Surgical Management

Open Surgery

Significant work has been done in recent years regarding evaluation of multiple strategies for surgical evacuation of intracerebral hemrorhage. Conceptually, removing the clot should improve outcomes by reducing the risk of herniation, reducing elevations in ICP, by removing the sustained toxicity of the blood products on surrounding parenchyma, and if performed early enough, mitigating hematoma expansion by addressing active bleeding. The following review of open surgical clinical trials for ICH reveals the inherent difficulty in improving functional outcomes in these patients and the recent advances that may in the near future yield an evidence-based strategy for hematoma removal.

One of the earliest studies of surgical intervention for spontaneous ICH was a prospective RCT published in 1966 from McKissock et al. that compared outcomes of open craniotomy vs. conservative medical management in 180 patients [109]. They observed that there was an overall mortality of 51% with males exhibiting worse outcomes than females (58% mortality vs. 30%, respectively. Surgical intervention was not found to have a significant benefit on outcomes compared to medical management in hypertensive patients (70% vs. 47% mortality, respectively). However, normotensive patients appeared to have a small improvement in mortality rate with surgical treatment compared to medical management (43% vs. 66%, respectively), although the numbers of patients in these subgroups was much smaller than in the hypertensive groups. Some of the risks relating to worsened outcomes were increased age and decreased level of consciousness on admission. The surgical interventions in this study were predominantly performed within 3 days of ictus which established a timeframe on which other subsequent studies could be compared against.

The advent of computerized tomography (CT) allowed for more specific and robust studies exploring treatment options in ICH. The first large scale study using CT scanning in a comparison of craniotomy vs. medical management for primary supratentorial ICH was by Juvela et al [110] This prospective randomized study enrolled 52 patients, with equal division of patients into surgical vs. medical arms. Overall, mortality between the groups at 6 months was relatively equal (38% in the medical group vs. 46% in the surgical group. In patients that presented in either semicomatose or stuporous states (GCS 7–10), there was a statistically significant survival benefit to surgical intervention, where mortality occurred in 80% of patients managed medically but 0% in patients managed with surgery. However, the numbers in these subgroups were small (5 medical arm patients and 4 surgical arm patients), and as such the overall power of this analysis is low. Importantly, even with a proposed survival benefit with surgical intervention in this subgroup, all of the patients were completely disabled at 1 year after ICH, suggesting that no improvements in quality of life were afforded by the intervention. For comatose patients GCS 3–6 there was no difference statistically in mortality at 6 months between the medical and surgical groups (83% vs. 82%, respectively, with all patients being completely disabled at 1 year. Similar results were observed in another smaller prospective randomized trial comparing medical management with open craniotomy in patients with primary supratentorial ICH [111].

Multiple subsequent trials examined the efficacy of surgery to improve outcomes in spontaneous ICH, however, a meta-analysis of this data continued to show no definitive conclusions regarding benefit compared to medical management alone [112]. In an effort to help answer this question, the International Surgical Trial in Intracerebral Hemorrhage (STICH) was conducted to assess the efficacy of early surgical ICH evacuation on morbidity and mortality [1]. This prospective randomized trial enrolled 83 centers with 1033 patients split into early surgery (503 patients) and medical management (530 patients), with an intention-to-treat analysis performed on the available data. Of the 468 patients randomized to surgery, the primary study outcome of favorable outcome at 6 months on the extended Glasgow outcome scale was met in 122 patients (26%). Of the 497 patients randomized to initial conservative treatment, 118 (24%) had a favorable outcome, with a nonsignificant absolute benefit of 2.3% and a relative benefit of 10% for surgery compared to medical management. There were no statistically significant differences in mortality at 6 months between the surgical vs. medical groups (36% vs 37%, respectively). Patients presenting with GCS less than 8 were uniformly found to have poor outcomes, with early surgery conferring an increased relative risk suggesting that in these patients an operation is more likely harmful. One of the most important findings of the study was in patients who had lobar ICH within 1 cm of the cortical surface, there was a statistically significant 29% relative benefit for early surgery. While conceptually the relative benefit and lesser risk of lobar clot evacuation compared to deeper thalamic/basal ganglia ICH is self-evident, this finding helped to lay the foundation for subsequent trials such as STICH II and the adaptive design of the Early Minimally Invasive Removal of Intracerebral Hemorrhage Trial (ENRICH) [113].

STITCH II was an international multicenter prospective randomized trial designed to test the hypothesis that early surgery in patients with superficial lobar ICH without IVH would improve outcomes [114]. A total of 601 patients from 78 centers were enrolled, with 307 allocated to early surgery and 294 to initial medical management. The results were analyzed on an intention-to-treat basis, ultimately demonstrating again that early surgery did not improve outcomes in patients with superficial ICH of 10–100 mL with no IVH compared to medical management. Unlike the first SITCH trial, mortality rate at 6 months remained lower with early surgery than with initial medical management (18% vs. 24% respectively), although this was not ultimately significant statistically. Patients with an expected poor prognosis based on a pre-randomization algorithm that incorporated GCS, age, and hemorrhage volume were more likely to have a favorable outcome with early surgery (OR 0·49, 95% CI 0·26–0·92; $p = 0{\cdot}02$) compared to medical management, however, this was not observed in patients with a good, expected prognosis. It was felt that this survival advantage in poor prognosis patients was lost in patients with better prognosis due to a greater time of initial observation and proceeding with surgery only if the patients deteriorated. Importantly, the majority of the operative procedures performed in STICH II were craniotomies or decompressive craniectomies, with some minimal access procedures performed. While STICH and STICH II failed to establish a benefit for improved outcomes, the increasing use of minimally invasive techniques has provided promising new data in the surgical management of ICH.

Minimally Invasive Surgical Evacuation

While trials evaluating open surgical evacuation of ICH have overall not demonstrated a benefit for surgical evacuation, trials and meta-analyses evaluating minimally invasive evacuation techniques have provided some positive information that certain techniques in certain subgroups may improve outcomes. One of the first major randomized clinical trials exploring minimally invasive evacuation of ICH was published by Auer et al. in 1989 [115], with 100 patients with primary supratentorial ICH split equally rolled into either surgical or medical arms. The surgical technique was evacuation of the ICH through a burr hole with a neuroendoscope, preferentially introducing the scope through the shortest distance of parenchyma. Artificial CSF was used as continuous irrigation and the clot and irrigation were suctioned at regular intervals. Patients with subcortical ICH who underwent surgery had a significantly lower mortality than those treated medically alone (30% vs. 70%, respectively. Functional outcomes were also improved in the surgical group compared to medical management alone, with 40% of those undergoing surgery having a good outcome with minimal or no deficits compared to 25% in the medical group. Additionally, ICH size significantly impacted recovery, where patients with surgical hematomas smaller than 50 mL had improved functional outcomes versus those in the medical group despite similar mortality rates. The significant difference in improved functional outcomes was also found only in those with age less than 60 as well as non-comatose admission neurological status. These promising results were all in patients with cortical hematomas; in patients with basal ganglia or thalamic hemorrhages, no significant differences in outcomes or mortality were found between the surgical or medical groups, although there was a trend towards improvement in the surgical group. These encouraging results led to further minimally invasive ICH studies.

Early studies utilizing a combined stereotactic aspiration and thrombolysis procedure, such as the Stereotactic Treatment of Intracerebral Hematoma by Means of a Plasminogen Activator (SICHPA) trials [116] failed to show any beneficial effect of this technique on functional outcomes or mortality at 180 days. The technique was subsequently refined and in the Minimally Invasive Surgery Plus Rt-PA for ICH Evacuation (MISTIE) trials [117], where a 14F sheath was advanced through a burr hole into ICH using image guidance. The clot was then manually aspirated until meeting resistance, at which point a catheter was placed and the sheath removed. Injections of rtPA were administered for up to 3 days into the clot. Initial reports of the MISTIE protocol demonstrated enhanced clot volume reduction compared to medical management, followed by the results of MISTIE-II trial which showed similar safety outcomes, possible improvement in functional outcomes at 180 days, increased clot volume reduction, and reduced perihematomal edema compared to medical management [118, 119]. While similar safety outcomes were observed, the use of the MISTIE protocol in this phase of the study was associated with a higher rebleed rate at 72 h (27.8% vs. 9.5% in the medical group. The results of MISTIE II were followed in 2019 by MISTIE III [117], which failed to show a difference in the primary outcome of mRS at 1 year. There was a significant increase in survival at 1 year for the MISTIE protocol arm at 1 year, and subgroup analysis of patients with an ICH volume reduction below 15 mL was observed to have a significant improvement in MRS at 1 year compared to the medical arm. This subgroup analysis demonstrated an indirect relationship between the volume of the hematoma left at the end of treatment, and long-term functional outcome, providing a surgical goal and suggesting that more effective methods of hematoma evacuation may be able to demonstrate improvement over medical management. In the MISTIE III trial, this surgical endpoint of 15 mL was achieved in 58% of patients in the surgical arm. MISTIE III, like the STICH trials, provided evidence that surgical evacuation may yield improvements in outcome if certain procedural goals are met, but further trials with newer MIS techniques are necessary to refine the approach.

Within the MISTIE trial, the efficacy of endoscopic evaluation was evaluated in Intraoperative Stereotactic Computed Tomography-Guided Endoscopic Surgery (ICES) for Brain Hemorrhage study [120]. A comparison of functional outcomes between endoscopic evacuation and medical management revealed that over 40% of the surgically treated patients had mRS below 4 at 6 months and 1 year while only 20% of

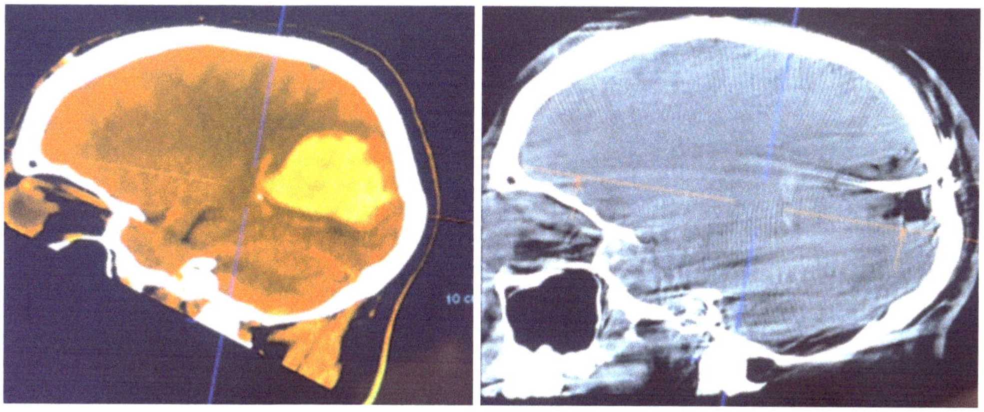

Fig. 21.4 SCUBA evacuation of left occipital hemorrhage. Left: Pre-evacuation. Right: Post evacuation with complete removal of ICH and drain left in hematoma cavity

the medical group met that criterion over the same time-frame. Further meta-analyses have been performed which also suggest endoscopic evacuation may be more beneficial as a surgical technique compared to craniotomy both in regard to mortality and complication rates [121, 122]. With these results, new protocols based on endoscopic-assisted evacuation techniques have been conducted with promising results. The Stereotactic Intracerebral Hemorrhage Underwater Blood Aspiration (SCUBA) technique for minimally invasive endoscopic ICH evacuation was a novel approach utilizing neuroendoscopy and continuous irrigation to visualize residual clot burden during evacuation and clearly identify and cauterize bleeding vessels (Fig. 21.4) [123]. Using this technique, an 88.2% reduction in clot volume was demonstrated in a study of 100 patients in whom the surgical goal of ≤15 mL remaining after evacuation was achieved in 86% of patients [124]. While this study and others have often waited to evacuate the clot until multiple scans demonstrated stability of the clot size, recent evidence in support of early evacuation has been reported [125].

Time to evacuation in surgical trials has been a topic of active debate. Does time equal brain in ICH as it does in ischemic stroke? One complicating factor is that while earlier evacuation may be physiologically beneficial, it may be technically more challenging as the probability of encountering active bleeding in the procedure increases. Morgenstern et al. in 2001 reported preliminary results of a trial evaluating ultra-early (≤ 4 h from ictus) and early evacuation (4–12 h from ictus) that was stopped early due to a high rate of rebleeding after ultra-early evacuation resulting in higher mortality in that group [126]. This study, however, utilized open surgical evacuation, which may not provide the improved visibility and other technology that facilitates hemostasis in endoscopic and endoport-mediated evacuations. There is a plethora of preclinical, clinical, and randomized data supporting early evacuation of ICH [127]. In a single-center series of 90 patients evacuated with the SCUBA technique between 6 and 72 h, time to evacuation was an independent predictor of long-term functional outcome (OR 0.95; CI 0.92–0.98) in addition to age, presence of IVH, and hematoma location, suggesting that operating an hour earlier increased the probability of achieving a good outcome at 6 months by 5%. In an RCT by Pantazis et al. reported in 2008, 108 patients were randomized to craniotomy for ICH evacuation within 8 h or medical management for cortical and putaminal hemorrhages ≥30 mL. 33% of the surgical group and 9% of the medical group ($p = 0.02$) achieved a GOS of >3 at 1 year [128]. In addition, a patient-level meta-analysis combining data from 8 RCTs performed prior to 2012 demonstrated that there appeared to be a benefit to surgery in patients who were enrolled in the study within 8 h after ictus (OR 0.53; CI 0.42–0.84) while there did not appear to be a benefit to surgery for patients enrolled at later time points [129].

Information gleaned from these earlier trials powered a new generation of RCTs focused on early evacuation with novel minimally invasive evacuation techniques. The Dutch Intracerebral Hemorrhage Trial (DIST, NCT03608423) studied the safety and feasibility of early (≤ 8 h from ictus) endoscopic minimally invasive ICH evacuation demonstrating a mean evacuation percentage of 78% (IQR 50–89) at 24 h after evacuation, median postoperative ICH volume of 10.5 mL (IQR 5.1–23.8) and a 30-day mortality of 10%. The Ultra-Early, Minimally Invasive Intracerebral Haemorrhage Evacuation Versus Standard Treatment trial (EVACUATE, NCT04434807) is an early (≤ 12 h from ictus) evacuation trial comparing minimally invasive evacuation with a surgiscope versus medical management funded by the Australian government. Finally, the Early Minimally Invasive Removal of Intracerebral Hemorrhage trial (ENRICH, NCT02880878) was an adaptive RCT comparing evacuation within 24 h with an endoport-mediated technique versus medical management that completed enrollment of 300 patients with 6 months follow up. According to data presented at the American Association of the Neurological Surgeons 2023 meeting, the trial was positive with a posterior probability of 0.9813, having reached the pre-specified threshold of 0.98. The trial was adaptive in that after an interim analysis after 175 patients were enrolled, the population of lobar hemorrhages was enriched by no longer enrolling anterior basal ganglia hemorrhages (ABG). The scientific community eagerly awaits the peer-reviewed publication.

Cerebellar Hemorrhage

The posterior fossa tolerates similarly sized ICH less than the supratentorial compartment owing to its narrower anatomical confines. There are no large-scale randomized trials assessing the efficacy of decompressive surgery and clot evacuation in cerebellar hemorrhage compared to medical management [10].. Multiple nonrandomized studies show that outcomes are improved following surgical decompression in patients with cerebellar hemorrhages greater than 3 cm in diameter or significant brainstem compression/hydrocephalus. Consensus guidelines regarding the placement of an EVD in cerebellar ICH suggest that ventricular drainage alone is insufficient to reduce ICP and may prove harmful in cases where the cisterns are compressed [130]. Mortality in multiple studies has been shown to approach 50–60%, but interestingly compared to data from supratentorial ICH the preoperative neurological exam does not correlate as strongly with poor prognosis [131]. In a recent meta-analysis by Kuramatsu et al. [132], surgical evacuation of cerebellar ICH in 152 patients was compared with conservative treatment in 152 patients. There were no differences between the two groups in functional outcomes at 3 months, but surgical management had a great probability of survival at that time (78.3% vs. 61.2%, respectively). The survival benefits in this analysis were driven by patients with larger hematoma volumes, further confirming the utility of decompression for large bleeds in the treatment guidelines above. The surgical modality of choice is suboccipital craniectomy with or without placement of an EVD, however, some small studies have explored stereotactic burr hole aspiration in smaller hemorrhages [133]. Current guidelines recommend urgent surgical evacuation of cerebellar hematoma over conservative medical management in patients whose neurological exam is deteriorating, who have evidence of brain stem compression or hydrocephalus, or cerebellar ICH > 15 mL in volume [2]. Overall, the evidence supports surgical decompression for cerebellar hemorrhage given its impact on survival benefit, but large-scale studies are necessary to help demonstrate these effects using more rigorous testing (Fig. 21.5).

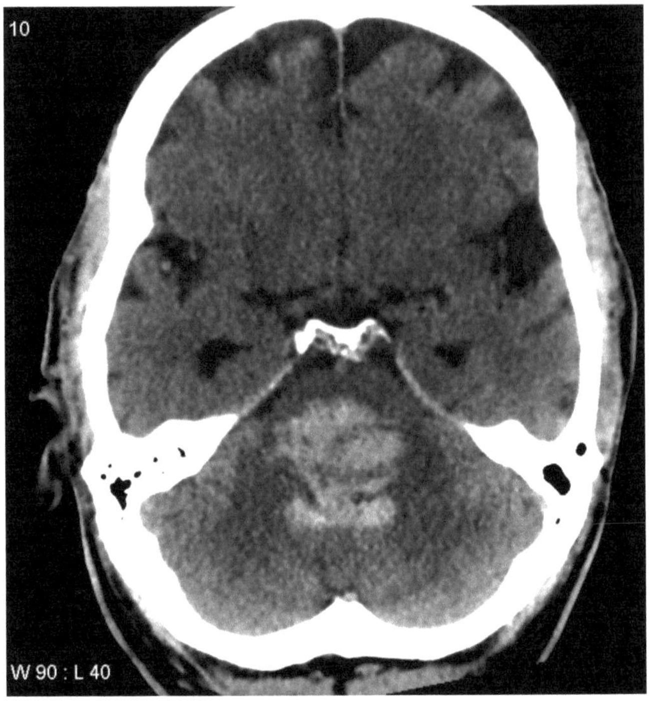

Fig. 21.5 Cerebellar ICH causing significant compression on the brainstem

ICH with IVH

When ICU occurs at deep intracranial sites near the ventricles the hemorrhage can lead to early rupture into the CSF space and compromise normal flow dynamics. Larger hemorrhages further away from the ventricles can also extend to the ventricles leading to rupture and IVH as their size increases [134]. Most IVH is secondary to hypertensive hemorrhages occurring within the basal ganglia or thalamus, although primary IVH unrelated to ICH can also occur [135, 136]. The presence of IVH in patients with spontaneous ICH is associated with a substantial increase in mortality [33, 137], with up to 79% mortality in these patients [134]. Additionally, fewer than 20% of survivors recover to a good functional outcome [137, 138], emphasizing the harmful effect when the ventricular space is violated by hemorrhage. This significant impact of IVH on ICH outcomes was why trials such as STICH II excluded those patients with this pathology (see above section on Open Surgery for ICH). Standard practice for IVH is to place an EVD to facilitate clearance of blood from the CSF space to aid in controlling ICP and preventing hydrocephalus. Despite providing adequate control of ICP in patients with IVH, the placement of an EVD in these patients that also developed hydrocephalus did not yield improvements in overall mortality in retrospective studies [139, 140]. However, a systematic review and meta-analysis examining the evacuation of IVH on survival and functional outcomes showed a significant improvement due to reduction in rates of hydrocephalus and neurotoxicity [141, 142]

The CLEAR III trial was a randomized, double-blinded study designed to test whether a combination of CSF diversion through an EVD and low-dose alteplase treatment would improve functional outcomes in IVH [143]. They randomized 500 patients into a treatment arm with alteplase and another with saline administration. The primary outcome of functional status was similar between groups, with no significant difference after adjusting for IVH size and the presence of thalamic ICH. There was a significant mortality benefit at 180 days in the alteplase group (18%) vs. the saline group (29%), however, the alteplase group has significantly more individuals with severely disabled functional status (mRS 5), suggesting that while survival may be improved there was unlikely to be a meaningful change in the quality of life with the alteplase treatment. Further trials exploring different measures of functional outcomes and stratifying experimental design to account for a more robust subgroup analysis may yield a clearer picture of the use of CSF diversion and thrombolytic therapy in ICH with associated IVH. Nevertheless, the use of EVD in patients with ICH and associated IVH patients (or lumbar drainage in non-obstructive IVH) is standard practice and recommended by consensus guidelines at this time despite the absence of large-scale trials [2].

Conclusion

ICH remains a devastating disease despite numerous trials and attempts to improve outcomes. Recent advances in minimally invasive ICH evacuation have provided a surgical target of 15 mL from the MISTIE III data and the ENRICH trial results suggest there may be a benefit to evacuation of lobar hemorrhages through a minimally invasive parafascicular approach within 24 h of ictus. Multiple ongoing trials emphasizing early and sometimes emergent intervention for ICH may provide tools to treat this challenging and dangerous disease.

References

1. Mendelow AD, et al. Early surgery versus initial conservative treatment in patients with spontaneous supratentorial intracerebral haematomas in the International Surgical Trial in Intracerebral Haemorrhage (STICH): a randomised trial. Lancet. 2005;365:387–97.
2. Greenberg SM, Ziai WC, Cordonnier C, Dowlatshahi D, Francis B, Goldstein JN, Hemphill JC 3rd, Johnson R, Keigher KM, Mack WJ, Mocco J, Newton EJ, Ruff IM, Sansing LH, Schulman S, Selim MH, Sheth KN, Sprigg N, Sunnerhagen KS, American Heart Association/American Stroke Association. 2022 guideline for the management of patients with spontaneous intracerebral hemorrhage: a guideline from the american heart association/american stroke association. Stroke. 2022;53(7):e282–361. https://doi.org/10.1161/STR.0000000000000407.
3. van Asch CJJ, et al. Incidence, case fatality, and functional outcome of intracerebral haemorrhage over time, according to age, sex, and ethnic origin: a systematic review and meta-analysis. Lancet Neurol. 2010;9:167–76. https://doi.org/10.1016/s1474-4422(09)70340-0.
4. Feigin VL, Lawes CMM, Bennett DA, Barker-Collo SL, Parag V. Worldwide stroke incidence and early case fatality reported in 56 population-based studies: a systematic review. Lancet Neurol. 2009;8:355–69.
5. Sacco S, Marini C, Toni D, Olivieri L, Carolei A. Incidence and 10-Year Survival of Intracerebral Hemorrhage in a Population-Based Registry. Stroke. 2009;40:394–9. https://doi.org/10.1161/strokeaha.108.523209.
6. Qureshi AI, et al. Spontaneous intracerebral hemorrhage. N Engl J Med. 2001;344:1450–60.
7. Qureshi AI, David Mendelow A, Hanley DF. Intracerebral haemorrhage. Lancet. 2009;373:1632–44. https://doi.org/10.1016/s0140-6736(09)60371-8.
8. Fewel ME, Gregory Thompson B, Hoff JT. Spontaneous intracerebral hemorrhage: a review. Neurosurg Focus. 2003;15:1–16. https://doi.org/10.3171/foc.2003.15.4.0.
9. Rincon F, Mayer SA. The epidemiology of intracerebral hemorrhage in the United States from 1979 to 2008. Neurocrit Care. 2013;19:95–102.
10. Ricardo Carhuapoma J, Mayer SA, Hanley DF. Intracerebral hemorrhage. Cambridge University Press; 2009.
11. Kleindorfer D, et al. The Unchanging Incidence and Case-Fatality of Stroke in the 1990s. Stroke. 2006;37:2473–8. https://doi.org/10.1161/01.str.0000242766.65550.92.
12. O'Donnell MJ, et al. Global and regional effects of potentially modifiable risk factors associated with acute stroke in 32 countries (INTERSTROKE): a case-control study. Lancet. 2016;388:761–75.
13. Sturgeon JD, et al. Risk factors for intracerebral hemorrhage in a pooled prospective study. Stroke. 2007;38:2718–25.
14. Sallinen H, Pietilä A, Salomaa V, Strbian D. Risk factors of intracerebral hemorrhage: a case-control study. J Stroke Cerebrovasc Dis. 2020;29:104630.
15. Thrift AG, McNeil JJ, Forbes A, Donnan GA. Risk factors for cerebral hemorrhage in the era of well-controlled hypertension. Melbourne risk factor study (MERFS) group. Stroke. 1996;27:2020–5.
16. Feldmann E, et al. Major risk factors for intracerebral hemorrhage in the young are modifiable. Stroke. 2005;36:1881–5.
17. Woo D, et al. Effect of untreated hypertension on hemorrhagic stroke. Stroke. 2004;35:1703–8.
18. Woo D, et al. Genetic and environmental risk factors for intracerebral hemorrhage: preliminary results of a population-based study. Stroke. 2002;33:1190–5.
19. Zia E, et al. Blood pressure in relation to the incidence of cerebral infarction and intracerebral hemorrhage. Hypertensive hemorrhage: debated nomenclature is still relevant. Stroke. 2007;38:2681–5.
20. Martini SR, et al. Risk factors for intracerebral hemorrhage differ according to hemorrhage location. Neurology. 2012;79:2275–82.
21. Jackson CA, Sudlow CLM. Is hypertension a more frequent risk factor for deep than for lobar supratentorial intracerebral haemorrhage? J Neurol Neurosurg Psychiatry. 2006;77:1244–52.
22. Jolink WMT, et al. Location-specific risk factors for intracerebral hemorrhage: Systematic review and meta-analysis. Neurology. 2020;95:e1807–18.
23. Samarasekera N, Smith C, Al-Shahi Salman R. The association between cerebral amyloid angiopathy and intracerebral haemorrhage: systematic review and meta-analysis. J Neurol Neurosurg Psychiatry. 2012;83:275–81.
24. Knudsen KA, Rosand J, Karluk D, Greenberg SM. Clinical diagnosis of cerebral amyloid angiopathy: validation of the Boston criteria. Neurology. 2001;56:537–9.

25. McCarron MO, Nicoll JAR. Cerebral amyloid angiopathy and thrombolysis-related intracerebral haemorrhage. Lancet Neurol. 2004;3:484–92.
26. Olichney JM, et al. The apolipoprotein E epsilon 4 allele is associated with increased neuritic plaques and cerebral amyloid angiopathy in Alzheimer's disease and Lewy body variant. Neurology. 1996;47:190–6.
27. O'Donnell HC, et al. Apolipoprotein E genotype and the risk of recurrent lobar intracerebral hemorrhage. N Engl J Med. 2000;342:240–5.
28. Tuhrim S, et al. Intracerebral hemorrhage: External validation and extension of a model for prediction of 30-day survival. Ann Neurol. 1991;29:658–63. https://doi.org/10.1002/ana.410290614.
29. Juvela S. Risk factors for impaired outcome after spontaneous intracerebral hemorrhage. Arch Neurol. 1995;52:1193–200.
30. Lisk DR, Pasteur W, Rhoades H, Putnam RD, Grotta JC. Early presentation of hemispheric intracerebral hemorrhage: Prediction of outcome and guidelines for treatment allocation. Neurology. 1994;44:133. https://doi.org/10.1212/wnl.44.1.133.
31. Ironside N, et al. Fully Automated Segmentation Algorithm for Hematoma Volumetric Analysis in Spontaneous Intracerebral Hemorrhage. Stroke. 2019;50:3416–23.
32. Flaherty ML, et al. Racial variations in location and risk of intracerebral hemorrhage. Stroke. 2005;36:934–7.
33. Hemphill JC, et al. The ICH Score. Stroke. *2001*;32:891–7. https://doi.org/10.1161/01.str.32.4.891.
34. Hemphill JC 3rd. The intracerebral hemorrhage score: what it is and what it is not. World Neurosurg. 2019;123:157–8.
35. Wang W, et al. Prognostic value of ICH score and ICH-GS score in Chinese intracerebral hemorrhage patients: analysis from the China National Stroke Registry (CNSR). PLoS One. 2013;8:e77421.
36. Cheung RTF, Zou L-Y. Use of the original, modified, or new intracerebral hemorrhage score to predict mortality and morbidity after intracerebral hemorrhage. Stroke. 2003;34:1717–22.
37. Falcone GJ, et al. Predictors of hematoma volume in deep and lobar supratentorial intracerebral hemorrhage. JAMA Neurol. 2013;70:988–94.
38. Anderson CS, et al. Intensive blood pressure reduction in acute cerebral haemorrhage trial (INTERACT): a randomised pilot trial. Lancet Neurol. 2008;7:391–9.
39. Anderson CS, et al. Effects of early intensive blood pressure-lowering treatment on the growth of hematoma and perihematomal edema in acute intracerebral hemorrhage: the Intensive Blood Pressure Reduction in Acute Cerebral Haemorrhage Trial (INTERACT). Stroke. 2010;41:307–12.
40. Anderson CS, et al. Rapid blood-pressure lowering in patients with acute intracerebral hemorrhage. N Engl J Med. 2013;368:2355–65.
41. Qureshi AI, Palesch YY. Antihypertensive treatment of acute cerebral hemorrhage (ATACH) II: design, methods, and rationale. Neurocrit Care. 2011;15:559–76.
42. Qureshi AI, et al. Intensive Blood-Pressure Lowering in Patients with Acute Cerebral Hemorrhage. N Engl J Med. 2016;375:1033–43.
43. Butcher KS, et al. The Intracerebral Hemorrhage Acutely Decreasing Arterial Pressure Trial. Stroke. 2013;44:620–6.
44. Steiner T, et al. Fresh frozen plasma versus prothrombin complex concentrate in patients with intracranial haemorrhage related to vitamin K antagonists (INCH): a randomised trial. Lancet Neurol. 2016;15:566–73.
45. Frontera JA, et al. Guideline for Reversal of Antithrombotics in Intracranial Hemorrhage: A Statement for Healthcare Professionals from the Neurocritical Care Society and Society of Critical Care Medicine. Neurocrit Care. 2016;24:6–46.
46. Pollack CV Jr, et al. Idarucizumab for Dabigatran Reversal – Full Cohort Analysis. N Engl J Med. 2017;377:431–41.
47. Connolly SJ, et al. Full study report of Andexanet Alfa for bleeding associated with Factor Xa inhibitors. N Engl J Med. 2019;380:1326–35.
48. Kuramatsu JB, Sembill JA, Huttner HB. Reversal of oral anticoagulation in patients with acute intracerebral hemorrhage. Crit Care. 2019;23:206.
49. Baharoglu MI, et al. Platelet transfusion versus standard care after acute stroke due to spontaneous cerebral haemorrhage associated with antiplatelet therapy (PATCH): a randomised, open-label, phase 3 trial. Lancet. 2016;387:2605–13.
50. Szaflarski JP, et al. Incidence of seizures in the acute phase of stroke: a population-based study. Epilepsia. 2008;49:974–81.
51. Vespa P. Continuous EEG monitoring for the detection of seizures in traumatic brain injury, infarction, and intracerebral hemorrhage: "To Detect and Protect". J Clin Neurophysiol. 2005;22:99–106. https://doi.org/10.1097/01.wnp.0000154919.54202.e0.
52. Vespa PM, et al. Acute seizures after intracerebral hemorrhage: A factor in progressive midline shift and outcome. Neurology. 2003;60:1441–6. https://doi.org/10.1212/01.wnl.0000063316.47591.b4.
53. Messé SR, et al. Prophylactic antiepileptic drug use is associated with poor outcome following ICH. Neurocrit Care. 2009;11:38–44.
54. Angriman F, et al. Antiepileptic Drugs to Prevent Seizures After Spontaneous Intracerebral Hemorrhage. Stroke. 2019;50:1095–9.
55. Haapaniemi E, et al. The CAVE score for predicting late seizures after intracerebral hemorrhage. Stroke. 2014;45:1971–6.
56. Gilmore E, Choi HA, Hirsch LJ, Claassen J. Seizures and CNS hemorrhage: spontaneous intracerebral and aneurysmal subarachnoid hemorrhage. Neurologist. 2010;16:165–75.
57. Caceres JA, Goldstein JN. Intracranial hemorrhage. Emerg Med Clin North Am. 2012;30:771–94.
58. Huisman TAGM. Intracranial hemorrhage: ultrasound, CT and MRI findings. Eur Radiol. 2005;15:434–40.
59. Kothari RU, et al. The ABCs of measuring intracerebral hemorrhage volumes. Stroke. 1996;27:1304–5.
60. Wada R, et al. CT angiography 'spot sign' predicts hematoma expansion in acute intracerebral hemorrhage. Stroke. 2007;38:1257–62.
61. Morotti A, et al. CT Angiography Spot Sign, Hematoma Expansion, and Outcome in Primary Pontine Intracerebral Hemorrhage. Neurocrit Care. 2016;25:79–85.
62. Delgado Almandoz JE, et al. The spot sign score in primary intracerebral hemorrhage identifies patients at highest risk of in-hospital mortality and poor outcome among survivors. Stroke. 2010;41:54–60.
63. Yang H, et al. The predictive accuracy of satellite sign for hematoma expansion in intracerebral hemorrhage: A meta-analysis. Clin Neurol Neurosurg. 2020;197:106139.
64. Deng L, et al. Comparison of Satellite Sign and Island Sign in Predicting Hematoma Growth and Poor Outcome in Patients with Primary Intracerebral Hemorrhage. World Neurosurg. 2019;127:e818–25.
65. Xiong X, et al. Comparison of Swirl Sign and Black Hole Sign in Predicting Early Hematoma Growth in Patients with Spontaneous Intracerebral Hemorrhage. Med Sci Monit. 2018;24:567–73.
66. Li Q, et al. Black Hole Sign: Novel Imaging Marker That Predicts Hematoma Growth in Patients With Intracerebral Hemorrhage. Stroke. 2016;47:1777–81.
67. Li Q, et al. Blend Sign on Computed Tomography: Novel and Reliable Predictor for Early Hematoma Growth in Patients With Intracerebral Hemorrhage. Stroke. 2015;46:2119–23.
68. Singer OC, Sitzer M, du Mesnil de Rochemont R, Neumann-Haefelin T. Practical limitations of acute stroke MRI due to patient-related problems. Neurology. 2004;62:1848–9.
69. Kidwell CS, Wintermark M. Imaging of intracranial haemorrhage. Lancet Neurol. 2008;7:256–67.

70. Greenberg SM, et al. Outcome markers for clinical trials in cerebral amyloid angiopathy. Lancet Neurol. 2014;13:419–28.
71. Linn J, et al. Prevalence of superficial siderosis in patients with cerebral amyloid angiopathy. Neurology. 2010;74:1346–50.
72. Charidimou A, Boulouis G, Frosch MP, et al. The Boston criteria version 2.0 for cerebral amyloid angiopathy: a multicentre, retrospective, MRI-neuropathology diagnostic accuracy study. Lancet Neurol. 2022;21(8):714–25. https://doi.org/10.1016/S1474-4422(22)00208-3.
73. Delgado Almandoz JE, et al. Practical scoring system for the identification of patients with intracerebral hemorrhage at highest risk of harboring an underlying vascular etiology: the Secondary Intracerebral Hemorrhage Score. AJNR Am J Neuroradiol. 2010;31:1653–60.
74. Zhu XL, Chan MS, Poon WS. Spontaneous intracranial hemorrhage: which patients need diagnostic cerebral angiography? A prospective study of 206 cases and review of the literature. Stroke. 1997;28:1406–9.
75. Chaudhary N, et al. Diffusion tensor imaging in hemorrhagic stroke. Exp Neurol. 2015;272:88–96.
76. Wang D-M, Li J, Liu J-R, Hu H-Y. Diffusion tensor imaging predicts long-term motor functional outcome in patients with acute supratentorial intracranial hemorrhage. Cerebrovasc Dis. 2012;34:199–205.
77. Koyama T, Uchiyama Y, Domen K. Associations of diffusion-tensor fractional anisotropy and FIM outcome assessments after intracerebral hemorrhage. J Stroke Cerebrovasc Dis. 2018;27:2869–76.
78. Fujii Y, et al. Hematoma enlargement in spontaneous intracerebral hemorrhage. J Neurosurg. 1994;80:51–7.
79. Fujii Y, Takeuchi S, Sasaki O, Minakawa T, Tanaka R. Multivariate analysis of predictors of hematoma enlargement in spontaneous intracerebral hemorrhage. Stroke. 1998;29:1160–6.
80. Broderick JP, et al. Determinants of intracerebral hemorrhage growth: an exploratory analysis. Stroke. 2007;38:1072–5.
81. Yaghi S, et al. Hematoma expansion in spontaneous intracerebral hemorrhage: predictors and outcome. Int J Neurosci. 2014;124:890–3.
82. Huynh TJ, et al. Validation of the 9-Point and 24-Point Hematoma Expansion Prediction Scores and Derivation of the PREDICT A/B Scores. Stroke. 2015;46:3105–10.
83. Barras CD, et al. Density and shape as CT predictors of intracerebral hemorrhage growth. Stroke. 2009;40:1325–31.
84. Ciura VA, et al. Spot sign on 90-second delayed computed tomography angiography improves sensitivity for hematoma expansion and mortality: prospective study. Stroke. 2014;45:3293–7.
85. Goldstein JN, et al. Contrast extravasation on CT angiography predicts hematoma expansion in intracerebral hemorrhage. Neurology. 2007;68:889–94.
86. Orito K, et al. Leakage Sign for Primary Intracerebral Hemorrhage: A Novel Predictor of Hematoma Growth. Stroke. 2016;47:958–63.
87. Dowlatshahi D, et al. Predicting Intracerebral Hemorrhage Growth With the Spot Sign: The Effect of Onset-to-Scan Time. Stroke. 2016;47:695–700.
88. Xu X, et al. Accuracy of spot sign in predicting hematoma expansion and clinical outcome: A meta-analysis. Medicine. 2018;97:e11945.
89. Al-Shahi Salman R, et al. Absolute risk and predictors of the growth of acute spontaneous intracerebral haemorrhage: a systematic review and meta-analysis of individual patient data. Lancet Neurol. 2018;17:885–94.
90. Brott T, et al. Early hemorrhage growth in patients with intracerebral hemorrhage. Stroke. 1997;28:1–5.
91. Kazui S, Naritomi H, Yamamoto H, Sawada T, Yamaguchi T. Enlargement of spontaneous intracerebral hemorrhage. Incidence and time course. Stroke. 1996;27:1783–7.
92. Li Z, et al. Hematoma Expansion in Intracerebral Hemorrhage: An Update on Prediction and Treatment. Front Neurol. 2020;11:702.
93. Venkatasubramanian C, et al. Natural history of perihematomal edema after intracerebral hemorrhage measured by serial magnetic resonance imaging. Stroke. 2011;42:73–80.
94. Arima H, et al. Significance of perihematomal edema in acute intracerebral hemorrhage: the INTERACT trial. Neurology. 2009;73:1963–8.
95. Appelboom G, et al. Volume-dependent effect of perihaematomal oedema on outcome for spontaneous intracerebral haemorrhages. J Neurol Neurosurg Psychiatry. 2013;84:488–93.
96. Suga S, Sato S, Yunoki K, Mihara B. Sequential change of brain edema by semiquantitative measurement on MRI in patients with hypertensive intracerebral hemorrhage. Acta Neurochir Suppl. 1994;60:564–7.
97. Carhuapoma JR, Hanley DF, Banerjee M, Beauchamp NJ. Brain edema after human cerebral hemorrhage: a magnetic resonance imaging volumetric analysis. J Neurosurg Anesthesiol. 2003;15:230–3.
98. Cook AM, et al. Guidelines for the Acute Treatment of Cerebral Edema in Neurocritical Care Patients. Neurocrit Care. 2020;32:647–66.
99. Kamel H, Claude Hemphill J. Characteristics and sequelae of intracranial hypertension after intracerebral hemorrhage. Neurocrit Care. *2012*;17:172–6. https://doi.org/10.1007/s12028-012-9744-7.
100. Le Roux P, et al. Consensus summary statement of the International Multidisciplinary Consensus Conference on Multimodality Monitoring in Neurocritical Care : a statement for healthcare professionals from the Neurocritical Care Society and the European Society of Intensive Care Medicine. Intensive Care Med. 2014;40:1189–209.
101. Diedler J, et al. Autoregulation and brain metabolism in the perihematomal region of spontaneous intracerebral hemorrhage: an observational pilot study. J Neurol Sci. 2010;295:16–22.
102. Ko S-B, et al. Multimodality monitoring for cerebral perfusion pressure optimization in comatose patients with intracerebral hemorrhage. Stroke. 2011;42:3087–92.
103. Lindner A, et al. Individualized blood pressure targets in the postoperative care of patients with intracerebral hemorrhage. J Neurosurg. 2021;135(6):1656–65.
104. Schiefecker AJ, et al. Clusters of cortical spreading depolarizations in a patient with intracerebral hemorrhage: a multimodal neuromonitoring study. Neurocrit Care. 2015;22:293–8.
105. Schiefecker AJ, et al. Brain temperature but not core temperature increases during spreading depolarizations in patients with spontaneous intracerebral hemorrhage. J Cereb Blood Flow Metab. *2018*;38:549–58. https://doi.org/10.1177/0271678x17703940.
106. Helbok R, et al. Spreading depolarizations in patients with spontaneous intracerebral hemorrhage: Association with perihematomal edema progression. J Cereb Blood Flow Metab. 2017;37:1871–82.
107. Fernandes HM, et al. Continuous monitoring of ICP and CPP following ICH and its relationship to clinical, radiological and surgical parameters. Acta Neurochir Suppl. 2000;76:463–6.
108. Al-Kawaz MN, et al. Intracranial Pressure and Cerebral Perfusion Pressure in Large Spontaneous Intracranial Hemorrhage and Impact of Minimally Invasive Surgery. Front Neurol. 2021;12:729831.
109. Mckissock W, Richardson A, Taylor J. Primary intracerebral HÆMORRHAGE. Lancet. 1961;278:221–6. https://doi.org/10.1016/s0140-6736(61)90353-1.
110. Juvela S, et al. The treatment of spontaneous intracerebral hemorrhage. A prospective randomized trial of surgical and conservative treatment. J Neurosurg. 1989;70:755–8.

111. Batjer HH, Reisch JS, Allen BC, Plaizier LJ, Su CJ. Failure of surgery to improve outcome in hypertensive putaminal hemorrhage. A prospective randomized trial. Arch Neurol. 1990;47:1103–6.
112. Fernandes HM, Gregson B, Siddique S, Mendelow AD. Surgery in intracerebral hemorrhage. The uncertainty continues. Stroke. 2000;31:2511–6.
113. Ratcliff JJ, et al. Early Minimally Invasive Removal of Intracerebral Hemorrhage (ENRICH): Study protocol for a multi-centered two-arm randomized adaptive trial. Front Neurol. 2023;14:1126958.
114. Mendelow AD, et al. Early surgery versus initial conservative treatment in patients with spontaneous supratentorial lobar intracerebral haematomas (STICH II): a randomised trial. Lancet. 2013;382:397–408.
115. Auer LM, et al. Endoscopic surgery versus medical treatment for spontaneous intracerebral hematoma: a randomized study. J Neurosurg. 1989;70:530–5.
116. Teernstra OPM, et al. Stereotactic treatment of intracerebral hematoma by means of a plasminogen activator: a multicenter randomized controlled trial (SICHPA). Stroke. 2003;34:968–74.
117. Hanley DF, et al. Efficacy and safety of minimally invasive surgery with thrombolysis in intracerebral haemorrhage evacuation (MISTIE III): a randomised, controlled, open-label, blinded endpoint phase 3 trial. Lancet. 2019;393:1021–32.
118. Hanley DF, et al. Safety and efficacy of minimally invasive surgery plus alteplase in intracerebral haemorrhage evacuation (MISTIE): a randomised, controlled, open-label, phase 2 trial. Lancet Neurol. 2016;15:1228–37.
119. Morgan T, et al. Preliminary findings of the minimally-invasive surgery plus rtPA for intracerebral hemorrhage evacuation (MISTIE) clinical trial. Acta Neurochir Suppl. 2008;105:147–51.
120. Vespa P, et al. ICES (Intraoperative Stereotactic Computed Tomography-Guided Endoscopic Surgery) for Brain Hemorrhage: A Multicenter Randomized Controlled Trial. Stroke. 2016;47:2749–55.
121. Ye Z, Ai X, Hu X, Fang F, You C. Comparison of neuroendoscopic surgery and craniotomy for supratentorial hypertensive intracerebral hemorrhage. Medicine. 2017;96:e7876. https://doi.org/10.1097/md.0000000000007876.
122. Nam TM, Kim YZ. A meta-analysis for evaluating efficacy of Neuroendoscopic surgery versus craniotomy for Supratentorial hypertensive intracerebral hemorrhage. J Cerebrovasc Endovasc Neurosurg. 2019;21:11–7.
123. Kellner CP, et al. The Stereotactic Intracerebral Hemorrhage Underwater Blood Aspiration (SCUBA) technique for minimally invasive endoscopic intracerebral hemorrhage evacuation. J Neurointerv Surg. 2018;10:771–6.
124. Kellner CP, et al. Long-term functional outcome following minimally invasive endoscopic intracerebral hemorrhage evacuation. J Neurointerv Surg. 2020;12(5):489–94. https://doi.org/10.1136/neurintsurg-2019-015528.
125. Ali M, et al. Early Minimally Invasive Endoscopic Intracerebral Hemorrhage Evacuation. World Neurosurg. 2021;148:115.
126. Morgenstern LB, Demchuk AM, Kim DH. Rebleeding leads to poor outcome in ultra-early craniotomy for intracerebral hemorrhage. Neurology. 2001;56(10):1294–9.
127. Kellner CP, Schupper AJ, Mocco J. Surgical evacuation of intracerebral hemorrhage: the potential importance of timing. Stroke. 2021;52:3391–8.
128. Pantazis G, et al. Early surgical treatment vs conservative management for spontaneous supratentorial intracerebral hematomas: A prospective randomized study. Surg Neurol. 2006;66:492–501; discussion 501–2.
129. Gregson BA, et al. Individual patient data subgroup meta-analysis of surgery for spontaneous supratentorial intracerebral hemorrhage. Stroke. 2012;43:1496–504.
130. van Loon J, Van Calenbergh F, Goffin J, Plets C. Controversies in the management of spontaneous cerebellar haemorrhage. A consecutive series of 49 cases and review of the literature. Acta Neurochir. 1993;122:187–93.
131. Dahdaleh NS, et al. Clinical and radiographic predictors of neurological outcome following posterior fossa decompression for spontaneous cerebellar hemorrhage. J Clin Neurosci. 2012;19:1236–41.
132. Kuramatsu JB, et al. Association of Surgical Hematoma Evacuation vs Conservative Treatment With Functional Outcome in Patients With Cerebellar Intracerebral Hemorrhage. JAMA. 2019;322:1392–403.
133. Lee JH, Kim DW, Kang SD. Stereotactic burr hole aspiration surgery for spontaneous hypertensive cerebellar hemorrhage. J Cerebrovasc Endovasc Neurosurg. 2012;14:170–4.
134. Hanley DF. Intraventricular hemorrhage: severity factor and treatment target in spontaneous intracerebral hemorrhage. Stroke. 2009;40:1533–8.
135. Hallevi H, et al. Intraventricular hemorrhage: Anatomic relationships and clinical implications. Neurology. 2008;70:848–52.
136. Engelhard HH, Andrews CO, Slavin KV, Charbel FT. Current management of intraventricular hemorrhage. Surg Neurol. 2003;60:15–21; discussion 21–2.
137. Tuhrim S, Horowitz DR, Sacher M, Godbold JH. Volume of ventricular blood is an important determinant of outcome in supratentorial intracerebral hemorrhage. Crit Care Med. 1999;27:617–21.
138. Hansen BM, et al. Intraventricular extension of supratentorial intracerebral hemorrhage: the modified graeb scale improves outcome prediction in lund stroke register. Neuroepidemiology. 2016;46:43–50. https://doi.org/10.1159/000442575.
139. Diringer MN, Edwards DF, Zazulia AR. Hydrocephalus: a previously unrecognized predictor of poor outcome from supratentorial intracerebral hemorrhage. Stroke. 1998;29:1352–7.
140. Adams RE, Diringer MN. Response to external ventricular drainage in spontaneous intracerebral hemorrhage with hydrocephalus. Neurology. 1998;50:519–23.
141. Nieuwkamp DJ, de Gans K, Rinkel GJE, Algra A. Treatment and outcome of severe intraventricular extension in patients with subarachnoid or intracerebral hemorrhage: a systematic review of the literature. J Neurol. 2000;247:117–21. https://doi.org/10.1007/pl00007792.
142. Gaberel T, et al. Intraventricular Fibrinolysis Versus External Ventricular Drainage Alone in Intraventricular Hemorrhage. Stroke. 2011;42:2776–81. https://doi.org/10.1161/strokeaha.111.615724.
143. Hanley DF, et al. Thrombolytic removal of intraventricular haemorrhage in treatment of severe stroke: results of the randomised, multicentre, multiregion, placebo-controlled CLEAR III trial. Lancet. 2017;389:603–11. https://doi.org/10.1016/s0140-6736(16)32410-2.

Arteriovenous Malformations: Evidence-Based Medicine, Diagnosis, Treatment, and Complications

22

Muhammad M. Abd-El-Barr, Seth F. Oliveria, Rashad Jabarkheel, Brian Jankowitz, Brian L. Hoh, and J. D. Mocco

Contents

M. M. Abd-El-Barr
Department of Neurosurgery, Duke School of Medicine, Durham, NC, USA
e-mail: m.abdelbarr@duke.edu

S. F. Oliveria
The Oregon Clinic, Portland, OR, USA
e-mail: seth.oliveria@neurosurgery.ufl.edu

R. Jabarkheel · B. Jankowitz
Department of Neurosurgery, Perelman School of Medicine, University of Pennsylvania, Philadelphia, PA, USA
e-mail: rashad.jabarkheel@pennmedicine.upenn.edu; brian.jankowitz@pennmedicine.upenn.edu

B. L. Hoh (✉)
Department of Neurosurgery, University of Florida School of Medicine, Gainesville, FL, USA
e-mail: brian.hoh@neurosurgery.ufl.edu

J. D. Mocco
Department of Neurosurgery, Icahn School of Medicine at Mount Sinai, New York, NY, USA
e-mail: j.mocco@mountsinai.org

Abstract

Cerebral arteriovenous malformations (AVMs) are complex lesions that require specialized, multidisciplinary treatment. Patients may be encountered in the intensive care unit either following intracranial hemorrhage (ICH) from AVM rupture or following elective surgical resection of an unruptured AVM. This chapter reviews all aspects of critical care management of AVMs.

Definition

Arteriovenous malformations are a complex tangle of abnormal arteries and veins, with an anatomic absence of an intervening capillary bed. This absence of a capillary bed can lead to high-flow shunting through various fistulae which are

E. Mahanna Gabrielli et al. (eds.), *Textbook of Neurointensive Care: Volume 1*, https://doi.org/10.1007/978-3-031-62220-5_22

susceptible to rupture [1]. Cerebral AVMs are relatively rare, complex entities to diagnose and treat.

Epidemiology and Natural History

It is unclear when the time of onset of cerebral AVMs is, but certain features, such as their presentation in younger patients, including infants, and their abnormal architecture, suggest that at least some are due to a developmental derangement [1, 2]. Other evidence of their early incidence is the fact that in the presence of an AVM, there are clear rearrangements of neuronal networks, such as the translocation of eloquent areas, a phenomenon seldom seen in other etiologies of acute intracranial hemorrhage [3]. A point of evidence against an embryonic disturbance is that, whereas there are numerous reports of in utero diagnosis of other vascular abnormalities, the number of AVMs diagnosed in utero is limited to single-digit case reports [4, 5].

Genetic predisposition to cerebral AVMs has been difficult to prove, with only a few candidate genes having been identified to this point [6, 7]. There are a number of germline mutations that have been found to be particularly important in the pathogenesis of AVMs. Some of these candidate proteins include transforming growth factor-beta (TGF-β), vascular endothelial growth factor (VEGF), and the angiopoietin receptor Tie-2 [8–12]. Recent work using single-cell RNA sequencing has made great strides in uncovering the molecular basis of AVMs [13].

The prevalence of AVMs has been difficult to pinpoint, with ranges from 5 to 600 per 100,000 persons [14, 15]. A retrospective analysis of symptomatic AVMs yielded a rate of 1.1 per 100,000 [16], though this figure may be falsely elevated due to the concurrent existence of other vascular malformations. A prospective, population-based survey yielded an incidence of 1.34 per 100,000 person-years, with approximately one-half presenting with a first-ever hemorrhage (0.51 per 100,000 person-years) [17].

Much of what is known about the natural history of cerebral AVMs is based on a cohort study of 262 symptomatic patients that presented to a central referral center in Finland [18]. In that study, 40% of the patients were excluded because they received a treatment upfront, but, for the remaining 160 patients, the incidence of hemorrhage averaged approximately 4% per year. A recent update to this data set revealed a somewhat similar risk of hemorrhage (2.4% per year), but this risk was higher in the first 5 years after diagnosis [19]. The "Medical management with or without interventional therapy for unruptured brain arteriovenous malformations (ARUBA): a multicenter, non-blinded, randomized trial" reported a 2.2% risk of rupture per year among 109 patients with unruptured AVMs randomized to medical management [20]. Some multivariate analyses have suggested that previous rupture, large AVMs (>50 mm nidus size), and infratentorial and deep locations were independent risk factors for higher hemorrhage rates [19]. Other studies have suggested that small AVM size and exclusive deep venous drainage and AVM-related aneurysms are risk factors associated with higher rates of AVM hemorrhage [21, 22]. Ultimately, the most definitive risk factor for AVM hemorrhage is prior hemorrhage.

Critical Care Management

Acute Evaluation

The most common clinical presentation of cerebral AVMs is hemorrhage (70%), followed by seizures (25%), and headaches (5%) [18, 19].

Because hemorrhage is the most common presentation, the hallmark characteristics of hemorrhage must be recognized readily by the medical team. These include the sudden onset of headache, focal neurologic symptoms, and changes in the level of consciousness.

As with all acute presentations, the "ABCs" of intensive care must be secured. This refers to the airway, breathing or blood pressure, and circulation or coagulation. It is estimated that approximately 30% of all patients with ICH will need to be mechanically ventilated [23]. It has been suggested that any patient with a Glasgow Coma Scale (GCS) of eight or below should be intubated [24]. Importantly, an arterial blood gas (ABG) should be drawn, as making sure that the patient is well-oxygenated is not enough, since hypercapnia can worsen intracranial hypertension (discussed later in this chapter).

In patients presenting with spontaneous ICH, acutely lowering systolic blood pressure (SBP) to a goal of 140 and maintaining it in the range of 130 to 150 is safe and may improve functional outcomes. Acutely lowering SBP to less than 130 in spontaneous ICH may be potentially harmful [25–27].

It is estimated that approximately 15% of patients with any ICH are on oral anticoagulation (OAC) [28, 29]. Rapid reversal of OAC in the setting of ICH is imperative. The traditional agents for the reversal of Vitamin K-related coagulopathy or all-cause coagulopathy have been Vitamin K and fresh frozen plasma (FFP). Vitamin K provides delayed yet durable reversal of coagulopathy while FFP provides rapid reversal. Importantly, recent American Heart Association (AHA)/American Stroke Association (ASA) guidelines now recommend prothrombin complex concentrate (PCC) over FFP for rapid reversal of all-cause coagulopathy. Additionally, with the advent of newer classes of OAC such as factor Xa inhibitors and direct thrombin inhibitors, direct reversal agents (Andexanet Alfa, Idarucizumab) are now recommended as reasonable alternatives to PCC for rapid reversal of coagulopathy [27].

Intracranial pressure (ICP) and cerebral perfusion pressures (CPP) are important parameters in many patients with severe neurologic injury. CPP is defined as the mean arterial pressure (MAP) minus ICP (CPP = MAP—ICP). Elevated ICP is usually defined as greater than 20 mmHg for greater than 5 min. Goal CPP is typically 60–80 mmHg. To measure ICP, a fiberoptic ICP wire or an external ventricular drain (EVD) can be placed. Placement of ICP monitors or EVDs can be considered in patients with a GCS of eight or below. An EVD can not only measure ICP and CPP but also provide direct therapy via drainage of cerebrospinal fluid (CSF).

Lowering ICP can be accomplished either by decreasing the occupied volume of the various intracranial constituents or by sedation, which acts to decrease brain tissue metabolism. The Kellie-Monro hypothesis states that the cranial compartment is incompressible and the volume of the intracranial contents is fixed. Thus, any increase in any of the three main constituents of cranial contents—namely, brain tissue, CSF, and blood—must be accompanied by a decrease in one of the others [30]. It is because of this principle that CSF drainage with the use of an EVD is helpful in the setting of hemorrhage from an AVM. An EVD can also help to control hydrocephalus that may develop secondary to AVM rupture-related intraventricular hemorrhage (IVH) or subarachnoid hemorrhage (SAH). Brain tissue volume can be decreased by the administration of mannitol or hypertonic saline. Mannitol and hypertonic saline, which are osmotic diuretics, work by drawing water out of brain parenchyma [31]. A recent meta-analysis comparing the two agents suggested that hypertonic saline may be more efficacious in lowering ICP, though the number of patients (112) was relatively small [31–33].

Another mechanism used to decrease ICP is causing vasoconstriction through hypocarbia. This can be accomplished by mild hyperventilation with a goal of $PaCO_2$ of 25–30 mmHg. Severe hypocarbia should be avoided as it can cause decreased cerebral blood flow. This therapy is effective when used intermittently, but chronic hyperventilation may cause rebound increased ICP when normocapnia is achieved [34]. Therefore, prolonged hypocarbia should not be pursued and instead used only to control refractory ICP elevation for brief periods of time.

Increased ICP can also be lowered using sedative agents which directly decrease brain tissue metabolic demands and also decrease agitation to indirectly lower ICP. If typical agents (propofol, benzodiazepines, opioids) are unable to control ICPs, an induced barbiturate coma with continuous electroencephalogram (EEG) can be considered. This is usually done until burst suppression is achieved [24]. The last resort for increased ICPs is decompressive craniectomy, discussed elsewhere (Chaps. 27 and 35). Many of the techniques for ICP management in the case of AVM rupture are borrowed from the traumatic brain injury (TBI) literature. Below is a detailed algorithm for ICP management that is used in the case of severe TBI which has relevance for AVM rupture-related ICP management (Fig. 22.1).

As stated earlier, approximately one-third of patients with AVMs present with seizures [35]. A retrospective analysis of 424 patients who presented with cerebral AVMs showed that male sex, age less than 65, AVM size greater than 3 cm, and location in the temporal lobe were significantly associated with seizure incidence [36]. In patients with ruptured AVMs who present with seizures, anti-epileptic drugs should be initiated. According to AHA/ASA guidelines, in patients with ruptured AVMs who do not present with seizures, prophylactic anti-epileptic drugs do not improve functional outcomes or long-term seizure control [27]. With that said, the recent PEACH trial found that 43% of patients with non-traumatic ICH had electroencephalographic seizures within the first 72 h as compared to 16% of patients who received prophylactic levetiracetam [37]. It remains unclear if preventing electroencephalographic seizures in acute ICH improves functional outcomes.

Important in the management of patients with AVMs are the systemic complications of neurological insult. Subendocardial ischemia, which has been shown to be in proportion to the neurological insult, may result in a myriad of symptoms from benign elevations in cardiac enzymes to life-threatening dysrhythmias and pulmonary edema [38, 39]. It is important to note preexisting cardiac conditions of these ill patients and monitor their progress.

Another organ system at risk in these situations is the pulmonary system. Patients with neurological compromise are at higher risk for atelectasis, aspiration, and pulmonary embolism [24]. Oftentimes, patients with neurological decline with AVMs require a pulmonary catheter to keep track of their central venous pressures (CVPs) to avoid pulmonary hypertension, a potential consequence of hypervolemia for patients undergoing "triple H" therapy for vasospasm, an infrequent but possible complication of SAH from an AVM or feeding artery aneurysm associated with an AVM (see Chap. 24 on SAH).

Electrolyte abnormalities must also be monitored in patients with AVMs. The most common abnormality is hyponatremia [40]. The two most common etiologies for hyponatremia, after exclusion of diuretic use, is cerebral salt wasting (CSW) and the syndrome of inappropriate antidiuretic hormone (SIADH). It is important to distinguish between these two etiologies, as the treatment for each is different. The most important laboratory value to differentiate between the two diagnoses is the patient's volume status. Greatly simplified, patients that are hypovolemic are most likely to have CSW, while those patients with euvolemia or hypervolemia are more likely to harbor SIADH. SIADH is treated with

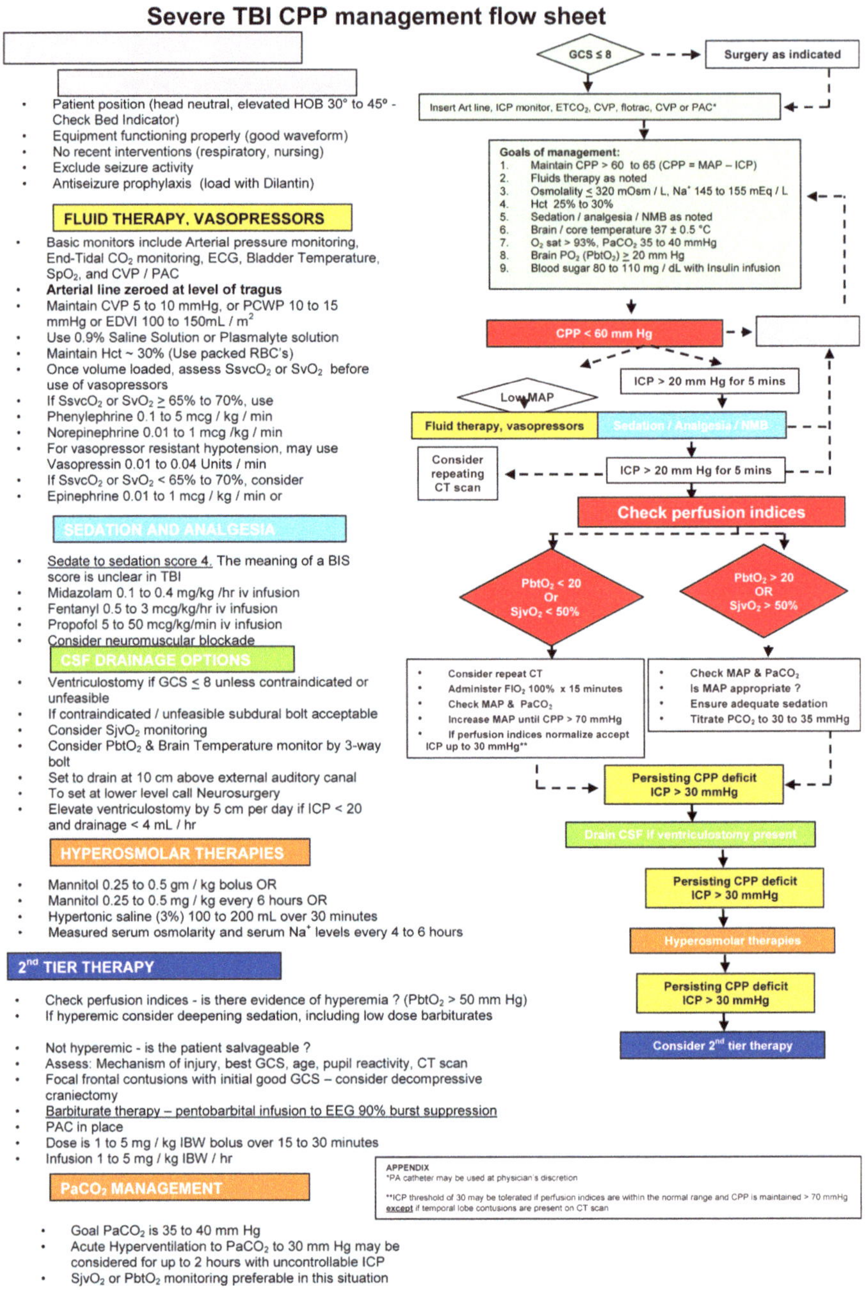

Fig. 22.1 Algorithm for management of patient's decreased Glasgow Coma Scale (GCS ≤8). Although this algorithm is used for patients with traumatic brain injury (TBI), many of the same methods are used in critically ill patients harboring AVMs or other vascular abnormalities

water and volume restriction, while CSW is treated with replacing Na and intravenous fluids [40]. Importantly, patients that are vulnerable to cerebral vasospasm due to SAH from AVM rupture may suffer irreversible infarcts if heavily volume depleted, so fluid restriction should be avoided in these patients.

Radiographic Assessment

Once the patient has been stabilized, it is important for radiographic imaging to take place. A non-contrast CT of the brain is the initial imaging modality of choice in a patient with an acute neurologic exam change. A CT can quickly differentiate between an ischemic versus hemorrhagic lesion. The addition of a CT angiogram (CTA) provides immediate and vital information about the possibility of an underlying vascular pathology.

For patients with AVMs who present with hemorrhage, approximately 60% will have an intraparenchymal hemorrhage (IPH) (Fig. 22.2), 30% will have a SAH (Fig. 22.3), and 10% will have IVH (Fig. 22.4) [41].

Although cerebral aneurysms are the major etiology responsible for SAH, AVMs constitute approximately 10%

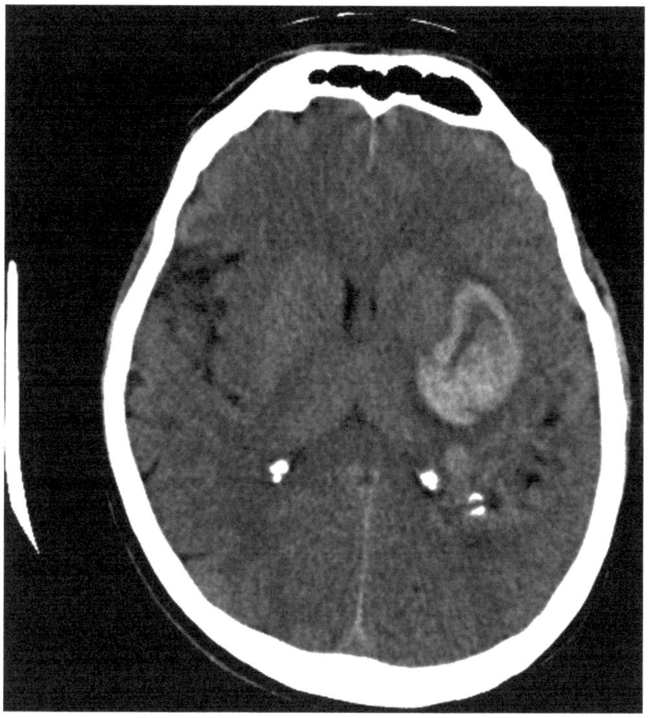

Fig. 22.2 Intracerebral hemorrhage (ICH) from an underlying AVM

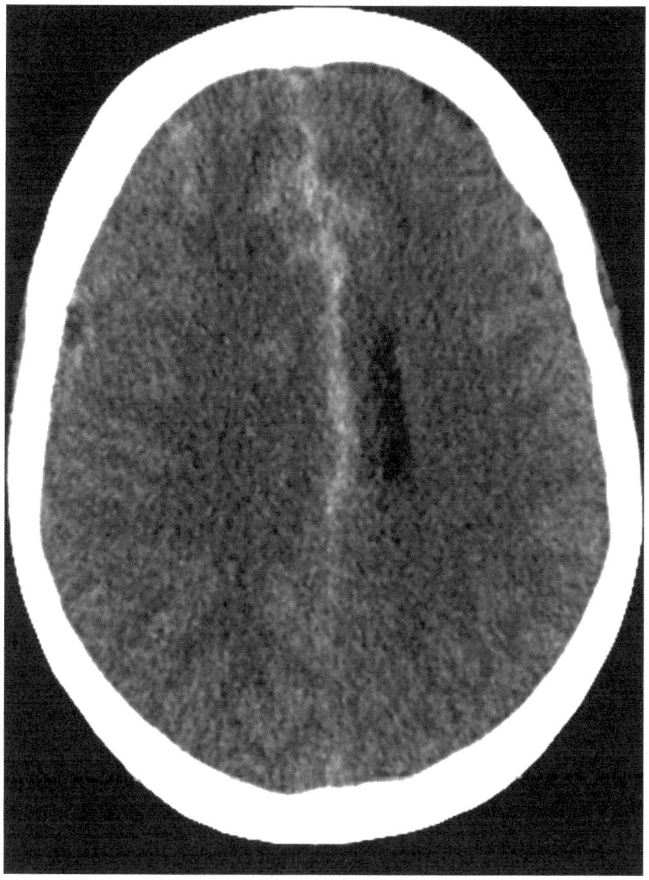

Fig. 22.3 Subarachnoid hemorrhage (SAH) from underlying AVM

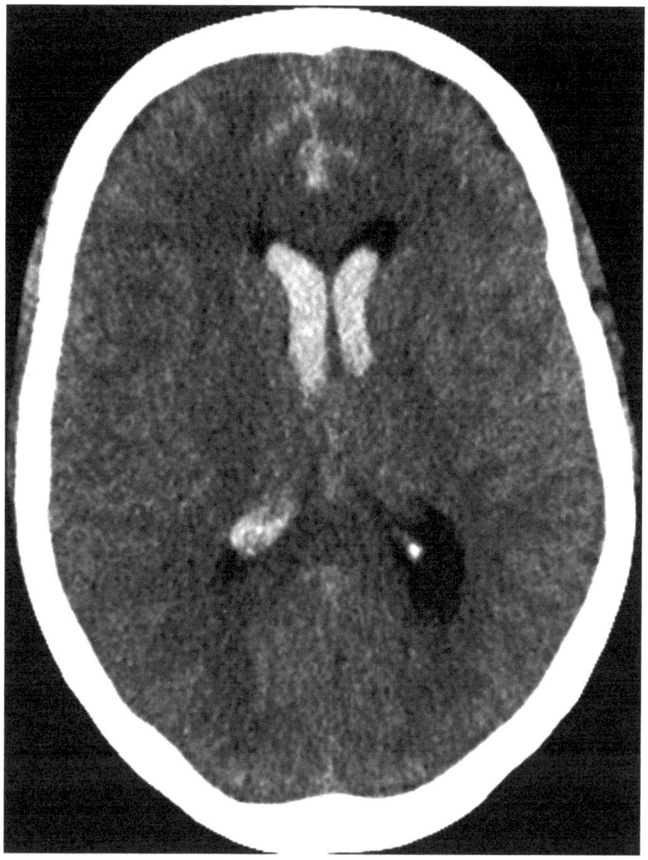

Fig. 22.4 The same patient from Fig. 22.3 also had evidence of intraventricular hemorrhage (IVH)

of cases of SAH. Importantly, approximately 10% of AVMs will have a feeding arterial aneurysm related to the AVM [42]. Importantly, the occurrence of cerebral vasospasm, which can be defined by various clinical and radiographic means but usually entails acute neurological decline in the face of focal or global decreases in cerebral vasculature, does not occur frequently with SAH-related AVM rupture [43, 44].

Catheter angiography is the gold standard for detecting AVMs [45] (Fig. 22.5) and should be pursued once the patient is stable. Per AHA/ASA guidelines, catheter angiography should be pursued in patients with (1) a CTA suggesting an underlying vascular lesion, (2) spontaneous IVH and no detectable IPH, (3) lobar IPH who are less than 70 years of age, (4) deep/posterior fossa IPH who are less than 45 years of age, or (5) deep/posterior fossa IPH and age 45–70 without a history of hypertension [27]. In addition to merely detecting AVMs, catheter angiography allows for the evaluation of possible feeding artery or intranidal aneurysms, direct AV shunts, venous outflow stenosis, (Fig. 22.6) and assessment of possible endovascular treatment options (discussed later in this chapter).

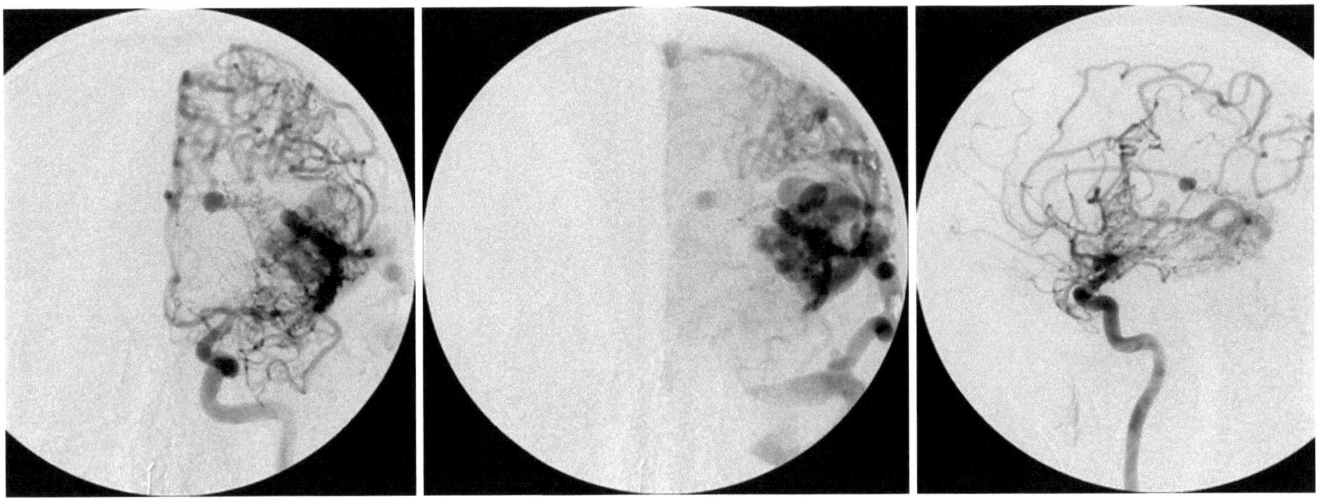

Fig. 22.5 Cerebral angiogram reveals a left frontal AVM with a large nidus and multiple arterial feeders and both superficial and deep venous drainage

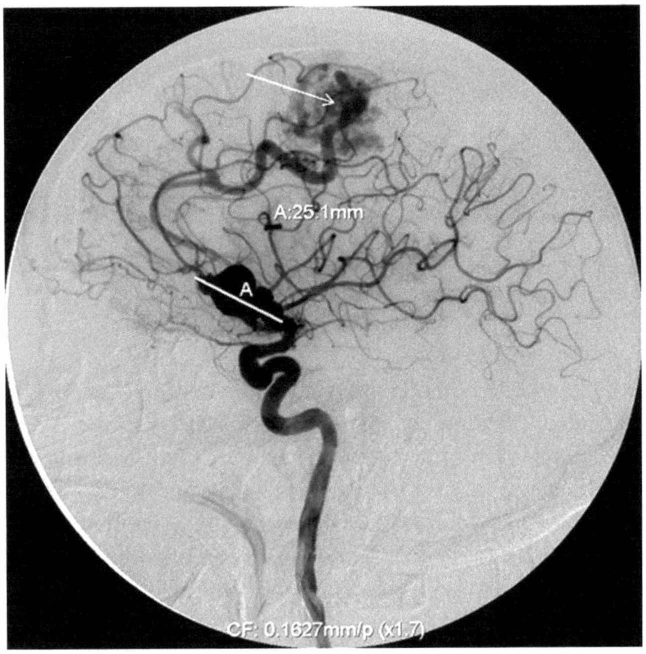

Fig. 22.6 Lateral view of a cerebral angiogram reveals a large (25 mm) feeding artery aneurysm to the AVM, whose nidus is seen (*white arrow*)

Anesthetic Considerations

Anesthesia plays an important role in the management of AVMs including for preoperative investigation, embolization, stereotactic radiosurgery, surgical resection, or long-term ICU care.

Both intravenous and inhaled anesthetics work to decrease the cerebral metabolic rate. However, most inhaled anesthetics, except N_2O, increase cerebral blood flow (CBF), while intravenous agents cause an increase in cerebral resistance and, hence, a decrease in CBF.

Sedation and monitoring are all that are usually required for CT or CTA. A common combination of midazolam and/or fentanyl, with some premedication with glycopyrrolate, usually suffices [46].

For catheter angiography, either conscious sedation or general anesthesia is used, depending on the neurological status of the patient and their ability to cooperate. For embolization, most centers use general anesthesia with endotracheal intubation.

Blood pressure control is of utmost importance in the management of patients with ruptured AVMs undergoing treatment as previously described in the preoperative context. In certain situations, deliberate hypotension is required, especially in the application of glue or onyx for AVM embolization to prevent systemic spread of the embolic material [46].

Grading and Surgical Management

AVM Grading

The Spetzler-Martin grading system for estimating the risk of morbidity or mortality following AVM resection was proposed in 1986 and remains well-known and widely referenced [47]. Under this system, lesions are graded based on size, venous drainage pattern, and eloquence of adjacent brain tissue using available imaging modalities including CT, MRI, and cerebral angiography. Lesion grade is calculated by summing a numerical value for each of the three categories described previously as follows: nidus size 1–3 points (small <3 cm, medium 3–6 cm, or large >6 cm, respectively), venous drainage 0–1 point (1 point for drainage into internal cerebral veins, basal veins, or precentral cerebellar vein), and eloquence 0–1 point (1 point for lesions near the sensorimotor, language, and visual cortex, the hypothalamus and thalamus, the internal capsule, the brain stem, the cerebellar peduncles, or the deep cerebellar nuclei). The graded variables of this system address the major issues influencing the overall technical difficulty of AVM resection. Since correlation between AVM grade and incidence of postoperative neurological complications is good, Spetzler-Martin Grade has become a reliable tool for use in preoperative counseling. Both the original manuscript by Spetzler and Martin and subsequent studies [48–53] reveal that resection of Grade I and II lesions was deemed relatively safe with a low incidence of neurologic complications, while Grade IV and V lesions resulted in a significant number of surgically induced neurologic deficits. Indeed, more recently it has been proposed that the Spetzler-Martin grading system be collapsed from a five-tiered (i.e., Grades I–V) to a three-tiered (i.e., Grades A–C) system since the difference in surgical results between Grades I and II and between Grades IV and V are small [54]. Of note, multiple other AVM grading systems have been devised [55–57] that incorporate additional variables—including patient age, diffuseness, nature of feeding artery supply, and clinical status at presentation—to improve surgical risk prediction and patient selection. Nevertheless, the Spetzler-Martin grading remains entrenched as a function of its simplicity and robust applicability.

The primary neurosurgical interventions available for AVM treatment include microsurgical resection, endovascular embolization, and stereotactic radiosurgery. AVM grading prominently influences which of these options are available for any individual patient. In general, low-grade lesions that are small and accessible are often resected directly; small, less accessible lesions are typically treated with radiosurgery; in contrast, high-grade, complex lesions frequently require multidisciplinary management with reductive embolization followed by another definitive treatment modality. These treatment modalities will be considered individually in the following section.

Treatment Modalities for AVM Management

Endovascular Embolization

There are two distinct treatment indications for endovascular AVM embolization. First, for a small number of lesions, AVM nidus embolization may be employed as a definite treatment. While this strategy is desirable because of potential decreased morbidity and mortality relative to open resection, it is essentially limited to small lesions supplied by one or very few feeding arteries. Embolization may fail to completely obliterate an AVM nidus, and it is also subject to late recurrence as a result of either recruitment of additional feeding vessels or true recanalization [58–60]. Partial embolization fails to protect against subsequent hemorrhage [61, 62] and carries the theoretical risk of precipitating hemorrhage via altered flow properties. Therefore, definitive AVM embolization should only be attempted if there is a high likelihood of successful nidus obliteration.

The second indication for endovascular intervention is strategic partial AVM embolization to facilitate subsequent definitive treatment with either open resection or radiosurgery. This adjunctive role for embolization is performed with the intent to reduce the size and/or volume of an AVM nidus. When followed by microsurgical resection, AVM embolization creates a more desirable dissection plane by preemptively occluding fragile vessels at the nidus periphery that can complicate microsurgical dissection [63, 64]. By reducing intraoperative blood loss and limiting unintended damage to adjacent tissue, endovascular embolization is generally considered to improve surgical outcomes.

The efficacy and safety of stereotactic radiosurgery decreases as AVM size increases [65–69]. Reductive endovascular embolization can potentially reduce the volume of large AVMs to a size that is amenable to stereotactic radiosurgery, reducing radiation exposure to adjacent normal tissue and potentially reducing the latency period of malformation obliteration [70–72]. However, embolization material can obscure the AVM nidus when imaging is performed for stereotactic radiosurgery treatment planning, and some reports suggest that prior embolization is a significant predictor of radiological failure following SRS treatment of AVMs [73–76]. Therefore, the use of combined endovascular embolization and stereotactic radiosurgery remains institution-dependent.

Finally, it should be noted that AVM embolization itself poses several risks including embolization of normal vessels and arterial perforation that can cause ischemia and/or hemorrhage, thus compounding the overall risk of patient morbidity or mortality during a staged procedure. For this reason, endovascular embolization may not be indicated prior to definitive treatment of low-grade AVMs.

Stereotactic Radiosurgery

Gamma knife (GK), particle beam (PB), and linear accelerator (LINAC) radiosurgical systems have all successfully been used to treat AVMs in large series, with reported obliteration rates of 60–80% and complication rates of approximately 2% [68, 77–80]. Pollock and Flickinger [73] developed the radiosurgery-based arteriovenous malformation (AVM) score (RBAS) from a multivariate analysis of predictive factors of outcome after radiosurgery. The RBAS is calculated as (0.1 × volume in cm ^{3}) + (0.02 × age in years) + (0.3 × location), with these location values: frontal/temporal = 0, parietal/occipital/corpus callosum/cerebellar = 1, and basal ganglia/thalamus/brain stem = 2. This score has been validated using GK, PB, and LINAC systems to accurately predict the likelihood of complete obliteration with no new neurological deficit after single-treatment radiosurgery; patients with an AVM score less than 1.0 are more likely to experience excellent results than those individuals with an AVM score greater than 2.0.

With careful dose planning, stereotactic radiosurgery can avoid injury to critical structures adjacent to an AVM nidus [66, 81]. This treatment modality is therefore potentially ideal for small, deep AVMs that are challenging to resect safely. However, there are several limitations to radiosurgical treatment of AVMs that must be considered: first, there is a well-documented latent period from radiosurgical treatment to complete AVM obliteration of approximately 1–3 years [66, 82, 83]; second, radiosurgery provides no apparent protective effect until complete AVM obliteration is achieved [84, 85]; finally, the probability of AVM obliteration following radiosurgery declines, and complication risk increases with larger AVM nidus volumes, as predicted by the RBAS equation. Taken together, this suggests that small, surgically inaccessible AVMs should be treated with radiosurgery since the risk of surgical complications outweighs that of hemorrhage during the latent period. In contrast, lesions amenable to resection should often be treated surgically to immediately eliminate the threat of hemorrhage. Complex lesions require multimodal therapy, as described earlier, potentially involving staged radiosurgery [80, 86, 87]. Some authors have described staged radiosurgery as a method of transforming high-grade AVMs into lower grade AVMs with more acceptable surgical risk [88].

Microsurgical Resection

Surgical resection remains the gold standard for obliteration of AVMs because the benefit of surgical therapy is immediate and definitive. The details of AVM resection are largely beyond the scope of this discussion [89, 90], but microsurgical resection generally proceeds as follows: exposure; then subarachnoid, pial, parenchymal, and periventricular dissection; and then finally resection. Wide exposure via a relatively large craniotomy and durotomy is preferred to permit close inspection of vessels feeding and draining the AVM nidus. While feeding arteries are meticulously dissected and ligated, great care is taken to preserve venous outflow to avoid intraoperative AVM rupture. This eventually results in gradual AVM involution, until the last venous pedicles can be safely ligated. Prior to closure, the resection bed must be carefully examined for residual AVM and for complete hemostasis. Microsurgery is often performed with the assistance of frameless stereotactic navigation and intraoperative neuromonitoring.

For patients presenting with hemorrhage, there is an increased predilection for possible curative surgical intervention, if possible, over other treatment modalities. A preexisting neurologic deficit after hemorrhage favors surgical intervention because the risk of a surgically induced deficit is lower [64]. Additionally, hemorrhage may facilitate surgery since an intraparenchymal hematoma can create a surgical corridor to better access some lesions by allowing entry into the clot cavity [64, 91, 92]. When the clinical situation permits, subacute microsurgical AVM resection is usually favored to allow time for hematoma organization, relief of brain edema, and resolution of transient neurological deficits [64, 89, 93]. For these reasons and because the risk of nonaneurysmal rebleeding from a ruptured AVM with intact venous drainage is low, the goal of acute surgery for hematoma evacuation when necessary is brain decompression, not AVM resection [90].

AVMs and Pregnancy

The risk of AVM hemorrhage is significantly increased during pregnancy. While the overall rate of hemorrhage of AVMs is estimated to be between 2% and 4% per year, during pregnancy one study of 54 pregnant women with AVMs found the rate of hemorrhage to be approximately 10.8% per year. Given the increased risk for hemorrhage of AVMs during pregnancy, many neurosurgeons recommend intervention for an unruptured AVM prior to pregnancy. If an unruptured AVM is discovered during pregnancy it is important to have a comprehensive discussion with the patient and their obstetrician regarding the risks and benefits of continuing pregnancy without intervention versus pursuing intervention during pregnancy. Cesarean section is the preferred method of delivery in pregnant patients with AVMs for tighter control of blood pressure [94].

Intraoperative and Postoperative Care

The brain parenchyma surrounding AVMs is well known to be subject to hemodynamic perturbations, which may account for both the vascular steal-associated symptoms experienced by some patients with AVMs preoperatively, as well as feared hyperemic complications postoperatively. Chronic arterial hypotension surrounding AVMs has been theorized to induce a loss of cerebrovascular autoregulatory capability, such that perfusion pressure elevation to normal range following AVM shunt obliteration results in reperfusion injury and/or hemorrhage ("normal perfusion pressure breakthrough") [95, 96]. Thus, the cornerstone of perioperative care during and after AVM treatment is strict blood pressure control with absolute prevention of hypertension. Careful administration of anesthesia is paramount, with smooth induction, intubation, and emergence of utmost importance; standard practices of neuroanesthesia otherwise apply, including careful ICP management, though the anesthesiologist should also be prepared for the possibility of sudden, profuse blood loss. Early postoperative complications are often attributed to inadequate blood pressure control [89, 90]. To avoid intra- or postoperative swelling or hemorrhage, systemic hypotension/normotension is typically pursued for 48–72 h postoperatively and then gradually liberalized.

When postoperative bleeding occurs despite adequate blood pressure control, residual malformation should be considered. For this reason, many surgeons perform either intraoperative or postoperative catheter angiography to document complete resection of the AVM nidus. More rarely, cerebral vasospasm has also been identified as a cause of delayed neurologic decline, perhaps as a result of either SAH or intraoperative vessel manipulation [43]; evaluation with CT or conventional catheter angiography should therefore be considered for neurologic deterioration once postoperative hemorrhage has been excluded as a cause. In addition to these measures, vigilant postoperative critical care management is necessary, employing the same principles described earlier in the chapter.

Conclusions

Critical care for patients with AVMs is a multidisciplinary challenge, often requiring the close collaboration of neurosurgeons, anesthesiologists, neuroradiologists, and intensivists. It is only with the close collaboration of these different entities that the best care can be administered to these usually critically ill patients.

References

1. Stapf C, Mohr JP, Pile-Spellman J, Solomon RA, Sacco RL, Connolly ES Jr. Epidemiology and natural history of arteriovenous malformations. Neurosurg Focus. 2001;11:e1.
2. Lasjaunias PL. Vascular diseases in neonates, infants, and children: interventional neuroradiology management. New York: Springer; 1996.
3. Lazar RM, Marshall RS, Pile-Spellman J, Hacein-Bey L, Young WL, Mohr JP, Stein BM. Anterior translocation of language in patients with left cerebral arteriovenous malformation. Neurology. 1997;49:802–8.
4. Campi A, Scotti G, Filippi M, Gerevini S, Strigimi F, Lasjaunias P. Antenatal diagnosis of vein of Galen aneurysmal malformation: MR study of fetal brain and postnatal follow-up. Neuroradiology. 1996;38:87–90.
5. DeCesare B, Omojola MF, Fogarty EF, Brown JC, Taylon C. Spontaneous thrombosis of congenital cerebral arteriovenous malformation complicated by subdural collection: in utero detection with disappearance in infancy. Br J Radiol. 2006;79:e140–4.
6. Oikawa M, Kuniba H, Kondoh T, Kinoshita A, Nagayasu T, Niikawa N, Yoshiura K. Familial brain arteriovenous malformation maps to 5p13-q14, 15q11-q13 or 18p11: linkage analysis with clipped fingernail DNA on high-density SNP array. Eur J Med Genet. 2010;53:244–9.
7. Zabel-du Bois A, Wagner-Ecker M, Milker-Zabel S, Schwager C, Wirkner U, Debus J, Abdollahi A, Huber PE. Gene expression signatures in the peripheral blood after radiosurgery of human cerebral arteriovenous malformations. Strahlenther Onkol. 2010;186:91–8.
8. Moftakhar P, Hauptman JS, Malkasian D, Martin NA. Cerebral arteriovenous malformations. Part 1: cellular and molecular biology. Neurosurg Focus. 2009;26:E10.
9. Hatva E, Jaaskelainen J, Hirvonen H, Alitalo K, Haltia M. Tie endothelial cell-specific receptor tyrosine kinase is upregulated in the vasculature of arteriovenous malformations. J Neuropathol Exp Neurol. 1996;55:1124–33.
10. Rothbart D, Awad IA, Lee J, Kim J, Harbaugh R, Criscuolo GR. Expression of angiogenic factors and structural proteins in central nervous system vascular malformations. Neurosurgery. 1996;38:915–24; discussion 924–5.
11. Hashimoto T, Emala CW, Joshi S, Mesa-Tejada R, Quick CM, Feng L, Libow A, Marchuk DA, Young WL. Abnormal pattern of Tie-2 and vascular endothelial growth factor receptor expression in human cerebral arteriovenous malformations. Neurosurgery. 2000;47:910–8; discussion 918–9.
12. Hirschi KK, Rohovsky SA, D'Amore PA. PDGF, TGF-beta, and heterotypic cell-cell interactions mediate endothelial cell-induced recruitment of 10T1/2 cells and their differentiation to a smooth muscle fate. J Cell Biol. 1998;141:805–14.
13. Winkler EA, Kim CN, Ross JM, Garcia JH, Gil E, Oh I, et al. A single-cell atlas of the normal and malformed human brain vasculature. Science. 2022;375(6584):eabi7377.
14. Jellinger K. Vascular malformations of the central nervous system: a morphological overview. Neurosurg Rev. 1986;9:177–216.
15. Sacco RL, Boden-Albala B, Gan R, Chen X, Kargman DE, Shea S, Paik MC, Hauser WA. Stroke incidence among white, black, and Hispanic residents of an urban community: the northern Manhattan stroke study. Am J Epidemiol. 1998;147:259–68.
16. Jessurun GA, Kamphuis DJ, van der Zande FH, Nossent JC. Cerebral arteriovenous malformations in The Netherlands Antilles. High prevalence of hereditary hemorrhagic telangiectasia-related single and multiple cerebral arteriovenous malformations. Clin Neurol Neurosurg. 1993;95:193–8.
17. Stapf C, Labovitz DL, Sciacca RR, Mast H, Mohr JP, Sacco RL. Incidence of adult brain arteriovenous malformation hemorrhage in a prospective population-based stroke survey. Cerebrovasc Dis. 2002;13:43–6.
18. Ondra SL, Troupp H, George ED, Schwab K. The natural history of symptomatic arteriovenous malformations of the brain: a 24-year follow-up assessment. J Neurosurg. 1990;3:387–91.
19. Hernesniemi JA, Dashti R, Juvela S, Vaart K, Niemela M, Laakso A. Natural history of brain arteriovenous malformations: a long-term follow-up study of risk of hemorrhage in 238 patients. Neurosurgery. 2008;63:823–9.
20. Mohr JP, Parides MK, Stapf C, Moquete E, Moy CS, Overbey JR, et al. Medical management with or without interventional therapy for unruptured brain arteriovenous malformations (Aruba): a multicentre, non-blinded, randomised trial. Lancet. 2014;383(9917):614–21.
21. Marks MP, Lane B, Steinberg GK, Chang PJ. Hemorrhage in intracerebral arteriovenous malformations: angiographic determinants. Radiology. 1990;176:807–13.
22. Stapf C, Mast H, Sciacca RR, Choi JH, Khaw AV, Connolly ES, Pile-Spellman J, Mohr JP. Predictors of hemorrhage in patients with untreated brain arteriovenous malformation. Neurology. 2006;66:1350–5.
23. Gujjar AR, Deibert E, Manno EM, Duff S, Diringer MN. Mechanical ventilation for ischemic stroke and intracerebral hemorrhage: indications, timing, and outcome. Neurology. 1998;51:447–51.

24. Jabbour PAIHD. Hemorrhagic cerebrovascular disease. In: Layon AGA, Friedman WA, editors. Textbook of neurocritical care. Philadelphia: Saunders; 2004. p. 155–81.
25. Arima H, Anderson CS, Wang JG, Huang Y, Heeley E, Neal B, Woodward M, Skulina C, Parsons MW, Peng B, Tao QL, Li YC, Jiang JD, Tai LW, Zhang JL, Xu E, Cheng Y, Morgenstern LB, Chalmers J. Lower treatment blood pressure is associated with greatest reduction in hematoma growth after acute intracerebral hemorrhage. Hypertension. 2010;56:852–8.
26. Delcourt C, Huang Y, Wang J, Heeley E, Lindley R, Stapf C, Tzourio C, Arima H, Parsons M, Sun J, Neal B, Chalmers J, Anderson C. The second (main) phase of an open, randomised, multicentre study to investigate the effectiveness of an intensive blood pressure reduction in acute cerebral haemorrhage trial (INTERACT2). Int J Stroke. 2010;5:110–6.
27. Greenberg SM, Ziai WC, Cordonnier C, Dowlatshahi D, Francis B, Goldstein JN, et al. 2022 guideline for the Management of Patients with Spontaneous Intracerebral Hemorrhage: a guideline from the American Heart Association/American Stroke Association. Stroke. 2022;53(7):e282–361.
28. Nilsson OG, Lindgren A, Stahl N, Brandt L, Saveland H. Incidence of intracerebral and subarachnoid haemorrhage in southern Sweden. J Neurol Neurosurg Psychiatry. 2000;69:601–7.
29. Morgenstern LB, Hemphill JC 3rd, Anderson C, Becker K, Broderick JP, Connolly ES Jr, Greenberg SM, Huang JN, MacDonald RL, Messe SR, Mitchell PH, Selim M, Tamargo RJ. Guidelines for the management of spontaneous intracerebral hemorrhage: a guideline for healthcare professionals from the American Heart Association/American Stroke Association. Stroke. 2010;41:2108–29.
30. Mokri B. The Monro-Kellie hypothesis: applications in CSF volume depletion. Neurology. 2001;56:1746–8.
31. Diringer MN, Zazulia AR. Osmotic therapy: fact and fiction. Neurocrit Care. 2004;1:219–33.
32. Schwartz ML, Tator CH, Rowed DW, Reid SR, Meguro K, Andrews DF. The University of Toronto head injury treatment study: a prospective, randomized comparison of pentobarbital and mannitol. Can J Neurol Sci. 1984;11:434–40.
33. Kamel H, Navi BB, Nakagawa K, Hemphill JC 3rd, Ko NU. Hypertonic saline versus mannitol for the treatment of elevated intracranial pressure: a meta-analysis of randomized clinical trials. Crit Care Med. 2011;39:554–9.
34. Broderick J, Connolly S, Feldmann E, Hanley D, Kase C, Krieger D, Mayberg M, Morgenstern L, Ogilvy CS, Vespa P, Zuccarello M. Guidelines for the management of spontaneous intracerebral hemorrhage in adults: 2007 update: a guideline from the American Heart Association/American Stroke Association stroke council, high blood pressure research council, and the quality of care and outcomes in research interdisciplinary working group. Circulation. 2007;116:e391–413.
35. Hofmeister C, Stapf C, Hartmann A, Sciacca RR, Mansmann U, terBrugge K, Lasjaunias P, Mohr JP, Mast H, Meisel J. Demographic, morphological, and clinical characteristics of 1289 patients with brain arteriovenous malformation. Stroke. 2000;31:1307–10.
36. Hoh BL, Chapman PH, Loeffler JS, Carter BS, Ogilvy CS. Results of multimodality treatment for 141 patients with brain arteriovenous malformations and seizures: factors associated with seizure incidence and seizure outcomes. Neurosurgery. 2002;51:303–9; discussion 309–11.
37. Peter-Derex L, Philippeau F, Garnier P, André-Obadia N, Boulogne S, Catenoix H, et al. Safety and efficacy of prophylactic levetiracetam for prevention of epileptic seizures in the acute phase of intracerebral haemorrhage (PEACH): a randomised, double-blind, placebo-controlled, phase 3 trial. The Lancet Neurology. 2022;21(9):781–91.
38. Lanzino G, Kongable GL, Kassell NF. Electrocardiographic abnormalities after nontraumatic subarachnoid hemorrhage. J Neurosurg Anesthesiol. 1994;6:156–62.
39. Wells C, Cujec B, Johnson D, Goplen G. Reversibility of severe left ventricular dysfunction in patients with subarachnoid hemorrhage. Am Heart J. 1995;129:409–12.
40. Rahman M, Friedman WA. Hyponatremia in neurosurgical patients: clinical guidelines development. Neurosurgery. 2009;65:925–35; discussion 935–6.
41. Zhao J, Wang S, Li J, Qi W, Sui D, Zhao Y. Clinical characteristics and surgical results of patients with cerebral arteriovenous malformations. Surg Neurol. 2005;63:156–61; discussion 161.
42. Cunha e Sa MJ, Stein BM, Solomon RA, PC MC. The treatment of associated intracranial aneurysms and arteriovenous malformations. J Neurosurg. 1992;77:853–9.
43. Morgan MK, Sekhon LH, Finfer S, Grinnell V. Delayed neurological deterioration following resection of arteriovenous malformations of the brain. J Neurosurg. 1999;90:695–701.
44. Yokobori S, Watanabe A, Nakae R, Onda H, Fuse A, Kushimoto S, Yokota H. Cerebral vasospasms after intraventricular hemorrhage from an arteriovenous malformation: case report. Neurol Med Chir (Tokyo). 2010;50:320–3.
45. Kokkinis C, Vlychou M, Zavras GM, Hadjigeorgiou GM, Papadimitriou A, Fezoulidis IV. The role of 3D-computed tomography angiography (3D-CTA) in investigation of spontaneous subarachnoid haemorrhage: comparison with digital subtraction angiography (DSA) and surgical findings. Br J Neurosurg. 2008;22:71–8.
46. Sinha PK, Neema PK, Rathod RC. Anesthesia and intracranial arteriovenous malformation. Neurol India. 2004;52:163–70.
47. Spetzler RF, Martin NA. A proposed grading system for arteriovenous malformations. J Neurosurg. 1986;65:476–83.
48. Heros RC, Korosue K, Diebold PM. Surgical excision of cerebral arteriovenous malformations: late results. Neurosurgery. 1990;26:570–7; discussion 577–8.
49. Hamilton MG, Spetzler RF. The prospective application of a grading system for arteriovenous malformations. Neurosurgery. 1994;34:2–6; discussion 6–7.
50. Schaller C, Schramm J, Haun D. Significance of factors contributing to surgical complications and to late outcome after elective surgery of cerebral arteriovenous malformations. J Neurol Neurosurg Psychiatry. 1998;65:547–54.
51. Hartmann A, Stapf C, Hofmeister C, Mohr JP, Sciacca RR, Stein BM, Faulstich A, Mast H. Determinants of neurological outcome after surgery for brain arteriovenous malformation. Stroke. 2000;31:2361–4.
52. Davidson AS, Morgan MK. How safe is arteriovenous malformation surgery? A prospective, observational study of surgery as first-line treatment for brain arteriovenous malformations. Neurosurgery. 2010;66:498–504; discussion 504–5.
53. Lawton MT, Kim H, McCulloch CE, Mikhak B, Young WL. A supplementary grading scale for selecting patients with brain arteriovenous malformations for surgery. Neurosurgery. 2010;66:702–13; discussion 713.
54. Spetzler RF, Ponce FA. A 3-tier classification of cerebral arteriovenous malformations. Clinical article. J Neurosurg. 2011;114:842–9.
55. Tamaki N, Ehara K, Lin TK, Kuwamura K, Obora Y, Kanazawa Y, Yamashita H, Matsumoto S. Cerebral arteriovenous malfor-

mations: factors influencing the surgical difficulty and outcome. Neurosurgery. 1991;29:856–61; discussion 861–3.
56. Hollerhage HG. Cerebral arteriovenous malformations: factors influencing surgical difficulty and outcome. Neurosurgery. 1992;31:604–5.
57. Spears J, Terbrugge KG, Moosavian M, Montanera W, Willinsky RA, Wallace MC, Tymianski M. A discriminative prediction model of neurological outcome for patients undergoing surgery of brain arteriovenous malformations. Stroke. 2006;37:1457–64.
58. Goodkin R, McKhann GM 2nd, Haynor DR, Mayberg MR, Eskridge JM, Winn HR. Persistent feeding arteries to angiographically completely embolized arteriovenous malformation demonstrated by intraoperative color-flow Doppler testing: report of two cases. Surg Neurol. 1995;44:326–32; discussion 332–3.
59. Standard SC, Guterman LR, Chavis TD, Hopkins LN. Delayed recanalization of a cerebral arteriovenous malformation following angiographic obliteration with polyvinyl alcohol embolization. Surg Neurol. 1995;44:109–12; discussion 112–3.
60. Gobin YP, Laurent A, Merienne L, Schlienger M, Aymard A, Houdart E, Casasco A, Lefkopoulos D, George B, Merland JJ. Treatment of brain arteriovenous malformations by embolization and radiosurgery. J Neurosurg. 1996;85:19–28.
61. Hurst RW, Berenstein A, Kupersmith MJ, Madrid M, Flamm ES. Deep central arteriovenous malformations of the brain: the role of endovascular treatment. J Neurosurg. 1995;82:190–5.
62. Paulsen RD, Steinberg GK, Norbash AM, Marcellus ML, Lopez JR, Marks MP. Embolization of rolandic cortex arteriovenous malformations. Neurosurgery. 1999;44:479–84; discussion 484–6.
63. Deruty R, Pelissou-Guyotat I, Morel C, Bascoulergue Y, Turjman F. Reflections on the management of cerebral arteriovenous malformations. Surg Neurol. 1998;50:245–55; discussion 255–6.
64. Gross BA, Duckworth EA, Getch CC, Bendok BR, Batjer HH. Challenging traditional beliefs: microsurgery for arteriovenous malformations of the basal ganglia and thalamus. Neurosurgery. 2008;63:393–410; discussion 410–1.
65. Steinberg GK, Fabrikant JI, Marks MP, Levy RP, Frankel KA, Phillips MH, Shuer LM, Silverberg GD. Stereotactic heavy-charged-particle Bragg-peak radiation for intracranial arteriovenous malformations. N Engl J Med. 1990;323:96–101.
66. Lunsford LD, Kondziolka D, Flickinger JC, Bissonette DJ, Jungreis CA, Maitz AH, Horton JA, Coffey RJ. Stereotactic radiosurgery for arteriovenous malformations of the brain. J Neurosurg. 1991;75:512–24.
67. Friedman WA. Radiosurgery for arteriovenous malformations. Clin Neurosurg. 1995;42:328–47.
68. Ellis TL, Friedman WA, Bova FJ, Kubilis PS, Buatti JM. Analysis of treatment failure after radiosurgery for arteriovenous malformations. J Neurosurg. 1998;89:104–10.
69. Chang JH, Chang JW, Park YG, Chung SS. Factors related to complete occlusion of arteriovenous malformations after gamma knife radiosurgery. J Neurosurg. 2000;93(Suppl 3):96–101.
70. Guo WY. Radiological aspects of gamma knife radiosurgery for arteriovenous malformations and other non-tumoural disorders of the brain. Acta Radiol Suppl. 1993;388:1–34.
71. Yoshimoto T, Takahashi A, Kinouchi H, Mizoi K, Jokura H. Role of embolization in the management of arteriovenous malformations. Clin Neurosurg. 1995;42:313–27.
72. Henkes H, Nahser HC, Berg-Dammer E, Weber W, Lange S, Kuhne D. Endovascular therapy of brain AVMs prior to radiosurgery. Neurol Res. 1998;20:479–92.
73. Pollock BE, Flickinger JC, Lunsford LD, Maitz A, Kondziolka D. Factors associated with successful arteriovenous malformation radiosurgery. Neurosurgery. 1998;42:1239–44. discussion 1244–7
74. Miyawaki L, Dowd C, Wara W, Goldsmith B, Albright N, Gutin P, Halbach V, Hieshima G, Higashida R, Lulu B, Pitts L, Schell M, Smith V, Weaver K, Wilson C, Larson D. Five year results of LINAC radiosurgery for arteriovenous malformations: outcome for large AVMS. Int J Radiat Oncol Biol Phys. 1999;44:1089–106.
75. Schlienger M, Atlan D, Lefkopoulos D, Merienne L, Touboul E, Missir O, Nataf F, Mammar H, Platoni K, Grandjean P, Foulquier JN, Huart J, Oppenheim C, Meder JF, Houdart E, Merland JJ. Linac radiosurgery for cerebral arteriovenous malformations: results in 169 patients. Int J Radiat Oncol Biol Phys. 2000;46:1135–42.
76. Andrade-Souza YM, Ramani M, Scora D, Tsao MN, terBrugge K, Schwartz ML. Embolization before radiosurgery reduces the obliteration rate of arteriovenous malformations. Neurosurgery. 2007;60:443–51; discussion 451–2.
77. Betti OO, Munari C, Rosler R. Stereotactic radiosurgery with the linear accelerator: treatment of arteriovenous malformations. Neurosurgery. 1989;24:311–21.
78. Friedman WA, Bova FJ, Bollampally S, Bradshaw P. Analysis of factors predictive of success or complications in arteriovenous malformation radiosurgery. Neurosurgery. 2003;52:296–307; discussion 307–8.
79. Andrade-Souza YM, Ramani M, Scora D, Tsao MN, TerBrugge K, Schwartz ML. Radiosurgical treatment for rolandic arteriovenous malformations. J Neurosurg. 2006;105:689–97.
80. Liscak R, Vladyka V, Simonova G, Urgosik D, Novotny J Jr, Janouskova L, Vymazal J. Arteriovenous malformations after Leksell gamma knife radiosurgery: rate of obliteration and complications. Neurosurgery. 2007;60:1005–14; discussion 1015–6.
81. Steiner L, Lindquist C, Cail W, Karlsson B, Steiner M. Microsurgery and radiosurgery in brain arteriovenous malformations. J Neurosurg. 1993;79:647–52.
82. Colombo F, Pozza F, Chierego G, Francescon P, Casentini L, De Luca G. Linear accelerator radiosurgery of cerebral arteriovenous malformations: current status. Acta Neurochir Suppl. 1994;62:5–9.
83. Bollet MA, Anxionnat R, Buchheit I, Bey P, Cordebar A, Jay N, Desandes E, Marchal C, Lapeyre M, Aletti P, Picard L. Efficacy and morbidity of arc-therapy radiosurgery for cerebral arteriovenous malformations: a comparison with the natural history. Int J Radiat Oncol Biol Phys. 2004;58:1353–63.
84. Pollock BE, Lunsford LD, Kondziolka D, Maitz A, Flickinger JC. Patient outcomes after stereotactic radiosurgery for "operable" arteriovenous malformations. Neurosurgery. 1994;35:1–7; discussion 7–8.
85. Friedman WA, Blatt DL, Bova FJ, Buatti JM, Mendenhall WM, Kubilis PS. The risk of hemorrhage after radiosurgery for arteriovenous malformations. J Neurosurg. 1996;84:912–9.
86. Firlik AD, Levy EI, Kondziolka D, Yonas H. Staged volume radiosurgery followed by microsurgical resection: a novel treatment for giant cerebral arteriovenous malformations: technical case report. Neurosurgery. 1998;43:1223–8.
87. Pollock BE, Kline RW, Stafford SL, Foote RL, Schomberg PJ. The rationale and technique of staged-volume arteriovenous malformation radiosurgery. Int J Radiat Oncol Biol Phys. 2000;48:817–24.
88. Abla AA, Rutledge WC, Seymour ZA, Guo D, Kim H, Gupta N, et al. A treatment paradigm for high-grade brain arteriovenous malformations: volume-staged radiosurgical downgrading followed by microsurgical resection. J Neurosurg. 2015;122(2):419–32.
89. Tew JM Jr, Lewis AI, Reichert KW. Management strategies and surgical techniques for deep-seated supratentorial arteriovenous malformations. Neurosurgery. 1995;36:1065–72.

90. O'Shaughnessy BA, Getch CC, Bendok BR, Batjer HH. Microsurgical resection of infratentorial arteriovenous malformations. Neurosurg Focus. 2005;19:E5.
91. Batjer H, Samson D. Surgical approaches to trigonal arteriovenous malformations. J Neurosurg. 1987;67:511–7.
92. Lee JP. Surgical treatment of thalamic arteriovenous malformations. Neurosurgery. 1993;32:498–503; discussion 503–4.
93. Lewis AI, Tew JM Jr. Management of thalamic-basal ganglia and brain-stem vascular malformations. Clin Neurosurg. 1994;41:83–111.
94. Gross BA, Du R. Hemorrhage from arteriovenous malformations during pregnancy. Neurosurgery. 2012;71(2):349–56.
95. Kader A, Young WL. The effects of intracranial arteriovenous malformations on cerebral hemodynamics. Neurosurg Clin N Am. 1996;7:767–81.
96. Hacein-Bey L, Young WL. Hemodynamic perturbations in cerebral arteriovenous malformations and management implications. Interv Neuroradiol. 1999;5:177–82.

Central Nervous System Vasculitis

23

Victor J. Del Brutto, Faddi Saleh Velez, and Jorge G. Ortiz

Contents

Abstract

Vasculitis is a group of disorders characterized by the inflammation of blood vessels resulting in occlusion and ischemia. The central nervous system (CNS) is a common target for vasculitis. CNS vasculitis can be classified according to the size of the vessels affected (small-, medium-, and large-vessel vasculitis), as well as the underlying etiology including primary vasculitis and vasculitis secondary to either systemic diseases, infections, neoplasms, or drugs. The clinical presentation is heterogeneous, the course may vary from insidious to fulminant, and the manifestations include headache, seizures, encephalopathy, and focal neurological deficits. Diagnosis of CNS vasculitis is challenging. A presumptive diagnosis is usually achieved by the combination of signs and symptoms, neuroimaging features, and serological or cerebrospinal fluid markers, whereas a definitive diagnosis usually requires tissue biopsy. Primary angiitis of the CNS is particularly difficult to diagnose due to the absence of pathognomonic findings. In this chapter, we review common causes of CNS vasculitis and provide an overview of their clinical presentation, diagnostic approach and therapeutic considerations.

Chapter Goals

- Review the etiologic classification of common vasculitis of the central nervous system.
- Describe the clinical manifestations and clinical course of common vasculitis of the central nervous system.
- Provide an overview of the diagnosis of common vasculitis of the central nervous system.

V. J. Del Brutto (✉)
Miller School of Medicine, University of Miami, Miami, FL, USA
e-mail: vjd30@med.miami.edu

F. Saleh Velez · J. G. Ortiz
University of Oklahoma Health Science Center,
Oklahoma, OK, USA

E. Mahanna Gabrielli et al. (eds.), *Textbook of Neurointensive Care: Volume 1*, https://doi.org/10.1007/978-3-031-62220-5_23

- Provide an overview of the management of patients with vasculitis of the central nervous system.
- Address potential toxicities related to vasculitis treatment with immunosuppressants.

Introduction

Vasculitis conveys a heterogeneous group of diseases characterized by inflammation and necrosis of blood vessels resulting in vessel occlusion and tissue ischemia. Primary vasculitides occur without a definitive cause, whereas secondary vasculitides develop from underlying recognized disorders such as infections, connective tissue disorders, neoplasms, or drugs. The central nervous system (CNS) is a common target for primary and secondary vasculitides. The true burden of CNS vasculitis is unknown. However, it is estimated that 3–5% of cerebrovascular events in patients aged <50 years are related to CNS vasculitis [1]. Diverse pathogenic mechanisms may lead to immune-mediated damage of blood vessels, which most commonly occurs with the formation and deposition of immune complex, the production of anti-neutrophilic cytoplasmic antibodies (ANCA), and the activation of pathogenic T-cell lymphocytes with granuloma formation [2]. Clinical presentation is characterized by headaches, seizures, encephalopathy, and stroke-like features [1, 3]. Neurological compromise may be severe or coexist with systemic critical illnesses. Therefore, is expected that many of these patients will be managed in a neurocritical care unit.

Guided by the Revised Chapel Hill Consensus Conference nomenclature [4], CNS vasculitides can be classified according to the size of the affected vessel (Table 23.1). Diagnosis of specific causes of CNS vasculitis is challenging. However, a presumptive diagnosis is possible based on the combination of symptoms and signs, disease-specific serologies, and neurovascular imaging features, while histopathological studies are generally required for diagnosis confirmation. Isolated CNS vasculitis, nowadays termed primary angiitis of the central nervous system (PACNS), is particularly difficult to diagnose due to the absence of systemic signs or symptoms [2]. In this chapter, we summarize the clinical features of vasculitides that frequently affect the CNS and provide an overview for the evaluation and therapeutic management of patients with CNS vasculitis admitted to the neurocritical care unit.

Table 23.1 Classification of vasculitides affecting the central nervous system

• Large-vessel vasculitis
– Giant cell arteritis
– Takayasu arteritis
• Medium- and small-vessel vasculitis
– Polyarteritis nodosa
– ANCA-associated vasculitis
Microscopic polyangiitis
Granulomatosis with polyangiitis
Eosinophilic granulomatosis with polyangiitis
– Immune complex small vasculitis
Cryoglobulinemia
• Variable-vessel vasculitis
– Behçet's disease
• Single-organ vasculitis
– Primary angiitis of the central nervous system (PACNS)
– Idiopathic aortitis (IgG4)
• Vasculitis associated with systemic diseases
– Systemic lupus erythematosus
– Rheumatoid arthritis vasculitis
– Sarcoid vasculitis
• Vasculitis associated with probable etiology
– Malignancy-induced vasculitis
– Drug-induced vasculitis
– Radiation-induced vasculitis
• Infectious vasculitis
– Human immunodeficiency virus (HIV)/AIDS
– Varicella zoster virus
– Acute bacterial meningitis
– Mycobacterium tuberculosis
– Spirochete disease (Neurosyphilis, Neuroborreliosis, leptospirosis)
– Fungal pathogens (Aspergillosis, Coccidiomycosis, Cryptococcosis, histoplasmosis, Mucormycosis)
– Parasitic pathogens (Neurocysticercosis)

Abbreviations: *AIDS* acquired immunodeficiency syndrome, *ANCA* antineutrophil cytoplasmatic antibody

Secondary CNS Vasculitides

Large-Vessel Vasculitides

Giant Cell Arteritis

Giant cell arteritis (GCA) is the most common large-vessel vasculitis that affects the aorta and its branches. GCA (formerly temporal arteritis) is mostly seen in adults aged >50 years. GCA is common in North America and Western Europe, and rare in people of African and Asian descent. In the US, the estimated incidence is 17–20 per 100,000 patients-years, and women-to-men ratio is 3:1 [5]. GCA has been associated with HLA-DBR1*04 allele in Caucasians [6]. In addition, a potential correlation with infections has been suggested based on the presence of microorganisms such as varicella-zoster virus (VZV) in biopsies of affected individuals. GCA pathogenesis involves the activation of dendritic cells in the adventitia media, followed by migration of macrophages into the media forming multinucleated giant cells. Simultaneously, the intimal proliferation reduces blood flow causing ischemia [7].

GCA clinical presentation is characterized by headaches, scalp tenderness, visual loss, and jaw claudication, and is commonly associated with systemic symptoms such as fatigue, anorexia, weight loss, and low-grade fever [3]. Headaches occur in 70–80% of cases and may be unilateral or bilateral in the temporal area. Scalp tenderness is characterized as a severe sharp and burning sensation. Visual loss occurs in 30% of patients and is permanent in 10–15% of cases. Other symptoms include deafness, dysphagia, and tongue and limb claudication. Polymyalgia rheumatica is present in 50% of patients [5]. Common features of systemic inflammation are found in 40–100% of patients including elevated erythrocyte sedimentation rate, C-reactive protein, interleukin-6 level, as well as transaminitis, thrombocytosis, and anemia. The gold standard for diagnosis is temporal artery biopsy, but it can be negative in 30% of patients. Temporal artery biopsy should not delay treatment and is recommended to be obtained within 2 weeks of starting steroids [8].

GCA is a medical emergency and needs immediate treatment when suspected. Glucocorticoids are the treatment of choice. The recommended regimen is a course of 0.5–1.0 g of IV methylprednisolone for 3–5 days, followed by 40–60 mg prednisone daily for the first month continued by a slow taper [7, 8]. Methotrexate has been used in refractory GCA cases. Other immunosuppressants like cyclophosphamide, mycophenolate, and leflunomide have shown promising results in small case series [8]. Tocilizumab, a monoclonal interleukin-6 receptor blocker, has shown benefits in clinical improvement as well [9].

Takayasu Arteritis

Takayasu arteritis (TA) is an idiopathic granulomatous large-vessel panarteritis of the aorta and its branches. TA is common in eastern Asia and Mexico, and women aged <40 years constitute the majority of cases [3]. In the U.S., TA prevalence is 2.6 per million people [3]. TA pathogenesis is poorly understood, but its association with HLA complex supports a genetic contribution. TA is associated with HLA-B52 in the Japanese population, whereas HLA-DR4 is associated with TA in North America [10]. The presence of circulating anti-endothelial cell antibodies and autoantibody-producing B-cells in the vessel wall suggests a role of humoral immunity. Several inflammatory markers are released, but interleukin-6, interleukin-12, and interleukin-18 have shown to correlate with disease activity [10].

TA manifests with hypertension, headaches, fever, weight loss, and myalgia, lasting for weeks to months. The chronic phase is known as the "pulseless" stage and is characterized by ischemic complications due to arterial occlusion. Blood pressure discrepancy of >10 mmHg between limbs is present in 50% of patients [10]. Neurological symptoms include headaches, stroke, meningitis, encephalitis, and seizures. Intracranial aneurysms have also been reported. Visual manifestations like retinal ischemia, vitreous hemorrhage, and retinal detachment may lead to blindness. Cardiovascular manifestations include aortic valve insufficiency and congestive heart failure. Cutaneous features include livedo reticularis, erythema nodosum, subcutaneous edema, purpura, urticaria, and digital gangrene. A common gastrointestinal feature is acute or chronic abdominal pain caused by mesenteric ischemia. Finally, nephrotic syndrome, IgA nephropathy, alveolar hemorrhage, and pulmonary hypertension have been reported in case series [10].

The American College of Rheumatology (ACR) criteria for TA diagnosis include: age < 40 years, extremities claudication, decreased brachial arterial pulse, blood pressure difference > 10 mmHg between arms, auscultatory bruits over the subclavian arteries or the aorta, and arteriographic narrowing or occlusion of the aorta or its branches not due to other causes [11]. TA is diagnosed if at least three of the six aforementioned criteria are present. The treatment is oral prednisone, 1 mg/kg daily, followed by tapering over weeks to months. About 50% of patients do not achieve remission with glucocorticoid therapy alone and require maintenance therapy with disease-modifying antirheumatic drugs (DMARDs) such as methotrexate, mycophenolate or azathioprine. Cases refractory to DMARDs are treated with biological agents such as infliximab, tocilizumab, or rituximab, but the evidence is limited to small case series [11].

Medium-to-Small Vessel Vasculitides

Polyarteritis Nodosa

Polyarteritis nodosa (PAN) is a systemic necrotizing vasculitis of medium-sized vessels. PAN is a sporadic disease but can be secondary to hepatitis B virus (HBV) infection, drug reactions, familial Mediterranean fever, or adenosine deaminase-2 deficiency (DADA2). The prevalence of PAN is about 30.7 per million adults [12]. PAN prevalence peaks between 40 and 60 years of age [3]. The pathogenesis of PAN is unclear. There are defective regulatory T-cells that contribute to vessel inflammation. The pathophysiology of HBV-related necrotizing vasculitis is related to immune complexes deposition in medium-sized vessels, while DADA2 demonstrates loss-of-function mutations in the CECR1 gene, resulting in a vasculopathy that resembles the classic PAN [13]. PAN predominantly affects the renal, mesenteric, and coronary circulation, and manifests clinically with fever, fatigue, skin eruptions and ulcers, mucosal ulcers, abdominal pain, anorexia, nausea and vomiting, diarrhea and melena, testicular pain, hypertension, and myocardial infarction [14]. Approximately 80% of PAN cases have neurological manifestations). Compared to the CNS, the peripheral nervous system is more frequently affected by mononeuritis multiplex, polyneuritis, or peripheral neuropathy. CNS involvement may result in headaches, seizures, spinal cord infarction, and encephalopathy [14]. Cerebrovascular events are infrequent, and lobar hemorrhages are more common than ischemic strokes [3].

Proposed PAN diagnostic criteria include weight loss >4 kg, livedo reticularis, testicular pain or tenderness, myalgias, mononeuropathy or polyneuropathy, diastolic blood pressure > 90 mmHg, elevated blood urea nitrogen or serum creatinine levels, serological HBV reactants, arteriographic abnormalities), and presence of granulocyte or mixed leukocyte infiltrate in arterial wall biopsy. The presence of 3 or more of these 10 criteria was associated with a sensitivity of 82.2% and specificity of 86.6% [15]. However, the validity of the aforementioned diagnostic criteria has been challenged and establishing a modern PAN diagnostic classification is a work in progress [16].

Glucocorticoids are the first-line treatment for PAN) management, but remission is achieved in only 50% of patients. For patients with active and severe PAN, initiating treatment with cyclophosphamide and high-dose glucocorticoids is recommended [16]. The use of other non-glucocorticoid immunosuppressants such as azathioprine, mycophenolate, or methotrexate may be considered in those unable to tolerate cyclophosphamide. For HBV-related PAN, anti-viral agents are recommended.

ANCA-Associated Vasculitis

Granulomatosis with polyangiitis (GPA), formerly known as "Wegener's granulomatosis," is characterized by necrotizing granulomatous inflammation and pauci-immune vasculitis of small- and medium-sized vessels. The prevalence of GPA in the US is 3 cases per 100,000 people, and GPA typically starts at the age of 35–55 years [17]. The cause of GPA is unknown. However, environmental factors (i.e., dust inhalation, silica) and infectious processes may trigger the disease. Some familial cases have been reported as well [17].

GPA) results in necrotizing granulomas in the respiratory tract, vasculitis, and glomerulonephritis. The nasal cavity and the paranasal sinuses are affected in 85–100% of cases; symptoms include nasal discharge, epistaxis, mucosal ulceration, nasal bridge collapse, nasal granulomas, sinusitis, stridor, pulmonary nodules, cavitating lung lesions, pleuritis, mesenteric vasculitis, diffuse pauci-immune crescentic necrotizing glomerulonephritis, headache, meningitis, cerebrovascular events, spinal cord lesions, cranial nerve palsies, and sensory-motor peripheral neuropathy [3, 18]. GPA diagnosis is based on the combination of clinical features, positive ANCA serology, and histological findings of necrotizing vasculitis, necrotizing glomerulonephritis, or granulomatous inflammation from organ biopsy (skin, lung, or kidney). The combination of glucocorticoids and cyclophosphamide is the standard of treatment for GPA [17].

Eosinophilic granulomatosis with polyangiitis (EGPA), formerly known as "Churg-Strauss syndrome," is a systemic vasculitis affecting small- and medium-sized vessels. The incidence of EGPA is estimated to be 2–6 cases per 100,000 adults per year [3]. The pathogenesis is unknown. However, the inflammatory process is characterized by hypergammaglobulinemia, increased Ig-E levels, elevated rheumatoid factor, and positive ANCA. Clinical manifestations include fatigue, flu-like symptoms, weight loss, fever, and myalgias. Asthma is a central feature and may precede vasculitis by up to 10 years. Other respiratory features include paranasal sinusitis, allergic rhinitis, cough, and hemoptysis. Patients may also experience heart failure, myocarditis, pericarditis, constrictive pericarditis, myocardial infarction, and eosinophilic gastritis/colitis [19]. CNS manifestations include dementia, encephalopathy, peripheral neuropathy, and mononeuritis multiplex. Stroke in EGPA is attributed to the eosinophilic release of a major basic protein that damages the endothelium causing thrombosis [20].

The ACR established 6 diagnostic criteria for EGPA): asthma, >10% eosinophils on complete blood count, neuropathy (mononeuropathy, mononeuritis multiplex, or polyneuropathy), migratory or transient pulmonary opacities, paranasal sinus abnormalities, and biopsy containing extravascular eosinophilic accumulation [21]. The presence of 4 or more of these criteria has a sensitivity of 85% and a specificity of 99.7% [21]. Treatment includes oral prednisone 1 mg/kg daily, followed by a slow taper for 12–18 months. High-dose IV methylprednisolone for 3–5 days before oral steroids may be considered for acute severe multiorgan disease. Mepolizumab, a humanized monoclonal antibody against interleukin-5, has shown clinical benefit in patients with EGPA [22].

Cryoglobulinemia

Cryoglobulinemia is a rare disorder characterized by abnormal immunoglobulins that precipitate at low temperatures. Cryoglobulins deposit in vessel walls, activate the complex cascade and induce vasculitis [23]. Cryoglobulins may be composed only of monoclonal immunoglobulins (type I cryoglobulinemia), monoclonal immunoglobulins bound to a constant domain of polyclonal heavy chains (type II cryoglobulinemia), or only polyclonal immunoglobulins (type III cryoglobulinemia) [23]. Cryoglobulinemia prevalence is related to the endemic presence of hepatitis C virus (HCV) infection within a population. Other disorders associated with cryoglobulins are Human Immunodeficiency Virus (HIV), HBV, autoimmune diseases, and lymphoproliferative disorders. The main clinical manifestations are purpura, livedo reticularis, Raynaud phenomenon, and necrotic ulcers. Other features include arthralgias, renal immune-complex disease, and peripheral neuropathy. CNS involvement is rare and includes encephalopathy, stroke, and intracranial hemorrhage [23, 24]. Hyperviscosity syndrome and moyamoya-type vasculopathy may also present as a complication of cryoglobulinemia. Treatment depends on the underlying cause of cryoglobulinemia. Glucocorticoids followed by either rituximab or cyclophosphamide is often used in patients with severe symptoms. In severe cases, plasmapheresis may be considered [23].

Behcet's Disease

Behcet's disease (BD) is a systemic inflammatory variable-sized vessel vasculitis characterized by oral aphthous ulcers, genital ulcers, skin lesions, ocular lesions, and other systemic manifestations [25]. BD prevalence is 0.12–0.33 cases per 100,000 adults-year. BD is common in Asian and Middle Eastern populations. The pathogenesis remains unclear, but genetic and environmental factors may play a role. The HLA-B51 genetic marker is seen in about 60% of cases [25]. International criteria for BD diagnosis include recurrent oral ulcerations with at least two of the following: genital ulcerations, anterior uveitis, posterior uveitis, retinal vasculitis, erythema nodosum, pseudo folliculitis, papulopustular lesions, acneiform nodules, and positive pathergy test. Patients can experience pulmonary vasculitis manifested by hemoptysis, dyspnea, and cough. Venous thrombosis with Budd-Chiari syndrome or superior vena-cava syndrome is also seen. The CNS is involved in 5–10% of cases, either through the development of immune-mediated meningoencephalitis, mainly affecting the brainstem and basal ganglia, or by cerebral venous thrombosis with intracranial hypertension [26]. Treatment includes the use of glucocorticoids, DMARDs (azathioprine, mycophenolate, methotrexate, tacrolimus), and biological therapies (infliximab, rituximab, and alemtuzumab) [27].

CNS Vasculitides Associated with Systemic Diseases

Systemic Lupus Erythematosus

Systemic Lupus Erythematosus (SLE) is a complex autoimmune disease that may affect any organ and has a broad spectrum of clinical and serological manifestations. Neuropsychiatric manifestations of SLE are present in nearly 37–90% of cases, being higher among those with early-onset disease [28]. CNS manifestations are heterogeneous and include cognitive dysfunction, headaches, mood disorders, seizures, and cerebrovascular events. CNS involvement in SLE is most commonly associated with non-inflammatory vasculopathies, thromboembolic events, and the presence of CNS auto-antibodies, whereas the occurrence of true CNS vasculitis is rare [29]. CNS vasculitis in SLE results from the deposition of immune complexes in the vascular path. In addition, the presence of anti-endothelial cell antibodies is responsible) for vascular inflammation. SLE-related CNS vasculitis lacks specific serum or cerebrospinal fluid (CSF) markers and angiographic studies are often negative due to isolated involvement of small vessels. Therefore, biopsy is usually required to differentiate from other disorders such as infections or lymphoma, SLE patients with CNS manifestations, including those with CNS vasculitis, require treatment with high-dose IV glucocorticoids followed by cyclophosphamide for 2 years rather than glucocorticoids alone [30]. Other treatments frequently employed for severe cases include rituximab, plasmapheresis, and intravenous immunoglobulins [28].

Rheumatoid Arthritis

Rheumatoid vasculitis (RV) is the most serious extra-articular complication of rheumatoid arthritis, mostly affecting medium- and small-sized vessels, and can affect a variety of organs [31]. Immune complex deposition and activation of the complement system play a role in the pathogenesis [31]. RV is more frequent in men, smokers, those with seropositive nodular erosive disease, and those with a disease duration longer than 10 years [32]. The widespread use DMARDs for rheumatoid arthritis has resulted in a significant drop in the incidence of RV [33, 34]. RV onset is characterized by fever, malaise, weight loss, and escalation of acute-phase markers. The skin is involved in 90% of cases with purpura, nail fold infarcts, digital ischemia, and cutaneous ulcers. Ocular manifestations include ulcerative keratitis and retinal vasculitis. Non-CNS manifestations include pericarditis, myocarditis, coronary vasculitis, pulmonary angiitis with alveolar hemorrhage, pauci-immune glomerulonephritis, mesenteric vasculitis, mononeuritis multiplex, and polyneuropathy [31]. CNS involvement is rare and carries a poor prognosis. CNS manifestations of RV include hypertrophic pachymeningitis, stroke, cranial nerve palsies, and seizures [31]. The diagnosis requires a combination of medical history, laboratory tests, and tissue biopsy of the affected organ. Treatment includes high doses of glucocorticoids followed by immunosuppression with cyclophosphamide. Plasma exchange has been used, but relapses may occur. The use of azathioprine, methotrexate, and mycophenolate, as well as biological agents such as rituximab, abatacept, and anakinra have been reported in case series [35]. Hydroxychloroquine and low-dose aspirin have demonstrated a protective effect for RV in patients with rheumatoid arthritis [36].

Infectious CNS Vasculitides

Viral

Human Immunodeficiency Virus

CNS vasculitis is a rare complication of HIV infection, and should be differentiated from other HIV-related cerebrovascular disorders such as HIV vasculopathy, accelerated atherosclerosis, cardioembolism, and HIV-associated coagulopathies [37]. Hospital-based series have reported <1% prevalence of CNS vasculitis among HIV patients [38, 39]. On the other hand, 13–28% of strokes in HIV patients are attributed to vasculitis [37]. Most cases of CNS vasculitis in HIV patients are associated with opportunistic infections, lymphoproliferative disorders, or autoimmune diseases, and may exist in almost every pattern affecting small, medium, and large vessels [40]. Common opportunistic infections associated with CNS vasculitis in HIV include VZV, cytomegalovirus (CMV), toxoplasmosis, pneumocystis, salmonella, and tuberculosis (TB). HIV patients may develop PAN-like vasculitis in the absence of HBV, as well as mixed cryoglobulinemia with negative HCV serology [41, 42].

After the exclusion of secondary causes of CNS vasculitis, HIV-related angiitis of the CNS (HIV-ACNS) should be considered. Pathogenic mechanisms involved in HIV-ACNS include direct vascular injury by HIV replication, molecular mimicry leading to immune complexes deposition, immune activation resulting in vascular inflammatory reaction, and immune restoration syndrome during antiretroviral therapy (HAART) [40]. Clinical manifestations are analogous to PACNS including headache, cognitive dysfunction, and focal neurological deficits [43]. The gold standard for HIV-ACNS diagnosis is histological evidence of vessel wall inflammation. However, brain biopsy is usually omitted due to procedure invasiveness and high rate of false negatives. Thus, diagnosis is frequently based on clinical-radiological patterns. Prognosis is generally considered poor [40].

Treatment of CNS vasculitis in HIV patients is challenging due to competing pathogenic mechanisms and lack of evidence-based therapies. Recognizing opportunistic infections is important to institute appropriate antibiotic therapy. Immune restoration with HAART is recommended to slow disease progression [44]. Although paradoxical, conjunct immunosuppression with glucocorticoids and DMARDs such as cyclophosphamide have been proposed for the treatment of severe cases [45, 46]. To avoid opportunistic infections, immunosuppressive therapy requires CD4+ T cells counts >200 cells/mm^3, suppressed viral activity (<60 k copies/mm^3), and antibiotic prophylactic therapy [46].

Varicella Zoster Virus

VZV is a neurotropic enveloped DNA virus that belongs to the Herpes virus family. Acute VZV infection causes chickenpox. Afterward, the virus remains latent in neural ganglion cells. In the absence of proper cell-mediated immunity, VZV may reactivate and spread peripherally causing a painful rash (i.e., shingles). Rarely, VZV can spread to the cerebral and spinal cord arteries resulting in large- and small-vessel vasculitis [47]. The true incidence of VZV vasculitis is unknown. One retrospective study across stroke patients admitted to a neurocritical care unit found that 0.05% of cases were diagnosed with VZV vasculitis [48]. This may be an underestimation as not all patients underwent CSF analysis for VZV.

VZV vasculitis often causes cerebral ischemia, whereas intracerebral hemorrhage and cerebral sinus thrombosis are less common. Large-vessel abnormalities include focal narrowing, dissection, ectasia, and aneurysm formation. Clinically, VZV vasculitis manifests with focal neurological deficits, headache, and monocular vision loss. VZV vasculitis should be suspected in stroke patients with history of recent zoster rash, immunocompromised states, absence of traditional vascular risk factors, and stroke recurrence despite optimal medical therapy [49]. Radiographic findings include well-defined ovoid infarcts typically located at the gray-white matter junction. Vascular imaging is abnormal in 70% of cases [49]. CSF mononuclear pleocytosis is found in two-thirds of cases, and diagnosis requires CSF virologic studies confirmation. The polymerase chain reaction (PCR) for VZV DNA is detectable within 2 weeks of the infection but disappears shortly after. Anti-VZV immunoglobulin G antibody (anti-VZV IgG) is a more sensitive test and persists after VZV PCR becomes negative. Decreased serum-to-CSF anti-VZV IgG ratio indicates intrathecal antibody production [49]. Recommended treatment for VZV vasculitis includes IV acyclovir 10–15 mg/kg three times per day for at least 14 days in immunocompetent patients, whereas immunocompromised patients may require prolonged acyclovir treatment or transition to oral valcyclovir [50]. A short course of IV glucocorticoids without taper is recommended in selected cases [50, 51].

Although less common than VZV, other viruses from the Herpesvirus family including Herpes simplex virus (types 1 and 2), Epstein-Barr virus, and CMV have been associated with CNS vasculitis. Diagnosis is reached by positive CSF PCR in the appropriate clinical setting. CMV, specifically, is known to replicate in vascular endothelial cells and may cause occlusive arteritis, mainly in HIV-positive or immunocompromised individuals. Anti-viral therapy includes IV ganciclovir, foscarnet, or a combination of both [51].

Bacterial

Pyogenic Bacterial Meningitis

Vascular complications occur in approximately one-fifth of bacterial meningitis cases including arterial infarction, subarachnoid and intraparenchymal hemorrhage, and venous thrombosis [51]. Compared to other bacterial meningitis, pneumococcal meningitis (streptococcus pneumoniae) has a particularly high risk of vascular compromise resulting in higher rates of death and severe neurological sequalae [52]. Cerebrovascular complications in bacterial meningitis may occur early in the course of illness, or present later secondary to a delayed immunological response [53]. Pathogenic mechanisms of vascular compromise include true CNS vasculitis, subarachnoid inflammatory exudate encasing of large vessels at the base of the cranium, hypercoagulability with intra-arterial thrombosis, vasospasm, and embolism associated with bacterial endocarditis [54, 55]. Clinically, focal neurological deficits may be evident in addition to typical manifestations of bacterial meningitis including fever, headaches, neck stiffness and altered mental status. CSF typically shows polymorphonuclear pleocytosis, an elevated protein with low glucose, and gram stain, CSF cultures, or bacterial antigen testing is required for definitive diagnosis [51]. Angiography typically reveals segmental narrowing and dilation of large- and medium-sized vessels. None of the above is considered specific for CNS vasculitis in the setting of bacterial meningitis and brain biopsy is considered the gold standard to confirm the diagnosis. However, brain biopsy is rarely pursued. No standardized guidelines exist for management of vascular complications in bacterial meningitis. Glucocorticoids have been proposed to be beneficial in improving outcomes among patients with bacterial meningitis [54–56]. Although often recommended, the use of glucocorticoids to treat vascular complications of bacterial meningitis is controversial [51].

Mycobacteria

TB continues to be prevalent worldwide with approximately nine million new cases and two million deaths each year [57]. In developing countries, high-risk populations include those with immunosuppression (i.e., HIV infection, alcoholism, use of immunosuppressants) and those coming from endemic areas. Hematogenous dissemination of TB to the CNS is the most devastating extrapulmonary complication, occurs in 1–2% of cases, and manifests either as a subacute-to-chronic meningitis, intracranial tuberculoma, or spinal tuberculous arachnoiditis [57]. TB meningitis is the result of tubercles ("Rich foci") rupture into the subarachnoid space leading to an intense cytokine-mediated inflammatory reaction. The latter leads to proliferative arachnoiditis with cranial nerve entrapment, CSF flow obstruction with hydrocephalus, and encroachment of arteries and veins resulting in large-vessel vasculitis [58]. The most common vessel pathologies in TB meningitis are infiltrative, proliferative, and necrotizing, either pure or in combination [59]. Stroke is found in 20–60% of patients with TB meningitis depending on the imaging method utilized [59].

Diagnosis should be suspected in high-risk populations and those with extrapulmonary TB. Pulmonary involvement is seen in 50–80% of adults with CNS TB. The tuberculin test and interferon-gamma are relatively insensitive. Neuroimaging may reveal clinical and subclinical infarctions classically affecting the anterior basal ganglia, as well as other typical TB findings such as basal leptomeningeal enhancement, parenchymal tuberculomas, and hydrocephalus. CSF studies usually reveal elevated intracranial pressure, mononuclear pleocytosis, elevated protein, and normal-to-low glucose. CSF acid-fast stain and mycobacterial cultures have inadequate sensitivity, which improves if sequential samples are analyzed. The nucleic acid-based amplification PCR is an alternative method to detect mycobacterial PCR in CSF. The prognosis of patients with TB affecting the CNS depends on early initiation on anti-TB therapy. Anti-TB therapy appears to be relatively ineffective in preventing vascular complications, perhaps suggesting an immune mechanism. Adjunctive glucocorticoids may have some benefit in preventive vascular complications in TB [60, 61].

Spirochetes

Syphilis is a spirochetal, sexually transmitted disease caused by *Treponema Pallidum*. Worldwide, there are approximately 12 million new cases every year [62]. *T. Pallidum* can be isolated in the CSF in about one-fourth of syphilis cases, and nearly 10% of untreated patients will develop CNS clinical manifestations [54, 55]. Neurosyphilis may manifest as meningitis or meningovascular syphilis in the early phase, or tabes dorsalis and neuropsychiatric syndromes in the late phase. Classical pathological findings in meningovascular syphilis include an inflammatory infiltrate on the adventitia and media of large and medium-sized vessels, with secondary fibroblastic intima proliferation leading to luminal narrowing and thrombosis (Heubner endarteritis); small cortical and pial vessels may also be involved (Nissl endarteritis) [63]. Stroke in meningovascular syphilis usually presents with either prodromal symptoms such as headache, vertigo, and behavioral changes, or as subacute progressive stroke syndromes rather than maximal deficits at onset [63]. In addition to treponemal and nontreponemal serologic tests, diagnosis is made based on the presence of either rapid plasma regain (RPR) or Venereal Disease Research Laboratory (VDRL) in the CSF. Both RPR and VDRL are positive in the early phase when most cases of meningovascular syphilis occur. The treponemal test Fluorescent Treponemal Antibody Absorption (FTA-ABS) in CSF is highly sensitive but may lead to false-positive results. Treatment consists of IV crystalline penicillin G for 10–14 days, and it is recommended to examine CSF every 6 months until pleocytosis normalizes and VDRL becomes negative. HIV testing is advised in stroke patients with syphilis [64].

Leptospira and *Borrelia burgdorferi*, the causative agents of leptospirosis and Lyme disease, are two additional spirochetes that may involve the CNS causing meningitis or meningoencephalitis. CNS vasculitis secondary to leptospirosis and Lyme neuroborreliosis are unusual but can result in either stroke, hemorrhage, or cerebral venous thrombosis [54, 55].

Fungal

Aspergillus fumigatus, *Aspergillus niger*, and *Aspergillus flavus* species are the causative agents of invasive aspergillosis. This opportunistic infection classically affects immunocompromised hosts including stem cell and solid organ transplant recipients, patients with neutropenia, renal and liver failure, HIV infection, diabetes, and alcohol abusers [65]. CNS involvement results from hematogenous dissemination from the lung or from direct spread from paranasal sinuses and orbits. CNS involvement occurs in 10–50% of cases and may present in the form of meningoencephalitis, mycotic aneurysms, intraparenchymal hemorrhage and necrosis, or vasculitis resulting in stroke [51]. Vessel pathology reveals vessel wall necrosis with inflammatory infiltrate, granuloma formation, and positive fungal stain [51]. Clinical presentation and neuroimaging features are variable and depend on the immune status of the host. Common brain MRI findings include Ischemic and hemorrhagic strokes, meningeal enhancement, and ring-enhancing lesions. *Aspergillus* species can be detected in CSF by cultures or DNA PCR, while the galactomannan and beta-D-glucan antigen essays in bronchoalveolar lavage or serum may help support the diagnosis [66]. Treatment consists of oral voriconazole and surgical resection of focal lesions. Mortality rate with CNS aspergillosis is as high as 85–99% [67].

Mucormycosis is an opportunistic infection caused by *Zygomytes* class fungi such as *Rhizopus* and *Mucor*. Mucormycosis is classically associated with poorly controlled diabetes, but can also occur in other immunocompromised conditions [68]. Rhinocerebral disease is the result of direct CNS invasion from paranasal sinus or orbits. Microorganisms invade cerebral blood vessels causing endothelial injury, thrombosis, and vessel rupture. Common structures involved are the cavernous sinus and the supraclinoid internal carotid artery. Initial clinical manifestations include headache, face pain and swelling, and fever, followed by infarction and hemorrhagic necrosis in complicated cases [51]. Early diagnosis and treatment are critical for a favorable outcome. Liposomal amphotericin B is the first-line therapy, whereas posaconazole and isavuconazole are antifungal alternatives [69].

Coccidiomycosis is caused by the soil-based fungus *Coccidioides immitis* and usually presents as a mild respiratory illness. Endemic areas include southwestern United States. Extrapulmonary disease is rare but may occur in immunocompromised individuals [70]. CNS involvement is a potentially devastating complication among disseminated cases. CNS coccidiomycosis manifests as meningitis or meningoencephalitis and, similar to other fungal meningitis, may invade the vessels at the base of the brain causing vasculitis and cerebral infarction [71]. CSF studies reveal either lymphocytic or eosinophilic pleocytosis, elevated protein, and low glucose. Diagnosis requires CSF culture, antibody detection, or complement fixation. However, CSF testing sensitivity is suboptimal [70]. High-dose fluconazole is the first-line treatment, whereas voriconazole is indicated for refractory cases. The use of glucocorticoids has been postulated as beneficial to reduce vascular inflammation in cases of coccidiomycosis-related stroke [70].

Histoplasma capsulatum is endemic in central United States including Ohio and Mississippi, as well as areas of Latin America, Asia, and Africa. Disseminated histoplasmosis may occur in those with impaired cellular immunity. CNS is involved in 10–20% of cases of disseminated disease [72]. Cerebral histoplasmosis can present as a chronic meningitis or ring-enhancing lesions causing mass effect. In addition, cerebrovascular complications can result from vascular granulomatous inflammation or embolism from histoplasma endocarditis [72]. Liposomal amphotericin B is the recommended therapy for disseminated disease followed by itraconazole for 1 year [73].

Cryptococcus neoformans is the most common cause of fungal meningitis. Cryptococcus meningitis commonly affects HIV patients but may occur in immunocompetent individuals as well [74]. Presentation is characterized by subacute headaches, fever, and altered mental status. CSF studies typically show opening pressure > 200 mmH_2O, pleocytosis, elevated protein, and normal glucose, diagnosis is confirmed either by yeast visualization with Indian ink staining or positive cryptococcal antigen titers [51]. The base of the brain is often bathed in a dense inflammatory exudate resulting in cranial nerve palsies, hydrocephalus, and vascular compromise. Stroke is found in nearly one-fourth of cases, with subcortical infarcts in the basal ganglia are the most common findings [75]. Stroke is associated with higher mortality rate and worse neurological outcomes [75]. Antifungal therapy includes a 2-week course of intravenous flucytosine and amphotericin followed by consolidation therapy with fluconazole [76]. Glucocorticoids may improve outcomes in those with cerebrovascular compromise.

Parasites

Human cysticercosis occurs when human beings act as the intermediate host for the larval stage of *Taenia soilum*. Neurocysticercosis (NCC) is the most common CNS helminthic infection and a leading cause of acquired epilepsy in endemic areas [77]. Cysticerci invade the brain parenchyma and undergo involution including the vesicular, colloidal, granular, and finally the calcified stage. Alternatively, cysticerci may occupy the subarachnoid space and undergo hydropic degeneration (racemose form) [77]. Clinical presentation is heterogeneous and depends on the number, location, and stage of cysticerci, as well as the host's immune response. Cerebrovascular complications occur in 3–12% of NCC cases, being more common in those with the racemose form, in which nearly 50% have angiographic evidence of vasculitis [78]. NCC diagnosis is established by widely accepted criteria that include absolute (i.e., histological confirmation of parasites), neuroimaging, and clinical/exposure findings [79]. In cases of cerebrovascular compromise, antiparasitic treatment with albendazole and praziquantel is recommended for longer periods, and adjunctive glucocorticoids is necessary to avoid worsening vessel inflammation in response to the accelerated death of parasites [77].

Other Specific Causes of CNS Vasculitis

Lymphomatoid granulomatosis is a hematological disorder characterized by vessel wall inflammatory infiltrate of neoplastic cells of T-lymphocytes derivation. Patients may present with a vasculitis clinical picture affecting the lungs and skin, and less commonly the CNS (20–30%) [80]. Malignant angioendotheliomatosis is another distinct intravascular neoplastic disorder from B-cell-derived lymphomatous cells that may present with CNS vasculitis [81]. CNS vasculitis secondary to idiopathic hypereosinophilic syndrome has also been reported [82]. Finally, various cancers (i.e., Hodgkin's disease) may trigger CNS vasculitis as a paraneoplastic phenomenon indistinguishable from PACNS [83]. Paraneoplastic CNS vasculitis should be differentiated from radiation-induced vascular injury, and a brain biopsy is usually required to confirm the diagnosis.

CNS vasculitis has also been associated with drug abuse. Amphetamine, methamphetamine, and their derivatives have a potent effect on the elevation of blood pressure, heart rate, increased level of alertness, insomnia, excitability, and aggressive behavior. Amphetamines increase the risk of hemorrhagic stroke four-fold, but its association with ischemic stroke is less clear [84]. CNS necrotizing vasculitis in the setting of IV methamphetamine abuse has been reported [85]. Cocaine is another highly addictive, highly potent CNS stimulant. Cocaine abuse doubles the risk of ischemic and hemorrhagic stroke [84]. Histologically-verified CNS vasculitis secondary to cocaine has been reported [86]. Most patients presented with acute-onset headaches and altered mental status immediately after intranasal cocaine consumption. CSF studies typically showed lymphocytic pleocytosis and angiographic studies revealed large-vessel irregularities with segmental narrowing. Pathology is consistent with either non-necrotizing vasculitis associated with transmural mononuclear infiltrate or necrosis of small cerebral vessels associated with polymorphonuclear cell inflammation [86]. CSN vasculitis in the setting of cocaine abuse should be differentiated from other mechanisms of cocaine-related stroke such as vasospasm, hypertensive emergency, and cardioembolism. Management is based on removing the offending agent and glucocorticoids are recommended when a vasculitic process is confirmed.

Primary Angiitis of the Central Nervous System

PACNS is a rare inflammatory disease characterized by isolated compromise of small- and medium-sized vessels of the brain, leptomeninges, and/or spine cord [2]. PACNS is a diagnosis of exclusion. Therefore, other systemic inflammatory disorders must be excluded. Based on a large cohort study from the Mayo Clinic, PACNS annual incidence was estimated to be 2.4 cases per 100.000 persons based on a North American White population [43]. PACNS incidence peaks in the fourth decade of life and the prevelance is similar between men and women [43]. Pathogenic mechanisms in PACNS are not well established. The presence of memory T-cells within the inflammatory infiltrate suggests an antigen-specific immune response occurring at the vessel wall [87]. Although no antigen triggers have been fully identified, it has been suggested that B-amyloid and infectious agents such as VZV or mycoplasma organisms may play a role in PACNS pathogenesis [2]. Histopathology in PACNS is characterized by vasculocentric transmural inflammation, with or without fibrinoid mural necrosis [88]. The three inflammatory patterns recognized are granulomatous, lymphocytic, and necrotizing, with granulomatous vasculitis being the most common [88].

PACNS lacks pathognomonic signs or symptoms, and diagnostic tests have modest sensitivity and specificity. Therefore, PACNS can be under- and over-diagnosed. The clinical course is usually insidious and gradually progressive, but may also present with an abrupt onset and rapid neurological deterioration [43]. Headache is the most common symptom followed by cognitive decline and focal neurological deficits related to cerebral infarction, whereas seizures, acute encephalopathy, and intracerebral hemorrhage are less frequent [43]. Constitutional symptoms such as fever, weight loss, and night sweats are uncommon and should suggest other systemic inflammatory conditions. CSF is abnormal in 80–90% of cases and typically shows mild lymphocytic pleocytosis and elevated proteins [43]. Abnormal brain MRI is found in the majority of patients. However, the pattern of brain MRI lesions is highly variable including ischemic lesions, signs of microangiopathy, intracerebral hemorrhage, parenchymal and leptomeningeal contrast enhancement, and tumor-like lesions [43, 89].

Cerebral digital subtraction angiogram (DSA) is superior than non-invasive techniques to detect features compatible with vasculitis and is considered the radiological gold standard to identify PACNS [2]. Multifocal areas of narrowing and dilation ("arterial beading") of intracranial vessels are classic findings in PACNS [43]. Other angiographic features include fusiform arterial dilations, development of collateral circulation, and delayed contrast enhancement. Arterial beading is non-specific for PACNS and can be seen in other conditions such as vasospasm, atherosclerosis, CNS infections, post-radiation, and in neurofibromatosis [90]. Moreover, DSA has limited sensitivity (40–90%) to detect vasculitis-related changes in isolated small-vessel PACNS [43]. High-resolution vessel wall imaging is an emerging technique that may help differentiate PACNS from atherosclerosis and other non-inflammatory vasculopathies [91]. For suspected PACNS cases with non-diagnostic vessel imaging, histopathological confirmation is required. Brain biopsy has low sensitivity (53–63%) due to sampling errors related to the focal and segmental distribution of PACNS pathology [90, 92]. Therefore, sampling of a specific radiologic target is advised.

Proposed diagnostic criteria include (1) unexplained neurological deficits, (2) classic angiographic or histopathological findings consistent with PACNS, and (3) no evidence of other disorders that could cause or mimic angiographic or pathological findings [93]. More recently, a level of certainty has been proposed as "definite" or "probable" diagnosis based on the presence or absence of histological verification [94, 95]. A diagnostic approach for PACNS is proposed in Fig. 23.1.

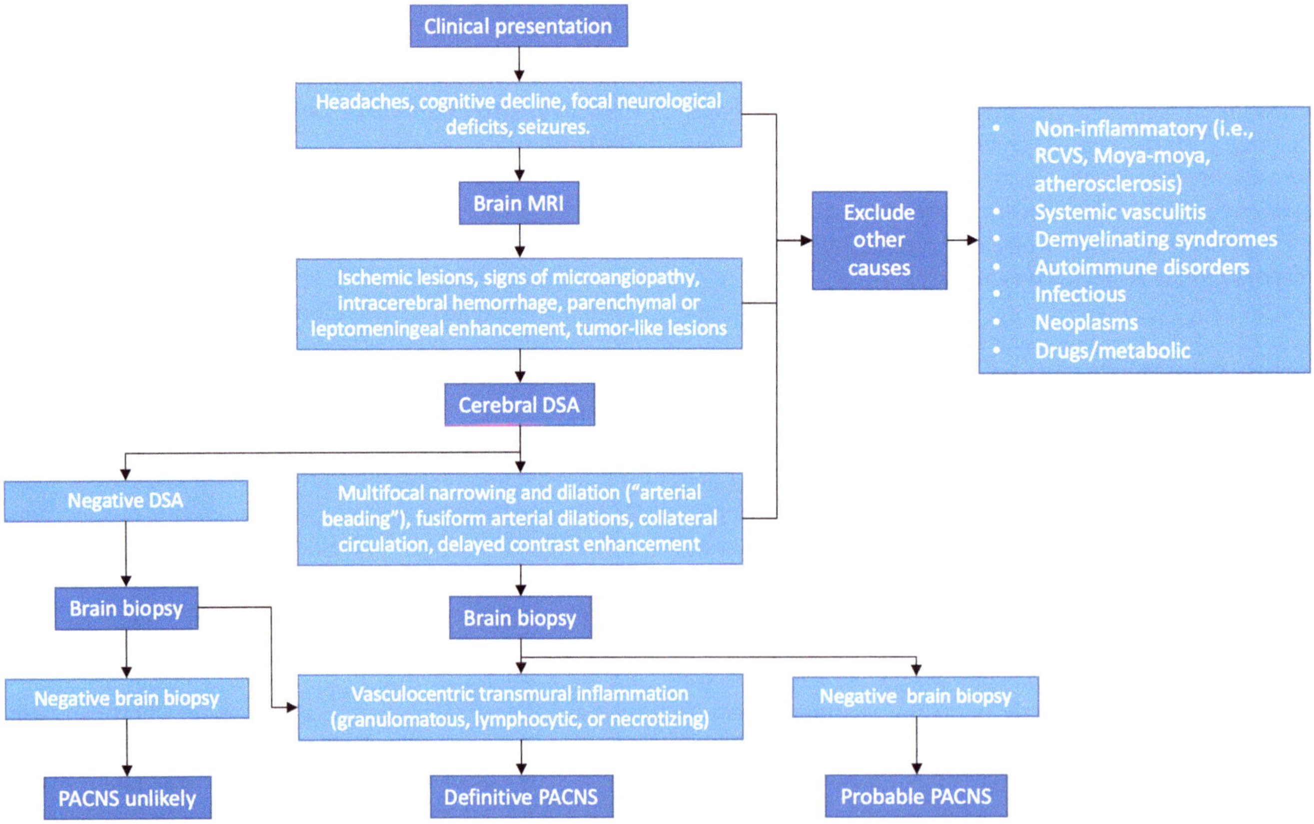

Fig. 23.1 Diagnostic approach to Primary Angiitis of the Central Nervous System. *DSA* digital subtraction angiogram, PACNS primary angiitis of the central nervous system, *RCVS* reversible cerebral vasoconstriction syndrome

Table 23.2 Therapeutic considerations and adverse effects profile for immunosuppressants commonly used to treat central nervous system vasculitis

Agent	Dose	Adverse effects/considerations
Glucocorticoids	Oral: Prednisone 1 mg/kg daily; Intravenous: Methylprednisolone 1 g daily for 3–5 days	Hyperglycemia, psychosis, osteopenia, immunosuppression, adrenal crisis.
Cyclophosphamide	Oral: 2 mg/kg/day for 3–6 months; Intravenous: 0.75 g/m^2 monthly for 6 months	Surveillance and treatment of the adverse effects of cyclophosphamide, such as infections, hemorrhagic cystitis, myelosuppression, and malignant neoplasms.
Azathioprine	Oral: 1–2 mg/kg daily	Skin rash, acute pancreatitis, leukopenia, anemia, thrombocytopenia.
Methotrexate	Oral, subcutaneously, intramuscular: 15–25 mg weekly	Oral ulcers, headache, hair loss, nausea, pneumonitis, leukopenia, transaminitis, hyperbilirubinemia.
Mycophenolate mofetil	Oral: 750 mg-1.5 g twice a day	Oral ulcers, diarrhea, nausea, emesis, gastrointestinal bleed, leukopenia.
Biological agents		
Rituximab	Intravenous: 375 mg/m^2 weekly for 4 doses or 1 g every 2 weeks for 2 doses.	Fevers, tachycardia, chills, hypotension, leukopenia, neutropenia, agammaglobulinemia.
Tumor necrosis alpha blockers		
Infliximab	Intravenous: 5 mg/kg at 0, 2, and 6 weeks.	Urticaria, hypotension, heart failure, immunosuppression, hepatotoxicity, leukopenia, thrombocytopenia, anemia, pancytopenia, demyelination.
Etanercept	Subcutaneous: 50 mg weekly or 25 mg twice weekly	Runny nose, nasal congestion, skin papilloma, immunosuppression, infusion reaction, upper respiratory infections, demyelination.

No evidence-based guidelines exist for PACNS treatment. Anecdotal reports suggest the use of glucocorticoids in combination with cyclophosphamide [43, 94, 95]. Initial prednisone dose is 1 mg/kg per day, which could be preceded by a 3–5-day course of high-dose IV methylprednisolone in patients with severe symptoms [2]. Cyclophosphamide can be administered either IV (0.75 g/m^2 per month for 6 months) or oral (2 mg/kg per day for 3–6 months), without a clear advantage of one route versus the other. Common adverse effects related to cyclophosphamide include infertility and malignancy (i.e., bladder cancer). The use of other immunosuppressants such as azathioprine, methotrexate, or mycophenolate is advised to maintain remission [2]. Route of administration and the adverse effects profile of immunosuppressants commonly used in PACNS and other CNS vasculitis are summarized in Table 23.2. Response rate to treatment is near 80%. Relapses and recurrences occurred in 27% of cases in the Mayo cohort [43].

References

1. Ferro JM. Vasculitis of the central nervous system. J Neurol. 1998;245(12):766–76. https://doi.org/10.1007/s004150050285.
2. Salvarani C, Brown RD Jr, Hunder GG. Adult primary central nervous system vasculitis. Lancet. 2012;380(9843):767–77. https://doi.org/10.1016/S0140-6736(12)60069-5.
3. Adams HP Jr. Cerebral vasculitis. Handb Clin Neurol. 2014;119:475–94. https://doi.org/10.1016/B978-0-7020-4086-3.00031-X.
4. Jennette JC, Falk RJ, Bacon PA, Basu N, Cid MC, Ferrario F, Flores-Suarez LF, Gross WL, Guillevin L, Hagen EC, Hoffman GS, et al. 2012 revised international Chapel Hill consensus conference nomenclature of Vasculitides. Arthritis Rheum. 2013;65(1):1–11. https://doi.org/10.1002/art.37715.
5. Sharma A, Mohammad AJ, Turesson C. Incidence and prevalence of giant cell arteritis and polymyalgia rheumatica: a systematic literature review. Semin Arthritis Rheum. 2020;50(5):1040–8. https://doi.org/10.1016/j.semarthrit.2020.07.005.
6. Carmona FD, Mackie SL, Martín JE, Taylor JC, Vaglio A, Eyre S, Bossini-Castillo L, Castañeda S, Cid MC, Hernández-Rodríguez J, Prieto-González S, et al. A large-scale genetic analysis reveals a strong contribution of the HLA class II region to giant cell arteritis susceptibility. Am J Hum Genet. 2015;96(4):565–80. https://doi.org/10.1016/j.ajhg.2015.02.009.
7. Ninan J, Lester S, Hill C. Giant cell arteritis. Best Pract Res Clin Rheumatol. 2016;30(1):169–88. https://doi.org/10.1016/j.berh.2016.05.001.
8. Ponte C, Rodrigues AF, O'Neill L, Luqmani RA. Giant cell arteritis: current treatment and management. World J Clin Cases. 2015;3(6):484–94. https://doi.org/10.12998/wjcc.v3.i6.484.
9. Unizony S, Arias-Urdaneta L, Miloslavsky E, Arvikar S, Khosroshahi A, Keroack B, Stone JR, Stone JH. Tocilizumab for the treatment of large-vessel vasculitis (giant cell arteritis, Takayasu arteritis) and polymyalgia rheumatica. Arthritis Care Res (Hoboken). 2012;64(11):1720–9. https://doi.org/10.1002/acr.21750.
10. Russo RAG, Katsicas MM. Takayasu Arteritis. Front Pediatr. 2018;6:265. https://doi.org/10.3389/fped.2018.00265.
11. Maz M, Chung SA, Abril A, Langford CA, Gorelik M, Guyatt G, Archer AM, Conn DL, Full KA, Grayson PC, Ibarra MF, et al. 2021 American College of Rheumatology/Vasculitis Foundation guideline for the Management of Giant Cell Arteritis and Takayasu Arteritis. Arthritis Rheumatol. 2021;73(8):1349–65. https://doi.org/10.1002/art.41774.
12. Mahr A, Guillevin L, Poissonnet M, Aymé S. Prevalences of polyarteritis nodosa, microscopic polyangiitis, Wegener's granulomatosis, and Churg-Strauss syndrome in a French urban multiethnic population in 2000: a capture-recapture estimate. Arthritis Rheum. 2004;51(1):92–9. https://doi.org/10.1002/art.20077.
13. Caorsi R, Penco F, Grossi A, Insalaco A, Omenetti A, Alessio M, Conti G, Marchetti F, Picco P, Tommasini A, Martino S, Malattia

C, Gallizzi R, Podda RA, Salis A, Falcini F, Schena F, Garbarino F, Morreale A, Pardeo M, Ventrici C, Passarelli C, Zhou Q, Severino M, Gandolfo C, Damonte G, Martini A, Ravelli A, Aksentijevich I, Ceccherini I, Gattorno M. ADA2 deficiency (DADA2) as an unrecognised cause of early onset polyarteritis nodosa and stroke: a multicentre national study. Ann Rheum Dis. 2017;76(10):1648–56. https://doi.org/10.1136/annrheumdis-2016-210802; Erratum in: Ann Rheum Dis. 2019;78(7):e73.
14. Pagnoux C, Seror R, Henegar C, Mahr A, Cohen P, Le Guern V, Bienvenu B, Mouthon L, Guillevin L, French Vasculitis Study Group. Clinical features and outcomes in 348 patients with polyarteritis nodosa: a systematic retrospective study of patients diagnosed between 1963 and 2005 and entered into the French Vasculitis study group database. Arthritis Rheum. 2010;62(2):616–26. https://doi.org/10.1002/art.27240.
15. Lightfoot RW Jr, Michel BA, Bloch DA, Hunder GG, Zvaifler NJ, McShane DJ, Arend WP, Calabrese LH, Leavitt RY, Lie JT, et al. The American College of Rheumatology 1990 criteria for the classification of polyarteritis nodosa. Arthritis Rheum. 1990;33(8):1088–93. https://doi.org/10.1002/art.1780330805.
16. Chung SA, Gorelik M, Langford CA, Maz M, Abril A, Guyatt G, Archer AM, Conn DL, Full KA, Grayson PC, Ibarra MF, et al. 2021 American College of Rheumatology/Vasculitis Foundation guideline for the Management of Polyarteritis Nodosa. Arthritis Rheumatol. 2021;73(8):1384–93. https://doi.org/10.1002/art.41776.
17. Comarmond C, Cacoub P. Granulomatosis with polyangiitis (Wegener): clinical aspects and treatment. Autoimmun Rev. 2014;13(11):1121–5. https://doi.org/10.1016/j.autrev.2014.08.017.
18. Kühn D, Hospowsky C, Both M, Hey M, Laudien M. Manifestation of granulomatosis with polyangiitis in head and neck. Clin Exp Rheumatol. 2018;36 Suppl 111(2):78–84.
19. Noth I, Strek ME, Leff AR. Churg-Strauss syndrome. Lancet. 2003;361(9357):587–94. https://doi.org/10.1016/S0140-6736(03)12518-4.
20. Wolf J, Bergner R, Mutallib S, Buggle F, Grau AJ. Neurologic complications of Churg-Strauss syndrome--a prospective monocentric study. Eur J Neurol. 2010;17(4):582–8. https://doi.org/10.1111/j.1468-1331.2009.02902.x.
21. Masi AT, Hunder GG, Lie JT, Michel BA, Bloch DA, Arend WP, Calabrese LH, Edworthy SM, Fauci AS, Leavitt RY, et al. The American College of Rheumatology 1990 criteria for the classification of Churg-Strauss syndrome (allergic granulomatosis and angiitis). Arthritis Rheum. 1990;33(8):1094–100. https://doi.org/10.1002/art.1780330806.
22. Wechsler ME, Akuthota P, Jayne D, Khoury P, Klion A, Langford CA, Merkel PA, Moosig F, Specks U, Cid MC, Luqmani R, Brown J, Mallett S, Philipson R, Yancey SW, Steinfeld J, Weller PF, Gleich GJ, EGPA Mepolizumab Study Team. Mepolizumab or placebo for eosinophilic granulomatosis with Polyangiitis. N Engl J Med. 2017;376(20):1921–32. https://doi.org/10.1056/NEJMoa1702079.
23. Cacoub P, Comarmond C, Domont F, Savey L, Saadoun D. Cryoglobulinemia Vasculitis. Am J Med. 2015;128(9):950–5. https://doi.org/10.1016/j.amjmed.2015.02.017.
24. Zaidan M, Mariotte E, Galicier L, Arnulf B, Meignin V, Vérine J, Mahr A, Azoulay E. Vasculitic emergencies in the intensive care unit: a special focus on cryoglobulinemic vasculitis. Ann Intensive Care. 2012;2(1):31. https://doi.org/10.1186/2110-5820-2-31.
25. Saip S, Akman-Demir G, Siva A. Neuro-Behçet syndrome. Handb Clin Neurol. 2014;121:1703–23. https://doi.org/10.1016/B978-0-7020-4088-7.00110-3.
26. Al-Araji A, Kidd DP. Neuro-Behçet's disease: epidemiology, clinical characteristics, and management. Lancet Neurol. 2009;8(2):192–204. https://doi.org/10.1016/S1474-4422(09)70015-8.
27. Borhani-Haghighi A, Kardeh B, Banerjee S, Yadollahikhales G, Safari A, Sahraian MA, Shapiro L. Neuro-Behcet's disease: an update on diagnosis, differential diagnoses, and treatment. Mult Scler Relat Disord. 2019;39:101906. https://doi.org/10.1016/j.msard.2019.101906.
28. Barile-Fabris L, Hernández-Cabrera MF, Barragan-Garfias JA. Vasculitis in systemic lupus erythematosus. Curr Rheumatol Rep. 2014;16(9):440. https://doi.org/10.1007/s11926-014-0440-9.
29. Brey RL, Holliday SL, Saklad AR, Navarrete MG, Hermosillo-Romo D, Stallworth CL, Valdez CR, Escalante A, del Rincón I, Gronseth G, Rhine CB, Padilla P, McGlasson D. Neuropsychiatric syndromes in lupus: prevalence using standardized definitions. Neurology. 2002;58(8):1214–20. https://doi.org/10.1212/wnl.58.8.1214.
30. Barile-Fabris L, Ariza-Andraca R, Olguín-Ortega L, Jara LJ, Fraga-Mouret A, Miranda-Limón JM, Fuentes de la Mata J, Clark P, Vargas F, Alocer-Varela J. Controlled clinical trial of IV cyclophosphamide versus IV methylprednisolone in severe neurological manifestations in systemic lupus erythematosus. Ann Rheum Dis. 2005;64(4):620–5. https://doi.org/10.1136/ard.2004.025528.
31. Makol A, Matteson EL, Warrington KJ. Rheumatoid vasculitis: an update. Curr Opin Rheumatol. 2015;27(1):63–70. https://doi.org/10.1097/BOR.0000000000000126.
32. Voskuyl AE, Zwinderman AH, Westedt ML, Vandenbroucke JP, Breedveld FC, Hazes JM. Factors associated with the development of vasculitis in rheumatoid arthritis: results of a case-control study. Ann Rheum Dis. 1996;55(3):190–2. https://doi.org/10.1136/ard.55.3.190.
33. Myasoedova E, Crowson CS, Turesson C, Gabriel SE, Matteson EL. Incidence of extraarticular rheumatoid arthritis in Olmsted County, Minnesota, in 1995-2007 versus 1985-1994: a population-based study. J Rheumatol. 2011;38(6):983–9. https://doi.org/10.3899/jrheum.101133.
34. Bartels C, Bell C, Rosenthal A, Shinki K, Bridges A. Decline in rheumatoid vasculitis prevalence among US veterans: a retrospective cross-sectional study. Arthritis Rheum. 2009;60(9):2553–7. https://doi.org/10.1002/art.24775.
35. de Cerqueira DPA, Pedreira ALS, de Cerqueira MG, Santiago MB. Biological therapy in rheumatoid vasculitis: a systematic review. Clin Rheumatol. 2021;40(5):1717–24. https://doi.org/10.1007/s10067-020-05459-9.
36. Makol A, Crowson CS, Wetter DA, et al. Vasculitis associated with rheumatoid arthritis: a case–control study. Rheumatology (Oxford). 2014;53:890–9.
37. Benjamin LA, Bryer A, Emsley HC, Khoo S, Solomon T, Connor MD. HIV infection and stroke: current perspectives and future directions. Lancet Neurol. 2012;11(10):878–90. https://doi.org/10.1016/S1474-4422(12)70205-3.
38. Vega LE, Espinoza LR. Vasculitides in HIV infection. Curr Rheumatol Rep. 2020;22(10):60. https://doi.org/10.1007/s11926-020-00945-0.
39. Zhang X, Li H, Li T, Zhang F, Han Y. Distinctive rheumatic manifestations in 98 patients with human immunodeficiency virus infection in China. J Rheumatol. 2007;34(8):1760–4.
40. Chetty R. Vasculitides associated with HIV infection. J Clin Pathol. 2001;54(4):275–8. https://doi.org/10.1136/jcp.54.4.275.
41. Font C, Miró O, Pedrol E, Masanés F, Coll-Vinent B, Casademont J, Cid MC, Grau JM. Polyarteritis nodosa in human immunodeficiency virus infection: report of four cases and review of the literature. Br J Rheumatol. 1996;35(8):796–9. https://doi.org/10.1093/rheumatology/35.8.796.
42. Scotto G, Cibelli DC, Saracino A, Prato R, Palumbo E, Fazio V, Scarabaggio T, Monno L, Angarano G. Cryoglobulinemia in subjects with HCV infection alone, HIV infection and HCV/HIV coinfection. J Infect. 2006;52(4):294–9. https://doi.org/10.1016/j.jinf.2005.05.025.

43. Salvarani C, Brown RD Jr, Christianson T, Miller DV, Giannini C, Huston J 3rd, Hunder GG. An update of the Mayo Clinic cohort of patients with adult primary central nervous system vasculitis: description of 163 patients. Medicine (Baltimore). 2015;94(21):e738. https://doi.org/10.1097/MD.0000000000000738.
44. Cheron J, Wyndham-Thomas C, Sadeghi N, Naeije G. Response of human immunodeficiency virus-associated cerebral Angiitis to the combined antiretroviral therapy. Front Neurol. 2017;8:95. https://doi.org/10.3389/fneur.2017.00095.
45. Melica G, Brugieres P, Lascaux AS, Levy Y, Lelièvre JD. Primary vasculitis of the central nervous system in patients infected with HIV-1 in the HAART era. J Med Virol. 2009;81(4):578–81. https://doi.org/10.1002/jmv.21462.
46. Fink DL, Hedley L, Miller RF. Systematic review of the efficacy and safety of biological therapy for inflammatory conditions in HIV-infected individuals. Int J STD AIDS. 2017;28(2):110–9. https://doi.org/10.1177/0956462416675109.
47. Bakradze E, Kirchoff KF, Antoniello D, Springer MV, Mabie PC, Esenwa CC, Labovitz DL, Liberman AL. Varicella Zoster Virus Vasculitis and Adult Cerebrovascular Disease. Neurohospitalist. 2019;9(4):203–8. https://doi.org/10.1177/1941874419845732.
48. Katchanov J, Siebert E, Klingebiel R, Endres M. Infectious vasculopathy of intracranial large- and medium-sized vessels in neurological intensive care unit: a clinico-radiological study. Neurocrit Care. 2010;12(3):369–74. https://doi.org/10.1007/s12028-010-9335-4.
49. Nagel MA, Cohrs RJ, Mahalingam R, Wellish MC, Forghani B, Schiller A, Safdieh JE, Kamenkovich E, Ostrow LW, Levy M, Greenberg B, Russman AN, Katzan I, Gardner CJ, Häusler M, Nau R, Saraya T, Wada H, Goto H, de Martino M, Ueno M, Brown WD, Terborg C, Gilden DH. The varicella zoster virus vasculopathies: clinical, CSF, imaging, and virologic features. Neurology. 2008;70(11):853–60. https://doi.org/10.1212/01.wnl.0000304747.38502.e8.
50. Nagel MA, Gilden D. Neurological complications of varicella zoster virus reactivation. Curr Opin Neurol. 2014;27(3):356–60. https://doi.org/10.1097/WCO.0000000000000092.
51. Chow FC, Marra CM, Cho TA. Cerebrovascular disease in central nervous system infections. Semin Neurol. 2011;31(3):286–306. https://doi.org/10.1055/s-0031-1287658.
52. Kastenbauer S, Pfister HW. Pneumococcal meningitis in adults: spectrum of complications and prognostic factors in a series of 87 cases. Brain. 2003;126(Pt 5):1015–25. https://doi.org/10.1093/brain/awg113.
53. Schut ES, Brouwer MC, de Gans J, Florquin S, Troost D, van de Beek D. Delayed cerebral thrombosis after initial good recovery from pneumococcal meningitis. Neurology. 2009;73(23):1988–95. https://doi.org/10.1212/WNL.0b013e3181c55d2e.
54. Younger DS, Coyle PK. Central nervous system Vasculitis due to infection. Neurol Clin. 2019;37(2):441–63. https://doi.org/10.1016/j.ncl.2019.01.002.
55. van de Beek D, Farrar JJ, de Gans J, Mai NT, Molyneux EM, Peltola H, Peto TE, Roine I, Scarborough M, Schultsz C, Thwaites GE, Tuan PQ, Zwinderman AH. Adjunctive dexamethasone in bacterial meningitis: a meta-analysis of individual patient data. Lancet Neurol. 2010;9(3):254–63. https://doi.org/10.1016/S1474-4422(10)70023-5.
56. Brouwer MC, McIntyre P, Prasad K, van de Beek D. Corticosteroids for acute bacterial meningitis. Cochrane Database Syst Rev. 2013;6:CD004405. https://doi.org/10.1002/14651858.CD004405.pub4. Update in: Cochrane Database Syst Rev. 2015;(9):CD004405.
57. Leonard JM. Central Nervous System Tuberculosis. Microbiol Spectr. 2017;5:2. https://doi.org/10.1128/microbiolspec.TNMI7-0044-2017.
58. Dastur DK, Manghani DK, Udani PM. Pathology and pathogenetic mechanisms in neurotuberculosis. Radiol Clin North Am. 1995;33(4):733–52.
59. Lammie GA, Hewlett RH, Schoeman JF, Donald PR. Tuberculous cerebrovascular disease: a review. J Infect. 2009;59(3):156–66. https://doi.org/10.1016/j.jinf.2009.07.012.
60. Thwaites GE, Nguyen DB, Nguyen HD, Hoang TQ, Do TT, Nguyen TC, Nguyen QH, Nguyen TT, Nguyen NH, Nguyen TN, Nguyen NL, Nguyen HD, Vu NT, Cao HH, Tran TH, Pham PM, Nguyen TD, Stepniewska K, White NJ, Tran TH, Farrar JJ. Dexamethasone for the treatment of tuberculous meningitis in adolescents and adults. N Engl J Med. 2004;351(17):1741–51. https://doi.org/10.1056/NEJMoa040573.
61. Prasad K, Singh MB. Corticosteroids for managing tuberculous meningitis. Cochrane Database Syst Rev. 2008;1:CD002244. https://doi.org/10.1002/14651858.CD002244.pub3. Update in: Cochrane Database Syst Rev. 2016;4:CD002244.
62. Cordato DJ, Djekic S, Taneja SR, Maley M, Beran RG, Cappelen-Smith C, Griffith NC, Hanna IY, Hodgkinson SJ, Worthington JM, McDougall AJ. Prevalence of positive syphilis serology and meningovascular neurosyphilis in patients admitted with stroke and TIA from a culturally diverse population (2005-09). J Clin Neurosci. 2013;20(7):943–7. https://doi.org/10.1016/j.jocn.2012.08.011.
63. Holmes MD, Brant-Zawadzki MM, Simon RP. Clinical features of meningovascular syphilis. Neurology. 1984;34(4):553–6. https://doi.org/10.1212/wnl.34.4.553.
64. Workowski KA, Berman S, Centers for Disease Control and Prevention (CDC). Sexually transmitted diseases treatment guidelines, 2010. MMWR Recomm rep. 2010;59(RR-12):1–110; Erratum in: MMWR Recomm rep. 2011;60(1):18. Dosage error in article text.
65. Denning DW. Invasive aspergillosis. Clin Infect Dis. 1998;26(4):781–803.; quiz 804-5. https://doi.org/10.1086/513943.
66. Wheat LJ. Rapid diagnosis of invasive aspergillosis by antigen detection. Transpl Infect Dis. 2003;5(4):158–66. https://doi.org/10.1111/j.1399-3062.2003.00031.x.
67. Denning DW. Therapeutic outcome in invasive aspergillosis. Clin Infect Dis. 1996;23(3):608–15. https://doi.org/10.1093/clinids/23.3.608.
68. Hong HL, Lee YM, Kim T, Lee JY, Chung YS, Kim MN, Kim SH, Choi SH, Kim YS, Woo JH, Lee SO. Risk factors for mortality in patients with invasive mucormycosis. Infect Chemother. 2013;45(3):292–8. https://doi.org/10.3947/ic.2013.45.3.292.
69. Tissot F, Agrawal S, Pagano L, Petrikkos G, Groll AH, Skiada A, Lass-Flörl C, Calandra T, Viscoli C, Herbrecht R. ECIL-6 guidelines for the treatment of invasive candidiasis, aspergillosis and mucormycosis in leukemia and hematopoietic stem cell transplant patients. Haematologica. 2017;102(3):433–44. https://doi.org/10.3324/haematol.2016.152900.
70. Mathisen G, Shelub A, Truong J, Wigen C. Coccidioidal meningitis: clinical presentation and management in the fluconazole era. Medicine (Baltimore). 2010;89(5):251–84. https://doi.org/10.1097/MD.0b013e3181f378a8.
71. Williams PL, Johnson R, Pappagianis D, Einstein H, Slager U, Koster FT, Eron JJ, Morrison J, Aguet J, River ME. Vasculitic and encephalitic complications associated with Coccidioides immitis infection of the central nervous system in humans: report of 10 cases and review. Clin Infect Dis. 1992;14(3):673–82. https://doi.org/10.1093/clinids/14.3.673.
72. Saccente M. Central nervous system histoplasmosis. Curr Treat Options Neurol. 2008;10(3):161–7. https://doi.org/10.1007/s11940-008-0017-x.
73. Azar MM, Loyd JL, Relich RF, Wheat LJ, Hage CA. Current concepts in the epidemiology, diagnosis, and Management

of Histoplasmosis Syndromes. Semin Respir Crit Care Med. 2020;41(1):13–30. https://doi.org/10.1055/s-0039-1698429.
74. Mitchell DH, Sorrell TC, Allworth AM, Heath CH, McGregor AR, Papanaoum K, Richards MJ, Gottlieb T. Cryptococcal disease of the CNS in immunocompetent hosts: influence of cryptococcal variety on clinical manifestations and outcome. Clin Infect Dis. 1995;20(3):611–6. https://doi.org/10.1093/clinids/20.3.611.
75. Vela-Duarte D, Nyberg E, Sillau S, Pate A, Castellanos P, Chastain DB, Franco-Paredes C, Henao-Martínez AF. Lacunar stroke in Cryptococcal meningitis: clinical and radiographic features. J Stroke Cerebrovasc Dis. 2019;28(6):1767–72. https://doi.org/10.1016/j.jstrokecerebrovasdis.2018.12.043.
76. Perfect JR, Dismukes WE, Dromer F, Goldman DL, Graybill JR, Hamill RJ, Harrison TS, Larsen RA, Lortholary O, Nguyen MH, Pappas PG, Powderly WG, Singh N, Sobel JD, Sorrell TC. Clinical practice guidelines for the management of cryptococcal disease: 2010 update by the infectious diseases society of america. Clin Infect Dis. 2010;50(3):291–322. https://doi.org/10.1086/649858.
77. Del Brutto OH. Neurocysticercosis. Continuum (Minneap Minn). 2012;18(6 Infectious Disease):1392–416. https://doi.org/10.1212/01.CON.0000423853.47770.90.
78. Marquez JM, Arauz A. Cerebrovascular complications of neurocysticercosis. Neurologist. 2012;18(1):17–22. https://doi.org/10.1097/NRL.0b013e31823d7a80.
79. Del Brutto OH, Nash TE, White AC Jr, Rajshekhar V, Wilkins PP, Singh G, Vasquez CM, Salgado P, Gilman RH, Garcia HH. Revised diagnostic criteria for neurocysticercosis. J Neurol Sci. 2017;372:202–10. https://doi.org/10.1016/j.jns.2016.11.045.
80. Scolding N. CNS involvement in systemic vasculitides. J Neurol Sci. 2021;424:117423. https://doi.org/10.1016/j.jns.2021.117423.
81. Sienknecht CW, Whetsell WO Jr, Pollock P. Intravascular malignant lymphoma ("malignant angioendotheliomatosis") mimicking primary angiitis of the central nervous system. J Rheumatol. 1995;22(9):1769–70.
82. Rice CM, Kurian KM, Renowden S, Whiteway A, Price C, Scolding NJ. Idiopathic hypereosinophilic syndrome: a new cause of vasculitis of the central nervous system. J Neurol. 2015;262(5):1354–9. https://doi.org/10.1007/s00415-015-7720-9.
83. Lopez-Chiriboga AS, Yoon JW, Siegel JL, Harriott AM, Pirris S, Eidelman BH, Freeman WD. Granulomatous Angiitis of the central nervous system associated with Hodgkin's lymphoma: case report and literature review. J Stroke Cerebrovasc Dis. 2018;27(1):e5–8. https://doi.org/10.1016/j.jstrokecerebrovasdis.2017.08.029.
84. Westover AN, McBride S, Haley RW. Stroke in young adults who abuse amphetamines or cocaine: a population-based study of hospitalized patients. Arch Gen Psychiatry. 2007;64(4):495–502. https://doi.org/10.1001/archpsyc.64.4.495.
85. Citron BP, Halpern M, McCarron M, Lundberg GD, McCormick R, Pincus IJ, Tatter D, Haverback BJ. Necrotizing angiitis associated with drug abuse. N Engl J Med. 1970;283(19):1003–11. https://doi.org/10.1056/NEJM197011052831901.
86. Younger DS. Central nervous system Vasculitis due to substance abuse. Neurol Clin. 2019;37(2):425–40. https://doi.org/10.1016/j.ncl.2019.01.012.
87. Iwase T, Ojika K, Mitake S, Katada E, Katano H, Mase M, Yoshida S, Ueda R. Involvement of CD45RO+ T lymphocyte infiltration in a patient with primary angiitis of the central nervous system restricted to small vessels. Eur Neurol. 2001;45(3):184–5. https://doi.org/10.1159/000052120.
88. Giannini C, Salvarani C, Hunder G, Brown RD. Primary central nervous system vasculitis: pathology and mechanisms. Acta Neuropathol. 2012;123(6):759–72. https://doi.org/10.1007/s00401-012-0973-9.
89. Beuker C, Schmidt A, Strunk D, Sporns PB, Wiendl H, Meuth SG, Minnerup J. Primary angiitis of the central nervous system: diagnosis and treatment. Ther Adv Neurol Disord. 2018;11:1756286418785071. https://doi.org/10.1177/1756286418785071.
90. Duna GF, Calabrese LH. Limitations of invasive modalities in the diagnosis of primary angiitis of the central nervous system. J Rheumatol. 1995;22(4):662–7.
91. Mandell DM, Matouk CC, Farb RI, Krings T, Agid R, terBrugge K, Willinsky RA, Swartz RH, Silver FL, Mikulis DJ. Vessel wall MRI to differentiate between reversible cerebral vasoconstriction syndrome and central nervous system vasculitis: preliminary results. Stroke. 2012;43(3):860–2. https://doi.org/10.1161/STROKEAHA.111.626184.
92. Miller DV, Salvarani C, Hunder GG, Brown RD, Parisi JE, Christianson TJ, Giannini C. Biopsy findings in primary angiitis of the central nervous system. Am J Surg Pathol. 2009;33(1):35–43. https://doi.org/10.1097/PAS.0b013e318181e097.
93. Calabrese LH, Mallek JA. Primary angiitis of the central nervous system. Report of 8 new cases, review of the literature, and proposal for diagnostic criteria. Medicine (Baltimore). 1988;67(1):20–39. https://doi.org/10.1097/00005792-198801000-00002.
94. Birnbaum J, Hellmann DB. Primary angiitis of the central nervous system. Arch Neurol. 2009;66(6):704–9. https://doi.org/10.1001/archneurol.2009.76.
95. Cupps TR, Moore PM, Fauci AS. Isolated angiitis of the central nervous system. Prospective diagnostic and therapeutic experience. Am J Med. 1983;74(1):97–105. https://doi.org/10.1016/0002-9343(83)91125-7.

Acute Ischemic Stroke[1]

24

Raquel Romero, Catherine Albin, and Dangayach Neha

Contents

Abstract

By 2030, 3.9% of the US adult population will have had a stroke. Ischemic strokes represent 87% of all strokes, and stroke is the fifth cause of death when considered separately from other cardiovascular diseases. Stroke remains one of the leading causes of serious long-term disability in the United States. Herein, we discuss the causes, acute treatment, hemodynamic goals and complications of acute ischemic stroke.

Introduction

According to the 2021 update report from the American Heart Association, the median stroke prevalence in adults is 3.4% in the United States. Projections show that by 2030, 3.9% of the US adult population will have had a stroke. Ischemic strokes represent 87% of all strokes. Stroke is the fifth cause of death among all causes when considered separately from other cardiovascular diseases. Stroke remains one of the leading causes of serious long-term disability in the United States [1].

Among patients with ischemic stroke that required ICU admission, the 30-day mortality rate is 31%; those who survived the first 30 days had a favorable outcome [2].

A dedicated neurocritical care unit under direct care of a neurointensivist has a positive impact on outcome in stroke patients with decreased length of intensive care and hospital stay, and more discharges home [3, 4].

Indications for ICU admission might include, a depressed level of alertness, bulbar weakness that could compromise airway patency, patients with large hemispheric infarcts at risk for developing cerebral edema and hemorrhagic transformation, patients with large cerebellar infarcts at risk for brainstem compression and acute hydrocephalus, infarcts with hemorrhagic transformation, patients with ongoing seizure activity, and post endovascular care [5].

R. Romero · D. Neha (✉)
Icahn School of Medicine at Mount Sinai, Neurocritical Care, New York, NY, USA
e-mail: raquel.romero@mountsinai.org; Neha.Dangayach@mountsinai.org

C. Albin
Neurocritical Care, Emory University, Atlanta, GA, USA
e-mail: catherine.sw.albin@emory.edu

E. Mahanna Gabrielli et al. (eds.), *Textbook of Neurointensive Care: Volume 1*, https://doi.org/10.1007/978-3-031-62220-5_24

Hyperacute Management of Ischemic Stroke

Sudden onset of a focal neurological sign/symptom should immediately raise suspicion of an acute ischemic stroke. The goal is rapid diagnosis and assessment of candidacy for intravenous thrombolytic treatment and/or endovascular therapy. Assessment of airway, breathing, circulation, obtaining a rapid medical history, and neurological assessment is critical. The use of a standardized scale for the assessment of neurological deficit severity is recommended. Use of the NIHSS score system is preferred as it is rapid and facilitates communication among providers.

Emergent CTA or MRA of the head and neck to evaluate the intracranial circulation and extracranial carotid and vertebral arteries is recommended to assess for large vessel occlusion and eligibility for endovascular treatment. AHA guidelines emphasize the importance of early neuroimaging within the first 20 min of arrival. While a plain non-contrasted head CT can be used for decision-making about thrombolysis, a CT angiogram provides important information about stroke mechanism. Many institutions have shifted to CTA for all acute strokes [6].

The AHA/ASA recommends the use of intravenous alteplase within a 3–4.5 h window. MRI with positive diffusion restriction and negative FLAIR sequences can help decide candidacy for IV fibrinolysis in patients presenting beyond the 4.5 h window or for those whose time of symptom onset is unknown (COR IIa/LOE B-R). The only laboratory test recommended to be performed prior to administration of IV fibrinolysis is blood glucose. Coagulation panel and platelet count should be obtained if there is suspicion of coagulopathy. Intravenous alteplase, which is the only FDA-approved thrombolytic, is administered at 0.9 mg/kg, with a maximum dose of 90 mg over 60 min. 10% of the total dose should be administered initially as a bolus over 1 min [7].

Although alteplase has long been the standard thrombolytic, Tenecteplase, a genetically modified recombinant tissue-type plasminogen activator, has advantages as a thrombolytic agent and is already being used for acute myocardial infarction patients. This drug can be administered as a single bolus and has greater fibrin specificity [8]. The EXTEND-IA TNK trial (Tenecteplase Versus Alteplase Before Endovascular Therapy for Ischemic Stroke) compared IV Tenecteplase (0.25 mg/kg bolus, maximum 25 mg) with IV alteplase (0.9 mg/kg over 60 min, maximum 90 mg). The trial randomized 202 patients within 4.5 h of symptom onset. Reperfusion of >50% of the ischemic territory or an absence of retrievable thrombus at the time of the initial cerebral angiography was achieved by 22% of patients treated with Tenecteplase versus 10% of those treated with alteplase ($P = 0.002$ for noninferiority and 0.03 for superiority). Symptomatic intracerebral hemorrhoage (ICH) was similar in both groups (1%). There is no strong evidence for the use of other fibrinolytics or sonothrombolysis [7].

There is Level I evidence (MR CLEAN, SWIFT PRIME, EXTEND-IA, ESCAPE, REVASCAT, THRACE) that mechanical thrombectomy has a favorable effect on outcomes for patients with occlusion of the internal carotid artery or first segment of the middle cerebral artery. For patients who present within 6 h of symptom onset and have a CT angiogram-verified large vessel occlusion, decisions about thrombectomy can be made based on the ASPECT score alone. For patients whose last known well is within 6–24 h, landmark trials have used MRI or CT perfusion in order to determine which patients might benefit from endovascular therapy. In these trials, imaging was used to discriminate between tissue that was already infarcted (core infarct) and tissue that was still viable but ischemic (ischemic penumbra) and to use the relative sizes of the core and penumbra (the "mismatch") to select patients for edovascular therapy. However, the CLEAR trial demonstrated that even patients presenting in the late window could be appropriately triaged to endovascular therapy using only the ASPECT score. The cut off score was an ASPECTS >6. It is worth noting that RESCUE-Japan LIMIT was recently presented. In this trial, for patients presenting with low ASPECTS score [1–3], endovascular therapy doubled the number of stroke patients who achieved an mRS of 3 at 90 days. Although this work will need to be validated, the criteria for endovascular therapy will likely shift to be more inclusive based on this work [7, 9–12].

Intra-arterial fibrinolytic therapy is used as second-line treatment after mechanical thrombectomy is attempted [13].

Hemodynamic Goals

Optimizing cerebral perfusion in the penumbra might limit stroke progression. However, to date, there is no strong evidence guiding blood pressure parameters in patients with acute ischemic stroke.

There is no evidence that hemodilution with fluid administration or volume expansion with albumin is beneficial for acute ischemic stroke [14, 15].

There is a high degree of uncertainty regarding the optimal blood pressure target in hyperacute management of acute ischemic stroke. Current AHA guidelines, based on The ESCAPE and DAWN protocols, suggest SBP ≥150 mmHg for cases in which reperfusion could not be achieved and SBP <140 once reperfusion has been achieved. BP TARGET is an open-label randomized controlled trial that enrolled patients with acute stroke due to large vessel occlusion in the anterior circulation, and who underwent endovascular treatment with successful recanalization (TICI 2b and TICI 3), to a systolic blood pressure (SBP) goal of 100–129 mm Hg (intervention) or an SBP goal of 130–185 mm Hg (control, standard of care) for 24 hours. The primary outcome was radiographic intraparenchymal hemorrhage on routine CT at 24–36 h. There was no significant difference between the two groups (42% in the intensive systolic blood pressure target group vs. 43% in the standard systolic blood pressure target group, aOR 0·96, 95% CI 0·60 to 1·51; $p = 0{\cdot}8$) Functional outcome at 90 days (mRS) did not differ between the groups [16].

Head position after stroke has also been a topic of investigation. Multiple observational studies and randomized trials have shown an increase in cerebral blood flow (CBF) velocities (by transcranial Doppler) in the affected hemisphere with head of bed flat positioning. The HeadPoST (Head Positioning in Acute Stroke Trial) randomized patients with acute stroke to flat head position (0°) vs. elevated head position (≥30°) for 24 h. There was no difference in outcome between groups; however, most patients enrolled had small strokes (median NIHSS score 4) which could mean that these patients did not have a large penumbras, and median times from the onset of symptoms to head positioning was 14 h, which may be too late to improve perfusion in the penumbra [7, 17].

Measurement of dynamic cerebral perfusion in response to blood pressure changes is still under investigation with use of transcranial Doppler and near-infrared spectroscopy [18].

Complications of Acute Ischemic Stroke

Cerebral Edema

Malignant MCA Stroke

Large hemispheric infarctions are associated with high morbidity and mortality of approximately 80%. This poor prognosis is not only related to the ischemic tissue itself, but also to secondary brain injury. Complete MCA territory infarction causing space-occupying brain edema is considered a "malignant" hemispheric infarction [19].

Predictors of complete MCA stroke include: hypodensity of >1/3 of the MCA territory on CT scan, a hyperdense MCA sign, brain edema, initial National Institutes of Health Stroke Scale (NIHSS) score ≥ 17, and stroke in progression during the first 5 days of admission [20].

Predictors of progression to a malignant MCA stroke include, an admission ASPECTS score ≤7, a hyperdense MCA sign, and mass effect with midline shift >4 mm at the level of the pineal gland with neurological deterioration within 48 h of symptom onset [21–24].

Pathophysiology

Cerebral ischemia with irreversible damage develops when cerebral blood flow decreases to <8 mL/100 g/min; this results in a cascade of events including failure of energy-dependent regulators of neuroglial cell homeostasis leading sequentially to cytotoxic edema, disruption of tight junctions and endothelial cell linings of the blood-brain barrier, and vasogenic edema. The amount of cytotoxic edema is directly proportional to the size of the ischemic tissue. Cytotoxic edema is the primary contributor to mass effect on surrounding structures and raised intracranial pressure [5, 25, 26].

Management

Management of a malignant MCA infarction is focused on treating intracranial hypertension and minimizing secondary brain damage. While hyperosmolar therapy (mannitol, hypertonic saline) has theoretical benefits, there is no evidence that it improves outcomes in patients with mlignant strokes and is generally used as a temporizing measure until definitive therapy is administered (e.g. craniectomy). There is no role for prophylactic administration of osmotic agents and some data suggest harm [27, 28].

Theoretically, reducing body temperature decreases the metabolic demand, alleviating the ischemic effects and possibly reducing cerebral edema; however, there is no good quality evidence that therapeutic hypothermia improves outcomes in malignant stroke.

Early decompressive hemicraniectomy (within 48 h of presentation) reduces mortality and improves functional outcomes in patients younger than 60 years of age. Pooled analysis from three randomized control trials addressing the effect of decompressive hemicraniectomy (DHC) on functional outcomes showed a number needed to treat of 4 for the prevention of 1 poor outcome and a number needed to treat of 2 for survival (with an absolute risk reduction in mortality of 50% (95% CI, 34–66) at 12 months). The patients in the DHC group had double the number who ultimately achieved a moderately good outcome, mRS of 2–3 (43% vs. 21%); however, a significant number of patients (31%) were left with a moderately severe disability (mRS of 4). The risk of severe disability was not increased. Since what constitutes an "acceptable" outcome is patient-specific, surgical decisions should be made on a case-by-case basis [29, 30].

Despite undergoing aggressive medical management and early decompressive hemicraniectomy, some patients progress to brain herniation and death. One study found an association between progression to herniation in large MCA infarcts after DHC and the presence of large volumes of infarct tissue not included within the craniectomy bed [31].

Given the morbidity of this condition, early recognition of patients at risk for malignant cerebral edema is essential.

Assessment of cerebral edema and intracranial pressure is typically indirect and relies on surrogate markers. Transcranial Doppler can be of value when assessing risk for increased intracranial pressure related to the development of malignant cerebral edema. Asymmetry in pulsatility index values (PI) with elevated ratios of ipsilateral-to-contralateral PI may correlate with hemispheric lesion volume [32].

Optic Nerve Sheath Diameter (ONSD) of more than 5.25 mm may identify MCA stroke patients at high risk of developing malignant MCA syndrome [33].

There is insufficient data regarding the role of invasive monitoring of intracranial pressure in large acute ischemic stroke, and a treatment threshold for ICP has not been established in this population [34].

Furthermore, monitoring of ICP in patients with ischemic stroke canbe misleading; studies have shown progression to brain herniation despite normal ICP values, and in many of the cases clinical signs of herniation appeared before elevated ICP was observed. Possible hypotheses explaining this include stroke being a focal process and the effects of decreased cerebral blood volume [35–37].

While DHC should be discussed with families of young stroke patients, for elderly patients (aged >60), DESTINY II demonstrated that surgical decompression was unlikely to offer a significant reduction in disability. As such, these patients are less often treated with surgical interventions. In the elderly treated with medical management alone, an NIHSS >20 on presentation and need for mechanical ventilation within 48 of admission have been associated with poor outcomes [38].

Malignant Cerebellar Infarction

Cytotoxic edema from large cerebellar strokes can cause compression of the braintem, effacement of the fourth ventricle with consequent acute hydrocephalus, downward or upward cerebellar herniation. Suboccipital craniectomy decompresses the posterior fossa (cerebellum and brainstem) thereby mitigating the complications of malignant cerebellar infarction. Suboccipital craniectomy is considered standard of care for large cerebellar infarcts. There is a conflicting opinion regarding use of external ventricular drains with or without suboccipital craniectomy; there is fear of the possibility of upwards herniation with placement of external ventricular drain without decompressive surgery. Hence, size of the infarct should be taken into consideration prior to placing an external ventricular drain without decompressive surgery [39].

Hemorrhagic Transformation

Bleeding into the infarcted tissue can be part of the natural history of acute ischemic stroke. However, there is an increased risk of hemorrhagic transformation in patients who received systemic fibrinolytics. Alteplase has a short chemical half-life of approximately 4 min, but its fibrinolytic effects (biological half-life) can last for over 24 h, likely related to a consumptive coagulopathy with hypofibrinogenemia and elevated PT and PTT [40].

A meta-analysis from 9 randomized control trials of rtPA-treated stroke patients ($n = 6756$) showed an increased risk of hemorrhagic transformation when compared to placebo; the rate of symptomatic intracranial hemorrhage was 3.7 to 6.8% depending on the definition of symptomatic hemorrhage used. Hemorrhagic transformation after thrombolysis has been classified based on radiographic and clinical findings based on NINDS and ECASS trials criteria [40, 41].

Risk factors associated with hemorrhagic conversion (with or without neurological deterioration) include older age, hyperglycemia, stroke severity, atrial fibrillation, congestive heart failure, renal impairment, prior antiplatelet use, leukoaraiosis, and ischemic changes visible in neuroimaging prior to alteplase treatment [42].

There are limited data regarding the management of asymptomatic hemorrhagic conversion. Hemorrhagic transformation should be managed according to the same recommendations for spontaneous intracranial hemorrhage and includes reversal of tPA with cryoprecipitate [40].

Angioedema

Rapidly progressing edema involving the oropharynx, larynx and/or palate can occur after rtPA therapy and requires intubation. Awake fiberoptic intubation is recommended. There is a fear of bleeding with nasal intubation if fibrinolytic therapy was administered. ACE inhibitors must be discontinued. Treatment includes methylprednisolone 125 mg IV, diphenhydramine 50 mg IV, and ranitidine 50 mg IV or famotidine 20 mg IV [7].

Icatibant is a selective bradykinin B2 receptor antagonist that can be administered at a dose of 3 mL (30 mg) subcutaneously with repeated 30 mg doses at 6 h to a maximum of 3 injections in 24 h. C1 esterase inhibitors at a dose of 20 IU/kg can also be used. These data are extrapolated from patients with hereditary angioedema [7].

Secondary Stroke Prevention

The CHANCE trial (Clopidogrel in High Risk Patients With Acute Nondisabling Cerebrovascular Events) conducted in China, enrolled patients with minor stroke (NIHSS ≤ 3) and high-risk TIA (ABCD2 ≥ 4) to treatment with dual antiplatelet regimen with aspirin (load of 75–300 mg followed by 75 mg daily) and clopidogrel (300 mg load followed by 75 daily) versus aspirin alone; results showed a decrease in the 90-day risk of stroke in the group treated with dual antiplatelet agents [hazard ratio (HR), 0.68 (95% CI, 0.57–0.81; $P < 0.001$)]. A one-year outcome report showed benefit of early dual antiplatelet without significant difference in major hemorrhagic events [43].

The POINT trial (Platelet-Oriented Inhibition in New TIA and Minor Ischemic Stroke), performed in North America, Europe, Australia, and New Zealand randomized subjects into a group treated with clopidogrel (600 mg loading dose followed by 75 mg daily) plus aspirin (50–325 mg daily) or a group treated with aspirin alone (50–325 mg/day) for 90 days. Dual antiplatelet treatment lowered the risk of ischemic events (HR, 0.75 [95% CI, 0.59–0.95]; $P = 0.02$) but was associated with more major hemorrhages (HR, 2.32 [95% CI, 1.10–4.87]; $P = 0.02$) [7].

A pooled analysis of the CHANCE and POINT trial suggested that the benefit of treatment with dual antiplatelet therapy for minor stroke and TIA is confined to the first 21 days [44].

Intracranial atherosclerosis is associated with a high stroke recurrence rate. The WASID trial (Warfarin-Aspirin Symptomatic Intracranial Disease), compared treatment with aspirin (650 mg twice daily to a minimum dose of 325 mg daily) to treatment with warfarin (target international normalized ratio, 2.0–3.0) for secondary stroke prevention in patients with intracranial atherosclerosis. The trial was terminated early due to safety concerns; warfarin provided no benefit over aspirin and was associated with more adverse events [45].

The SAMMPRIS trial (Stenting and Aggressive Medical Management for Preventing Recurrent Stroke in Intracranial Stenosis) compared Wingspan stenting plus aggressive medical therapy to aggressive medical therapy alone. Aggressive medical management included treatment with aspirin 325 mg per day and clopidogrel 75 mg per day for 90 days, lifestyle modification program, management of risk factors (target SBP <140 mm Hg, SBP <130 mm Hg in diabetic patients, and an LDL cholesterol level < 70 mg per deciliter). There was no benefit to stenting ompared to medical management. As such, intracranial atherosclerosis is most often managed medically [46].

In patients with moderate (50–69%) to severe (70–99%) extracranial carotid stenosis ipsilateral to the hemisphere involved in stroke/TIA, carotid endarterectomy (CAE) or carotid artery stenting (CAS) is recommended depending on the patient's risk factors. In patients ≥70 years of age CAE is recommended given less periprocedural stroke risk. In patients with significant cardiovascular comorbidities, CAS is preferred [47].

Cardiac monitoring for at least 24 h and echocardiography is recommended to rule out potential cardioembolic sources. Long-term cardiac rhythm monitoring can also be considered to improve atrial fibrillation detection.

Post-ICU Care

Critical care survivors are at increased risk of suffering from post-intensive care unit syndrome; these patients can suffer from a myriad of symptoms and syndromes including anxiety, depression, post-traumatic stress syndrome, cognitive impairment, and physical manifestations [48].

Use of neurostimulants in the acute setting could improve functional outcomes in patients; however, there are no large, randomized trials in this patient population, studies are needed evaluating outcomes and type of stimulant [49].

References

1. Varelas PN, Schultz L, Conti M, Spanaki M, Genarrelli T, Hacein-Bey L. The impact of a neuro-intensivist on patients with stroke admitted to a neurosciences intensive care unit. Neurocrit Care. 2008;9(3):293–9. https://doi.org/10.1007/s12028-008-9050-6.
2. Bershad EM, Feen ES, Hernandez OH, Suri MFK, Suarez JI. Impact of a specialized Neurointensive care team on outcomes of critically ill acute ischemic stroke patients. Neurocrit Care. 2008;9(3):287–92. https://doi.org/10.1007/s12028-008-9051-5.
3. McDermott M, Jacobs T, Morgenstern L. Critical care in acute ischemic stroke. Handb Clin Neurol. 2017;140:153–76. https://doi.org/10.1016/B978-0-444-63600-3.00010-6.
4. Virani SS. Et al; American Heart Association Council on epidemiology and prevention statistics committee and stroke statistics subcommittee. Heart disease and stroke Statistics-2021 update: a report from the American Heart Association. Circulation. 2021;143(8):e254–743. https://doi.org/10.1161/CIR.0000000000000950.
5. Van Valburg MK, et al. Long-term mortality among ICU patients with stroke compared with other critically ill patients. Crit Care Med. 2020;48(10):e876–83. https://doi.org/10.1097/CCM.0000000000004492.
6. Mayer SA, Viarasilpa T, Panyavachiraporn N, Brady M, Scozzari D, Van Harn M, Miller D, Katramados A, Hefzy H, Malik S, Marin H, Kole M, Chebl A, Lewandowski C, Mitsias PD. CTA-for-All: Impact of Emergency Computed Tomographic Angiography for All Patients With Stroke Presenting Within 24 Hours of Onset. Stroke. 2020;51(1):331–4. https://doi.org/10.1161/STROKEAHA.119.027356.
7. Powers WJ, Rabinstein AA, Ackerson T, et al. Guidelines for the early Management of Patients with Acute Ischemic Stroke: 2019 update to the 2018 guidelines for the early Management of Acute Ischemic Stroke: a guideline for healthcare professionals from the American Heart Association/American Stroke Association. Stroke. 2019;50(12):e344–418. https://doi.org/10.1161/STR.0000000000000211.
8. Huang X, et al. Tenecteplase versus alteplase in stroke thrombolysis: an individual patient data meta-analysis of randomized controlled trials. Int J Stroke. 2016;11(5):534–43. https://doi.org/10.1177/1747493016641112.
9. Jadhav AP, et al. Thrombectomy With and Without Computed Tomography Perfusion Imaging in the Early

Time Window: A Pooled Analysis of Patient-Level Data. Stroke. 2022;53(4):1348–53. https://doi.org/10.1161/STROKEAHA.121.034331.
10. Nogueira RG. Et al; DAWN trial investigators. Thrombectomy 6 to 24 hours after stroke with a mismatch between deficit and infarct. N Engl J Med. 2018;378(1):11–21. https://doi.org/10.1056/NEJMoa1706442.
11. Albers GW, et al. DEFUSE 3 Investigators. Thrombectomy for Stroke at 6 to 16 Hours with Selection by Perfusion Imaging. N Engl J Med. 2018;378(8):708–18. https://doi.org/10.1056/NEJMoa1713973.
12. Nguyen TN, et al. Noncontrast computed tomography vs. computed tomography perfusion or magnetic resonance imaging selection in late presentation of stroke with large-vessel occlusion. JAMA Neurol. 2022;79(1):22–31. https://doi.org/10.1001/jamaneurol.2021.4082. Erratum in: JAMA Neurol 2022 Jan 1;79(1):93.
13. Renú A, Millán M, San Román L, et al. Effect of intra-arterial Alteplase vs placebo following successful Thrombectomy on functional outcomes in patients with large vessel occlusion acute ischemic stroke: the CHOICE randomized clinical trial. JAMA. 2022;327:826. https://doi.org/10.1001/jama.2022.164.
14. Chang TS, Jensen MB. Haemodilution for acute ischaemic stroke. Cochrane Database Syst Rev. 2014;2014(8):CD000103. https://doi.org/10.1002/14651858.CD000103.pub2.
15. Ginsberg MD, Palesch YY, Hill MD, et al. High-dose albumin treatment for acute ischaemic stroke (ALIAS): a phase 3, randomised, double-blind, placebo-controlled trial. Lancet Neurol. 2013;12(11):1049–58. https://doi.org/10.1016/S1474-4422(13)70223-0.
16. Mazighi M, Richard S, Lapergue B, et al. Safety and efficacy of intensive blood pressure lowering after successful endovascular therapy in acute ischaemic stroke (BP-TARGET): a multicentre, open-label, randomized controlled trial. Lancet Neurol. 2021;20(4):265–74. https://doi.org/10.1016/S1474-4422(20)30483-X.
17. Anderson CS, Olavarría VV. Head Positioning in Acute Stroke: Down but Not Out. Stroke. 2019;50(1):224–8. https://doi.org/10.1161/STROKEAHA.118.020087.
18. Nogueira RC, Aries M, Minhas JS, et al. Review of studies on dynamic cerebral autoregulation in the acute phase of stroke and the relationship with clinical outcome. J Cereb Blood Flow Metab. 2022;42(3):430–53. https://doi.org/10.1177/0271678X211045222.
19. Hacke W, Schwab S, Horn M, Spranger M, De Georgia M, von Kummer R. 'Malignant' middle cerebral artery territory infarction: clinical course and prognostic signs. Arch Neurol. 1996;53(4):309–15. https://doi.org/10.1001/archneur.1996.00550040037012.
20. Chen CF, Lin RT, Lin HF, Chao AC. A multiparameter model predicting in-hospital mortality in malignant cerebral infarction. Medicine (Baltimore). 2017;96(28):e7443. https://doi.org/10.1097/MD.0000000000007443.
21. Maccallum C, Churilov L, Mitchell P, Dowling R, Yan B. Low Alberta stroke program early CT score (ASPECTS) associated with malignant middle cerebral artery infarction. Cerebrovasc Dis. 2014;38(1):39–45. https://doi.org/10.1159/000363619.
22. Muscari A, Faccioli L, Lega MV, et al. Predicting cerebral edema in ischemic stroke patients. Neurol Sci. 2019;40(4):745–52. https://doi.org/10.1007/s10072-019-3717-y.
23. Pullicino PM, Alexandrov AV, Shelton JA, Alexandrova NA, Smurawska LT, Norris JW. Mass effect and death from severe acute stroke. Neurology. 1997;49(4):1090–5. https://doi.org/10.1212/WNL.49.4.1090.
24. Qureshi AI, Suarez JI, Yahia AM, Mohammad Y, Uzun G, Suri MF, Zaidat OO, Ayata C, Ali Z, Wityk RJ. Timing of neurologic deterioration in massive middle cerebral artery infarction: a multicenter review. Crit Care Med. 2003;31(1):272–7. Cited in: Journals@Ovid Full Text at http://ovidsp.ovid.com/ovidweb.cgi?T=JS&PAGE=reference&D=ovftf&NEWS=N&AN=00003246-200301000-00043. Accessed 04 Dec 2021
25. Khanna A, Kahle KT, Walcott BP, Gerzanich V, Simard JM. Disruption of ion homeostasis in the Neurogliovascular unit underlies the pathogenesis of ischemic cerebral edema. Transl Stroke Res. 2014;5(1):3–16. https://doi.org/10.1007/s12975-013-0307-9.
26. Baron JC. Perfusion thresholds in human cerebral ischemia: historical perspective and therapeutic implications. Cerebrovasc Dis. 2001;11(1):2–8. https://doi.org/10.1159/000049119.
27. Papagianni M, Tziomalos K, Kostaki S, et al. Treatment with mannitol is associated with increased risk for in-hospital mortality in patients with acute ischemic stroke and cerebral edema. Am J Cardiovasc Drugs. 2018;18(5):397–403. https://doi.org/10.1007/s40256-018-0285-0.
28. Cook AM, Morgan Jones G, Hawryluk GWJ, et al. Guidelines for the acute treatment of cerebral edema in Neurocritical care patients. Neurocrit Care. 2020;32(3):647–66. https://doi.org/10.1007/s12028-020-00959-7.
29. Vahedi K, Hofmeijer J, Juettler E, Vicaut E, George B, Algra A, Amelink GJ, Schmiedeck P, Schwab S, Rothwell PM, Bousser MG, van der Worp HB, Hacke W, DECIMAL, DESTINY, and HAMLET investigators. Early decompressive surgery in malignant infarction of the middle cerebral artery: a pooled analysis of three randomised controlled trials. Lancet Neurol. 2007;6(3):215–22. https://doi.org/10.1016/S1474-4422(07)70036-4.
30. Beez T, Munoz-Bendix C, Steiger HJ, Beseoglu K. Decompressive craniectomy for acute ischemic stroke. Crit Care. 2019;23:209. https://doi.org/10.1186/s13054-019-2490-x.
31. Hinduja A, Samant R, Feng D, Hannawi Y. Herniation despite Decompressive Hemicraniectomy in large hemispherical ischemic strokes. J Stroke Cerebrovasc Dis. 2018;27(2):418–24. https://doi.org/10.1016/j.jstrokecerebrovasdis.2017.09.016.
32. Barrozo HG, De Guzman MA, Navarro J, Venketasubramanian N. Asymmetric TCD findings in malignant MCA infarction, resolution after Decompressive Hemicraniectomy: a case report. Case Rep Neurol. 2020;12(Suppl 1):127–36. https://doi.org/10.1159/000508589.
33. Albert AF, Kirkman MA. Clinical and radiological predictors of malignant middle cerebral artery infarction development and outcomes. J Stroke Cerebrovasc Dis. 2017;26(11):2671–9. https://doi.org/10.1016/j.jstrokecerebrovasdis.2017.06.041.
34. Hernández-Durán S, Meinen L, Rohde V, von der Brelie C. Invasive monitoring of intracranial pressure after Decompressive Craniectomy in malignant stroke. Stroke. 2021;52(2):707–11. https://doi.org/10.1161/STROKEAHA.120.032390.
35. Poca MA, Benejam B, Sahuquillo J, et al. Monitoring intracranial pressure in patients with malignant middle cerebral artery infarction: is it useful?: clinical article. J Neurosurg. 2010;112(3):648–57. https://doi.org/10.3171/2009.7.JNS081677.
36. Frank JI. Large hemispheric infarction, deterioration, and intracranial pressure. Neurology. 1995;45(7):1286–90.
37. Schwab S, Aschoff A, Spranger M, Albert F, Hacke W. The value of intracranial pressure monitoring in acute hemispheric stroke. Neurology. 1996;47(2):393–8. https://doi.org/10.1212/WNL.47.2.393.
38. Datar S, McLouth C, Reynolds P. Factors associated with the outcome of very elderly patients with large hemispheric infarction treated with medical management only. Neurocrit Care. 2018;28(3):322–9. https://doi.org/10.1007/s12028-017-0484-6.
39. Pallesen LP, Barlinn K, Puetz V. Role of Decompressive Craniectomy in ischemic stroke. Front Neurol. 2019;9:1119. https://doi.org/10.3389/fneur.2018.01119.
40. Yaghi S, et al. Treatment and Outcome of Hemorrhagic Transformation After Intravenous Alteplase in Acute Ischemic Stroke: A Scientific Statement for Healthcare Professionals From the American Heart Association/American Stroke Association.

Stroke. 2017;48(12):e343–61. https://doi.org/10.1161/STR.0000000000000152.
41. Emberson J, Lees KR, Lyden P, et al. Effect of treatment delay, age, and stroke severity on the effects of intravenous thrombolysis with alteplase for acute ischaemic stroke: a meta-analysis of individual patient data from randomised trials. Lancet. 2014;384(9958):1929–35. https://doi.org/10.1016/S0140-6736(14)60584-5.
42. Whiteley WN, Slot KB, Fernandes P, Sandercock P, Wardlaw J. Risk factors for intracranial hemorrhage in acute ischemic stroke patients treated with recombinant tissue plasminogen activator: a systematic review and meta-analysis of 55 studies. Stroke. 2012;43(11):2904–9. https://doi.org/10.1161/STROKEAHA.112.665331.
43. Wang Y, Pan Y, Zhao X, et al. Clopidogrel with aspirin in acute minor stroke or transient ischemic attack (CHANCE) trial: one-year outcomes. Circulation. 2015;132(1):40–6. https://doi.org/10.1161/CIRCULATIONAHA.114.014791.
44. Pan Y, Elm JJ, Li H, et al. Outcomes associated with Clopidogrel-aspirin use in minor stroke or transient ischemic attack. JAMA Neurol. 2019;76(12):1466–73. https://doi.org/10.1001/jamaneurol.2019.2531.
45. Chimowitz MI, Lynn MJ, Howlett-Smith H, Stern BJ, Hertzberg VS, Frankel MR, Levine SR, Chaturvedi S, Kasner SE, Benesch CG, Sila CA, Jovin TG, Romano JG. Warfarin-Aspirin Symptomatic Intracranial Disease Trial Investigators. Comparison of warfarin and aspirin for symptomatic intracranial arterial stenosis. N Engl J Med. 2005;352(13):1305–16. https://doi.org/10.1056/NEJMoa043033.
46. Chimowitz MI, Lynn MJ, Derdeyn CP, et al. Stenting versus aggressive medical therapy for intracranial arterial stenosis. N Engl J Med. 2011;365(11):993–1003. https://doi.org/10.1056/NEJMoa1105335.
47. Kleindorfer DO, Towfighi A, Chaturvedi S, Cockroft KM, Gutierrez J, Lombardi-Hill D, Kamel H, Kernan WN, Kittner SJ, Leira EC, Lennon O. 2021 Guideline for the Prevention of Stroke in Patients With Stroke and Transient Ischemic Attack: A Guideline From the American Heart Association/American Stroke Association. Stroke. 2021;52(7):e364–467. https://doi.org/10.1161/STR.0000000000000375.
48. LaBuzetta JN, Rosand J, Vranceanu AM. Review: post-intensive care syndrome: unique challenges in the Neurointensive care unit. Neurocrit Care. 2019;31(3):534–45. https://doi.org/10.1007/s12028-019-00826-0.
49. Leclerc AM, Riker RR, Brown CS, et al. Amantadine and Modafinil as Neurostimulants following acute stroke: a retrospective study of intensive care unit patients. Neurocrit Care. 2021;34:102–11. https://doi.org/10.1007/s12028-020-00986-4.

Cerebral Venous Sinus Thrombosis

25

Arooshi Kumar, Jonah Zuflacht, and Brett Cucchiara

Contents

Abstract

Cerebral venous sinus thrombosis (CVST) is a relatively uncommon but important condition to be aware of in neuro-critical care practice. CVST refers to thrombosis of a cerebral venous sinus which can lead to venous ischemia, edema, and hemorrhage. Diagnosis of CVST can be challenging given the broad range of presenting symptoms that overlap with many common benign conditions. CVST is an important and often unrecognized cause of coma and intracerebral hemorrhage. CT or MR venography can accurately confirm the diagnosis. Prompt treatment with anticoagulation, even in the setting of intracerebral hemorrhage, may improve outcomes.

A. Kumar · B. Cucchiara (✉)
Department of Neurology, University of Pennsylvania, Philadelphia, PA, USA
e-mail: cucchiar@pennmedicine.upenn.edu

J. Zuflacht
Department of Neurology, Beth Israel Deaconess Medical Center, Boston, MA, USA

E. Mahanna Gabrielli et al. (eds.), *Textbook of Neurointensive Care: Volume 1*, https://doi.org/10.1007/978-3-031-62220-5_25

Introduction

This chapter discusses the clinical presentation, diagnosis, and management of cerebral venous sinus thrombosis (CVST). The cerebral venous system consists of multiple large connected venous sinuses into which cortical veins drain, providing egress of blood from the intracranial compartment (Fig. 25.1). Key goals of the chapter include the following: (1) review the broad range of clinical symptoms that may be caused by CVST, (2) review the potential causes and risk factors for CVST, (3) explain how to optimally and rapidly diagnose CVST, (4) provide consensus recommendations for acute treatment for CVST and long-term treatment to prevent recurrence, and 5) review the common complications of CVST and how to approach them.

Key Clinical Questions
The chapter will answer

- What are the typical clinical presentations of cerebral venous sinus thrombosis (CVST)?
- What factors increase the risk for CVST?
- What imaging modalities are useful to diagnose CVST?
- What additional testing should patients with confirmed CVST undergo?
- How should patients with CVST be treated?
- What radiographic features can help identify CVST?

Clinical Presentation

Cerebral venous sinus thrombosis constitutes about 0.5% - 1% of all strokes [1]. In the largest prospective observational study, the International Study on Cerebral and Dural Venous Thrombosis (ISCVT), CVST was more common in younger patients (78% of patients presenting under age of 50) and almost twice as prevalent in women compared to men under 60 years of age [2].

The clinical presentations of CVST are highly variable and protean. Patients can present with isolated headaches, seizures, non-focal neurologic impairment, or focal neurologic deficits. Importantly, many patients present subacutely, often with prodromal headache for days or weeks, and this provides an important clue to the diagnosis. Delays in the diagnosis of CVST are common. In ISCVT, symptom onset was acute (less than 48 h) in 37% of patients, subacute (greater than 48 h to 30 days) in 56% of patients, and chronic (greater than 30 days) in 7% of patients. The median delay from symptom onset to hospital admission was 4 days and from symptom onset to diagnosis was 7 days [2]. This underscores the need for a high level of clinical suspicion and a careful history from the patient or family about antecedent symptoms prior to presentation.

Headache is one of the most common presenting symptoms of CVST. The reported prevalence of headache as a presenting symptom ranges from 50% to 90% [2–4]. In ISCVT, up to 90% of patients presented with headache, and

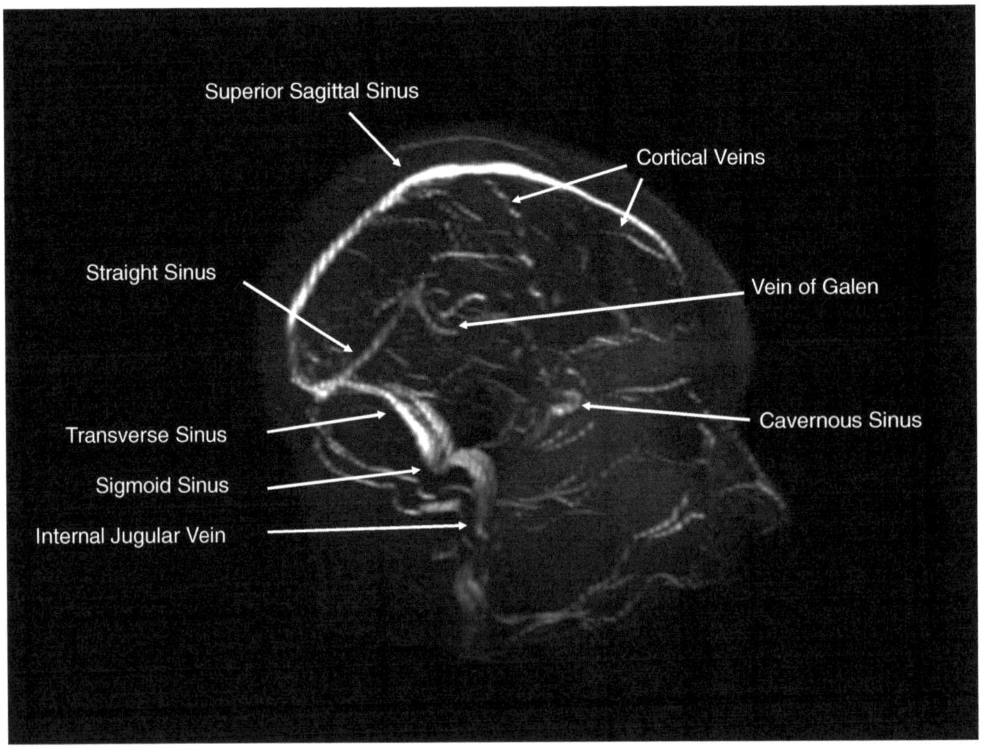

Fig. 25.1 MR venography showing anatomy of the cerebral venous sinuses

for 25% of patients it was the only symptom [2]. Headache may be more common in younger patients and women [5]. A broad range of headache types may be seen in CVST. Often patients present with gradually escalating headache intensity that is usually persistent and can be focal or diffuse, but "thunderclap" (sudden) headache can also occur [3] [6]. Given the frequent association with elevated intracranial pressure (ICP) from venous congestion, patients may report headaches with features consistent with intracranial hypertension, such as worsening of headaches with recumbent positioning and with coughing or other Valsalva equivalents. Additionally, exacerbation of pre-existing migraine headaches may occur, a situation which can be diagnostically very challenging.

The second most common symptom in CVST is seizure, present in nearly 40% of cases [2]. These may be focal or generalized. When CVST leads to venous infarction, edema, or hemorrhage, focal neurologic deficits referable to the affected brain region occur, such as hemiparesis, aphasia, neglect, or visual field defects. In ISCVT, 63% of patients (394/624) patients presented with focal deficits. Importantly, since sagittal sinus thrombosis impacts venous drainage to both hemispheres, bilateral focal deficits may occur. Papillaedema may be seen in over a quarter of patients due to venous hypertension, and CVST may mimic idiopathic intracranial hypertension, including causing diplopia due to sixth cranial nerve palsies and causing pulsatile tinnitus [7]. Stupor or coma may occur, typically with thrombosis of the deep venous system. In such cases, venous edema or infarction affecting the thalami and other deep structures are invariably seen on brain imaging. Less common presentations of CVST include psychosis associated with focal neurological symptoms, multiple lower cranial nerve abnormalities causing Collett-Sicard syndrome associated with transverse and sigmoid sinus and jugular vein occlusion, and orbital pain, proptosis, ptosis, and oculomotor nerve palsy associated with cavernous sinus thrombosis [8, 9] [10].

CVST presenting symptom complexes may be categorized into three broad syndromes which correlate with involvement of specific venous sinuses: 1) intracranial hypertension, 2) focal neurologic deficits, and 3) encephalopathy/coma [3, 11]. Patients with intracranial hypertension typically have involvement of the superior sagittal sinus and/or bilateral transverse sinuses and often present with positional headache and visual symptoms from papillaedema or sixth nerve palsies. In these cases, there are often no parenchymal abnormalities on brain imaging. In contrast, patients with focal neurologic deficits almost always have identified parenchymal abnormalities consistent with venous infarction, edema, or hemorrhage on brain imaging with the affected brain regions correlating with the area of venous drainage of the occluded venous sinus. For instance, patients with hemiparesis typically have thrombosis of the superior sagittal sinus with frontal lobe parenchymal abnormalities; patients with aphasia often have involvement of the left transverse sinus and/or vein of Labbe with corresponding temporal lobe abnormalities. These patients also frequently have seizures. Finally, patients with encephalopathy or coma typically have involvement of the deep venous system with bilateral thalamic injury. Such patients with thrombosis of the deep venous system can rapidly deteriorate neurologically, and thus very close monitoring and aggressive treatment is indicated [12–14].

Risk Factors/Causes

Similar to deep vein thrombosis (DVT) in the peripheral veins, hypercoagulability is an important cause of CVST and is present in roughly one-third of patients [2]. Unlike peripheral DVT, immobilization is not a contributor to CVST. However, dehydration is felt to be an important factor increasing the risk of CVST. A careful history inquiring about recent gastrointestinal illness or decreased fluid intake should be conducted in all patients. Additionally, local infections, particularly in parameningeal locations, are an uncommon but important cause of CVST and should always be considered.

Inherited Thrombophilias

The factor V Leiden and prothrombin G20210A gene mutations increase the risk of CVST. A meta-analysis including 469 CVST patients reported a greater than three-fold odds of CVST in patients with the factor V Leiden mutation compared to those without [15]. A more recent case-control study found factor V Leiden mutations were present in 16.8% of patients with cerebral sinus venous thrombosis (CVT) and in 17.8% of patients with arterial ischemic stroke (AIS) [16]. In a case-control study of separate patients with CVST, lower extremity DVT, and healthy controls, the prothrombin G20210A gene mutation was present in 20% of CVST patients, 18% of leg DVT controls, and only 3% of normal controls [17]. Patients with a combination of the prothrombin gene mutation and oral contraceptive pill (OCP) use appear to be at even higher risk for CVST. A pooled meta-analysis analysis demonstrated that the prothrombin G20210A mutation was associated with a nearly ten-fold increased risk of CVTS (OR 9.27,95% CI 5.85–14.67) for CVST [15]. Testing for factor V Leiden and prothrombin gene mutations can be performed in the acute phase of CVST as they are genetic tests.

Deficiencies of antithrombin III, protein C, and protein S, while uncommon, may be associated with an increased risk of CVST. Genetic mutations leading to protein C and S deficiencies have been associated with a 2 to 11-fold increased risk of CVT [18]. Levels of these factors may be altered in the acute phase of a thrombotic event, as well as by other medical conditions such as liver disease, nephrotic syndrome, surgery, pregnancy, and certain infections. Therefore, measurement should generally be deferred until after the acute phase of CVST has resolved. Given the relative rarity of abnormalities in these factors, testing may be best reserved for patients with a significant family history of thrombosis.

Hyperhomocysteinemia, which can be inherited or acquired, has been associated with DVT and may also be associated with an increased risk of CVST. In one case-control study, hyperhomocysteinemia was present in 27% of CVST patients and 8% of control patients [19]. Of note, low levels of serum folate and the 677TT methylenetetrahydrofolate reductase genotype were not associated with CVT risk independent of homocysteine level. Whether lowering homocysteine levels reduces the risk of recurrent thrombosis remains uncertain. North American and European studies have found no benefit for homocysteine-lowering vitamin therapy in reducing the risk of ischemic stroke [20, 21] while a more recent Chinese study demonstrated a reduction with treatment [22]. This may correspond to varying background levels of nutrient fortification in food products in different countries. No studies testing homocysteine lowering therapy specifically in CVST have been conducted.

Acquired Pro-Thrombotic Conditions

Antiphospholipid Antibody Syndrome (APLS)

APLS, an important pro-thrombotic condition associated with both arterial and venous thrombosis, was present in 6% of patients in ISCVT [2]. Testing for APLS should include measurement of anti-cardiolipin and anti-beta 2 glycoprotein antibodies as well as testing for the presence of a lupus anticoagulant. To confirm APLS, one or more of these must be positive on two separate occasions 12 weeks apart. Identification of APLS is of particular importance as two randomized trials suggest superiority of warfarin over direct oral anticoagulants for prevention of recurrent events in patients with APLS-related thrombosis [23, 24].

Cancer

Cancer associated hypercoagulability is an important cause of venous and arterial clots. In a large case-control study, a history of cancer increased the risk of CVST approximately five-fold, with the highest risk seen in patients with hematological cancers, particularly leukemia [25]. Among solid cancers the highest risk was seen in subjects with lung cancer. A careful history and examination should be done in all patients with CVST to investigate for signs or symptoms suggestive of malignancy, and patients should be counseled to be sure they are up to date on all age-appropriate cancer screening. Patients with a history of treated cancer should be carefully assessed for signs of active recurrence.

Pregnancy and Puerperium

The frequency of peripartum and postpartum CVST is about 12 cases per 100,000 deliveries [26]. The third trimester and up to 12 weeks post-delivery are associated with the highest risk [27, 28]. In ISCVT about 6% of patients with CVST presented during pregnancy and about 14% in the puerperium. The increased risk of CVST associated with pregnancy is postulated to be due to transient hypercoagulability. Fortunately, the risk of recurrent venous thrombosis during subsequent pregnancies appears to be low [29].

Oral Contraceptives

Use of oral contraceptives has been shown in multiple observational studies to increase the odds of CVST by 5- to 22-fold [15]. A systematic review reported the pooled odds of developing CVST in women aged 15–50 years taking OCPs was 7.59 times higher compared to women not taking OCPs [30]. The association between newer third-generation progestin oral contraceptives and risk of CVST has not yet been established. Women with CVST should be counseled to permanently avoid oral contraceptives and use alternative means of birth control.

Heparin-Induced Thrombocytopenia/ Vaccine-Induced Thrombotic Thrombocytopenia

CVST is a rare thrombotic manifestation in patients with heparin-induced thrombocytopenia (HIT) [31, 32]. A recent systematic review reported an overall rate of CVST in patients with HIT was 1.6% as compared to 0.002% in the general population. HIT-related CVST appears to be associated with higher rates of intracerebral hemorrhage and a higher mortality rate when compared with historical CVST controls from the ISCVT study. Patients with CVST due to HIT should be treated with non-heparin anticoagulants. The advent of adenoviral vector vaccines (particularly the ChAdOx1 nCoV-19 vaccine) targeting SARS-CoV-2 infection has introduced a unique syndrome of Vaccine-induced Thrombotic Thrombocytopenia (VITT) which shares many mechanistic similarities with HIT. CVST is a prominent feature of this condition. Recognition of this syndrome is critical as treatment typically involves avoidance of heparin, use of an alternative anticoagulant, and administration of intravenous immunoglobulin [33].

Other Pro-Thrombotic Conditions

In addition to the above conditions, a number of other disease states have rarely been associated with CVST. These include paroxysmal nocturnal hemoglobinuria, thrombotic thrombocytopenic purpura, inflammatory bowel disease, systemic lupus erythematosus, and Behçcet disease [34]. Hematology consultation may be useful if any of these are suspected contributors to CVST in an individual patient.

Infections

Relatively unique to CVST, as opposed to peripheral DVT, is the causal association with local infection. In ISCVT, 12% of CVST cases were associated with infection [2]. Typical infections whose course can be complicated by CVST include otitis and mastoiditis, which can affect the nearby sigmoid and transverse sinuses. Large observational studies suggest the prevalence of infectious causes of CVST has declined over time, likely due to more effective antibiotics and timely delivery of treatment [1]. The association between CVST and infection may be more common in children [35]. Identification of infection is important, as antibiotic treatment, and occasionally surgical intervention, is needed.

A unique type of infectious CVST is septic cavernous sinus thrombosis (SCST), which is associated with relatively high morbidity and mortality despite modern antibiotic treatment. SCST develops from the local spread of infection, from an oral, sinus, or maxillofacial source, to the cavernous sinus via contiguous phlebitis or ensnared septic emboli [36]. Common clinical manifestations include signs of systemic infection plus periorbital edema, ptosis, chemosis, proptosis, and ophthalmoplegia, and possible loss of vision associated with painful eye movements. Importantly, patients with the common anatomic variant of a hypoplastic transverse sinus can be more symptomatic if the dominant sinus is affected.

Mechanical and Procedural Factors

An association between head injury and CVST has been observed [37]. While the mechanisms underlying this association are uncertain, it has been proposed that CSVT could be caused by venous compression associated with external or internal cranial injuries leading to swelling and mass effect [38]. One small study found CSVT in 4–6.5% of patients with penetrating head trauma [37]. In addition to head injury, head and neck, and neurosurgical procedures have been associated with a risk of CVST. For example, in one study, skull base surgery was associated with a 9% risk of venous sinus thrombosis, though only 11% of patients were symptomatic [39].

Lumbar puncture (LP) has also been reported as a precipitant of CVST, both in the setting of intrathecal injections for myelography or other treatments [40, 41] and with diagnostic dural puncture [42]. A proposed mechanism for post-LP CSVT is a creation of a negative cranial-spinal pressure gradient created by intracranial hypotension leading to traction on meninges and stretching of cerebral veins.

Essential Management Priorities

Early: Immediate/First 24 h

The initial priority in a patient with possible CVST is to confirm the diagnosis. This is particularly important in cases where intracerebral hemorrhage (ICH) is present, as the main targeted treatment for ICH in the setting of CVST is therapeutic anticoagulation, a treatment specifically contraindicated with other causes of ICH. Diagnosis may initially be suggested by clinical history. However, in a critically ill patient unable to provide history, prodromal symptoms of headache for days to weeks prior to presentation may be unrecognized. Contacting the patient's family or friends to obtain a reliable and complete history may provide important clues raising one's level of suspicion for CVST. When suspected, confirmation of the diagnosis of CVST rests on neuroimaging. While the diagnosis may sometimes be apparent on non-contrast CT or MRI, often MR or CT venography is required (see "Key Radiographic Findings" section below). As mentioned above, given the key management implications of diagnosing CVST, urgent imaging needs to be pursued to ensure accurate diagnosis and early implementation of therapy.

Once CVST is confirmed, the main management goals are 1) to prevent further clot propagation and facilitate vessel recanalization, 2) to prevent other thrombotic events, 3) to effectively manage venous hypertension and elevated intracranial pressure if present, and 4) to promptly diagnose and manage medical or neurological complications. Expert consensus strongly recommends the use of parenteral anticoagulation acutely to treat CVST, even in the face of intracerebral hemorrhage [34]. This is based on data from two small randomized controlled trials comparing anticoagulation to placebo. The first trial compared unfractionated intravenous heparin (with a bolus followed by continuous infusion) to placebo in 20 patients with CVST. In the group randomized to heparin, 80% of patients had complete recovery and none had ICH, while in the placebo arm, only 10% had complete recovery, 60% had residual deficits and 20% had ICH [43]. The second trial enrolled 59 patients and compared subcutaneous nadroparin (a low molecular weight heparin) to placebo. In this trial, death or dependence at 12 weeks was seen in 13% of patients treated with nadroparin and 21% of patients treated with placebo [44]. Notably, in patients with intracerebral hemorrhage at the time of enrolment, anticoagulation was not associated with hemorrhage expansion. Other studies have also demonstrated low rates of new hemorrhage after anticoagulation for CVT [43, 45]. In general, full-dose parenteral anticoagulation should be started as soon as possible once the diagnosis of CVST is confirmed.

In addition to anticoagulation, measures to optimize venous drainage are important. These include nursing with the head of bed in an elevated and neutral position and avoidance of factors that might increase systemic venous pressure. Dehydration may contribute to CVST and must be rigorously avoided. Patients should receive sufficient fluids to maintain a euvolemic state.

Unlike acute ischemic stroke, the role of endovascular intervention in CVST is limited at present. While such intervention may accelerate recanalization of the venous sinuses, the sole randomized trial testing endovascular intervention for CVST showed no benefit and possible harm. This trial, the TO-ACT trial, randomized 67 patients to endovascular intervention (including mechanical thrombectomy and/or pharmacological thrombolysis) versus heparin [46]. Only high-risk patients were eligible for enrollment. This was defined as at least one of the following features: altered mental status, coma, intracerebral hemorrhage, or deep cerebral venous thrombosis. At 1-year follow-up, excellent outcome was seen in 67% of patients assigned endovascular intervention and 68% assigned heparin (RR 0.99, 95% CI 0.71–1.38). Mortality was 12% in the endovascular arm compared to 3% in the anticoagulation arm, though this was not statistically significant. Based on this trial, most experts feel endovascular intervention should not be used as first-line therapy in CVST. However, for patients with neurological deterioration despite therapeutic anticoagulation, or in whom anticoagulation is contraindicated, it may be considered.

In addition to these immediate management priorities, testing to identify a potential cause of CVST should start promptly, noting that some conditions require additional early treatment interventions (i.e., hematological malignancies, VITT, infectious causes). Current AHA/ASA guidelines recommend sending a complete blood count, comprehensive chemistry panel, sedimentation rate, and coagulation studies in all patients. Additional studies, such as hypercoagulable testing, should be individualized based on the patient's clinical history.

Subsequent Inpatient Management

Once the patient is clinically stable and approaching discharge, parenteral anticoagulation should be transitioned to a long-term oral anticoagulant. Traditionally, warfarin has been used, although there is increasing evidence supporting use of direct oral anticoagulants. In the RE-SPECT CVT trial, 120 patients with CVST were randomized to 6 months of treatment with dose-adjusted warfarin versus dabigatran [47]. No recurrent venous thrombotic events occurred in either study arm; there was 1 major bleeding event in the dabigatran arm and 2 in the warfarin arm. Overall, the study concluded that both warfarin and dabigatran were safe and effective treatments for CSVT. The ACTION-CVT study, a multicenter retrospective observational study including 1025 patients with CVST, found that patients on any direct oral anticoagulant had similar rates of recurrent venous thrombosis, death, and partial/complete recanalization of the venous sinuses compared to those on warfarin, but with a lower risk of hemorrhage [48]. Given these data and the many practical advantages of direct oral anticoagulants compared to warfarin, it is reasonable to use direct oral anticoagulants for prevention of recurrent VTE in patients with CVST. Treatment is generally continued for at least 6 months; the decision about whether to treat beyond that depends on the underlying cause of the CVST.

Long-Term Clinical Course

Despite its variable presentation and often progressive nature if not treated appropriately, most patients with CVST have a favorable outcome, with only about 15% dying or having persistent deficits limiting functional independence [2]. Risk factors associated with poor outcomes include older age, presence of CNS infection, any malignancy, deep vein thrombosis, ICH on admission imaging, and coma or altered mental status. Predictors of 30-day mortality from ISCVT included depressed consciousness, altered mental status, thrombosis of the deep venous system, right hemisphere hemorrhage, and posterior fossa lesions. Risk of recurrent CVST is approximately 2% in the first year, with an additional 4% having some other thrombotic event during this period [2]. A 2018 systematic review and meta-analysis of 19 studies demonstrated favorable recanalization rates in 85% of 818 patients with CVST who had follow-up imaging, with partial recanalization in 35% and complete recanalization in 49% [49].

Near Misses

Failure to identify ICH as due to CVST

Patients with intracranial hemorrhage due to a variety of underlying causes are commonly admitted to the neurointensive care unit. Though often overlooked, CVST is an important cause of ICH that requires very different management from other causes of ICH. In ISCVT, roughly 40% of patients with CVST had ICH [2]. Hemorrhages are typically lobar, though subarachnoid hemorrhage may also occur, and may at times be bilateral. Isolated thrombosis of the vein of

Labbe, with or without dural sinus involvement, is an important cause of posterior-lateral temporal lobe hemorrhage [50]; a high index of suspicion for CVST should always be maintained for hemorrhage in this location. Thrombosis of other cortical veins, such as the vein of Trolard, can also lead to intraparenchymal hemorrhage [51] as well as to convexity subarachnoid hemorrhage [52]. Given the treatment implications (i.e., systemic anticoagulation), early venous imaging is essential in patients presenting with lobar ICH in whom CVST is a clinical consideration.

Deep CVST and Coma

Patients with thrombosis of the deep cerebral veins may present in stupor or coma without any accompanying focal neurological signs or evidence of increased ICP. The presentation is often fulminant, although some patients will experience a more mild course depending on the degree of venous congestion, extent of collateral vessels, and the territories involved [13]. In patients with deep cerebral vein thrombosis causing stupor or coma, neuroimaging (both CT and MRI) almost always shows bilateral deep parenchymal lesions. Failure to recognize that deep cerebral vein thrombosis may cause this pattern can lead to delayed diagnosis and initiation of anticoagulation.

CVST Mimicking Idiopathic Intracranial Hypertension (IIH)

Many patients with CVST will develop the syndrome of idiopathic intracranial hypertension (IIH) without focal neurological findings. In ISCVT, 22.9% of patients presented in this manner (defined as any combination of headache, vomiting, and papilledema with or without associated vision impairment or sixth nerve palsies) [2]. IIH can present with nearly identical clinical features. As such, it can be quite challenging to distinguish between the two based only on the history and examination. Among those patients with a presumptive diagnosis of IIH, between 9.4 and 26% will subsequently be diagnosed with CVST after dedicated venous imaging (MRI/MRV or angiography) [53, 54]. Cerebral venous imaging should therefore be performed in all patients with a presumed diagnosis of IIH to exclude the possibility of CVST.

CVST from Underlying Infection

CVST may occur in the setting of underlying head, neck, or central nervous system infections, and identification and treatment of these infections are of obvious importance. Suspicion should be particularly elevated in patients with fever or systemic symptoms suggestive of infection, ear drainage or pain suggestive of middle ear infection, or localizing signs suggesting cavernous sinus involvement (e.g., chemosis, proptosis, and ophthalmoplegia) [55]. Appropriate antibiotic therapy should be administered promptly in those with suspected septic CVST and surgical treatment (such as drainage) considered early where appropriate.

Adenoviral-Vector COVID-19 Vaccination and CVST

CVST has been reported as a rare complication after administration of the ChAdOx1 nCoV-19 (Oxford/AstraZeneca) and the Ad26.COV2.S (Janssen/Johnson & Johnson) COVID-19 vaccines [56, 57]. Nearly all patients have severe thrombocytopenia and markedly elevated levels of heparin-platelet factor 4 HIT antibodies [58]. As such, these cases are felt to represent a vaccine-related variant of heparin-induced thrombocytopenia and are therefore referred to as "vaccine-induced immune thrombotic thrombocytopenia" (VITT) [56]. While CVST has also been reported following the mRNA-based vaccines [59, 60], large population studies suggest that the mRNA-based vaccines do not increase the risk of CVST above the estimated background risk [61]. Dedicated venous imaging should be considered in patients with persistent headaches following COVID-19 vaccination, particularly those who received adenovirus-based vaccines.

Treatment of VITT is similar to that of heparin-induced thrombocytopenia. All heparin products, including heparinized IV flushes, should be promptly discontinued. Platelet transfusions, if possible, should be avoided [62]. Treatment with an alternative non-heparin anticoagulant, such as bivalirudin, argatroban, or fondaparinux, is essential—particularly in those with confirmed thromboses such as CVST. Adjunctive treatment with intravenous immunoglobin should be initiated along with anticoagulation [33]. Hematology consultation is advised.

Key Radiographic Findings

Given the protean clinical presentations of CVST, diagnostic imaging is critical to establishing the diagnosis. Radiologic findings in CVST may be categorized by modality (CT, MR, etc.), invasiveness (invasive or non-invasive), and whether there is direct or indirect evidence of venous thrombosis [34, 63]. Table 25.1 summarizes the most important radiologic findings based on these parameters.

It is important to note several unique radiologic features of brain injury from CVST, regardless of the given imaging modality. First, the pattern of injury often does not follow that of typical arterial territories [34]. Infarction, hemor-

Table 25.1 Key Radiologic Findings in CVST

Key finding	Description	Modality/modalities	Invasiveness	Direct or indirect sign
Dense clot sign	Hyperdensity within dural venous sinus	Non-contrast head CT	Non-invasive	Direct
Cord sign	Linear hyperdensity representing thrombosed cortical vein	Non-contrast head CT, "hyperintense vein sign" on MRI	Non-invasive	Direct
Empty delta sign [64]	Intrasinus filling defect with peripheral enhancement, most commonly seen in the superior sagittal sinus	Contrast-enhanced head CT	Non-invasive	Direct
Sigmoid notch sign [65]	"Negative" when there is loss of signal within the sigmoid plate notch, "Positive" when asymmetrically smaller sigmoid notch suggestive of congenital atresia	Non-contrast head CT	Non-invasive	Direct
Filling defect	Incomplete or absent filling of venous structure (cortical vein or dural venous sinus) representing thrombus	Contrast-enhanced CT, CTV, MRV, conventional venography	Non-invasive or invasive	Direct
Flow void	Absence of normal flow void suggestive of thrombus	MRI	Non-invasive	Direct
Edema	Focal or diffuse parenchymal swelling	CT (hypodensity) or MRI (FLAIR hyperintensity)	Non-invasive	Indirect
Venous infarction	Cerebral infarction with atypical features including: extension over more than one arterial territories/not conforming to typical arterial distribution, sparing of overlying cortex, early hemorrhage, marked edema [66]	CT (hypodensity) or MRI (restricted diffusion)	Non-invasive	Indirect
Venous hemorrhage	Intracerebral hemorrhage, often near the site of thrombosed venous sinus/cortical vein, may be multifocal	CT or MRI	Non-invasive	Indirect

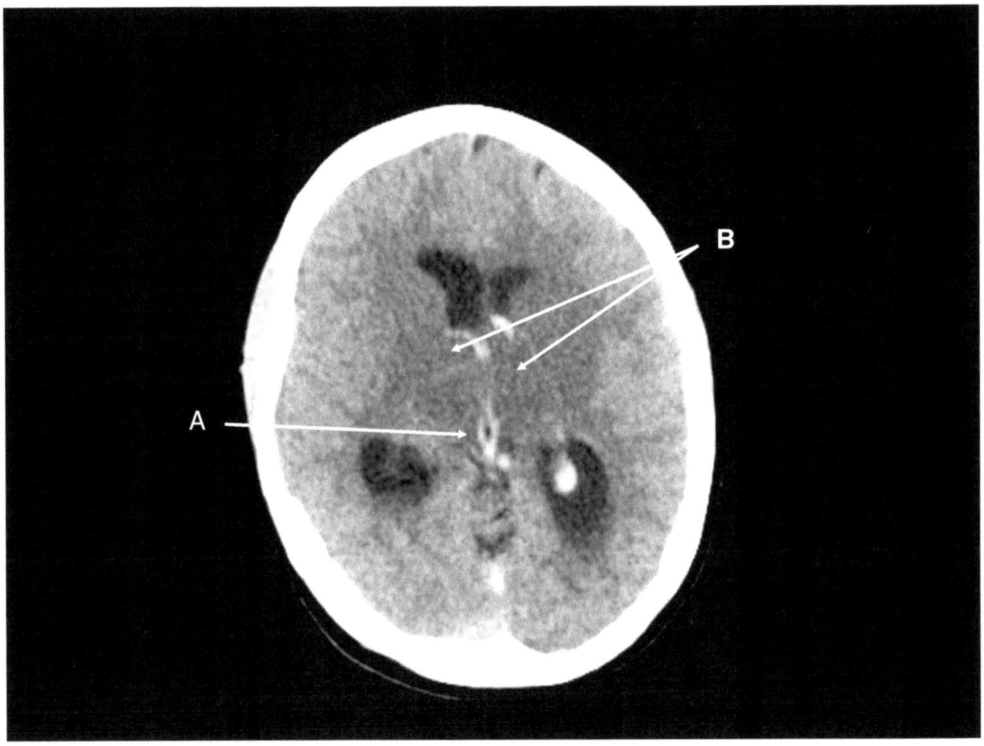

Fig. 25.2 Non-contrast head CT demonstrating hyperdensity in the deep cerebral veins consistent with thrombosis (**a**) and bilateral thalamic and subcortical hypodensity consistent with deep cerebral edema due to impaired venous drainage (**b**)

rhage, or swelling in an unusual location (e.g., posterior temporal lobe) or crossing arterial territories should prompt consideration of CVST. Second, given the distinct anatomy of the cerebral venous circulation, bilateral lesions are common. Specific examples include bithalamic infarction from deep cerebral vein thrombosis (Fig. 25.2) and bilateral parasagittal injury from superior sagittal sinus thrombosis [34]. Third, unlike arterial infarct, venous infarction often results in significant edema with sparing of the overlying cortex [67].

Even with advanced imaging techniques, several diagnostic pitfalls should be considered when evaluating patients with suspected CVST. Congenitally hypoplastic or atretic venous sinuses are common anatomic variants and can be confused with thrombosis of the sinus. Asymmetric transverse sinuses, in particular, may be seen in nearly half of patients [68]. Complete absence of one transverse sinus is not infrequent. Filling defects may result from normal intrasinus structures such as arachnoid granulations or intrasinus septae and thus do not always represent thrombus [69]. Consultation with an experienced neuroradiologist can help distinguish between these CVST mimics and cases of true venous thrombosis.

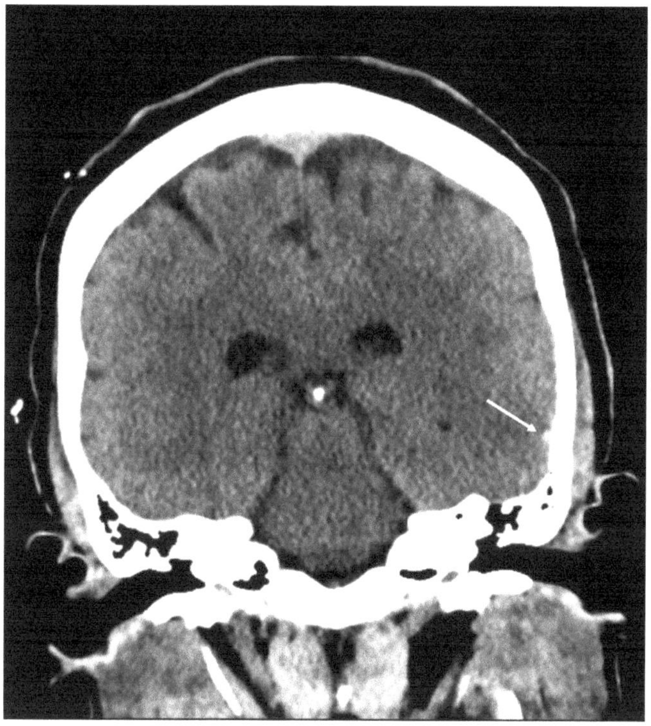

Fig. 25.3 Non-contrast head CT demonstrating hyperdensity consistent with acute thrombosis of the vein of Labbe (arrow)

Imaging Modalities

While findings on non-contrast head CT may sometimes suggest CVST (see Key Radiological Features Table and Figs. 25.3 and 25.4), sensitivity of CT alone is poor. Contrast-enhanced brain MRI has reasonable sensitivity for detection of CVST when interpreted by an experienced neuroradiologist, but in general dedicated imaging of the venous system is necessary to confirm the diagnosis. We prefer CT venography (CTV) over MR venography (MRV) given rapid image acquisition/interpretation and high sensitivity/specificity (ranging from 75% to 100% depending on the site of thrombosis), although either approach is reasonable and choice may vary depending on the clinical scenario [70, 71]. CTV may be more sensitive in detecting small cortical vein thromboses (Fig. 25.5) than MRV [70]. Unenhanced MRV (Fig. 25.6), though potentially useful in those with impaired renal function or other contraindications to IV contrast media, is particularly susceptible to artifactual flow gaps [71]. Contrast-enhanced MRV leads to better visualization of the venous system and is less prone to artifact than unenhanced MRV, and is therefore generally preferred. Brain MRI without venography may allow for direct visualization

Fig. 25.4 Non-contrast head CT showing hyperdense left transverse sinus consistent with thrombosis (**a**) and left temporal lobar hemorrhage (**b**)

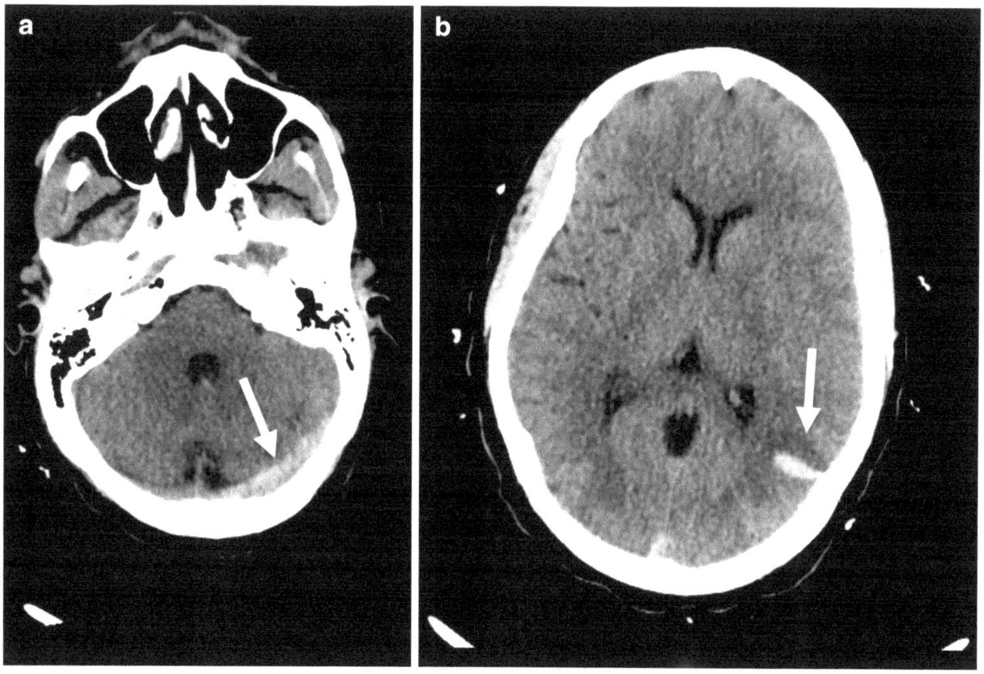

of the thrombus itself while also revealing subtle parenchymal lesions undetected on other sequences. Given the evolution of hemoglobin degradation products over time, MRI is more sensitive to venous thrombus in the subacute stage since acute thrombus may mimic normal venous flow voids on both T1 and T2 weighted images. As such, contrast-enhanced brain MRI is generally necessary. Catheter cerebral angiography may be considered in those with ambiguous non-invasive imaging findings or when there is concern for underlying dural arteriovenous fistula. However, given the high sensitivity of both CTV and MRV, catheter angiography is rarely needed for diagnosis.

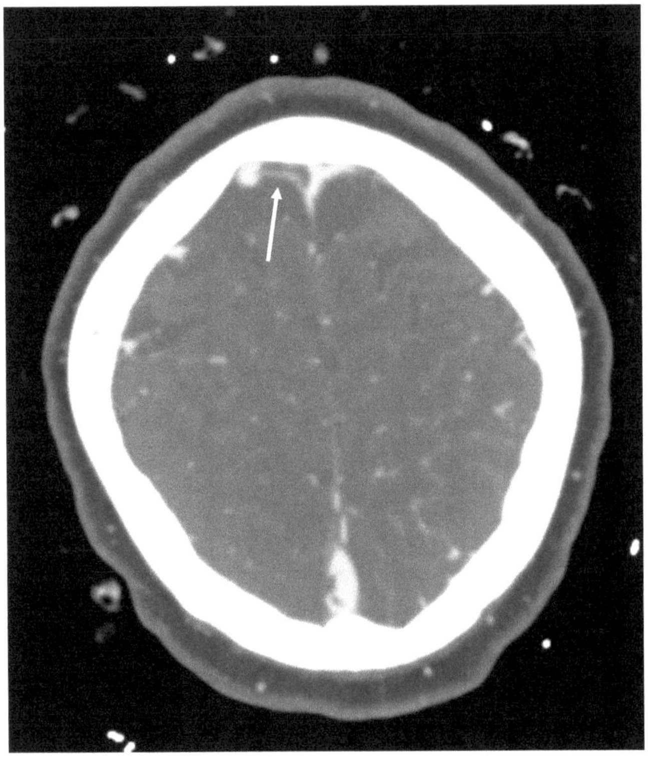

Fig. 25.5 CT venography showing filling defect in a cortical vein draining into the superior saggital sinus, consistent with cortical vein thrombosis (arrow)

Key Monitoring

If clinically stable, patients with newly diagnosed CVST should be admitted to a dedicated stroke unit for close neurological monitoring. Those with evidence of elevated intracranial pressure, intracerebral hemorrhage, recurrent seizures, or early deterioration should be admitted to an intensive care unit.

Intracranial Hypertension

In ISCVT, nearly 23% of patients presented with isolated intracranial hypertension [2]. Treatment of intracranial hypertension—either by improving venous outflow, removing CSF, or reducing CSF production—should be guided by the patient's clinical status as no optimal treatments have been identified. In the rare patient who develops non-communicating hydrocephalus from CVST-related intraventricular hemorrhage, neurosurgical consultation, and early ventriculostomy may be required [34].

Acetazolamide is a carbonic anhydrase inhibitor commonly used to treat intracranial hypertension in patients with

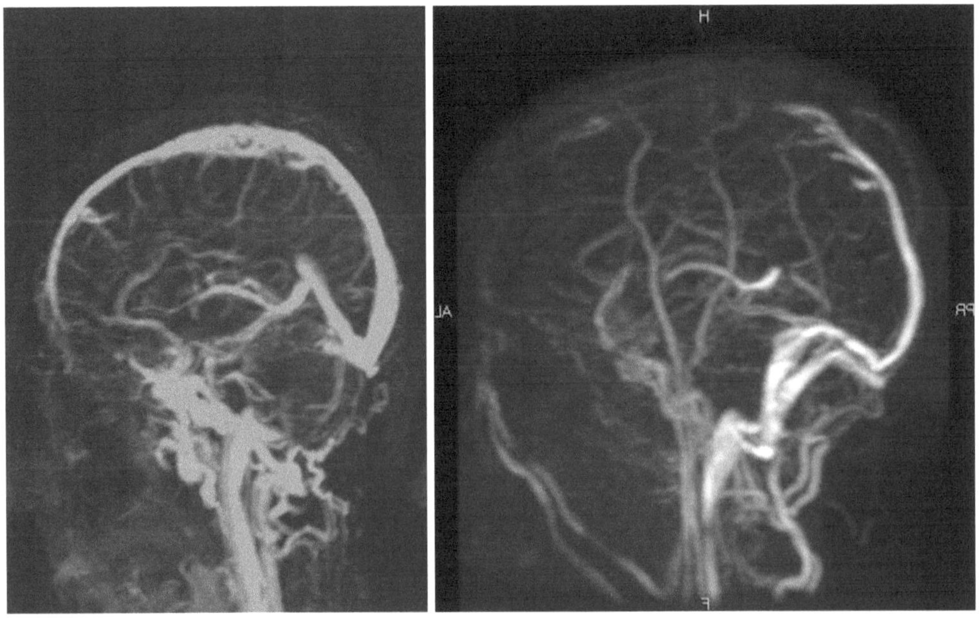

Fig. 25.6 MR venography without contrast demonstrating superior sagittal sinus thrombosis (right panel). A normal study for comparison purposes is shown in the left panel

CVST. Though reasonable to consider for symptomatic relief in those with severe headaches and/or papilledema, data supporting its use are anecdotal. The European Stroke Organization recommends against using acetazolamide in acute CVST to prevent death or improve outcome [70].

Papilledema

More than one-quarter of patients in ISCVT present with papilledema [2]. Severe vision loss, although rare, is among the most dreaded complications of CVST. The length of time between CVST diagnosis and documentation of papilledema is highly variable but may be delayed by as many as several weeks [72]. When present, the severity of papilledema and degree of associated visual field loss should be monitored early and serially with the assistance of an ophthalmologist [34].

Seizures

Nearly 40% of patients of patients in the ISCVT trial presented with seizures. More than 10% of these patients experienced a recurrent seizure within 2 weeks of establishing the diagnosis of CVST [73]. Thus close monitoring for early and recurrent seizures is paramount. Continuous EEG monitoring may be required in those with otherwise unexplained depressed consciousness to assess for non-convulsive status epilepticus. Prophylactic anticonvulsant therapy is generally not indicated in the absence of seizures; however, once a seizure has occurred, anticonvulsant therapy should be started and continued for at least several months given the high risk of seizure recurrence.

Therapeutic Anticoagulation

As most patients with CVST are started on therapeutic anticoagulation with heparin, close monitoring of coagulation studies in general—and partial thromboplastin time and platelet count in particular—is important to both ensure therapeutic dosing and monitor for dangerous complications (such as heparin-induced thrombocytopenia, bleeding, etc.).

Herniation

Though most patients with CVST experience a favorable outcome, a small subset will develop large parenchymal hematomas and/or edematous venous infarcts leading to herniation and death. Decompressive craniectomy, either with or without clot evacuation, may be necessary for such instances. Retrospective data from a large multinational registry indicate that surgical treatment is lifesaving and often leads to good functional outcomes. Importantly, even older patients and those with poor exams, appear to benefit from surgical intervention [74].

Take Home Message

CVST is a rare but important cause of cerebrovascular disease, particularly affecting young adults and those without traditional vascular risk factors. While many patients experience only minor symptoms, others will require admission to an intensive care unit due to severe neurological injury from intracerebral hemorrhage, intracranial hypertension, or seizures. As such, it is important for physicians to be aware of the protean clinical manifestations, key diagnostic studies, and preferred treatment strategies.

Further Reading

1. Stam J. Thrombosis of the cerebral veins and sinuses. N Engl J Med. 2005;352:1791–8.
2. Ferro JM, Canhao P, Stam J, Bousser MG, Barinagarrementeria F, Investigators I. Prognosis of cerebral vein and dural sinus thrombosis: Results of the international study on cerebral vein and dural sinus thrombosis (iscvt). Stroke. 2004;35:664–70.
3. Agrawal K, Burger K, Rothrock JF. Cerebral sinus thrombosis. Headache. 2016;56:1380–9.
4. Song SY, Lan D, Wu XQ, Meng R. The clinical characteristic, diagnosis, treatment, and prognosis of cerebral cortical vein thrombosis: A systematic review of 325 cases. J Thromb Thrombolysis. 2021;51:734–40.
5. Coutinho JM, Stam J, Canhao P, Barinagarrementeria F, Bousser MG, Ferro JM, et al. Cerebral venous thrombosis in the absence of headache. Stroke. 2015;46:245–7.
6. Dodick DW. Thunderclap headache. Curr Pain Headache Rep. 2002;6:226–32.
7. Essibayi MA, Oushy SH, Lanzino G, Brinjikji W. Venous causes of pulsatile tinnitus: Clinical presentation, clinical and radiographic evaluation, pathogenesis, and endovascular treatments: A literature review. Neurosurgery. 2021;89:760–8.
8. Appenzeller S, Zeller CB, Annichino-Bizzachi JM, Costallat LT, Deus-Silva L, Voetsch B, et al. Cerebral venous thrombosis: Influence of risk factors and imaging findings on prognosis. Clin Neurol Neurosurg. 2005;107:371–8.
9. Otto M, Otto V, Gotzinger R, Cordes P, Wessel K. Collet-sicard's syndrome as a result of jugular vein thrombosis. J Neurol. 2001;248:143–4.
10. Desa V, Green R. Cavernous sinus thrombosis: Current therapy. J Oral Maxillofac Surg. 2012;70:2085–91.
11. Bousser MG, Barnett HJM. Cerebral venous thrombosis. Stroke: Pathophysiology, diangosis and management. New York: Churchill-Livingstone; 1992. p. 517–37.
12. Sagduyu A, Sirin H, Mulayim S, Bademkiran F, Yunten N, Kitis O, et al. Cerebral cortical and deep venous thrombosis without sinus thrombosis: Clinical mri correlates. Acta Neurol Scand. 2006;114:254–60.
13. van den Bergh WM, van der Schaaf I, van Gijn J. The spectrum of presentations of venous infarction caused by deep cerebral vein thrombosis. Neurology. 2005;65:192–6.

14. Yamini B, Loch Macdonald R, Rosenblum J. Treatment of deep cerebral venous thrombosis by local infusion of tissue plasminogen activator. Surg Neurol. 2001;55:340–6.
15. Dentali F, Crowther M, Ageno W. Thrombophilic abnormalities, oral contraceptives, and risk of cerebral vein thrombosis: A meta-analysis. Blood. 2006;107:2766–73.
16. Beye A, Pindur G. Clinical significance of factor v leiden and prothrombin g20210a-mutations in cerebral venous thrombosis - comparison with arterial ischemic stroke. Clin Hemorheol Microcirc. 2017;67:261–6.
17. Martinelli I, Sacchi E, Landi G, Taioli E, Duca F, Mannucci PM. High risk of cerebral-vein thrombosis in carriers of a prothrombin-gene mutation and in users of oral contraceptives. N Engl J Med. 1998;338:1793–7.
18. Bombeli T, Basic A, Fehr J. Prevalence of hereditary thrombophilia in patients with thrombosis in different venous systems. Am J Hematol. 2002;70:126–32.
19. Martinelli I, Battaglioli T, Pedotti P, Cattaneo M, Mannucci PM. Hyperhomocysteinemia in cerebral vein thrombosis. Blood. 2003;102:1363–6.
20. Toole JF, Malinow MR, Chambless LE, Spence JD, Pettigrew LC, Howard VJ, et al. Lowering homocysteine in patients with ischemic stroke to prevent recurrent stroke, myocardial infarction, and death: The vitamin intervention for stroke prevention (visp) randomized controlled trial. JAMA. 2004;291:565–75.
21. Bonaa KH, Njolstad I, Ueland PM, Schirmer H, Tverdal A, Steigen T, et al. Homocysteine lowering and cardiovascular events after acute myocardial infarction. N Engl J Med. 2006;354:1578–88.
22. Huo Y, Li J, Qin X, Huang Y, Wang X, Gottesman RF, et al. Efficacy of folic acid therapy in primary prevention of stroke among adults with hypertension in china: The csppt randomized clinical trial. JAMA. 2015;313:1325–35.
23. Pengo V, Banzato A, Bison E, Zoppellaro G, Padayattil Jose S, Denas G. Efficacy and safety of rivaroxaban vs warfarin in high-risk patients with antiphospholipid syndrome: Rationale and design of the trial on rivaroxaban in antiphospholipid syndrome (traps) trial. Lupus. 2016;25:301–6.
24. Ordi-Ros J, Saez-Comet L, Perez-Conesa M, Vidal X, Riera-Mestre A, Castro-Salomo A, et al. Rivaroxaban versus vitamin k antagonist in antiphospholipid syndrome: A randomized noninferiority trial. Ann Intern Med. 2019;171:685–94.
25. Silvis SM, Hiltunen S, Lindgren E, Jood K, Zuurbier SM, Middeldorp S, et al. Cancer and risk of cerebral venous thrombosis: A case-control study. J Thromb Haemost. 2018;16:90–5.
26. Lanska DJ, Kryscio RJ. Risk factors for peripartum and postpartum stroke and intracranial venous thrombosis. Stroke. 2000;31:1274–82.
27. Cantu C, Barinagarrementeria F. Cerebral venous thrombosis associated with pregnancy and puerperium. Review of 67 cases. Stroke. 1993;24:1880–4.
28. Kamel H, Navi BB, Sriram N, Hovsepian DA, Devereux RB, Elkind MS. Risk of a thrombotic event after the 6-week postpartum period. N Engl J Med. 2014;370:1307–15.
29. Aguiar de Sousa D, Canhao P, Crassard I, Coutinho J, Arauz A, Conforto A, et al. Safety of pregnancy after cerebral venous thrombosis: Results of the iscvt (international study on cerebral vein and dural sinus thrombosis)-2 pregnancy study. Stroke. 2017;48:3130–3.
30. Amoozegar F, Ronksley PE, Sauve R, Menon BK. Hormonal contraceptives and cerebral venous thrombosis risk: A systematic review and meta-analysis. Front Neurol. 2015;6:7.
31. Aguiar de Sousa D, Romoli M, Sanchez Van Kammen M, Heldner MR, Zini A, Coutinho JM, et al. Cerebral venous thrombosis in patients with heparin-induced thrombocytopenia a systematic review. Stroke. 2022;53(6):1892–903.
32. Greinacher A, Thiele T, Warkentin TE, Weisser K, Kyrle PA, Eichinger S. Thrombotic thrombocytopenia after chadox1 ncov-19 vaccination. N Engl J Med. 2021;384:2092–101.
33. Rizk JG, Gupta A, Sardar P, Henry BM, Lewin JC, Lippi G, et al. Clinical characteristics and pharmacological management of covid-19 vaccine-induced immune thrombotic thrombocytopenia with cerebral venous sinus thrombosis: A review. JAMA Cardiol. 2021;6:1451–60.
34. Saposnik G, Barinagarrementeria F, Brown RD Jr, Bushnell CD, Cucchiara B, Cushman M, et al. Diagnosis and management of cerebral venous thrombosis: A statement for healthcare professionals from the american heart association/american stroke association. Stroke. 2011;42:1158–92.
35. deVeber G, Andrew M, Adams C, Bjornson B, Booth F, Buckley DJ, et al. Cerebral sinovenous thrombosis in children. N Engl J Med. 2001;345:417–23.
36. Caranfa JT, Yoon MK. Septic cavernous sinus thrombosis: A review. Surv Ophthalmol. 2021;66:1021–30.
37. Ochagavia AR, Boque MC, Torre C, Alonso S, Sirvent JJ. Dural venous sinus thrombosis due to cranial trauma. Lancet. 1996;347:1564.
38. Holzmann D, Huisman TA, Linder TE. Lateral dural sinus thrombosis in childhood. Laryngoscope. 1999;109:645–51.
39. Arnone GD, Kunigelis KE, Gurau A, Coulter I, Thompson J, Youssef AS. Acute sigmoid sinus compromise following skull base procedures: Is a "laissez-faire" approach best? J Neurol Surg B Skull Base. 2021;82:652–8.
40. Brugeilles H, Penisson-Besnier I, Pasco A, Oillic P, Lejeune P, Mercier P. Cerebral venous thrombosis after myelography with iopamidol. Neuroradiology. 1996;38:534–6.
41. Bienfait HP, Gijtenbeek JM, van den Bent MJ, de Bruin HG, Voogt PJ, Pillay M. Cerebral venous and sinus thrombosis with cerebrospinal fluid circulation block after the first methotrexate administration by lumbar puncture. Neuroradiology. 2002;44:929–32.
42. Ghatge S, Uppugonduri S, Kamarzaman Z. Cerebral venous sinus thrombosis following accidental dural puncture and epidural blood patch. Int J Obstet Anesth. 2008;17:267–70.
43. Einhaupl KM, Villringer A, Meister W, Mehraein S, Garner C, Pellkofer M, et al. Heparin treatment in sinus venous thrombosis. Lancet. 1991;338:597–600.
44. de Bruijn SF, Stam J. Randomized, placebo-controlled trial of anticoagulant treatment with low-molecular-weight heparin for cerebral sinus thrombosis. Stroke. 1999;30:484–8.
45. Preter M, Tzourio C, Ameri A, Bousser MG. Long-term prognosis in cerebral venous thrombosis. Follow-up of 77 patients. Stroke. 1996;27:243–6.
46. Coutinho JM, Zuurbier SM, Bousser MG, Ji X, Canhao P, Roos YB, et al. Effect of endovascular treatment with medical management vs standard care on severe cerebral venous thrombosis: The to-act randomized clinical trial. JAMA Neurol. 2020;77:966–73.
47. Ferro JM, Coutinho JM, Dentali F, Kobayashi A, Alasheev A, Canhao P, et al. Safety and efficacy of dabigatran etexilate vs dose-adjusted warfarin in patients with cerebral venous thrombosis: A randomized clinical trial. JAMA Neurol. 2019;76:1457–65.
48. Yaghi S, Shu L, Bakradze E, Salehi Omran S, Giles JA, Amar JY, et al. Direct oral anticoagulants versus warfarin in the treatment of cerebral venous thrombosis (action-cvt): A multicenter international study. Stroke. 2022;53:728–38.
49. Aguiar de Sousa D, Lucas Neto L, Canhao P, Ferro JM. Recanalization in cerebral venous thrombosis. Stroke. 2018;49:1828–35.
50. Thomas B, Krishnamoorthy T, Purkayastha S, Gupta AK. Isolated left vein of labbe thrombosis. Neurology. 2005;65:1135.
51. Singh R, Cope WP, Zhou Z, De Witt ME, Boockvar JA, Tsiouris AJ. Isolated cortical vein thrombosis: Case series. J Neurosurg. 2015;123:427–33.

52. Chang R, Friedman DP. Isolated cortical venous thrombosis presenting as subarachnoid hemorrhage: A report of three cases. AJNR Am J Neuroradiol. 2004;25:1676–9.
53. Lin A, Foroozan R, Danesh-Meyer HV, De Salvo G, Savino PJ, Sergott RC. Occurrence of cerebral venous sinus thrombosis in patients with presumed idiopathic intracranial hypertension. Ophthalmology. 2006;113:2281–4.
54. Leker RR, Steiner I. Features of dural sinus thrombosis simulating pseudotumor cerebri. Eur J Neurol. 1999;6:601–4.
55. Ebright JR, Pace MT, Niazi AF. Septic thrombosis of the cavernous sinuses. Arch Intern Med. 2001;161:2671–6.
56. Schultz NH, Sorvoll IH, Michelsen AE, Munthe LA, Lund-Johansen F, Ahlen MT, et al. Thrombosis and thrombocytopenia after chadox1 ncov-19 vaccination. N Engl J Med. 2021;384:2124–30.
57. See I, Su JR, Lale A, Woo EJ, Guh AY, Shimabukuro TT, et al. Us case reports of cerebral venous sinus thrombosis with thrombocytopenia after ad26.Cov2.S vaccination, march 2 to april 21, 2021. JAMA. 2021;325:2448–56.
58. Sharifian-Dorche M, Bahmanyar M, Sharifian-Dorche A, Mohammadi P, Nomovi M, Mowla A. Vaccine-induced immune thrombotic thrombocytopenia and cerebral venous sinus thrombosis post covid-19 vaccination; a systematic review. J Neurol Sci. 2021;428:117607.
59. Yagi Y, Asami Y, Kyoya M, Yokota T. Cerebral venous sinus thrombosis after mrna-based covid-19 vaccination. Neurol Sci. 2022;43:41–3.
60. Krzywicka K, Heldner MR, Sanchez van Kammen M, van Haaps T, Hiltunen S, Silvis SM, et al. Post-sars-cov-2-vaccination cerebral venous sinus thrombosis: An analysis of cases notified to the european medicines agency. Eur J Neurol. 2021;28:3656–62.
61. Krzywicka K, van de Munckhof A, Sanchez van Kammen M, Heldner MR, Jood K, Lindgren E, et al. Age-stratified risk of cerebral venous sinus thrombosis after sars-cov-2 vaccination. Neurology. 2022;98:e759–68.
62. Arepally GM, Ortel TL. Vaccine-induced immune thrombotic thrombocytopenia: What we know and do not know. Blood. 2021;138:293–8.
63. Wasay M, Azeemuddin M. Neuroimaging of cerebral venous thrombosis. J Neuroimaging. 2005;15:118–28.
64. Virapongse C, Cazenave C, Quisling R, Sarwar M, Hunter S. The empty delta sign: Frequency and significance in 76 cases of dural sinus thrombosis. Radiology. 1987;162:779–85.
65. Chik Y, Gottesman RF, Zeiler SR, Rosenberg J, Llinas RH. Differentiation of transverse sinus thrombosis from congenitally atretic cerebral transverse sinus with ct. Stroke. 2012;43:1968–70.
66. Forbes KP, Pipe JG, Heiserman JE. Evidence for cytotoxic edema in the pathogenesis of cerebral venous infarction. AJNR Am J Neuroradiol. 2001;22:450–5.
67. Poon MT, Fonville AF, Al-Shahi SR. Long-term prognosis after intracerebral haemorrhage: Systematic review and meta-analysis. J Neurol Neurosurg Psychiatry. 2014;85:660–7.
68. Zouaoui A, Hidden G. Cerebral venous sinuses: Anatomical variants or thrombosis? Acta Anat (Basel). 1988;133:318–24.
69. Leach JL, Fortuna RB, Jones BV, Gaskill-Shipley MF. Imaging of cerebral venous thrombosis: Current techniques, spectrum of findings, and diagnostic pitfalls. Radiographics. 2006;26(Suppl 1):S19–41; discussion S42–13.
70. Ferro JM, Bousser MG, Canhao P, Coutinho JM, Crassard I, Dentali F, et al. European stroke organization guideline for the diagnosis and treatment of cerebral venous thrombosis - endorsed by the european academy of neurology. Eur Stroke J. 2017;2:195–221.
71. Ghoneim A, Straiton J, Pollard C, Macdonald K, Jampana R. Imaging of cerebral venous thrombosis. Clin Radiol. 2020;75:254–64.
72. Liu KC, Bhatti MT, Chen JJ, Fairbanks AM, Foroozan R, McClelland CM, et al. Presentation and progression of papilledema in cerebral venous sinus thrombosis. Am J Ophthalmol. 2020;213:1–8.
73. Ferro JM, Canhao P, Bousser MG, Stam J, Barinagarrementeria F, Investigators I. Early seizures in cerebral vein and dural sinus thrombosis: Risk factors and role of antiepileptics. Stroke. 2008;39:1152–8.
74. Ferro JM, Crassard I, Coutinho JM, Canhao P, Barinagarrementeria F, Cucchiara B, et al. Decompressive surgery in cerebrovenous thrombosis: A multicenter registry and a systematic review of individual patient data. Stroke. 2011;42:2825–31.

Key/Landmark References

Coutinho JM, Zuurbier SM, Bousser MG, Ji X, Canhao P, Roos YB, et al. Effect of endovascular treatment with medical management vs standard care on severe cerebral venous thrombosis: The to-act randomized clinical trial. JAMA Neurol. 2020;77:966–73.

de Bruijn SF, Stam J. Randomized, placebo-controlled trial of anticoagulant treatment with low-molecular-weight heparin for cerebral sinus thrombosis. Stroke. 1999;30:484–8.

Ferro JM, Canhao P, Stam J, Bousser MG, Barinagarrementeria F, Investigators I. Prognosis of cerebral vein and dural sinus thrombosis: Results of the international study on cerebral vein and dural sinus thrombosis (iscvt). Stroke. 2004;35:664–70.

Ferro JM, Coutinho JM, Dentali F, Kobayashi A, Alasheev A, Canhao P, et al. Safety and efficacy of dabigatran etexilate vs dose-adjusted warfarin in patients with cerebral venous thrombosis: A randomized clinical trial. JAMA Neurol. 2019;76:1457–65.

Saposnik G, Barinagarrementeria F, Brown RD Jr, Bushnell CD, Cucchiara B, Cushman M, et al. Diagnosis and management of cerebral venous thrombosis: A statement for healthcare professionals from the american heart association/american stroke association. Stroke. 2011;42:1158–92.

Traumatic Brain Injury: Evidence-Based Medicine, Diagnosis, and Treatment

26

Jeff Vitt, Ryan Martin, and Lara L. Zimmermann

Contents

Abstract

Traumatic brain injury (TBI) is a major cause of death and disability worldwide. The initial trauma triggers a complex cascade of cellular and tissue changes with subsequent secondary injury to the vulnerable brain. Injury can result from derangements of multiple physiological parameters including blood pressure, brain oxygenation, intracranial pressure, and temperature. The monitoring and treatment of the multiple physiological derangements that often occur after TBI are important aspects of the intensive care management of this patient population, but the specific treatment thresholds for each variable and their relationship to outcome are varied. The focus of this chapter is on severe traumatic brain injury and its treatment with an emphasis on the updated recommendations

J. Vitt · R. Martin · L. L. Zimmermann (✉)
Department of Neurological Surgery, UC Davis Health, Sacramento, CA, USA
e-mail: LLZimmermann@ucdavis.edu

E. Mahanna Gabrielli et al. (eds.), *Textbook of Neurointensive Care: Volume 1*, https://doi.org/10.1007/978-3-031-62220-5_26

from the Fourth Edition of the "Brain Trauma Foundation's Guidelines for the Management of Severe Traumatic Brain Injury."

Epidemiology

Traumatic brain injury (TBI) is a major public health concern in the U.S. and globally. While the incidence of TBI is highest in North America and Europe, the largest burden of disease occurs in low- and middle-income countries [1]. Worldwide, over 27 million people suffered a TBI in 2016 [2]. Another published model estimates that 69 million people may experience a TBI annually, of which over five million may suffer a severe TBI [1]. In the US, the latest report from the Centers for Disease Control and Prevention (CDC) estimates 2.87 million people suffered a TBI in 2014, including over 837,000 children. This is a 53% increase from 2006 when there was approximately 1.88 million TBI-related emergency department (ED) visits, hospitalizations, and deaths. Of those individuals who present to the ED with TBI, 288,000 are hospitalized and 56,800 die, including over 2500 deaths in children [3].

While CDC data show increased rates of TBI and TBI hospitalization among all common mechanisms of injury, age-adjusted rates of hospitalization and death have decreased by 8% and 6% respectively, from 2006 to 2014 [3]. These changes likely reflect decreased age-adjusted rates of TBI-related hospitalizations and deaths from motor vehicle crashes indicating real progress in motor vehicle safety. Unfortunately, over this same period, rates of TBI deaths due to intentional self-harm increased, mirroring the increasing US suicide rate.

The most common mechanisms of TBI are falls (47.9%), being stuck by or against an object (17.1%), and motor vehicle crashes (13.2%). Falls (52%) and motor vehicle crashes (20%) are the most common mechanisms leading to hospitalization. Unfortunately, intentional self-harm (32.5%), falls (28%), and motor vehicle crashes (18.7%) are the most common mechanisms leading to TBI-related deaths. Adults older than 75 years, followed by children (ages 0–4 years) and young adults (15–24 years) are most likely to sustain a TBI. Rates of TBI-related hospitalizations and deaths were highest among adults 75 years and older [3, 4].

Several limitations and challenges involved in the study of the epidemiology of TBI have been described in the literature [5–8]. These limitations include different study methods, underestimation of TBI due to exclusion of individuals who did not or could not seek medical attention or who were treated in the outpatient setting, exclusion of TBI cases from federal, military, or VA hospitals, and limitations relating to the coding used to identify the TBI cases [5, 6].

Pathophysiology

Severe head trauma occurs and triggers cascade of cellular and tissue derangements that lead to ongoing or secondary brain injury. Shear forces damage vascular structures, causing direct axonal injury as well as cell membrane depolarization with neurotransmitter release and resulting excitotoxicity [9]. Oxidative stress, inflammation, and calcium-mediated mitochondrial dysfunction play an important role [10, 11]. Intracellular levels of calcium are elevated in neurons after TBI, leading to the activation of multiple intracellular enzymes that impair mitochondrial function and result in energy failure, apoptosis, and necrotic cell death [12, 13]. Cerebral blood flow is frequently decreased in the first days after severe TBI, which puts patients at risk for episodes of critical brain ischemia. Optimizing cerebral blood flow and reducing brain ischemia are priorities in the critical care management of patients with TBI [14]. In addition to decreased cerebral blood flow, disruptions in brain glucose metabolism are common and can lead to metabolic crisis [15, 16]. This dynamic metabolic impairment serves to heighten brain tissue vulnerability after trauma. These alterations of metabolism and blood flow can be demonstrated at the bedside by low brain tissue oxygen tension and deranged brain chemistry seen with cerebral microdialysis.

This environment of high energy requirements in the setting of impaired substrate delivery caused by systemic hypotension, hypoxia, and local mass effect from elevated intracranial pressure has potentially disastrous consequences. In total, these factors lead to secondary insults that are often fatal to exquisitely vulnerable neural tissue.

Diagnosis

Traumatic brain injury (TBI) has a broad spectrum of severity, pathology, physiology, and sequelae. Because of this, there are numerous ways in which to describe and classify TBI.

Primary brain injury is commonly described as those events associated with the acute impact or event. This includes acute depolarization of neuronal membranes and efflux of excitatory neurotransmitters such as glutamate as well as shearing injury to axons and vascular structures.

Secondary injury includes a constellation of hemodynamic, electrical, and metabolic events which can impair the adequate delivery of metabolic substrate and may increase tissue demand. These include hypotension, hypoxia, fever, seizures, elevated intracranial pressure, and anemia.

Mechanistic descriptions of TBI are common: for example, blunt force as opposed to penetrating or blast injury. The terms "mild," "moderate," and "severe" are often used to categorize patients. This is a clinical approach that uses the

Table 26.1 Glasgow Coma Scale

Eye opening	
Spontaneous	4
To sound	3
To pain	2
None	1
Verbal response	
Oriented	5
Confused conversation	4
Inappropriate words	3
Incomprehensible sounds	2
None	1
Motor response	
Obeys commands	6
Localize to pain	5
Flexion (withdrawal)	4
Flexion (abnormal)	3
Extension	2
None	1

Adapted with kind permission of Springer Science + Business Media from Teasdale and Jennett [17]

Glasgow Coma Scale (GCS, Table 26.1) [17] to stratify patients with mild GCS 13–15, moderate GCS 9–12, and severe GCS 3–8.

Categorization of TBI based on the initial CT scan can use an imaging grading system such as the Marshall CT score or the Rotterdam score [18, 19] or describe the structural lesions seen on CT such as subdural, epidural, intraparenchymal hematomas, traumatic subarachnoid hemorrhage, or axonal shearing injury.

In reality, each of these approaches has distinct strengths and weaknesses, and none are able to completely encompass the heterogeneity of clinical TBI. A combination of a clinical and image-based description is often helpful. For example, a patient with a "severe TBI with an acute subdural hematoma and midline shift" would be likely to need urgent surgical therapy.

Patients who sustain a TBI often have associated injuries to the chest, abdomen, or extremities. The Injury Severity Scale (ISS) [20] is used to document the combined impact of multiple injuries. Patients with TBI and polytrauma are at risk for hypoxic and ischemic complications that may increase their risk of secondary brain injury. Such patients are among the most challenging for the neuro-intensivist to treat, yet their outcomes maybe excellent.

Treatment of Severe TBI

The Brain Trauma Foundation (BTF) has five sets of published guidelines on the management of TBI [21]. These include guidelines on medical management, surgical management, field management of combat-related injury, prehospital management, and management of pediatric TBI. These form the foundation of evidence-based clinical therapy for patients with acute traumatic brain injuries.

A key aspect in the intensive care management of patients with severe TBI relates to the monitoring, maintenance, and treatment of derangements of multiple physiological parameters that are potential causes for secondary injury in the vulnerable TBI brain. The specific treatment thresholds to target for these variables and the relationship of the different physiological parameters—individually or in combination—to outcome vary depending on the particular variable and at times are not well defined.

Some of the physiological parameters that have been studied in the severe TBI population include blood pressure (BP), intracranial pressure (ICP), cerebral perfusion pressure (CPP), systemic oxygenation, brain tissue oxygen tension ($PbtO_2$), brain chemistry (measured with cerebral microdialysis), and brain temperature (Table 26.2). It is intuitive that derangements in the physiological variables such as hypotension, hypoxia, high ICP, and fever should be avoided, but the range of values in which to maintain the different parameters is not always well defined. Other variables such as CPP, brain oxygen, and brain chemistry also lack consistent treatment threshold values.

Blood pressure, temperature, and oxygenation (PaO_2 and SaO_2) monitoring should be routinely performed in patients with severe TBI, and ICP monitoring is indicated in most cases. Specifically, patients in coma, with an abnormal CT scan, or those with a nonrevealing CT scan and older age, hypotension, or posturing on exam should receive ICP monitoring. Other variables such as indexes of autoregulation, $PbtO_2$, and measures of brain chemistry by microdialysis may be useful in directing and optimizing the clinical management of these patients. The advent of multimodality monitoring has opened an avenue for exploring the impact of multiple physiological measures on secondary injury and outcome after TBI.

Table 26.2 Key physiological parameters in severe TBI (based on the BTF guidelines)

Blood pressure	Target SBP > = 110 mmHg in patients 15–49 or > 70 years Target SBP > = 100 mmHg in patients 50–69 years Avoid systolic blood pressure < 90 mmHg
	Hypotension is associated with poor outcome
Oxygenation	Avoid PaO_2 < 60 mmHg and SaO_2 < 90%
	Hypoxia is associated with poor outcome
Temperature	Avoid fever (temp >38.3)
Intracranial pressure	Treatment of ICP above 22 mmHg is recommended
Cerebral perfusion pressure (CPP)	A CPP value of approximately 60 mmHg is recommended
	Attempts to keep CPP above 70 mmHg with fluids and pressors are discouraged due to the risk of ARDS
	CPP <50 mmHg should be avoided
Brain oxygen	$PbtO_2$ < 20 mmHg and SjO_2 < 50% are recommended as treatment thresholds

Blood Pressure

Hemodynamic monitoring after severe TBI for the avoidance and timely treatment of systemic hypotension is standard-of-care. Prehospital and in-hospital hypotension (SBP < 90 mmHg) is strongly associated with increased morbidity and mortality in TBI and must be avoided [22, 23]. The BTF Guidelines, fourth Edition, provide a level III recommendation to maintain SBP ≥ 100 mmHg for patients 50–69 years or ≥ 110 mmHg for patients 15–49 or over 70 years to decrease mortality and improve outcomes [21]. These systolic BP thresholds were identified in a large retrospective cohort study of 15,733 patients with moderate-severe TBI as the thresholds associated with reduced mortality in each prespecified age groups [24]. Based on this and other prospective observational and retrospective studies [25, 26], the prior recommendation to maintain SBP > 90 mmHg was revised.

Individualized care using dynamic blood pressure and cerebral perfusion pressure (CPP) thresholds determined by an individual patient's pressure autoregulatory status and calculated 'optimal CPP' is feasible and safe [27]. A trial powered for clinical outcome has not yet been performed.

Systemic Oxygenation

Systemic hypoxia is a predictor of mortality and poor neurological outcome after TBI. Analysis of the large, prospectively collected data set of 717 patients with severe TBI from the Trauma Coma Data Bank demonstrated that hypoxia (defined as Pa02 < =60 mmHg or apnea or cyanosis in the field) was significantly associated with increased morbidity and mortality [28]. While the influence of hypoxia was less than the influence of hypotension on mortality, hypoxia occurred more frequently than hypotension in the early post-traumatic period in this cohort. McHugh and colleagues analyzed secondary insults (hypotension, hypoxia, and hypothermia) occurring prior to or on admission and their association with outcomes in TBI. They reported an overall prevalence of 20% for hypoxia on admission and identified it as a significant predictor for adverse outcomes [29]. A retrospective analysis of 13,151 patients with moderate-severe TBI showed that the adjusted odds of death for patients who suffer both hypotension and hypoxia were more than 2 times greater than those with hypotension or hypoxemia alone [30]. Post-TBI hypoxia is associated with prolonged neuroinflammation, which is one possible mechanism of secondary brain injury [31]. Monitoring oxygenation using pulse oximetry and avoiding systemic hypoxia (PaO_2 < 60 mmHg or SaO_2 < 90%) is considered good trauma care and is particularly important to prevent secondary brain injury in patients with TBI.

Intracranial Pressure (Table 26.3)

Table 26.3 ICP management protocol. Targets: Overall aim is to optimize brain perfusion and avoid secondary injury. CPP 60–70 mmHg; ICP < = 22 mmHg; Temperature < 37.5 C; CVP 6–10; maintain CPP with fluids and vasopressors as needed

Stage 1[a]
Head of the bed to 30°
Optimize sedation
Optimize analgesia
Ventilation to normocarbia
Normothermia
Vent ventricular drain for 5 min at a time if ICP >22 mmHg for >5 min
Stage 2[a]
Osmotherapy (see text for discussion)
Stage 3[a]
Mild hyperventilation (use as temporizing measure only and avoid in first 24 h after TBI)
Neuromuscular paralysis
Stage 4[a]
Barbiturates
Decompressive craniectomy for refractory ICP

Adapted from the NSICU University of Miami/Jackson Memorial Hospital protocol. Reproduced with kind permission of Springer Science + Business Media from O'Phelan et al. [32]

[a] Consider obtaining a CT Head at any stage to assess for surgically treatable changes (see discussion on surgical decompression)

Monitoring

The BTF guidelines give a level II recommendation to use ICP data to manage patients with severe TBI to reduce in-hospital and 2-week mortality [21]. While there was insufficient evidence to support a level I recommendation on this topic, the BTF guideline emphasizes that intracranial hypertension is an important cause of secondary brain injury after TBI and should be managed aggressively to optimize patient outcomes.

ICP Treatment

The fourth Edition of the BTF guidelines provides a level II recommendation to treat ICP above 22 mmHg [21]. The management of elevated ICP generally follows a tiered approach. Initial steps include general measures such as positioning the neck midline and head of the bed at 30°, providing adequate analgesia and sedation, normalizing pCO_2 pH, and temperature, and CSF drainage. If ICP is not controlled after this initial stage, potential therapies include osmotherapy, hyperventilation, paralysis, and consideration of surgical decompression and/or barbiturates.

Osmotherapy

Mannitol and hypertonic saline are hyperosmolar therapies used to treat cerebral edema and lower ICP. Both drugs work by generating an osmotic gradient between the intracellular and extracellular compartments of the brain, driving fluid from endothelial cells into the cerebral vasculature and thereby decreasing total brain water content and intracranial pressure. The two pharmacotherapies have not been compared to each other in a prospective randomized study to determine comparative efficacy on ICP control or clinical outcome. The authors of the fourth Edition of the BTF Guidelines agreed that mannitol and hypertonic saline are useful in the treatment of patients with TBI but concluded that while hyperosmolar therapy lowers ICP, there was insufficient data on the effects of hyperosmolar therapy on clinical outcomes to make a recommendation for its use in severe TBI [21].

The Neurocritical Care Society published Guidelines for the Acute Treatment of Cerebral Edema in Neurocritical Care Patients in 2020 [33]. Regarding the treatment of cerebral edema in patients with TBI, they suggested using hypertonic sodium solutions over mannitol for the early management of cerebral edema/high ICP due to its non-inferior safety profile and slight advantage related to fluid resuscitation and increased cerebral perfusion benefits. Mannitol is an effective alternative. Neither mannitol nor hypertonic saline is suggested in the prehospital setting due to studies showing no potential benefit in the prehospital setting [33].

There is a lack of evidence to support the recommendations on whether hypertonic saline (HTS) treatment should be used as a bolus or continuous infusion and what the optimal concentration used should be [23]. In general, serum osmolality and sodium should be measured every 6 h to guide osmotic therapy. Mannitol should not be administered if the serum osmolality exceeds 320 mOsm. If hypertonic saline is being administered concomitantly, the osmolar gap can be calculated to monitor renal clearance of mannitol. Mannitol doses should be held if the osmolar gap exceeds 20 mmol/L.

Sorani and colleagues [34] reported that mannitol lowers ICP in a dose-dependent fashion with 100 gm doses resulting in a larger and more long-lasting reduction in ICP than a 50 gm dose. Interestingly, patients with ICP lower than 20 mmHg at the time of mannitol administration had a lower decrease in ICP, which they conclude argues against prophylactic mannitol administration [34]. Ideally, mannitol dosing should be individualized according to each patient's potential for complications and their need for ICP control. Oddo and coworkers [35] compared hypertonic saline to mannitol for refractory ICP elevation. They found that hypertonic saline reduced ICP as well as improved brain oxygen, CPP, and cardiac output when given as a second-tier therapy for refractory ICP in patients with severe TBI. They analyzed 12 patients who had severe TBI, ICP, and $PbtO_2$ monitoring and were treated with mannitol (25%, 0.75 g/kg) for ICP >20 mmHg or hypertonic saline (7.5%, 250 mL) if mannitol did not control ICP. Hypertonic saline was associated with an improvement in $PbtO_2$, whereas mannitol was not. They also observed lower ICP and higher CPP and cardiac output with hypertonic saline. The impact of HTS on $PbtO_2$ was thought to be possibly due to its effects on CBF or due to cardiac output augmentation with subsequent increase in oxygen delivery or improvement of flow in the cerebral microcirculation. The authors acknowledge that the question of the superiority of HTS vs. mannitol cannot be drawn from their study given limitations that include small numbers and the treatments not being compared in parallel (HTS was administered after mannitol in all patients); also, there may have been a cumulative effect and the fact that the treatments were not given in equi-osmolar doses [35]. Other studies have also shown the effects of HTS on CPP, brain oxygenation, and ICP. Pascual and coworkers [36] reported a study of 12 hypotensive patients with severe TBI who had CPP and $PbtO_2$ monitoring and received HTS infusions (250 cc of 7.5% saline over 30 min). HTS administration resulted in ICP reductions by more than 45% and elevation of CPP and brain oxygen [36]. In another study examining the role of 23.4% hypertonic saline in patients with severe TBI, Rockswold and colleagues reported 25 patients who received 30 mL of 23.4% hypertonic saline boluses for ICP >20 mmHg after having failed mild hyperventilation, CSF drainage, and sedation. There was a decrease in ICP with increase in CPP levels and $PbtO_2$ values, with a more significant response in patients with higher baseline ICP and lower CPP [37].

There is currently no definitive data to support the use of one osmotic agent over another (mannitol vs. HTS) for the treatment of elevated ICP. Given the different potential benefits and complication profiles for each therapy, the patient's renal, cardiac, electrolyte, and hemodynamic status may play a role in the determination of which therapy to use in a given patient, e.g., HTS in the setting of hypotension and renal failure vs. mannitol in the setting of hypernatremia or volume overload. Neuro-intensivists should be aware of the potential for cumulative nephrotoxicity in septic patients, those on aminoglycoside antibiotics, the elderly, and those with a history of renal disease, and avoid high osmolarity (>320 mOsm) in those cases in particular.

Hyperventilation

It is important to avoid hyperventilation in patients with severe TBI unless there are signs of brain herniation such as a dilated or non-reactive pupil, Cushing reflex (hypertension plus bradycardia), or extensor/decerebrate posturing. Hyperventilation reduces cerebral blood flow and is associated with increased mortality [38]. The BTF Guidelines, fourth Edition, provide a level IIb recommendation that prolonged prophylactic hyperventilation driving the partial pressure of carbon dioxide in arterial blood to 25 mm or less is not recommended. Hyperventilation may be used as a temporizing measure to reverse brain herniation or elevated ICP until definitive surgical treatment can be provided. Monitoring of brain oxygen with the use of a brain tissue oxygen monitor or jugular venous oxygen saturation monitor should be considered if a hyperventilation strategy is used [23].

Paralysis

Pharmacological neuromuscular paralysis is a strategy for the management of high ICP refractory to first-line therapies such as head-of-bed elevation, CSF diversion, hyperosmolar therapy, and sedation. Therapeutic pharmacological paralysis may be considered in the clinical setting of an intubated patient with high ICP associated with coughing/suctioning or other patient-ventilator asynchrony to blunt the asynchrony-associated increases in intrathoracic pressure, which may lead to elevated venous pressures, increased cerebral blood volume, reduced cerebral venous outflow, increased ICP and reduced cerebral blood flow [39]. While experience suggests that initiation of neuromuscular paralysis is sometimes effective to lower ICP, there is limited data showing benefits on cerebral edema/ICP, mortality, or functional outcome in traumatic brain injury.

In a retrospective review of 514 patients from the traumatic coma data bank, Hsiang and colleagues compared patients that had pharmacological paralysis early in the ICU course and lasting for at least 12 h to patients that did not receive paralytics. They published that early routine use of paralytics for ICP management does not improve overall outcomes and can lead to greater ICU stay and higher rate of complications such as pneumonia [40]. Sanfilippo and colleagues performed a systematic review of neuromuscular paralysis for management of elevated ICP in TBI and reported a paucity of evidence on the effect of neuromuscular paralysis on the outcome of patients with TBI [41]. Currently, the use of paralytics for the management of elevated ICP should be reserved for cases refractory to first-line therapies.

Hypothermia

The fourth Edition of the BTF guidelines recommends against early, prophylactic hypothermia in patients with blunt head trauma [21]. While, a large number of preclinical experimental data supports the use of therapeutic hypothermia for neuroprotection in TBI [42], high-quality clinical trials in humans have failed to show translation into a clinical benefit [43–46].

The Hypothermia for Intracranial Hypertension after Traumatic Brain Injury (Eurotherm 3235 Trial) randomized 387 adults with severe TBI and ICP greater than 20 mmHg despite stage 1 treatments to hypothermia (32–35 °C) plus standard care or standard care alone. Hypothermia was maintained for at least 48 h and continued as long as necessary to keep ICP less than 20 mmHg. The primary outcome was neurological function measured by the Extended Glasgow Outcome Scale at 6 months. Therapeutic hypothermia plus standard care did not result in better outcomes than standard care alone. There was also an increased risk of death at 6 months in the hypothermia group [45].

The Prophylactic Hypothermia Trial to Lessen Traumatic Brain Injury (POLAR-RCT) randomized 511 patients with severe TBI to prophylactic hypothermia (33–35 °C) or normothermia (37 °C) for at least 72 h and up to 7 days followed by gradual rewarming. The primary outcome was neurological function measured by the Extended Glasgow Outcome Scale at 6 months. Early prophylactic hypothermia did not improve neurological outcomes at 6 months [46]. A meta-analysis of the effects of therapeutic hypothermia in adults with severe TBI, largely influenced by the results of these two high-quality randomized controlled trials, found that hypothermia does not reduce and may increase mortality in severe TBI [47]. In summary, neither prophylactic hypothermia nor the use of early hypothermia for treatment of high ICP is beneficial for adults with severe TBI and is not currently recommended.

Surgical Decompression

Some patients will require surgical therapy for their traumatic brain injury. The available literature suggests that the speed and aggressiveness of surgical management will greatly impact patient outcomes [48, 49]. To this end, the Brain Trauma Foundation published guidelines in 2006 for the surgical management of traumatic brain injury based on the available literature published between 1975 and 2001 [50]. As of this writing, these have not been revised. Additionally, the guidelines for management of severe TBI fourth edition added a new section addressing recommendation for decompressive craniectomy in 2016 [21]. The Rescue ICP [51] Trial was published later that year examining the effect of decompressive craniectomy in patients with traumatic brain injury and refractory ICP elevation. We will briefly review the major recommendations and their supporting rationale:

- *Epidural hematoma*: 10% of patients with severe traumatic brain injury have acute epidural hematomas requiring craniotomy [52, 53]. It is recommended that lesions measuring greater than 30 cc in volume should be surgically evacuated. Nonoperative management is appropriate in awake patients without focal deficits and lesions less than 30 cc, less than 15 mm thickness with less than 5 mm midline shift. The timing of therapy is also important. Comatose patients with pupillary changes should have surgical evacuation as soon as possible. Ipsilateral mydriasis is not associated with adverse outcomes if surgical evacuation is performed within 70 min [54]. However, bilateral mydriasis is associated with poor outcomes related to brainstem injury.
- *Acute subdural hematoma*: 15–30% of severe TBI patients have an acute subdural hematoma on imaging. Surgical evacuation is recommended for lesions that are greater than 10 mm in thickness or associated with a greater than 5 mm midline shift. It is also recommended to perform intracranial pressure monitoring in patients with acute subdural hematomas and a Glasgow Coma Scale score of less than nine. Indications for surgical management of lesions less than 10 mm in thickness or with less than 5 mm shift are recommended if patients deteriorate by two points on the GCS or have an elevated ICP >20.
- *Traumatic parenchymal hemorrhage*: These account for 20% of operative lesions in patients with severe TBI [55, 56]. Because the mass effect from large parenchymal lesions may cause secondary injury, some patients with this type of injury would likely benefit from surgical therapy. However, the particular characteristics of this group are as yet unclear. The majority of available data is taken from case series and one prospective trial [57]. Thus, the decision to proceed with surgical therapy is often based on a pattern of progressing deficit or uncontrolled ICP. Surgical therapy is recommended for patients with progressive clinical deterioration referable to the lesion, medically refractory elevation in ICP, or evidence of mass effect on CT imaging. Surgical treatment is also recommended for frontotemporal lesions >20 cc in volume associated with midline shift >5 mm or compressed basal cisterns.
- *Posterior fossa lesions*: Extra-axial lesions in the posterior fossa are relatively rare in severe TBI with the potential to produce rapid clinical deterioration because of the limited size of the posterior fossa and the risks of brainstem compression and hydrocephalus. Surgical therapy of posterior fossa lesions is recommended if there is evidence of progressive clinical deterioration referable to the lesion or mass effect referable to the lesions such as distortion of the fourth ventricle, compression of the basal cisterns, or obstructive hydrocephalous. Surgical therapy in these patients typically involves evacuation of the hematoma and a suboccipital craniectomy.
- *Decompressive Craniectomy*: Surgical removal of a portion of the skull is performed in order to decrease intracranial pressure. Various surgical techniques exist. A large frontotemporoparietal decompressive craniectomy with a diameter not less than 12 x 15 cm is recommended over a small frontotemporal craniectomy to reduce mortality in patients with severe TBI [21]. Reduction in mortality and in ICP has been consistently found in patients treated with decompressive craniectomy. However improved functional outcome has not been supported by high quality evidence [51].

Steroids

Steroids are not recommended in TBI for reducing ICP or improving outcomes [21]. The corticosteroid randomization after significant head injury (CRASH) trial randomized 10,008 head injury patients within 8 h of injury to a 48-h methylprednisolone infusion or placebo. The risk of death and death or severe disability was higher in the steroid group [58]. For this reason, high-dose methylprednisolone is contraindicated in severe TBI. This is the only Level 1 recommendation in the Fourth Edition of the Brain Trauma Foundation's Guidelines for the Management of Severe TBI.

Sedation

Sedation with propofol or pentobarbital may be used to lower ICP by reducing cerebral metabolism coupled with reduced cerebral blood flow and thereby lower cerebral blood volume and ICP. The BTF guidelines provide a level II recommendation for use of propofol to control ICP and high-dose barbiturate to reduce high ICP refractory to standard medical and surgical treatment. Studies do not demonstrate an improvement in survival or functional outcome with use of propofol or barbiturates [59] and barbiturates to induce burst suppression on EEG as prophylaxis against high ICP is not recommended. Blood pressure must be monitored closely because both high-dose propofol and barbiturates can cause hypotension.

CPP/Autoregulation

The fourth Edition of the BTF guidelines recommends using a guideline-based recommendation for CPP monitoring [21] but does not suggest a CPP threshold. The previous third Edition BTF guidelines made a level III recommendation to keep CPP between 50–70 mmHg, with a general CPP target of 60 mmHg [23]. It remains common practice to keep a CPP target of 60 mm Hg. They note that the parameters used to calculate CPP (blood pressure and ICP) have been shown to individually correlate to outcome after TBI since both hypotension and elevated ICP have been associated with poor outcome. They also state that there is no defined critical lower threshold of CPP that is associated with cerebral ischemia or poor outcome, but suggest that a CPP of 50–60 mmHg appears to be a critical lower threshold range for ischemia [23].

The target CPP in a given patient may ultimately vary depending on the individual's autoregulatory status. (For a discussion on the methods and indices used to measure autoregulation, refer to the neuromonitoring chapters: Chaps. 7 and 8.) A study by Jaeger and colleagues supports the concept of determining individual optimal cerebral perfusion pressure based on measures of cerebrovascular pressure reactivity [60]. Howells and colleagues analyzed a group of patients treated with ICP-oriented vs. CPP-oriented protocols in two different centers. They concluded that the pressure reactivity index can identify the most appropriate treatment strategy in a given patient. They found that in pressure-passive patients, ICP-oriented therapy resulted in better outcomes, and in pressure-active and pressure-stable TBI patients, the CPP-oriented therapy was more beneficial [61]. In a study by Johnson and colleagues, patients with impaired cerebral pressure autoregulation with lower CPP had a more favorable outcome compared to patients with higher CPP. No difference in outcome was seen with different CPP levels in patients with intact autoregulation [62].

Brain Tissue Oxygen Tension ($PbtO_2$)

Low brain tissue oxygen tension ($PbtO_2$) is associated with poor outcomes following severe TBI. Brain tissue oxygen tension is measured with a probe placed directly into the brain parenchyma, usually into the frontal lobe subcortical white matter, approximately 3 cm below the inner table of the skull. Brain tissue oxygen tension is determined by cerebral blood flow as well as the arteriovenous oxygen tension difference and reflects diffusion of dissolved plasma oxygen across the blood–brain barrier more than total oxygen delivery or cerebral oxygen metabolism [63]. Brain tissue oxygen tension monitoring is used in addition to, but not in place of, ICP monitoring for patients with severe TBI. When $PbtO_2$ monitoring is used, a treatment threshold of $PbtO_2 < 20$ mmHg for 5 min warrants intervention. If ICP is elevated, then treatments to lower ICP should be prioritized as this often results in improved brain tissue oxygen tension via improvement in CPP. Medical therapies to improve brain tissue oxygen tension include interventions to (1) decrease cerebral oxygen demand, (2) increase cerebral oxygen supply, or both. Interventions that decrease cerebral oxygen demand include preventing fever, controlling shivering, preventing seizures, and optimizing sedation. Interventions that increase oxygen supply include optimizing ventilation, CPP augmentation and increasing arterial oxygen content [64]. Treatment of patients with severe TBI guided by $PbtO_2$ plus ICP monitoring is safe, feasible, and reduces brain tissue hypoxia with a trend toward improved outcomes [65]. **B**rain tissue **O**xygen **O**ptimization in **S**evere **T**BI (BOOST-3) is a phase III randomized controlled trial currently in process to determine whether treatment guided by $PbtO_2$ and ICP leads to better neurological outcomes compared to treatment guided by ICP monitoring alone [66].

Brain Chemistry (Microdialysis)

Assessment of brain chemistry by microdialysis has the potential to aid in the management of severe TBI patients in conjunction with the other physiological variables discussed previously. Cerebral microdialysis measures brain metabolism by directly sampling the extracellular metabolites, lactate, pyruvate, glycerol, and glucose. Metabolic crisis is an impaired redox state in the brain, defined as an increased lactate/pyruvate ratio with low extracellular glucose. In one observational study of 76 patients with severe TBI, adequately resuscitated with well-controlled ICP, 74% experienced metabolic crisis in the first 72 h after injury [67]. In one of the largest TBI studies to date on microdialysis monitoring, Timofeev and coworkers studied 223 patients (75% with severe TBI) and found on multivariate analysis that metabolic crisis had a significant association with increased mortality. Also, higher cerebral glucose was associated with increased mortality, and higher pyruvate was associated with reduced mortality [68]. Definitive data are currently lacking regarding the potential impact that targeting the different derangements in the measured brain chemistry parameters would have on patients with TBI, but future research will likely shed light on the subject.

Seizure Prophylaxis

Posttraumatic seizures (PTS) are commonly defined as 'early' if they occur within 7 days of injury and 'late' if they occur more than 7 days after injury. Early PTS are not benign and may result in secondary brain injury through cerebral metabolic crisis [69], cerebral edema [70], and increased intracranial pressure [71]. Seizure prophylaxis is recommended for the first 7 days after TBI to reduce the risk of early post-traumatic seizures [21]. This recommendation is largely based on the randomized, double-blind trial performed by Temkin and colleagues that evaluated the effectiveness of phenytoin for the prevention of posttraumatic seizures in 404 adult patients with moderate-severe

TBI. Treatment with phenytoin reduced the incidence of early posttraumatic seizures (3.6% vs. 14.2%) but did not reduce the risk of late PTS or post-traumatic epilepsy [72]. Other studies of valproate, phenobarbital, carbamazepine, and magnesium also failed to show benefit in the prevention of posttraumatic epilepsy. Therefore, prophylactic administration of antiseizure medications beyond 7 days is not recommended unless a patient experiences a late post-traumatic seizure. Patients who experience a late posttraumatic seizure are at high risk of seizure recurrence and antiseizure treatment must be resumed.

Neurocritical care practice shifted from using phenytoin to using levetiracetam to prevent early PTS, likely due to leviteracitam's safety profile, lack of requirement for serum drug level monitoring, limited drug interactions, and emerging data that levetiracetam is an effective alternative to phenytoin/fosphenytoin for seizure prophylaxis after TBI [73, 74]. Recent meta-analyses [75, 76] identified no significant difference in the incidence of early seizures with levetiracetam versus phenytoin. Unfortunately, no treatment has been identified to reduce the risk of late post-traumatic seizures, or post-traumatic epilepsy.

Nutrition

Severe TBI is associated with an increase in whole body energy metabolism, but recent data suggest that there is a high degree of variability in resting energy expenditure. Furthermore, modern critical care treatments, such as sedation and temperature management, likely influence and may blunt this response. The BTF guidelines provide a level II recommendation to feed patients to achieve basal caloric replacement by the fifth to seventh day post-injury to decrease mortality. Transgastric jejunal feeding is recommended over gastric feeds to reduce the incidence of ventilator-associated pneumonia [21]. In children, early enteral nutrition within 72 h of injury is suggested to decrease mortality and improve outcomes (level III recommendation) [77].

Conclusion

Overall, outcomes after traumatic brain injury have improved significantly over the past several decades. This is likely due to a combination of improvements in emergency response and prehospital care, early triage, and improved critical care. Because of the brain's exquisite vulnerability to small insults after trauma, excellent critical care is enormously important to mitigate secondary injury and improve long-term outcomes.

References

1. Dewan MC, et al. Estimating the global incidence of traumatic brain injury. J Neurosurg. 2018;130:1080–97.
2. Injury GBDTB, C. Spinal cord Injury, global, regional, and national burden of traumatic brain injury and spinal cord injury, 1990-2016: a systematic analysis for the global burden of disease study 2016. Lancet Neurol. 2019;18(1):56–87.
3. Centers for Disease Control and Prevention. Surveillance Report of Traumatic Brain Injury-related Emergency Department Visits, H., and Deaths—United States, 2014. Centers for Disease Control and Prevention, U.S. Department of Health and Human Services; 2019.
4. Centers for Disease Control and Prevention. Surveillance report of traumatic brain Injury-related deaths by age group, S., and mechanism of Injury—United States, 2018 and 2019. Centers for Disease Control and Prevention, U.S. Department of Health and Human Services; 2022.
5. Faul M, Xu L, Wald MM, Coronado VG. Traumatic brain injury in the United States: emergency department visits, hospitalizations and deaths 2002–2006. Centers for Disease Control and Prevention, National Center for Injury Prevention and Control: Atlanta; 2010.
6. Langlois JA, Rutland-Brown W, Wald MM. The epidemiology and impact of traumatic brain injury: a brief overview. J Head Trauma Rehabil. 2006;21(5):375–8.
7. Jennett B. Epidemiology of head injury. J Neurol Neurosurg Psychiatry. 1996;60(4):362–9.
8. Bruns J Jr, Hauser WA. The epidemiology of traumatic brain injury: a review. Epilepsia. 2003;44(Suppl 10):2–10.
9. Zauner A, Bullock R. The role of excitatory amino acids in severe brain trauma: opportunities for therapy: a review. J Neurotrauma. 1995;12:547–54.
10. Bullock R, Zauner A, Woodward JJ, Myseros J, Choi SC, Ward JD, Marmarou A, Young HF. Factors affecting excitatory amino acid release following severe human head injury. J Neurosurg. 1998;89:507–18.
11. Reinert MM, Bullock R. Clinical trials in head injury. Neurol Res. 1999;21:330–8.
12. Clausen T, Bullock R. Medical treatment and neuroprotection in traumatic brain injury. Curr Pharm Des. 2001;7:1517–32.
13. Fiskum G. Mechanisms of neuronal death and neuroprotection. J Neurosurg Anesthesiol. 2004;16:108–10.
14. Robertson CS, Valadka AB, Hannay HJ, Contant CF, Gopinath SP, Cormio M, Uzura M, Grossman RG. Prevention of secondary ischemic insults after severe head injury. Crit Care Med. 1999;27:2086–95.
15. Bergsneider M, Hovda DA, Shalmon E, Kelly DF, Vespa PM, Martin NA, Phelps ME, McArthur DL, Caron MJ, Kraus JF, Becker DP. Cerebral hyperglycolysis following severe traumatic brain injury in humans: a positron emission tomography study. J Neurosurg. 1997;86(2):241–51.
16. Giza CC, Hovda DA. The neurometabolic cascade of concussion. J Athl Train. 2001;36(3):228–35.
17. Teasdale G, Jennett B. Assessment and prognosis of coma after head injury. Acta Neurochir. 1976;34(1–4):45–55.
18. Marshall LF, Marshall SB, Klauber MR, Clark MB, Eisenberg HM, Jane JA, Luerssen TG, Marmarou A, Foulkes MA. A new classification of head injury based on computerized tomography. J Neurosurg. 1991;75:S14–20.
19. Maas AI, Hukkelhoven CW, Marshall LF, Steyerberg EW. Prediction of outcome in traumatic brain injury with computed tomographic characteristics: a comparison between the computed tomographic classification and combinations of computed tomographic predictors. Neurosurgery. 2005;57(6):1173–82.

20. Baker SP, O'Neill B, Haddon W Jr, Long WB. The injury severity score: a method for describing patients with multiple injuries and evaluating emergency care. J Trauma. 1974;14:187–96.
21. Carney N, et al. Guidelines for the Management of Severe Traumatic Brain Injury, Fourth Edition. Neurosurgery. 2017;80(1):6–15.
22. Butcher I, Maas AI, Lu J, Marmarou A, Murray GD, Mushkudiani NA, McHugh GS, Steyerberg EW. Prognostic value of admission blood pressure in traumatic brain injury: results from the IMPACT study. J Neurotrauma. 2007;24(2):294–302.
23. Brain Trauma Foundation; American Association of Neurological Surgeons; Congress of Neurological Surgeons; Joint Section on neurotrauma and Critical Care, AANS/CNS. Guidelines for the management of severe traumatic brain injury. J Neurotrauma. 2007;24(Suppl 1):S1–106.
24. Berry C, et al. Redefining hypotension in traumatic brain injury. Injury. 2012;43(11):1833–7.
25. Murray GD, et al. Multivariable prognostic analysis in traumatic brain injury: results from the IMPACT study. J Neurotrauma. 2007;24(2):329–37.
26. Brenner M, et al. Traditional systolic blood pressure targets underestimate hypotension-induced secondary brain injury. J Trauma Acute Care Surg. 2012;72(5):1135–9.
27. Tas J, Beqiri E, van Kaam RC, et al. Targeting autoregulation-guided cerebral perfusion pressure after traumatic brain Injury (COGiTATE): a feasibility randomized controlled clinical trial. J Neurotrauma. 2021;38(20):2790–800.
28. Chesnut RM, et al. The role of secondary brain injury in determining outcome from severe head injury. J Trauma. 1993;34(2):216–22.
29. McHugh GS, Engel DC, Butcher I, Steyerberg EW, Lu J, Mushkudiani N, Hernández AV, Marmarou A, Maas AI, Murray GD. Prognostic value of secondary insults in traumatic brain injury: results from the IMPACT study. J Neurotrauma. 2007;24(2):287–93.
30. Spaite DW, et al. The effect of combined out-of-hospital hypotension and hypoxia on mortality in major traumatic brain Injury. Ann Emerg Med. 2017;69(1):62–72.
31. Yan EB, et al. Post-traumatic hypoxia is associated with prolonged cerebral cytokine production, higher serum biomarker levels, and poor outcome in patients with severe traumatic brain injury. J Neurotrauma. 2014;31(7):618–29.
32. O'Phelan KH, Mangat HS, Olvey SE, Bullock MR. Multimodal monitoring in acute brain injury. In: Bhardwaj A, Mirski MA, editors. Handbook of neurocritical care. 2nd ed. New York: Springer Science + Business Media; 2011.
33. Cook AM, et al. Guidelines for the acute treatment of cerebral edema in Neurocritical care patients. Neurocrit Care. 2020;32(3):647–66.
34. Sorani MD, Morabito D, Rosenthal G, Giacomini KM, Manley GT. Characterizing the dose-response relationship between mannitol and intracranial pressure in traumatic brain injury patients using a high-frequency physiological data collection system. J Neurotrauma. 2008;25(4):291–8.
35. Oddo M, Levine JM, Frangos S, Carrera E, Maloney-Wilensky E, Pascual JL, Kofke WA, Mayer SA, LeRoux PD. Effect of mannitol and hypertonic saline on cerebral oxygenation in patients with severe traumatic brain injury and refractory intracranial hypertension. J Neurol Neurosurg Psychiatry. 2009;80(8):916–20.
36. Pascual JL, Maloney-Wilensky E, Reilly PM, Sicoutris C, Keutmann MK, Stein SC, LeRoux PD, Gracias VH. Resuscitation of hypotensive head-injured patients: is hypertonic saline the answer? Am Surg. 2008;74(3):253–9.
37. Rockswold GL, Solid CA, Paredes-Andrade E, Rockswold SB, Jancik JT, Quickel RR. Hypertonic saline and its effect on intracranial pressure, cerebral perfusion pressure, and brain tissue oxygen. Neurosurgery. 2009;65(6):1035–41; discussion 1041–2.
38. Muizelaar JP, et al. Adverse effects of prolonged hyperventilation in patients with severe head injury: a randomized clinical trial. J Neurosurg. 1991;75(5):731–9.
39. Perry BG, et al. Cerebral hemodynamics during graded Valsalva maneuvers. Front Physiol. 2014;5:349.
40. Hsiang JK, Chesnut R, et al. Early, routine paralysis for intracranial pressure control in severe head injury: is it necessary? Crit Care Med. 1994;22:1471–6.
41. Sanfilippo F, et al. The role of neuromuscular blockade in patients with traumatic brain injury: a systematic review. Neurocrit Care. 2015;22(2):325–34.
42. Dietrich WD, Bramlett HM. The evidence for hypothermia as a neuroprotectant in traumatic brain injury. Neurotherapeutics. 2010;7(1):43–50.
43. Clifton GL, Valadka A, Zygun D, Coffey CS, Drever P, Fourwinds S, Janis LS, Wilde E, Taylor P, Harshman K, Conley A, Puccio A, Levin HS, McCauley SR, Bucholz RD, Smith KR, Schmidt JH, Scott JN, Yonas H, Okonkwo DO. Very early hypothermia induction in patients with severe brain injury (the National Acute Brain Injury Study: hypothermia II): a randomised trial. Lancet Neurol. 2011;10(2):131–9.
44. Andrews PJ, Sinclair HL, Battison CG, Polderman KH, Citerio G, Mascia L, Harris BA, Murray GD, Stocchetti N, Menon DK, Shakur H, De Backer D. Eurotherm3235Trial collaborators. European society of intensive care medicine study of therapeutic hypothermia (32–35°C) for intracranial pressure reduction after traumatic brain injury (the Eurotherm3235Trial). Trials. 2011;12:8.
45. Andrews PJD, et al. Hypothermia for intracranial hypertension after traumatic brain Injury. N Engl J Med. 2015;373(25):2403–12.
46. Cooper DJ, et al. Effect of early sustained prophylactic hypothermia on neurologic outcomes among patients with severe traumatic brain Injury: the POLAR randomized clinical trial. JAMA. 2018;320(21):2211–20.
47. Chen H, et al. A meta-analysis of the effects of therapeutic hypothermia in adult patients with traumatic brain injury. Crit Care. 2019;23(1):396.
48. Concensus conference: rehabilitation of persons with traumatic brain injury. NIH consensus development panel on rehabilitation of persons with traumatic brain Injury. JAMA. 1999;282:974–83.
49. Picard J, Bailey S, Sanderson H, Reese M, Garfeld JS. Steps towards cost benefits analysis of regional neurosurgical care. BMJ. 1990;301:629–35.
50. Bullock MR, Chesnut R, Ghajar J, Gordon D, Hartl R, Newell DW, Servadei F, Walters BC, Wilberger J. Guidelines for the surgical management of traumatic brain injury. Neurosurgery. 2006;58(Suppl 3):S21–62.
51. Hutchinson PJ, et al. Trial of Decompressive Craniectomy for traumatic intracranial hypertension. N Engl J Med. 2016;375(12):1119–30.
52. Gennarelli T, Spielman G, Langfitt T, Gildenberg P, Harrington T, Jane J, Marshall L, Miller J, Pitts L. Influence of the type of intracranial lesion on outcome from severe head injury. J Neurosurg. 1982;56:26–32.
53. Seelig J, Marshall L, Toutant S, Toole B, Klauber M, Bowers S, Varnell J. Traumatic acute epidural hematoma: unrecognized high lethality in comatose patients. Neurosurgery. 1984;15:167–620.
54. Cohen J, Montero A, Israel Z. Prognosis and clinical relevance of anisocoriacraniotomy lantency for epidural hematoma in comatose patients. J Trauma. 1996;41:120–2.
55. Miller JD, Butterworth JF, Gudeman SK, Faulkner JE, Choi SC, Selhorst JB, Harbison JW, Lutz HA, Young HF, Becker DP. Further experience in the management of severe head injury. J Neurosurg. 1981;54:289–99.
56. Wu J, Hsu C, Liao S, Wong Y. Surgical outcome of traumatic intracranial hematoma at a regional hospital in Taiwan. J Trauma. 1999;47:39–43.
57. Taylor A, Butt W, Rosenfeld J, Shann F, Ditchfield M, Lewis E, Klug G, Wallace D, Henning R, Tibballs J. A randomized trial of very early decompressive craniectomy in children with traumatic

brain injury and sustained intracranial hypertension. Childs Nerv Syst. 2001;17:154–62.

58. Edwards P, Arango M, Balica L, Cottingham R, El-Sayed H, Farrell B, Fernandes J, Gogichaisvili T, Golden N, Hartzenberg B, Husain M, Ulloa MI, Jerbi Z, Khamis H, Komolafe E, Laloë V, Lomas G, Ludwig S, Mazairac G, Muñoz SanchézMde L, Nasi L, Olldashi F, Plunkett P, Roberts I, Sandercock P, Shakur H, Soler C, Stocker R, Svoboda P, Trenkler S, Venkataramana NK, Wasserberg J, Yates D, Yutthakasemsunt S. CRASH trial collaborators. Final results of MRC CRASH, a randomised placebo-controlled trial of intravenous corticosteroid in adults with head injury-outcomes at 6 months. Lancet. 2005;365(9475):1957–9.
59. Roberts I, Sydenham E. Barbiturates for acute traumatic brain injury. Cochrane Database Syst Rev. 1999:(3):CD000033. https://doi.org/10.1002/14651858.CD000033.
60. Jaeger M, Dengl M, Meixensberger J, Schuhmann MU. Effects of cerebrovascular pressure reactivity-guided optimization of cerebral perfusion pressure on brain tissue oxygenation after traumatic brain injury. Crit Care Med. 2010;38(5):1343–7.
61. Howells T, Elf K, Jones PA, Ronne-Engström E, Piper I, Nilsson P, Andrews P, Enblad P. Pressure reactivity as a guide in the treatment of cerebral perfusion pressure in patients with brain trauma. J Neurosurg. 2005;102(2):311–7.
62. Johnson U, Nilsson P, Ronne-Engström E, Howells T, Enblad P. Favorable outcome in traumatic brain injury patients with impaired cerebral pressure autoregulation when treated at low cerebral perfusion pressure levels. Neurosurgery. 2011;68(3):714–21; discussion 721–2.
63. Rosenthal G, et al. Brain tissue oxygen tension is more indicative of oxygen diffusion than oxygen delivery and metabolism in patients with traumatic brain injury. Crit Care Med. 2008;36(6):1917–24.
64. Bohman LE, Heuer GG, Macyszyn L, Maloney-Wilensky E, Frangos S, Le Roux PD, Kofke A, Levine JM, Stiefel MF. Medical management of compromised brain oxygen in patients with severe traumatic brain injury. Neurocrit Care. 2011;14(3):361–9.
65. Okonkwo DO, et al. Brain oxygen optimization in severe traumatic brain Injury phase-II: a phase II randomized trial. Crit Care Med. 2017;45(11):1907–14.
66. Bernard F, et al. Brain oxygen optimization in severe traumatic brain Injury (BOOST-3): a multicentre, randomised, blinded-endpoint, comparative effectiveness study of brain tissue oxygen and intracranial pressure monitoring versus intracranial pressure alone. BMJ Open. 2022;12(3):e060188.
67. Stein NR, et al. Early cerebral metabolic crisis after TBI influences outcome despite adequate hemodynamic resuscitation. Neurocrit Care. 2012;17(1):49–57.
68. Timofeev I, Carpenter KL, Nortje J, Al-Rawi PG, O'Connell MT, Czosnyka M, Smielewski P, Pickard JD, Menon DK, Kirkpatrick PJ, Gupta AK, Hutchinson PJ. Cerebral extracellular chemistry and outcome following traumatic brain injury: a microdialysis study of 223 patients. Brain. 2011;134(Pt 2):484–94.
69. Vespa P, et al. Metabolic crisis occurs with seizures and periodic discharges after brain trauma. Ann Neurol. 2016;79(4):579–90.
70. Vespa PM, et al. Acute seizures after intracerebral hemorrhage: a factor in progressive midline shift and outcome. Neurology. 2003;60(9):1441–6.
71. Vespa PM, et al. Nonconvulsive electrographic seizures after traumatic brain injury result in a delayed, prolonged increase in intracranial pressure and metabolic crisis. Crit Care Med. 2007;35(12):2830–6.
72. Temkin NR, Dikmen SS, Wilensky AJ, Keihm J, Chabal S, Winn HR. A randomized, double-blind study of phenytoin for the prevention of post-traumatic seizures. N Engl J Med. 1990;323(8):497–502.
73. Jones KE, Puccio AM, Harshman KJ, Falcione B, Benedict N, Jankowitz BT, Stippler M, Fischer M, Sauber-Schatz EK, Fabio A, Darby JM, Okonkwo DO. Levetiracetam versus phenytoin for seizure prophylaxis in severe traumatic brain injury. Neurosurg Focus. 2008;25(4):E3.
74. Szaflarski JP, Sangha KS, Lindsell CJ, Shutter LA. Prospective, randomized, single-blinded comparative trial of intravenous levetiracetam versus phenytoin for seizure prophylaxis. Neurocrit Care. 2010;12(2):165–72.
75. Khan NR, et al. Should Levetiracetam or phenytoin be used for posttraumatic seizure prophylaxis? A systematic review of the literature and meta-analysis. Neurosurgery. 2016;79(6):775–82.
76. Xu JC, et al. The safety and efficacy of levetiracetam versus phenytoin for seizure prophylaxis after traumatic brain injury: a systematic review and meta-analysis. Brain Inj. 2016;30(9):1054–61.
77. Kochanek PM, et al. Guidelines for the Management of Pediatric Severe Traumatic Brain Injury, third edition: update of the brain trauma foundation guidelines. Pediatr Crit Care Med. 2019;20(3S Suppl 1):S1–S82.

Traumatic Neurovascular Injury

27

Walter L. Biffl

Contents

Abstract

The management of traumatic neurovascular injuries has changed dramatically over the past 25 years. Advances in imaging and technology have allowed early recognition of asymptomatic injuries, therapy to prevent stroke, and endovascular interventions to both prevent and treat potentially devastating injuries. There are signs and symptoms, as well as known risk factors, that should prompt diagnostic evaluation. Computed tomographic angiography is a reliable imaging test, and antithrombotic therapy provides effective stroke prevention. Endovascular interventions require further study.

W. L. Biffl (✉)
Scripps Clinic Medical Group, La Jolla, CA, USA
e-mail: Biffl.Walter@scrippshealth.org

Introduction

Over the past 25 years there has been a tremendous change in the diagnosis and management of traumatic neurovascular injuries (TNVI). As recently as the early 1990s, a stroke resulting from blunt carotid or vertebral artery injury (BCVI) was essentially a fait accompli, as the diagnosis was typically made based on the discovery of an ischemic neurologic deficit. With recognition that BCVI could be diagnosed and treated prior to the occurrence of stroke, screening of asymptomatic patients has become routine. The management of penetrating injuries has evolved as well, given advances in noninvasive imaging and endovascular capabilities. In this chapter we will provide answers to the key clinical questions regarding TNVI (Table 27.1).

Table 27.1 Key clinical questions

What are the signs and symptoms of TNVI?
What patients are at risk for TNVI?
What is the optimal diagnostic test for TNVI?
What is the best treatment strategy for TNVI?
What follow-up should be performed for TNVI?

E. Mahanna Gabrielli et al. (eds.), *Textbook of Neurointensive Care: Volume 1*, https://doi.org/10.1007/978-3-031-62220-5_27

Epidemiology

Traumatic neurovascular injuries refers to injuries of the carotid and vertebral arteries; the basilar artery; the anterior (ACA), middle (MCA), and posterior (PCA) cerebral arteries; and other intracranial vessels. The most common of these injuries involve the carotid and vertebral arteries, and the most common mechanism of injury is blunt. Consequently, blunt carotid and vertebral artery injuries (BCVI) are the subject of the large majority of literature in this area, and will be the focus of this chapter. Blunt carotid and vertebral artery injuries have historically been considered rare but potentially devastating events. As of 1980, there were only 113 reported cases of blunt carotid artery injuries [1]. Multicenter reviews in the early 1990s[2] established the incidence to be approximately 1 in 1000 (0.1%) blunt trauma admissions to major trauma centers. In these early series, blunt carotid injury was associated with mortality rates ranging from 23% to 28%, with 48–58% of survivors suffering permanent severe neurologic deficits [1]. Clinical studies in the early 1990s suggested that these injuries were being underdiagnosed [2]. In the current era of screening based upon specific clinical criteria, the reported incidence of BCVI is 1–2% of blunt trauma admissions in major trauma centers [3].

Penetrating injuries to the carotid and vertebral arteries are much less common, occurring in only 8% of penetrating neck injuries [4]. Non-lethal penetrating injuries to intracranial arteries are very rare.

Pathophysiology

In 1974, Crissey and Bernstein [5] described four fundamental pathophysiologic mechanisms of blunt carotid artery injury. Type I injuries result from direct trauma to the neck (eg, seat belt, strangulation, near-hanging) and account for up to 10% of blunt carotid injuries. Type II injuries, the most common, are due to hyperextension and contralateral rotation of the head and neck, with stretch injury to the vessel. The lateral articular processes and pedicles of the upper three cervical vertebrae (C1 to C3) project more anteriorly than those of the lower four cervical (C4 to C7) vertebrae. Thus, in the upper region, the cervical internal carotid artery (ICA) can be stretched across the lateral processes with cervical hyperextension. Rotation at the atlantoaxial joint aggravates stretch injury because it can cause anterior movement of the contralateral C1 transverse process [6]. Cervical hyperflexion injury may result in a crushing injury of the artery between the angle of the mandible and the bony cervical spine.Type III injuries involve intraoral trauma that impacts the internal carotid artery at the angle of the jaw. This type of injury is seen in patients who fall with a hard object in the mouth, such as children who have fallen with a toothbrush in their mouth. Type IV injuries involve a laceration of the carotid artery resulting from basilar skull fracture, most commonly in the region of the carotid canal.

The vertebral arteries are most often injured in the setting of cervical spine fracture or distraction injury. High-risk injury patterns include fractures to the upper cervical vertebral bodies or transverse foramina; subluxation or distraction injuries; and ligamentous disruption. Approximately 70% of vertebral artery injuries occur in the setting of a cervical spine injury [7].

Regardless of the underlying mechanism of injury, the pathologic insult in most cases is an intimal tear. The exposed subendothelial collagen promotes platelet aggregation and thrombus formation, which may occlude the vessel altogether or embolize to the cerebral circulation. The intimal tear may remain static or there may be a subintimal dissection that progresses cranially, which can cause luminal narrowing or acute vessel occlusion as the false lumen collapses against the true lumen. Less commonly, partial or complete transection of the artery occurs, resulting in pseudoaneurysm formation or free rupture. A pseudoaneurysm may increase in size to compress and occlude the vessel lumen, or rupture; if it contains thrombus, it may be a source of platelet thromboembolism. Rupture may result in intracranial or extracranial hemorrhage, or formation of an arteriovenous fistula.

Other TNVI mechanisms have been reported. For example, numerous case reports document blunt injuries (mostly dissection) following mechanisms that would not typically raise a suspicion for injury, so-called "trivial trauma." These mechanisms include chiropractic manipulation, hyperflexion or hyperextension during hair washing, "head banging" to music, "bottoms-up" drinking, rapid head turning, virtually any athletic endeavor, and everyday activities such as coughing, shaving, vomiting, and nose-blowing [1].

"Spontaneous" carotid and vertebral artery dissections occur in the absence of apparent etiologic factors and account for approximately 2–3% of primary strokes. Risk factors include hypertension, Marfan syndrome, fibromuscular dysplasia, syphilis, arteriopathies, and Erdheim's cystic medial necrosis. Some speculate that the presence of these medical risk factors predisposes patients to BCVI following lesser degrees of trauma.

Disease Subtypes

A grading scale for blunt cerebrovascular injury was created to standardize clinical communication and to guide therapy (Table 27.2) [8]. The injury grades given below apply to carotid or vertebral artery lesions.

Table 27.2 Injury grades

Grade	Description
Grade I	Intimal irregularity or dissection with <25% luminal narrowing
Grade II	Dissection or intramural hematoma with ≥25% luminal narrowing, intraluminal clot, or a visible intimal flap
Grade III	Pseudoaneurysm or hemodynamically insignificant arteriovenous fistula
Grade IV	Complete occlusion
Grade V	Transection with active extravasation (hemorrhage) or hemodynamically significant arteriovenous fistula

This grading scale was initially developed based on arteriographic findings, but it has been validated using CT angiography [9]. For the carotid artery, stroke rates increase with increasing injury grade. In contrast, stroke incidence following vertebral injury are independent of injury grade [10]. In a study of 171 patients found to have 236 blunt cerebrovascular injuries, the distribution of injury is representative: grade I (58%), grade II (22%), grade III (14%), grade IV (11%), and grade V (3%) [10].

The grading scale has been widely used in its original form, but recently it was suggested that within the grade II and III classifications, there may be incremental risk based on the degree of luiminal narrowing [11]. This is worthy of further study.

Essential Management Priorities

Early: Immediate/ First 24 h (Table 27.3)

Table 27.3 Immediate/early priorities checklist

Apply principles of ATLS
Make the diagnosis of TNVI
Determine optimal treatment strategy
Assess contraindications for treatment, and timing

Making the Diagnosis (Fig. 27.1)

Given the catastrophic potential of TNVI, the first priority is to make the diagnosis. Signs and symptoms generally relate to bleeding or ischemia, and will vary depending upon the site (i.e., which vessel and at what level) and type (i.e., grade) of injury. The neurologic manifestations will vary based on the adequacy of collateral circulation (e.g., intact Circle of Willis) and the presence of underlying arterial disease.

Signs that should be considered arterial injury until proven otherwise include acute arterial hemorrhage from the neck, mouth, nose, or ear; expanding cervical hematoma; cervical bruit in a patient younger than 50 years of age; and focal or lateralizing neurologic deficits (e.g., hemiparesis, transient ischemic attack, vertebrobasilar insufficiency). These warrant emergent diagnostic evaluation. There may be more subtle signs associated with local arterial injury in the neck. For example, blunt carotid artery trauma can disrupt the periarterial sympathetic plexus, leading to Horner's syndrome (ptosis, myosis, anhidrosis) or oculosympathetic paresis, i.e., ptosis and miosis, or "partial Horner's syndrome". Symptoms such as neck, ear, face, or periorbital pain occur in up to 60% of patients with carotid or vertebral artery dissection in the neck. However, pain may be difficult to elicit in the multiply injured patient, or may be attributed to other injuries. Thus, any patient with neck pain or headache following blunt trauma should be suspected of having cerebrovascular injury.

In the current era, the majority of patients with blunt cerebrovascular injury have no obvious neurologic manifestations at presentation. In these patients, TNVI are diagnosed based on screening evaluation.

Screening

In the early 1990s, it was believed that there were many clinically occult blunt carotid artery injuries that were not being identified [2]. It was also recognized that a latent period existed between the time of injury and the onset of symptoms. Unless the vessel immediately occludes, time is required for thrombus formation that might limit flow or lead to distal embolization. In various studies, 25–50% of patients first developed signs or symptoms of blunt carotid injury more than 12 h after the traumatic event [1]. A recent multicenter study of the Western Trauma Association [12] found that of all patients suffering a stroke related to BCVI, only 37% of patients had signs or symptoms at the time of initial presentation. The diagnosis in the remaining 63% was made at a median of 48 h. It was felt that this delay provides a window of opportunity during which patients at risk for adverse outcomes can be identified and stroke prevention therapy initiated.

Based on this premise, the Denver group performed the first screening study for blunt carotid artery injuries [13]. A consecutive series of 171 patients undergoing digital subtraction arteriography to exclude thoracic aortic injury also underwent carotid arteriography. Carotid artery injuries were found in 3.5% of patients, and half of them were unsuspected on clinical grounds. This study was followed by implementation of a systematic screening protocol for BCVI in mid-1996. After 1.5 years, the incidence at the Denver Health Medical Center had increased from 0.2% to 0.9% of all blunt trauma admissions [14]; 4 years later, the Denver group reported BCVI in 1.6% of blunt trauma admissions [10]. This was replicated at other centers in the early 2000s.

Who to Screen

Selection of patients for screening was initially based on the common mechanisms of injury [14]. A list of high risk criteria was published in 1999, and included Glasgow Coma

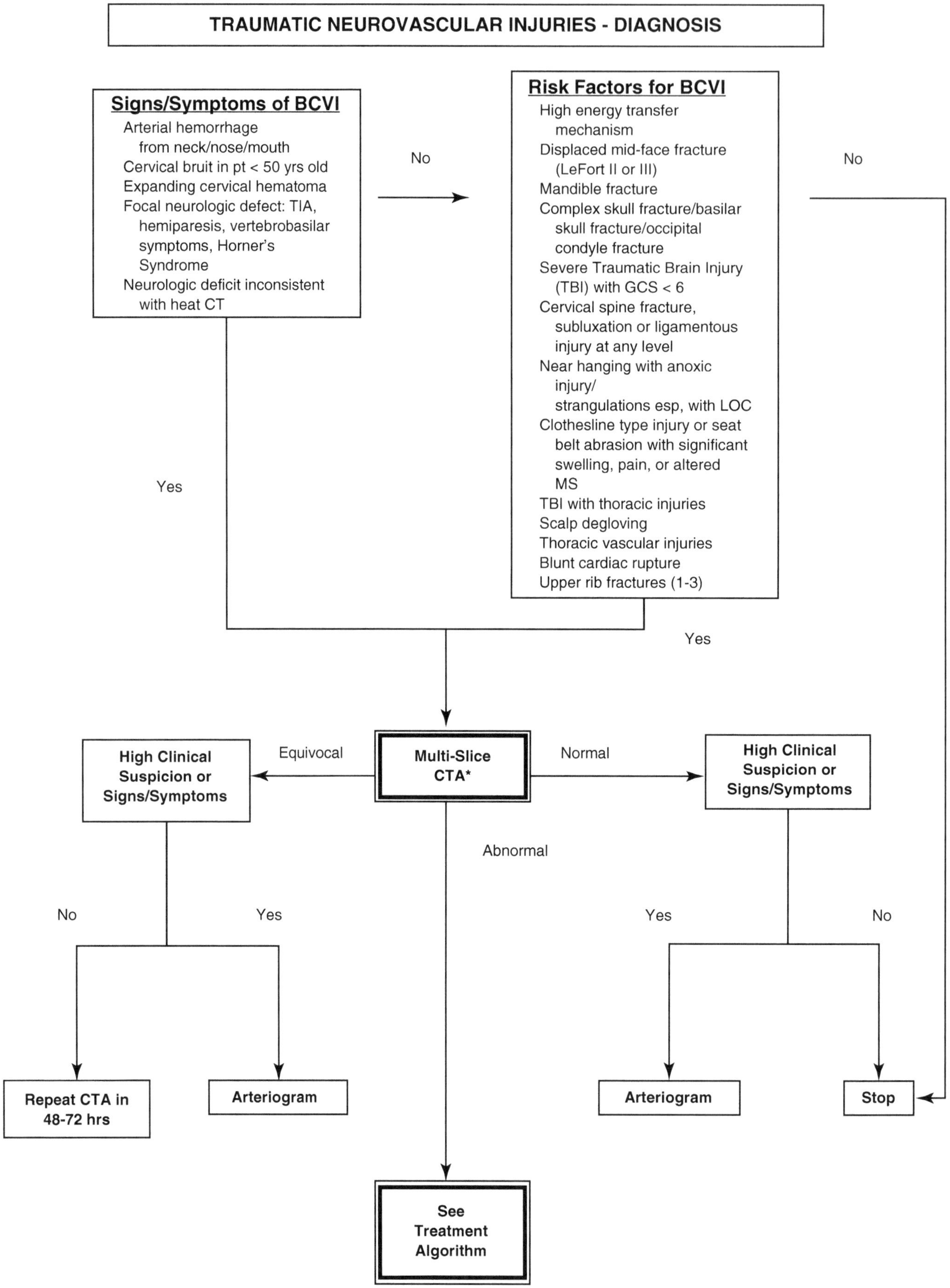

Fig. 27.1 Diagnostic flow diagram

Scale score ≤ 6, petrous bone fracture, diffuse axonal injury of the brain, LeFort II or III fracture, and cervical spine fractures [15]. However, 20% of patients with BCVI had none of these risk factors. Over the ensuing years, additional criteria were added to the list, resulting in the current "expanded Denver criteria." [3] Recent guidelines from the Western Trauma Association (WTA) and Eastern Association for the Surgery of Trauma (EAST) recommend more liberal screening, even based on low risk criteria [16, 17]. The current debate is focused on the implementation of "universal screening." Proponents of this approach point out that there continue to be a large percentage of blunt TNVI identified in patients who do not meet the expanded Denver criteria, or other published screening criteria [18, 19]. Two studies of universal screening have identified BCVI in 2.7% [18] and 7.6% [19] of patients. Implementation of universal screening protocols is likely to yield more injuries, but the additional cost, radiation, and intravenous contrast should be considered along with the mechanism of injury. This should be studied on a broader scale.

How to Screen

Digital Subtraction Arteriography (DSA)

The original screening studies were performed using four-vessel biplanar cerebral DSA [13, 14]. It is still considered the criterion standard for the diagnosis of BCVI, but it is invasive and associated with access site complications (eg, hematoma, pseudoaneurysm), contrast nephropathy, contrast allergy, and stroke [10, 20]. In addition, DSA is expensive and interventional radiology is a precious resource in many centers. Consequently, a search for an accurate noninvasive alternative has continued over the past 20 years. The current role for DSA is to make a definitive diagnosis in a symptomatic patient with equivocal or normal-appearing CT angiogram, or to plan interventions.

Duplex Ultrasonography

Duplex ultrasonography was the first noninvasive study considered for the evaluation of BCVI, as it is considered a reliable means of evaluating other pathology (e.g., atherosclerosis) of the extracranial carotid arteries. However, it is not recommended as first-line imaging for a number of reasons. First, it is user-dependent and a skilled ultrasonographer may not be readily available during off-hours. Second, removal of the cervical collar is required to perform the examination and this is often contraindicated in the at-risk group. Third, the technique has limitations for visualizing arteries within the bony spine or as they enter the base of the skull. Although duplex ultrasound can provide indirect evidence of distal injuries, such findings are not reliable when the degree of stenosis is less than 60%. Thus, grade I, grade III, and many grade II injuries could potentially be missed. In clinical studies, the accuracy is not sufficiently high enough to recommend it as the primary screening test [21]. Duplex ultrasonography may have a limited role in evaluating select cases that involve direct blows to the anterior neck, follow-up of proximal lesions, and possibly in children, in whom other imaging techniques might require conscious sedation.

Magnetic Resonance Angiography (MRA)

Advantages of MRA include the avoidance of iodinated contrast agents, lack of bony artifact, and earlier detection of cerebral infarction. However, screening studies have found poor specificity at 67% with sensitivities ranging from 50–75% compared with catheter-based arteriography [22, 23]. A recent meta-analysis reported overall sensitivity of 55% [24]. Given issues such as the time required for the study and incompatibility with implanted devices, MRA is not used for routine screening. It may have a role in follow-up imaging especially with equivocal CTA results or in the setting of other injuries requiring MR imaging.

Computed Tomographic Angiography (CTA)

Computed tomographic (CT) angiography has become the screening test of choice under both urgent and emergency circumstances (Fig. 27.1). This is primarily because patients who are candidates for screening typically have indications for scanning other regions of the body. The volume of contrast can be less than one half that needed for DSA. The sensitivity and specificity of CT angiography for blunt cerebrovascular injury has increased with improvements in CT technology, and 16-channel or greater multidetector row CT appears to be reliable in detecting clinically-important BCVI [20, 22, 23, 25, 26]. Whole-body multidetector-row CT has now been adopted in some centers. It offers more rapid imaging, with a single dose of intravenous contrast. A preliminary report suggests an accuracy equivalent to 16-slice CT angiography, but further evaluation is needed [27].

The same imaging principles apply in the setting of penetrating trauma, in which bleeding problems are more common than thrombotic problems. The diagnostic approach is similar, with MDCT and DSA used most commonly.

Treatment (Fig. 27.2)

The three primary treatment options for TNVI are surgical repair, antithrombotic therapy, and endovascular therapy. There are limited prospective data to guide management. Treatment is based upon reduced neurologic morbidity and mortality in treated patients compared with those who are untreated (and to historical controls); indirect evidence derived from the penetrating neck injury literature, and strategies used in the management of nontraumatic cerebrovascular disorders (eg, spontaneous cerebrovascular dissection). Factors that determine the treatment strategy for a specific patient include symptoms, site of injury, severity or grade of injury, and associated injuries that may contraindicate a specific therapy. The rationale and recommendations for anti-

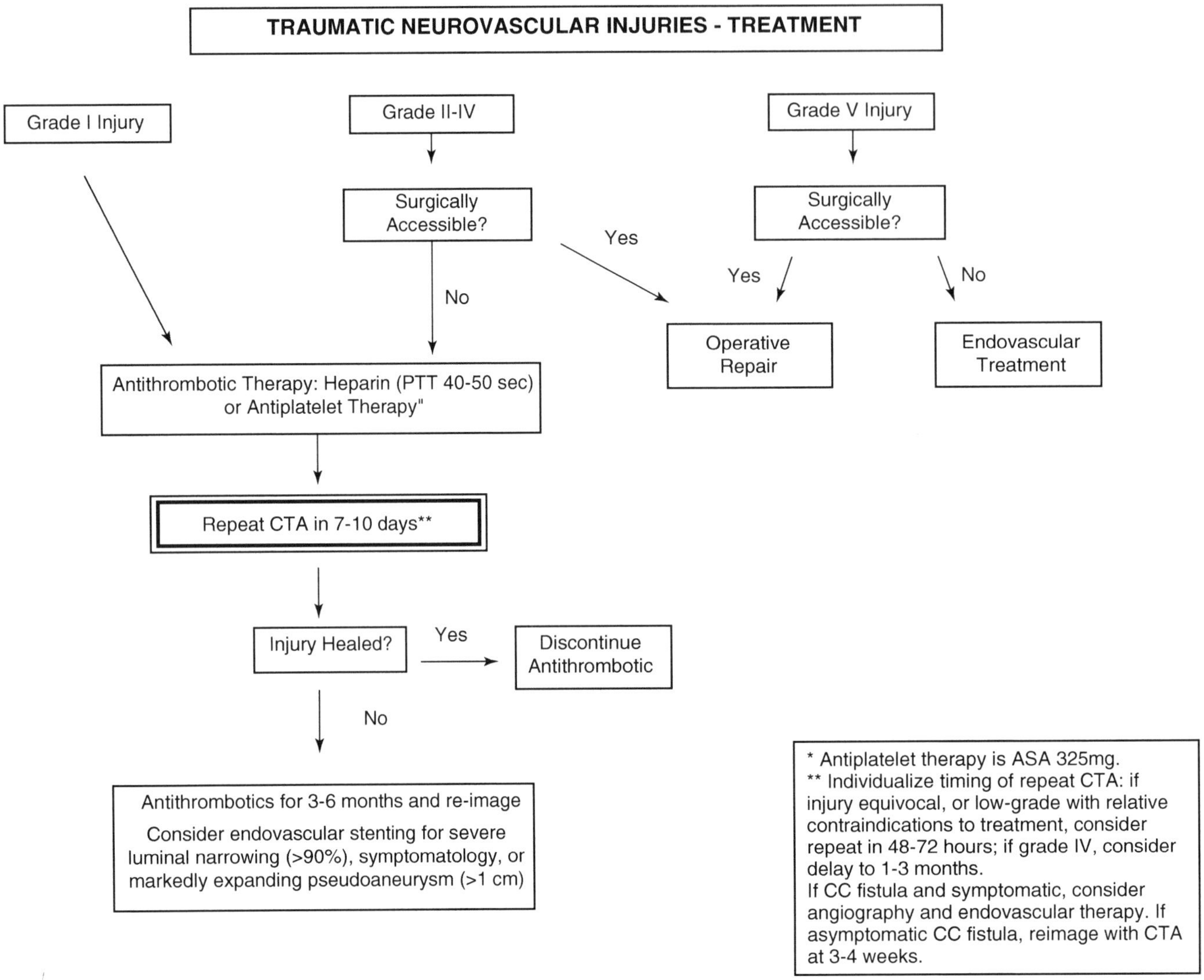

Fig. 27.2 Treatment flow diagram

thrombotic therapy or other intervention, follow-up, and injury grade-specific recommendations are discussed below.

Antithrombotic Therapy

Antithrombotic therapy (heparin or antiplatelet therapy) is recommended for essentially all patients with TNVI who do not have contraindications (e.g., active hemorrhage from the vessel). Stroke rates in case series from the era prior to screening were considerably higher than contemporary series, as injuries were previously not diagnosed until the ischemic neurologic event occurred [14]. The rationale for using antithrombotic therapy is based on retrospective reviews reporting reduced rates of ischemic neurologic events and better neurologic outcomes among patients treated with heparin or antiplatelet agents compared with untreated patients [10, 28, 29]. However, patients who are not treated are usually more severely injured, with contraindications to treatment, such as head injury, which influences the comparison. The first-line therapy in major society guidelines is currently unfractionated heparin [16, 17, 29]. Heparin is administered at 15 units/kg per hour without bolus dosing, to achieve an activated partial thromboplastin time (aPTT) of 40–50 s. This is a lower target range compared with other indications and was selected based on its efficacy and attempted minimization of bleeding complications [10, 28]. Heparin is preferred in the acute setting because it is reversible. The literature is mixed on which treatment is superior. Retrospective studies lack granularity to indicate the timing of treatment after injury; transitions from one treatment to another; or interruptions in treatment [1, 9, 10, 30, 31].

For patients who have contraindications to heparin, antiplatelet agents (aspirin 325 mg daily or clopidogrel 75 mg daily) are recommended. The 325 mg dose of aspirin is recommended based on the rate of nonresponders, which in one study was 36% for doses <101 mg, as compared with 19% for doses >299 mg [32]. Although dual antiplatelet therapy may be indicated for other conditions, it is not recommended for primary management of TNVI due to potential increased risk of bleeding and undemonstrated benefit [33]. There are currently no data regarding the treatment of TNVI with direct thrombin inhibitors or factor Xa inhibitors. Given the data supporting the safety and efficacy of these medications in other scenarios (eg, stroke prevention with atrial fibrillation, treatment and prevention of venous thromboembolism), they warrant study in this patient population.

The treatment of patients who suffer stroke after blunt cerebrovascular injury has not been well studied. The seminal work by Fabian and colleagues [28] reported significant improvement in neurologic outcomes following heparin therapy, but no patients were treated with antiplatelet medications. A trial among patients with cervical arterial dissection with stroke or transient ischemic attack, found that antiplatelet therapy was not inferior to heparin followed by warfarin for preventing recurrent stroke [34]. These were not trauma patients, so whether these results can be generalized to patients with TNVI is unclear.

Surgical Repair

Surgical management is recommended for patients with surgically accessible penetrating injury in the absence of completed hemiplegic deficits. This is based on lower rates of neurologic morbidity and mortality for patients undergoing neck exploration and vascular repair compared with carotid artery ligation or nonoperative management [35–39]. The recommendation for management of blunt TNVI is extrapolated from these data: surgically accessible grade II-V injuries should be repaired (Fig. 27.2) [16, 17, 29]. However, many BCVI involve the vessel at the base of the skull and are therefore not surgically accessible. In the experience at Denver Health Medical Center, only 2 of the first 700 patients with BCVI had a surgically accessible lesion.

Endovascular Treatment

Endovascular interventions appear to be the best option to manage active hemorrhage, arteriovenous fistulae, and stroke, particularly if not surgically-accessible [40–42]. On the other hand, there are limited data supporting prophylactic endovascular interventions in the setting of asymptomatic dissections or occlusions [43]. Current recommendations for endovascular treatment include placing stents for severe flow-limiting stenoses, symptomatic arteriovenous fistulae, or enlarging pseudoaneurysms greater than 1.0–1.5 cm in diameter [29]. Prospective studies are needed in this area, as complication rates must be weighed against the benefit beyond that of antithrombotic therapy [44–46]. Complications with sequelae occur in approximately 15% of patients undergoing mechanical thrombectomy [47], and are reported in 5–6% of patients undergoing carotid artery stenting and embolization of unruptured aneurysms [48].

Long-Term Clinical Course

There are no good long-term outcome data to guide the duration of antithrombotic therapy. Follow-up imaging has been recommended 7–10 days after the injury has been identified because a significant number of injuries evolve in a manner that alters treatment [10]. If complete healing has been demonstrated by follow-up imaging, antithrombotic therapy can be discontinued. In some cases with equivocal imaging or significant potential contraindications to treatment, early repeat imaging is warranted to inform the risk:benefit discussion.

For long-term antithrombotic therapy, antiplatelet therapy may be preferable to warfarin due to its potential equivalent efficacy, better safety profile, and lower cost [50]. However, this recommendation may change in the future. An analysis of the Nationwide Readmission Database reported that the rate of readmission with new stroke in patients with blunt cerebrovascular injury was 3.8% [30]. Patients treated with antiplatelet medications had a higher rate of readmission for stroke compared with those treated with other anticoagulant medications (5.7% vs. 1.8%).

Key Monitoring

The most devastating complications of TNVI are intracranial or paraspinal bleeding, and stroke. Monitoring for neurologic deterioration is important. Extracranial hemorrhage is a potential complication of antithrombotic therapy, especially in patients with multiple injuries. Monitoring for this is important as well.

The selection and timing of treatment interventions is based on a risk:benefit assessment, and the equation evolves as neurologic status and bleeding status are assessed. Microemboli burden, as assessed by transcranial Doppler, is associated with higher risk of stroke due to internal carotid (but not vertebral) artery injuries [49]. Such testing may prove to be a useful tool in the risk/benefit assessment for anticoagulation in the setting of associated injuries.

Take Home Message

The majority of TNVI are asymptomatic at the time of presentation. Recognition of patients at risk, and early imaging, will identify the injuries when there is an opportunity to provide prophylactic antithrombotic treatment. In the setting of active hemorrhage or stroke, timely endovascular or open surgical interventions offer the best chance for favorable outcomes. An institutional screening and treatment algorithm is recommended. Treatment pearls are listed in (Table 27.4).

Table 27.4 Treatment pearls

Suspect TNVI based on mechanism of injury and associated injuries
Obtain CT angiography early during trauma evaluation
Treat bleeding or stroke immediately
Initiate stroke prevention therapy as soon as possible
Assess risk:Benefit at least daily
Repeat imaging at 7–10 days to assess evolution of injury
Provide long-term stroke prevention therapy

References

1. Biffl WL, Moore EE, Elliott JP, et al. Blunt cerebrovascular injuries. Curr Prob Surg. 1999;36:507–99.
2. Cogbill TH, Moore EE, Meissner M, et al. The spectrum of blunt injury to the carotid artery: a multicenter perspective. J Trauma. 1994;37:473.
3. Biffl WL, Burlew CC, Moore EE. Blunt cerebrovascular injury: mechanisms, screening, and diagnostic evaluation. In: Collins KA, editor. UpToDate. Waltham, MA: UpToDate; 2011. Last updated May 2021.
4. Biffl WL, Moore EE, Rehse DH, et al. Selective management of penetrating neck trauma based on cervical level of injury. Am J Surg. 1997;174:678–82.
5. Crissey MM, Bernstein EF. Delayed presentation of carotid intimal tear following blunt craniocervical trauma. Surgery. 1974;75:543–8.
6. Zelenock GB, Kazmers A, Whitehouse WM Jr, et al. Extracranial internal carotid artery dissections: noniatrogenic traumatic lesions. Arch Surg. 1982;117:425–30.
7. Biffl WL, Moore EE, Elliott JP, et al. The devastating potential of blunt vertebral arterial injuries. Ann Surg. 2000;231:672–81.
8. Biffl WL, Moore EE, Offner PJ, et al. Blunt carotid arterial injuries: implications of a new grading scale. J Trauma. 1999;47:845–51.
9. Foreman PM, Griessenauer CJ, Kicielinski KP, et al. Reliability assessment of the Biffl scale for blunt traumatic cerebrovascular injury as detected on computer tomography angiography. J Neurosurg. 2017;127:32–5.
10. Biffl WL, Ray CE Jr, Moore EE, et al. Treatment-related outcomes from blunt cerebrovascular injuries: importance of routine follow-up arteriography. Ann Surg. 2002;235:699–706.
11. Lauerman MH, Irizarry K, Sliker C, et al. Influence of luminal stenosis in aneurysmal and non-aneurysmal blunt traumatic cerebrovascular injury. Injury. 2019;50(1):131–6.
12. Burlew CC, Sumislawski JJ, Behnfield CD, et al. Time to stroke: a Western trauma association multicenter study of blunt cerebrovascular injuries. J Trauma Acute Care Surg. 2018;85:858–66.
13. Prall JA, Brega KE, Coldwell DM, et al. Incidence of unsuspected blunt carotid artery injury. Neurosurgery. 1998;42:495.
14. Biffl WL, Moore EE, Ryu RK, et al. The unrecognized epidemic of blunt carotid arterial injuries: early diagnosis improves neurologic outcome. Ann Surg. 1998;228:462–8.
15. Biffl WL, Moore EE, Offner PJ, et al. Optimizing screening for blunt cerebrovascular injuries. Am J Surg. 1999;178:517–23.
16. Biffl WL, Cothren CC, Moore EE, et al. Western trauma association critical decisions in trauma: screening for and treatment of blunt cerebrovascular injuries. J Trauma. 2009;67:1150–6.
17. Kim DY, Biffl W, Bokhari F, et al. Evaluation and management of blunt cerebrovascular injury: a practice management guideline from the eastern Association for the Surgery of trauma. J Trauma Acute Care Surg. 2020;88:875–81.
18. Leichtle SW, Banerjee D, Schrader R, et al. Blunt cerebrovascular injury: the case for universal screening. J Trauma Acute Care Surg. 2020;89:880–6.
19. Black JA, Abraham PJ, Abraham MN, et al. Universal screening for blunt cerebrovascular injury. J Trauma Acute Care Surg. 2021;90:224–31.
20. Paulus EM, Fabian TC, Savage SA, et al. Blunt cerebrovascular injury screening with 64-channel multidetector computed tomography: more slices finally cut it. J Trauma Acute Care Surg. 2014;76:279–85.
21. Mutze S, Rademacher G, Matthes G, et al. Blunt cerebrovascular injury in patients with blunt multiple trauma: diagnostic accuracy of duplex Doppler US and early CT angiography. Radiology. 2005;237:884–90.
22. Biffl WL, Ray CE Jr, Moore EE, et al. Noninvasive diagnosis of blunt cerebrovascular injuries: a preliminary report. J Trauma. 2002;53:850–5.
23. Miller PR, Fabian TC, Croce MA, et al. Prospective screening for blunt cerebrovascular injuries: analysis of diagnostic modalities and outcomes. Ann Surg. 2002;236:386–91.
24. Karagiorgas GP, Brotis AG, Giannis T, et al. The diagnostic accuracy of magnetic resonance angiography for blunt vertebral artery injury detection in trauma patients: a systematic review and meta-analysis. Clin Neurol Neurosurg. 2017;160:152–63.
25. Eastman AL, Chason DP, Perez CL, et al. Computed tomographic angiography for the diagnosis of blunt cervical vascular injury: is it ready for primetime? J Trauma. 2006;60:925–30.
26. Berne JD, Reuland KS, Villarreal DH, et al. Sixteen-slice multi-detector computed tomographic angiography improves the accuracy of screening for blunt cerebrovascular injury. J Trauma. 2006;60:1204–9.
27. Sliker CW, Shanmuganathan K, Mirvis SE. Diagnosis of blunt cerebrovascular injuries with 16-MDCT: accuracy of whole-body MDCT compared with neck MDCT angiography. AJR Am J Roentgenol. 2008;190:790–5.
28. Fabian TC, Patton JH Jr, Croce MA, et al. Blunt carotid injury. Importance of early diagnosis and anticoagulant therapy. Ann Surg. 1996;223:513–9.
29. Biffl WL, Burlew CC, Moore EE. Blunt cerebrovascular injury: treatment and outcomes. In: Collins KA, editor. UpToDate. Waltham, MA: UpToDate; 2011. Last updated May 2021.
30. Hanna K, Douglas M, Asmar S, et al. Treatment of blunt cerebrovascular injuries: anticoagulants or antiplatelet agents? J Trauma Acute Care Surg. 2020;89:74–81.
31. Bonow RH, Witt CE, Mossa-Basha M, et al. Aspirin versus anticoagulation for stroke prophylaxis in blunt cerebrovascular injury: a propensity-matched retrospective cohort study. J Neurosurg. 2021;135(5):1413–20. https://doi.org/10.3171/2020.10.JNS201836.
32. Hovens MMC, Snoep JD, Eikenboom JCJ, et al. Prevalence of persistent platelet reactivity despite use of aspirin: a systematic review. Am Heart J. 2007;153:175–81.
33. Hermosillo AJ, Spinler SA. Aspirin, clopidogrel, and warfarin: is the combination appropriate and effective or inappropriate and too dangerous? Ann Pharmacother. 2008;42:79–84.
34. CADISS trial investigators, Markus HS, Hayter E, et al. Antiplatelet treatment compared with anticoagulation treatment for cervical artery dissection (CADISS): a randomised trial. Lancet Neurol. 2015;14:361–6.
35. Ledgerwood AM, Mullins RJ, Lucas CE. Primary repair vs. ligation for carotid artery injuries. Arch Surg. 1980;115:488–93.
36. Karlin RM, Marks C. Extracranial carotid artery injury. Current surgical management. Am J Surg. 1983;146:225–9.
37. Richardson JD, Simpson C, Miller FB. Management of carotid artery trauma. Surgery. 1988;104:673–7.

38. Ramadan F, Rutledge R, Oller D, et al. Carotid artery trauma: a review of contemporary trauma center experiences. J Vasc Surg. 1995;21:46–50.
39. Tisherman SA, Bokhari F, Collier B, et al. Clinical practice guideline: penetrating zone II neck trauma. J Trauma. 2008;64:1392–5.
40. Higashida RT, Halbach VV, Tsai FY, et al. Interventional neurovascular treatment of traumatic carotid and vertebral artery lesions: results in 234 cases. AJR Am J Roentgenol. 1989;153:577–82.
41. Ray CE Jr, Biffl WL. Neurovascular interventions in the trauma patient. Semin Interv Radiol. 2002;19:377–87.
42. Bell RS, Vo AH, Roberts R, et al. Wartime traumatic aneurysms: acute presentation, diagnosis, and multimodal treatment of 64 craniocervical arterial injuries. Neurosurgery. 2010;66:66–79.
43. Indo M, Oya S, Shojima M, et al. Prevention of thromboembolic infarction after surgery for traumatic cervical fracture with vertebral artery occlusion by preoperative endovascular coil embolization. World Neurosurg. 2019;129:e838–44.
44. Cothren CC, Moore EE, Ray CE Jr, et al. Carotid artery stents for blunt cerebrovascular injury: risks exceed benefits. Arch Surg. 2005;140:480–5.
45. Burlew CC, Biffl WL, Moore EE, et al. Endovascular stenting is rarely necessary for the management of blunt cerebrovascular injuries. J Am Coll Surg. 2014;218:1012–6.
46. Shahan CP, Sharpe JP, Stickley SM, et al. The changing role of endovascular stenting for blunt cerebrovascular injuries. J Trauma Acute Care Surg. 2018;84:308–13.
47. Balami JC, White PM, McMeekin PJ, et al. Complications of endovascular management for ischemic stroke: prevention and management. Int J Stroke. 2018;13:348–61.
48. Pasarikovski CR, Tanner BK, Marques AJP, et al. Neurointerventional procedural complications in a growing Canadian regional stroke center: single hospital experience analysis in the context of recommended case volumes. World Neurosurg. 2019;127:e94–e100. https://doi.org/10.1016/j.wneu.2019.02.137.
49. Bonow RH, Witt CE, Mosher BP, et al. Transcranial Doppler microemboli monitoring for stroke risk stratification in blunt cerebrovascular injury. Crit Care Med. 2017;45:e1011–5.
50. Cothren CC, Biffl WL, Moore EE, et al. Treatment for blunt cerebrovascular injuries: equivalence of anticoagulation and antiplatelet agents. Arch Surg. 2009;144:685–90.

Key/Landmark References

Biffl WL, Moore EE, Ryu RK, et al. The unrecognized epidemic of blunt carotid arterial injuries: early diagnosis improves neurologic outcome. Ann Surg. 1998;228:462.

Biffl WL, Moore EE, Offner PJ, et al. Blunt carotid arterial injuries: implications of a new grading scale. J Trauma. 1999;47:845.

Biffl WL, Ray CE Jr, Moore EE, et al. Treatment-related outcomes from blunt cerebrovascular injuries: importance of routine follow-up arteriography. Ann Surg. 2002;235:699.

Fabian TC, Patton JH Jr, Croce MA, et al. Blunt carotid injury. Importance of early diagnosis and anticoagulant therapy. Ann Surg. 1996;223:513.

Acute Traumatic Spinal Cord Injury

28

François Mathieu and Michael G. Fehlings

Contents

F. Mathieu
Division of Neurosurgery and Spinal Program, Department of Surgery, University of Toronto, Toronto, ON, Canada

Interdepartmental Division of Critical Care Medicine, Faculty of Medicine, University of Toronto, Toronto, ON, Canada

Division of Neurosurgery, St. Michael's Hospital, Toronto, Canada
e-mail: Francois.Mathieu@mail.utoronto.ca

M. G. Fehlings (✉)
Division of Neurosurgery and Spinal Program, Department of Surgery, University of Toronto, Toronto, ON, Canada

Division of Genetics and Development, Krembil Brain Institute, University Health Network, Toronto, ON, Canada

Division of Neurosurgery, Krembil Neuroscience Centre, University Health Network, Toronto, ON, Canada
e-mail: Michael.Fehlings@uhn.ca

Abstract

Spinal cord injury remains one of the most important causes of trauma-related mortality as well as morbidity worldwide and imposes a substantial economic burden on society. Survivors not only suffer from life-altering motor and sensory deficits but are also vulnerable to acute and chronic complications affecting many organ systems. Since there currently exists no effective treatment to reverse the primary neurological injury, mitigation of secondary injury and avoidance of complications constitute the main goals of clinical management. Increasing evidence that timely intervention—including prompt transfer to specialized centers, early decompressive surgery, and emergent restoration of adequate oxygenation, ventilation, and mean arterial pressure—translate into improved long-term functional outcomes has led to growing recognition of the concept that "time is spine." A num-

E. Mahanna Gabrielli et al. (eds.), *Textbook of Neurointensive Care: Volume 1*, https://doi.org/10.1007/978-3-031-62220-5_28

ber of neuroprotective and neuroregenerative therapies have also emerged in recent years and are under active investigation in clinical trials. In this chapter, we review key assessment principles, propose evidence-based critical care and surgical treatment strategies, and review promising approaches to protect and regenerate the traumatically injured spinal cord.

Epidemiology

The Global Burden of Disease Study estimated that there were 0.93 million (0.78–1.16 million) new cases of traumatic spinal cord injury (SCI) worldwide in 2016, translating into an age-standardized incidence rate of 13 per 100,000 [1]. According to the National SCI Statistical Center (NSCISC), there are approximately 17,800 new cases of SCI each year in the United States, with a total of 250,000 to 368,000 persons currently living with a SCI [2]. Motor vehicle accidents (39%), falls (32%), violence (14%), and recreation (8%) represent the main causes of traumatic SCI in the United States [2]. There is substantial variation in these proportions and in overall incidence rates between countries; reflecting population demographics, degree of socioeconomic development, rates of violence, and gunshot injuries amongst other factors, although cross-country comparisons have been limited by lack of uniformity in data collection and reporting [3, 4].

The average age of the acute traumatic SCI victim in the United States has increased from 22 in the 1970s to 43 in 2020, reflecting the ageing population and the increasing proportion of injuries attributed to falls in the elderly [5, 6]. The current age distribution is bimodal with a large peak observed between 15 and 29 years of age and a second peak occurring after age 60. Males remain about three to four times more likely to suffer from SCI; however, there has been a rising incidence among women in recent years [7].

The cervical spine is affected in approximately 59.5% of cases, with incomplete tetraplegia currently being the most frequent neurological category (47.2%) [2]. While the incidence of complete injuries has been decreasing relative to incomplete injuries, potentially stemming from improved vehicle safety devices and regulatory efforts, the proportion of high cervical SCI has increased [7]. This trend has been in part attributed to the concomitant increase in fall-related injuries in the elderly and to improvements in prehospital care translating to a greater number of victims surviving the early respiratory and cardiac compromise associated with high-cervical injuries. Several underlying spinal conditions increase individual susceptibility to traumatic SCI, including degenerative cervical myelopathy or spondylosis, osteoporosis, and spinal arthropathies such as ankylosing spondylitis or rheumatoid arthritis. The shifting demographics of SCI have important critical care implications as many patients are older with associated medical comorbidities that require concomitant management [8].

Annual health care costs and other living expenses attributable to SCI vary considerably depending on the level and severity of the injury, with expenses associated with high tetraplegia (C1-C4) estimated at over one million dollars in the first year following injury and approximately $200,000 for each subsequent year, compared to about half these figures for paraplegic with ASIA Impairment Scale (AIS) score A, B, or C [2, 9]. Aggregate costs for the acute and chronic care of individuals living with SCI in the United States amount to over $9.7 billion annually [10].

Despite these concerning figures, the formation of organized trauma networks, optimization of prehospital and critical care management strategies, advances in surgical treatment, and dissemination of evidence-based guidelines have led to improved overall clinical outcomes for survival and recovery.

Pathophysiology

Traumatic SCIs usually occur in association with disruption of the vertebral column. Injurious forces are transmitted to the spinal cord through bony element fractures, facet joint dislocation, ligamentous tears, and/or traumatic disc herniation. In patients with pre-existing central canal stenosis, particularly in the cervical region, SCI can occur with minor trauma and in the absence of radiographically conspicuous bony or disco-ligamentous injury. Less frequently, spinal cord tissue is directly transected by a penetrating object or indirectly damaged from the kinetic energy emitted by bullet fragments in cases of gunshot injuries [11]. The initial damage produced from combinations of these mechanical forces has been referred to as the primary injury.

The primary injury is immediately followed by a complex and progressive pathophysiological cascade comprising the secondary injury (Fig. 28.1). Mechanisms implicated in this phenomenon include cord ischemia, microhemorrhage, edema, inflammation, excitotoxicity, disturbances of ion homeostasis, and apoptosis [12–14]. Damage to the spinal cord microvascular supply results in cord edema, hemorrhage, and ischemia within minutes of injury, while also allowing for an influx of vasoactive peptides and cytokines such as tumor necrosis factor (TNF) and IL-1β via disruption of the blood-spinal cord barrier [15, 16]. Recruitment of inflammatory cells follows, further contributing to cord edema, which can extend to adjacent segments and exacerbate neurological deficits. Death of neurons and glia due to ischemia and inflammation causes the accumulation of excess extracellular glutamate, which promotes excitotoxicity. The ensuing release of pro-apoptotic signals and cyto-

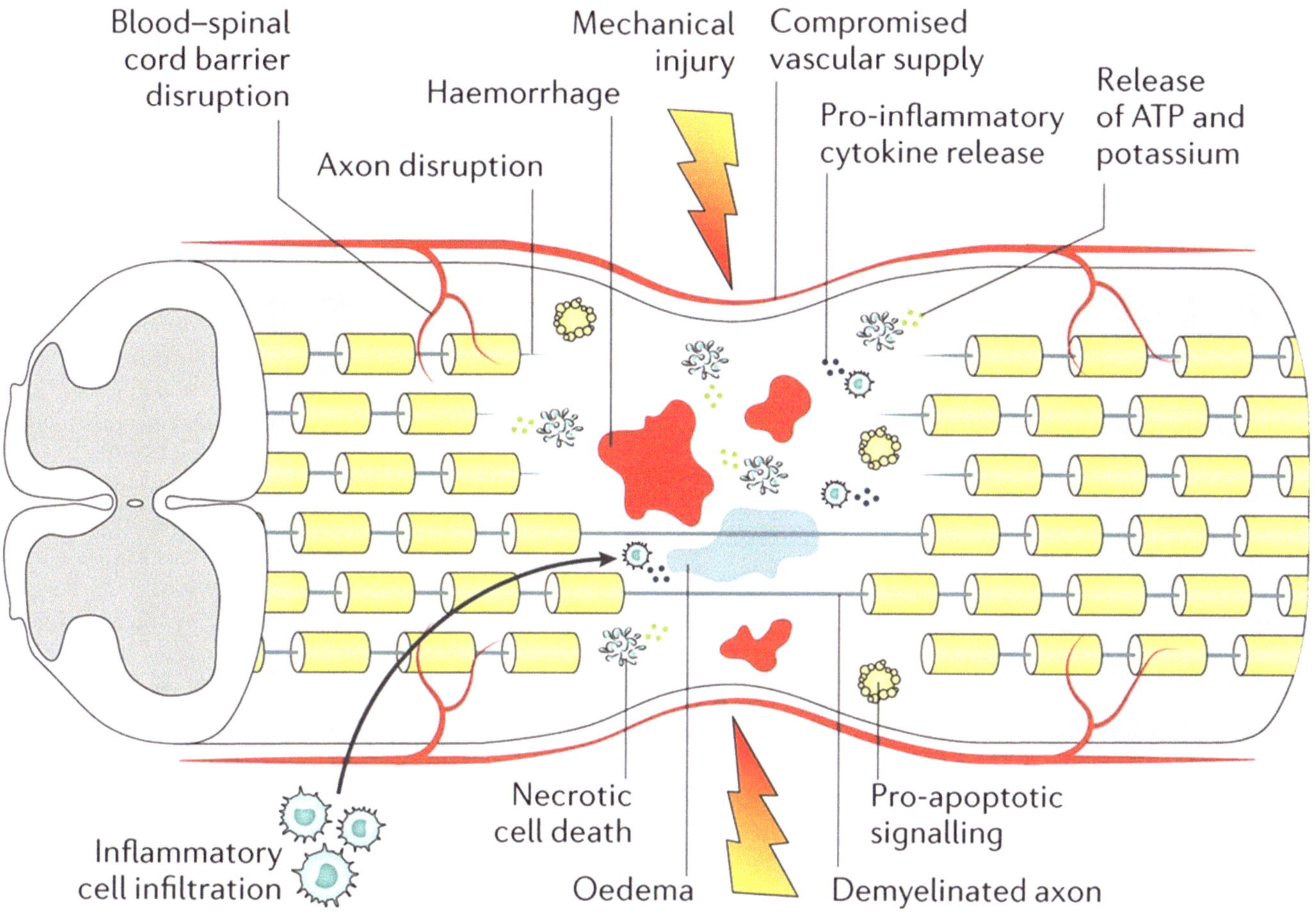

Fig. 28.1 Pathophysiology of traumatic spinal cord injury. The initial mechanical trauma to the spinal cord initiates a secondary injury cascade that is characterized in the acute phase by edema, hemorrhage, ischemia, inflammatory cell infiltration, the release of cytotoxic products and cell death. This secondary injury leads to necrosis and/or apoptosis of neurons and glial cells, such as oligodendrocytes, which can lead to demyelination and the loss of neural circuits. (Republished with permission. Republished with permissions of Macmillan Publishers Limited, Traumatic spinal cord injury. Reproduced with permission from Ahuja C.S et al. *Nature Reviews Disease Primers*. 3:17019, 2017)

toxic by-products into the local microenvironment propagates neuronal cell damage and death [15].

This local metabolic crisis is rapidly compounded by systemic hypotension and hypoxia if cardiovascular and respiratory compromise are not promptly addressed. Mitigation of this secondary injury cascade with expeditious medical and surgical interventions represents the central goal of clinical management during the acute phase. The rest of this chapter will focus on key management strategies that must be implemented in the early post-injury period to optimize neurological and functional outcomes for patients.

Initial Evaluation and Resuscitation

The initial management and resuscitation of trauma patients, including those with suspected spinal trauma and/or SCI, should follow the Advanced Trauma Life Support (ATLS) protocols outlined by the American College of Surgeons (ACS). First responders should prioritize the "ABCs"—airway, breathing, and circulation—while ensuring maintenance of spinal alignment. Initial stabilization efforts in the field should be followed by complete primary and secondary surveys upon arrival at the emergency department. However, early transfer (within 24 h) of patients with acute SCI to specialized care centers has been associated with improved long-term outcomes and should not be delayed by non-essential investigations [17].

Whether in the prehospital or hospital setting, any evidence of airway compromise requires immediate attention. After mechanical obstruction by a foreign body, blood or emesis has been relieved, an initial jaw thrust maneuver can be performed as long as neutral cervical alignment is maintained. An oropharyngeal airway can also be inserted as a temporizing measure in patients with a depressed level of consciousness and a diminished gag reflex. Rapid-sequence intubation may be necessary for individuals presenting with a Glasgow Coma Scale score less than or equal to 8 or patients presenting with obvious respiratory distress. Intubation should be performed by the most experienced provider and preferably using video laryngoscopy or fiberoptic techniques to help minimize neck motion. If these techniques are not readily available, direct laryngoscopy with manual in-line stabilization by a second care provider is an acceptable alternative [18]. After securing the airway, a cervical collar should be applied, if not already in place, and additional spinal protection techniques should include a backboard and lateral support device for patients requiring transfer or transportation.

After establishment of a protected airway, the second most important step is to assess for sufficient breathing and ventilation. Mid- to upper cervical SCI can significantly compromise spontaneous breathing efforts, with loss of diaphragmatic innervation leading to severe hypoventilation and potentially apnea in patients with injuries above C4. Even lower cervical and thoracic SCI can compromise ventilatory function via dysfunction of the intercostal and abdominal musculature, resulting in atelectasis as well as ineffective cough and secretion clearance. Up to one-third of patients with cervical spine injuries will require intubation, most of these in the first 24 h [19]. Close respiratory monitoring is therefore essential in any patient with a suspected cervical SCI. End-tidal CO_2 monitoring should be considered to facilitate early identification of patients developing ventilatory failure. Patients with thoracic spinal trauma are especially prone to concomitant chest injuries including pneumo- as well as hemothoraces, and these should be identified and addressed during the primary survey if contributing to respiratory compromise. Supplemental oxygen should be supplied to maintain saturation $\geq 92\%$ given that hypoxemia can adversely affect neurological outcomes in SCI [18].

Adequate cardiovascular support with avoidance and correction of hypotension is the third critical component of the initial assessment, but depending on the medical personnel available, the "A, B and Cs" should ideally be assessed and managed in parallel using a team-based approach while neurogenic shock is an important consideration in the patient with a suspected SCI, hypovolemia and hemorrhage should always be ruled out in the setting of polytrauma and immediately addressed with fluid resuscitation and/or blood products and source control if applicable. A systemic assessment of other potential causes of hemodynamic instability, such as tension hemothorax and cardiac tamponade, should be performed during the primary survey using adjuncts such as chest radiography and a FAST ultrasound examination. Neurogenic shock—a syndrome characterized by a sudden loss of vasomotor tone and sympathetic innervation to the heart—should be suspected in the patient presenting with bradycardia and distributive features of shock. Volume resuscitation alone is usually inadequate for treating neurogenic shock even in polytrauma patients with concomitant hypovolemia. Vasoactive agents which augment chronotropy and vascular resistance should be considered early with norepinephrine being a first-line option [20]. Persistent bradycardia may require atropine or temporary pacing to prevent further cardiovascular collapse. Maintaining normotension is essential to reduce secondary ischemic neural tissue injury, which has been consistently associated with worse neurologic outcomes [21].

The rapid neurological evaluation obtained during the "disability" component of the primary trauma survey should be supplemented with a focused history and the International Standards for Neurological Classification of the Spinal Cord Injury (ISNCSCI) examination once life-threatening injuries have been identified and addressed [22]. The ISNCSCI comprises three neurological summary scores: the American Spinal Injury Association (ASIA) motor score grading muscle power in key myotomes, the ASIA sensory score which assesses light touch and pinprick sensation in 28 dermatomes, and the ASIA Impairment Scale (AIS) grade; a five-letter classification system reflecting the degree of motor and sensory loss below the injury level. An AIS grade of A represents a complete SCI with absence of motor and sensory function below the injury level including the sacral segments S4–5, while the spectrum of incomplete injury is described in AIS grades of B, C, D with an AIS grade of E representing normal cord function. The specific criteria corresponding to each category of the AIS grade are provided in Table 28.1 and key dermatomes and myotomes are shown in Fig. 28.2. Logrolling of the patient must be performed to maintain alignment while assessing sensory and motor function in sacral segments. While the validity and reliability of the ASIA scale is well-established, a full assessment may not be possible in the presence of distracting injuries, intoxication or altered level of consciousness.

The AIS exam is ideally performed once the patient has been stabilized and within 72 h of injury at the latest to reliably serve as a baseline for treatment decisions, clinical trial

Table 28.1 American Spinal Injury Association Impairment Scale

Grade	Type	Description
A	Complete	No motor or sensory function is preserved in the sacral segments S4-S5
B	Incomplete	Sensory but not motor function is preserved below the neurological level and includes the sacral segments S4-S5
C	Incomplete	Motor function is preserved below the neurological level, and more than half of key muscles below the neurological level have a muscle grade less than 3
D	Incomplete	Motor function is preserved below the neurological level, and at least half of key muscles below the neurological level have a muscle grade of 3 or more
E	Normal	Motor and sensory function are normal

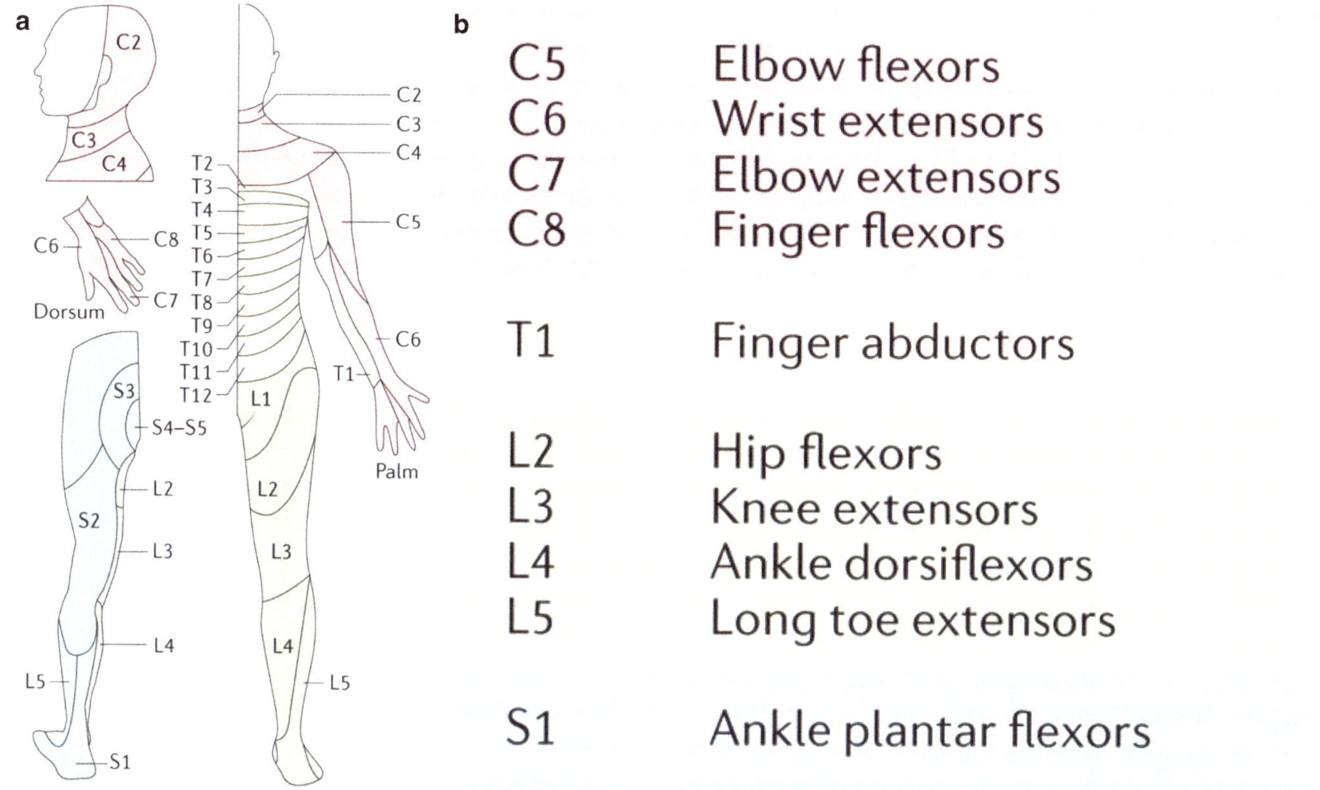

Fig. 28.2 Key dermatomes (**a**) and myotomes (**b**) described in the International Standards for Neurological Classification of Spinal Cord Injury. (Republished with permissions of Macmillan Publishers Limited, Traumatic spinal cord injury. Reproduced with permission from Ahuja C.S et al. *Nature Reviews Disease Primers*. 3:17019, 2017)

eligibility, prognostication, and for monitoring or recovery. It is important to keep in mind that the initial neurological exam can be confounded by the presence of spinal shock: a clinical syndrome characterized by transient physiologic loss of spinal cord function, including spinal reflexes, below the level of injury, often seen in patients with severe SCI. Reappearance of the bulbocavernosus reflex (BCR) has traditionally defined the resolution of spinal shock, but more recent research suggests a multiphasic process spanning from the onset of injury and lasting up to 12 months in some patients [23]. For the purpose of classifying an injury as complete or incomplete in the acute stage, the presence or return of a BCR or deep tendon reflexes is deemed sufficient to obtain an assessment which is predictive of the final neurological outcome. A notable exception to this paradigm would be direct injury to lower motor neurons involved in the bulbocavernosus reflex arc which is seen in some injuries at the bony thoracolumbar junction involving the distal conus medullaris and/or cauda equina.

Incomplete SCIs can be further described in terms of specific patterns of neurological deficits, which reflect the anatomical regions of the spinal cord that have been predominantly damaged. Central cord syndrome is the most common incomplete SCI pattern and is characterized by disproportionate motor impairment in the upper extremities compared to the lower extremities, with varying degrees of bladder dysfunction and sensory disturbance, most commonly hyperalgesia [24, 25]. Central cord syndrome is often caused by a hyperextension injury in the setting of preexisting cervical stenosis, but can also present in younger individuals with traumatic cervical disc herniations and/or fracture dislocations [26]. Less commonly encountered patterns of incomplete SCI include Brown-Séquard syndrome, anterior cord syndrome, and posterior cord syndrome. Brown-Séquard syndrome most commonly occurs with penetrating trauma causing hemisection of the spinal cord and presents with ipsilateral loss of motor function, light touch, proprioception and vibration sense, as well as contralateral loss of pain and temperature sensation. Isolated anterior and posterior cord syndromes are rare in the traumatic setting and are usually seen with vascular, metabolic, or inflammatory etiologies [25]. Anterior cord syndrome occurs with injury or occlusion of the anterior spinal artery and results in a pattern of neurological deficit dominated by motor paralysis as well as loss of pain and temperature sensation below the level of injury. Posterior cord syndrome is extremely rare and is characterized by isolated loss of proprioception and vibratory sensation from dorsal column pathology with occasional mild paresis in the upper extremities with larger lesions extending to the lateral corticospinal tract [27].

Imaging Assessment

After completion of the primary and secondary trauma survey, as well as initial stabilization of the patient, adjunctive evaluations are obtained. High-quality computed tomography (CT) imaging has now largely supplanted plain films as the initial diagnostic imaging modality of choice in patients with suspected spinal injuries. A number of prospective case series have demonstrated the superior sensitivity of CT over plain radiographs for the detection of spinal injury after trauma, particularly for the cervical spine [28, 29]. These studies have provided the evidence base for a Level 1 recommendation supporting the use of CT as the initial imaging modality of choice in the symptomatic and in the obtunded or unevaluable trauma patient [28]. Given concerns related to increased health care costs and radiation exposure associated with the liberal use of CT, two validated decision-making tools have been developed to facilitate clinical cervical spine clearance in the awake and asymptomatic patient: the Canadian C-Spine Rule and the NEXUS criteria [30, 31]. Both tools have demonstrated a near perfect sensitivity for the identification of clinically significant cervical spine injuries in awake patients. Patients meeting either set of criteria can therefore have their cervical spine cleared without reliance on radiographic workup. For patients with indications for imaging, CT angiography of the head and neck to detect blunt cerebrovascular injury (BCVI) should be considered if certain screening criteria are met (see Table 28.2) [32, 33]. Although some groups have advocated for more selective use of CTA based on high-risk features identified on non-contrast imaging, defined by the Denver group as upper cervical spine (C1–3) subluxation, and cervical spine fractures extending into the transverse foramen, a number of studies have demonstrated a similar incidence of BCVI in patients with and without high-risk criteria [34]. In the 2020 iteration of their BCVI guidelines, the Eastern Association for the Surgery of Trauma conditionally recommends also performing CTA in patients with low-risk injury patterns based on their meta-analysis of the literature showing an incidence of BCVI ranging from 2 to 9% in this subgroup [34].

CT imaging is limited in its ability to assess the spinal cord itself and surrounding soft tissue structures. While magnetic resonance imaging (MRI) is the modality of choice for evaluation of ligamentous and nervous tissue, its role in acute SCI has been debated owing to concerns about availability, cost-effectiveness and due to the risks associated with subjecting potentially unstable patients to prolonged scanning protocols [35, 36]. However, it needs to be recognized that MRI should be obtained when medically and logistically feasible to evaluate a patient with SCI. If the patient's clinical status permits and if timely access is feasible so as to not delay further interventions, MRI can provide valuable information with regards to the presence and specific pathoanatomy of ongoing spinal cord compression and the extent of disco-ligamentous injury, which can influence surgical treatment. In a single-center prospective study of 91 patients with acute SCI, outcomes for patients who had a pre-treatment MRI improved on average an additional 7/tenth of a Frankel grade compared to a reference group in which MRI could not be performed due to contraindications [37]. Based on their systematic review of the literature and on the clinical expertise of its multidisciplinary guideline development group, the AO Spine Foundation provided a weak recommendation for the use of MRI in patients with acute SCI prior to surgical intervention, when feasible, to facilitate surgical decision-making [38]. MRI may also provide important prognostic information in the setting of SCI [36]. Longer cord hemorrhage length on MRI and cord swelling (increased spinal cord diameter) in the acute phase have been associated worse neurological recovery [39, 40]. In a recent analysis based on a sample of 459 SCI patients from the prospective North American Clinical Trials Network registry, the presence of intrinsic spinal cord signal change on T2-weighted MRI was associated with an increased rate of in-hospital adverse events and prolonged length of stay

Table 28.2 Screening Criteria for BCVI

Denver Criteria	Memphis Criteria
Signs/symptoms of BCVI	Unexplained neurological deficit
Potential arterial hemorrhage from neck/nose/mouth	Horner's syndrome
Cervical bruit in patient <50 yrs. old	Lefort II or III fracture
Expanding cervical hematoma	Cervical spine injury
Focal neurological deficit	Skull base fractures involving the foramen laacerum
Stroke on CT or MRI	Neck soft tissue injury (e.g., seatbelt injury or hanging)
Risk factor for BCVI	
High-energy transfer mechanism	
Displaced midface fracture (Lefort II or III)	
Mandible fracture	
Complex skull base or occipital condyle fracture	
Severe TBI with GCS < 6	
Cervical spine fracture, subluxation or ligamentous injury	
Near hanging with anoxic brain injury	
Clothesline type injury or seat belt avrasing with siginficant swelling, pain, or altered mental status	
TBI with thoracic injuries	
Scalp degloving	
Thoracic vascular injuries	
Blunt cardiac rupture	
Upper rib fractures	

[41]. While there is growing interest in incorporating data from advanced neuroimaging modalities such as diffusion tensor imaging into prognostic models, current limitations of these techniques preclude widespread clinical use in SCI [42].

Surgical Management of SCI

There currently exists no effective surgical means for direct repair of the injured spinal cord. Surgical management of SCI is therefore primarily focused on expeditious relief of mechanical compression on spinal cord tissue in order to curtail the secondary injury cascade and optimize the potential for neurological recovery. Concomitant stabilization of the vertebral column allows for early mobilization and rehabilitation while preventing delayed neurological deterioration from pathological displacement of unstable spinal elements. Surgical techniques and instrumentation are constantly evolving to provide better spinal column stabilization, reconstruction, and restoration of normal alignment. Fixation devices are available for stabilization of the full neuraxis ranging from the occiput to the sacrum and pelvis. Implants are designed to be used in a variety of surgical approaches including anterior, posterior, and lateral exposures depending on the primary location of injury, instability, or mechanical failure. Further discussion of complex spine surgical techniques and instrumentation for the treatment of spinal column injuries is presented in a separate chapter.

In patients with cervical fracture-dislocation injuries, closed reduction can provide a way to rapidly restore spinal alignment and decompress the spinal cord. This is usually accomplished by applying longitudinal traction with incremental weights using skull tongs or a halo ring. Fluoroscopy or serial cervical spine radiographs should be used to monitor the progress and prevent overdistraction. Administration of muscle relaxants may facilitate reduction. A combined case series totalling over 1200 patients showed that successful reduction was achieved in approximately 80% of patients with acute cervical spine fracture-dislocation, with neurological complication rates under 1% [43]. Contraindications to closed reduction include an uncooperative or unexaminable patient and the presence of rostral spinal injuries or skull fractures at the intended halo or tong fixation site. Earlier concerns that closed reduction in the presence of an associated disc herniation could exacerbate neurological injury have not been corroborated in the literature. As such, as long as the patient is awake and examinable, a pre-reduction MRI has not been deemed necessary. Patients who cannot be assessed during reduction maneuvers (open or closed) are at higher risk for neurological deterioration and pre-reduction MRI is recommended as an option in this setting [44].

The last few decades have witnessed somewhat of a paradigm shift with respect to the timing of surgical management for patients with spinal cord injury. Historically, an initial conservative approach with bedrest and external immobilization was favored to avoid higher risk of surgical complications in acutely injured patients [45]. Spinal decompression was performed in a delayed fashion, if at all. However, mounting preclinical data pointing to a time-dependent effect of early surgical decompression on spinal cord recovery after SCI motivated the Surgical Timing in Acute Spinal Cord Injury Study (STASCIS), a multicenter prospective cohort study evaluating the relative effectiveness of early (<24 h after injury) vs. late (≥24 h after injury) decompressive surgery after cervical SCI [46]. 313 patients with acute cervical SCI were enrolled in 6 participating North American centers, 182 of which underwent early surgery. After controlling for baseline group differences in a multivariate analysis, the odds of at least a 2 grade AIS score at 6-month follow-up were 2.8 times higher for those who underwent early surgical intervention [46]. A growing body of literature alongside STASCIS favors early surgical decompression in traumatic SCI and has led to the concept that "time is spine" [47]. In a recent pooled analysis of individual data from 1548 patients enrolled in four prospective multicenter studies, surgical decompression within 24 h of acute SCI was associated with significantly improved sensorimotor recovery and AIS grades at 1-year follow-up [48]. In light of increasing evidence pointing to the benefits of early surgical and neuroprotective interventions, the concept that "time is spine" has become a key principle in the management of patients with acute SCI [49]. A large multicenter prospective observational study sponsored by AO Spine Europe (SCI-POEM) comparing the efficacy and safety of surgical intervention within 12 h of traumatic SCI versus >12 h and < 14 days found no statistically significant or clinically meaningful neurological improvements 12 months after surgery [50].

One subpopulation in which timing and indications for surgery have traditionally been more controversial is patients with central cord syndrome (CCS). CCS is characterized by more prominent weakness of the upper extremities compared to the lower extremities, with varying degrees of sensory disturbance, and commonly, hyperalgesia [24]. Proposed criteria to operationalize this definition have included ASIA lower extremity motor scores that are at least 10 points greater compared to upper extremity motor scores, but this definition has not been universally accepted [51, 52]. The prototypical central cord syndrome is an older individual with pre-existing cervical stenosis sustaining an incomplete cervical SCI after a fall or low-energy trauma without clear evidence of fracture or dislocation on imaging. However, it is now recognized that CCS encompasses a more heterogeneous spectrum of clinical phenotypes, including acute cervical disc herniation in younger age groups and cervical column fracture and/or dislocation after higher energy trauma [26]. While early surgical intervention in cases with clear mechanical instability or an acutely herniated disc has been encouraged and generally accepted, the role of early surgical intervention in CCS patients without these imaging findings has been more controversial. Previous reports suggesting a favorable natural history with conservative management in this subgroup of patients have contributed to hesitancy in decompressing these patients early [53]. However, more recent evidence suggests that natural recovery is not the rule in CCS and is largely influenced by the initial severity of the injury. Moreover, there are mounting data suggesting that surgical decompression within 24 h can enhance the potential for neurological recovery in CCS patients with ongoing compression [26, 47, 54, 55]. In accordance with these findings, clinical practice guidelines have suggested that early surgical decompression (≤24 h after injury) be considered as a treatment option in adult patients with traumatic central cord syndrome [56].

Despite global surveys showing that a majority of spinal surgeons now prefer to decompress the spinal cord within 24 h in most SCI cases [45], existing prehospital logistics and in-hospital care structures pose persisting barriers to early decompression. Studies conducted in North America and Europe have estimated that only 20 to 50% of patients are transferred to an appropriate care center early enough to be eligible for surgical decompression within 24 h of their initial trauma [57, 58]. Similarly, a recent analysis of data from 2862 cervical SCI patients included in the Trauma Quality and Improvement Program between 2010 and 2016, and who underwent decompressive surgery, showed that less than two-thirds of patients received surgery within the recommended timeframe [59]. Besides delays in transport to an appropriate care facility, timely access to operating room resources, local hospital practice patterns, as well as patient characteristics including race, and the presence of severe head or abdominal injuries, have been cited as factors contributing to these delays [53, 58–61]. A concerted effort to address these barriers is urgently needed to increase the proportion of SCI patients who can achieve their greatest potential for neurological recovery.

Acute Medical Management of SCI

Patients with traumatic SCI are prone to a number of life-threatening systemic and neurological complications. Close monitoring of respiratory, hemodynamic, and neurological function in the early period after SCI is therefore required and is best accomplished in the intensive care unit (ICU) setting. Prevention and early recognition of these multisystem issues are crucial in optimizing the potential for recovery.

Respiratory Management

Intubation and Mechanical Ventilation

Respiratory complications represent the most common causes of early and late morbidity and mortality after SCI and are a major contributor to prolonged ICU stay [62–64]. The risk of respiratory complications directly correlates with the anatomic level and severity of the injury, with an incidence reaching up to 84% in patients with higher cervical lesions (C1–4) and in 60% of those with C5–8 injuries [65–67]. Patients with lesions above C5 typically require early endotracheal intubation and mechanical ventilation due to complete or partial failure of all major muscles of respiration, including the diaphragm. Patients with lower cervical and thoracic injury can also develop progressive respiratory insufficiency and must be monitored closely in the acute stages. Even with an intact phrenic nerve, intercostal muscle dysfunction can reduce forced vital capacity (FVC) and maximum negative inspiratory force (NIF) by approximately two-thirds of normal [68–70]. Direct chest trauma and pulmonary injury also often frequently contribute to reduced respiratory reserve in patients with thoracic SCI. A declining forced vital capacity, increasing pCO_2, or falling pO_2 predict impending respiratory failure and should prompt strong consideration for intubation and mechanical ventilation regardless of injury level [67]. Optimal ventilator settings in patients with respiratory failure secondary to acute SCI have not been firmly established. The 2005 Consortium for Spinal Cord Medicine's Clinical Practice Guidelines on Respiratory Management Following Spinal Cord Injury recommended the use of high tidal volumes (20 mL/kg of ideal body weight) as a means of preventing atelectasis and facilitating ventilator weaning [71]. This recommendation stands in sharp contrast with the low tidal volume approach used as part of a lung protective strategy in ICU patients at risk for acute respiratory distress syndrome (ARDS). There is a large body of Class I evidence supporting a low tidal volume strategy in conjunction with positive end expiratory pressure (PEEP) to prevent atelectasis in this setting to reduce the risk of ventilator-associated lung injury and improve survival [72, 73]. An approach favouring lung protective ventilation in the acute phase of the injury, when the risk of ARDS is highest, followed by a gradual increase in tidal volumes during the weaning phase is used in many specialized centres. Prospective trials are needed to reconcile these diverging viewpoints and to determine optimal ventilation parameters in acute SCI patients. Similarly, the role of non-invasive ventilation in treating respiratory failure patients or in optimizing extubation success in SCI has not been well studied and remains to be clearly defined [66, 74, 75].

Pneumonia

Pneumonia accounts for the majority of respiratory-related deaths in SCI [65, 76]. As with other respiratory complications, the risk of pneumonia is closely correlated with the level of injury, with a greater than 60% incidence in patients with SCI at C4 or above [62, 65, 77, 78]. Weakness of the diaphragm, chest wall, and abdominal muscles leads to ineffective cough and secretion clearance, contributing to a significantly elevated risk of respiratory infection. In a retrospective analysis of 197 patients with complete traumatic SCI, surgical timing >24 h after injury was also strongly associated with the development of pneumonia in the acute period [79]. Sustained hypoxia from moderate and severe pneumonia may also impact neurological outcomes by contributing to the secondary injury burden. Vigilant attention to secretion management, chest physiotherapy as well as prompt recognition and antibiotic treatment of pneumonias is therefore crucial to minimize the adverse consequences of respiratory infections in this patient population [80].

Tracheostomy

As the initial flaccidity of respiratory muscles associated with spinal shock transitions to a more spastic state, spontaneous ventilation may improve sufficiently to allow for liberation from mechanical ventilation in some patients. However, tracheostomy should be considered in patients in which prolonged intubation is anticipated or in those who fail to wean from mechanical ventilation. Tracheostomy offers several advantages including facilitation of ventilation weaning by reducing airway resistance, easier tracheal access for secretion management, improved patient comfort and phonation, while minimizing complications of prolonged mechanical ventilation, such as vocal cord ulceration, subglottic edema, and tracheal stenosis. Age, level and completeness of injury, higher injury severity score (ISS), preexisting lung disease, presence of pneumonia, and poor PaO_2/FiO_2 ratios have been identified as potential predictors of tracheostomy requirement, although most studies on this topic are retrospective [81, 82]. The optimal timing of tracheostomy in this patient population remains unclear owing to the lack of class I and class II studies. In a retrospective analysis of 5980 patients with cervical SCI in the American College Trauma Quality Improvement Program database, early tracheostomy patients (≤4 days from initial intubation) showed lower rates of respiratory complications, higher ventilator- and ICU-free days and a shorter hospital length of stay compared with those receiving late tracheostomy (>4 days) [83]. A recent meta-analysis of 17 studies looking at tracheostomy timing in SCI reached similar conclusions with respect to the benefits of early tracheostomy on duration of mechanical ventilation and ICU or hospital length of stay, with most studies defining early tracheostomy as within 7 days of injury or intubation [84]. This study also demonstrated an association between early tracheostomy and decreased incidence of ventilator-associated pneumonia and tracheostomy-related complications, but there was no short-term mortality benefit. Despite a perceived risk of cross-contamination when tracheostomy is performed in close temporal proximity to anterior cervical spinal surgery, early tracheostomy prior to, or just after, anterior surgery has not been associated with increased rates of surgical site infection [85–88].

Hemodynamic Management

Neurogenic Shock

Patients with severe cervical and upper thoracic SCI are at risk for developing neurogenic shock. Neurogenic shock refers to the combination of bradycardia, hypotension, and vasoplegia attributed to the interruption of sympathetic fibers innervating the heart and peripheral vascular beds. It should be differentiated from spinal shock, which is a phenomenon characterized by hypotonia and areflexia below the injury level after acute SCI. In neurogenic shock, the interruption of preganglionic input to efferent cardiac sympathetic fibers arising from upper thoracic spinal cord segments results in decreased chronotropy, inoptropy, and dromotropy. Because the vagal nerve originates at the brainstem level, descending parasympathetic cardiac inputs to the sinoatrial and atrioventricular nodes are left unopposed and relative bradycardia ensue (Fig. 28.3). The resulting drop in cardiac output is compounded by a concomitant loss of sympathetic vascular tone below the neurological level, contributing to a further reduction in mean arterial pressure and risk of circulatory collapse. As described in previous sections of this chapter, adequate mean arterial pressure (MAP) should be promptly restored with a combination of volume expansion and vasopressors to avoid the detrimental effects of hypotension on spinal cord perfusion and longer-term neurological recovery [78]. With the exception of significant hemorrhage from polytrauma, most patients are relatively euvolemic and excessive fluid administration should generally be avoided to minimize cord swelling and the risk of precipitating pulmonary edema [89]. Appropriate management of neurogenic shock involves the use of vasoactive agents to counteract the loss of systemic vasoconstriction and dysregulation of cardiac function (Table 28.3). Norepinephrine is a first-line agent for the treatment of neurogenic shock as it combines alpha vasoconstrictive properties with beta-chronotropic and inotropic effects. Dopamine has also traditionally been used in this setting but suffers from a worse side-effect profile and safety profile [20, 90]. Phenylephrine should generally be avoided in this context given the rebound bradycardia that in some instances can lead to sinus arrest and asystole. Bradyarrhythmia secondary to loss of sympathetic tone can

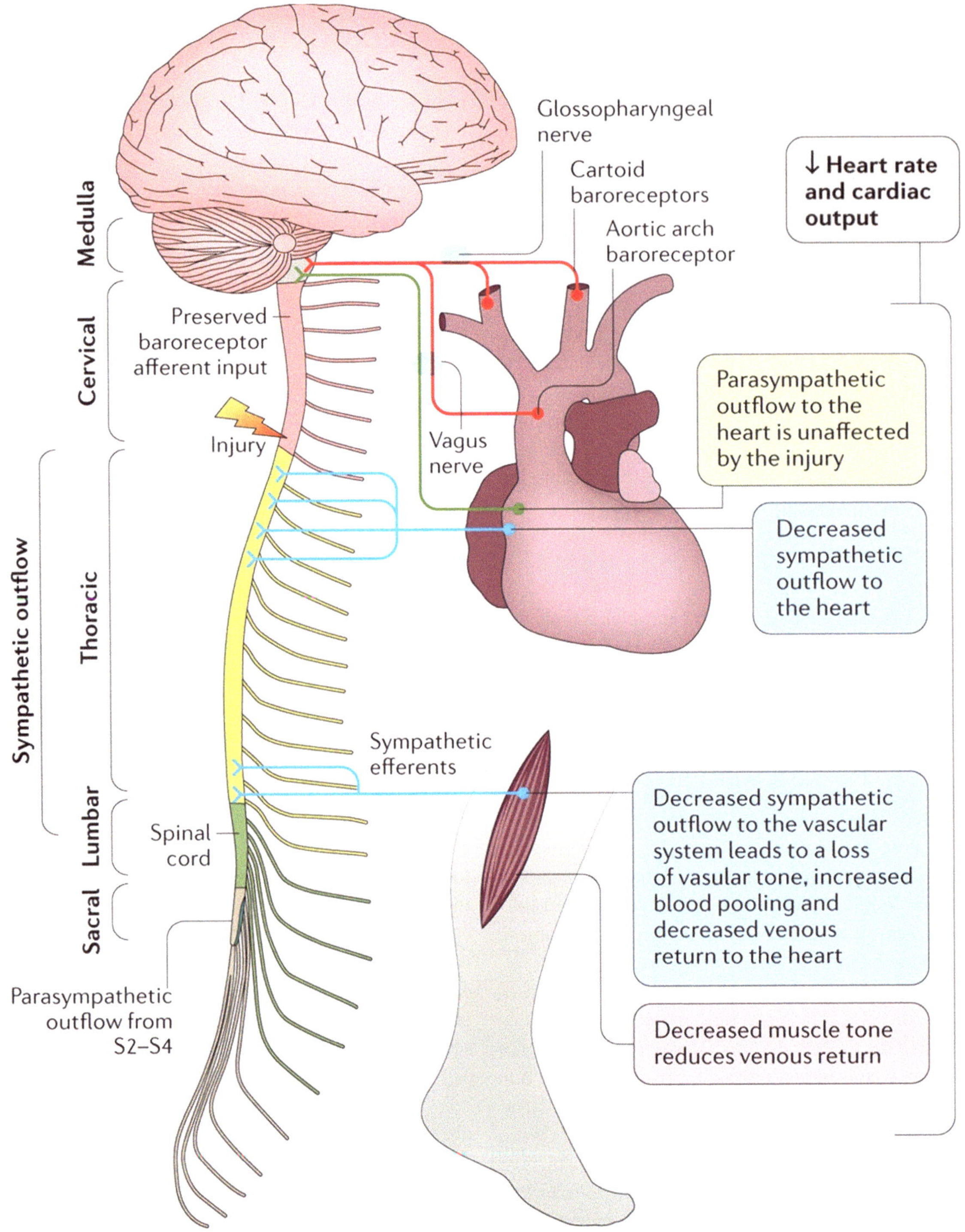

Fig. 28.3 Cervical and high thoracic spinal cord injuries disrupt the outflow of the sympathetic nervous system. Injuries in the cervical and high thoracic cord can disrupt the sympathetic outflow (blue line) to the heart and the peripheral vascular system, while preserving baroreceptor inputs (red line) and parasympathetic output (green line). As a result, parasympathetic innervation to the heart dominates in patients with cervical and upper thoracic injuries, which causes bradycardia and decreased cardiac output. This is further compounded by the loss of peripheral muscular and vascular tone, which promotes a redistribution of blood to the periphery with reduced venous return. Consequently, patients often experience hypotensive symptoms, particularly with exertion or upright positioning. The parasympathetic–sympathetic imbalance can also allow unchecked reflex spinal sympathetic stimulation as a consequence of noxious triggers (such as bladder distension or pressure sores), which leads to sudden peripheral vasoconstriction and acute hypertension. As a response, parasympathetic outflow above the injury level increases, leading to vasodilation, headaches, sweating and sinus congestion. This dangerous acute syndrome is known as autonomic dysreflexia. S2–S4, sacral levels 2–4. (Republished with permissions of Macmillan Publishers Limited, Traumatic spinal cord injury. Republished with permissions of Macmillan Publishers Limited, Traumatic spinal cord injury. Reproduced with permission from Ahuja C.S et al. *Nature Reviews Disease Primers*. 3:17019, 2017)

Table 28.3 Vasoactive agents for refractory hypotention and neurogenic shock in traumatic spinal cord injury

Agent	Typical dose	Activity	Considerations
Norepinephrine	0.05–0.4 μg/kg/min	αααβ	Generally considered first line option
Epinephrine	0.01–0.5 μg/kg/min	αβββ	Arrhythmogenic potential
Dopamine	2–20 μg/kg/min	αβββD	Dose-dependent action, myocardial ischemia, arrhythmogenic potential, increased mortality with use in septic shock
Phenylephrine	0.25–5 μg/kg/min	αβ	Reflex bradycardia
Vasopressin	0.01–0.04 units/min	V1&V2	Pure vasopressor effect, antidiuretic effect and theoretical risk of worsened spinal cord edema
Dobutamine	1.5–20 μg/kg/min	ββββ	Variable effect on mean arterial pressure

be managed either by anticholinergics, such as atropine, or with chronotropic agents, such as norepinephrine and epinephrine. In refractory cases, temporary or permanent pacing may be necessary.

MAP Augmentation and Spinal Cord Perfusion

The joint guideline from the American Association of Neurological Surgeons/Congress of Neurological Surgeons (AANS/CNS) recommends maintaining a mean arterial pressure (MAP) goal of 85 to 90 mmHg for the first 7 days after injury [78]. This recommendation was based on Class III evidence, and while there is general agreement that hypotension after acute neurological injury is harmful and should be avoided, the optimal target and duration of blood pressure management remains uncertain. A systematic review which included additional data that became available after the publication of the 2013 AANS/CNS guidelines, concluded that despite a lack of high-quality data, MAP goals of 85–90 mmHg for 5–7 days should be considered based on 2 prospective studies suggesting stable to improved neurological outcomes [20]. The first step in achieving these targets is ensuring adequate intravascular fluid status by a combination of clinical examination, point-of-care transthoracic echocardiography, and other non-invasive cardiac output monitors if available. Fluid overload should be avoided given the increased risk of pulmonary edema in these patients secondary to autonomic nervous system dysregulation. The routine use of pulmonary artery catheters has fallen out of favor after a series of randomized controlled trials demonstrating possible harm and lack of a clear benefit in various ICU subpopulations [91]. Other common causes of hemodynamic instability in trauma patients, such as hemorrhagic shock, tension pneumothorax, pericardial tamponade and sepsis, should be considered and expeditiously treated if present. Use of blood products should be considered depending on the overall systemic injury pattern and guided by hemodynamic status, blood counts, and coagulation profile. After taking the aforementioned steps, vasoactive agents should be initiated if the MAP remains below the target range. The Consortium for Spinal Cord Medicine recommends selection of vasopressor agent according to level of injury [92]. Given the risk of bradydysrhythmias in cervical and high thoracic injuries, they recommend agents with chronotropic and inotropic properties as well as vasoconstrictor effects such as dopamine and norepinephrine in this patient subgroup. For lower thoracic lesions where hypotension is primarily mediated by peripheral vasodilation, they recommend a pure vasoconstrictor such as phenylephrine (Table 28.3). However, there is growing evidence that dopamine use is associated with higher mortality in the critical care literature [93, 94]. It has also been linked to an increased incidence of arrythmias and myocardial ischemia in SCI patients [20, 95, 96]. Therefore, norepinephrine has been gaining acceptance as the initial vasopressor of choice in SCI, especially in patients in which both alpha and beta-adrenergic effects are desired. Phenylephrine remains an acceptable choice for patients in whom reflex bradycardia is less of a concern, and theoretically holds less arrhythmogenic potential as a pure alpha agonist, although adequate comparisons between phenylephrine and norepinephrine have not been performed. There is a paucity of data to support the use of epinephrine and vasopressin in SCI. Regardless of vasopressor choice, the minimum dose required to achieve MAP targets should be used to minimize the potential harmful effects of hemodynamic augmentation.

During the last decade, there has been interest in using spinal cord perfusion pressure (SCPP) rather than MAP as a target for hemodynamic management in SCI. This is analogous to controlling cerebral perfusion pressure in severe traumatic brain injury via simultaneous measurements of arterial and intracranial pressure. In the spine, this could potentially be accomplished via insertion of a lumbar drain, allowing for measurement of cerebrospinal fluid (CSF) pressure in the intrathecal compartment. In a multicenter prospective study of 92 patients with acute SCI, maintaining an SCPP (MAP—CSF pressure) above 50 mmHg was a strong independent predictor of improved neurological recovery [97]. Critics of this approach have suggested that CSF pressure measured in the lumbar compartment may not accurately reflect intraspinal pressure (ISP) when circumferential occlusion of CSF space at the injury site from cord swelling is present [98]. Alternative ISP measurement methods include intraparenchymal or subdural probes placed at the injury site during surgical decompression. Autoregulatory failure has been implicated as a potential secondary injury mechanism in SCI and measurements of ISP via either method also allow for calculation of spinal cerebrovascular reactivity indices [21]. The spinal pressure reactivity index (sPRX), calculated as the moving correlation coefficient between ISP and MAP, has been proposed as a surrogate of spinal cord autoregulation, with more negative values representing better autoregulatory capacity. This index, in turn, allows for calculation of the continuous optimal SCPP, that is, the SCPP value at which the sPRx is minimized. In a small preliminary study on 14 patients with severe traumatic SCI, the mean SCPP deviation from the optimal SCPP correlated with worse neurological outcomes at 9–12 months [99].

Autonomic Dysreflexia

Patients with injury above the T6 level are at risk of autonomic dysreflexia. While it is usually a later complication of traumatic SCI, it can occasionally present while the patient is still hospitalized in an acute care setting. It is characterized by an exaggerated sympathetic response to noxious stimuli below the injury level leading to vasocontriction and severe hypertension, with a compensatory parasympathetic response above the injury level causing bradycardia and vasodilation. Clinically, this manifests as hypertension associated with headache, diaphoresis and facial flushing, nasal congestion, visual disturbances, nausea, or anxiety. In some cases, elevation of blood pressure can be severe and life-threatening. Management principles during acute attacks include close monitoring of vital signs, sitting the patient upright if possible, prompt recognition and elimination of the trigger and pharmacological control of blood pressure. In up to 85% of cases, the culprit stimulus is urological such as a distended bladder or urinary tract infection (UTI) [100]. Bladder drainage should be promptly performed and if an indwelling catheter is in place, it should be evaluated for obstruction. If bladder distention has been ruled out, evaluation for UTI should be considered. Fecal impaction is another common trigger and should be appropriately relieved [101]. In cases in which the hypertensive response is severe or persistent, rapid onset short-acting antihypertensive such as nitrates, nifedipine, or intravenous hydralazine or labetalol should be used.

Venous Thromboembolism

Spinal cord injury patients have been shown to have the highest risk of venous thromboembolism (VTE) among major trauma patients [102]. Rates vary according to surveillance technique, ranging from 18% to 100% in SCI patients undergoing routine screening [103–105]. A more recent study of patients treated with leg compression devices but no anticoagulant thromboprophylaxis reported deep venous thrombosis (DVT) rates of 41% in acute SCI patients undergoing serial ultrasonography [106]. When considering the subgroup of patients with ASIA A or B injuries only, the rate of DVT was 73%. The greatest risk period appears to be between 72 h and 2 weeks after injury [104, 105, 107]. The risk decreases significantly after the first 3 months but remains elevated compared to the general population [108]. The risk of pulmonary embolism after acute SCI has been estimated at 4 to 14% (see NCC guidelines). The Consortium for Spinal Cord Medicine (2016), the Neurocritical Care Society (2016), AO Spine (2017), and the AANS/CNS (2013) have each published their own set of guidelines for VTE prophylaxis in SCI patients [102, 104, 105, 109]. There is general agreement that pharmacological prophylaxis with low-molecular-weight heparin (LMWH) should be initiated as soon as possible, provided bleeding risk is acceptable and there are no other contraindications. Mechanical methods including intermittent pneumatic compression devices and/or graduated compression stockings can be used as adjuncts, but should not be used in isolation unless a contraindication to pharmacological prophylaxis is present. The routine use of inferior vena cava filters is not recommended and should only be considered in patients with contraindications to anticoagulation after ultrasonographic confirmation of a DVT [105].

Other Acute Care Considerations

Gastrointestinal

Dysfunction of the enteric nervous system after SCI may lead to gastrointestinal complications including impaired gastric emptying, gastroduodenal ulceration, paralytic ileus, and constipation [89, 110]. Gastric ulceration prophylaxis should be considered, especially in patients requiring mechanical ventilation with contraindication to enteral feeding [111–113]. Nutritional support should be initiated within 72 h if feasible. Multimodal bowel management regimens, which include a combination of high dietary fiber intake, stool softeners and laxatives, promotility agents, digital rectal stimulation as well as manual disimpaction, should be implemented early to improve patient comfort and reduce the incidence of autonomic dysreflexia [114].

Genitourinary

Interruption of the micturition reflex pathways during the spinal shock phase invariably causes urinary retention requiring catheterization to avoid bladder overdistention [115]. During this phase, indwelling catheterization also allows for closer monitoring of overall fluid status, particularly in polytrauma patients. However, continuous bladder catheterization poses an increased risk of urinary tract infections, prostatitis, epididymitis, and renal impairment [110, 115]. Early transition to clean intermittent catheterization or suprapubic cystostomy is recommended to reduce the risk of developing urinary tract infections and other renal complications [116]. A meta-analysis of 15 clinical trials examining the use of antimicrobial prophylaxis for UTI in SCI failed to show a reduced rate of symptomatic infections [117]. Prophylaxis was also associated with a twofold increase in the risk of developing bacterial resistance.

Pressure Ulcers

Patients with severe SCI are at high risk for developing pressure ulcers. Inadequate tissue perfusion, prolonged maintenance on a spine backboard, immobilization with inadequate logrolling, and the patient's impaired sensation of tissue injury contribute to increased risk for skin ulceration [118]. Standard care should include manual logrolling, use of rotating beds if available, and meticulous skin care with frequent inspection and hygiene. Occupational and physical therapy should be initiated as soon as the patient is stable and able to participate.

Pain

A majority of SCI patients report musculoskeletal and/or neuropathic pain, which should be managed with a multimodal and opioid-sparing approach, particularly in patients with concomitant head injuries requiring frequent neurological reassessments, or non-intubated SCI patients at risk of ventilatory compromise. Prompt realignment and stabilization of fractures may help alleviate pain originating from the primary injury site. Between 26% and 96% of SCI patients may develop chronic pain refractory to conventional pharmacological as well as allopathic treatments, and may benefit from surgical and/or neuromodulatory approaches including spinal cord stimulation, deep brain stimulation, and dorsal root entry lesioning [119–121].

Psychosocial

Given the life-altering consequences of SCI, sensitivity to the patient's and family's emotional reactions is essential. As with any grieving process, patients progress through the typical stages of grief including denial, anger, depression, and finally acceptance. The role of critical care providers in caring for these patients must include an awareness of these stages of grief and fostering completion of the grieving process. While there is no clear ideal method for helping patients through this extraordinary time, in general, compassion and honesty in discussing care and prognosis, education, and counseling are advocated.

Neuroprotection and Neuroregeneration

The role of neuroprotective agents and neuroregenerative therapies designed to treat SCI and improve functional recovery is currently limited. Several clinical trials have investigated the role of neuroprotective drugs in curtailing secondary injury mechanisms. A number of neuroregenerative strategies have also emerged and are under active investigation in preclinical and clinical studies. The most promising therapies are discussed below and summarized in Table 28.4.

Neuroprotective Drugs

Methylprednisolone Sodium Succinate (MPSS)

Administration of intravenous high-dose methylprednisolone sodium succinate (MPSS) for the treatment of acute SCI has been the subject of considerable scrutiny and debate. The rationale for the use of corticosteroids in SCI is derived from preclinical studies showing potential benefits in attenuating the inflammatory cascade contributing to secondary injury [122–126]. A series of randomized controlled trials (RCTs), the National Acute Spinal Cord Injury Study (NASCIS) I, II, and III, have been conducted to study the safety and efficacy of MPSS therapy [127–130]. While no significant benefits in terms of sensorimotor or functional

Table 28.4 Selected trials and emerging therapies in traumatic spinal cord injury

Treatment	Stage	ClinicalTrials.gov identifier
Pharmacological neuroprotection/ neuroregeneration		
Minocycline	Phase III	NCT01828203
Riluzole	Phase IIb/III	NCT01597518
Acidic fibroblast growth factor	Phase III	NCT03229031
Granulocute colony-stimulating factor	Phase I/ II	N/A
Rho-ROCK inhibition	Phasse IIb/III	NCT02669849
Anti-Nogo-A antibody	Phase II	NCT03935321
Non-pharmacological neuroprotection		
Therapeutic hypothermia	Phase II/ III	NCT02991690
Cell-based strategies		
Oligodendrocytes precursors cells	Phase I/ II	NCT02302157
Schwann cells	Phase I	NCT01739023
Mesenchymal stem cells	Phase II	NCT02570932
Biomaterial scaffolds		
Bioresorbable polymers hyaluronan/methylcellulose	Phase I	N/A
Neuromodulation		
Electrical spinal cord stimulation	Phase I/ II	N/A
Brain-spinal cord interfaces	Phse I/II	N/A

Adapted with permissions of Macmillan Publishers Limited, Traumatic spinal cord injury. Ahuja C.S et al. *Nature Reviews Disease Primers*. 3:17019, 2017 recovery were seen in the primary outcome analysis, post-hoc analysis of the NASCIS II data showed that patients who received MPSS within 8 h of injury demonstrated a modest but statistically significant (16.0 vs. 11.2 ASIA motor score, $p = 0.033$ at 6 months) improvement in motor function at 6 months compared to placebo [129]. Similarly, a post-hoc analysis of the NASCIS III data showed greater motor recovery within a 48 h compared to a 24 h MPSS protocol if corticosteroid treatment was initiated within 3–8 h of injury, however, the 48 h protocol was associated with a significantly higher rate of pneumonia and a trend toward higher rates of sepsis [131]. In the aftermath of the NASCIS studies, administration of MPSS within 8 h of SCI became commonplace in many centers. However, a shift away from the use of MPSS occurred after the AANS/CNS 2013 included a level 1 recommendation against the administration of MPSS for the treatment of acute SCI [132]. This recommendation represented a departure from their 2002 guidelines despite the lack of a commensurate shift in the body of evidence. Given the extensive debate about the methodology and subgroup analyses from the NASCIS series, a comprehensive Cochrane review encompassing six RCTs and key observational studies on the use of intravenous corticosteroids in SCI was performed in 2012 [133]. This analysis demonstrated a modest but significant 4-point ASIA motor score improvement for patients receiving MPSS within 8 h of injury. Based on an updated systematic review of the literature including this analysis, in their 2017 Clinical Practice Guideline for the Management of Patients with Acute Spinal Cord Injury, AO Spine suggested that a 24 h infusion of high-dose MPSS be offered as a treatment option for acute SCI patient without contraindications [134, 135]. While the use of steroids in the treatment of acute SCI remains controversial and should not be viewed as standard of care, it remains an option after carefully balancing the risks and benefits in individual patients given that small motor gains in key myotomes can lead to meaningful improvement in function and quality of life in selected patients.

Minocycline

The antibiotic minocycline is a tetracycline derivative that has been shown to reduce oligodendrocyte and microglial apoptosis in animal models of SCI [136, 137]. In a phase II trial published in 2012, acute cervical SCI patients treated with minocycline ($N = 27$) compared to placebo ($N = 25$) demonstrated an improvement in ASIA motor score at 1 year, which approached significance (14 points, $p = 0.05$) [138]. This led to the phase III Minocycline in Acute Spinal Cord Injury (MASC) trial that tested the effect of twice daily IV minocycline versus placebo for 7 days in cervical SCI patients with a target enrollment of 248 (NCT01828203).

Riluzole

Riluzole is a benzothiazole voltage-gated sodium-channel-blocker that modulates glutamatergic neurotransmission and has been shown to reduce motor neuron degeneration and improve survival in patients with Amyotrophic Lateral Sclerosis [139]. A phase I/II trial that enrolled 36 SCI patients demonstrated improved ASIA motor scores (15.5 points) in riluzole-treated patients with cervical SCI with a similar complication profile compared to matched controls from the North American Clinical Trials Network SCI Registry [140]. These findings set the stage for the phase IIb/III Riluzole in Acute Spinal Cord Injury (RISCIS) study designed to further assess the efficacy of riluzole in patients with C4–8 level injuries [141]. Unfortunately, the trial was recently terminated early due to slow enrollment.

Acidic Fibroblast Growth Factor

Acidic fibroblast growth factor (aFGF) has been shown to stimulate axonal regeneration and promote neuronal survival in animal studies [142]. In a trial of 49 chronic SCI patients, surgical application of fibrin glue containing aFGF with booster treatments via lumbar puncture at 3 and 6 months resulted in significant improvements in ASIA motor and sensory scores, AIS grade, and Functional Independence Measure at 24 months after treatment [143]. A phase III placebo-controlled RCT started the recruitment process in 2017 with a target enrollment of 100 patients with an AIS grade A SCI (NCT03229031).

Granulocyte Colony-Stimulating Factor

Granulocyte colony-stimulating factor (G-CSF) is a cytokine glycoprotein that stimulates bone marrow to produce neutrophils and promotes their survival and mobilization. It has also been shown to have neuroprotective effects in SCI animal models via suppression of neuronal and oligodendroglial apoptosis, affecting myelin repair, and by modulating the expression of inflammatory cytokines such as TNF-α and IL-1β [144, 145]. A phase III RCT in which 120 chronic SCI patients were randomized to 300 μg/day of G-CSF for one week compared to placebo showed significant improvements in AIS motor scores in the treatment arm [146]. A second phase III trial, G-SPIRIT, investigated the benefits of 400 μg/day of intravenous G-CSF for 5 days in patients with acute AIS grade A or B SCIs. This trial completed recruitment in 2019 and publication of the results is pending (umin.ac.jp/ctr/, UMIN000018752).

Non-Pharmacological Neuroprotective Strategies

Therapeutic Hypothermia

The neuroprotective effects of hypothermia have long been documented. Putative mechanisms through which hypothermia affords neuroprotection include a reduction in metabolic rate, decreased generation of free radicals, mitigation of the inflammatory response and inhibition of excitotoxity [147–149]. Targeted temperature management with a target of 32–36 °C is currently advocated to improve neurological outcomes in patients who remain comatose after cardiac arrest [150]. A pilot study of 14 acute AIS grade A patients in which therapeutic hypothermia was induced with systemic intravascular cooling showed AIS grade conversion in 6/14 of the participants (42.8%) [151]. The Miami Project to Cure Paralysis is currently sponsoring a phase II/III trial to further evaluate the safety and efficacy of modest (33 °C) hypothermia for 48 h in acute cervical AIS A-C patients (ARCTIC, NCT02991690).

Neuroregenerative Therapies

Rho-ROCK Inhibition

Preclinical data suggest that upregulation of the Rho/Rho-associated kinase (ROCK) signaling pathway after SCI promotes inhibition of axonal regeneration [152]. C3 transferase, an enzyme produced by *Clostridium botulinum*, has been shown to counteract Rho-mediated inhibition of axonal growth and promote neural regeneration in animal models of SCI. In a phase I/IIa clinical trial, a cell-permeable recombinant version of C3 transferase, BA-210, was applied locally on the dural surface at the site of injury during decompressive surgery in 48 patients with acute complete SCI [153]. Patients who received BA-210 treatment demonstrated increased motor recovery and AIS-grade conversion at 12 months in comparison to historical controls. This motivated the Spinal Cord Injury Rho Inhibition Investigation (SPRING) trial, a phase IIb/III study, led by Vertex Pharmaceuticals, to test the efficacy of VX-210 (formerly BA-210) delivered epidurally in a fibrin sealant at the injury site during decompressive surgery. This trial began recruiting in 2016 (NCT02669849), but was ended prematurely after an interim analysis failed to show improvement in upper-extremity motor scores at 6 months between the treatment and placebo arm.

Anti-Nogo-A Antibody

Nogo-A, a protein found in central nervous system myelin, is an important inhibitor of neurite growth after injury. In preclinical studies, Anti-Nogo-A antibodies have shown promising results in terms of promoting axonal regeneration and recovery during locomotor training [154, 155]. A phase II RCT testing safety, feasibility, and preliminary efficacy of intrathecally-delivered antibodies against Nogo-A in ameliorating upper extremity motor function in patients with acute cervical SCI is currently underway (NCT03935321).

Anti-RGMa-Antibody

The glycoprotein, repulsive guidance molecule A (RGMa), is upregulated in various cell types around the SCI lesion site and plays an important role in the inhibition of neurite growth [156]. Systematic or intrathecal administration of Anti-RGMa antibodies in animal models of SCI has been associated with enhanced neuronal survival, regeneration of the corticospinal tract, and motor recovery [157–160]. These findings prompted a phase II RCT investigating the safety and efficacy of intravenously administered Elezanumab—a monoclonal antibody that neutralizes RGMa—for improving upper extremity motor score after AIS A or B cervical SCI (NCT04295538).

Cell-Based Therapies

A number of neuroprotective and neurodegenerative approaches based on exogenous cell-based therapies are also currently being investigated. Specific strategies include transplantation of autologous Schwann cells, mesenchymal stem cells, olfactory ensheathing cells, neural precursor cells, oligodendrocyte progenitor cells, and activated macrophages. Despite significant challenges associated with delivery, safety, and cost-effectiveness, many of these strategies have demonstrated positive results in Phase 1 and II trials [161–163].

Biomaterial Scaffolds

The use of biological scaffolds to provide structural guidance for growing axons, optimize local drug delivery, and support cell-based therapies is another avenue of active research. The bioresorbable polymers hyaluronan/methylcellulose (HAMC) and the Neuron-Spinal Scaffold (InVIvoTherapeutics) have been used to support engraftment of neural stem cells with promising results in preclinical and Phase I studies [164–166].

Neuromodulation

Spinal cord stimulation (SCS) is currently approved as a treatment option for a variety of chronic pain conditions refractory to conventional therapies. Within the realm of SCI research, it has been applied to exploit the activity-dependent plasticity of spinal networks in conjunction with neurorehabilitation protocols. Improvements in weight-bearing capacity and locomotion have been reported when applying transcutaneous or epidural stimulation in animal models and human SCI subjects undergoing rehabilitation training [167, 168]. Similarly, implantation of lumbosacral SCS was recently associated with improved ambulation in a series of chronic SCI patients when combined with an intense rehabilitation program [169–171]. Stimulation technologies have also been coupled with brain-spine interfaces to bypass the disrupted spinal cord tissue in the generation of volitional movements. The use of such interfaces was shown to restore locomotion in rodent and monkey models of SCI [172, 173]. Several trials are currently underway to further delineate the role of electrical spinal cord stimulation and other neuromodulatory technologies in optimizing functional recovery after SCI.

Conclusion

Although traumatic SCI continues to have devastating consequences for patients and their families, progress in our understanding of its pathophysiology has led to improved diagnostic and therapeutic approaches during the last few decades. The development of specialized SCI centers, along with recognition of the importance of early surgery, has translated into improved functional outcomes and quality of life for SCI patients. Early intubation and ventilatory support with lung-protective strategies in patients developing signs of respiratory failure is a key component of the acute management of SCI in the intensive care unit. From a cardiovascular standpoint, vasoactive agents with alpha- and beta-agonist properties, such as norepinephrine, should be used to treat neurogenic shock and maintain the mean arterial pressure between 85 and 90 mmHg. Promising research into the use of spinal cord perfusion and spinal vascular reactivity monitoring should allow for the development of individualized hemodynamic targets. Better awareness, prevention and management of the multisystemic complications associated with this diagnosis, including avoidance of thromboembolism, urinary tract infections, gastric and pressure ulceration and autonomic dysreflexia, are also crucial to mitigate the longer-term morbidity and mortality associated with SCI. Further work to enhance knowledge translation and remove barriers to early intervention is needed to maximize the number of patients achieving their greatest rehabilitation potential. More systematic efforts to gather large-scale datasets via the development and implementation of common data elements will also be crucial to better understand the heterogeneity between patient subgroups and develop more personalized treatment pathways. Ultimately, evidence-based medical, surgical, and pharmacological treatments, cell-based therapies, and other evolving neuroprotective and neurogenerative interventions will need to be used in combination to optimally reduce the impact of SCI on patients and society.

Acknowledgement The authors acknowledge the work and contributions of Alexander Taghva and Daniel J. Hoh in the previous edition of this chapter, which inspired this new third edition.

References

1. Injury GBDTB, Spinal Cord Injury C. Global, regional, and national burden of traumatic brain injury and spinal cord injury, 1990-2016: a systematic analysis for the global burden of disease study 2016. Lancet Neurol. 2019;18(1):56–87. https://doi.org/10.1016/S1474-4422(18)30415-0.
2. The National Spinal Cord Injury Statistical Center. Accessed Nov 28 2021. https://www.nscisc.uab.edu. Accessed 28 Nov 2021.
3. Ackery A, Tator C, Krassioukov A. A global perspective on spinal cord injury epidemiology. J Neurotrauma. 2004;21(10):1355–70. https://doi.org/10.1089/neu.2004.21.1355.
4. Lee BB, Cripps RA, Fitzharris M, Wing PC. The global map for traumatic spinal cord injury epidemiology: update 2011, global incidence rate. Spinal Cord. 2014;52(2):110–6. https://doi.org/10.1038/sc.2012.158.
5. Fehlings MG, Tetreault L, Nater A, et al. The aging of the global population: the changing epidemiology of disease and Spinal disorders. Neurosurgery. 2015;77(Suppl 4):S1–5. https://doi.org/10.1227/NEU.0000000000000953.
6. van den Berg ME, Castellote JM, Mahillo-Fernandez I, de Pedro-Cuesta J. Incidence of spinal cord injury worldwide: a systematic review. Neuroepidemiology. 2010;34(3):184–92.; discussion 192. https://doi.org/10.1159/000279335.
7. Devivo MJ. Epidemiology of traumatic spinal cord injury: trends and future implications. Spinal Cord. 2012;50(5):365–72. https://doi.org/10.1038/sc.2011.178.
8. Badhiwala JH, Wilson JR, Fehlings MG. Global burden of traumatic brain and spinal cord injury. Lancet Neurol. 2019;18(1):24–5. https://doi.org/10.1016/S1474-4422(18)30444-7.
9. Malekzadeh H, Golpayegani M, Ghodsi Z, et al. Direct cost of illness for Spinal Cord injury: a systematic review Global. Spine J. 2021;92(1):223–31. https://doi.org/10.1177/21925682211031190.
10. DeVivo MJ. Causes and costs of spinal cord injury in the United States. Spinal Cord. 1997;35(12):809–13. https://doi.org/10.1038/sj.sc.3100501.
11. Mirovsky Y, Shalmon E, Blankstein A, Halperin N. Complete paraplegia following gunshot injury without direct trauma to the cord. Spine (Phila Pa 1976). 2005;30(21):2436–8. https://doi.org/10.1097/01.brs.0000184588.54710.61.
12. Agrawal SK, Fehlings MG. Mechanisms of secondary injury to spinal cord axons in vitro: role of Na+, Na(+)-K(+)-ATPase, the Na(+)-H+ exchanger, and the Na(+)-Ca2+ exchanger. J Neurosci. 1996;16(2):545–52.
13. Choo AM, Liu J, Lam CK, Dvorak M, Tetzlaff W, Oxland TR. Contusion, dislocation, and distraction: primary hemorrhage and membrane permeability in distinct mechanisms of spinal cord injury. J Neurosurg Spine. 2007;6(3):255–66. https://doi.org/10.3171/spi.2007.6.3.255.
14. Tator CH, Fehlings MG. Review of the secondary injury theory of acute spinal cord trauma with emphasis on vascular mechanisms. J Neurosurg. 1991;75(1):15–26. https://doi.org/10.3171/jns.1991.75.1.0015.
15. Ulndreaj A, Chio JC, Ahuja CS, Fehlings MG. Modulating the immune response in spinal cord injury. Expert Rev Neurother. 2016;16(10):1127–9. https://doi.org/10.1080/14737175.2016.1207532.
16. Pineau I, Lacroix S. Proinflammatory cytokine synthesis in the injured mouse spinal cord: multiphasic expression pattern and identification of the cell types involved. J Comp Neurol. 2007;500(2):267–85. https://doi.org/10.1002/cne.21149.
17. Ahn H, Singh J, Nathens A, et al. Pre-hospital care management of a potential spinal cord injured patient: a systematic review

of the literature and evidence-based guidelines. J Neurotrauma. 2011;28(8):1341–61. https://doi.org/10.1089/neu.2009.1168.
18. Stein DM, Knight WAt. Emergency neurological life support: traumatic spine injury. Neurocrit Care. 2017;27(Suppl 1):170–80. https://doi.org/10.1007/s12028-017-0462-z.
19. Gardner BP, Watt JW, Krishnan KR. The artificial ventilation of acute spinal cord damaged patients: a retrospective study of forty-four patients. Paraplegia. 1986;24(4):208–20. https://doi.org/10.1038/sc.1986.30.
20. Saadeh YS, Smith BW, Joseph JR, et al. The impact of blood pressure management after spinal cord injury: a systematic review of the literature. Neurosurg Focus. 2017;43(5):E20. https://doi.org/10.3171/2017.8.FOCUS17428.
21. Lee YS, Kim KT, Kwon BK. Hemodynamic Management of Acute Spinal Cord Injury: a literature review. Neurospine. 2021;18(1):7–14. https://doi.org/10.14245/ns.2040144.072.
22. Kirshblum SC, Waring W, Biering-Sorensen F, et al. Reference for the 2011 revision of the international standards for neurological classification of Spinal Cord injury. J Spinal Cord Med. 2011;34(6):547–54. https://doi.org/10.1179/107902611X13186000420242.
23. Ditunno JF, Little JW, Tessler A, Burns AS. Spinal shock revisited: a four-phase model. Spinal Cord. 2004;42(7):383–95. https://doi.org/10.1038/sj.sc.3101603.
24. Schneider RC, Cherry G, Pantek H. The syndrome of acute central cervical spinal cord injury; with special reference to the mechanisms involved in hyperextension injuries of cervical spine. J Neurosurg. 1954;11(6):546–77. https://doi.org/10.3171/jns.1954.11.6.0546.
25. McKinley W, Santos K, Meade M, Brooke K. Incidence and outcomes of spinal cord injury clinical syndromes. J Spinal Cord Med. 2007;30(3):215–24. https://doi.org/10.1080/10790268.2007.11753929.
26. Badhiwala JH, Wilson JR, Fehlings MG. The case for revisiting central cord syndrome. Spinal Cord. 2020;58(1):125–7. https://doi.org/10.1038/s41393-019-0354-5.
27. Kunam VK, Velayudhan V, Chaudhry ZA, Bobinski M, Smoker WRK, Reede DL. Incomplete Cord syndromes: clinical and imaging review. Radiographics. 2018;38(4):1201–22. https://doi.org/10.1148/rg.2018170178.
28. Ryken TC, Hadley MN, Walters BC, et al. Radiographic assessment. Neurosurgery. 2013;72(Suppl 2):54–72. https://doi.org/10.1227/NEU.0b013e318276edee.
29. Solis MM, Ayoub MM, Rogers JJ, Ashley DW, Harvey RL, Dalton ML. Limitations of cervical radiography in the evaluation of acute cervical trauma. J Trauma. 1994;36(3):458–9.
30. Hoffman JR, Mower WR, Wolfson AB, Todd KH, Zucker MI. Validity of a set of clinical criteria to rule out injury to the cervical spine in patients with blunt trauma. National Emergency X-radiography utilization study group. N Engl J Med. 2000;343(2):94–9. https://doi.org/10.1056/NEJM200007133430203.
31. Stiell IG, Wells GA, Vandemheen KL, et al. The Canadian C-spine rule for radiography in alert and stable trauma patients. JAMA. 2001;286(15):1841–8. https://doi.org/10.1001/jama.286.15.1841.
32. Biffl WL, Cothren CC, Moore EE, et al. Western trauma association critical decisions in trauma: screening for and treatment of blunt cerebrovascular injuries. J Trauma. 2009;67(6):1150–3. https://doi.org/10.1097/TA.0b013e3181c1c1d6.
33. Geddes AE, Burlew CC, Wagenaar AE, et al. Expanded screening criteria for blunt cerebrovascular injury: a bigger impact than anticipated. Am J Surg. 2016;212(6):1167–74. https://doi.org/10.1016/j.amjsurg.2016.09.016.
34. Kim DY, Biffl W, Bokhari F, et al. Evaluation and management of blunt cerebrovascular injury: a practice management guideline from the eastern Association for the Surgery of trauma. J Trauma Acute Care Surg. 2020;88(6):875–87. https://doi.org/10.1097/TA.0000000000002668.
35. Lammertse D, Dungan D, Dreisbach J, et al. Neuroimaging in traumatic spinal cord injury: an evidence-based review for clinical practice and research. J Spinal Cord Med. 2007;30(3):205–14. https://doi.org/10.1080/10790268.2007.11753928.
36. Miyanji F, Furlan JC, Aarabi B, Arnold PM, Fehlings MG. Acute cervical traumatic spinal cord injury: MR imaging findings correlated with neurologic outcome—prospective study with 100 consecutive patients. Radiology. 2007;243(3):820–7. https://doi.org/10.1148/radiol.2433060583.
37. Papadopoulos SM, Selden NR, Quint DJ, Patel N, Gillespie B, Grube S. Immediate spinal cord decompression for cervical spinal cord injury: feasibility and outcome. J Trauma. 2002;52(2):323–32. https://doi.org/10.1097/00005373-200202000-00019.
38. Fehlings MG, Martin AR, Tetreault LA, et al. A clinical practice guideline for the Management of Patients with Acute Spinal Cord Injury: recommendations on the role of baseline magnetic resonance imaging in clinical decision making and outcome prediction. Global Spine J. 2017;7(3 Suppl):221S–30S. https://doi.org/10.1177/2192568217703089.
39. Boldin C, Raith J, Fankhauser F, Haunschmid C, Schwantzer G, Schweighofer F. Predicting neurologic recovery in cervical spinal cord injury with postoperative MR imaging. Spine (Phila Pa 1976). 2006;31(5):554–9. https://doi.org/10.1097/01.brs.0000201274.59427.a4.
40. Selden NR, Quint DJ, Patel N, d'Arcy HS, Papadopoulos SM. Emergency magnetic resonance imaging of cervical spinal cord injuries: clinical correlation and prognosis. Neurosurgery. 1999;44(4):785–92.; discussion 792-3. https://doi.org/10.1097/00006123-199904000-00057.
41. Jentzsch T, Cadotte DW, Wilson JR, et al. Spinal Cord signal change on magnetic resonance imaging may predict worse clinical in- and outpatient outcomes in patients with Spinal Cord injury: a prospective multicenter study in 459 patients. J Clin Med. 2021;10(20):4778. https://doi.org/10.3390/jcm10204778.
42. Zaninovich OA, Avila MJ, Kay M, Becker JL, Hurlbert RJ, Martirosyan NL. The role of diffusion tensor imaging in the diagnosis, prognosis, and assessment of recovery and treatment of spinal cord injury: a systematic review. Neurosurg Focus. 2019;46(3):E7. https://doi.org/10.3171/2019.1.FOCUS18591.
43. Hadley MN, Walters BC, Grabb BC, et al. Initial closed reduction of cervical spine fracture-dislocation injuries. Neurosurgery. 2002;50(3 Suppl):S44–50. https://doi.org/10.1097/00006123-200203001-00010.
44. Gelb DE, Hadley MN, Aarabi B, et al. Initial closed reduction of cervical spinal fracture-dislocation injuries. Neurosurgery. 2013;72(Suppl 2):73–83. https://doi.org/10.1227/NEU.0b013e318276ee02.
45. Fehlings MG, Rabin D, Sears W, Cadotte DW, Aarabi B. Current practice in the timing of surgical intervention in spinal cord injury. Spine (Phila Pa 1976). 2010;35(21 Suppl):S166–73. https://doi.org/10.1097/BRS.0b013e3181f386f6.
46. Fehlings MG, Vaccaro A, Wilson JR, et al. Early versus delayed decompression for traumatic cervical spinal cord injury: results of the surgical timing in acute Spinal Cord injury study (STASCIS). PLoS One. 2012;7(2):e32037. https://doi.org/10.1371/journal.pone.0032037.
47. Anderson KK, Tetreault L, Shamji MF, et al. Optimal timing of surgical decompression for acute traumatic central Cord syndrome: a systematic review of the literature. Neurosurgery. 2015;77(Suppl 4):S15–32. https://doi.org/10.1227/NEU.0000000000000946.
48. Badhiwala JH, Wilson JR, Witiw CD, et al. The influence of timing of surgical decompression for acute spinal cord injury: a pooled analysis of individual patient data. Lancet

Neurol. 2021;20(2):117–26. https://doi.org/10.1016/S1474-4422(20)30406-3.

49. Ramakonar H, Fehlings MG. 'Time is Spine': new evidence supports decompression within 24 h for acute spinal cord injury. Spinal Cord. 2021;59(8):933–4. https://doi.org/10.1038/s41393-021-00654-0.
50. Hosman AJF, Barbagallo G, Popescu EC, et al. Neurological recovery after early versus delayed surgical decompression for acute traumatic spinal cord injury. Bone Joint J. 2023;105-B(4):400–11. https://doi.org/10.1302/0301-620X.105B4.BJJ-2022-0947.R2.
51. Pouw MH, van Middendorp JJ, van Kampen A, Curt A, van de Meent H, Hosman AJ. Diagnostic criteria of traumatic central cord syndrome. Part 3: descriptive analyses of neurological and functional outcomes in a prospective cohort of traumatic motor incomplete tetraplegics. Spinal Cord. 2011;49(5):614–22. https://doi.org/10.1038/sc.2010.171.
52. van Middendorp JJ, Pouw MH, Hayes KC, et al. Diagnostic criteria of traumatic central cord syndrome. Part 2: a questionnaire survey among spine specialists. Spinal Cord. 2010;48(9):657–63. https://doi.org/10.1038/sc.2010.72.
53. Wilson JR, Witiw CD, Badhiwala J, Kwon BK, Fehlings MG, Harrop JS. Early surgery for traumatic Spinal Cord injury: where are we now? Global Spine J. 2020;10(1 Suppl):84S–91S. https://doi.org/10.1177/2192568219877860.
54. Wilson JR, Tetreault LA, Kwon BK, et al. Timing of decompression in patients with acute Spinal Cord injury: a systematic review. Global Spine J. 2017;7(3 Suppl):95S–115S. https://doi.org/10.1177/2192568217701716.
55. Lenehan B, Fisher CG, Vaccaro A, Fehlings M, Aarabi B, Dvorak MF. The urgency of surgical decompression in acute central cord injuries with spondylosis and without instability. Spine (Phila Pa 1976). 2010;35(21 Suppl):S180–6. https://doi.org/10.1097/BRS.0b013e3181f32a44.
56. Fehlings MG, Tetreault LA, Wilson JR, et al. A clinical practice guideline for the Management of Patients with Acute Spinal Cord Injury and Central Cord Syndrome: recommendations on the timing (</=24 hours versus >24 hours) of Decompressive surgery. Global Spine J. 2017;7(3 Suppl):195S–202S. https://doi.org/10.1177/2192568217706367.
57. Botel U, Glaser E, Niedeggen A. The surgical treatment of acute spinal paralysed patients. Spinal Cord. 1997;35(7):420–8. https://doi.org/10.1038/sj.sc.3100407.
58. Glennie RA, Bailey CS, Tsai EC, et al. An analysis of ideal and actual time to surgery after traumatic spinal cord injury in Canada. Spinal Cord. 2017;55(6):618–23. https://doi.org/10.1038/sc.2016.177.
59. Balas M, Prommel P, Nguyen L, et al. Reality of accomplishing surgery within 24 hours for complete cervical Spinal Cord injury: clinical practices and safety. J Neurotrauma. 2021;38(21):3011–9. https://doi.org/10.1089/neu.2021.0177.
60. Wilson JR, Voth J, Singh A, et al. Defining the pathway to definitive care and surgical decompression after traumatic Spinal Cord injury: results of a Canadian population-based cohort study. J Neurotrauma. 2016;33(10):963–71. https://doi.org/10.1089/neu.2015.4258.
61. Dru AB, Reichwage B, Neal D, et al. Race and socioeconomic disparity in treatment and outcome of traumatic cervical spinal cord injury with fracture: Nationwide inpatient sample database, 1998-2009. Spinal Cord. 2019;57(10):858–65. https://doi.org/10.1038/s41393-019-0280-6.
62. Jackson AB, Groomes TE. Incidence of respiratory complications following spinal cord injury. Arch Phys Med Rehabil. 1994;75(3):270–5. https://doi.org/10.1016/0003-9993(94)90027-2.
63. Claxton AR, Wong DT, Chung F, Fehlings MG. Predictors of hospital mortality and mechanical ventilation in patients with cervical spinal cord injury. Can J Anaesth. 1998;45(2):144–9. https://doi.org/10.1007/BF03013253.
64. Winslow C, Bode RK, Felton D, Chen D, Meyer PR Jr. Impact of respiratory complications on length of stay and hospital costs in acute cervical spine injury. Chest. 2002;121(5):1548–54. https://doi.org/10.1378/chest.121.5.1548.
65. Brown R, DiMarco AF, Hoit JD, Garshick E. Respiratory dysfunction and management in spinal cord injury. Respir Care. 2006;51(8):853–68; discussion 869–70.
66. Berney S, Bragge P, Granger C, Opdam H, Denehy L. The acute respiratory management of cervical spinal cord injury in the first 6 weeks after injury: a systematic review. Spinal Cord. 2011;49(1):17–29. https://doi.org/10.1038/sc.2010.39.
67. Berney SC, Gordon IR, Opdam HI, Denehy L. A classification and regression tree to assist clinical decision making in airway management for patients with cervical spinal cord injury. Spinal Cord. 2011;49(2):244–50. https://doi.org/10.1038/sc.2010.97.
68. Linn WS, Adkins RH, Gong H Jr, Waters RL. Pulmonary function in chronic spinal cord injury: a cross-sectional survey of 222 southern California adult outpatients. Arch Phys Med Rehabil. 2000;81(6):757–63. https://doi.org/10.1016/s0003-9993(00)90107-2.
69. Winslow C, Rozovsky J. Effect of spinal cord injury on the respiratory system. Am J Phys Med Rehabil. 2003;82(10):803–14. https://doi.org/10.1097/01.PHM.0000078184.08835.01.
70. Baydur A, Adkins RH, Milic-Emili J. Lung mechanics in individuals with spinal cord injury: effects of injury level and posture. J Appl Physiol (1985). 2001;90(2):405–11. https://doi.org/10.1152/jappl.2001.90.2.405.
71. Cosortium for Spinal Cord M. Respiratory management following spinal cord injury: a clinical practice guideline for health-care professionals. J Spinal Cord Med. 2005;28(3):259–93. https://doi.org/10.1080/10790268.2005.11753821.
72. Walkey AJ, Goligher EC, Del Sorbo L, et al. Low tidal volume versus non-volume-limited strategies for patients with acute respiratory distress syndrome. A systematic review and meta-analysis. Ann Am Thorac Soc. 2017;14(Supplement_4):S271–9. https://doi.org/10.1513/AnnalsATS.201704-337OT.
73. Korupolu R, Stampas A, Uhlig-Reche H, et al. Comparing outcomes of mechanical ventilation with high vs. moderate tidal volumes in tracheostomized patients with spinal cord injury in acute inpatient rehabilitation setting: a retrospective cohort study. Spinal Cord. 2021;59(6):618–25. https://doi.org/10.1038/s41393-020-0517-4.
74. Tromans AM, Mecci M, Barrett FH, Ward TA, Grundy DJ. The use of the BiPAP biphasic positive airway pressure system in acute spinal cord injury. Spinal Cord. 1998;36(7):481–4. https://doi.org/10.1038/sj.sc.3100676.
75. Bach JR. Noninvasive respiratory management of high level spinal cord injury. J Spinal Cord Med. 2012;35(2):72–80. https://doi.org/10.1179/2045772311Y.0000000051.
76. Savic G, DeVivo MJ, Frankel HL, Jamous MA, Soni BM, Charlifue S. Causes of death after traumatic spinal cord injury-a 70-year British study. Spinal Cord. 2017;55(10):891–7. https://doi.org/10.1038/sc.2017.64.
77. Zimmer MB, Nantwi K, Goshgarian HG. Effect of spinal cord injury on the respiratory system: basic research and current clinical treatment options. J Spinal Cord Med. 2007;30(4):319–30. https://doi.org/10.1080/10790268.2007.11753947.
78. Ryken TC, Hurlbert RJ, Hadley MN, et al. The acute cardiopulmonary management of patients with cervical spinal cord injuries. Neurosurgery. 2013;72(Suppl 2):84–92. https://doi.org/10.1227/NEU.0b013e318276ee16.
79. Bourassa-Moreau E, Mac-Thiong JM, Ehrmann Feldman D, Thompson C, Parent S. Complications in acute phase hospitalization of traumatic spinal cord injury: does surgical timing mat-

ter? J Trauma Acute Care Surg. 2013;74(3):849–54. https://doi.org/10.1097/TA.0b013e31827e1381.
80. Arora S, Flower O, Murray NP, Lee BB. Respiratory care of patients with cervical spinal cord injury: a review. Crit Care Resusc. 2012;14(1):64–73.
81. Yugue I, Okada S, Ueta T, et al. Analysis of the risk factors for tracheostomy in traumatic cervical spinal cord injury. Spine (Phila Pa 1976). 2012;37(26):E1633–8. https://doi.org/10.1097/BRS.0b013e31827417f1.
82. Scantling D, Granche J, Williamson J, Gracely E, Thosani D, McCracken B. Development of clinical tracheostomy score to identify cervical spinal cord injury patients requiring prolonged ventilator support. J Trauma Acute Care Surg. 2019;87(1):195–9. https://doi.org/10.1097/TA.0000000000002286.
83. Anand T, Hanna K, Kulvatunyou N, et al. Time to tracheostomy impacts overall outcomes in patients with cervical spinal cord injury. J Trauma Acute Care Surg. 2020;89(2):358–64. https://doi.org/10.1097/TA.0000000000002758.
84. Foran SJ, Taran S, Singh JM, Kutsogiannis DJ, McCredie V. Timing of tracheostomy in acute traumatic spinal cord injury: a systematic review and meta-analysis. J Trauma Acute Care Surg. 2021;92(1):223–31. https://doi.org/10.1097/TA.0000000000003394.
85. Northrup BE, Vaccaro AR, Rosen JE, Balderston RA, Cotler JM. Occurrence of infection in anterior cervical fusion for spinal cord injury after tracheostomy. Spine (Phila Pa 1976). 1995;20(22):2449–53. https://doi.org/10.1097/00007632-199511001-00014.
86. O'Keeffe T, Goldman RK, Mayberry JC, Rehm CG, Hart RA. Tracheostomy after anterior cervical spine fixation. J Trauma. 2004;57(4):855–60. https://doi.org/10.1097/01.ta.0000083006.48501.b2.
87. Berney S, Opdam H, Bellomo R, et al. An assessment of early tracheostomy after anterior cervical stabilization in patients with acute cervical spine trauma. J Trauma. 2008;64(3):749–53. https://doi.org/10.1097/.TA.0b013e31802c8234.
88. Babu R, Owens TR, Thomas S, et al. Timing of tracheostomy after anterior cervical spine fixation. J Trauma Acute Care Surg. 2013;74(4):961–6. https://doi.org/10.1097/TA.0b013e3182826ea4.
89. Lo V, Esquenazi Y, Han MK, Lee K. Critical care management of patients with acute spinal cord injury. J Neurosurg Sci. 2013;57(4):281–92.
90. Ploumis A, Yadlapalli N, Fehlings MG, Kwon BK, Vaccaro AR. A systematic review of the evidence supporting a role for vasopressor support in acute SCI. Spinal Cord. 2010;48(5):356–62. https://doi.org/10.1038/sc.2009.150.
91. Marik PE. Obituary: pulmonary artery catheter 1970 to 2013. Ann Intensive Care. 2013;3(1):38. https://doi.org/10.1186/2110-5820-3-38.
92. Consortium for Spinal Cord M. Early acute management in adults with spinal cord injury: a clinical practice guideline for health-care professionals. J Spinal Cord Med. 2008;31(4):403–79. https://doi.org/10.1043/1079-0268-31.4.408.
93. De Backer D, Biston P, Devriendt J, et al. Comparison of dopamine and norepinephrine in the treatment of shock. N Engl J Med. 2010;362(9):779–89. https://doi.org/10.1056/NEJMoa0907118.
94. Du Y, Wang L, Shi H, Gao M. Comparison of clinical effect of dopamine and norepinephrine in the treatment of septic shock. Pak J Pharm Sci. 2015;28(4 Suppl):1461–4.
95. Inoue T, Manley GT, Patel N, Whetstone WD. Medical and surgical management after spinal cord injury: vasopressor usage, early surgerys, and complications. J Neurotrauma. 2014;31(3):284–91. https://doi.org/10.1089/neu.2013.3061.
96. Readdy WJ, Whetstone WD, Ferguson AR, et al. Complications and outcomes of vasopressor usage in acute traumatic central cord syndrome. J Neurosurg Spine. 2015;23(5):574–80. https://doi.org/10.3171/2015.2.SPINE14746.
97. Squair JW, Belanger LM, Tsang A, et al. Spinal cord perfusion pressure predicts neurologic recovery in acute spinal cord injury. Neurology. 2017;89(16):1660–7. https://doi.org/10.1212/WNL.0000000000004519.
98. Saadoun S, Papadopoulos MC. Targeted perfusion therapy in Spinal Cord trauma. Neurotherapeutics. 2020;17(2):511–21. https://doi.org/10.1007/s13311-019-00820-6.
99. Chen S, Smielewski P, Czosnyka M, Papadopoulos MC, Saadoun S. Continuous monitoring and visualization of optimum Spinal Cord perfusion pressure in patients with acute Cord injury. J Neurotrauma. 2017;34(21):2941–9. https://doi.org/10.1089/neu.2017.4982.
100. Blackmer J. Rehabilitation medicine: 1. Autonomic dysreflexia. CMAJ. 2003;169(9):931–5.
101. Krassioukov A, Warburton DE, Teasell R, Eng JJ. Spinal Cord injury rehabilitation evidence research T. A systematic review of the management of autonomic dysreflexia after spinal cord injury. Arch Phys Med Rehabil. 2009;90(4):682–95. https://doi.org/10.1016/j.apmr.2008.10.017.
102. Dhall SS, Hadley MN, Aarabi B, et al. Deep venous thrombosis and thromboembolism in patients with cervical spinal cord injuries. Neurosurgery. 2013;72(Suppl 2):244–54. https://doi.org/10.1227/NEU.0b013e31827728c0.
103. Geerts WH, Pineo GF, Heit JA, et al. Prevention of venous thromboembolism: the seventh ACCP conference on antithrombotic and thrombolytic therapy. Chest. Sep 2004;126(3 Suppl):338S–400S. https://doi.org/10.1378/chest.126.3_suppl.338S.
104. Prevention of venous thromboembolism in individuals with spinal cord injury: Clinical Practice Guidelines for Health Care Providers, 3rd ed.: consortium for spinal cord medicine. Top Spinal Cord Inj Rehabil. 2016;22(3):209–40. https://doi.org/10.1310/sci2203-209.
105. Nyquist P, Bautista C, Jichici D, et al. Prophylaxis of venous thrombosis in Neurocritical care patients: an evidence-based guideline: a statement for healthcare professionals from the Neurocritical care society. Neurocrit Care. 2016;24(1):47–60. https://doi.org/10.1007/s12028-015-0221-y.
106. Matsumoto S, Suda K, Iimoto S, et al. Prospective study of deep vein thrombosis in patients with spinal cord injury not receiving anticoagulant therapy. Spinal Cord. 2015;53(4):306–9. https://doi.org/10.1038/sc.2015.4.
107. Arnold PM, Harrop JS, Merli G, et al. Efficacy, safety, and timing of anticoagulant Thromboprophylaxis for the prevention of venous thromboembolism in patients with acute Spinal Cord injury: a systematic review. Global Spine J. 2017;7(3 Suppl):138S–50S. https://doi.org/10.1177/2192568217703665.
108. Chung WS, Lin CL, Chang SN, Chung HA, Sung FC, Kao CH. Increased risk of deep vein thrombosis and pulmonary thromboembolism in patients with spinal cord injury: a nationwide cohort prospective study. Thromb Res. 2014;133(4):579–84. https://doi.org/10.1016/j.thromres.2014.01.008.
109. Fehlings MG, Tetreault LA, Aarabi B, et al. A clinical practice guideline for the Management of Patients with Acute Spinal Cord Injury: recommendations on the type and timing of anticoagulant Thromboprophylaxis. Global Spine J. 2017;7(3 Suppl):212S–20S. https://doi.org/10.1177/2192568217702107.
110. Benevento BT, Sipski ML. Neurogenic bladder, neurogenic bowel, and sexual dysfunction in people with spinal cord injury. Phys Ther. 2002;82(6):601–12.
111. Barletta JF, Erstad BL, Fortune JB. Stress ulcer prophylaxis in trauma patients. Crit Care. 2002;6(6):526–30. https://doi.org/10.1186/cc1831.
112. Simons RK, Hoyt DB, Winchell RJ, Holbrook T, Eastman AB. A risk analysis of stress ulceration after trauma. J

Trauma. 1995;39(2):289–93; discussion 293–4. https://doi.org/10.1097/00005373-199508000-00017.
113. Wuermser LA, Ho CH, Chiodo AE, Priebe MM, Kirshblum SC, Scelza WM. Spinal cord injury medicine. 2. Acute care management of traumatic and nontraumatic injury. Arch Phys Med Rehabil. 2007;88(3 Suppl 1):S55–61. https://doi.org/10.1016/j.apmr.2006.12.002.
114. Johns J, Krogh K, Rodriguez GM, et al. Management of Neurogenic Bowel Dysfunction in adults after Spinal Cord injury: clinical practice guideline for health care providers. Top Spinal Cord Inj Rehabil. 2021;27(2):75–151. https://doi.org/10.46292/sci2702-75.
115. Taweel WA, Seyam R. Neurogenic bladder in spinal cord injury patients. Res Rep Urol. 2015;7:85–99. https://doi.org/10.2147/RRU.S29644.
116. Weld KJ, Dmochowski RR. Effect of bladder management on urological complications in spinal cord injured patients. J Urol. 2000;163(3):768–72.
117. Morton SC, Shekelle PG, Adams JL, et al. Antimicrobial prophylaxis for urinary tract infection in persons with spinal cord dysfunction. Arch Phys Med Rehabil. 2002;83(1):129–38. https://doi.org/10.1053/apmr.2002.26605.
118. Consortium for Spinal Cord Medicine Clinical Practice G. Pressure ulcer prevention and treatment following spinal cord injury: a clinical practice guideline for health-care professionals. J Spinal Cord Med. 2001;24(Suppl 1):S40–101. https://doi.org/10.1080/10790268.2001.11753592.
119. Cardenas DD, Felix ER. Pain after spinal cord injury: a review of classification, treatment approaches, and treatment assessment. PM R. 2009;1(12):1077–90. https://doi.org/10.1016/j.pmrj.2009.07.002.
120. Michailidou C, Marston L, De Souza LH, Sutherland I. A systematic review of the prevalence of musculoskeletal pain, back and low back pain in people with spinal cord injury. Disabil Rehabil. 2014;36(9):705–15. https://doi.org/10.3109/09638288.2013.808708.
121. Dijkers M, Bryce T, Zanca J. Prevalence of chronic pain after traumatic spinal cord injury: a systematic review. J Rehabil Res Dev. 2009;46(1):13–29.
122. Ducker TB, Hamit HF. Experimental treatments of acute spinal cord injury. J Neurosurg. 1969;30(6):693–7. https://doi.org/10.3171/jns.1969.30.6.0693.
123. Black P, Markowitz RS. Experimental spinal cord injury in monkeys: comparison of steroids and local hypothermia. Surg Forum. 1971;22:409–11.
124. Campbell JB, DeCrescito V, Tomasula JJ, Demopoulos HB, Flamm ES, Ransohoff J. Experimental treatment of spinal cord contusion in the cat. Surg Neurol. 1973;1(2):102–6.
125. Lewin MG, Hansebout RR, Pappius HM. Chemical characteristics of traumatic spinal cord edema in cats. Effects of steroids on potassium depletion. J Neurosurg. 1974;40(1):65–75. https://doi.org/10.3171/jns.1974.40.1.0065.
126. Green BA, Kahn T, Klose KJ. A comparative study of steroid therapy in acute experimental spinal cord injury. Surg Neurol. 1980;13(2):91–7.
127. Bracken MB, Collins WF, Freeman DF, et al. Efficacy of methylprednisolone in acute spinal cord injury. JAMA. 1984;251(1):45–52.
128. Bracken MB, Shepard MJ, Collins WF, et al. A randomized, controlled trial of methylprednisolone or naloxone in the treatment of acute spinal-cord injury. Results of the second national acute Spinal Cord injury study. N Engl J Med. 1990;322(20):1405–11. https://doi.org/10.1056/NEJM199005173222001.
129. Bracken MB, Shepard MJ, Collins WF Jr, et al. Methylprednisolone or naloxone treatment after acute spinal cord injury: 1-year follow-up data. Results of the second National Acute Spinal Cord Injury Study. J Neurosurg. 1992;76(1):23–31. https://doi.org/10.3171/jns.1992.76.1.0023.
130. Bracken MB, Shepard MJ, Holford TR, et al. Administration of methylprednisolone for 24 or 48 hours or tirilazad mesylate for 48 hours in the treatment of acute spinal cord injury. Results of the Third National Acute Spinal Cord Injury Randomized Controlled Trial. National Acute Spinal Cord Injury Study. JAMA. 1997;277(20):1597–604.
131. Bracken MB, Shepard MJ, Holford TR, et al. Methylprednisolone or tirilazad mesylate administration after acute spinal cord injury: 1-year follow up. Results of the third National Acute Spinal Cord Injury randomized controlled trial. J Neurosurg. 1998;89(5):699–706. https://doi.org/10.3171/jns.1998.89.5.0699.
132. Hurlbert RJ, Hadley MN, Walters BC, et al. Pharmacological therapy for acute spinal cord injury. Neurosurgery. 2013;72(Suppl 2):93–105. https://doi.org/10.1227/NEU.0b013e31827765c6.
133. Bracken MB. Steroids for acute spinal cord injury. Cochrane Database Syst Rev. 2012;1:CD001046. https://doi.org/10.1002/14651858.CD001046.pub2.
134. Fehlings MG, Wilson JR, Harrop JS, et al. Efficacy and safety of methylprednisolone sodium succinate in acute Spinal Cord injury: a systematic review. Global Spine J. 2017;7(3 Suppl):116S–37S. https://doi.org/10.1177/2192568217706366.
135. Fehlings MG, Wilson JR, Tetreault LA, et al. A clinical practice guideline for the Management of Patients with Acute Spinal Cord Injury: recommendations on the use of methylprednisolone sodium succinate. Global Spine J. 2017;7(3 Suppl):203S–11S. https://doi.org/10.1177/2192568217703085.
136. Lee SM, Yune TY, Kim SJ, et al. Minocycline reduces cell death and improves functional recovery after traumatic spinal cord injury in the rat. J Neurotrauma. 2003;20(10):1017–27. https://doi.org/10.1089/089771503770195867.
137. Wells JE, Hurlbert RJ, Fehlings MG, Yong VW. Neuroprotection by minocycline facilitates significant recovery from spinal cord injury in mice. Brain. 2003;126(Pt 7):1628–37. https://doi.org/10.1093/brain/awg178.
138. Casha S, Zygun D, McGowan MD, Bains I, Yong VW, Hurlbert RJ. Results of a phase II placebo-controlled randomized trial of minocycline in acute spinal cord injury. Brain. 2012;135(Pt 4):1224–36. https://doi.org/10.1093/brain/aws072.
139. Miller RG, Mitchell JD, Moore DH. Riluzole for amyotrophic lateral sclerosis (ALS)/motor neuron disease (MND). Cochrane Database Syst Rev. 2012;3:CD001447. https://doi.org/10.1002/14651858.CD001447.pub3.
140. Grossman RG, Fehlings MG, Frankowski RF, et al. A prospective, multicenter, phase I matched-comparison group trial of safety, pharmacokinetics, and preliminary efficacy of riluzole in patients with traumatic spinal cord injury. J Neurotrauma. 2014;31(3):239–55. https://doi.org/10.1089/neu.2013.2969.
141. Fehlings MG, Nakashima H, Nagoshi N, Chow DS, Grossman RG, Kopjar B. Rationale, design and critical end points for the Riluzole in acute Spinal Cord injury study (RISCIS): a randomized, double-blinded, placebo-controlled parallel multi-center trial. Spinal Cord. 2016;54(1):8–15. https://doi.org/10.1038/sc.2015.95.
142. Lee YS, Hsiao I, Lin VW. Peripheral nerve grafts and aFGF restore partial hindlimb function in adult paraplegic rats. J Neurotrauma. 2002;19(10):1203–16. https://doi.org/10.1089/08977150260338001.
143. Wu JC, Huang WC, Chen YC, et al. Acidic fibroblast growth factor for repair of human spinal cord injury: a clinical trial. J Neurosurg Spine. 2011;15(3):216–27. https://doi.org/10.3171/2011.4.SPINE10404.
144. Koda M, Nishio Y, Kamada T, et al. Granulocyte colony-stimulating factor (G-CSF) mobilizes bone marrow-derived cells into injured spinal cord and promotes functional recovery after compression-

induced spinal cord injury in mice. Brain Res. 2007;1149:223–31. https://doi.org/10.1016/j.brainres.2007.02.058.

145. Nishio Y, Koda M, Kamada T, et al. Granulocyte colony-stimulating factor attenuates neuronal death and promotes functional recovery after spinal cord injury in mice. J Neuropathol Exp Neurol. 2007;66(8):724–31. https://doi.org/10.1097/nen.0b013e3181257176.
146. Derakhshanrad N, Saberi H, Yekaninejad MS, Joghataei MT, Sheikhrezaei A. Granulocyte-colony stimulating factor administration for neurological improvement in patients with postrehabilitation chronic incomplete traumatic spinal cord injuries: a double-blind randomized controlled clinical trial. J Neurosurg Spine. 2018;29(1):97–107. https://doi.org/10.3171/2017.11.SPINE17769.
147. Dietrich WD. Therapeutic hypothermia for acute severe spinal cord injury: ready to start large clinical trials? Crit Care Med. 2012;40(2):691–2. https://doi.org/10.1097/CCM.0b013e318236eacb.
148. Wang J, Pearse DD. Therapeutic hypothermia in Spinal Cord injury: the status of its use and open questions. Int J Mol Sci. 2015;16(8):16848–79. https://doi.org/10.3390/ijms160816848.
149. Batchelor PE, Skeers P, Antonic A, et al. Systematic review and meta-analysis of therapeutic hypothermia in animal models of spinal cord injury. PLoS One. 2013;8(8):e71317. https://doi.org/10.1371/journal.pone.0071317.
150. Nolan JP, Morley PT, Hoek TL, Hickey RW. Advancement life support task force of the international liaison committee on R. Therapeutic hypothermia after cardiac arrest. An advisory statement by the advancement life support task force of the international liaison committee on resuscitation. Resuscitation. 2003;57(3):231–5. https://doi.org/10.1016/s0300-9572(03)00184-9.
151. Levi AD, Green BA, Wang MY, et al. Clinical application of modest hypothermia after spinal cord injury. J Neurotrauma. 2009;26(3):407–15. https://doi.org/10.1089/neu.2008.0745.
152. Dubreuil CI, Winton MJ, McKerracher L. Rho activation patterns after spinal cord injury and the role of activated rho in apoptosis in the central nervous system. J Cell Biol. 2003;162(2):233–43. https://doi.org/10.1083/jcb.200301080.
153. Fehlings MG, Theodore N, Harrop J, et al. A phase I/IIa clinical trial of a recombinant rho protein antagonist in acute spinal cord injury. J Neurotrauma. 2011;28(5):787–96. https://doi.org/10.1089/neu.2011.1765.
154. Buchli AD, Schwab ME. Inhibition of Nogo: a key strategy to increase regeneration, plasticity and functional recovery of the lesioned central nervous system. Ann Med. 2005;37(8):556–67. https://doi.org/10.1080/07853890500407520.
155. Chen K, Marsh BC, Cowan M, et al. Sequential therapy of anti-Nogo-a antibody treatment and treadmill training leads to cumulative improvements after spinal cord injury in rats. Exp Neurol. 2017;292:135–44. https://doi.org/10.1016/j.expneurol.2017.03.012.
156. Schwab JM, Conrad S, Monnier PP, Julien S, Mueller BK, Schluesener HJ. Spinal cord injury-induced lesional expression of the repulsive guidance molecule (RGM). Eur J Neurosci. 2005;21(6):1569–76. https://doi.org/10.1111/j.1460--9568.2005.03962.x.
157. Nakagawa H, Ninomiya T, Yamashita T, Takada M. Treatment with the neutralizing antibody against repulsive guidance molecule-a promotes recovery from impaired manual dexterity in a primate model of Spinal Cord injury. Cereb Cortex. 2019;29(2):561–72. https://doi.org/10.1093/cercor/bhx338.
158. Mothe AJ, Coelho M, Huang L, et al. Delayed administration of the human anti-RGMa monoclonal antibody elezanumab promotes functional recovery including spontaneous voiding after spinal cord injury in rats. Neurobiol Dis. 2020;143:104995. https://doi.org/10.1016/j.nbd.2020.104995.
159. Hata K, Fujitani M, Yasuda Y, et al. RGMa inhibition promotes axonal growth and recovery after spinal cord injury. J Cell Biol. 2006;173(1):47–58. https://doi.org/10.1083/jcb.200508143.
160. Mothe AJ, Tassew NG, Shabanzadeh AP, et al. RGMa inhibition with human monoclonal antibodies promotes regeneration, plasticity and repair, and attenuates neuropathic pain after spinal cord injury. Sci Rep. 2017;7(1):10529. https://doi.org/10.1038/s41598-017-10987-7.
161. Ekberg JA, St John JA. Olfactory ensheathing cells for spinal cord repair: crucial differences between subpopulations of the glia. Neural Regen Res. 2015;10(9):1395–6. https://doi.org/10.4103/1673-5374.165504.
162. Li L, Adnan H, Xu B, et al. Effects of transplantation of olfactory ensheathing cells in chronic spinal cord injury: a systematic review and meta-analysis. Eur Spine J. 2015;24(5):919–30. https://doi.org/10.1007/s00586-014-3416-6.
163. Assinck P, Duncan GJ, Hilton BJ, Plemel JR, Tetzlaff W. Cell transplantation therapy for spinal cord injury. Nat Neurosci. 2017;20(5):637–47. https://doi.org/10.1038/nn.4541.
164. Teng YD, Lavik EB, Qu X, et al. Functional recovery following traumatic spinal cord injury mediated by a unique polymer scaffold seeded with neural stem cells. Proc Natl Acad Sci USA. 2002;99(5):3024–9. https://doi.org/10.1073/pnas.052678899.
165. Pritchard CD, Slotkin JR, Yu D, et al. Establishing a model spinal cord injury in the African green monkey for the preclinical evaluation of biodegradable polymer scaffolds seeded with human neural stem cells. J Neurosci Methods. 2010;188(2):258–69. https://doi.org/10.1016/j.jneumeth.2010.02.019.
166. Theodore N, Hlubek R, Danielson J, et al. First human implantation of a Bioresorbable polymer scaffold for acute traumatic Spinal Cord injury: a clinical pilot study for safety and feasibility. Neurosurgery. 2016;79(2):E305–12. https://doi.org/10.1227/NEU.0000000000001283.
167. Ragnarsson KT. Functional electrical stimulation after spinal cord injury: current use, therapeutic effects and future directions. Spinal Cord. 2008;46(4):255–74. https://doi.org/10.1038/sj.sc.3102091.
168. Harkema S, Gerasimenko Y, Hodes J, et al. Effect of epidural stimulation of the lumbosacral spinal cord on voluntary movement, standing, and assisted stepping after motor complete paraplegia: a case study. Lancet. 2011;377(9781):1938–47. https://doi.org/10.1016/S0140-6736(11)60547-3.
169. Gill ML, Grahn PJ, Calvert JS, et al. Neuromodulation of lumbosacral spinal networks enables independent stepping after complete paraplegia. Nat Med. 2018;24(11):1677–82. https://doi.org/10.1038/s41591-018-0175-7.
170. Angeli CA, Boakye M, Morton RA, et al. Recovery of overground walking after chronic motor complete Spinal Cord injury. N Engl J Med. 2018;379(13):1244–50. https://doi.org/10.1056/NEJMoa1803588.
171. Wagner FB, Mignardot JB, Le Goff-Mignardot CG, et al. Targeted neurotechnology restores walking in humans with spinal cord injury. Nature. 2018;563(7729):65–71. https://doi.org/10.1038/s41586-018-0649-2.
172. Capogrosso M, Milekovic T, Borton D, et al. A brain-spine interface alleviating gait deficits after spinal cord injury in primates. Nature. 2016;539(7628):284–8. https://doi.org/10.1038/nature20118.
173. Pena Pino I, Hoover C, Venkatesh S, et al. Long-term Spinal Cord stimulation after chronic complete Spinal Cord injury enables volitional movement in the absence of stimulation. Front Syst Neurosci. 2020;14:35. https://doi.org/10.3389/fnsys.2020.00035.

The Management of Brain Tumor Patients in the Neurointensive Care Unit

29

Vaidya Govindarajan, Alexis A. Morell, Nitesh V. Patel, and Ricardo J. Komotar

Contents

Abstract

Brain Tumor patients are regularly admitted into the Neurointensive Care Unit (NICU), generally in the context of neurologic deterioration or perioperative care. This chapter summarizes practical concepts that can be easily adopted in most NICUs. Although surgical intervention for brain tumors is common, each patient requires a personalized approach. Prevention and recognition of post-operative complications are critical points for the neurointensivist. Moreover, balancing a safe approach with care optimization and early discharge can be challenging. In this chapter, we summarize our institutional experience as well as the current evidence for patient management in each phase of care.

V. Govindarajan · A. A. Morell (✉) · N. V. Patel
R. J. Komotar (✉)
Department of Neurosurgery, University of Miami, Miller School of Medicine, Miami, FL, USA
e-mail: alexis.morell@jhsmiami.org; rkomotar@med.miami.edu

Introduction

Epidemiology

Despite constituting less than 2% of all primary tumors, primary brain tumors still demonstrate an incidence of 23.8 per 100,000 persons per year, with 83,830 cases of primary brain tumors estimated in 2020 alone [1]. Approximately 30% of primary brain tumors are malignant, with glioblastoma multiforme (GBM) constituting the majority of malignant brain tumors [1]. Recent demographic analyses have shown no significant differences in incidence of primary brain tumors between patient sexes or races, though there have been notable yearly increases in brain tumor incidence as the population ages [1].

Primary brain tumors are classified based on the World Health Organization (WHO) grading system, in which tumors are assessed on histological criteria and the presence of particular genetic alterations, such as the presence of isocitrate dehydrogenase (IDH) mutations and O-methylguanine DNA methyltransferase (MGMT) hypermethylation [2]. The addition of novel genetic and epigenetic features to the WHO classification has greatly improved the prognostic value of the scale, as a notable early criticism of the WHO system was its inability to adequately assign tumor features that affected patient survival [2].

E. Mahanna Gabrielli et al. (eds.), *Textbook of Neurointensive Care: Volume 1*, https://doi.org/10.1007/978-3-031-62220-5_29

The incidence of primary brain tumors is largely surpassed by the incidence of metastatic brain tumors, with the overall incidence of brain metastases increasing in recent years [3]. The increase in incidence is likely due to a combination of an aging population and increased survival among cancer patients overall; thus, patients may simply be living with cancer for a duration sufficient to develop brain metastases [3]. The most frequent source of brain metastases are lung cancers, with breast cancer and melanoma following closely behind [3].

Regardless of the type of brain tumor, the surgical management of these lesions is often indicated when all conservative measures either fail or are not sufficient to provide benefit. This chapter will briefly review the characterization of brain tumors and then review the typical surgical approaches. This introduction will serve as a primer for the rest of this chapter, which will focus on the intensive care unit (ICU) management of brain tumor patients. The section on ICU management will be organized by phases of perioperative care.

Characterization

Primary Versus Metastatic Tumors

Brain tumors are frequently classified by whether they are primary (originating in the brain) or metastatic. With respect to primary brain tumors, the largest subclass of these tumors are gliomas, which comprise 75% of all primary lesions and are defined as neuroectodermal tumors arising either directly from glial cells or their precursors [2]. This includes oligodendrogliomas and meningiomas [2]. In contrast, secondary or metastatic brain tumors are a direct consequence of an underlying primary malignancy [3, 4]. As stated previously, large-scale studies have stratified primary malignancies by their propensity to cause metastatic intracranial disease, with lung, breast cancers, and melanomas forming the most frequent primary foci [3, 4].

With respect to clinical presentation, there are relatively few key features that allow for reliable differentiation between primary and secondary brain tumors, largely due to the inherent variability in clinical presentation that is generally seen in brain malignancy. Patients may present with focal or generalized symptoms, typically dependent on whether the lesions impinge upon discrete functional brain regions [2]. Symptom onset is dependent on several features, such as rate of tumor growth and location [2]. Differentiation between primary and secondary malignancy is therefore challenging based on physical exam findings alone. Nevertheless, there are several common findings that may raise suspicion for CNS involvement of malignancy, such as headache, paresis, and behavioral changes, some combination of which may be present in approximately half of all patients [2].

Imaging findings in conjunction with patient history are frequently used to differentiate primary from metastatic brain tumors. Namely, primary tumors frequently present as solitary lesions, while metastatic tumors typically present with multiple focal lesions on imaging [2, 4]. However, solitary metastatic lesions are not uncommon. Tissue diagnosis is typically necessary to formally elucidate the etiology of a discovered mass. Nonetheless, in a case of multiple intracranial lesions with a known primary cancer diagnosis, metastasis is most often the diagnosis.

Intra-Axial Versus Extra-Axial Tumors

Another means of categorization involves distinguishing intra-axial versus extra-axial malignancies. Intra-axial tumors refer to malignancies that directly arise from and impact the brain parenchyma, while extra-axial tumors primarily affect intracranial structures external to the parenchyma, primarily the meninges [5]. Meningiomas constitute the largest class of extra-axial tumors and are among the most common primary brain malignancies overall [6]. These lesions also tend to be well-circumscribed and are usually distinct from the rest of the brain [7]. Vestibular schwannomas are also considered extra-axial lesions, as involvement of cranial nerves does not constitute the brain parenchyma [7]. It is critical to recognize that metastatic lesions may be extra-axial as they do not originate from the brain parenchyma [5, 7].

Ventricular Tumors

Another unique subtype of primary tumors is ventricular tumors, typically affecting the lateral and third ventricles [8]. These tumors are most common in the pediatric population, with approximately 41% of ventricular tumors occurring in children [9]. In adults, ventricular tumors comprise a mere 7% of all primary malignancies, with over half of adult ventricular tumors occurring in the lateral ventricles [8, 9]. It is critical to note that many ventricular tumors are not derived from cells native to the ventricular system (e.g., choroid plexus papillomas and ependymomas) and that astrocytomas, glioblastomas, and meningiomas can extend into into ventricular spaces [10].

Approaches to Treatment

Open Surgery

Surgical intervention of CNS malignancies centers on three fundamental goals: oncological benefit, preservation of function, and quality of life—with surgical intervention considered beneficial when at least one of these objectives can be reasonably met [11]. Usage of open surgical approaches is also greatly affected by the nature of the malignancy. For example, glioblastoma is typically managed with the Stupp protocol, which involves maximal safe open resection followed by a combination of radiotherapy and temozolomide [12]. Typically, the extent of resection (EOR) in open techniques has a significant impact on patient survival. Supramaximal resection, defined as resection of a contrast-enhancing lesion and its surrounding non-enhancing tissue, is an evolving technique for open resection of CNS malignancy [13, 14]. Unfortunately, most open resection techniques are limited in their ability to treat multiple metastatic lesions. In these cases, targeted or whole-brain radiotherapy is considered [15].

Minimally Invasive Techniques

Minimally invasive techniques have gained traction in all surgical fields, including neurosurgery. Endoscopic resection methods have been well-described in the neurosurgical literature, with endoscopic resection of pituitary tumors being the most well-known [16]. However, minimally invasive techniques are not the exclusive approach to resection of skull-base tumors, as open techniques may still be used depending on the size and anatomical location of the tumors.

Another increasingly common minimally invasive technique is tubular retraction. Tubular retractors offer a minimally invasive and much more benign means of accessing parenchymal tumors. By shifting brain tissue radially and utilizing natural pathways through sulci, stereotactically placed tubular retractors offer a promising alternative to traditional methods of brain retraction by reducing perioperative complications and resultant brain trauma [17].

Laser Interstitial Thermal Therapy (LITT)

In poorly accessible or recurrent malignancies, laser interstitial thermal therapy (LITT) offers a promising alternative to traditional open or minimally invasive techniques [18]. Typically, LITT involves inducing targeted hyperthermic therapy in malignant tissue via a thermally active probe [11]. LITT has demonstrated substantial efficacy in halting tumor progression when utilized on metastatic lesions [18].

Non-Surgical Approaches

Non-surgical approaches are typically considered salvage therapies in the context of CNS malignancy. Typically, these approaches are considered when surgical intervention will likely have little benefit in reducing disease burden or significantly improve quality of life [11]. This is especially true of metastatic tumors, which typically present with multiple lesions and are thus not amenable to resection. Traditionally, whole-brain radiation therapy (WBRT) has been used, with advances in stereotactic radiosurgery largely supplanting WBRT [19]. Brachytherapy has also recently been shown to be well-tolerated. Initial use of brachytherapy for the management of metastatic lesions was poorly adopted given concerns of radiation necrosis and prolonged half-life of radioactive iodine [20]. However, there has been recent adoption of radioactive cesium (Cs-131) due to its more benign side-effect profile [21].

The Patient with a Brain Tumor in the Neuro ICU

The vast majority of brain tumor patients are admitted into the Neuro ICU in the context of a surgical intervention. These patients require special care, and management guidelines from other types of diseases (traumatic brain injury, stroke, subarachnoid hemorrhage, etc.) should not be used for patients with brain tumors.

Pre-Operative Phase of Care

Admission for Preoperative Monitoring or Optimization

The most common clinical scenario in which a brain tumor patient is admitted into the ICU before surgery is acute neurologic deterioration. However, patients may also be admitted for medical optimization to reduce surgical risks.

1. *Monitoring*—In some instances, patients may be transferred to the ICU when more frequent neurological monitoring (q2 h or less) or other diagnostic / therapeutic interventions are needed. Obviously, there is a wide spectrum of neurological exam change that may trigger this transfer. From a therapeutic standpoint, neuromonitoring devices such as intracranial pressure monitors, external ventricular drains, lumbar drain catheters, and endovascular sheaths, are all typically handled in an ICU setting.
   (a) *Neurological Exam Changes*—Rapidly deteriorating patients with brain tumors should be evaluated as any other neurologic patient. Nonetheless, it is important to avoid certain assumptions, as neurological deterioration related to brain tumors will need specific management. Figure 29.1 addresses some of these important points. For patients that are hemodynamically stable, typical changes can include new onset altered mental status, seizures, aphasia, confusion, or new motor and/or sensory deficit. For patients who are unable to communicate (e.g. due to seizures) the patient's family, or the previous care providers (primary care physician, neuro-oncologist, neurosurgeon, etc.) should be contacted to provide an overview of the patient's history. If possible, discussing the status of the patient with the primary treating team should be pursued and might provide extremely useful information, including prognosis, previous treatments, complications, or possible obstacles to patient

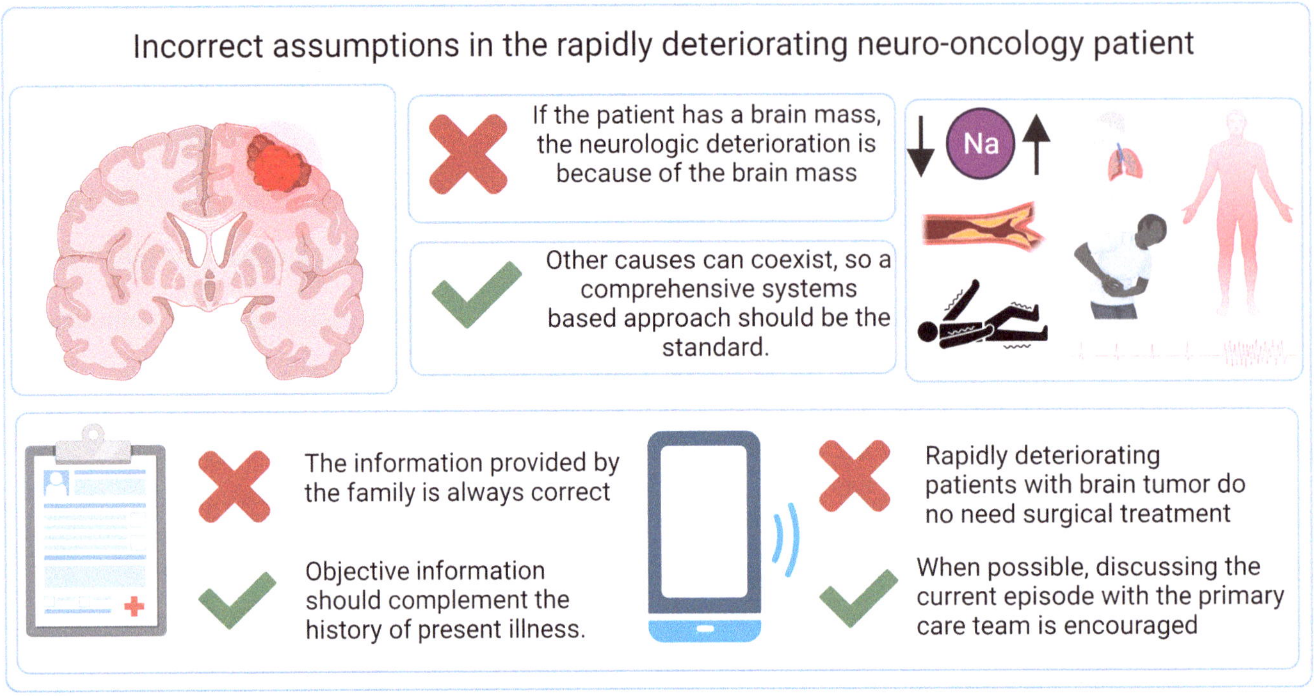

Fig. 29.1 Incorrect assumptions in the rapidly deteriorating neuro-oncology patient. (Created with biorender.com)

care. In the case of seizures, priority should be placed on immediate seizure control to avoid permanent neurological injury or conversion to grand mal seizures in the case of an initial partial seizure. It is important to note, sometimes the cause is not the mass: just because a patient has a brain mass does not mean that the patient's neurologic deterioration is because of that mass. Patients with undiagnosed slow-growing tumors can withstand a large mass effect without presenting any symptoms. Although the finding of a brain mass always requires specific assessment, other possible causes should be considered. Electrolyte imbalances, infectious diseases, stroke, myocardial infarctions, and organ failure can produce non-focal neurologic deficits such as altered mental status or confusion. A comprehensive systems-based approach should be the standard, even in patients with a known history of brain tumors.

2. *Therapeutic/Diagnostic Neuromonitoring*—Often, patients may stay in the ICU setting prior to their main surgical intervention for careful electrolyte, hemodynamic, or intracranial/thecal pressure monitoring. In regards to electrolytes, sodium balance in the context of pituitary dysfunction is a very common factor to be considered. However, sodium derangements can also be seen in cases of acute brain injury such as traumatic brain injury or subarachnoid hemorrhage. In either case, the optimal approach involves careful monitoring of fluid intake/output, judicious use of intravascular fluids, and serial measurements of serum and urine electrolytes. Hemodynamic monitoring is an important part of preoperative management for patients in whom preoperative embolization is used to devascularize a tumor. In these cases, an endovascular sheath may be left in place for further access and careful blood pressure monitoring is essential. Patients who need frequent or invasive neuromonitoring are often admitted to the ICU preoperatively.

   (a) *External Ventricular Drains (EVD)*—These drains may be placed for both diagnostic and therapeutic purposes. EVDs allow for simultaneous cerebrospinal fluid (CSF) drainage and measurement of intracranial pressure (ICP). Typically, these drains are placed from a frontal trajectory into the lateral ventricles; however, they can also be placed using other trajectories when appropriate. Some important points to note for the intensivist regarding EVDs include accurate and timely evaluation of ICP with nursing instruction for regular interval ICP checks, ensuring ICP values and waveforms are documented, and quantitative as well as qualitative evaluation of CSF output from drains. Brain tumor patients may sometimes receive EVDs prior to brain tumor resection—this is more likely with a ventricular tumor or one which causes ventricular obstruction (such as a posterior fossa lesion).

(b) *Intra-Thecal or Lumbar Drains*—For intracranial lesions, lumbar drains are not commonly used as there can be a risk for downward herniation. However, in cases of CSF leaks, there may be a need for CSF diversion. CSF leaks can occur spontaneously in cases of encephaloceles or pituitary / sellar pathology. Nursing staff should be well-versed in drain management. Unlike most EVDs, the resting state of a lumbar drain is usually in the closed position—drains are only opened at specified intervals to drain a specified volume. If a drain remains in the open position, there can be devastating consequences as over-drainage of CSF can occur very easily. Additionally, care must be taken during patient repositioning or transport to ensure drains do not become dislodged.

Post-Operative Phase of Care

After brain tumor surgery patients should be assessed comprehensively. The objectives of this care phase are primarily to (1) recognize potential postoperative complications, (2) continue medical treatment, and (3) advance patient care with the goal of successful discharge. Post-operative brain tumor patients can often be categorized by whether their tumor (and surgery) was supratentorial or infratentorial.

1. *Supratentorial Craniotomies*—Supratentorial compartment refers to the intracranial compartment above the tentorium. From a pain management standpoint, balancing pain control and patient arousal status is important. Patients should be counseled preoperatively and reminded postoperatively that a certain degree of discomfort and pain is to be expected with any surgery. This discussion often leads to patients being less likely to request pain control at even the slightest discomfort or soreness. When medication is required, avoiding opiates and non-steroidal anti-inflammatory drugs (NSAIDS), and instead, utilizing acetaminophen (oral or intravenous) can be highly effective. For supratentorial cases, antiepileptics are typically given for a minimum of 7 days; however, surgeon preference and individual ICU protocols may have some variability. Initiation of oral intake will likely vary as well, nonetheless, patients often tolerate liquids and solids within a few hours of brain tumor surgery. Post-operative imaging is commonly necessary. Not all brain tumor patients will get the same imaging protocols, however, surgeons may often want to review imaging prior to transferring out of the ICU. Priority should be placed on obtaining post operative imaging along with timely review by the ICU and surgical teams. Table 29.1 and Fig. 29.2 summarizes these points.
   (a) *Hemorrhage*—The most feared complication after supratentorial surgery is postoperative hemorrhage at the surgical bed. Its incidence after brain tumor resection is between 4–6%, with half of those patients requiring surgical intervention [25]. Patients presenting with neurological deterioration, resistant headache or new neurologic deficits should be screened for postoperative bleeding with non-contrast head CT. Head CT Scan is fast and accurate for excluding hemorrhage MRI takes more time but can also be used to evaluate for cerebral edema and ischemia.

Table 29.1 General postoperative management of brain tumor patients

	Initial regimen	Remember
Pain management	– Acetaminophen (Tylenol™) p.r.n – Oxycodone – Using local anesthetics before wound closure in a multilayered fashion can reduce postoperative pain after brain tumor surgery[22, 23]	– Postoperative pain after craniotomy is frequent, and many times undermanaged [24]
Anti-seizure prophylaxis	– Levetiracetam (Keppra™) in non-epileptic patients 500 mg BID to 1000 mg BID – Maintain the previous regimen in epileptic patients	– 7 days is generally sufficient for non-epileptic patients
Diet	– Liquids: 1 h after surgery if there is no vomiting or nausea – Foods: 2 h after surgery if there is no vomiting or nausea	– Vomiting increases ICP and can be detrimental in patients with a high risk of CSF leak
Postopereratíve imaging	– Brain tumor resection: MRI < 24 hs after surgery – Brain needle biopsy: CT scan <24 after surgery	– In case of new neurologic deficits or altered mental status, new brain imaging should not be delayed
Vasogenic edema	– Steroids are generally administered for 24–48 h after surgery	– For supratentorial surgeries, 7 days is the initial regimen. Then taper if asymptomatic – For infratentorial surgeries, 14 days is the initial regimen. Then taper if asymptomatic

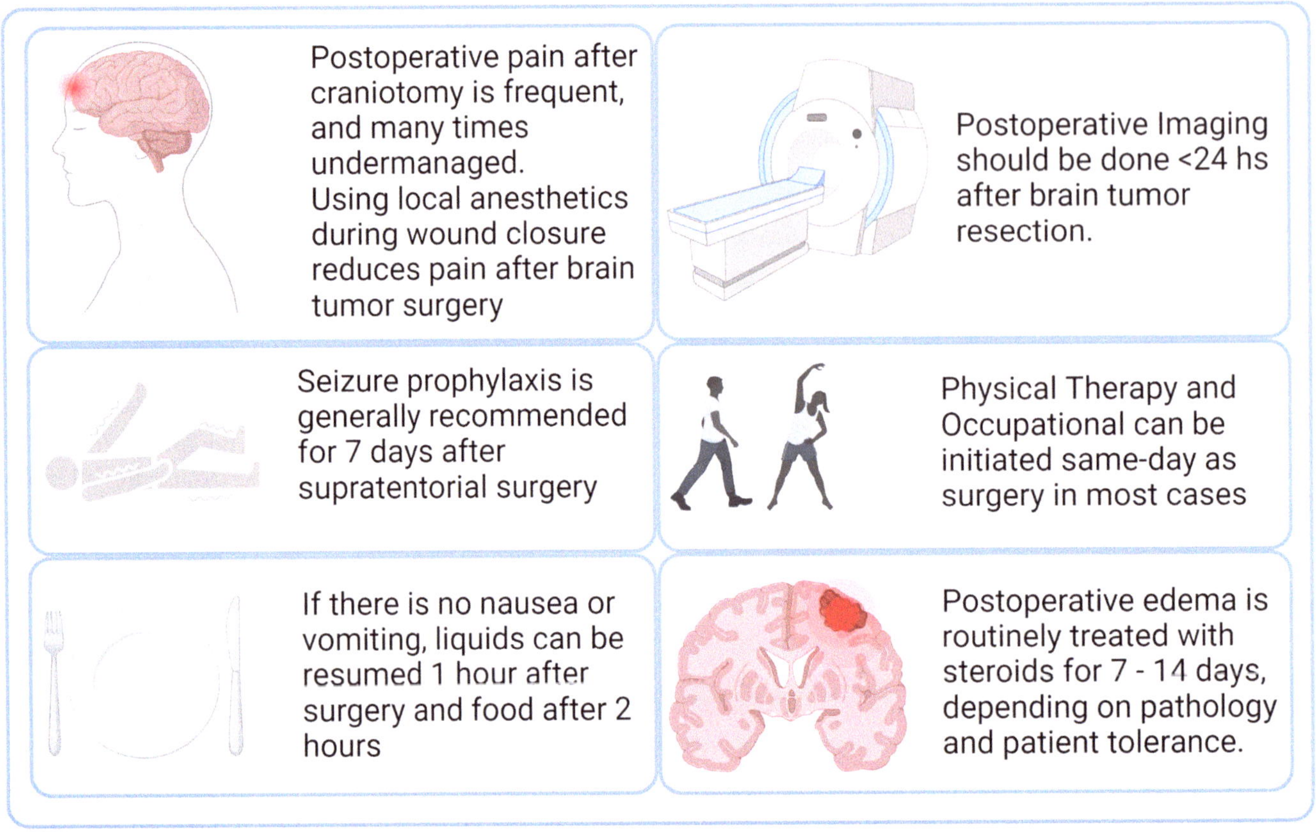

Fig. 29.2 General recommendations after supratentorial surgery. (Created with biorender.com)

Most brain tumor programs have specific protocols regarding postoperative imaging to assess for residual tumor and postoperative bleeding before discharging the patient. Early imaging (< 24 hs) does not totally eliminate the possibility of having a postoperative cavity hematoma, as more than 50% of hemorrhages appear more than 24 h after surgery [25].

(b) *Cerebral Edema*—Patients with significant perilesional edema after surgery should be carefully managed. General measures include head position at 30°, avoidance of neck compression, hypoxia, hypercapnia, hypotension, fever, and hyponatremia. Pharmacologic management is generally needed in patients with significant mass effects and mainly includes the use of steroids. Osmotherapy agents such as mannitol and hypertonic saline are not routinely used in vasogenic edema. Long-term use of mannitol has been associated with paradoxical exacerbation of vasogenic edema, probably by leakage into the brain parenchyma in patients with disrupted blood-brain barrier [26].

(c) *Cerebral Ischemia*—iatrogenic strokes after brain tumor surgery have a reported incidence of 14.1–19.8 per 1000 cases [27]. These cases range from a small asymptomatic lacunar infarct due to injury of a penetrating artery, to a life-threatening large territorial stroke from damage to a large vessel, such as the carotid artery. Postoperative imaging is recommended to confirm the etiology, however, there may be few effective therapeutic options.

2. *Infratentorial Craniotomies*—The region of the brain below the tentorium includes the brainstem, cerebellum, and fourth ventricle. The small volume of the posterior fossa does not accomodate significant mass lesions without life-threatening consequences (acute hydrocephalus, brainstem compression, cerebellar tonsilar herniation). Postoperative hemorrhage, edema, or ischemia can block the normal flow of CSF, with subsequent development of obstructive hydrocephalus. New postoperative hydrocephalus after posterior fossa surgery has an incidence of 1–2% [28].

Preoperative hydrocephalus may be present in over 20% of patients with posterior fossa tumors and up to 15% of these patients might require postoperative ventriculoperitoneal shunting because of persistent hydrocephalus [29]. It is important to attend to patient positioning and to monitor the patient's pillow for CSF leakage. Infratentorial surgical access is usually through a posterior or lateral trajectory. As these areas become dependent and subject to pressure, wound breakdown and fluid egress (including CSF leaks) can place the patient at increased risk for infection, including meningitis.

3. *Endoscopic Endonasal Approaches*—Approaches to the pituitary gland and sellar region are often through an endoscopic endonasal approach. This approach may be used alone or in combination with a transcranial route for resection of certain types of brain tumors. The above-mentioned pearls for supratentorial and infratentorial craniotomies still apply; however, special consideration should be given to the following:
   (a) *CSF Leakage*—The overall rate of postoperative CSF leakage after transsphenoidal resection is approximately 5.6% [30]. Patients with intraoperative CSF leakage, larger tumor size or who undergo revision or endoscopic surgery are at increased risk for postoperative CSF leak. While early diagnosis and adequate management are paramount to avoid significant morbidity, all possible measures to prevent the development of a CSF fistula should be pursued [31]. A summary of the general measures and checklist can be found in Table 29.2.
   (b) *Pneumocephalus*—Postoperative abnormal communication of the subarachnoid space with the external space can allow for air to replace the space normally occupied by CSF, causing pneumocephalus. Tension pneumocephalus is a rare but serious complication, and occurs when a valvular mechanism is formed in a dural defect, allowing for air to enter the skull in a unidirectional fashion, with subsequent intradural air expansion. This type of complication can produce severe neurologic deterioration, and once diagnosed, it constitutes a true neurosurgical emergency. Before addressing the primary dural valvular defect, intracranial pressure should be decreased by needle aspiration, burr hole, or ventriculostomy. Non-tension pneumocephalus is a more benign condition, that can be managed conservatively in most cases. Some providers may utilize protocols involving steady-state or cycling of oxygen, however, evidence is limited and is based primarily on retrospective studies. In the presence of an evolving or new postoperative pneumocephalus, an occult CSF leakage should be excluded.
4. *Laser Ablation*—Laser ablation is a minimally invasive procedure that uses a stereotactically placed probe that delivers thermal energy to induce cell death. While the complication rate is very low (3–4%), superficial wound infections, seizures, and postoperative hemorrhages have been reported [32]. In many patients, the postoperative MRI can show an increased volume of perilesional edema, which should not be considered a complication. Asymptomatic increase in the perilesional edema is expected as part of the lesional mechanism and is well managed with steroids in most cases [33].

Table 29.2 General postoperative management of transsphenoidal surgery

Checklist	General measures
– Intake & Output registry – Steroids – Diabetes insipidus / SIADH monitoring – Screen for panhypopituitarism – Patient education and general measures for CSF leak prevention	– Bed rest with the head of bed at 30° – Do not drink using a straw – No incentive spirometry – Empiric antibiotics until nasal packaging is removed – No straining – Coughing with an open mouth

Conclusion

The management of the brain tumor patient in the neurosurgical ICU should take into account several factors unique to this patient population. A systems-based approach should be used in conjunction with a phase-of-care plan. In the event that a brain tumor patient is admitted to the ICU preoperatively, the goal may be for close monitoring and/or medical optimization. In the post-operative phase of care, hemorrhage, ischemia, and CSF leak should be always kept in mind as possible complications. Additionally, patient nutrition, physical and occupational therapy, and imaging should be prioritized to ensure timely discharge from the ICU and hospital. For special circumstances, such as endoscopic endonasal surgeries and laser ablation cases, a few additional factors should be kept in mind. Finally, as the intensive care unit team prepares the plan of care for brain tumor patients, each body system should be taken into consideration to optimize the patient's neurological recovery. Using a carefully planned approach, the care of brain tumor patients in the ICU can be accomplished efficiently and effectively.

References

1. Ostrom QT, et al. CBTRUS statistical report: primary brain and other central nervous system tumors diagnosed in the United States in 2013-2017. Neuro-Oncology. 2020;22(12 Suppl 2):iv1–iv96.
2. Lapointe S, Perry A, Butowski NA. Primary brain tumours in adults. Lancet. 2018;392(10145):432–46.
3. Singh R, et al. Epidemiology of synchronous brain metastases. Neuro Oncol Adv. 2020;2(1):vdaa041.

4. Soffietti R, et al. Diagnosis and treatment of brain metastases from solid tumors: guidelines from the European Association of Neuro-Oncology (EANO). Neuro-Oncology. 2017;19(2):162–74.
5. Rapalino O, Smirniotopoulos JG. Extra-axial brain tumors. Handb Clin Neurol. 2016;135:275–91.
6. Buerki RA, et al. An overview of meningiomas. Future Oncol (London, England). 2018;14(21):2161–77.
7. Drevelegas A. Extra-axial brain tumors. Eur Radiol. 2005;15(3):453–67.
8. Pendl G, Oztürk E, Haselsberger K. Surgery of tumours of the lateral ventricle. Acta Neurochir. 1992;116(2–4):128–36.
9. Elwatidy SM, et al. Tumors of the lateral and third ventricle: surgical management and outcome analysis in 42 cases. Neurosciences (Riyadh, Saudi Arabia). 2017;22(4):274–81.
10. Zuccaro G, et al. Lateral ventricle tumors in children: a series of 54 cases. Childs Nerv Syst. 1999;15(11–12):774–85.
11. Rivera M, et al. Updates on surgical management and advances for brain tumors. Curr Oncol Rep. 2021;23(3):35.
12. Stupp R, et al. Radiotherapy plus concomitant and adjuvant temozolomide for glioblastoma. N Engl J Med. 2005;352(10):987–96.
13. Lally M, Johnston KW, Cobbold RS. Limitations in the accuracy of peak frequency measurements in the diagnosis of carotid disease. J Clin Ultrasound. 1984;12(7):403–9.
14. Li YM, et al. The influence of maximum safe resection of glioblastoma on survival in 1229 patients: can we do better than gross-total resection? J Neurosurg. 2016;124(4):977–88.
15. Hatiboglu MA, Akdur K, Sawaya R. Neurosurgical management of patients with brain metastasis. Neurosurg Rev. 2020;43(2):483–95.
16. Govindarajan V, et al. Perioperative complications in endoscopic Endonasal versus transcranial resections of adult Craniopharyngiomas. World Neurosurg. 2021;152:e729–37.
17. Jackson C, Gallia GL, Chaichana KL. Minimally invasive biopsies of deep-seated brain lesions using tubular retractors under exoscopic visualization. J Neurol Surg A Cent Eur Neurosurg. 2017;78(06):588–94.
18. Chaunzwa TL, et al. Laser thermal ablation for metastases failing radiosurgery: a multicentered retrospective study. Neurosurgery. 2018;82(1):56–63.
19. Iorio-Morin C, et al. Repeat stereotactic radiosurgery for the management of locally recurrent brain metastases. J Neuro-Oncol. 2019;145(3):551–9.
20. Shafiq AR, et al. Placement of cesium-131 permanent brachytherapy seeds using the endoscopic endonasal approach for recurrent anaplastic skull base meningioma: case report and technical note. J Neurosurg. 2019;132(3):921–6.
21. Wernicke AG, et al. Surgical technique and clinically relevant resection cavity dynamics following implantation of cesium-131 brachytherapy in patients with brain metastases. Oper Neurosurg. 2016;12(1):49–60.
22. Potters J-W, Klimek M. Local anesthetics for brain tumor resection: current perspectives. Local Reg Anest. 2018;11:1–8.
23. Song J, et al. Preemptive scalp infiltration with 0.5% ropivacaine and 1% lidocaine reduces postoperative pain after craniotomy. Acta Neurochir. 2015;157(6):993–8.
24. Vadivelu N, et al. Options for perioperative pain management in neurosurgery. J Pain Res. 2016;9:37–47.
25. Viken HH, et al. When are complications after brain tumor surgery detected? World Neurosurg. 2018;112:e702–10.
26. Esquenazi Y, Lo VP, Lee K. Critical Care Management of Cerebral Edema in brain tumors. J Intensive Care Med. 2017;32(1):15–24.
27. De la Garza-Ramos R, et al. Surgical complications following malignant brain tumor surgery: an analysis of 2002–2011 data. Clin Neurol Neurosurg. 2016;140:6–10.
28. Marx S, et al. Frequency and treatment of hydrocephalus prior to and after posterior fossa tumor surgery in adult patients. Acta Neurochir. 2018;160(5):1063–71.
29. Chen T, et al. Risk factors for hydrocephalus following fourth ventricle tumor surgery: a retrospective analysis of 121 patients. PLoS One. 2020;15(11):e0241853.
30. Zhou Z, et al. Risk factors for postoperative cerebrospinal fluid leakage after transsphenoidal surgery for pituitary adenoma: a meta-analysis and systematic review. BMC Neurol. 2021;21(1):417.
31. Ivan ME, et al. Risk factors for postoperative cerebrospinal fluid leak and meningitis after expanded endoscopic endonasal surgery. J Clin Neurosci. 2015;22(1):48–54.
32. Shah AH, et al. The role of laser interstitial thermal therapy in surgical neuro-oncology: series of 100 consecutive patients. Neurosurgery. 2020;87(2):266–75.
33. Luther E, et al. Supralesional ablation volumes are feasible in the posterior fossa and may provide enhanced symptomatic relief. Oper Neurosurg. 2021;21(6):418–25.

Autoimmune Encephalopathies Presenting in the ICU

30

Samantha A. Banks and Alejandro A. Rabinstein

Contents

Abstract

Autoimmune encephalitis (AE) is an increasingly recognized cause of encephalitis. Patients with AE often require admission to an intensive care unit (ICU). Early recognition and treatment are critical to improve outcomes. In this chapter, we will outline an approach to the diagnosis of AE in the ICU setting including bedside, serologic, and radiographic testing. We will describe common presentations of antibody-positive cases and discuss seronegative criteria. We will also present management strategies including immunotherapy and complications of AE, such as dysautonomia and seizures. We will finally discuss long-term outcomes and prognosis. Intensivists should be aware of these diseases and trained in the appropriate management of these conditions.

Introduction

Autoimmune or paraneoplastic diseases of the nervous system are potentially devastating and often treatable diseases that may necessitate care in an intensive care unit (ICU). Autoimmune disease may involve any aspect of the central or peripheral nervous system (Table 30.1), but this chapter will focus specifically on autoimmune and paraneoplastic encephalitis (PNE), which will be collectively referred to as autoimmune encephalitis (AE). Patients with AE may require intensive care due to seizures, respiratory failure, dysautonomia, or coma. These patients are complex, and physicians need a high index of suspicion to diagnose these disorders and ensure early and appropriate treatment to improve outcomes. The term autoimmune encephalitis encompasses a

S. A. Banks · A. A. Rabinstein (✉)
Mayo Clinic Department of Neurology, Rochester, MN, USA
e-mail: rabinstein.alejandro@mayo.edu

E. Mahanna Gabrielli et al. (eds.), *Textbook of Neurointensive Care: Volume 1*, https://doi.org/10.1007/978-3-031-62220-5_30

Table 30.1 Autoimmune disorders of the nervous system presenting to the intensive care unit

Muscle
Dermatomyositis
Polymyositis
Necrotizing autoimmune myopathy
Neuromuscular junction
Myasthenia gravis
Lambert Eaton Myasthenic syndrome
Lower motor neuron
Guillian-Barre syndrome (acute inflammatory demyelinating polyradiculopathy)
Spinal cord
Transverse myelitis
Brain or brainstem
Autoimmune encephalitis
Neuromyelitis Optica Spectrum disorder
Myelin oligodendrocyte glycoprotein antibody associated disorder

variety of disorders involving immune-mediated inflammation of the brain. AE should be considered in patients with progression over less than 3 months of working memory deficits, change in mental status, seizures, or psychiatric symptoms. Extra attention should be paid to patients with known systemic autoimmunity, cancer, and those being treated with immune checkpoint inhibitors.

Chapter Goals

- List autoimmune and paraneoplastic disorders that may result in critical illness.
- Describe a parsimonious approach to the diagnosis of autoimmune encephalopathies in the ICU, including when to order autoimmune panels and when and how much to investigate for underlying malignancy.
- Discuss the salient features of the main autoimmune encephalopathies that can be seen in the ICU.
- Highlight considerations specifically pertinent to the ICU management of autoimmune encephalopathies and its complications.
- Briefly discuss the prognosis of critically ill patients with autoimmune encephalopathies.

Key Clinical Questions

The chapter will answer the following questions:

- When should one suspect autoimmune encephalitis as the etiology of the patient's symptoms?
- What investigations should be done?
- In what cases does an underlying malignancy need to be excluded?
- What treatments should be used?

Epidemiology

The prevalence of autoimmune encephalitis is likely underestimated due to limited testing and the recent discovery of many antibodies. A population-based study in Olmstead County found the incidence of AE (0.8/100,000 person-years) was not significantly different from infectious encephalitis (1/100,000 person-years) [1], while a recent study in France found the incidence of PNE or AE to be 3.2 per million person-years [2]. Both studies have found an increasing incidence of antibody-positive cases in recent years, likely due to increased antibody testing and detection. Among large case series, anti-NMDA receptor is the most common antibody detected [2, 3]. When AE is taken as a group, there is variability in reported demographic characteristics as each antibody has unique demographic features (Tables 30.2 and 30.3). Patients with AE frequently require ICU level of care, with estimates as high as 55% of hospitalized cases requiring ICU [38–40].

Table 30.2 Demographic and clinical features of neuronal-specific antibodies to intracellular antigens according to largest case series published to date

Intracellular target	Female sex (%)	Typical age of onset	Common clinical accompaniments	Cancer risk (cancer types)
AK5 [4, 5]	25	60–80	LE; seizures; weight loss	0%
Amphiphysin [6]	60	60–70	LE; peripheral neuropathy; myelopathy; SPS; ataxia	80% (breast, SCLC)
ANNA-1 (Hu) [7, 8]	55–65	60–70	LE; sensory neuronopathy; GI dysmotility; ataxia	85–90% (SCLC)
ANNA-2 (Ri) [9]	65	60–70	Brainstem syndrome (opsoclonus-myoclonus, laryngospasm, jaw opening dystonia); ataxia; myelopathy; neuropathy	80% (breast, SCLC)
ANNA-3 [10]	50	50–60	LE; cerebellar ataxia; peripheral neuropathy; myelopathy	80–90% (SCLC)
CRMP5 (CV2) [11, 12]	30–60	60–70	LE; chorea; optic neuropathy/retinopathy; peripheral neuropathy; myelopathy; ataxia	90% (SCLC)
GAD-65 [13–15]	75–85	40–60	LE; SPS; ataxia; seizures	8% (lung, thymoma)
GFAP [16]	55	50–60	Meningo-encephalo-myelitis; optic disc edema; tremor; viral-like prodrome	35% (teratoma)
ITPR1 [17]	70	60–70	Cerebellar ataxia; peripheral neuropathy; encephalitis with seizures; myelopathy	35%(breast cancer)
Kelch11 [18]	0	30–50	Ataxia; brainstem dysfunction (hearing loss, diplopia, vertigo); seizure; encephalopathy	>70% (seminoma, lung)
Ma2 (ta) [19]	35	60–70	LE; diencephalic syndrome (narcolepsy/cataplexy); brainstem symptoms	90% (testicular germ-cell, lung)
NIF [20]	40	60–70	Ataxia; encephalopathy; myeloradiculoneuropathy	55% (SCLC, Merkel cell, adenocarcinoma)
PCA-1 (Yo) [21]	100	60–70	Ataxia; brainstem syndrome; myelopathy; peripheral neuropathy	>80% (fallopian, ovarian, breast)
PCA-2/ MAP1B [22]	70	60–70	Ataxia; LE; brainstem symptoms; peripheral neuropathy	90% (SCLC)
PCA-TR [23]	80	60–70	Cerebellar ataxia	90% (Hodgkin's lymphoma)

Abbreviations: *AK5* adenylate kinase 5, *ANNA-1/2* anti-neuronal nuclear antibodies type-1/2, *CRMP5* collapsin response-mediator protein-5, *GAD-65* glutamic acid decarboxylase-65, *GFAP* glial fibrillary acidic protein, *GI* gastrointestinal, *LE* limbic encephalitis, *NIF* neuronal intermediate filament, *PCA-TR* Purkinje cell antibody-TR, *PCA-1* purkinje cell antigen −1, *PCA-2/MAP1B* purkinje cell antigen-2/microtubule-associated protein 1B, *SCLC* small cell lung cancer, *SPS* stiff-person syndrome

Table 30.3 Demographic and clinical features of neuronal-specific antibodies to cell surface antigens according to largest case series published to date

Cell-surface target	Female sex (%)	Typical age of onset (years)	Common clinical accompaniments	Cancer risk (cancer types)
AMPAR [24]	65	50–60	LE; seizures; hyponatremia	65% (thymoma, SCLC)
AQP4 [25]	70–90	30–40	Optic neuritis; myelitis; area postrema syndrome; narcolepsy; cerebral lesion	<20%
CASPR2 [26]	25	60–70	LE; seizures; peripheral nerve hyperexcitability; ataxia	20% (thymoma, melanoma)
DPPX [27]	40	50–60	Encephalopathy; brainstem syndrome; sleep disturbances; GI dysmotility; weight loss; hyperexcitability	10%(hematologic malignancies)
$GABA_AR$ [28]	50	40–50	Encephalopathy; seizures; movement disorders	25%(thymoma)
$GABA_BR$ [29]	40	60–70	LE; seizures	50% (SCLC)
GlyRα1 [30]	45	40–50	SPS; PERM; brainstem syndrome	10–20% (thymoma, seminoma)
IgLON5 [31, 32]	50	60–70	Sleep disturbances; bulbar symptoms; ataxia; chorea	Rare
LGI1 [26, 33]	35–40	60–70	LE; FBDS; sleep disturbance; hyponatremia	10% (thymoma)
MOG [34]	50	30–40	ADEM; ON; myelitis; brainstem symptoms; viral-like prodromes	Rare
mGluR1 [34]	45	20–30	LE; sleep dysfunction; seizures; ataxia; movement disorder	45% (Hodgkin's lymphoma)
Neurexin 3α [35]	80	40–50	Encephalitis; viral-like prodrome; oro-facial dyskinesia; central hypoventilation	Unknown
NMDAR [36, 37]	80–90	20–30	LE; psychosis; viral-like prodrome; dyskinesias, central hypoventilation	40–60% (teratoma)

Abbreviations: *ADEM* acute disseminated encephalomyelitis, *AMPAR* α-amino-3-hydroxy-5-methyl-4-isoxazolepropionic acid receptor, *ANA* anti-nuclear antibody, *CASPR2* contactin associated protein 2, *DPPX* dipeptidyl aminopeptidase-like protein 6, *FBDS* facio-brachial dystonic seizures, *$GABA_AR$* γ-aminobutyric acid type-A receptor, *$GABA_BR$* γ-aminobutyric acid type-B receptor, *GI* gastrointestinal, *mGluR5* metabotropic glutamate receptor 5, *GlyRα1* glycine receptor subunit alpha-1, *IgLON5* immunoglobulin-like cell adhesion molecule IgLON family member 5, *LE* limbic encephalitis, *LGI1* leucine-rich glioma inactivated 1, *MOG* myelin oligodendrocyte glycoprotein, *NMDAR* N-methyl-D-aspartate receptor, *ON* optic neuritis, *PERM* progressive encephalopathy with rigidity and myoclonus, *SCLC* small cell lung cancer, *SPS* stiff-person syndrome

Pathophysiology

Antibodies are categorized into two groups based on the location of their antigenic target: cell surface or intracellular. Antibodies to cell surface or synaptic antigens are suspected to be directly pathogenic leading to receptor dysfunction or internalization, antibody-mediated cytotoxicity, or activation of complement (Fig. 30.1) [36, 41, 42]. These antibodies, including anti-NMDA-Receptor and anti-LGI1, have a weaker association with underlying cancer and are generally more responsive to immune therapy. In contrast, it is suspected though not proven that the antibodies directed to intracellular targets, such as ANNA-1 and CRMP-5, are not directly pathogenic and are more likely marker of disease that is mediated by CD8-T-cells (Fig. 30.1) [42–44]. These diseases more commonly are paraneoplastic and are less responsive to immunotherapy.

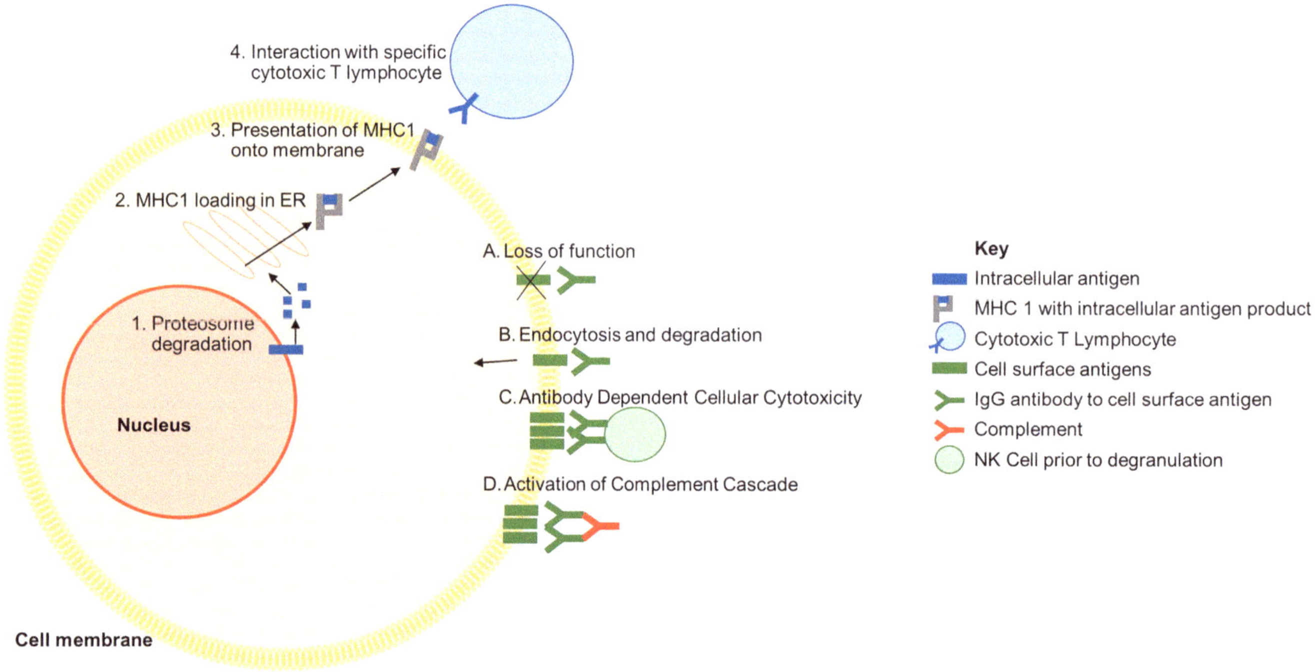

Fig. 30.1 **Mechanisms of Disease**. Antibodies are divided into two primary types, intracellular (blue) or cell surface (green). Intracellular antigens (blue) are degraded by proteosomes (1) and loaded onto major histocompatibility complex class 1 (MHC1) in endoplasmic reticulum (ER) (2). MHC1 is then presented onto the cell surface (3) allowing interaction with cytotoxic T-cells and cell destruction (4). Antibodies to cell surface antigens (green) result in direct loss of function of receptors (A), endocytosis and degradation (B), antibody dependent cellular cytotoxicity and cell destruction (C), or activation of complement cascade (D). Abbreviations: *MHC* major histocompatability complex

Disease Subtypes

Patients with AE may present with typical neurologic phenotypes dependent on what area of the brain is affected. Limbic encephalitis (LE) is a common phenotype of AE and can be caused by many different antibodies (Tables 30.2 and 30.3) including anti-NMDAR, LGI-1, ANNA-1 and GAD-65. LE is characterized by deficits in working memory, seizures, and personality changes. When LE is driven by anti-NMDAR antibody, patients may have orofacial dyskinesia. When associated with anti-LGI-1 antibodies patients may have faciobrachial dystonic seizures, which are negative on surface EEG [45]. Another common presentation of AE is a rapidly progressive cerebellar syndrome with ataxic gait, abnormal movements, and dysarthria. This presentation can be seen in association with many antibodies such as GAD-65, PCA-2, and IgLON-5. Brainstem encephalitis, also known as rhombencephalitis, may present with dysarthria, dysphagia, cranial nerve dysfunction, hearing loss, central hypoventilation, jaw dystonia, narcolepsy, or ataxia. Antibodies that may lead to rhombencephalitis include ANNA-2, Kelch11, or Ma2.

Many cases of AE end up being termed "seronegative" when testing does not result in discovery of a neuronal-specific antibody. This diagnosis must be made only after carefully excluding other etiologies such as degenerative, infectious, toxic, metabolic, and psychiatric causes. Refer to Fig. 30.3 for diagnostic criteria of seronegative AE [46].

Essential Management Priorities

Early: Immediate/First 24 h

Diagnosis

The most common reasons patients with AE present to critical care are status epilepticus, delirium, respiratory failure, and coma [47]. What is particularly difficult in these cases is identifying those patients with whom there should be concern for AE. By the time these patients present to the ICU they have likely already seen other providers, and the reason for their presentation will often have been misattributed to psychiatric, toxic, metabolic, or infectious etiologies. It is therefore critical that the clinician retake the history and pay close attention to the time course of the presentation, and prodromal symptoms (such as headache, respiratory or gastrointestinal symptoms), and attempt to differentiate what is part of the syndrome and what may be a side effect of prior management. Furthermore, a thorough history of prior autoimmune disease, cancers, and immune checkpoint inhibitor exposure should be obtained (Fig. 30.2) (Tables 30.4 and 30.5).

Early testing should include a bedside cognitive assessment to determine the severity of the cognitive impairment and to monitor its progression and treatment response over time. Extensive testing on serum and CSF should be performed (Fig. 30.2) to exclude more common etiologies of cognitive decline such as infectious, metabolic, or toxic causes. MRI imaging is important and described in further

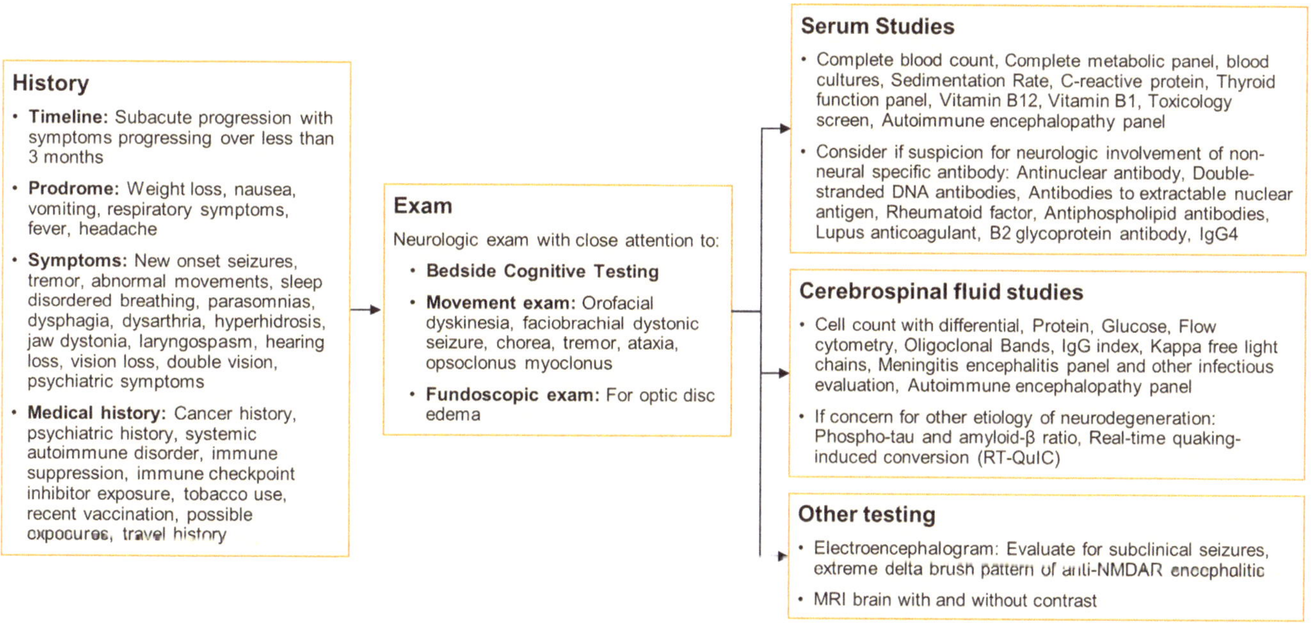

Fig. 30.2 Diagnostic Evaluation. Clinical history, exam, and testing should be completed in evaluation of patients with possible autoimmune encephalitis. Abbreviations: *anti-NMDAR* anti-N-methyl-D-aspartate receptor IgG, *MRI* magnetic resonance imaging

Table 30.4 Key clinical questions

History	What is the time course of the presentation?
	What symptoms does the patient have?
	What medical comorbidities does patient have?
Exam	Does patient have an abnormal neurologic exam?
	Does patient have abnormal movements?
Testing	Do serum studies show evidence of systemic inflammation?
	Do lab tests seem more consistent with a infectious, toxic, or metabolic cause?
	Does CSF show signs of inflammation?
	Is EEG or MRI abnormal?
	Is a neuronal specific antibody positive? Is it consistent with the clinical picture?
	Is patient at risk for cancer with positive antibody result?

Table 30.5 Immediate/early priorities checklist

Stabilize patient
Ensure airway patency, sufficient tissue perfusion, ventilation and oxygenation
Neurological evaluation
Focused history and neurologic exam
Emergency head CT if focal or lateralizing signs or concern for brain swelling
EEG monitoring in suspected seizures or status epilepticus
Consider sedation if patient on EEG for control of movements
Broad laboratory investigations on serum (Fig. 30.2)
Consider empiric coverage for CNS infection
Obtain CSF
When patient stabilized
Obtain thorough history and performed detailed chart review
MRI of the brain with and without contrast
Consider initiation of immunotherapy if AE deemed likely (Fig. 30.3) and infection is ruled out

detail in the section titled "Key radiologic findings." Electroencephalogram (EEG) can be helpful not only for monitoring patients with seizures but also because patients with NMDAR encephalitis may have a distinctive pattern of background slowing known as extreme delta brush [48]. One study evaluating AE patients in the ICU found 84% had abnormal EEGs, including generalized slowing, focal abnormalities, or epileptic discharges [49].

Autoimmune encephalopathy panels should only be tested when there is a reasonable pretest probability for the diagnosis of AE because false positive results can dangerously misguide therapy. A recently developed algorithm, Antibody-Prevalence-in-Epilepsy-and-Encephalopathy (APE [2]) score is useful in identifying patients with high likelihood of antibody-positive AE. Patients with a score ≥ 4 had 99% specificity and 93% sensitivity for a neural-specific antibody [50, 51]. In addition to clinical history and exam findings, this score utilizes testing including cerebrospinal fluid (CSF) and brain MRI. The antibody tests should be ordered in a panel as there is significant overlap across clinical syndromes and therefore it is difficult to accurately predict which individual antibody should be tested. Optimally, the panels should be ordered on serum and CSF as different antibody tests are more accurate on one or the other sample. When a patient has a positive antibody on serum but not CSF, or a low titer positivity and a clinical scenario that does not fit with the particular antibody, the clinician should consider the possibility of a false-positive result and discuss with the performing laboratory the option of retesting. Figure 30.3 presents a diagnostic flow algorithm for evaluation of patients with probable and definite AE; this is adapted from the 2016 diagnostic criteria [46] with the exception of Hashimoto's encephalopathy given an increasing body of evidence questioning this diagnosis [52].

Investigations for underlying cancer should be tailored to antibody results. Tables 30.2 and 30.3 display antibodies with reported risk of cancer association; however, it should be noted that more data are being published on these and other novel antibodies and we would recommend the reader to check the literature for the most updated guidelines on specific antibody associations. Clinicians should ensure all patients are up to date on age-appropriate cancer screening such as colonoscopy, mammogram, and low-dose chest CT in patients with significant smoking history. In patients with antibodies with high or moderate correlation to cancer (Tables 30.2, 30.3), cancer screening should be pursued starting with CT of the chest, abdomen, and pelvis, and if negative, whole-body FDG-PET CT. Evaluation should also include ovarian or testicular ultrasound and skin exam by Dermatology. If initial screening is negative and a patient has a high-risk antibody such as ANNA-1, subsequent screening at 6 months and then at 1-year intervals should be performed.

Treatment

Treatment of AE can be divided into three parts: immunotherapy, treatment of underlying cancer, and treatment of the sequelae of the disease (Table 30.6). When caring for patients with underlying cancer, clinicians should collaborate with Oncology to determine best treatment course. For patients who are already on immune checkpoint inhibitor therapy, a possible trigger for AE, consideration should be given to stopping the immune checkpoint inhibitor, though this decision should also be made in conjunction with Oncology. Further management recommendations regarding immune checkpoint inhibitor-related AE are beyond the scope of this chapter, please refer to the article by Valencia-Sanchez for a thorough review of presentation and treatment guidance [53].

Immunotherapy

There are currently no completed randomized controlled trials to help guide immunotherapy for patients with AE. Evidence is predominantly limited to retrospective

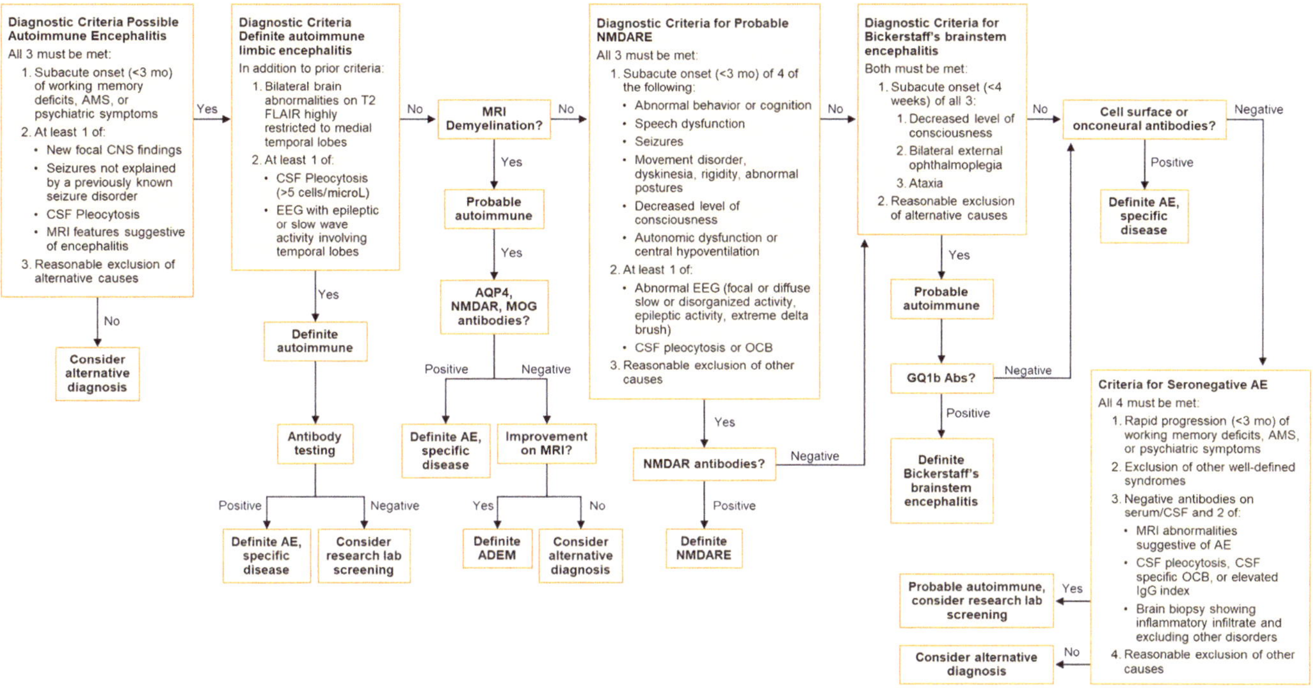

Fig. 30.3 Diagnostic flow diagram. Proposed diagnostic flow for diagnosis of probable and definite AE, adapted from diagnostic criteria [46]. Abbreviations: *ADEM* acute disseminated encephalomyelitis, *AE* autoimmune encephalitis, *AMS* altered mental status, *AQP4* anti-aquaporin-4 IgG, *CNS* central nervous system, *CSF* cerebrospinal fluid, *EEG* electroencephalogram, *FLAIR* fluid attenuated inversion recovery, *GQ1b* anti-ganglioside Q1b IgG, *mo* months, *MOG* anti-myelin oligodendrocyte glycoprotein IgG, *MRI* magnetic resonance imaging, *NMDAR* anti-N-methyl-D-aspartate receptor IgG, *NMDARE* N-methyl-D-aspartate receptor encephalitis, *OCB* oligoclonal bands

Table 30.6 Treatment pearls

• Thorough investigation for infection must be done before initiation of immunotherapy
• Patients may take prolonged time to respond to immunotherapy, and will often require second agent
• Complications including seizures and paroxysmal sympathetic hyperactivity must be treated aggressively
• Patients are at high risk of systemic complications such as pneumonia, urinary tract infection, and venous thromboembolism which should be diagnosed promptly and treated appropriately

observational studies. Before starting immunotherapy the treating clinician must identify an objective measure to determine if the patient has a therapeutic response—such as short test of mental status score, EEG findings, or MRI findings. Ideally, other medications should not be adjusted during the immunotherapy trial to be able to reliably evaluate the effect of immunotherapy itself. Further, serum and CSF tests should be performed prior to treatment as intravenous immunoglobulin (IVIg) can result in false positive results, while plasmapheresis can result in false negative results. Treatments may be used in combination, but IVIg will be removed with plasmapheresis. Typical first and second-line immunotherapies are summarized in Figure 30.4 [54, 55].

Many patients will respond to their first-line therapy particularly in the first week [56], though there are nearly 40% of patients who require second-line treatment. Patients with anti-LGI1 encephalitis typically have resolution of cognitive symptoms in the first few weeks of steroid initiation [57], while patients with anti-NMDAR encephalitis may also improve early but will take months to years to return to baseline and often require second line therapy [37]. Individual antibodies will likely respond better to different treatment regimens, for example, a retrospective study evaluating 118 patients with anti-LGI1 encephalitis found patients did significantly better when treated acutely with steroids than IVIg [58]. Patients who respond to acute therapy are typically treated with chronic immunosuppression for 2–5 years to prevent relapse. In general, we use antibody or B-cell targeted therapy for cell surface antibodies, and T-cell depleting agents for antibodies targeted to intracellular antigens (Fig. 30.1). These treatments include rituximab, azathioprine, methotrexate, and mycophenolate.

Management of Complications

In addition to managing the underlying problem with immune suppression and cancer treatment, management of the associated complications is important to optimize outcomes. These patients are frequently admitted to the ICU for status epilepticus, airway management, agitation, coma,

Fig. 30.4 Treatment of autoimmune encephalitis. Treatment is dependent on immunotherapy, treatment of underlying cancer if present, and management of complications. Abbreviations: *CSF* cerebrospinal fluid, *EEG* electroencephalogram, *IV* Intravenous

Immunotherapy

First line
- IV Methylprednisolone: 1000 mg daily 3-5 days; sometimes continued once weekly 6-12 weeks
- IV immunoglobulin: 0.4 g/kg/day for 5 days; sometimes followed by 0.4 g/kg once weekly for 6-12 w
- Plasmapheresis: 1 session every other day for 5-7 sessions

Second line
- IV Rituximab: 375 mg/m^2 infusion weekly for 4 weeks
- IV Cyclophosphamide: 0.6-1 g/m^2 monthly for 6 months

Cancer therapy

Treatment of underlying cancer in collaboration with Oncology

Sequelae of Disease

Status epilepticus
- Continuous EEG monitoring
- Manage according to local protocols

Paroxysmal sympathetic hyperactivity
- Intravenous morphine
- Gabapentin
- Non cardioselective beta blockers
- Clonidine

Airway protection
- Mechanical ventilation

Hyperkinetic movements
- Sedation to prevent rhabdomyolysis

Rigidity
- Diazepam
- Baclofen
- Dantrolene

Elevated intracranial pressure
- Consideration for CSF diversion

treatment of autonomic instability, hyperkinetic movements, and elevated intracranial pressure. Further, these critically ill patients are at high risk for systemic complications, including pneumonia, urinary tract infection, and venous thromboembolism [49, 59].

Status epilepticus is a frequent complication of AE and can often be refractory. In one cohort of 120 patients with AE, approximately one-third developed status epilepticus which could be either generalized or focal and often was nonconvulsive. These patients required a median of five antiseizure medications [49]. Following local hospital protocols for management of status epilepticus is appropriate and beyond the scope of this discussion. Once infectious etiologies have been ruled out, immunotherapy should be initiated as soon as possible because immunotherapy improves outcomes in patients with AE-related status epilepticus. For instance, in a series of 103 patients with faciobrachial dystonic seizures related to anti-LGI-1, only 10% had resolution of seizures with anti-seizure medications alone, while 50% had resolution with immunotherapy, and earlier immunotherapy led to better cognitive outcomes at 2 years [57].

Dysautonomia is another frequent problem in AE of all types, affecting up to 45% of patients [49]. It may manifest with hyperthermia, rigidity, fever, hyperventilation, tachy or bradyarrhythmia, hypo or hypertension, diarrhea, hyperhidroses, and sialorrhea. Episodes of paroxysmal sympathetic hyperactivity are relatively common while parasympathetic features are less frequent. Severe cases of sympathetic hyperactivity may even result in Takotsubo cardiomyopathy [60]. Autonomic dysfunction portends a worse outcome [49]. Paroxysmal sympathetic hyperactivity can be treated with intravenous morphine to abort the episodes and gabapentin with or without non-cardioselective beta blockers or clonidine to prevent them. Bradycardia is less common, but if present it requires avoidance of beta-blockers and other AV node blockers and availability of atropine at the bedside readily; a temporary pacemaker may be needed.

Mechanical ventilation may be required for airway protection (depressed level of consciousness, absent lower brainstem reflexes, or sedation related to treatment of seizures or psychosis) or respiratory failure from superimposed pneumonia or pulmonary embolism. In one series, intubation was required in 57% of patients, with a median duration of 28 days; 54% of these patients developed ventilator-associated pneumonia [49].

Hyperkinetic movement disorders, which may or may not be associated with seizure, may also require treatment with sedation due to hyperthermia and rhabdomyolysis. Extreme rigidity may be treated with diazepam, baclofen, or dantrolene.

Elevated intracranial pressure has been reported in some case series of anti-NMDAR encephalitis but is a less common complication [61]. In patients with cerebellitis or rhombencephalitis of any cause there needs to be close monitoring for hydrocephalus that may require urgent CSF diversion.

Long-Term Clinical Course

Outcomes and prognosis vary depending on antibody detected, underlying cancer, and severity of presentation. The Response-to-immunotherapy-in-epilepsy-and-encephalopathy (RITE [2]) score may be helpful in identifying patients who are more likely to respond to immunotherapy. A score ≥ 7 has high sensitivity (96%) and specificity (86%) for a positive response to immunotherapy, while a score < 7 is associated with immunotherapy refractory disease even with positive neural antibody [50]. Amongst patients with AE admitted to the ICU, mortality at 1 year has ranged from 82% to 93%, with 15–63% of patients requiring tracheostomy [47, 59, 62]. Prognostic factors for poor modified Rankin score on hospital discharge after ICU stay in one cohort included autonomic dysfunction, severe sepsis, tracheostomy, tumor, and mechanical ventilation [49].

Near Misses

Misdiagnosis

Antibody test results must be interpreted critically given the risk for false positive or negative results. All tests should be drawn prior to immunotherapy because IVIg can cause false positive results and plasmapheresis could cause false negative results. If a patient has a low positive titer or an antibody only positive on serum and not CSF, these results must be interpreted in the setting of the clinical scenario. Low positive titers of antibodies against GAD-65, voltage-gated potassium channel, voltage-gated calcium channels, and acetylcholine receptor should be deemed diagnostic only in patients with high pre-test probability (i.e. in whom the autoimmune disease suggested by the antibody positivity was considered highly likely a priori). In this chapter, we focused on neuronal-specific antibodies leading to autoimmune encephalitis. One must be cautious when diagnosing an autoimmune encephalitis based on a non-neural specific antibody. For example, the term Hashimoto's encephalopathy was used previously to categorize patients with encephalopathy and anti-TPO antibodies. A recent study evaluated 144 patients referred to a tertiary center with diagnosis of Hashimoto's encephalitis and found that 73% of these patients actually had an alternative non-immune mediated diagnosis, while over half did not have a primary neurologic disorder [52].

Insufficiently Aggressive Treatment

Many patients will respond to first-line immunotherapy, but up to 40% will require a second agent [56]. If the patient has not had an adequate response to the first-line agent, addition of another first-line or second-line agent should be considered. Further, patients with autoimmune encephalitis are at risk for relapse and prolonged immune suppression is most often necessary [63].

Key Radiologic Findings

MRI of the brain with and without contrast is an important part of the evaluation in patients with suspected AE. Oftentimes, the MRI will be unremarkable, but there are findings that can signal the diagnosis. A common finding in LE is unilateral or bilateral T2 hyperintensity of the mesial temporal lobe, sometimes with gadolinium enhancement (Fig. 30.6). However, this finding is non-specific and can also be seen in epilepsy or herpes simplex virus encephalitis [64]. Basal ganglia T2 hyperintensity may be seen in association with multiple antibodies including anti-LGI1, anti-NMDAR, anti-Ma2, and anti-CRMP5 [19, 65–67]. Thalamic hyperintensity can be seen with anti-Ma2 antibodies as well, particularly near the third ventricle [19]. GFAP-IgG typically shows radial perivascular enhancement [16], and $GABA_AR$ antibodies may have multiple areas of T2-hyperintensity in cortical and subcortical regions [28]. Patients with anti-KLHL11 may exhibit T2 hyperintensity of the temporal lobe, cerebellum, brainstem, or thalamus (Fig. 30.5), as well as changes in the spinal cord and leptomeninges [18].

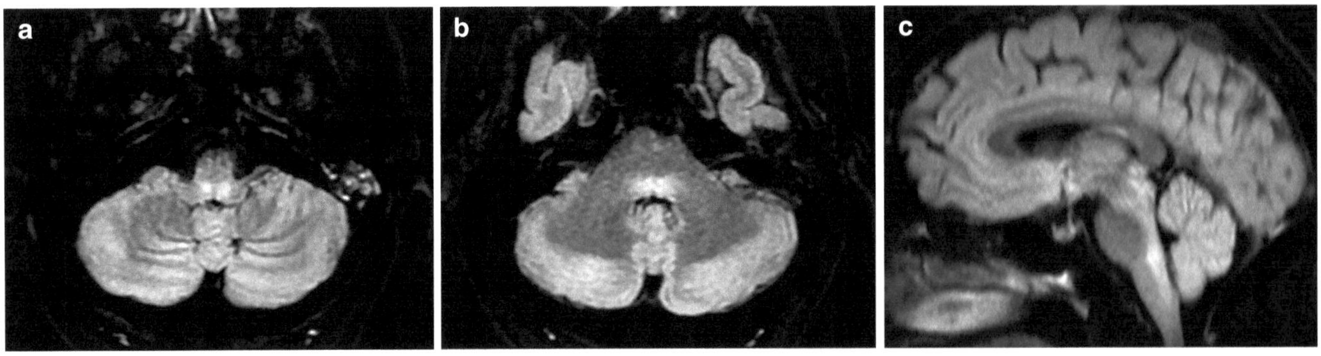

Fig. 30.5 KLHL-11 rhombencephalitis. A 45-year-old gentleman presented after 9 months of progressive ataxia, dysphagia, dysarthria, trismus, binocular diplopia, and unintentional 50 lb. weight loss. His initial MRI showed the findings above with a hyperintense lesion on T2 FLAIR sequences extending from the dorsal medulla (**a**) to the pons (**b**) and midbrain (**c**). He was ultimately diagnosed with anti-KLHL-11 rhombencephalitis. Scrotal ultrasound revealed a 1.1 cm left testicular mass, he underwent radical orchiectomy and pathology was consistent with a fibrous nodule. He underwent multiple rounds of immunotherapy including intravenous steroids, intravenous immunoglobulin, and rituximab. Despite immunotherapy, he developed central apnea requiring continuous BiPAP therapy. He underwent placement of tracheostomy. With placement of a diaphragmatic pacer, he was able to be independent from the ventilator during daytime hours. Twenty two months after his initial symptom development he was stabilized on this ventilation method and a prednisone taper. Unfortunately, he had a fall in the nighttime while off the ventilator and the pacer was not turned on, the patient suffered respiratory and cardiac arrest for an uncertain duration of time. Despite resuscitation attempts he suffered anoxic brain injury and goals of care were changed to comfort measures only

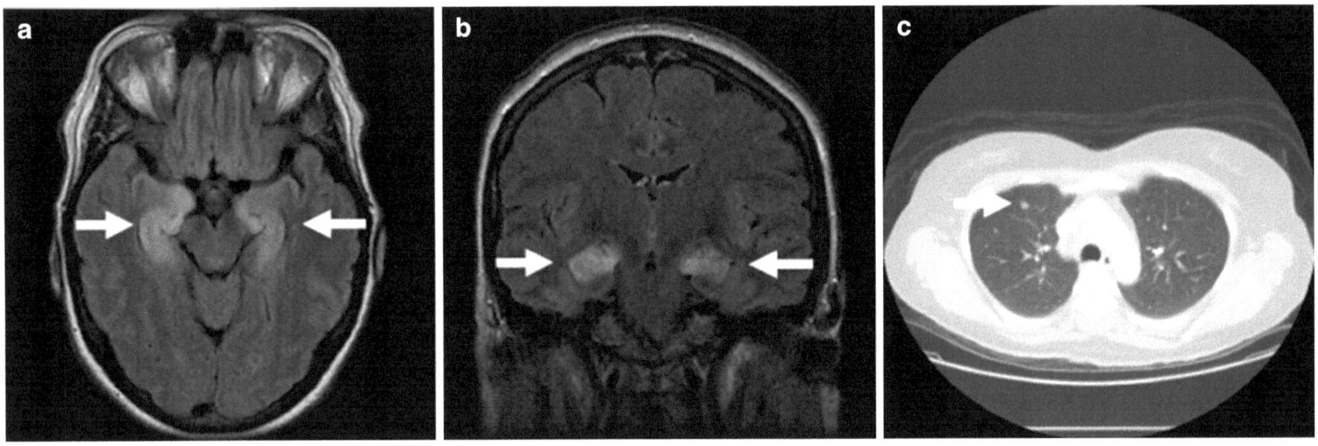

Fig. 30.6 Paraneoplastic Limbic Encephalitis. A 51-year-old female with 30 pack year history of smoking presented with 3 weeks of progressive confusion, behavioral change, disturbed sleep, impaired short-term memory, and new onset of seizures. MRI of her brain revealed typical findings of limbic encephalitis with hyperintensity on T2 FLAIR imaging in the mesial temporal lobe on axial (**a**) and coronal (**b**) sequences. This patient was found to have a highly positive N-type calcium channel antibody and underwent biopsy of a right upper lobe lung nodule found on CT (**c**) consistent with squamous cell carcinoma. Patient underwent a 5-day course of high-dose IV steroids and plasma exchange without improvement. The family opted for no further treatment of underlying cancer and patient ultimately died 2 years later

Key Monitoring

Monitoring while in the ICU and afterward is important to ensure cerebral and systemic complications of the disease are not missed and to evaluate patient outcomes. Serial cognitive evaluation is helpful in monitoring progression of the disease and response to treatment and clinicians should employ the same test of mental status across the disease course. Continuous EEG monitoring is important in patients with status epilepticus or suspected seizures. Serial MRI can be helpful in patients who are not improving or keep worsening, though it should be noted that improvement on MRI will often be delayed for weeks. Serial antibody monitoring may be useful in helping determine the need for prolonged immunosuppression, though clear guidelines have not been developed. For example, a patient with NMDAR encephalitis may have a declining antibody titer after initial response to immunotherapy but later may develop a recrudescence of the disease which is associated with an increase in titer [68]. There is however no clear evidence that treatment aggressiveness should be affected by ongoing antibody positivity and clinicians should prioritize clinical response when making those therapeutic decisions.

Take Home Message

AE should be suspected in any patient presenting to the ICU with newly progressive symptoms over less than 3 months consisting of seizures, mental status change, or behavioral disturbances. Yet, appropriate investigations should be pursued to rule out infectious, toxic, or psychiatric causes before making the diagnosis of AE. Antibody panels should be ideally checked in serum and CSF. Once the diagnosis of AE is confirmed or strongly suspected, it is critical to initiate immunotherapy treatment rapidly.

Neurointensivists should be adept at managing the most common neurological complications in patients with AE (hyperkinetic movement disorders, severe agitation, autonomic dysfunction, seizures, among others) and capable of directing the immunotherapy necessary to control the primary disease process. Patients with AE requiring ICU admission are at higher risk of morbidity and mortality, but aggressive and careful medical attention can result in good clinical outcomes.

References

1. Dubey D, Pittock SJ, Kelly CR, et al. Autoimmune encephalitis epidemiology and a comparison to infectious encephalitis. Ann Neurol. 2018;83:166–77.
2. Hébert J, Riche B, Vogrig A, et al. Epidemiology of paraneoplastic neurologic syndromes and autoimmune encephalitides in France. Neurol Neuroimmunol Neuroinflamm. 2020;7:e883.
3. Gu Y, Zhong M, He L, et al. Epidemiology of antibody-positive autoimmune encephalitis in Southwest China: a multicenter study. Front Immunol. 2019;10:2611.
4. Do L-D, Chanson E, Desestret V, et al. Characteristics in limbic encephalitis with anti–adenylate kinase 5 autoantibodies. Neurology. 2017;88:514–24.
5. Muñiz-Castrillo S, Hedou JJ, Ambati A, et al. Distinctive clinical presentation and pathogenic specificities of anti-AK5 encephalitis. Brain. 2021;144(9):2709–21.
6. Pittock SJ, Lucchinetti CF, Parisi JE, et al. Amphiphysin autoimmunity: paraneoplastic accompaniments. Ann Neurol. 2005;58:96–107.
7. Dalmau J, Graus F, Rosenblum MK, Posner JB. Anti-Hu—associated paraneoplastic encephalomyelitis/sensory neuronopathy. A clinical study of 71 patients. Medicine. 1992;71:59–72.
8. Lucchinetti CF, Kimmel DW, Lennon VA. Paraneoplastic and oncologic profiles of patients seropositive for type 1 antineuronal nuclear autoantibodies. Neurology. 1998;50:652–7.
9. Pittock SJ, Lucchinetti CF, Lennon VA. Anti-neuronal nuclear autoantibody type 2: paraneoplastic accompaniments. Ann Neurol. 2003;53:580–7.
10. Chan KH, Vernino S, Lennon VA. ANNA-3 anti-neuronal nuclear antibody: marker of lung cancer-related autoimmunity. Ann Neurol. 2001;50:301–11.
11. Yu Z, Kryzer TJ, Griesmann GE, Kim KK, Benarroch EE, Lennon VA. CRMP-5 neuronal autoantibody: marker of lung cancer and thymoma-related autoimmunity. Ann Neurol. 2001;49:146–54.
12. Honnorat J, Cartalat-Carel S, Ricard D, et al. Onco-neural antibodies and tumour type determine survival and neurological symptoms in paraneoplastic neurological syndromes with Hu or CV2/CRMP5 antibodies. J Neurol Neurosurg Psychiatry. 2009;80:412–6.
13. Pittock SJ, Yoshikawa H, Ahlskog JE, et al. Glutamic acid decarboxylase autoimmunity with brainstem, extrapyramidal, and spinal cord dysfunction. Mayo Clin Proceed. 2006;81:1207–14.
14. Saiz A, Blanco Y, Sabater L, et al. Spectrum of neurological syndromes associated with glutamic acid decarboxylase antibodies: diagnostic clues for this association. Brain. 2008;131:2553–63.
15. Ariño H, Höftberger R, Gresa-Arribas N, et al. Paraneoplastic neurological syndromes and glutamic acid decarboxylase antibodies. JAMA Neurol. 2015;72:874–81.
16. Flanagan EP, Hinson SR, Lennon VA, et al. Glial fibrillary acidic protein immunoglobulin G as biomarker of autoimmune astrocytopathy: analysis of 102 patients. Ann Neurol. 2017;81:298–309.
17. Alfugham N, Gadoth A, Lennon VA, et al. ITPR1 autoimmunity: frequency, neurologic phenotype, and cancer association. Neurol Neuroimmunol Neuroinflamm. 2018;5:e418.
18. Dubey D, Wilson MR, Clarkson B, et al. Expanded clinical phenotype, oncological associations, and immunopathologic insights of paraneoplastic kelch-like protein-11 encephalitis. JAMA Neurol. 2020;77:1420–9.
19. Dalmau J, Graus F, Villarejo A, et al. Clinical analysis of anti-Ma2-associated encephalitis. Brain. 2004;127:1831–44.
20. McKeon A, Shelly S, Zivelonghi C, et al. Neuronal intermediate filament IgGs in CSF: autoimmune Axonopathy biomarkers. Ann Clin Transl Neurol. 2021;8:425–39.
21. McKeon A, Tracy JA, Pittock SJ, Parisi JE, Klein CJ, Lennon VA. Purkinje cell cytoplasmic autoantibody type 1 accompaniments: the cerebellum and beyond. Arch Neurol. 2011;68:1282–9.
22. Vernino S, Lennon VA. New Purkinje cell antibody (PCA-2): marker of lung cancer–related neurological autoimmunity. Ann Neurol. 2000;47:297–305.
23. Bernal F, Shams'Ili S, Rojas I, et al. Anti-Tr antibodies as markers of paraneoplastic cerebellar degeneration and Hodgkin's disease. Neurology. 2003;60:230–4.
24. Laurido-Soto O, Brier MR, Simon LE, McCullough A, Bucelli RC, Day GS. Patient characteristics and outcome associations in AMPA receptor encephalitis. J Neurol. 2019;266:450–60.
25. Quek AM, McKeon A, Lennon VA, et al. Effects of age and sex on aquaporin-4 autoimmunity. Arch Neurol. 2012;69:1039–43.
26. Gadoth A, Pittock SJ, Dubey D, et al. Expanded phenotypes and outcomes among 256 LGI 1/CASPR 2-I g G–positive patients. Ann Neurol. 2017;82:79–92.
27. Tobin WO, Lennon VA, Komorowski L, et al. DPPX potassium channel antibody: frequency, clinical accompaniments, and outcomes in 20 patients. Neurology. 2014;83:1797–803.
28. Spatola M, Petit-Pedrol M, Simabukuro MM, et al. Investigations in GABAA receptor antibody-associated encephalitis. Neurology. 2017;88:1012–20.
29. Höftberger R, Titulaer MJ, Sabater L, et al. Encephalitis and GABAB receptor antibodies: novel findings in a new case series of 20 patients. Neurology. 2013;81:1500–6.
30. Carvajal-Gonzalez A, Leite MI, Waters P, et al. Glycine receptor antibodies in PERM and related syndromes: characteristics, clinical features and outcomes. Brain. 2014;137:2178–92.
31. Gaig C, Graus F, Compta Y, et al. Clinical manifestations of the anti-IgLON5 disease. Neurology. 2017;88:1736–43.
32. Honorat JA, Komorowski L, Josephs KA, et al. IgLON5 antibody: neurological accompaniments and outcomes in 20 patients. Neurol Neuroimmunol Neuroinflamm. 2017;4:e385.
33. van Sonderen A, Thijs RD, Coenders EC, et al. Anti-LGI1 encephalitis: clinical syndrome and long-term follow-up. Neurology. 2016;87:1449–56.

34. Cobo-Calvo A, Ruiz A, Maillart E, et al. Clinical spectrum and prognostic value of CNS MOG autoimmunity in adults: the MOGADOR study. Neurology. 2018;90:e1858–69.
35. Gresa-Arribas N, Planagumà J, Petit-Pedrol M, et al. Human neurexin-3α antibodies associate with encephalitis and alter synapse development. Neurology. 2016;86:2235–42.
36. Dalmau J, Gleichman AJ, Hughes EG, et al. Anti-NMDA-receptor encephalitis: case series and analysis of the effects of antibodies. Lancet Neurol. 2008;7:1091–8.
37. Titulaer MJ, McCracken L, Gabilondo I, et al. Treatment and prognostic factors for long-term outcome in patients with anti-NMDA receptor encephalitis: an observational cohort study. Lancet Neurol. 2013;12:157–65.
38. Yeshokumar AK, Gordon-Lipkin E, Arenivas A, et al. Neurobehavioral outcomes in autoimmune encephalitis. J Neuroimmunol. 2017;312:8–14.
39. Harutyunyan G, Hauer L, Dünser MW, et al. Risk factors for intensive care unit admission in patients with autoimmune encephalitis. Front Immunol. 2017;8:835.
40. de Montmollin E, Demeret S, Brulé N, et al. Anti–N-methyl-D-aspartate receptor encephalitis in adult patients requiring intensive care. Am J Respir Crit Care Med. 2017;195:491–9.
41. Martinez-Hernandez E, Horvath J, Shiloh-Malawsky Y, Sangha N, Martinez-Lage M, Dalmau J. Analysis of complement and plasma cells in the brain of patients with anti-NMDAR encephalitis. Neurology. 2011;77:589–93.
42. Vogrig A, Muñiz-Castrillo S, Desestret V, Joubert B, Honnorat J. Pathophysiology of paraneoplastic and autoimmune encephalitis: genes, infections, and checkpoint inhibitors. Ther Adv Neurol Disord. 2020;13:1756286420932797.
43. Tanaka M, Tanaka K, Tokiguchi S, Shinozawa K, Tsuji S. Cytotoxic T cells against a peptide of Yo protein in patients with paraneoplastic cerebellar degeneration and anti-Yo antibody. J Neurol Sci. 1999;168:28–31.
44. Roberts WK, Deluca IJ, Thomas A, et al. Patients with lung cancer and paraneoplastic Hu syndrome harbor HuD-specific type 2 CD8+ T cells. J Clin Invest. 2009;119:2042–51.
45. Diaz-Arias LA, Pardo CA, Probasco JC. Autoimmune encephalitis in the intensive care unit. In: Neurointensive Care Unit; 2020. p. 249.
46. Graus F, Titulaer MJ, Balu R, et al. A clinical approach to diagnosis of autoimmune encephalitis. Lancet Neurol. 2016;15:391–404.
47. Harutyunyan G, Hauer L, Dünser MW, et al. Autoimmune encephalitis at the neurological intensive care unit: etiologies, reasons for admission and survival. Neurocrit Care. 2017;27:82–9.
48. Schmitt SE, Pargeon K, Frechette ES, Hirsch LJ, Dalmau J, Friedman D. Extreme delta brush: a unique EEG pattern in adults with anti-NMDA receptor encephalitis. Neurology. 2012;79:1094–100.
49. Schubert J, Brämer D, Huttner HB, et al. Management and prognostic markers in patients with autoimmune encephalitis requiring ICU treatment. Neurol Neuroimmunol Neuroinflamm. 2019;6:e514.
50. Dubey D, Kothapalli N, McKeon A, et al. Predictors of neural-specific autoantibodies and immunotherapy response in patients with cognitive dysfunction. J Neuroimmunol. 2018;323:62–72.
51. Dubey D, Alqallaf A, Hays R, et al. Neurological autoantibody prevalence in epilepsy of unknown etiology. JAMA Neurol. 2017;74:397–402.
52. Valencia-Sanchez C, Pittock SJ, Mead-Harvey C, et al. Brain dysfunction and thyroid antibodies: autoimmune diagnosis and misdiagnosis. Brain commun. 2021;3:fcaa233.
53. Valencia-Sanchez C, Zekeridou A. Paraneoplastic neurological syndromes and beyond emerging with the introduction of immune checkpoint inhibitor cancer immunotherapy. Front Neurol. 2021;12:494.
54. Shin Y-W, Lee S-T, Park K-I, et al. Treatment strategies for autoimmune encephalitis. Ther Adv Neurol Disord. 2018;11:1756285617722347.
55. Banks SA, Sechi E, Flanagan EP. Autoimmune encephalopathies presenting as dementia of subacute onset and rapid progression. Ther Adv Neurol Disord. 2021;14:1756286421998906.
56. Flanagan EP, McKeon A, Lennon VA, et al. Autoimmune dementia: clinical course and predictors of immunotherapy response. Mayo Clin Proceed. 2010;85:881–97.
57. Thompson J, Bi M, Murchison AG, et al. The importance of early immunotherapy in patients with faciobrachial dystonic seizures. Brain. 2018;141:348–56.
58. Rodriguez A, Klein C, Sechi E, et al. LGI1 antibody encephalitis: acute treatment comparisons and outcome. Neurosurgery & Psychiatry: J Neurol; 2021.
59. Shah S, VanHaerents S. Autoimmune Encephalitis in the Neurologic Intensive Care Unit: Clinical Characteristics, Complications, and Outcomes.(P2. 2–005). Neurology. 2019;92(15_supplement):P2-2.
60. Kakinuma Y, Kimura T, Sakae Y, Kubota S, Ono K, Kinno R. Takotsubo syndrome associated with autoimmune limbic encephalitis: a case report. BMC Cardiovasc Disord. 2021;21:1–7.
61. Chi X, Wang W, Huang C, et al. Risk factors for mortality in patients with anti-NMDA receptor encephalitis. Acta Neurol Scand. 2017;136:298–304.
62. Mittal MK, Rabinstein AA, Hocker SE, Pittock SJ, Wijdicks EF, McKeon A. Autoimmune encephalitis in the ICU: analysis of phenotypes, serologic findings, and outcomes. Neurocrit Care. 2016;24:240–50.
63. Gabilondo I, Saiz A, Galán L, et al. Analysis of relapses in anti-NMDAR encephalitis. Neurology. 2011;77:996–9.
64. Oyanguren B, Sánchez V, González F, et al. Limbic encephalitis: a clinical-radiological comparison between herpetic and autoimmune etiologies. Eur J Neurol. 2013;20:1566–70.
65. Zhang T, Duan Y, Ye J, et al. Brain MRI characteristics of patients with anti-N-methyl-D-aspartate receptor encephalitis and their associations with 2-year clinical outcome. Am J Neuroradiol. 2018;39:824–9.
66. Kinirons P, Fulton A, Keoghan M, Brennan P, Farrell M, Moroney J. Paraneoplastic limbic encephalitis (PLE) and chorea associated with CRMP-5 neuronal antibody. Neurology. 2003;61:1623–4.
67. Flanagan EP, Kotsenas AL, Britton JW, et al. Basal ganglia T1 hyperintensity in LGI1-autoantibody faciobrachial dystonic seizures. Neurol Neuroimmunol Neuroinflamm. 2015;2:e161.
68. Gresa-Arribas N, Titulaer MJ, Torrents A, et al. Antibody titres at diagnosis and during follow-up of anti-NMDA receptor encephalitis: a retrospective study. Lancet Neurol. 2014;13:167–77.

Key/Landmark References

Dubey D, Kothapalli N, McKeon A, et al. Predictors of neural-specific autoantibodies and immunotherapy response in patients with cognitive dysfunction. J Neuroimmunol. 2018;323:62–72.
Graus F, Titulaer MJ, Balu R, et al. A clinical approach to diagnosis of autoimmune encephalitis. Lancet Neurol. 2016;15:391–404.
Mittal MK, Rabinstein AA, Hocker SE, Pittock SJ, Wijdicks EF, McKeon A. Autoimmune encephalitis in the ICU: analysis of phenotypes, serologic findings, and outcomes. Neurocrit Care. 2016;24:240–50.

Central Nervous System Infections

31

Lennox K. Archibald, Alaina Ritter,
and Gautam Kalyatanda

Contents

L. K. Archibald (✉)
The Malcom Randall VA Medical Center, Gainesville, FL, USA

Department of Medicine, College of Medicine, University of Florida College of Medicine, Gainesville, FL, USA
e-mail: lennox.archibald@medicine.ufl.edu

A. Ritter · G. Kalyatanda
Department of Medicine, College of Medicine, University of Florida College of Medicine, Gainesville, FL, USA

E. Mahanna Gabrielli et al. (eds.), *Textbook of Neurointensive Care: Volume 1*, https://doi.org/10.1007/978-3-031-62220-5_31

Abstract

Central nervous system (CNS) infections—i.e., infections involving the brain (cerebrum and cerebellum), spinal cord, optic nerves, and their covering membranes—are medical emergencies that are associated with substantial morbidity, mortality, and/or long-term sequelae that may have catastrophic quality of life implications for affected individuals. Acute CNS infections fall broadly into three categories: meningitis, encephalitis, and abscesses. These infections generally result from blood-borne spread of the respective microorganisms, but there are several mechanisms by which CNS infections may occur. Head trauma resulting in fractures at the base of the skull or the cribriform plate can cause CNS infections via the creation of an opening between the CNS and the sinuses, mastoid, middle ear, or nasopharynx. Extrinsic contamination of the CNS can also occur intraoperatively during neurosurgical procedures and as a result of bacterial entry via congenital malformations (e.g., spina bifida or sinus tracts). Implanted medical devices or hardware (e.g., shunts, ventriculostomies, deep brain stimulators, or external drainage tubes) can become colonized and serve as foci of infection. Viruses, such as rabies, herpes simplex virus (HSV), or poliovirus, can spread to the CNS via intraneural pathways resulting in encephalitis. If infection occurs at sites contiguous with the CNS, such as the middle ear or mastoid, infection may spread directly into the CNS causing brain abscesses. Amoebae, like *Naegleria fowleri,* can infect people when contaminated water enters the body through the nose. Once the ameba enters the nose, it travels to the brain where it causes primary *amebic* meningoencephalitis, which is usually fatal. These infections may in turn spread directly to the subarachnoid space, causing meningitis. Alternatively, the organism may reach the CNS indirectly via venous drainage or via the sheaths of cranial and spinal nerves.

An intact blood–brain barrier (BBB) is essential in preventing the development of CNS infections. Breaches in the BBB can be caused by damage to the surrounding tissue, overproduction of cytokines that degrade tight junction proteins, and microbe-specific interactions that facilitate transcellular passage of the microorganism. The microorganisms that cause CNS infections include a wide range of bacteria, mycobacteria, yeasts, fungi, viruses, ameba, spirochaetes (e.g., neurosyphilis), and parasites (e.g., cerebral malaria and strongyloidiasis). The clinical presentation of CNS infections can either be nonspecific or characterized by distinct, recognizable clinical syndromes. In severe cases, patients may require admission to the neuro-intensive care unit (NICU).

This chapter addresses a wide range of severe CNS infections that often require admission to the NICU. Topics covered include the epidemiology, pathophysiology, and clinical symptoms of CNS infections as well as diagnostic techniques, therapeutics, and prognosis. In addition, this chapter will discuss the relevant neuroanatomy as it relates to the pathogenesis of these infections.

Introduction

Acute infections of the central nervous system (CNS) are medical emergencies that, if not addressed promptly, may result in significant morbidity and mortality. To fully understand the pathogenesis, clinical implications, and management of CNS infections, some knowledge of applied neuroanatomy is essential.

The CNS is comprised of the brain (cerebrum and cerebellum), spinal cord, optic nerves, and their covering membranes. These structures are protected within the rigid confines of the skull and spinal canal of the vertebral column. The cerebral cortex (the outermost, gray tissue layer of the cerebrum) and the spinal cord are covered by three layers of continuous protective tissue called the meninges. The innermost meningeal layer that directly overlies the cerebral cortex is called the pia mater. The middle and outermost layers are known as the arachnoid and dura mater, respectively. The dura mater forms several intracranial compartments, including sinuses for venous drainage. Parts of the arachnoid—the arachnoid villi—project into these sinuses. The subpial space is continuous with the Virchow-Robin spaces. These two spaces transmit penetrating vessels to and from the brain parenchyma and do not connect with the subarachnoid space. The subarachnoid space lies between the pia mater and the arachnoid and is continuous in nature; the subdural space lies between the arachnoid and the dura mater. The epidural space lies between the dura and the skull. Certain infections can access the subpial and Virchow-Robin spaces, while most do not. Infections within the epidural spaces are usually caused by direct extension from adjacent infections and remain in close proximity to the inciting source. Subdural infections are often associated with an extracerebral source, but these infections can spread widely within the subdural space. It is not uncommon to develop serious subdural effusions in bacterial meningitis. Subarachnoid infections are most often caused by hematogenous dissemination of organisms or viruses. The term neuraxis defines the entire nervous system, from receptors in the periphery to spinal cord and the subcortical structures and cortex of the brain.

Cerebrospinal fluid (CSF) is continuously produced by the choroid plexus within the four ventricles of the brain. CSF fills the lateral and third ventricles and circulates to the fourth ventricle, which lies between the cerebellum and the midbrain. CSF flows from the fourth ventricle into the subarachnoid space, where it bathes the entire CNS and drains via the arachnoid villi into the superior sagittal sinus in the dura mater, where it is resorbed into the bloodstream.

A working knowledge of the blood supply is also essential for understanding the pathogenesis of CNS infections. The capillary supply to the brain and spinal cord is unique given that the outermost layers of endothelial cells are fused together. These specialized brain microvascular endothelial cells constitute the blood–brain barrier, which separates the brain and the meninges from the circulating blood and impedes the influx of microorganisms, toxic agents, and most other compounds while also regulating the flow of essential nutrients and molecules for normal neural function. Thus, pathogens that breach the blood–brain barrier can cause CNS infections. Breaches can occur due to damage (e.g., microhemorrhage or necrosis of surrounding tissue), mechanical obstruction of microvessels (via parasitized red blood cells, leukocytes, or platelets), overproduction of cytokines that degrade tight junction proteins, and/or microbe-specific interactions with the blood–brain barrier that facilitate transcellular passage (e.g., *Escherichia coli*, mycobacteria, and spirochaetes). Antimicrobials prescribed for CNS infections must be therefore able to cross the blood–brain barrier in order to be effective.

In patients with bacteremia or viremia, the organism may enter the venous sinuses, cross the blood–brain barrier, penetrate the dura and arachnoid, and gain access to the subarachnoid space. Fractures at the base of the skull or the cribriform plate can lead to an opening between the CNS and the sinuses, mastoid, middle ear, or nasopharynx. Since these sites are all contiguous with the upper respiratory tract, CSF leaks occurring at any of these sites may enable respiratory flora to track back up into the subarachnoid space. Extrinsic contamination of the CNS can also occur intraoperatively during neurosurgical procedures and as a result of bacterial entry via congenital malformations (e.g., spina bifida or sinus tracts). Implanted medical devices or hardware (e.g., shunts, ventriculostomies, deep brain stimulators, or external drainage tubes) can become colonized and serve as foci of infection. Viruses, such as rabies, HSV, or poliovirus, can spread to the CNS via intraneural pathways resulting in encephalitis.

If infection occurs at sites (e.g., middle ear or mastoid) contiguous with the CNS, infection may spread directly into the CNS causing brain abscesses. Alternatively, the organism may reach the CNS indirectly via venous drainage or via the sheaths of cranial and spinal nerves. Abscesses also may become localized in the subdural or epidural spaces and subsequently spread to the subarachnoid space, causing meningitis. CNS abscesses may result from septic emboli associated with endocarditis, lung abscesses, or other serious purulent infections, such as those caused by *Staphylococcus aureus* or the *Streptococcus milleri* group.

Routes of Infection

Acute CNS infections fall broadly into three categories: meningitis, encephalitis, and abscesses. These infections generally result from blood-borne spread of the causative microorganisms. Bacteremia or viremia can result from infection at sites adjacent or contiguous to the CNS, such as the mastoid, sinuses, or middle ear, or from primary infections at more remote anatomic sites, such as the lungs, heart, skin, gastrointestinal tract, or kidney. In children, the most common predisposing conditions are sinus or middle ear infections, which may lead to transient bacteremia and hematogenous seeding of the CNS [1–3]. Bacterial infections of the paranasal and otomastoid sinuses often produce phlebothrombosis of adjacent draining cortical (cerebral) veins. This thrombotic process can extend into regional dural sinuses and offer a direct route of transmission from the infected sinus to the adjacent extra-axial spaces or the brain via cortical venous drainage pathways. Venous obstruction can produce intra-axial brain swelling, which may complicate the interpretation of brain and spinal imaging studies and obscure the primary infectious source.

Acute Bacterial Meningitis

Bacterial meningitis can develop rapidly into a life-threatening infection even in previously healthy children or adults. Bacteria that cause meningitis enter the bloodstream and can penetrate the protective blood–brain barrier. Bacterial meningitis is associated with high mortality with an estimated 16 million cases worldwide in 2013 [4].

Definition

Bacterial meningitis is defined as an inflammatory response to bacterial invasion of the membranes surrounding the CNS. This infection typically involves the entire length of the neuraxis, including the brain (cerebrum, cerebellum), spinal cord, optic nerves, and their covering membranes because of the continuous nature of the subarachnoid space. Pyogenic meningitis is associated with a marked, acute inflammatory exudate; non-pyogenic microorganisms (e.g., mycobacteria or spirochetes like *Leptospira* spp.) are less commonly implicated. Clinically, onset is acute with the development of headache, fever, irritability, and stiff neck with or without focal neurological signs over hours to a few days. Although the overall annual incidence of pyogenic bacterial meningitis in the United States is decreasing, the outcome is invariably fatal if left untreated [1–6].

Epidemiology

The most common microorganisms causing bacterial meningitis in the United States include *Streptococcus pneumoniae*, *Neisseria meningitidis*, group B *Streptococcus* spp., *Listeria monocytogenes*, and *Haemophilus influenzae*. Collectively, these agents account for over 95% of cases (Table 31.1). The age distribution, predisposing conditions, and fatality rates for the most common agents are summarized in Fig. 31.1 and Table 31.1.

Streptococcus pneumoniae

Of the three predominant organisms (*S. pneumoniae*, *N. meningitidis*, and *H. influenzae*) implicated in community-associated meningitis in the United States, *S. pneumoniae* is the most common and affects all age groups, except infants in the immediate neonatal period. *S. pneumoniae* are lancet-shaped, gram-positive, facultative anaerobic bacteria with more than 100 known serotypes. Most *S. pneumoniae* serotypes can cause disease, but only a minority of serotypes produce the majority of pneumococcal infections. The estimated incidence of invasive *Streptococcus pneumoniae* infection is 38 per 100,000 population/year. The risk of pneumococcal meningitis varies with age but is significantly higher in infants than in young children and adults. Over the age of 70 years, the incidence rises again to approximately double the average incidence for young and middle-aged adults. In adults, the major predisposing factors for infection include alcoholism, splenectomy, human immunodeficiency virus (HIV) infection, other acquired immunodeficiency conditions, diabetes, underlying chronic conditions (e.g., chronic renal disease), and prior viral respiratory infection. Pneumococcal meningitis is the most common form of recurrent meningitis in patients who have CSF leaks. *S. pneumoniae* is spread by respiratory transmission in the general population and results in colonization of the nasopharynx with rates commonly in the range of 5–10% of healthy adults. During the wintertime, carriage rates can rise to 20–30% in certain populations depending on age and other factors. Overcrowding in daycare centers, military barracks, and prisons are well-recognized risk factor for transmission.

N. meningitidis

N. meningitidis is an aerobic, gram-negative diplococcus that colonizes the mucosal surface of the nasopharynx. The main mode of transmission is via direct contact with large droplet respiratory secretions from patients or asymptomatic carriers; humans are the only hosts. Invasive disease caused by this organism occurs in three clinical forms: meningitis (50% of cases), blood infection (30%), and pneumonia (10%);

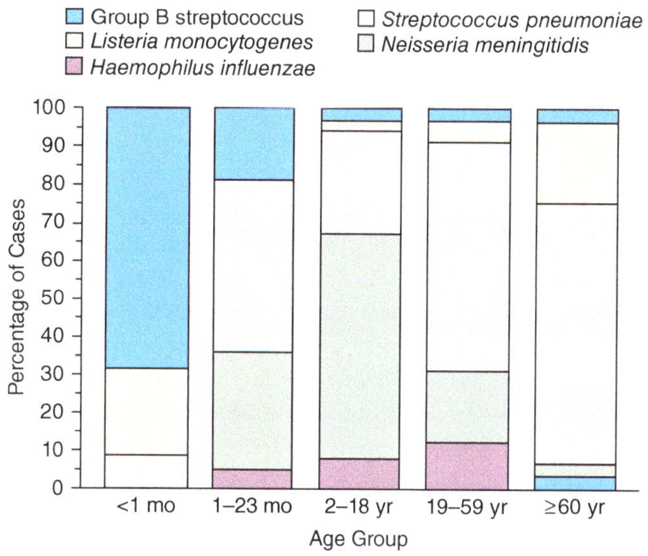

Fig. 31.1 Pathogenic agents of bacterial meningitis according to age group (Used with permission of the Massachusetts Medical Society from Schuchat et al. [1])

Table 31.1 Causes of bacterial meningitis and overall case fatality rate according to organism

Organism	% of total cases	Incidence	Predisposing conditions	Case fatality rate (%)
Streptococcus pneumoniae	47	1.1	Otitis media; sinusitis; alcoholism; cirrhosis; pneumococcal pneumonia; immunosuppression; skull fracture; CSF leak; myeloma; sickle cell disease	21
Neisseria meningitidis	25	0.6	"Closed" institutional setting; lack of specific antibody; complement deficiencies	3
Group B Streptococcus	12	0.3	Neonatal period; colonized mothers; preterm labor; prolonged rupture of membranes; intrapartum fever	7
Listeria monocytogenes	8	0.2	Neonatal period; immunosuppression; age; alcoholism/cirrhosis	15
Haemophilus influenzae	7	0.2	Lack of antibody to polysaccharide capsule; preceding otitis media	6

Adapted with permission of the Massachusetts Medical Society from Schuchat et al. [1]

other forms account for the remainder (10%) of the cases. Persons at risk include household contacts of infected patients, military recruits, college freshmen who live in dormitories, microbiologists who work with isolates of *N. meningitidis*, persons traveling to a country where meningococcal disease is epidemic or highly endemic, and patients without spleens or with terminal complement component deficiencies. Infants <1 year of age and adolescents ages 16–21 years have higher rates of disease than other age groups, although infection can occur in all age groups including the elderly.

Strains of *N. meningitidis* are characterized according to the serologic recognition of polysaccharide epitopes on their capsule and outer membrane and are classified into serogroups A, B, C, W135, and Y. In the United States, strains from serogroups B, C, and Y cause the majority (45%) of infections, whereas in economically less-developed countries serogroups A and C predominate; serogroup A has also been implicated in epidemics in sub-Saharan Africa.

H. influenza

This is a small, pleomorphic, aerobic or facultative anaerobic gram-negative coccobacillus that is classified according to six serologically distinct antigenic types based on capsular polysaccharides a–f. Of these, only *H. influenzae* type b (Hib) is pathogenic. Although the nonencapsulated form of *H. influenzae* is a common inhabitant of the upper respiratory tract of healthy humans and causes localized infection (e.g., conjunctivitis or otitis media in children) without bacteremia, the more virulent encapsulated Hib serotype causes more invasive disease and is an important cause of meningitis or epiglottitis. Hib meningitis is relatively uncommon during the first 2 months of life likely due to passively transferred maternal antibodies. By the fourth month of life, children lose these antibodies and are at increased risk of Hib meningitis. The occurrence of *H. influenzae* meningitis is directly associated with the presence and development of type-specific anticapsular antibodies to polyribosylribitol phosphate. Whether vaccine-induced or occurring naturally, presence of these antibodies is directly related to protection from invasive *H. influenzae* infection [7]. Various clinical studies have shown these antibodies to be opsonic and bactericidal against *H. influenzae* in vitro and protective in vivo. In the pre-vaccine era, colonization with nontypable strains of *H. influenzae* led to the development of cross-reacting antibodies that were largely protective against infection caused by type b strains. Before the introduction of the Hib conjugate polysaccharide capsular vaccine in 1986, *H. influenzae* was the most common cause of acute bacterial meningitis in children under the age of 5, with as many as 1 in 200 children acquiring invasive *H. influenzae* infection, including epiglottitis, septicemia, arthritis, and soft tissue infections in addition to meningitis. However, by 1995, the prevalence of meningitis caused by Hib had fallen 55% [6]. Risk factors for Hib meningitis include malignancy, chronic renal disease, sickle cell disease, immunoglobulin dyscrasias, HIV infections, and cystic fibrosis.

Listeria monocytogenes

Listeria monocytogenes is a facultative anaerobic, intracellular gram-positive bacillus that remains a significant cause of neonatal meningitis in the USA. Although the mode of transmission to humans is generally fecal-oral, transmission of the pathogen to the neonate generally occurs at the time of birth in mothers who had asymptomatic colonization of the genital or gastrointestinal tract prior to delivery. Domestic and wild animals are the main reservoirs for *L. monocytogenes*, but as the prevalence of stool carriage of this organism among asymptomatic adults is about 1%, humans remain a small but still significant reservoir.

Generally, healthy adults exposed to the organism do not become ill, unless exposed to high numbers of infectious organisms, such as during an outbreak. *L. monocytogenes* causes meningitis most often in adults with depressed cell-mediated immunity, patients on steroids or other immunosuppressive agents, HIV-infected individuals, transplant recipients, and other vulnerable populations, such as persons with diabetes, alcohol abuse, chronic liver disease, renal disease requiring hemodialysis, or age >60 years. Outbreaks of *L. monocytogenes* meningitis in the United States and elsewhere have been associated with unpasteurized milk products, such as Swiss or feta cheese, undercooked chicken or hot dogs, seafood, vegetables, or coleslaw.

Other Microorganisms

Gram-negative microorganisms are important causes of acute bacterial meningitis. Persons with diabetes, a history of alcohol abuse, hepatic cirrhosis, or chronic urinary tract infections are particularly susceptible. *E. coli* with the K1 capsular polysaccharide antigen accounts for most of the cases of gram-negative meningitis in the newborn [8]. Carriage rates of the *E. coli* K1 serotypes vary in different populations but range from 7% to 38% in women of childbearing age and may be as high as 50% in nursing personnel [9–11]. In a study of 231 children presenting with bacterial meningitis to the emergency department during the era of widespread heptavalent conjugate pneumococcal vaccination, *E. coli* was implicated in 4% and other gram-negative bacilli in 3.0% [12, 13]. Other gram-negative organisms such as *Klebsiella* spp., *Enterobacter* spp., *Pseudomonas* spp., *Citrobacter* spp., and *Salmonella* spp. may also cause meningitis in the neonatal period, with an epidemiology similar to that of the *E. coli* K1 strains. Gram-negative bacillary meningitis still carries a worse prognosis than meningitis with a gram-positive organism [14]. Beyond the neonatal period, most cases of gram-negative meningitis occur in the inpatient setting, especially following neurosurgery (e.g., craniotomy), spinal procedures, placement of devices (e.g., ventriculostomy tubes or shunts), surgical procedures that include placement of in situ hardware, or in patients who have suffered head trauma [15].

Group B Streptococcus (*Streptococcus agalactiae*) is the single most frequent cause of neonatal meningitis. This organism has been cultured from vaginal secretions in 30–40% of women prior to delivery. During pregnancy, labor, and delivery, the microorganism can be transmitted to amniotic fluid or the newborn may become colonized as it passes through the birth canal. Transmission to the infant during delivery can result in neonatal meningitis within the first week of life. Alternatively, the organism may be acquired within the first few days after birth and meningitis may develop during the first 1–2 months after birth even if the infant appeared healthy at the time of delivery. While the probability of transmission from mothers colonized with *S. agalactiae* to neonates delivered vaginally is approximately 50%, only 2% of colonized neonates go on to develop invasive group B streptococcal disease. Group B streptococci produce polysaccharide capsules that manifest ten antigenic serotypes (designated as Ia, Ib, II, III, IV, V, VI, VII, VIII, and IX). Serotypes Ia, Ib, II, III, and V account for most of the cases of neonatal meningitis in the US. A number of virulence factors have been identified and include the capsule and production of higher levels of neuraminidase, beta-haemolysin, and superoxide dismutase. Epidemiologically, the increase in occurrence over the past decade parallels the increasing prevalence of obesity and diabetes.

Almost any microorganism that crosses the blood–brain barrier can cause acute meningitis. Other bacterial agents include group A streptococci, non-pneumococcal alpha hemolytic streptococci, *Neisseria gonorrhea*, *Salmonella* species, *Flavobacterium meningosepticum*, non-influenzae *Haemophilus* species, and even *Bacillus anthracis* (anthrax). Although *S. aureus* and *Staphylococcus epidermidis* are rarely implicated as causes of primary bacterial meningitis, these organisms are relatively common causes of bacterial meningitis following trauma or associated with in situ CSF shunts or neurosurgical procedures. Other microorganisms, such as *Mycobacterium* spp., *Nocardia* spp., yeasts and fungi (e.g., *Coccidioides immitis*, *Histoplasma capsulatum*, or *Cryptococcus neoformans*), *Treponema* spp., *Brucella* spp., *Leptospira* spp., or *Toxoplasma gondii*, can also cause meningitis. Except for *Leptospira* spp., however, these microorganisms tend to produce a more chronic form of meningitis [16]. For example, *Mycobacterium* spp., *C. immitis*, *H. capsulatum*, and *C. neoformans* typically produce chronic granulomatous inflammatory changes rather than acute pyogenic infections. *Streptococcus suis* has been a common cause of meningitis in Asia, especially in populations involved in pig farming.

Pathogenesis of Meningeal Invasion

Colonization of the respiratory tract or nasopharynx is the critical first step preceding infection caused by the three microorganisms (*S. pneumoniae*, *N. meningitides*, and *H. influenzae*) most commonly associated with community-acquired meningitis. Biologically, colonization is mediated by affinity of these organisms for the nasopharyngeal mucosa. Colonization is facilitated by attachment and adherence of the microorganisms to cell surface receptors on nasopharyngeal epithelial cells, enabling them to replicate in the upper airway for prolonged periods. All three pathogens, typically, may colonize the upper airway without producing symptoms. Both host susceptibility and pathogen-specific factors (e.g., virulence and pathogenicity) are critical in the development of invasive disease. Many of these factors, though identified and characterized, are still not fully understood. For example, splenectomy predisposes the affected person to invasive disease by *S. pneumoniae*, while it appears to have relatively little effect on the occurrence of invasive *N. meningitidis* disease, even though both are encapsulated organisms.

Adherence to nasopharyngeal mucosa is mediated by fimbriae or pili, in the case of gram-negative organisms. The pili of *N. meningitidis* are filamentous glycoproteins which bind to specific receptors on nasopharyngeal cells, such as the CD4+ receptor [17, 18]. After receptor binding, further interaction with the host cell is established by outer membrane proteins on *N. meningitidis*, designated Opa and Opc [19]. Binding of the outer membrane proteins to specific receptors promotes engulfment of the *N. meningitidis* by the epithelial cells followed by transportation of the bacteria across the cell in membrane-bound vacuoles to the intravascular space. Organisms also gain access to the intravascular space by creating separations in the tight junctions of columnar epithelial cells. *N. meningitidis* possesses additional outer membrane proteins that function as IgA proteases, degrading the surface IgA antibodies on epithelial cells in order to facilitate invasive disease [20]. Once the mucosal barrier has been breached, the development of meningococcal disease is dependent upon the survival of the organism in the bloodstream.

The most important virulence factor for survival of meningococci is the polysaccharide capsule that protects the organism against complement-mediated phagocytosis by neutrophils in the reticular endothelial system [21, 22]. Host defense is dependent on existing humoral antibodies to specific polysaccharide capsular types as well as the cellular responses of the innate immune system.

Protective IgG antibody for meningococcal disease is acquired through maternal transmission and is protective for the first few months after birth. Colonization by nonpathogenic *Neisseria* species or a cross-reacting gram-negative organism such as *E. coli* K1 induces protective antibodies. Antibodies promoting optimization of phagocytosis through opsonization and specific lysis via complement activation. For this reason, patients who are deficient in complement factor C5 are particularly susceptible to repeated invasive infections by *N. meningitidis*. In fact, individuals with an inherited deficiency of any of the terminal components of complement C5, C6, C7, and C8 have a greater risk of invasive disease [23].

Virulence factors for the invasion of *S. pneumoniae* are primarily a function of the capsular polysaccharide type. There are at least 93 known capsular serotypes of *S. pneumoniae* with the various serotypes having different propensities for producing disease or developing antibiotic resistance [24, 25].

Colonization of the upper airway by *H. influenzae* is also mediated by fimbrial attachment to epithelial cells. Alpha fimbriae enhance the binding to the anterior nasopharynx and β fimbriae facilitate binding to the posterior ciliated nasopharyngeal cells [26]. Although *H. influenzae* type b strains that lack fimbriae are generally unable to colonize the nasopharynx, isolates from the CSF do not express fimbria, suggesting that while the presence of fimbriae on *H. influenzae* is important for colonization of and attachment to nasopharyngeal mucosa, fimbriae do not appear play a significant role in the development of meningitis [27, 28].

N. meningitis, *S. pneumoniae*, *H. influenzae* type b and other pathogens utilize a variety of virulence factors to facilitate infection of the meninges [29]. In addition, certain host characteristics and cellular processes may also be used to the advantage of the pathogen. For example, bacteria migrate through the brain microvascular endothelial cells in enclosed vacuoles via a mechanism that is dependent on F-actin. Cytoskeletal rearrangement involving both microfilaments and microtubules therefore plays an important role in pathogen transport. The CSF also contains lower levels of immunoglobulins, complement, and leukocytes as compared to the serum and interstitial fluid due to the BBB. Therefore, in the early phase of infection involving the subarachnoid space, bacterial replication may proceed virtually unchecked by host defense mechanisms. Opsonization of bacteria and subsequent phagocytosis by neutrophils are hindered by the relative paucity of complement and immunoglobulins, and leukocyte proteases derived from the initial influx of leukocytes further degrade whatever complement components are present in the CSF [30–32].

Lipopolysaccharide (LPS) molecules from gram-negative bacteria are known to stimulate a potent immune response [32, 33]. This response is likely mediated through the induction of inflammatory cytokines such as Interleukin 1 (IL-1) and tumor necrosis factor (TNF) [30, 33]. In vitro studies with LPS and with IL-1 and TNF show that incubation with endothelial cell monolayers leads to a rapid, transient increase in the expression of the intercellular adhesion molecules (ICAM-1 and ICAM-2) as well as the selectin molecules such as ELAM-1. As a result, neutrophils are able to bind to CNS vascular endothelial cells at vastly increased rates and then subsequently migrate by diapedesis into the subarachnoid space. At the same time, adherence of neutrophils to the capillary endothelium increases the permeability of the blood vessels enabling more protein leakage into the CSF and subarachnoid space, adding to the inflammatory exudate. Figure 31.2a, b shows the dense inflammatory infiltrate with neutrophils, lymphocytes, and macrophages seen in a patient with purulent meningitis caused by *S. pneumoniae*. IL-1 and TNF, in turn, stimulate leukocytes and

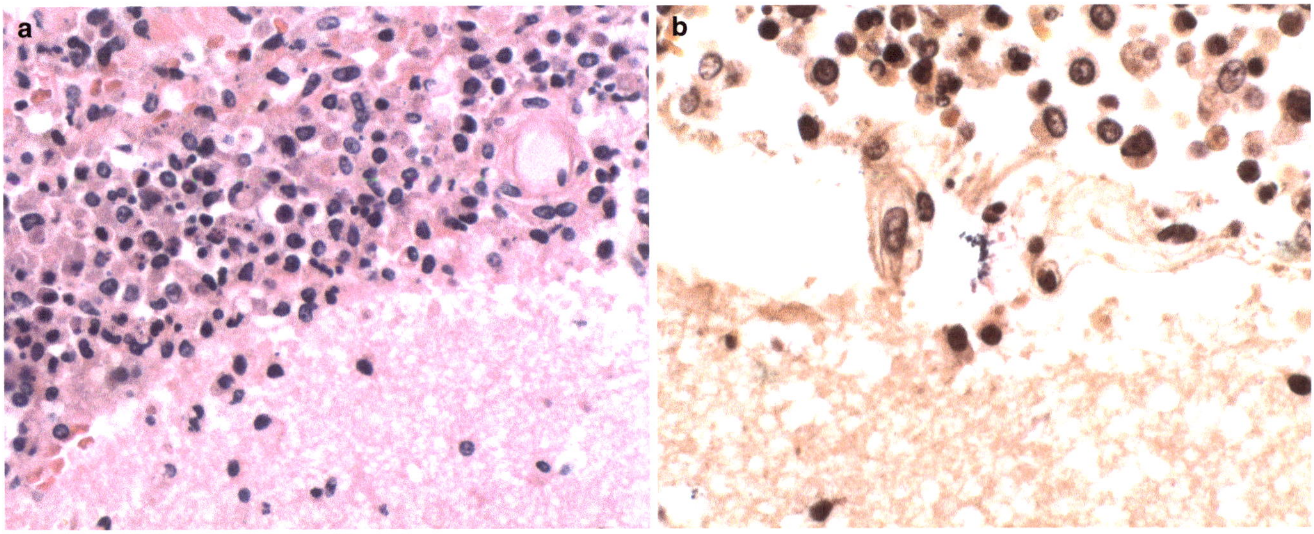

Fig. 31.2 (**a**) Acute purulent meningitis caused by the *Streptococcus pneumoniae*. Leptomeninges expanded by a dense necroinflammatory infiltrate with neutrophils, lymphocytes, and macrophages (H&E 40×). (**b**) Gram stain of exudate specimens showing gram-positive diplococci (Both courtesy of Anthony Yachnis, MD, and Kelly Devers, MD, University of Florida College of Medicine)

other categories of inflammatory cells to produce and secrete a host of other proinflammatory cytokines, proteolytic enzymes, free radicals, and nitric oxide. The result is edema of the surrounding tissues, cell injury, and tissue necrosis. Infiltration of the walls of small arteries and cortical veins also leads to a vasculitis with intimal thickening, narrowing and occlusion of small arteries, thrombophlebitis of the cortical veins, and thrombosis of the major venous sinuses, which leads to ischemia and infarction of brain tissues. Inflammation of the pia mater and arachnoid also inhibits glucose transport into the CSF, resulting in a decrease in CSF glucose levels.

This intense neutrophil response accounts for many of the clinical consequences of meningitis, including increased permeability of the blood–brain barrier, hydrocephalus, reduced cerebral blood flow, and increased intracranial pressure (ICP) [33]. The increase in ICP is multifactorial. The increased permeability of the blood-brain barrier results in vasogenic edema through increased intracellular water content, potassium leakage, and a shift in brain metabolism to anaerobic glycolysis with increased lactate production. In addition, inflammation in the subarachnoid space decreases reabsorption of CSF. Increased ICP may ultimately precipitate transtentorial brain herniation and death.

Clinical Manifestations

Meningitis typically presents with fever, headache, and stiff neck in adults. Varying degrees of altered consciousness may also be present, as well as vomiting, which is attributable to elevated ICP and inflammation affecting the midbrain. Clinical symptoms also vary depending on the causative organism. For example, patients with pneumococcal meningitis (*S. pneumoniae* being the most common etiologic agent in adult bacterial meningitis cases) may initially present with upper or lower respiratory tract symptoms prior to bacteremia and progression to meningitis.

In a review of 493 episodes of meningitis, Durand and colleagues found that 95% of patients with acquired meningitis had a temperature >37.7 °C on admission, while neck stiffness was present in 88%. Only 22% were alert, 51% were confused or lethargic, and 22% were responsive only to pain. Within the first 24–48 h of onset, 29% had suffered focal seizures or had exhibited focal neurologic signs [34]. The most common predisposing factors for acute meningitis included pneumonia, sinusitis, otitis media, alcoholism, diabetes, malignancy, connective tissue diseases, sickle cell disease, diabetes, organ transplantation, splenectomy, dialysis, steroid use, or other immunosuppressive conditions. Immunosuppressed patients may not always present with a classic clinical presentation.

Meningococcal meningitis often has a non-specific presentation but can rapidly progress to irreversible shock and death. Manifestations of meningococcal septicemia may precede symptoms of meningitis by 12–24 h. Early in meningococcemia, the patient may exhibit a subtle petechial rash (Fig. 31.3) that precedes progression to fulminant disseminated intravascular coagulation (DIC) and development of a more severe purpuric rash that may progress to necrosis of the fingers and toes (Fig. 31.3). Purpura fulminans in the patient with meningococcemia is classically associated with hemorrhagic necrosis of the adrenal gland, known as Waterhouse-Friderichsen syndrome. Thus, the clinical manifestation of meningococcal meningitis depends on the relative degree of meningococcemia and shock, as well as the severity of meningitis.

The presentation of meningitis in the elderly and the very young may be more insidious compared to those patients not at the extremes of age. For example, in a review of 54 cases, Gorse and coworkers found that confusion was a predominating symptom in presentation among the elderly compared with the younger age group, and pneumonia was also more likely to be present in the older age group [35]. Typical symptoms and signs are also less commonly reported in the elderly since these patients often have cervical rigidity due to osteoarthritis, cervical spondylosis, or existing cerebrovascular disease. In addition, there may be hypertonicity of the neck muscles in conditions such as Parkinson's disease. Among the elderly, meningitis itself may progress more rapidly, and patients are more likely to present with coma when compared with younger patient populations. With the development of coma, nuchal rigidity may be markedly less pronounced. Thus, when meningitis is suspected in the elderly, true nuchal rigidity has to be distinguished by careful physical examination. The absence of fever does not rule out the diagnosis of meningitis in the elderly patient.

In children, the presentation of meningitis is fundamentally similar to young and middle-aged adults, although nonspecific symptoms, such as irritability, nausea and vomiting, respiratory symptoms, and photophobia are more common in children. In neonates and infants, meningitis may present simply as fever or irritability. Generally, there is a tendency for fever to be higher in children as compared to that in adults. The classic physical signs of meningeal inflammation or irritation described in medical textbooks are Brudzinski's and Kernig's signs [36, 37]. Although Brudzinski originally described several signs of inflammation of the meninges, the best known of these is the so-called "nape of the neck" sign. This sign is elicited by flexing the neck forward. The stretching of the meninges induced by this movement results in involuntary flexion of the hips and knees. Kernig's sign is elicited with the patient in the supine position and the thigh flexed on the abdomen with the knee flexed at a 45° angle. Upon passive extension of the leg in the presence of meningeal irritation, the patient resists

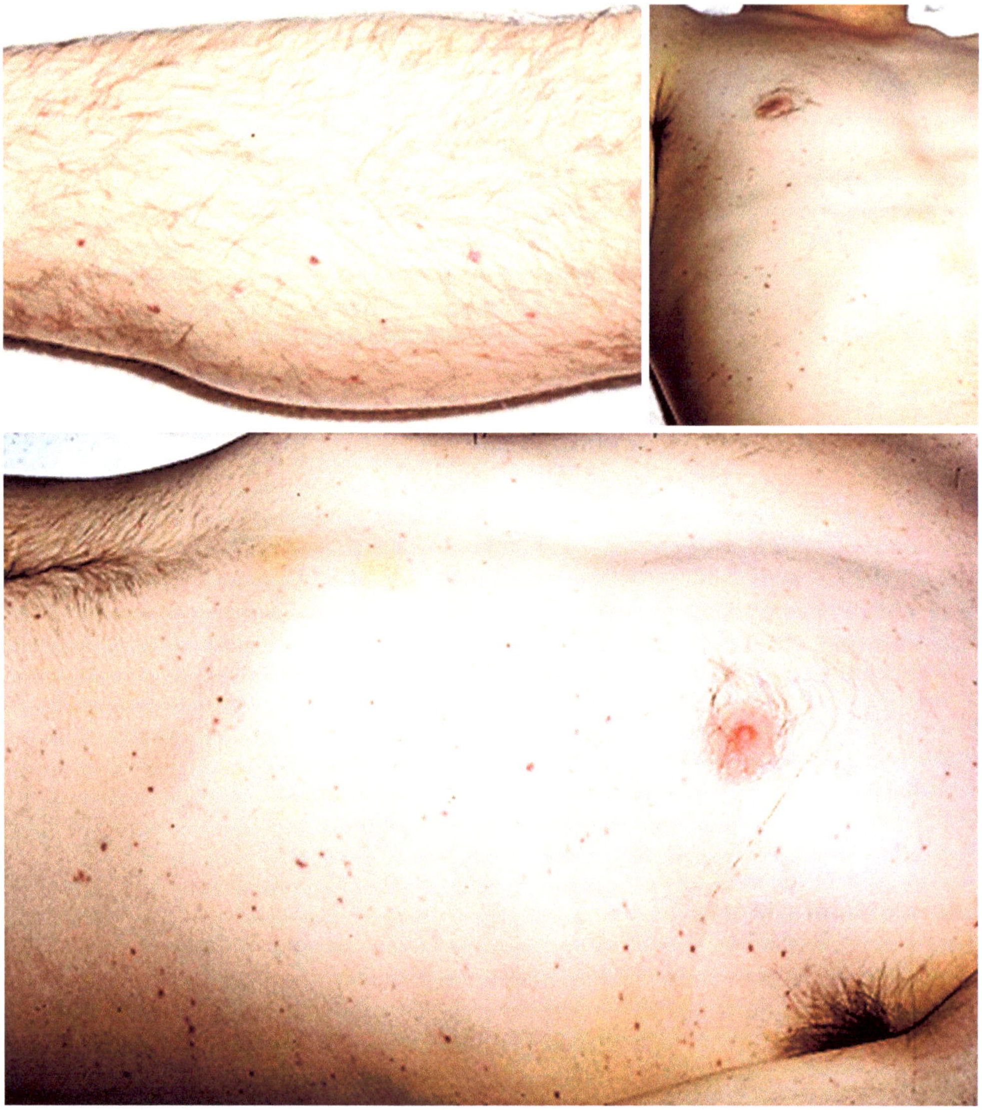

Fig. 31.3 Petechial rash associated with meningococcal meningitis

extension with complaints of lower back and hamstring pain. Kernig's and Brudzinski's signs are neither sensitive nor specific indicators of meningitis, however, and are potentially elicited in only about 50% of children and only 5% of adults with acute bacterial meningitis.

Diagnosis

An acute CNS infection is a medical emergency. Bacterial meningitis may have to be differentiated from aseptic meningitis, encephalitis, brain abscess, subdural empyema, or other noninfectious conditions affecting the CNS. Differentiation from encephalitis can be challenging. The classic features of meningitis (headache, neck stiffness, photophobia, fever, and vomiting) are often absent in neonates, patients who are immunocompromised—including persons with HIV infection—alcoholics, or the elderly. In encephalitis, an altered state of consciousness, confusion, convulsions, and obtundation predominate. As the level of consciousness declines in patients with meningitis or encephalitis, differentiation between the two may only be possible through laboratory and radiographic findings. Because acute bacterial meningitis is a medical emergency, therapy should be implemented empirically on clinical grounds without waiting for confirmatory laboratory or radiographic studies.

Meningism involves the triad of neck stiffness, photophobia, and headache. Meningismus is a constellation of signs and symptoms of meningism without objective findings of infection or inflammation. Fever and altered mental status with or without meningismus may occur in a variety of systemic infections as well as noninfectious conditions. For example, Rocky Mountain spotted fever (RMSF) can present with fever, shock, and a petechial rash (Fig. 31.4a–c), which must be differentiated from the rash associated with early meningococcemia (Fig. 31.3). Meningococcal disease may initially present simply as meningococcemia with shock and

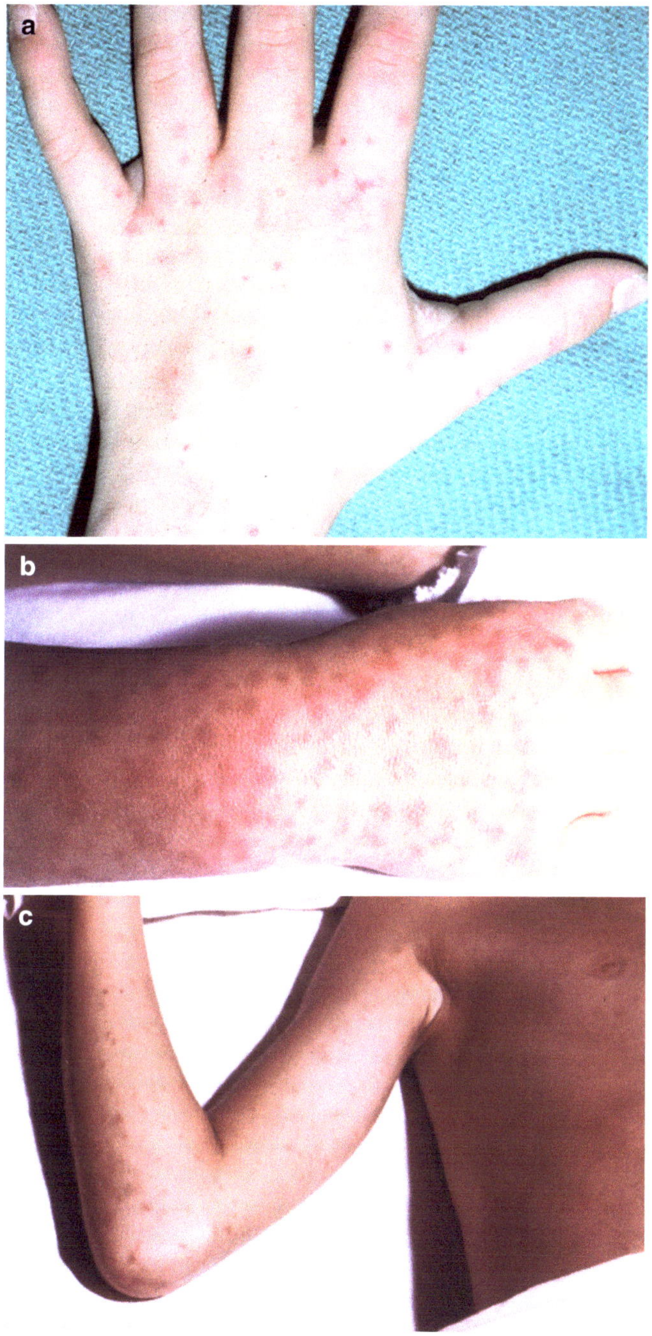

Fig. 31.4 (**a–c**) Rocky Mountain spotted fever rash (**a**: Courtesy of Daniel J. Sexton, MD, Duke University Medical Center; (**b**, **c**): Courtesy of the Centers for Disease Control and Prevention)

skin rash instead of meningeal signs. Other infections that present with headache and fever include brain abscesses, influenza, leptospirosis, dengue, typhoid, parameningeal infections, and Q fever. Noninfectious conditions may also present precipitously with severe headache, fever, or nuchal rigidity. Examples include subarachnoid hemorrhage, acute hemorrhagic or ischemic strokes, cerebral venous sinus thrombosis, autoimmune disorders (e.g., temporal arteritis), neuroleptic malignant syndrome, status epilepticus, or toxic encephalopathies of various etiologies.

Lumbar Puncture and CSF Analysis

A lumbar puncture with analysis of the CSF facilitates the diagnosis of meningitis and other conditions affecting the CNS. Before performing a lumbar puncture on a patient with meningitis, elevated ICP must first be ruled out to prevent uncal, midbrain, medullary, or cerebellar tonsillar herniation after the procedure, which can lead to irreversible brain injury or death. Cerebral herniation occurs in about 5% of patients with acute bacterial meningitis, accounting for about 30% of the mortality risk [38]. The role of a CT scan is primarily to ascertain whether a space-occupying lesion is present; a CT scan cannot rule out the presence of increased ICP. Clinical signs suggestive of impending herniation include deteriorating level of consciousness, brainstem signs (including pupillary changes, decorticate posturing, or irregular respirations), recent seizures, absent oculocephalic reflexes, or papilledema. Lumbar puncture should be delayed in such patients, even for those with a normal CT scan, until preventive measures can be implemented to decrease ICP [38–42]. Other relative contraindications to immediate lumbar puncture include clinical instability due to shock, presence of an epidural abscess, bleeding disorders, and infection or loss of skin (e.g., burns) over the lumbar spine.

If the clinical picture is suggestive of bacterial meningitis or other intracranial infection and the patient is critically ill, especially if there is a rash or altered mental status, blood cultures should be drawn immediately, and intravenous antimicrobial therapy initiated without delay. If the patient is not critically ill, antimicrobial therapy may potentially be withheld until radiographic studies and lumbar puncture can be performed. If raised ICP is suspected and no focal lesions are defined by radiographic studies, intravenous mannitol is sometimes used to reduce cerebral edema prior to lumbar puncture. Elective intubation and sedation of the patient may also be considered to reduce the ICP. These measures may decrease the risk of herniation.

After insertion of the needle, the opening CSF pressure should be measured with the patient in the supine position. Normal opening pressure ranges from 1 to 10 cm H_2O in young children, 6–20 cm H_2O after 8 years of age, and up to 25 cm H_2O in obese patients [43]. The level should fluctuate with respiration and can be elevated by the Valsalva maneuver. If the CSF pressure is measured again at the end of the procedure after appropriate volumes of CSF have been obtained and have dropped to zero, the possibility of a complete CSF block should be considered. CSF is normally crystal clear and colorless. A minimum of 200 white blood cells or 400 red blood cells/mm^3 is necessary to impart turbidity to the fluid. CSF will appear reddish if more than 6000 red blood cells/mm^3 are present [43].

Xanthochromia is a yellow, orange, or pink discoloration of the CSF and is caused by the lysis of red blood cells resulting in hemoglobin breakdown to oxyhemoglobin, methemoglobin, and bilirubin. Discoloration begins after RBCs have been in spinal fluid for about 2 h. In cases of subarachnoid hemorrhage, xanthochromia occurs within 2–4 h after the initial cerebral bleed; xanthochromia may develop in vitro if the CSF specimen contains increased numbers of red blood cells and is not centrifuged immediately upon arrival in the laboratory. Xanthochromia also occurs when CSF protein concentrations are greater than 150 mg/dL. Appearance alone is not enough to make a specific diagnosis of bacterial or viral meningitis, however.

In adults and children older than the neonatal age group, normal CSF generally contains <5 white cells/mm^3, usually small lymphocytes. In neonates, CSF may contain up to 25–30 white cells/mm^3 with up to 60% neutrophils; this falls after a few days to the range of 8–9 white cells/mm^3 [9]. Because red cells may be present in spinal fluid as a result of subarachnoid hemorrhage or through a traumatic tap, it is important to note whether red-tinged or bloody CSF clears as sequential specimen tubes of CSF are obtained. Such clearing suggests a traumatic tap and can be documented in the laboratory by counting the red cells in successive tubes. CSF cells should be counted in the laboratory within 1–2 h of collection; further delays may result in a falsely low cell count because of cell lysis or adherence of cells to the walls of the specimen tube.

Glucose enters the CSF by transport through the choroid plexus and capillary endothelium in the subarachnoid space. CSF glucose levels are therefore a function of both active transport of glucose into the CNS and its rate of consumption within the CNS. CSF glucose levels in normal subjects are, on average, 60–70% of the blood glucose levels. However, a study by Skipper and Davis showed the CSF to serum glucose ratio was most accurate when the serum glucose was between 89 and 115 mg/dL [44]. For blood glucose levels >125 mg/dL, the ratio was <60%; for blood glucose levels >192 mg/dL, the ratio fell to 50% even among normal patients with no evidence of meningitis.

CSF protein levels are generally <40 mg/dL due to the exclusion of larger proteins by the blood–brain barrier. When the barrier breaks down during meningitis, CSF protein tends to rise and increase with the duration of disease prior to initiation of therapy. Protein levels in newborn infants are significantly higher compared to older children and adults, averaging 90 mg/dL with normal levels up to 170 mg/dL. Extremely high levels (more than 1 g/dL) of CSF protein are suggestive of a CSF spinal block. Elevation of CSF protein on its own, however, is not specific for any specific type of meningitis.

Table 31.2 summarizes the CSF characteristics (macroscopic appearance, white cell count range and differential,

Table 31.2 CSF findings in acute and chronic meningitis and other CNS infectious conditions

Type of infection	Macroscopic appearance	Cells	Protein (mg/dL)	Glucose (mg/dL)	Other tests
Normal	Clear	<5 lymphocytes/mm ^{3}	15–45	50–75	Negative test results
Bacterial meningitis (*S. pneumoniae*; *N. meningitides*; *L. monocytogenes*)	Cloudy or turbid	*Increased (commonly > 200)* *Typically > 90% PMNs* Can be normal in meningococcemia	>100	Reduced (<40)	Gram stain, bacterial culture, and antigen tests may be positive
Viral meningitis (enteroviruses; herpes simplex; arboviral encephalitis)	Clear or rarely opalescent	Increased May have PMN predominance early in the course of infection; converts to lymphocytic predominance within 12–24 h	Usually <100	Normal	Gram stain, bacterial culture, and antigen tests negative PCR for HSV, VZV, arboviruses, and enteroviruses may be positive
Fungal meningitis (cryptococcus; histoplasmosis; coccidioidomycosis)	Cloudy or turbid	>100 (<50%) Usual range 100–400 usually lymphocytic predominance May be normal in cryptococcal meningitis	100–900	<40	Cryptococcus can be diagnosed from India ink preps, antigen tests, or culture; PCR
Tuberculous meningitis	Cloudy or turbid	Increased Typically >100 Usual range 100–400 PMN early but converts to lymphocytic predominance	100–900	<40	Acid-fast bacilli occasionally seen on CSF smear stained with Kinyoun or Ziehl-Neelsen stains
Parameningeal infections (sinusitis; epidural abscess; paraspinous abscess)	Clear	<100 (<50%) Occasionally PMN predominance If rupture into CSF, like acute meningitis	Increased	Normal	

Adapted with permission from Rand et al. [45]

protein and glucose levels) typically encountered in meningitis caused by various classes of organisms. In general, high CSF white cell counts are found in bacterial meningitis, where levels may be >10,000 cells/mm^3 with 95% polymorphonuclear leukocytes (PMNs). Typically, the WBC count in bacterial meningitis ranges between 500 and 5000 cells/mm^3, CSF glucose is <40 mg/dL, and protein levels are in the 100–500 mg/dL range. It is important to recognize that a predominance of PMNs may occur early in viral meningitis, within the first 24–48 h, but this gradually shifts to a mononuclear predominance over the next 8 h if the lumbar puncture is repeated [46, 47]. In patients with meningitis caused by *L. monocytogenes*, the organism grows and survives within the host cell cytoplasm, thereby stimulating a monocytic CSF response; in infants, there may be a monocytic predominance.

Once CSF specimens are obtained, a gram stain should be performed immediately in patients with suspected bacterial meningitis followed by plating on solid culture media. Centrifugation of CSF improves the yield for both gram stain smears and culture. In general, a CSF concentration >10^3 organisms/mL is required before organisms could be identified on light microscopy of the gram stain. With lower concentrations, there are simply too few organisms to detect by direct microscopy. Approximately 75% of patients with acute bacterial meningitis will have a positive gram stain, and this percentage may drop to about 50% among patients who have received significant doses of prior antimicrobial therapy. Generally, the gram stain is positive in 90% of untreated patients with pneumococcal meningitis, 86% of patients with meningitis due to *H. influenzae*, and approximately 75% of cases due to *N. meningitidis* [48]. Among children, the overall sensitivity of gram stain to detect bacterial meningitis is 67%. Most children without bacterial meningitis have a negative gram stain with a negative predictive value of 99.9%. Thus, CSF gram stain is useful in evaluating children for empiric therapy of bacterial meningitis [49].

In addition to gram stain, several rapid diagnostic tests have been developed for diagnosing acute bacterial meningitis. In the 1970s, counter immunoelectrophoresis (CIE) was used for direct detection of bacterial polysaccharide antigens; this test is quite insensitive and is no longer in use. Agglutination tests are commercially available for *H. influenza*, *S. pneumoniae*, and five serotypes of *N. meningitidis*. However, the sensitivity and specificity of these tests are no better than that of the gram stain, and they provide no additional diagnostic yield above and beyond the gram stain and the clinical picture and rarely influence the decision to treat empirically [50, 51]. Therefore, they are not currently recommended in the diagnosis of acute bacterial meningitis upon initial presentation.

Miscellaneous Testing

C-reactive protein (CRP) can be measured in CSF and, when >100 μg/mL, may be useful in differentiating bacterial from viral meningitis [52]. Extensive literature exists describing the application of real-time polymerase chain reaction (PCR) for detection and quantification of various bacterial and viral pathogens in CSF of patients with a putative diagnosis of bacterial meningitis. Real-time PCR is faster and more sensitive than previous technologies. This technique is expensive and not readily available in most hospital laboratories, however, clinicians are likely to initiate empiric antimicrobial therapy regardless in patients with typical CNS symptoms and signs.

Imaging Studies

Neuroimaging plays little role in the diagnosis of acute bacterial meningitis except to rule out the presence of mass lesions and raised ICP, which might increase the risk of herniation when lumbar puncture is performed. The major value of CT and MRI scans in patients with acute bacterial meningitis is in the investigation of complications, such as cerebral infarction, vasculitis, abscess, or hydrocephalus. Figure 31.5a–d shows the typical neuroradiological appearances of the brain in patients with meningitis caused by *L. monocytogenes*, *N. meningitidis*, *S. pneumoniae*, and *M. tuberculosis*. In patients with prolonged fever of 10 days duration or longer, up to 25% may have a subdural effusion (Fig. 31.6). In some cases, this may progress to a subdural empyema, which may account for the prolonged fever (Fig. 31.7). Cortical infarction is a common complication of bacterial meningitis and usually results from vasospasm of cerebral vasculature or vasculitis associated with meningitis itself. The MRI scan is more sensitive than CT imaging in detecting cerebritis and cortical infarction. Cerebritis is an early complication that may occur during the first 4 days (Fig. 31.8). Early necrotic regions filled with polymorphonuclear cells, lymphocytes, and plasma cells and with ill-defined parenchymal swelling characterize cerebritis. In late cerebritis (4–8 days), central necrosis increases, there is vascular proliferation and more inflammatory cells, and suppurative foci begin to breakdown and become encapsulated.

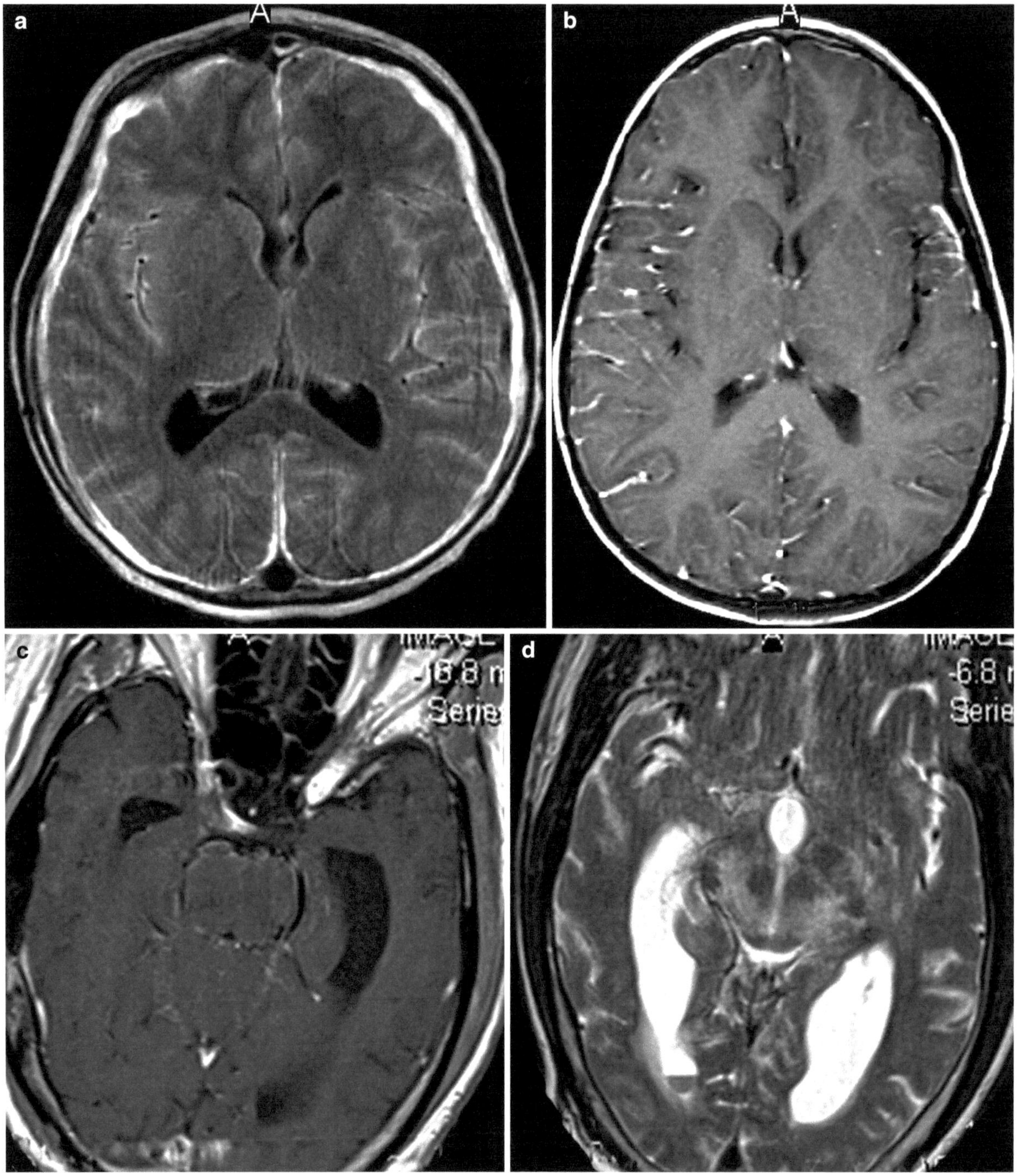

Fig. 31.5 (**a**, **b**) Acute meningitis; images include fluid-sensitive, FLAIR T2-w sequence (**a**) and post-contrast T1-w (**b**) axial sequences. Findings in acute meningitis are frequently subtle especially viral meningitis. The FLAIR sequence. A presents normal CSF within the ventricles and sulci as hypointense (dark) relative to the brain. With pial inflammation, there is a leak of proteinaceous fluid into the subpial and subdural spaces. This highly proteinaceous fluid is hyperintense (bright relative to the brain) and thus becomes visualized on fluid-sensitive MRI sequences. Serous subdural effusions are often present as well, which are imaged as high-intensity fluid outside the brain, as in this case, but without contrast enhancement along their surfaces. These types of fluid collections are considered noninfective and they typically clear spontaneously after medical treatment. The contrasted MRI (**b**) demonstrates pial hyperemia along the right lateral cerebral convexity (compared to *left side*). On the left, there is thickening of the pia probably early subpial empyema. (**c**, **d**) Listeria rhombencephalitis; images include post-contrast T1-w section (**c**) and a T2-w sequence (**d**). When the distribution of the inflammatory process involves mainly the upper brain stem, as in this instance, it is described as rhombencephalitis. Rhombencephalitis is uncommon but is one of the manifestations of Listeria-based meningitis, as in this case. Note there is relatively little abnormal enhancement in this case of Listeria infection. If there is a thick obvious enhancement in a similar distribution, findings would be more consistent with a granulomatous infection, as in fungal or tuberculous meningitis. Similar findings can also be part of noninfectious granulomatous pial disease, as in neurosarcoidosis and non-Langerhans histiocytosis; thus, tissue confirmation is usually necessary

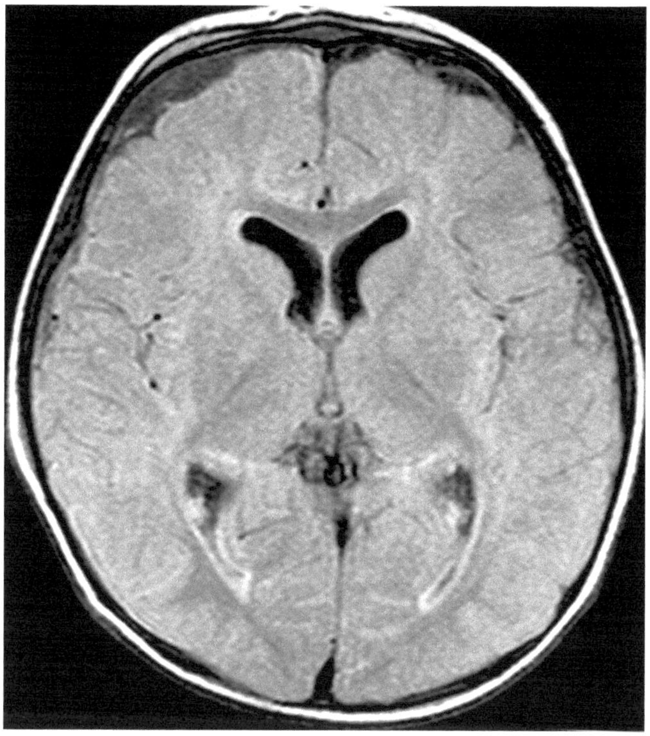

Fig. 31.6 Active meningitis and secondary subdural effusions. This FLAIR sequence, which emphasizes tissue edema, but deemphasizes bulk CSF signal, shows increased signal along the trigones of the lateral ventricular surfaces indicative of ependymitis, plus increased signal along the pial surfaces indicative of meningitis, plus minimal ventriculomegaly. All of these findings commonly occur in acute meningitis. Additionally, there are small bifrontal extra-axial fluid collections without any signal along their margins which are consistent with likely sterile subdural effusions. The fluid signal is minimally higher than CSF within the lateral ventricles indicating elevated CSF protein, a feature common to reactive subdural effusions

Treatment

The pathophysiology of the blood–brain barrier is of critical importance in determining the choice of antimicrobials for the treatment of acute bacterial meningitis. The permeability of the blood–brain barrier depends on the degree of inflammation of the meninges as well as the properties of the antimicrobial (e.g., lipid solubility, molecular size, and molecular structure). For example, chloramphenicol, which is highly lipid soluble, will readily penetrate uninflamed meninges. In inflamed meninges, therapeutic concentrations of penicillins, cephalosporins, and vancomycin can be achieved for the treatment of most cases of bacterial meningitis. Since only the free, unbound portion of an antimicrobial agent is capable of crossing the blood–brain barrier, the degree of protein binding of the antimicrobial in the serum is critical in determining how much of the agent eventually gets through to the CSF. As concentrations of protein increase in the CSF, protein binding becomes a significant factor in the effectiveness of those antimicrobials that are highly protein-bound.

The penetration of aminoglycosides is generally so poor that they are of little value in the treatment of acute meningitis when given intravenously, although they may be useful intrathecally. The penetration of the third-generation cephalosporins (e.g., ceftriaxone and cefotaxime) is significantly better than that of the first- and second-generation cephalosporins. Quinolones, tetracyclines, and macrolides do not penetrate the blood–brain barrier sufficiently to be useful first-line agents in the treatment of meningitis, whereas sulfa agents (e.g., trimethoprim-sulfamethoxazole) and vancomycin, in the presence of inflamed meninges, may reach sufficient concentrations to be of therapeutic value.

Treatment regimens for acute bacterial meningitis in children above the age of 3 months and in adults up to the age of 50 are geared towards treating the most common pathogens: *N. meningitidis*, *S. pneumoniae*, and, less commonly, *H. influenzae*. The prevalence of penicillin-resistant *S. pneumoniae* has risen so that more than 50% of strains may be resistant or exhibit intermediate resistance to penicillin in some parts of the United States and other countries. By definition, pneumococci are considered susceptible to penicillin if the minimum inhibitory concentration (MIC) < 0.06 μg/mL and resistant if >0.12 μg/mL. If penicillin-resistant but susceptible to third-generation cephalosporins (i.e., MIC <1.0 μg/mL) treatment with ceftriaxone would be appropriate. Among penicillin-resistant strains, resistance to the third-generation cephalosporins, including cefotaxime and ceftriaxone, has been increasing; resistance to ceftriaxone as high as 35–38% has been documented for *S. pneumoniae* isolates in some areas [53–56].

Once a clinical diagnosis of acute bacterial meningitis is suspected or made, institution of antimicrobial therapy should be immediate. If clinical evaluation is concerning for raised intracranial pressure, such as if the patient manifests signs of papilledema or focal neurological deficits, blood should be drawn for culture and baseline testing (e.g., white blood count and glucose) and empiric antimicrobial therapy initiated before imaging is obtained. Choice of empirical antimicrobial therapy is dictated by the age of the patient, vaccine status, and whether bacterial meningitis was acquired in the community or within the healthcare setting.

For community-associated meningitis, the microorganisms most commonly implicated are *S. pneumoniae*, *N. meningitidis*, *Listeria* spp., other *Streptococcus* spp., *S. aureus*, and *H. influenzae*. Healthcare-associated meningitis usually follows neurosurgical procedures, such as craniotomy, placement of ventriculostomy tubes, or deep brain stimulation of the brain for Parkinson's disease; pathogens most commonly implicated in healthcare settings include gram-negative microorganisms (e.g., *Enterobacteriaceae* and non-fermenters), *S. aureus*, and *Streptococcus* spp.

Initial empirical therapy for community-acquired meningitis: for adults and children 3 months–50 years, ceftriaxone

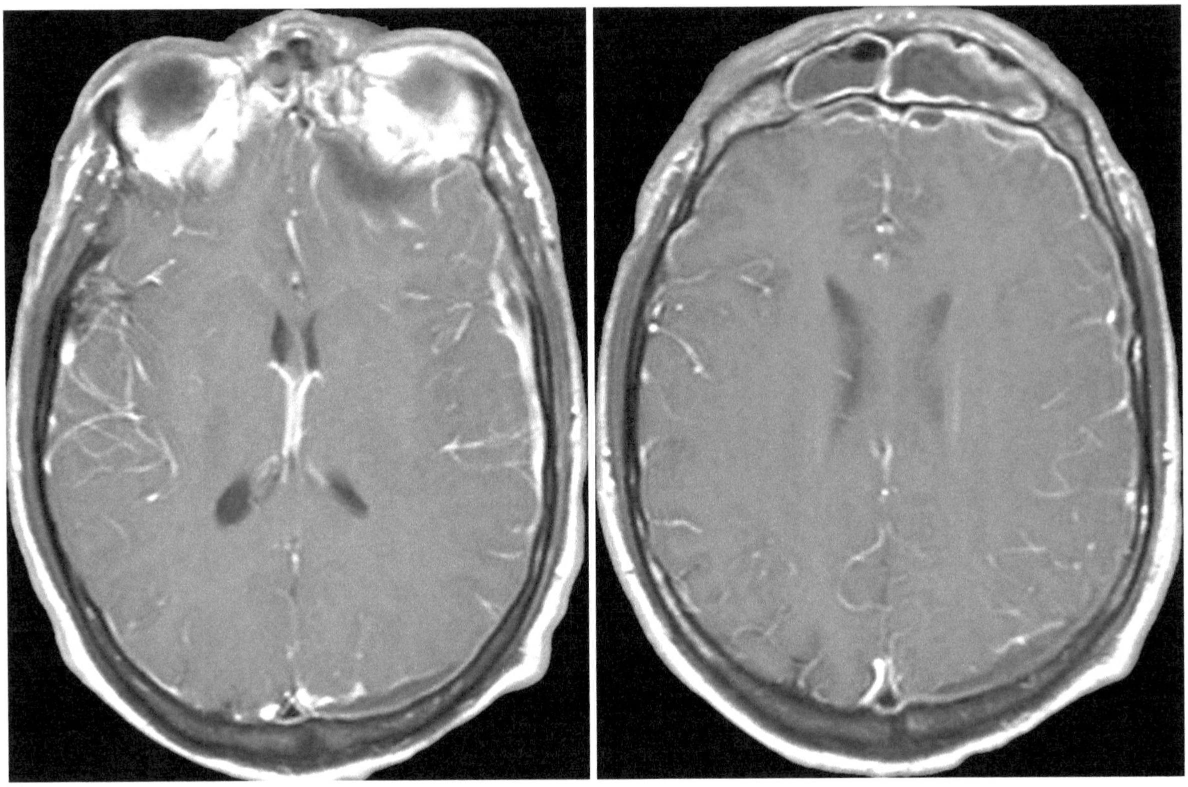

Fig. 31.7 Acute frontal sinusitis with secondary subdural empyema; images include contiguous post-contrast mid-convexity axial MRI sections. This case illustrates the spread pattern of subdural empyema. The source of the infection is the frontal sinus. Once the infection accesses the subdural space it can spread widely within the intracranial compartment. In this instance, it continues to the occipital region. These multicentric pockets of subdural empyema are often sequestered requiring multiple surgical drains. Thus, it is imperative that the full extent of the subdural empyema is appreciated

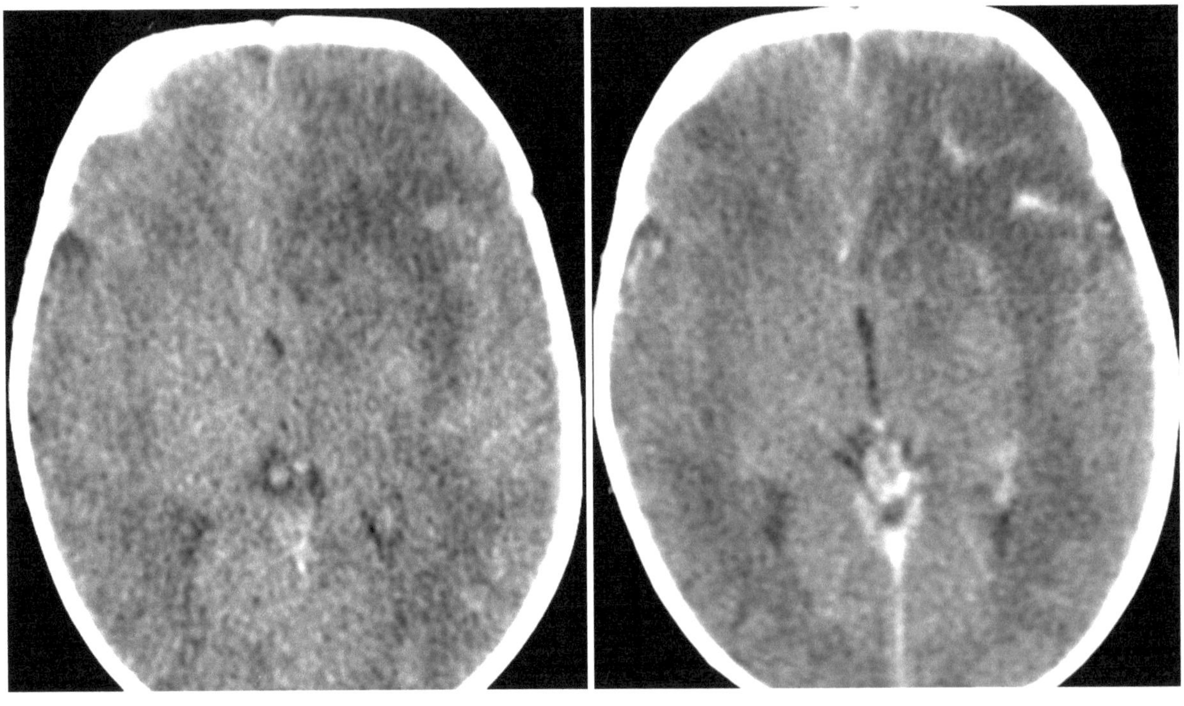

Fig. 31.8 Acute left frontal lobe bacterial cerebritis; images include pre and post-contrast CT sections sagittal projection lower thoracic area. The early phase of brain infection (early cerebritis) demonstrates nonspecific cerebral edema and poorly defined contrast enhancement. There is frequently reactive pial hyperemia. In later stages, the cerebritis will organize into early and then mature stages of brain abscess

or cefotaxime can be given, especially if risk factors (e.g., CSF leak, pneumonia, or sinusitis) for *S. pneumoniae* meningitis are present. If the patient is very sick or if gram-positive cocci are seen on CSF microscopy, vancomycin should be added to the therapeutic regimen to cover for penicillin-resistant *S. pneumoniae* in a dose of 2–3 g/day given every 8–12 h in adults and at 60 mg/kg for children in four divided doses, until it is known that the penicillin MIC is <0.1 µg/mL. For patients with a history of idiosyncratic reactions to penicillin or cephalosporins, vancomycin is recommended. In adults more than 60 years of age, patients with chronic alcoholism, immunosuppression, or other debilitating conditions, the possibility of *L. monocytogenes* meningitis should be considered. Empirical therapy to cover *L. monocytogenes* includes the addition of maximal doses of ampicillin (12 g daily dosed every 4 h) to the cephalosporin or vancomycin regimen until culture results for blood or CSF become available. For patients with penicillin allergy, the use of meropenem or trimethoprim/sulfamethoxazole can be considered as an alternative to cover for Listeria until culture results are available. Therapy may need to be broadened depending on the results of the gram stain. In cases where gram-negative diplococci are seen, it is prudent to wait until culture results confirm *N. meningitidis* before narrowing the bacterial coverage to penicillin because of the possibility that the gram stain might have been misinterpreted. Treatment of the most common etiologic agents of acute bacterial meningitis is summarized in Table 31.3.

The utility of adjunctive therapy with dexamethasone in the treatment of acute bacterial meningitis remains controversial. The use of dexamethasone as an adjunct to therapy in acute bacterial meningitis is complex. It has been shown clearly in animal models and in patient studies that dexamethasone reduces the level of inflammation and reduces the levels of the inflammatory cytokines IL1 beta and tumor necrosis factor-alpha [57]. However, in an animal model, administration of dexamethasone together with vancomycin reduced the penetration of vancomycin into the CSF by 29% and lowered the rate of bacterial clearance during the first 6 h in animals who received an intermediate dose of vancomy-

Table 31.3 Therapy of acute bacterial meningitis

Empirical treatment for patients with suspected meningitis but negative gram stain or culture		
Age group	Likely organisms	Empiric regimen
Preterm to <1 month	Group B Streptococcus; *Escherichia coli*; *Listeria* sp.	Ampicillin 100 mg/kg IV q6 h *plus* cefotaxime 50 mg/kg IV q6 h or ampicillin 100 mg/kg IV q6 h *plus* gentamicin 2.5 mg/kg IV q8 h
1 month–50 years	*Streptococcus pneumoniae*; *Neisseria meningitidis*; *Haemophilus influenzae*; *Listeria* sp.	Adult: ceftriaxone 2 g IV q12 h or cefotaxime 2 g IV q4–6 h *plus* vancomycin 15 mg/kg q6–8 h
		Child: ceftriaxone 100 mg/kg/day IV (doses given q12 h) or cefotaxime 200–300 mg/kg/day IV (doses given q6 h) *plus* vancomycin 60 mg/kg/day IV (doses given q6 h)
>50 years	*S. pneumoniae*; *N. meningitidis*; *H. influenzae*; *Listeria* sp.; aerobic gram-negative microorganisms	Ampicillin 2 g IV q4 h *plus* ceftriaxone 2 g IV q12 h or cefotaxime 2 g IV q6 h *plus* vancomycin 15 mg.kg IV q8–12 h
Trauma: skull fracture	*S. pneumoniae*; *H. influenzae*; Group B Streptococcus	Vancomycin 15 mg kg IV q8–12 h *plus* ceftriaxone 2 g IV q12 h
Trauma: penetrating	*Staphylococcus aureus*, coagulase-negative staphylococcus, *Enterobacteriaceae*, *Pseudomonas* spp.	Vancomycin 15 mg.kg IV q8–12 h *plus* cefepime 2 g IV q8 h
Meningitis associated with shunts	*S. aureus*, coagulase-negative staphylococcus, *Enterobacteriaceae*, *Pseudomonas* spp.	Vancomycin 15 mg kg IV q8–12 h *plus* cefepime 2 g IV q8 h
Neurosurgery (e.g., craniotomy)	*S. aureus*, coagulase-negative staphylococcus, *Enterobacteriaceae*, *Pseudomonas* spp.	Vancomycin 15 mg kg IV q8–12 h *plus* cefepime 2 g IV q8 h
Therapy for patients with acute bacterial meningitis (suggested by gram stain or culture)—by microorganism		
Microorganism	**Treatment**	**Duration of therapy (days)**
Streptococcus pneumoniae		
Penicillin-susceptible isolate (MIC <0.1 µg/mL)	Adults: penicillin G four million units IV q4h or ampicillin 2 g IV q4–6 h	10–14
	Children: 250,000–400,000 U/kg IV q4–6 h	
	Severe penicillin allergy: substitute cephalosporin agent with chloramphenicol 75–100 mg/kg/day in 4 divided doses	

(continued)

Table 31.3 (continued)

Empirical treatment for patients with suspected meningitis but negative gram stain or culture		
Age group	Likely organisms	Empiric regimen
Isolate with intermediate (MIC = 0.1–1 μg/mL) susceptibility to penicillin	Ceftriaxone 2 g IV q12 h or cefotaxime 2 g IV q4–6 h	
Isolate resistant (≥2 μg/mL) to penicillin	Ceftriaxone 2 g IV q12 h or cefotaxime 2 g IV q4–6 h *plus* vancomycin 15 mg/kg q6–8 h	
Neisseria meningitidis	Adults: penicillin G four million units IV q4 h or ampicillin 2 g IV q4–6 h or ceftriaxone 2 g IV q12 h or cefotaxime 2 g IV q4–6 h. Penicillin allergy: as for *S. pneumoniae* above	7
	Children: penicillin G 250,000–400,000 U/kg IV q4–6 h. Penicillin allergy: substitute with chloramphenicol 75–100 mg/kg/day in 4 divided doses	
Haemophilus influenzae		
Beta-lactamase positive	*Ceftriaxone 2 g IV q12 h or cefotaxime 2 g IV q6 h*	**7**
Beta-lactamase negative	*Ampicillin 2 g IV q q4–6 h*	
Group B Streptococcus (Streptococcus agalactiae)		
Suspected/empiric	Preterm: ampicillin 200–300 mg/kg/day IV in 3 divided doses *plus* cefotaxime	14–21
	Infants ≤7 days: ampicillin 200–300 mg/kg/day IV in 3 divided doses *plus* an aminoglycoside, adjusted for age and birth weight (BW), i.e., gentamicin 2.5 mg/kg IV q12 h; 2.5 mg/kg IV q8–12 h if BW < 2000 g; 2.5 mg/kg IV q8 h if BW > 2000 g	
	Infants >7 days: ampicillin 300 mg/kg/day iv in 4–6 doses/day *plus* an aminoglycoside, adjusted for age and BW, i.e., gentamicin 2.5 mg/kg IV q8–12 h if BW < 2000 g; 2.5 mg/kg IV q8 h if BW > 2000 g	
	Intraventricular treatment not recommended	
Known	Adults: penicillin G four million units IV q4h *plus* gentamicin 3–5 mg/kg IV daily, divided q8 h	14–21
	Infants ≤ 7 days: penicillin G 250,000–450,000 U/kg/day IV in 3 divided doses	
	Infants > 7 days: penicillin G 450,000 U/kg/day IV	
Listeria monocytogenes		
	Infants ≤ 7 days: ampicillin 200–300 mg/kg/day IV in 3 divided doses *plus* an aminoglycoside, adjusted for age and BW, i.e., gentamicin 2.5 mg/kg IV q12 h if BW < 2000 g; 2.5 mg/kg IVq12 h if BW > 2000 g	21 or longer
	Infants > 7 days: ampicillin 300 mg/kg/day IV in 4–6 doses/day plus an aminoglycoside, adjusted for age and BW, i.e., gentamicin 2.5 mg/kg IV q8–12 h if BW < 2000 g; 2.5 mg/kg IV q8h if BW > 2000 g	
	Adults >50, alcoholism, or other risk factors: ampicillin 2 g IV q4 h *plus* ceftriaxone 2 g IV q12 h or cefotaxime 2 g IV q6 h *plus* gentamicin 2 mg IV loading dose, then 1.7 mg/kg q8h *plus* dexamethasone 0.4 mg/kg IV q12 h × 2	
	Penicillin allergy: trimethoprim/sulfamethoxazole	
	Consider stopping gentamicin after 1 week	
	Where ampicillin is suggested, amoxicillin may be used	
Pseudomonas aeruginosa	Ceftazidime 1 g IV q8 h or cefepime 2 g IV q8 h *plus* gentamicin 3–5 mg/kg IV daily divided q8 h	21
Enterobacteriaceae (e.g., *Escherichia coli*)	Ceftriaxone 2 g IV q12 h or cefotaxime 2 g IV q4–6 h *plus* gentamicin 3–5 mh/kg IV daily divided q8 h	21

cin. Animals that received a higher dose had therapeutic peaks maintained despite steroid use, suggesting that the anti-inflammatory effect of the steroids, which reduce entry of antibiotics into the CSF, may be overcome to some extent by increasing the dose [58]. In animal studies of experimental pneumococcal meningitis, an antibiotic-induced secondary inflammatory response in the CSF was demonstrated only in animals with high initial CSF bacterial concentrations; these effects were modulated by dexamethasone therapy [59].

Human studies of the use of dexamethasone have clearly shown that there is a reduction in severe hearing loss in patients who have *H. influenza* type b meningitis and there is a similar reduction in overall neurologic complications although perhaps not as significant. In children with meningitis due to *S. pneumoniae*, there also appears to be a significant reduction in long-term hearing loss [60]. Major side effects from dexamethasone include secondary fever and a small incidence of gastrointestinal bleeding which is probably negligible if treatment is limited to 2 days but increases up to 3% in patients who receive 4 or more days of treatment or more.

In summary, dexamethasone probably should be used as an adjunct in children at a dose of 0.4 mg/kg IV every 12 h for no more than 2 days and probably should be given just before, or at the time of, the first antibiotic dose to block any increase in any inflammatory cytokine production following initial bacterial lysis. A 2015 Cochrane review of the use of corticosteroids in patients of all ages with bacterial meningitis showed insufficient evidence for a reduction in overall mortality but did show lower rates of hearing loss and neurological sequelae [61].

The duration of treatment of bacterial meningitis is based on empiric observation. In cases of *Streptococcus pneumoniae* meningitis treatment should stop in 10 days if patients have recovered, otherwise continue therapy for 14 days. In cases of penicillin or cephalosporin resistance, treat for 14 days. In patients with *Listeria monocytogenes* and *Enterobacteriaceae* meningitis treatment should be continued for 14 days [62].

In general, the minimum duration treatment is 7 days if the patient is afebrile for the last 4–5 days. Treatment of *S. pneumoniae* generally takes longer than *H. influenzae* and *N. meningitidis* and may be extended to 10–14 days, depending on the patient's response. Meningitis following trauma and neurosurgical procedures is discussed elsewhere.

Complications

Elevated ICP is a result of cerebral edema due to acute bacterial meningitis and should be anticipated. Clinical manifestations of raised ICP include bradycardia, hypertension, altered mental status, drowsiness, obtundation and coma, third cranial nerve palsies (including unilateral or bilateral dilated, poorly reactive, or nonreactive pupils), abnormal ocular movement, abnormal respiration, or decerebrate posturing. Papilledema is relatively uncommon and as such is an unreliable sign of raised ICP as it may take several hours to develop after the ICP has increased. Signs of herniation may supersede those of increased pressure and include unequal, dilated, or nonreactive pupils, dysconjugate eye movements, decorticate and decerebrate posturing, and bradycardia with abnormal respiratory patterns.

Patients who are awake and alert can be monitored closely. Patients who are obtunded or comatose, or who manifest other signs of increased ICP may benefit from ICP monitoring. Pressures exceeding 20 mmHg should be treated and some studies suggest that even pressures >15 mmHg may benefit from treatment [63]. An indication for treating at lower pressure levels is the phenomenon of "plateau waves" (Fig. 31.9), which are large elevations in pressure that occur spontaneously, or due to changes in cerebral blood flow, small shifts in intracranial blood volume resulting from hypoxia, fever, or otherwise innocuous events like tracheal suctioning. When these waves develop on a background of already increased ICP, herniation, and irreversible brain stem injury may ensue [62–64].

The treatment of increased ICP includes elevation of the head of the bed to 30° above the horizontal to facilitate venous drainage, intubation, and hyperventilation to reduce and maintain the arterial $PaCO_2$ concentrations to levels between 27 and 30 mmHg. Hypertonic osmotic agents, such as mannitol or hypertonic saline infusions, play a vital role in

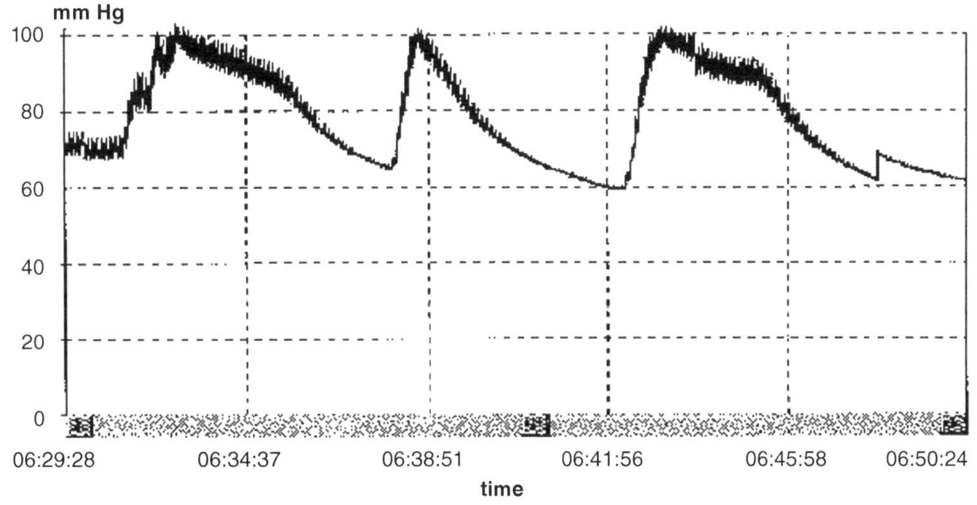

Fig. 31.9 Plateau waves: characterized by a sudden rapid elevation of intracranial pressure to 50–100 mmHg for 5–20 min. After a sustained period of elevation, the termination of the wave is characterized by a rapid decrease in ICP. These waves are thought to be caused by changes in cerebral blood flow

the reduction of elevated intracranial pressure and treatment of cerebral edema in patients with CNS infections [65–70]. Both mannitol and hypertonic saline reduce cerebral edema in many clinical syndromes [65–69]. However, data suggest that hypertonic saline appears to achieve a greater reduction in ICP than other osmotic agents [65, 67]. The objective in using osmotic agents is to achieve a sustained reduction in intracranial pressure by modifying the modes and rates of administration of the respective osmotic agent [65–69].

Phenobarbital therapy may be considered if raised ICP remains uncontrolled by the aforementioned interventions. Caution is advised in the use of hyperventilation to lower arterial $PaCO_2$ concentrations because overly vigorous treatment may cause these values to fall below 25 mmHg, running the risk of further reductions in cerebral blood flow causing cerebral ischemia. The dose of mannitol in children is 0.5–2.0 g/kg infused over 30 min and repeated as necessary; in adults, the usual dose is 0.25–1 g/kg bolus injection and 0.25 g/kg every 2–3 h as needed. Mannitol and hypertonic saline act as hyperosmolar agents and remain almost entirely within the intravascular space, producing an osmotic gradient that shifts intracranial fluid into this space. Serum osmolality should be frequently checked and kept between 315 and 320 mOsm/L [63–65, 69–73].

Dexamethasone has been used to reduce intracranial swelling in other settings primarily because of its effectiveness in vasogenic cerebral edema. Various clinical studies support the use of adjunctive dexamethasone in infants or children with *H. influenza* type b meningitis to reduce the risk of neurologic and audiologic complications, especially in those with raised ICP or coma. High-dose barbiturates may be helpful when other methods have failed to control increased ICP. Barbiturates decrease the CNS metabolic demand for oxygen thereby decreasing cerebral blood flow which, in turn, causes a fall in ICP. Phenobarbital is given at an initial dose of 5–10 mg/kg, at a rate of 1 mg/kg per minute followed by 1–3 mg/kg/h [63, 64]. Such therapies require regular ICP measurements and monitoring of cerebral electrical activity with electroencephalography. Phenobarbital is given until the ICP falls to levels 20 mmHg or until approximately 90% burst suppression on the EEG (i.e., nine out of the ten screens of the EEG are flat) has been achieved. Serum phenobarbital concentrations should be kept within the range of 20–40 μg/mL. Pentobarbital is preferred because of its relatively short half-life (24 h) versus phenobarbital with a relatively longer half-life. Side effects of high-dose barbiturate therapy include cardiac depression with dysrhythmias and hypotension, thus mandating invasive hemodynamic monitoring in these patients.

Seizures

Seizures occur in approximately 30–40% of children and adults with acute bacterial meningitis within the first few days of illness. If not treated, seizures may progress to status epilepticus, which in turn can lead to anoxic damage of the temporal lobe, cerebellum, and thalamus. The principles of therapy are to control seizure activity quickly and definitively. To initiate therapy, short-acting anticonvulsants, such as lorazepam or diazepam, are administered followed by a long-acting agent like phenytoin. Lorazepam is given IV in doses of 1–4 mg in adults, and 0.05 mg/kg in children. Phenytoin is given IV at a dose of 18–20 mg/kg and a rate of no more than 50 mg/min. The rate should be decreased if signs of toxicity, such as hypotension or a prolonged QT interval, develop. If phenytoin is not successful in controlling seizure activity, intubation and treatment with IV phenobarbital may be necessary. Patients must be watched and monitored carefully for signs of toxicity, such as hypotension and respiratory depression. Phenobarbital should be given IV at a rate of 100 mg/min until seizure activity stops, up to an initial dose of 20 mg/kg.

In children, the phenobarbital rate should be decreased to 30 mg/min. Should these measures fail to control seizures, general anesthesia, and additional phenobarbital therapy may have to be considered.

Vaccination for Meningitis

N. meningitidis became a leading cause of bacterial meningitis in the United States after dramatic reductions in the incidence of *S. pneumoniae* and *H. influenzae* type b infections had been achieved as a result of using conjugate vaccines [1, 3, 4, 74, 75]. However, since 2000, meningococcal disease incidence has decreased and incidence for serogroups C and Y, which represent the majority of cases of vaccine-preventable meningococcal disease, is at historic lows. In 2005, a quadrivalent meningococcal polysaccharide-protein conjugate vaccine (MenACWY, covering serogroups A, C, Y, and W-135) was licensed for use among persons aged 11–55 years. The most recent ACIP 2020 update recommends routine vaccination of adolescents aged 11–12 years with MenACWY followed by a booster at age 16 years. This update also provides additional dosing recommendations for individuals at higher risk of meningococcal disease. A 2-dose MenB vaccination series, which covers serogroup B, is recommended for adolescents and young adults ages 16–23 as well as those at increased risk of meningococcal disease [3].

Persons at increased risk for severe pneumococcal disease include those who are immunocompromised, asplenic or splenectomized, or patients with chronic illness such as chronic cardiovascular disease (e.g., congestive heart failure or cardiomyopathies), chronic pulmonary disease, diabetes mellitus, alcoholism, chronic liver disease (cirrhosis), or CSF leaks. CDC has updated recommendations from ACIP for prevention of invasive pneumococcal disease (i.e., bacteremia, meningitis, or infection of other normally sterile sites) through the use of the 23-valent pneumococcal polysaccharide vaccine among all adults aged ≥65 years and those adults aged 19–64 years with underlying medical conditions that put them at greater risk for serious pneumococcal infection [76].

Viral Meningitis and Encephalitis

Viral CNS infections may be classified as exogenous, due to infection with a viral agent acquired outside the host, or endogenous due to reactivation of viruses that have remained latent in the host. The majority of viral CNS infections are caused by exogenously acquired enteroviruses (Coxsackie virus A and B, echovirus, polio virus), arboviruses, and, less commonly, by HSV, mumps virus, varicella-zoster virus (VZV), cytomegalovirus (CMV), Epstein-Barr virus (EBV), adenovirus, human immunodeficiency virus (HIV), West Nile virus (WNV), rabies virus, or lymphocytic choriomeningitis virus. HSV encephalitis is unique in that it may occur as part of the primary infection or be seen in patients in whom the infection has been latent for many years. CNS infections due to the other herpes viruses, such as EBV, VZV, or CMV occasionally may be seen as part of the primary infection but may also occur as reactivated infections in patients who are immunosuppressed or HIV-infected.

Epidemiology

Meningitis and meningoencephalitis are the most common viral CNS infections encountered in the United States. The overwhelming majority of these infections are caused by enteroviruses, which produce disease in outbreaks occurring mainly during the summer months but may occur during May to October in warmer parts of the United States. The five most commonly reported serotypes (Enterovirus D68, Echovirus 30, Coxsackievirus A6, Echovirus 18, and Coxsackievirus B3) in descending order of frequency accounted for approximately 75% of all reports in the US between 2014 and 2016 [77]; CSF was the most common specimen type. The epidemiologic pattern is one in which certain strains cause disease endemically, while other strains occur in sporadic outbreaks varying from year to year in different regions. Enteroviruses are transmitted from person to person by the fecal-oral route and their activity tends to be increased in areas of overcrowding, poverty, and generally poor hygienic conditions.

Arboviruses account for most epidemic cases of encephalitis. Their occurrence follows an identical seasonal distribution to that of viral meningitis and meningoencephalitis associated with enteroviruses. However, the mode of transmission is completely different. Arboviruses are spread by the bite of infected mosquitoes, which are part of a complex cycle of enzootic transmission between birds, mosquitoes, and small mammals. The epidemiology of these diseases may be affected in part by prevention efforts from the public health authorities. For example, many states maintain surveillance systems that include testing of mosquitoes for the presence of virus, as well as sentinel chicken flocks to determine arbovirus activity. Such efforts lead to early recognition of an outbreak and warnings by public health authorities for the population to take precautions such as insect repellants, wearing long-sleeved shirts, and avoiding outdoor activity in the early evening hours when transmission is most likely to occur. In addition, mosquito control activities may contribute to reduction in rates of infection.

Although rabies is rare among humans in the United States, potential exposures to rabid animals lead to between 16,000 and 39,000 persons receiving post-rabies exposure prophylaxis each year [78]. Since the 1950s, the incidence of rabies in domestic animals has declined dramatically because of immunization of dogs and other domestic animals. Unlike the situation in developing countries, wild animals are the most important potential source of rabies for both humans and domestic animals in the United States; most reported cases of rabies occur among raccoons, skunks, and foxes and various species of bats [78, 79].

Pathogenesis

Viral infection of the CNS occurs via two distinct routes: hematogenous and neuronal. Enteroviruses and arboviruses are carried to the CNS via the blood stream, while HSV and the rabies virus are carried to the CNS via nerve cells themselves. Because viruses must replicate intracellularly, the ability to cause disease is largely determined by whether viral surface proteins can attach to specific receptors on specific cells in affected tissues—i.e., tissue trophism. An example of viral tissue tropism being determined by the combination of viral surface proteins and specific tissue receptors is the binding of the HIV GP120 to the CD4+ receptor on T4 lymphocytes. Other tissues with HIV tropism include monocytes and derived cells (macrophages), Langerhans cells, glial cells, and dendritic cells, all of which express the CD4+ receptor. Cells that do not express this receptor generally do not become infected with HIV [80]. Given the importance of these surface binding sites for their respective cellular receptors, several viruses such as rhinovirus, influenza virus, and poliovirus have evolved molecular mechanisms to protect these sites from the host immune response.

Enteroviruses are transmitted in human populations largely through fecal–oral transmission. These viruses survive stomach acid, replicate in the intestine, and an initial viremia leads to infection of multiple organs within the body. A secondary viremia from these sources can lead to CNS involvement. The prompt production of antibodies disrupts this second viremia and prevents invasion of the CNS. In the case of arboviruses, humans typically become infected when an infectious mosquito pierces the host epidermis to take a blood meal, depositing the virus principally in the extravascular tissue, although direct inoculation into the bloodstream can occur. Local replication is followed by viremia, and brain involvement is probably determined by viral tropism and the rapidity of the host immune response.

For CNS infections that occur following a viremia, invasion of the brain involves attachment of the virus to the endothelial cells, presumably via specific receptors. Following invasion, an acute inflammatory reaction occurs with a perivascular distribution within the brain parenchyma and varying degrees of involvement of the meninges, depending on the infecting viral agent. The perivascular inflammatory response is predominately mononuclear although polymorphonuclear leukocytes may be seen. Infection of neural cells results in degenerative changes and phagocytosis by tissue macrophages or microglial cells. Some pathologic features are unique to certain viruses: for example, cerebral atrophy and production of multinucleated giant cells and multiple nodules of infected microglia are seen in the white matter in patients with HIV encephalitis (Fig. 31.10), or the characteristic features of multinucleation, nuclear molding, chromatin margination, ground glass nuclei, and Cowdry type A intranuclear inclusion bodies seen in HSV infections (Fig. 31.11), with extensive asymmetrical necrosis in the temporal lobes, in the insulae, and in the cingulate gyri, typically seen in neuroimaging studies (Fig. 31.12a, b) [81]. In the case of rabies, histopathologic evidence of rabies encephalomyelitis (inflammation) in brain tissue and meninges includes mononuclear infiltration, perivascular cuffing of lymphocytes or polymorphonuclear cells, lymphocytic foci, Babes nodules consisting of glial cells, and the pathognomonic Negri body—an intracytoplasmic inclusion body within which the virus can be identified (Fig. 31.13a, b).

Some viral infections, most notably HSV and rabies, spread to the CNS via a neuronal route. In the case of HSV, the distribution involves the medial part of the temporal lobe bilaterally with one temporal lobe generally much more involved than the other. Autopsy studies carried out on patients who died during active HSV encephalitis show the presence of virus in the olfactory bulbs, olfactory tracts, and the tracts of the limbic system which end in the hippocampus, amygdala, insula, cingulate gyrus, and olfactory cortex [82]. Thus, the virus appears to gain access to the CNS from the nasal mucosa to the olfactory bulbs and olfactory tracts, although the mechanism by which the virus does this remains unknown. About two-thirds of cases of HSV encephalitis in adults and older children occur in patients who have antibodies to the virus at the time of infection. Many of these patients have a history of cold sores dating back 20–30 years. In the other one-third of patients, antibody to HSV is lacking at the time of onset of symptoms indicating that the encephalitis is likely part of the primary infection. Approximately 90–95% of the cases of HSV encephalitis in older children and adults are due to HSV type I, with the remaining 5–10% due to HSV type II. Neonatal herpes appears to be different, in that 90–95% of these cases are due to HSV type II acquired from maternal or other sources at the time of birth. Infection of the CNS in neonates generally follows systemic viremic spread; however, there is no temporal lobe localization.

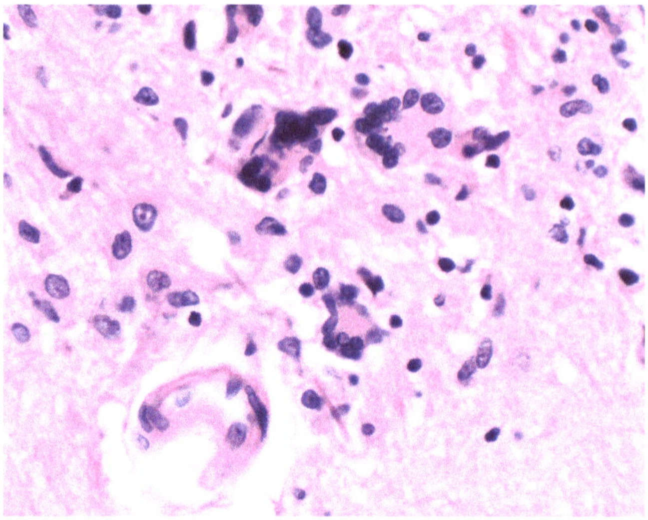

Fig. 31.10 Primary HIV infection of the CNS. The pathology specimen is from the brain of a 25-year-old male with recently diagnosed HIV. The patient developed pneumonia and died of respiratory failure. The figure shows perivascular inflammation with multiple giant cells involving a small vessel in the pons (H&E, 40×) (Courtesy of Anthony Yachnis, MD, and Kelly Devers, MD, University of Florida College of Medicine)

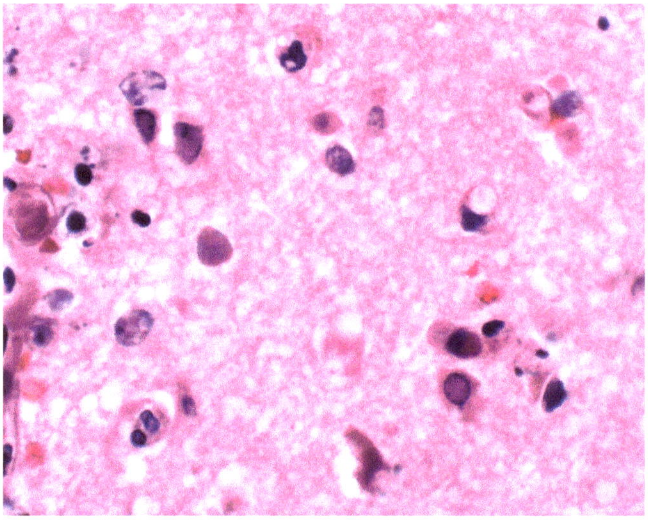

Fig. 31.11 Herpes encephalitis from an autopsy case: 32-year-old male patient with end-stage AIDS. Figure shows herpesvirus-infected neurons with marginated chromatin and glassy, smudged nuclei. H&E 60× (Courtesy of Anthony Yachnis, MD, and Kelly Devers, MD, University of Florida College of Medicine)

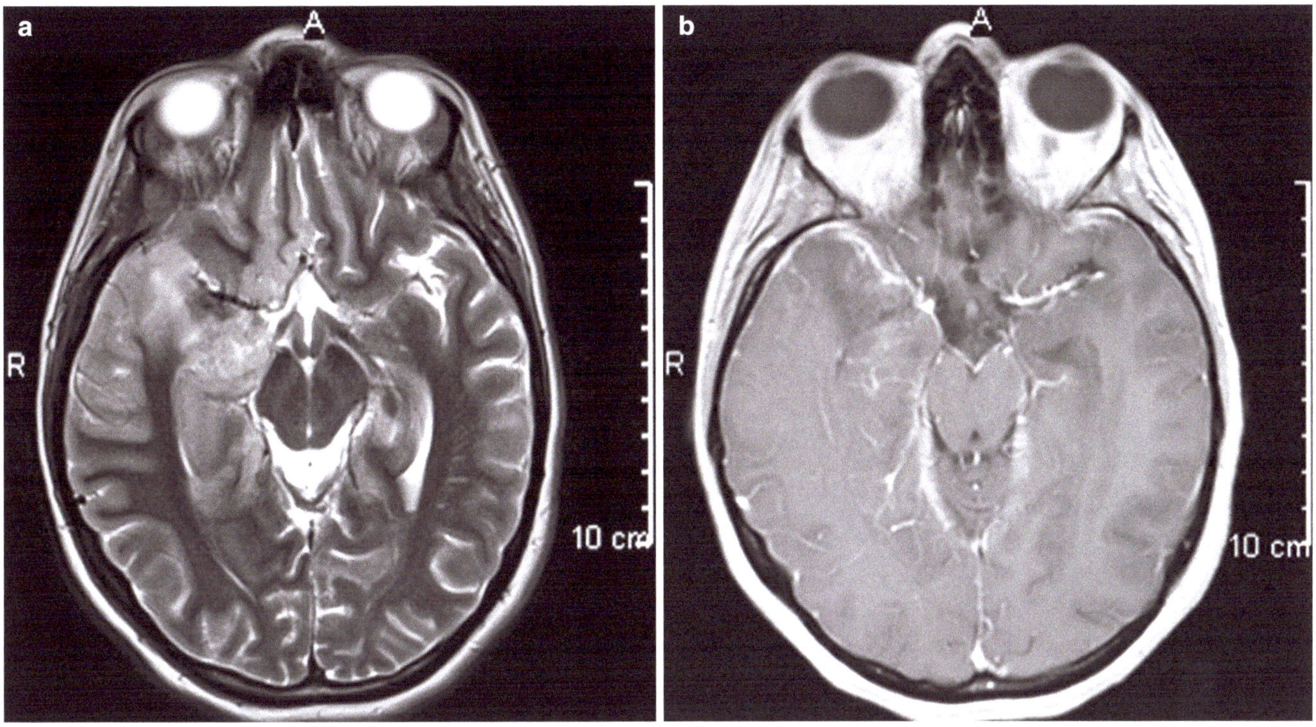

Fig. 31.12 (**a**, **b**) Herpes (HSV-1) encephalitis; images include low convexity axial T2-w sequence (**a**) and post-contrast T1-w sequence in the same brain section level. The T2-w image (**a**) illustrates cytogenic edema distributed not only within the anterior and mesial right temporal lobe but also within the frontotemporal association bundle and basi-frontal cortex. It involves gray and white matter. There is a less obvious change on the left. This pattern, in the right clinical context, is typical of HSV-1 cerebritis. It has a differential of tumoral gliomatosis, but the latter typically has a more prolonged presenting clinical course. The post-contrast T1-w image (**b**) demonstrates pial and perivascular enhancement. HSV-1 is an angiophilic organism that can produce a necrotizing intrinsic angiitis that can cause subarachnoid hemorrhage, although not in this case

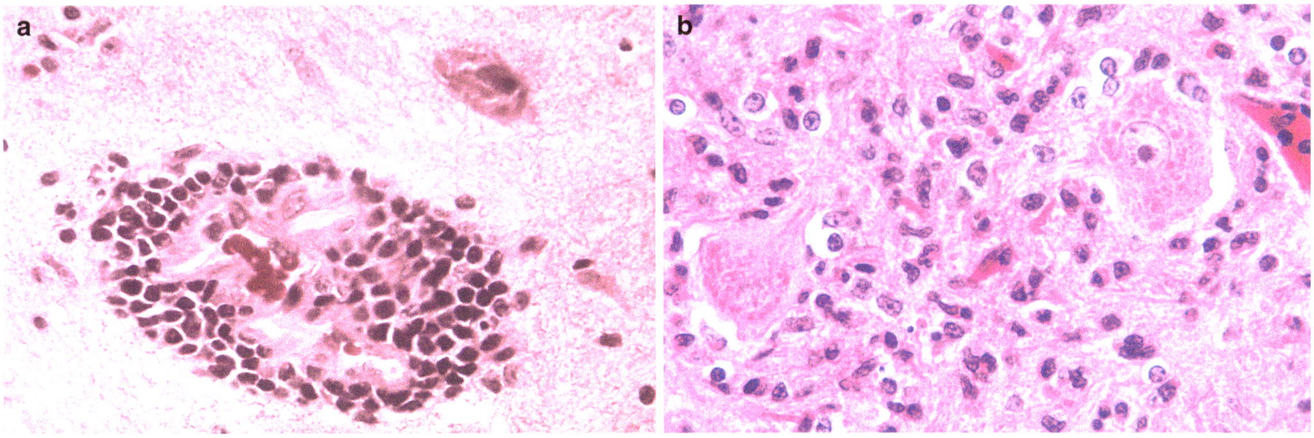

Fig. 31.13 (**a**) This micrograph depicts the histopathologic changes associated with rabies encephalitis prepared using an H&E stain. Note the perivascular cuffing due to the perivascular accumulation of inflammatory cell infiltrates (i.e., lymphocytes and polymorphonuclear leukocytes). Figure (**b**) is a photomicrograph of H&E stained brain tissue from a rabies encephalitis patient displaying the pathognomonic finding of Negri bodies within the neuronal cytoplasm (Both: Courtesy of the Centers for Disease Control and Prevention)

Rabies infection may result from contact with saliva or other secretions from infected animals as well as the animal bite itself. Rabies replicates initially at the local site of inoculation, and for this reason, emergency preventive measures, such as thorough cleansing of the wound and infiltration with human rabies immunoglobulin, can be effective in preventing infection. During local replication, the rabies virus invades the nerve sheaths and is transported via nerve cells to the CNS. The rapidity of the rabies virus in reaching the CNS is a function of the distance of the nerve endings from the CNS. Thus, bites on the lower extremities may take months to produce symptoms in the CNS, whereas bites in the face may reach the CNS within weeks. It is also important to recognize that the initial incident may be forgotten because of the length of time of the onset of CNS symptoms after the initial infecting event or because the inoculation event was not easily recognized, as has been reported for bats [83]. Therefore, a high index of suspicion for rabies is essential when managing patients with encephalitis of unknown cause, especially in patients who exhibit signs of hyperirritability.

Clinical Manifestations

Viral meningitis is an acute illness characterized by fever, headache, stiff neck, photophobia, and varying degrees of nonspecific symptoms such as malaise, myalgia, nausea, vomiting, abdominal pain, or diarrhea. Generally, neither disturbance of mental status nor abnormal neurological signs are characteristic of viral meningitis. The presence of obtundation, disorientation, seizures, or localized neurologic signs should suggest brain parenchymal involvement and a diagnosis of encephalitis or meningoencephalitis. Neck stiffness is generally less severe compared with bacterial meningitis. Clinical clues to an enteroviral etiology include the presence of a viral exanthem, pleuropericarditis, pleurodynia, painful oropharyngeal ulcers, or peripheral vesicular lesions suggestive of hand, foot, and mouth disease. The CSF in patients with viral meningitis is usually clear with an elevated white cell count; polymorphonuclear leukocytes may predominate within the first 24–48 h, although this number rarely exceeds 80% of total CSF white cells. CSF protein is generally mildly elevated, and the glucose is normal with the occasional exception in about 10–20% of patients with mumps and less often in patients with enterovirus or HSV infection. In viral meningitis, the CSF gram stain will be negative and routine CSF cultures will not yield bacterial growth. When the initial CSF analysis shows over 50% polymorphonuclear leukocytes, it is not uncommon for clinicians to repeat the lumbar puncture over the next 12–24 h to determine whether there is a shift towards a lymphocytic predominance, as one would expect in viral meningitis.

A parameningeal infectious focus (e.g., brain abscess) will characteristically be associated with a CSF pleocytosis, a likely elevated protein, and normal glucose. Thus, a patient with an epidural abscess or a brain abscess could present with mild headache, fever, and a CSF picture identical to that of viral meningitis. Some cases of sphenoid or frontal sinusitis may feature a CSF pleocytosis. Patients with fungal and tuberculous meningitis may also present with headache, fever, and stiff neck, but in general, the clinical course is longer than acute viral meningitis. The CSF in patients with fungal or tuberculous meningitis generally has a relatively low glucose level, usually <40 mg/dL.

The CSF in patients with cryptococcal meningitis may be completely normal. Fever, headache, and nonspecific CSF findings can also be seen in other infections, such as syphilis, ehrlichiosis, and noninfectious conditions, such as sarcoidosis, Behcet's disease, systemic lupus erythematosus, vasculitis, or uveoparotitis.

Viruses other than enteroviruses can also produce aseptic meningitis. For example, HSV type II produces very typical aseptic meningitis with low-grade fever, headache, stiff neck, and photophobia as part of primary genital herpes infection. Therefore, it is important to question the sexually active patient about a history of genital herpetic lesions and to perform a pelvic examination in women where indicated. Aseptic meningitis can also be seen as part of the syndrome of primary HIV infection. Certain strains of leptospirosis will typically present with aseptic meningitis; however, most cases present in conjunction with systemic disease and severe involvement of other organs such as lung, liver, and kidney. Lymphocytic choriomeningitis virus (LCMV) belongs to the family *Arenavirus* and is found globally [84]. LCMV meningitis is typically associated with exposure to rodents, such as common house mouse (*Mus musculus* and *M. domesticus*), hamsters, and guinea pigs. Transmission occurs by inhalation (aerosol and droplet), fomites, or direct contact with excreta or blood from infected rodents. The incubation period is 1–2 weeks; symptoms are nonspecific and include fever, chills, myalgia, headache, photophobia, anorexia, pharyngitis, and cough. CNS invasion is seen only in a few patients after an initial febrile illness. During the neurologic phase, patients acquire aseptic meningitis and peripheral leukocytosis. CSF leukocyte cell counts are often >1000 cells/μL, and glucose levels are low. LCMV meningitis may be associated with ascending paralysis, transverse myelitis, or encephalitis; overall case fatality is <1% [84].

The laboratory diagnosis of viral meningitis is generally one of exclusion. Viral cultures of CSF that yield growth of enteroviruses are diagnostic. However, these are positive in only 30–50% of cases. PCR has become available for the diagnosis of enteroviral meningitis, and these PCR platforms correlate very well with the results of viral culture. Unfortunately, PCR testing may not be routinely available at clinical microbiology laboratories for various reasons, including cost and lack of trained personnel. Sending specimens to reference laboratories or highly specialized research laboratories is an alternative but results generally will not be available during the acute phase of the patient's illness. In the case of HSV meningitis, the diagnosis is confirmed if HSV is cultured from CSF or detected by PCR. For aseptic meningitis associated with systemic infections, such as leptospirosis, syphilis, or ehrlichiosis, diagnosis can be confirmed through standard serologic testing generally available at state public health laboratories or reference laboratories.

Because there are over 75 different enterovirus serotypes, testing is only possible for a subset of these. In addition, there is tremendous overlap in the serologic response between the different serotypes such that seroconversion to one or more enterovirus serotypes can occur. Moreover, since there is no specific therapy, expensive laboratory testing is unlikely to affect patient outcomes. For these reasons, serologic studies for the diagnosis of enterovirus infections are generally not indicated.

A common diagnostic misconception is the usefulness of CSF antibodies. With the exception of the venereal disease research laboratory (VDRL) test, which indicates active CNS syphilis, and the ratio of measles antibodies in CSF to serum levels in extremely rare cases of subacute sclerosing panencephalitis (SSPE), routine CSF antibody testing does not affect patient outcomes. In general, infectious viral agents can more readily be diagnosed from serum rather than CSF studies. Tests for common viral infections and preferred diagnostic methods are outlined in Table 31.4.

Finally, certain drugs such as sulfa and nonsteroidal anti-inflammatory agents can produce acute syndromes of

Table 31.4 Laboratory diagnosis of selected viral diseases

Virus	CNS disease	Serology	Viral culture	Direct antigen	PCR/other
Herpes viruses					
Herpes simplex	Temporal lobe encephalitis	About 2/3 seropositive on admission, not helpful in Dx	Almost always negative in CSF, throat, etc.	None for CSF FA can be done on brain biopsy	≥90% sensitive on CSF—reference labs and some academic medical centers only
Varicella	Encephalitis in HIV patients	Not helpful diagnostically	Usually negative in CSF, throat, etc.	None for CSF FA can be done on brain biopsy	Reference labs only MRI may be suggestive
Cytomegalovirus	Encephalitis in HIV patients	Almost always positive	Urine, throat, blood may be positive—consistent with but not proof of encephalitis	Antigenemia test on blood, positive test consistent with but not proof of encephalitis	If CSF positive, encephalitis likely, but asymptomatic HIV patients may also be positive MRI may be suggestive
Epstein-Barr Virus	Rare encephalitis in mononucleosis	Monospot test good presumptive test, may be negative in up to 20% in first week VCA-IgG and IgM, positive IgM virtually diagnostic	Not available	Not available	Reference labs only, not needed for diagnosis
Human herpes virus 6 and 7 (HHV 6 and 7)	Seizures, encephalitis in 1–3 year olds	Reference labs only	Reference labs only	Not available	Reference labs only
Respiratory viruses					
Influenza A and B	Parainfluenza occasionally, others rarely cause encephalitis	Not useful	NP swabs; throat washings	Direct antigen ELISA available for RSV (excellent sensitivity), and Influenza (moderately sensitive)	Not available
Parainfluenza 1–3			Cultures via bronchoscopy		
Adenovirus			Excellent sensitivity, diagnostic if positive		
Respiratory syncytial virus (RSV)					

(continued)

Table 31.4 (continued)

Virus	CNS disease	Serology	Viral culture	Direct antigen	PCR/other
Enterovirus					
Coxsackie	Summertime outbreaks of meningitis, meningoencephalitis	Not useful: too many serotypes and too much cross-reactivity	Send stool, throat, CSF	None	Available in reference labs, picks up most serotypes, may take a week to get result
Echovirus			If throat or CSF culture positive—diagnostically definitive		
			If stool culture positive—presumptive (enteroviruses may be shed in stool for weeks)		
Arboviruses					
St. Louis encephalitis	Summertime outbreaks of encephalitis	Diagnostic, if positive	Generally not available	Not available	Not available
California encephalitis		Serum is preferred specimen; CSF not helpful			
Western equine		Done in reference laboratory and public health labs			
Eastern equine					
La Crosse					
West Nile virus					
HIV	Encephalopathy	ELISA	Research labs only	P 24 antigen in serum	Reference labs, many tertiary medical centers, used for following treatment
		Confirm with Western Blot			
Lymphocytic choriomeningitis virus	Meningitis	Reference laboratory	Not available	Not available	Not available
JC virus	Progressive multifocal leukoencephalopathy	Reference laboratory	Not available	Not available	Available in reference laboratories
	Mostly in HIV & other immunocompromised patients				Diagnostic if positive on CSF
					MRI highly suggestive
					Brain biopsy definitive
Rabies	Encephalitis	Reference or state public health labs	Research labs only	Direct fluorescent antibody staining of hair follicles in skin biopsy from nape of neck above the hairline—50% positive in first week, higher later	RT-PCR may be available in reference labs, state public health labs. Send saliva, CSF, or tissue
		Antibody is generally undetectable before day 6, 50% by day 8, and 100% by day 15			

Adapted with permission from Rand et al. [45]

aseptic meningitis (Table 31.5). Other noninfectious factors have been associated with an aseptic meningitis picture, including intravenous immunoglobulin, intrathecal administration of drugs, receipt of certain vaccines, malignancies, autoimmune conditions, and connective tissue disorders (Table 31.5) [85].

The hallmark of the presentation of viral encephalitis is fever, headache, confusion, drowsiness, and convulsions. Prominent signs include an altered level of consciousness with or without focal neurologic signs or meningism (i.e., the triad of neck stiffness, photophobia, and headache) in the setting of an acute febrile illness. By and large, the differential diagnosis is the same as for acute bacterial or viral meningitis. Varying degrees of nuchal rigidity can be present in patients with encephalitis. Lumbar puncture yields CSF with a picture similar to that of viral meningitis. HSV, VZV, arbo-

Table 31.5 Nonviral causes of aseptic meningitis and encephalomyelitis

Infective causes	
Ehrlichia spp.	Rocky Mountain spotted fever
Bacterial endocarditis	Brain abscess/cerebritis
Staphylococcus aureus	*Treponema pallidum* meningitis
Lyme disease	Leptospirosis
Mycoplasma pneumoniae	*Listeria monocytogenes* (rhomboid encephalitis)
Typhus	*Legionella* spp.
Cat-scratch disease	*Nocardia* spp.
Mycobacterium tuberculosis meningitis	*Cryptococcus neoformans meningitis*
Histoplasmosis	Coccidioidomycosis
Cerebral amebiasis	Cerebral malaria
Trypanosomiasis	Cerebral abscess and other parameningeal infections
Partially treated bacterial meningitis	CNS cysts (e.g., craniopharyngioma, dermoid/epidermoid)
Noninfective medical conditions	
Malignancy, especially lymphoma	Behçet's disease
Still's Disease	Systemic lupus erythematosus
Chronic subdural hematoma	Vasculitis
Intrathecal injections	Neurosurgery-related procedures
Drugs	
Certain nonsteroidal anti-inflammatory drugs	
Antimicrobial agents, including trimethoprim, cephalosporins, penicillin, amoxicillin, isoniazid, ciprofloxacin, metronidazole, and sulfonamides	
Carbamazepine	
Ranitidine, famotidine	
Azathioprine	
Sulfasalazine	
Indinavir	
Vaccines: measles, mumps, rubella (MMR), alone or in combination	
Monoclonal antibodies (e.g., muromonab-CD3) [OKT3] that targets the CD3 receptor	
Intravenous immunoglobulin	

Adapted with permission from Rand et al. [45]

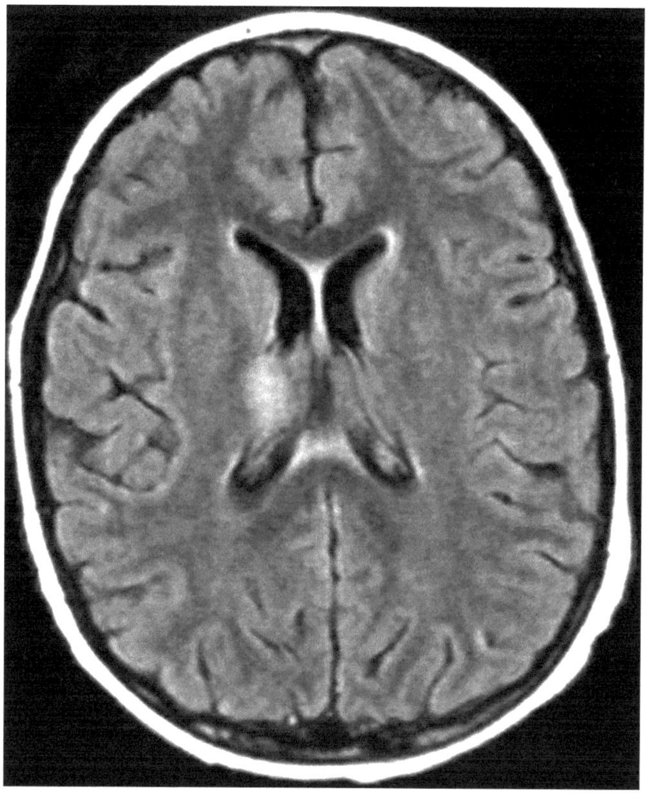

Fig. 31.14 West Nile viral thalamic encephalitis T2-w mid-convexity brain section. Arbovirus (West Nile virus in this example) encephalitis typically has multicentric areas of cytogenic edema, which typically involve gray matter both in the cortex and in the central nuclear structures. The lesions are usually multicentric but not symmetric between hemispheres. In this example, cytogenic edema is evident in the right thalamus and the splenium of the corpus callosum. The splenial abnormality can be from the virus but may also occur following recent seizure activity

viruses, and enteroviruses can now be diagnosed by PCR analyses of CSF specimens. MRI imaging is a useful test for ascertaining HSV encephalitis and for differentiating postinfectious encephalomyelitis from viral encephalitis. It is important to recognize that some patients with arbovirus encephalitis, particularly Eastern equine encephalitis and West Nile virus encephalitis, may have focal lesions by MRI (Fig. 31.14). However, the distribution of these lesions is not consistent and differs from the pattern seen in neuroimaging studies of HSV encephalitis (Fig. 31.12a, b). Diagnosis of arbovirus encephalitis can almost always be made by serological testing as antibody titers to all of the common arboviruses are generally present by the time the patient presents with symptoms. Because there is only a very low background frequency of these antibodies in the general healthy population, a positive arbovirus serology can be accepted as clinically definitive of exposure or infection.

The diagnosis of HSV encephalitis is of critical importance because of the effectiveness of acyclovir in improving patient outcomes. HSV is the most common cause of sporadic encephalitis. Patients with HSV type I encephalitis generally present with a 3- to 5-day history of fever, headache, and focal signs, including dysphasia and personality changes that may progress to obtundation and coma; the latter can occur abruptly and may be associated with the onset of seizures. HSV encephalitis can occur in any age group from childhood through old age at any time of the year—i.e., there is no characteristic seasonal variation pattern in occurrence. The incidence is estimated at 1 in 250,000 to 1 in

500,000 people per year; HSV encephalitis accounts for approximately 10–20% of viral encephalitides in the United States.

A diagnosis of HSV encephalitis is supported by MRI findings showing bilateral temporal lobe involvement that is generally asymmetrical (Fig. 31.12a, b). CT imaging may reveal frontotemporal changes in HSV encephalitis. In untreated patients, this may progress to hemorrhagic lesions; swelling of the more severely affected temporal lobe may result in a mass effect sufficient to produce a shift of the midline structures and tentorial herniation. PCR for HSV in the spinal fluid is almost uniformly positive in patients with HSV encephalitis, despite the fact that in 1–4% of cases, one cannot grow the virus from CSF or specimens from other anatomic sites in patients [86, 87]. The use of PCR in combination with the detection of a specific intrathecal antibody response to HSV currently represents the most reliable strategy for the diagnosis and monitoring of the treatment of adult patients with HSV encephalitis [86–89]. Serologic diagnosis is not particularly helpful early on, although generally, all patients with HSV encephalitis will show a significant rise in HSV titer both in the spinal fluid and serum. EEG studies may reveal focal features.

Conditions that mimic encephalitis include brain abscess, subdural empyema, cerebritis due to *Listeria* spp., mycoplasma, fungal infections, tuberculosis, cryptococcus, rickettsia, toxoplasmosis, mucor, and agents frequently associated with bacterial meningitis, such as pneumococcus and meningococcus (Fig. 31.5c, d) [90, 91]. Influenza A virus can cause encephalitis during epidemics; children are particularly affected. Tumors, subdural hematomas, CNS lupus, adrenal leukodystrophy, acute strokes, neuroleptic malignant syndrome, or Reye's syndrome can also mimic the symptoms and signs of encephalitis.

Encephalitis can sometimes occur as part of systemic infection with common viruses that do not normally produce encephalitis. For example, EBV infection can, on occasion, present with seizures and even coma; these patients generally recover completely. CNS involvement with toxoplasmosis, lymphoma, VZV, and CMV in HIV-infected patients can also mimic the features of encephalitis. Table 31.5 lists nonviral infections that may resemble viral encephalitis.

Although rare, rabies should be considered in atypical cases of encephalitis or in cases where the results of all investigations are negative. Because affected patients often do not have a clear history of an animal bite, a history of close contact with potentially infected animals, including bats, should be sought. Infection is almost always from inoculation but occasionally by inhalation. Rabies has been transmitted by corneal and solid organ allografts [92, 93]. The virus is transmitted to the CNS via nerve trunks. Proliferation in nerve cells in the brain and peripheral ganglia leads to fatal meningoencephalitis. The incubation period varies anywhere from 2 weeks to more than a year. Proximal bites with a relatively large inoculum of the virus tend to be associated with shorter incubation periods. The onset is rapid with fever, anxiety, insomnia, headache, malaise, myalgia, fatigue, anorexia, nausea, vomiting, sore throat, and cough. The patient may complain of symptoms suggestive of paresthesias or fasciculations at the site of the original animal bite due to viral replication at the site of inoculation or in the dorsal ganglia of the sensory nerve supplying that area. The disease quickly progresses to an encephalitic phase consisting of agitation, excitation, and excessive motor activity. Patients may experience hallucinations, become combative, and develop muscle spasms with opisthotonus and involvement of the respiratory muscles. Painful spasms of the throat muscles, precipitated by attempts to swallow, may follow, which may result in patients avoiding drinking or swallowing. Spasms may be precipitated by blowing air onto the face and seizures are common. Periods of hallucinations and aberrant mentation may alternate with lucid periods that get progressively shorter as the disease progresses. Hyperesthesias with excessive reactivity to normal stimulation of light, sound, and touch are very common; autonomic nervous system changes such as dilated pupils, increased salivation, lacrimation, perspiration, and postural hypotension also may occur. Ultimately, brain stem function is affected by cranial nerve palsies, optic neuritis, and the characteristic hydrophobia due to the painful, violent involuntary contractions of the muscles of respiration and those in the pharynx and the larynx, which are initiated by attempts to swallow. Eventually, the disease progresses to cardiorespiratory depression, coma, and death. Occasionally, rabies may present as an ascending paralysis clinically similar to the Guillain-Barré syndrome; corneal transplants from two patients presumed to have died from Guillain-Barré actually transmitted clinical rabies, resulting in the death of the recipients [94, 95]. The laboratory diagnosis of rabies requires viral isolation, positive serology (assuming the patient has not been immunized), or demonstration of the characteristic Negri bodies in brain tissue. Laboratory diagnostic evaluation for rabies includes serological testing plus demonstration of viral antigen by IFA in infected tissue, including corneal scrapings, skin biopsies or brain biopsies, and analysis of CSF or saliva specimens for rabies virus antigen or RNA [96]. Survival of patients with rabies is rare; most of the few who have survived received the rabies vaccine prior to the onset of illness.

In patients who have traveled overseas, encephalitis may be caused by various other infectious diseases, including Japanese B encephalitis, Murray Valley encephalitis, Omsk hemorrhagic fever, Kyasanur forest disease complex, Powassan virus, *louping ill*, Russian spring-summer encephalitis, Rift Valley fever, yellow fever, dengue, chikungunya,

Hantaan virus, Puumala virus (a species of hantavirus), and the highly fatal hemorrhagic fevers caused by the Marburg, Ebola, and Lassa fever viruses.

B virus infection is caused by Macacine herpesvirus 1 (formerly Cercopithecine herpesvirus 1 (CHV-1), an alpha-herpesvirus closely related to herpes simplex virus. B virus is also commonly referred to as herpes B, monkey B virus, herpesvirus simiae, and herpesvirus B. The virus is commonly found among macaque monkeys, including rhesus macaques, pig-tailed macaques, and cynomolgus monkeys (also called crab-eating or long-tailed macaques), any of which can harbor latent B virus infection and appear to be natural hosts for the virus. Monkeys infected with B virus usually have no or only mild symptoms. In addition, rabbits, guinea pigs, and mice can be experimentally infected with B virus. The virus is related to human HSV, but humans have little native ability to contain it in contrast to its natural host in whom it produces "cold sores." Human infection usually results from bites or scratches from macaques or mucocutaneous exposure to monkey saliva; laboratory personnel who work with ostensibly healthy monkeys or their tissues are particularly at risk. Indirect contact transmission, such as a needlestick injury with a contaminated needle has been documented. B virus is transmitted to humans from saliva in monkeys and reaches the brain via nerves at the site of the monkey bite. Patients acquire ascending myelitis and fulminant meningoencephalitis, which often leads to death. Infection is diagnosed by a rise in antibody titer or by isolating the virus from the CNS. There are seven different exposures for which post-exposure prophylaxis is recommended: if postexposure prophylaxis is administered, it should be started soon (within hours) after the exposure. Neurologic tests should include lumbar puncture and MRI of the brain; electroencephalography (EEG) should also be considered. CSF samples should be sent for culture, PCR detection of viral DNA, and serologic testing. While the use of intravenous acyclovir and ganciclovir therapy for patients with the early stages of B virus disease, including patients with early signs of CNS disease has been associated with increased survival for some patients, antiviral therapy is generally not effective in patients with advanced encephalomyelitis [97].

Treatment

No specific drug or serologic therapy is currently available for enterovirus or arbovirus infections. In general, viral meningitis due to enteroviruses is clinically mild, and most patients can be treated without admission to the hospital unless bacterial meningitis is a possibility in the differential diagnosis and needs to be ruled out. Patients with enteroviral meningitis usually recover within 7–10 days without antiviral therapy.

Intravenous acyclovir is indicated for patients with HSV or VZV meningitis. In patients with symptoms suggestive of encephalitis or brain parenchymal involvement, and in whom appropriate radiologic imaging studies have ruled out other pathology (such as brain abscess or subdural empyema), initiation of empiric intravenous acyclovir intravenously in doses appropriate for HSV encephalitis is indicated. The dose of acyclovir is 10 mg/kg IV every 8 h for 14–21 days. Timely diagnosis is of paramount importance since a successful outcome is largely associated with early initiation of acyclovir therapy. Brain biopsy is not indicated to prove the presence of herpes encephalitis prior to therapy. Before antiviral agents became available for the treatment of HSV encephalitis, the disease was fatal in approximately 70% of patients, with an additional 20–25% surviving with severe disabilities.

Brain Abscess

Brain abscesses have been recognized since the days of Hippocrates in 460 BC. By definition, a brain abscess is a localized suppurative infection of the brain parenchyma [98]. While the etiology and distribution of associated diseases have remained essentially unchanged over the years for pyogenic brain abscesses, the AIDS epidemic led to the occurrence of brain abscesses due to toxoplasmosis. The use of antiretroviral therapy (ART) has resulted in a reduction in morbidity and mortality in HIV-associated cerebral opportunistic infections.

Pathogenesis

Brain abscesses develop as localized areas of cerebritis (i.e., poorly demarcated areas of encephalitis), initially consisting of bacteria in the brain parenchyma together with inflammation and edema. This area of cerebritis subsequently becomes more localized with the development of necrosis in the middle and a ring-enhancing capsule. Ultimately, host defenses lead to the development of a well-formed fibrous capsule. The most common predisposing conditions for the development of a brain abscess are infections in the middle ear, paranasal sinuses, mastoids, and teeth (dental abscess). It is believed that bacteria reach the brain through valveless emissary veins, which traverse the cranium into the venous drainage system of the brain, or via retrograde spread through the venous system. Alternatively, direct extension through an area of osteitis or osteomyelitis adjacent to the sinus or middle ear infection provides access to the CNS. Chronic otitis media is a common predisposing factor with the abscesses most frequently forming in the temporal lobe or cerebellum. The other major mechanism by which the brain parenchyma becomes seeded is via metastatic transmission through the cerebral arteries from an extracranial focus of infection. Approximately 20% of brain abscesses arise from a contiguous focus; 25% are associated with hematogenous spread from a distant focus, such as a pyogenic lung abscess or bronchiectasis, and 25% occur following trauma [99–101].

Hematogenous brain abscesses generally tend to be multiple and are often located at the gray-white matter junction; they also tend to follow a vascular distribution within the brain. Hematogenous dissemination from a contiguous focus of infection has also been described. Other distant foci that have been associated with brain abscesses include wound infections, osteomyelitis, pelvic infections, cholecystitis, and other intra-abdominal foci. Any procedure that results in a transient bacteremia can on occasion be associated with the subsequent development of a brain abscess. Endocarditis accounts for only 1–5% of cases of brain abscess despite the relatively high frequency of bacteremia and involvement of the brain in 20–40% of cases [102, 103]. Patients with cyanotic congenital heart disease are at increased risk of acquiring brain abscesses. A significant number of brain abscesses are associated with penetrating trauma such as gunshot wounds, depressed skull fractures with retained bone fragments, and cranial penetration from objects such as pencils and animal bites. Cervical traction associated with pin-site infection can also pose a risk. In patients with HIV infection, reactivation of toxoplasmosis can lead to brain abscesses. In approximately 25% of cases, no underlying etiology can be established.

Microbiology

The bacterial etiology of brain abscesses is to a great extent dependent on the location of the abscess and the predisposing factors. Thus, aerobic, anaerobic, and microaerophilic streptococci are the most frequently isolated bacterial species. *Staphylococcus aureus* is the underlying cause of 25% of brain abscesses and is often associated with trauma, endocarditis, or following a neurosurgical procedure. In addition to streptococci, brain abscesses associated with paranasal sinus or chronic otitis media infection may be caused by *Haemophilus* species, *Bacteroides* species, other anaerobes, and *Pseudomonas aeruginosa*. If the source of bacteremia is intra-abdominal, *Enterobacteriaceae*, enterococci, and anaerobes are likely to be implicated. A urinary tract source is more likely associated with *Pseudomonas* spp. or *Enterobacteriaceae*, but not anaerobes. Brain abscesses caused by anaerobes, including actinomyces, may be associated with the spread from a lung abscess [104].

Although *S. aureus* is the most common organism complicating penetrating trauma, *Clostridium* species and *Enterobacteriaceae* are also commonly implicated. The nature of the precipitating trauma is important: for example, if trauma occurs in a water environment, *Pseudomonas* spp. and *Aeromonas* spp. may need to be considered. Microorganisms associated with postoperative infections include *S. aureus*, *Staphylococcus epidermidis* and *Enterobacteriaceae*, and *Pseudomonas* spp.

Nocardia species are uncommon but important causes of brain abscesses (Fig. 31.15a, b), especially in immunocompromised populations [105–107]. The clinical

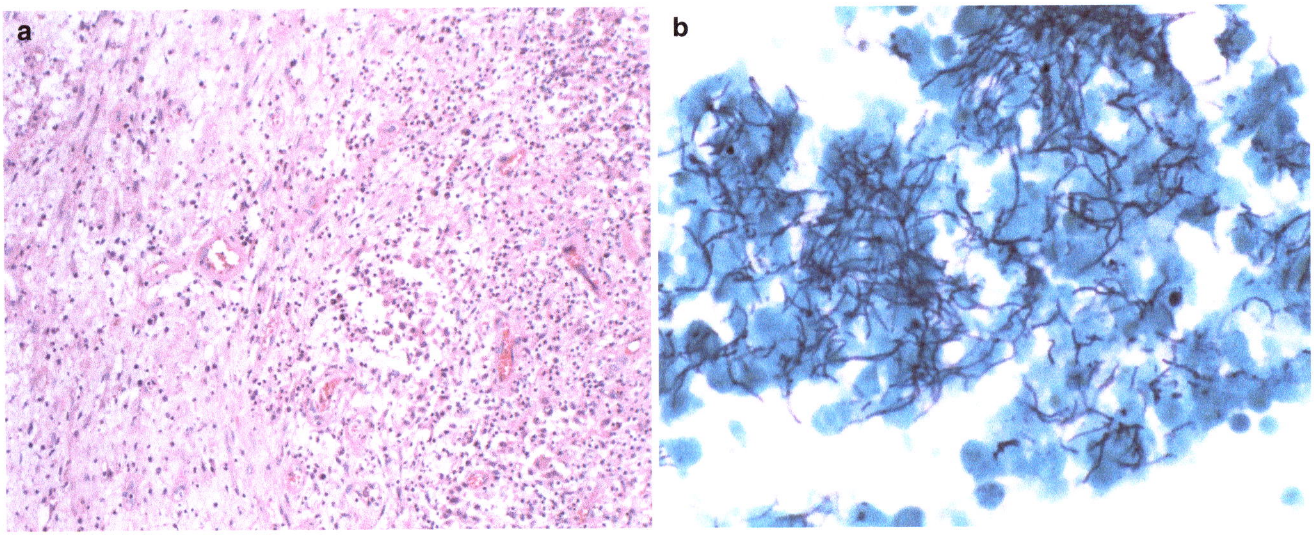

Fig. 31.15 (**a**, **b**) A 52-year-old female with a left frontal lobe intraparenchymal abscess caused by *Nocardia* sp. Figure (**a**) shows the thickened collagenous abscess wall with neovascularization adjacent to acute inflammatory infiltrate. H&E, 10×. In figure (**b**), Gomori methenamine silver (GMS) stain highlights numerous branching, filamentous bacteria. GMS, 60× (Both courtesy of Anthony Yachnis, MD, and Kelly Devers, MD, University of Florida College of Medicine)

presentation of Nocardia infections in the CNS is the same in normal and compromised hosts, although more frequent in compromised hosts. In a series of 11 cases and a review of 120 cases of nocardial brain abscess in the literature, concomitant pulmonary disease was present in 34%. Most of the brain abscesses were single; about one-third were multiple, and, overall, 38% of the cases occurred in patients who were immunocompromised by virtue of HIV or other causes [107]. Rarely, *Mycobacterium tuberculosis* may produce a space-occupying lesion (tuberculoma), and while uncommon in the United States, tuberculomas are relatively common causes of brain abscesses in some less-developed countries [108, 109].

Yeasts and fungi are important causes of brain abscess. *Candida albicans* almost never causes isolated brain abscesses but may cause microabscesses in association with disseminated candidiasis. Although cryptococcal infection of the CNS typically affects patients with HIV infection, cryptococcomas are rarely observed [110]. Agents of phaeohyphomycosis, such as *Cladosporium*, *Bipolaris*, *Curvularia*, and *Wangiella*, as well as the agents of chromoblastomycosis have all been reported as causes of brain abscesses.

Aspergillus spp. are well-recognized causes of brain abscess but are almost always limited to immunocompromised patient populations, and in particular, transplant patients. *Aspergillus fumigatus* is the most common species affecting humans; maxillary sinusitis of dental origin or the lungs are the most common sites of primary *Aspergillus* spp. infection [111]. Infection reaches the brain directly from the nasal sinuses via vascular channels or spreads through the blood from the lungs and gastrointestinal tract [111].

Zygomycoses such as Mucor, Rhizopus, and Rhizomucor produce brain infection by direct extension from the paranasal sinuses in poorly controlled diabetics. Cerebral mucormycosis without rhino-orbital or systemic involvement is an extremely rare condition mostly associated with parenteral drug abuse [112].

Protozoa and other parasites are important causes of brain abscess. The incidence of protozoal and helminthic infestations of the CNS is <1%, but these infestations tend to follow a fatal course and are more common among children, the elderly, and immunocompromised individuals. *Toxoplasma gondii* is probably the most frequent protozoal cause of brain abscess in the United States and is almost entirely associated with HIV infection. Strongyloides, entamoeba, echinococcus, paragonimus, trichinosis, sparganosis, and angiostrongylus have all been reported, particularly in less-developed nations. Rarely, brain abscesses due to naegleria and acanthamoeba occur in the United States.

Clinical Manifestations

Presentation, generally, is that of an intracranial mass lesion: subacute onset, headache, and focal neurological deficits [100, 101, 103]. However, the classic triad of focal neurological signs, fever, and headache is present in <50% of cases; nuchal rigidity is not prominent in patients with brain abscess. Similarly, patients with subdural empyema typically present with a more localized headache and focal neurologic symptoms. Other common signs and symptoms include fever, chills, seizures, nausea, vomiting, and altered sensorium [113]. Fever is present in 40–50% of cases, and focal neurologic symptoms and signs, such as hemiparesis, aphasia, ataxia, and sensory deficits, may be present in one-third to one-half of cases. Papilledema as a reflection of increased ICP is present in only a minority of cases [106, 113]. Likewise, seizures are observed in approximately 25–45% of patients by the time they present. The seizures are most often generalized and associated with frontal lobe lesions. The presenting signs and symptoms are often dependent on the location of the abscess. For example, cerebellar abscesses often present with nystagmus, ataxia in the ipsilateral extremities, vomiting, and dysmetria [114, 115]. Frontal lobe abscesses generally present with headache, drowsiness, and deterioration of mental status or aphasia together with hemiparesis and unilateral motor signs. Temporal lobe abscesses may present with or without aphasia or dysphasia, depending on whether the abscess is in the dominant hemisphere. Patients with occipital lobe abscesses may present with homonymous hemianopia, while typical features in parietal lobe abscesses include hemianesthesia, homonymous hemianopia, neglect of one-half of the body, alexia, or impaired spatial perception. Pituitary abscesses may simulate a tumor and can present with visual field defects and endocrine abnormalities. Brain stem abscesses typically exhibit facial weakness, fever, headache, hemiparesis, dysphasia, and vomiting.

The differential diagnosis includes a wide range of other CNS infections, such as meningitis, subdural empyema, epidural abscess, viral encephalitis, as well as noninfectious causes, such as migraine, intracerebral and subarachnoid hemorrhage, venous sinus thrombosis, or malignancy.

Diagnosis

The diagnosis of a brain abscess is best established by neuroimaging [116, 117]. MRI is more sensitive than CT scans and provides information on the size, location, and stage of the abscess together with the extent of surrounding edema and the presence or absence of mass effect, such as midline shift, hydrocephalus, and impending herniation. The timeline for bacterial brain abscess evolution is reasonably predictable and is divided into early cerebritis, late cerebritis, early abscess, mature abscess, and finally resolution (Fig. 31.8). Success of treatment is measured by progressively diminishing cross-sectional diameter of the abscess cavity. Radiologic changes in the abscess wall (i.e., thickness and contrast enhancement), surrounding edema, or status of internal contents are not reliable predictors of treatment success. Characteristic findings of a brain abscess are a ring-enhancing lesion in the contrast CT or MRI studies with a hypodense center reflecting the necrotic center of the abscess surrounded by a variable zone of edema [118] (Fig. 31.16a, b).

CT imaging studies are especially useful in defining contiguous head and neck pathology, which can be the source of infection. High-detail CT imaging can detect the bone lysis of aggressive sinusitis and otomastoiditis better than MRI. CT is also better at defining bone dehiscence associated with prior trauma, which can also be the source of intracranial infection. MRI and CT are comparable in defining retropharyngeal abscesses and chronic fungal sinus and skull base infections. CT is less sensitive than MRI for characterizing the stages of cerebritis and abscess formation and for excluding other causes of intra-axial necrotic masses in the brain [119, 120]. MRI, especially with diffusion brain imaging sequences, maintains a high degree of sensitivity and specificity. However, some abscesses remain in a chronic sequestered state and are difficult to differentiate from tumors; these are included in the category of tumefactive lesions along with others such as sequestered infarcts, thrombosed giant aneurysms, and the Balo variant of multiple sclerosis.

The major difficulty with neuroimaging studies, especially CT imaging, is their lack of sensitivity in differentiating an abscess from a tumor, including neuroblastomas and metastatic lesions. In one study, 8 out of 26 patients with a brain abscess were initially diagnosed as having a tumor [119]. MRI scanning provides soft tissue resolution and

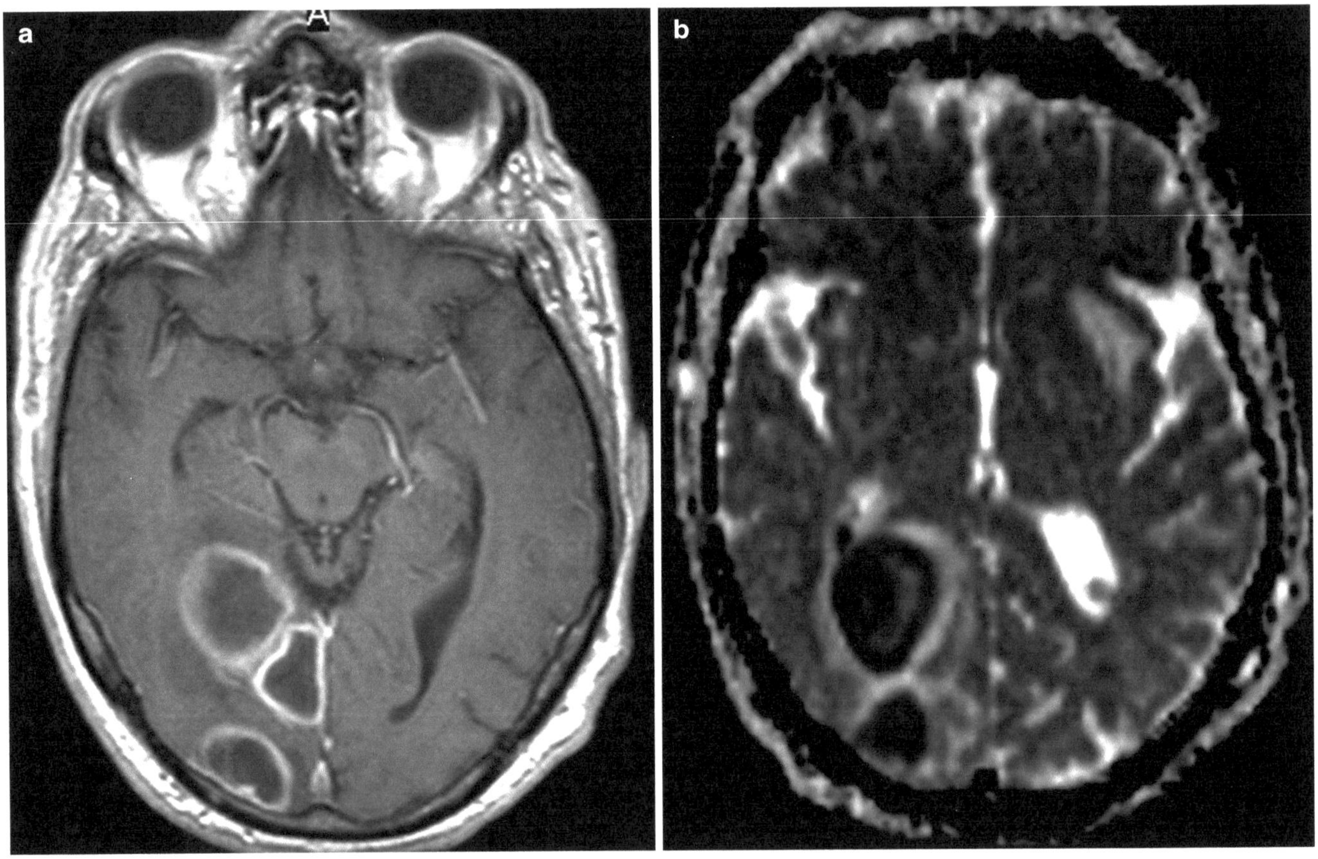

Fig. 31.16 (**a**, **b**) Occipital abscess with daughter abscesses; images include two MRI images in the low convexity region of brain. Figure (**a**) is a post-contrast T1-w sequence and the left image is an ADC map (apparent diffusion coefficient) sequence, which provides information as to the diffusibility of the free water in the area of abnormality. The post-contrast TD1-w sequence (**b**) demonstrates contiguous ring-enhancing lesions in the right occipital brain. These findings do not distinguish between tumors versus tumefactive lesions, especially abscess. The diffusion-sensitive imaging demonstrates free motion restriction within the central portions of the lesion. This in tandem with enhanced images is typical of brain abscess. The purulent material within the abscess contains increased water content (hyperintense of T2-w sequences), but it does not allow the water molecule to diffuse as well as fluid with the ventricles for instance. Hence, this ADC map shows the central water-restriction, often seen in pyogenic brain abscess

detail that is superior to that achieved with CT scanning [120]. In addition, there is no exposure to ionizing radiation, although the cost is substantially higher. On T1-weighted MRI scans, brain abscesses appear hypointense and show ring enhancement following administration of the contrast agent gadolinium. On T2-weighted sequences, the central area of necrosis appears hyperintense and is surrounded by a well-defined hypointense capsule and readily discernible surrounding area of low density, representing cerebral edema. Another major advantage of MRI imaging studies is their ability to detect the cerebritis stage before the formation of the abscess with a fully developed capsule. The most helpful MR sequence is the diffusion technique. This technique, most applicable once central necrosis has occurred, demonstrates the restriction of water movement within the forming fibrous abscess capsule. Other methods, such as magnetic resonance spectroscopy (MRS), can detect products of bacterial metabolism, such as lactate, acetate, or pyruvate, and may improve our ability to differentiate brain abscesses from malignancy [121–123]. Radionuclide brain scans using Indium-111-labeled leukocytes do not provide any advantage over conventional neuroimaging techniques. During the past several years, positron emission tomography (PET) with 18F-fluorodeoxyglucose (FDG) imaging have been playing larger roles in the diagnosis and management of patients with suspected brain abscesses [118, 124–127].

Routine laboratory studies are not particularly useful in the diagnosis of brain abscess. The white count is normal in 40% of patients; the erythrocyte sedimentation rate is elevated in about 60%, and C-reactive protein levels are not consistently elevated. If the sedimentation rate is elevated, it may be useful to follow this over time to document a therapeutic response. Lumbar puncture in a patient with a space-occupying lesion is absolutely contraindicated unless an MRI or CT scan has indicated that herniation is unlikely to occur following an LP and there is a clear clinical suspicion of meningitis or meningeal carcinomatosis to justify taking the risk. The CSF in patients with brain abscess generally shows findings similar to any other parameningeal focus of infection, i.e., a pleocytosis with mixed neutrophils and lymphocytes, elevated protein levels, normal glucose levels, and a negative gram stain. CSF cultures are generally sterile unless there is an anatomic connection between the abscess and the spinal fluid, such as from trauma or a postoperative complication. Blood cultures are positive in 10–20% of patients. While reasonable empiric therapy can be devised for most common brain abscesses, culture of the material and transport to the laboratory under strictly anaerobic conditions is essential for optimal identification of the causative microorganism(s). In addition, a biopsy can be obtained and sent for pathologic evaluation to rule out malignancy, fungal invasion, and for detection of unusual microorganisms using special stains.

Treatment

Therapy for brain abscesses requires a combined medical and surgical approach [128]. Stereotactic-guided needle aspiration of pus drains the collection and enables procurement of specimens for gram stain, culture, and histology. Open craniotomy may be considered in cases where the response to antimicrobial therapy is poor or the organism isolated from culture is antimicrobial-resistant. Antimicrobial therapy alone may be considered for patients with numerous abscesses that are not amenable to surgical drainage or for patients with small abscesses who have stable neurologic function. The choice of antimicrobials is determined both by the spectrum of microbiological agents known to cause brain abscess and the degree to which individual antimicrobials penetrate the blood–brain barrier and enter into the abscess cavity itself. For brain abscesses that develop in contiguity with frontal sinus infection, mixed aerobic and anaerobic flora may be assumed to be present. In this situation, even if anaerobic bacteria are not recovered, anaerobic coverage should be initiated with an agent such as metronidazole 500 mg every 6 h. If there is any suspicion that the abscess may have arisen from a dental focus, anaerobic cultures should be held for 7–14 days to enable detection of *Actinomyces* spp. growth. Brain abscesses that are related to chronic otitis media and mastoiditis should be treated with a combination of antimicrobials that will cover anaerobes, *Enterobacteriaceae*, and *Pseudomonas* spp. Thus, a combination of cefotaxime, cefepime, ceftazidime, or ceftriaxone plus metronidazole would work well in this clinical scenario. Although bacterial cultures may not always yield growth of anaerobes, particularly if the organisms are fastidious, the absence of growth of *Enterobacteriaceae* or *Pseudomonas* spp. on culturing abscess material from a patient who has not received prior intravenous antimicrobial therapy can be relied upon to rule out these organisms as the cause of infection. Similarly, the absence of *S. aureus* from culture of abscess matter would also be reassuring that this agent is not involved in the pathogenesis of the abscess. In general, *S. aureus* is much more likely to be implicated in endocarditis, metastatic infection to the CNS, or in the setting of trauma or postsurgical wound infection. If a brain abscess is associated with a neurosurgical procedure, vancomycin should be included in the empirical therapeutic regimen to cover both methicillin-resistant *S. aureus* (MRSA) and coagulase-negative *Staphylococcus* spp.

A 6- to 8-week course of parenteral antimicrobial therapy plus follow-up computed tomography or MRI scans to evaluate the therapeutic response is recommended. The antimicrobial regimen can be modified once antimicrobial susceptibility testing results become available. Patients with a brain abscess caused by *Nocardia* spp. should be treated with higher doses of trimethoprim/sulfamethoxazole (typically 15 mg/kg/day of the trimethoprim component) in three to five divided doses until the infection is controlled; thereafter, the dose can be reduced to one double-strength trimethoprim/sulfamethoxazole tablet orally twice daily for 3–6 months in non-immunocompromised patients and up to a year in immunocompromised patients. In severely immunocompromised patients, lifelong treatment for Nocardia CNS infections may be required. The method of surgical intervention depends on the patient's clinical status and the neuroradiographic characteristics of the abscess.

Spinal Epidural Abscess

The epidural space is defined as an area posterolateral to the spinal cord between the dura and the vertebral column. It extends from the foramen magnum to the sacrum; the space is largest in the midthoracic and lumbar regions. The epidural space contains lymphatics, spinal nerve roots, loose fatty tissue, and small arteries. An epidural abscess is a collection of pus between the dura and the vertebral column. A spinal epidural abscess is a medical emergency because of the risk of spinal cord compression and potential progression to irreversible paraplegia or quadriplegia.

Spinal epidural abscess is more common in the elderly with a peak incidence during the sixth and seventh decades [129]. The disease is rare among children and typically affects patients whose comorbid conditions predispose them to immunocompromised states [129–133]. Other populations at risk include IV drug abusers, immunocompromised patients, and patients who have undergone spinal surgical procedures [134].

Pathophysiology

The formation of spinal epidural abscesses can be spontaneous or secondary to direct inoculation of a pathogen into the epidural space. The most common cause of spontaneous infection in the epidural space is hematogenous spread from distant foci (50%), such as infections of the skin and oral cavity, pneumonia and other respiratory tract infections, endocarditis, intra-abdominal and pelvic sepsis, and urinary tract infections [129]. Other causes of spontaneous abscess formation include direct extension (i.e., contiguous spread) from preexisting discitis or osteomyelitis in an adjacent vertebral body, extension of a decubitus ulcer or paraspinal abscess, blunt spinal trauma, or penetrating injuries. Secondary causes include postoperative infections (16% of all spinal epidural abscesses) and infections associated with epidural anesthesia catheters [134–136]. An epidural hematoma resulting from trauma can also become secondarily infected and progress to an epidural abscess [129].

The location of an epidural abscess within the spinal canal is determined largely by the underlying cause of the epidural abscess [129, 133, 134]. The majority of spontaneous spinal epidural abscesses that result from hematogenous spread of bacteria are usually located posteriorly within the spinal canal; epidural abscesses secondary to preexisting vertebral osteomyelitis are usually confined to the anterior spinal canal [133–138]. The segregation and isolation of abscesses to the anterior or posterior spinal canal is thought to be secondary to septations within the epidural fat [133]. These septations not only divide the epidural space into anterior and posterior compartments but also divide the space longitudinally. The longitudinal septations usually limit the extent of epidural abscess formation to up to four vertebral levels [133]. Postsurgical spinal epidural abscesses often involve multiple compartments, extending several levels and circumferentially around the spinal cord, secondary to disruption of the epidural septations [137]. In addition to causing compression of the spinal cord, pus and granulation tissue in the epidural space can cause ischemia of the spinal cord by compromising and reducing arterial blood flow. The neurologic sequelae of epidural abscess formation can be slowly progressive or dramatically acute in nature; in the latter scenario, complete paralysis could occur within a matter of hours [134]. The neurological injury is thought to be secondary to both compression of the neural elements vascular thrombosis and ischemia [133, 134, 139, 140].

Risk Factors

The majority of patients who develop a spinal epidural abscess have one or more identifiable risk factors [134, 136]. Implicated comorbid conditions include osteomyelitis, discitis, diabetes, degenerative joint disease of the spine, IV drug abuse, alcoholism, chronic renal failure, immunodeficiency states, and cancer [141]. The spectrum of risk factors is fairly consistent between reports of other large case series [129, 130, 133. 136]. Risk factors, such as discitis and bacteremia associated with IV drug abuse, have a more direct role in the development of spinal epidural abscesses by directly seeding the epidural space with pathogens responsible for the epidural infection [134].

Microbiology of Spinal Epidural Abscess Formation

S. aureus is the microorganism most commonly isolated from spinal epidural abscesses followed by gram-negative organisms particularly *E. coli* and *Pseudomonas* spp. (18%), other gram-positive organisms including *Streptococcus* spp. (10%), or anaerobes (2%); polymicrobial growth is observed in 5–10% of cases. *Mycobacterium tuberculosis* has been implicated in various cases, especially in economically less-developed countries. Pathogens less frequently implicated as causes of spinal epidural abscesses include *Brucella* spp., *Actinomyces*, *Cryptococcus* spp., and *Aspergillus* spp. [129, 135, 136].

Clinical Features and Diagnostic Considerations

The classic clinical presentation of a patient with spinal epidural abscess is back pain and fever. Further progression to spinal cord compression may lead to motor weakness, bowel and bladder dysfunction, limb weakness, and paralysis [134]. In reality, the presentation is highly variable; other common clinical findings include fever (61%), paresis (53%), bowel or bladder dysfunction (36%), sepsis (17%), radiculopathy (12%), and plegia (14%) [142, 143]. Since symptoms and signs may be nonspecific, patients may initially be misdiagnosed [141]. Point tenderness over the involved vertebral levels is present in about one-quarter of patients and is associated with underlying bony involvement [141]. The most common location of spinal epidural abscess formation is in the lumbar region, but thoracic and cervical involvement is not uncommon [129].

Time between symptom onset and presentation is highly variable and does not correlate well with intraoperative findings [144]. Neurological deficits are present on physical examination in the majority of patients at the time of presentation [129, 130, 132, 134, 136, 141]. Neurological decline can occur chronically over months or precipitously over a few hours [130, 132, 134, 136–139, 142].

The most consistent laboratory abnormality is an elevated erythrocyte sedimentation rate (ESR), which is almost always present; ESR and C-reactive protein have been found to be highly sensitive and moderately specific in identifying patients in the emergency room with spinal epidural abscess [145, 146]. Leukocytosis is found in roughly 75% of patients [134, 141]. Results of CSF analysis are variable, ranging from normal to frank pus [137]. Blood cultures have been reported to be positive in up to 60% of cases [133]. Contrast-enhanced MRI scans give superior resolution of soft tissue, the spinal cord, and epidural space when compared to CT myelography and are the diagnostic procedure of choice in many facilities. An epidural abscess appears as a low-intensity image on T1-weighted MRI scans (Fig. 31.17). If MRI services are not available, myelography should be carried out. Lumbar puncture to determine CSF protein concentrations should not be performed as it may introduce bacteria into the subarachnoid space with consequent meningitis [147].

Treatment

Surgical intervention for removal of pus and granulation tissue forms the basis of therapy, followed by a prolonged course of parenteral antimicrobials. If the patient has neurological signs at presentation, immediate surgical decompres-

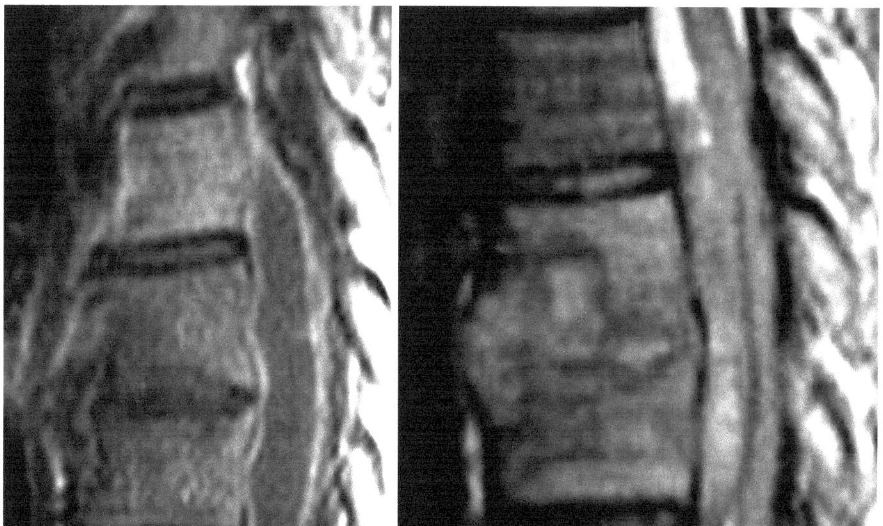

Fig. 31.17 Acute discitis with secondary osteomyelitis and anterior epidural empyema; images include post-contrast T1-w (on *left*) and T2-w (on *right*) sequences. In this instance, there is a central disc infection with adjacent osteomyelitis in vertebral bodies above and below the disc infection. This is the pattern usually associated with primary disc infection with secondary bone involvement and is usually of pyogenic causative agent. Additionally, there is an anterior epidural abscess that bridges the infected motion segment

sion of the spinal cord is essential. During the time that culture results are not available, and because *S. aureus* is a commonly implicated pathogen in spinal epidural abscesses, vancomycin should be included in the treatment regimen together with an agent that is active against gram-negative organisms, such as a third-generation cephalosporin. Spinal epidural abscess carries with it a high mortality rate and significant long-term sequelae, including paralysis. The mortality rate is estimated to be 14%, and 35–40% of patients will have neurological sequelae, such as residual weakness or permanent paralysis [129, 131, 133, 141]. Prognosis depends upon the clinical and neurological condition of the patient at the time of presentation [129, 134, 139, 142]. Patients presenting with sepsis or plegia have higher mortality and long-term morbidity rates [130, 131, 135, 137, 138, 141, 143, 147].

Some spinal epidural abscesses can be managed with medical therapy alone [140]. The majority of these cases fall into one of three categories: (1) infections not amenable to drainage; (2) patients who are poor operative candidates, such as those with chronic cardiac or pulmonary disease; or (3) complete paralysis for >24 h [148]. In order to treat patients nonoperatively, empiric antibiotics should be used or tailored to available culture data. In addition, serial neurological exams and imaging studies are often required [148]. Patients are treated for six to eight weeks with antibiotics or until the abscess has resolved on imaging.

Vertebral Osteomyelitis

Pyogenic spinal infections, including vertebral osteomyelitis, account for approximately 2–4% of all cases of osteomyelitis and is the most common type of hematogenously acquired osteomyelitis [149–152]. The incidence of vertebral osteomyelitis has increased over time, possibly due to an increase in the number of immunocompromised patients [149, 150, 152–155]. This condition occurs more frequently in men, especially those aged 50 years or older [150, 154, 156, 157]. Risk factors associated with spontaneous, acute vertebral osteomyelitis include diabetes mellitus, systemic steroid use, history of a genital or urinary infection, urinary tract procedures, bacteremia, protein-calorie malnutrition, IV drug abuse, malignancy, various immunodeficient states, and advanced age [149, 150, 157–160].

Vertebral osteomyelitis in younger populations is frequently associated with IV drug abuse [158]. In fact, drug abusers account for over half the cases of pyogenic spinal osteomyelitis in some large series [150, 154, 161]. The overall incidence of diabetes in patients with vertebral osteomyelitis is between 18% and 25% [149]. However, in one series, 43% of adult patients with hematogenous vertebral osteomyelitis at a tertiary care hospital had diabetes [162].

Prolonged steroid use is a risk factor for vertebral osteomyelitis caused by bacteria and atypical mycobacteria [158, 163]. The common denominator in each of these predisposing conditions appears to be a deficiency in some aspect of cellular or humoral immunity [158]. Postsurgical vertebral osteomyelitis accounts for approximately 2.5% of all spinal osteomyelitis and occurs more frequently in malnourished patients, diabetics, and patients on steroid therapy [157, 159, 161, 164]. As the prevalence of AIDS increased, there has been resurgence in the incidence of spinal tuberculosis and the emergence of other fungal causes of vertebral osteomyelitis in this population [151, 155, 158, 160].

Pathogenesis

Spontaneous vertebral osteomyelitis usually results from hematogenous spread of organisms through the segmental spinal arteries to the subchondral plate region of the vertebral body adjacent to the disc space [159, 160]. In adults, the nidus of infection begins in the vertebral bodies at the level of the end arteriolar arcades and, after endplate destruction, spreads secondarily into the avascular disc space [149, 160]. In children, the disc space contains vascular channels that allow primary seeding of the intervertebral disc [149, 160, 161]. Segmental spinal arteries typically bifurcate to supply adjacent vertebral segments, this bifurcation is thought to account for the fact that vertebral osteomyelitis typically involves two adjacent vertebrae and the intervening disc space [160]. Postoperative vertebral osteomyelitis usually occurs due to direct inoculation of the microorganism at the time of surgery [149, 150, 152, 156, 159, 161]. The principal sources of wound contamination are surgery personnel or the patient's own skin flora [159]. Unlike spontaneous vertebral osteomyelitis, the disc space is often the nidus of infection in patients who have undergone a surgical procedure [149, 159, 161]. Other sources or risk factors for vertebral osteomyelitis include inoculation via decubitus ulcers and trauma or IV drug abuse [157, 165–167].

Microbiology of Vertebral Osteomyelitis

Of the various microorganisms known to be associated with culture-positive, pyogenic vertebral osteomyelitis, gram-positive aerobic cocci are implicated 68% of the time with *S. aureus* isolated in up to 60% of cases, gram-negative aerobic bacilli in 29% of the patients, and anaerobic bacteria in 3% [149, 155, 157–159, 162, 168–174]. Radiological imaging is often unable to differentiate between vertebral osteomyelitis caused by mycobacteria and bacteria; thus, initial clinical assessment of a patient with spinal osteomyelitis should include tuberculosis in the differential diagnosis, especially in high-risk patients or in regions or countries with a high prevalence of mycobacterial infections [155, 157, 158]. *Coccidioides immitis*, *Blastomyces dermatitidis*, *Cryptococcus neoformans*, *Aspergillus* species, and other less common fungi have all been implicated as causes of vertebral osteomyelitis [157, 175]. *Pseudomonas aeruginosa* and *S. aureus* are the most commonly implicated pathogens in vertebral osteomyelitis in IV drug abusers and occur at roughly equal rates [168, 176].

In elderly males with urinary tract infections or following invasive urological procedures, the most common causes of vertebral osteomyelitis are *E. coli* and *Proteus* species [157]. Postoperative spinal infections are usually caused by *S. aureus* [155, 157, 159, 174–176]. Patients on long-term steroid treatment are susceptible to infections caused by atypical mycobacteria and *Aspergillus* spp. [111, 158, 163, 177–183]. Although vertebral osteomyelitis is generally caused by a single microorganism, contiguous sources of infection, such as a decubitus pressure ulcer or intra-abdominal abscess (e.g., psoas abscess), can lead to polymicrobial infection involving both aerobic and anaerobic microorganisms [157, 158].

Clinical Presentation and Diagnostic Considerations

Back pain is the most common (>90%) presentation of vertebral osteomyelitis [152, 158]. The pain is localized, continuous, and generally unrelated to movement or position [156]. Vertebral osteomyelitis acquired by the hematogenous mode tends to involve the lower dorsal and lumbar spine. Nearly all spine infections are associated with tenderness on palpation over the involved level [149, 150, 152, 158]. Involvement of the cervical vertebrae has been noted among IV drug abusers and patients with pulmonary tuberculous [149]. Neurologic impairment, such as sensory loss, weakness, or radiculopathy, is reported in one-third of cases. The presence of radiculopathy, positive straight leg raise, and neurological deficit is less reliable and often indicates the presence of epidural involvement [150, 158]. Fever is found in approximately half of patients with pyogenic spinal osteomyelitis, and constitutional symptoms, including malaise, night sweats, and anorexia, have been reported [150, 152, 159, 184].

Vertebral osteomyelitis has an insidious onset and may prove to be a diagnostic challenge because of the nonspecific nature of the symptoms and signs. For example, the differential diagnosis of back pain in a patient with fever includes various viral syndromes, aortitis, pyelonephritis, and pancreatitis [152]. In the absence of fever, other causes of back pain, such as an osteoporotic fracture, spondylarthritis, degenerative disc disease, or spinal stenosis, might have to be ruled out [152, 160]. In several large patient series, the delay between the onset of symptoms and eventual diagnosis has ranged from 3 weeks to 3 months [150, 154, 160, 185]. These delays in diagnosis can result in significant neurological morbidity [160]. Other complications arising from vertebral osteomyelitis include paraspinal abscesses, soft tissue extension, and spinal cord compression.

Leukocytosis is found in less than half of patients with vertebral osteomyelitis [150]. The most common laboratory abnormality is an elevated ESR. Blood cultures are critical in the workup of a patient with a putative diagnosis of vertebral osteomyelitis and, if positive—up to 78% of blood cultures are positive—might obviate the need for an invasive diagnostic procedure to procure a biopsy specimen [150, 157, 171]. Plain X-ray findings include disc space narrowing and vertebral end-plate changes that usually become apparent 2–4 weeks after symptom onset in approximately 80% of patients [149, 150, 159, 184]. Technetium 99 m bone scanning combined with gallium scanning has a 90% sensitivity and specificity for vertebral osteomyelitis [186]. MRI imaging is the most sensitive and specific imaging modality for vertebral osteomyelitis and has the added benefit of providing details regarding the presence of an epidural or paraspinal abscess and various other complications [149, 152, 187–189]. Characteristic MRI changes include decreased T1 signal and increased T2 signal of the involved vertebral endplates and disc space [149, 189] (Fig. 31.18). Positron emission tomographic (PET) scanning with 18F-fluorodeoxyglucose has a diagnostic accuracy similar to that of MRI and might be considered if the patient has metallic implants [188].

Optimal pharmacologic treatment requires that the causative microbe be identified, and the antimicrobial susceptibility profile determined [150]. If imaging is suggestive of vertebral osteomyelitis but blood cultures are negative for bacterial growth, then a biopsy of the infected vertebra is indicated [149, 150, 159, 184]. The procedure of choice would depend on the presence of underlying intrinsic patient risk factors with input from surgical and interventional radiology personnel regarding CT-guided versus open biopsy [160]. When blood cultures are negative, a CT-guided needle biopsy can be used to make a definitive microbiological diagnosis 60–90% of the time [150]. An open biopsy should be considered when both blood cultures and CT-guided aspirates are negative [159]. A skin test for tuberculosis should also be considered [159, 185]. To overcome the limitations of tuberculosis skin testing, interferon-gamma release assays, such as the T-cell spot of the TB assay or QuantiFERON-TB Gold In-Tube are now available in most tertiary care centers. It should be borne in mind, however, that neither skin testing nor interferon-gamma release assays can distinguish latent from active tuberculosis infection. If polymicrobial osteomyelitis is suspected (e.g., a patient with

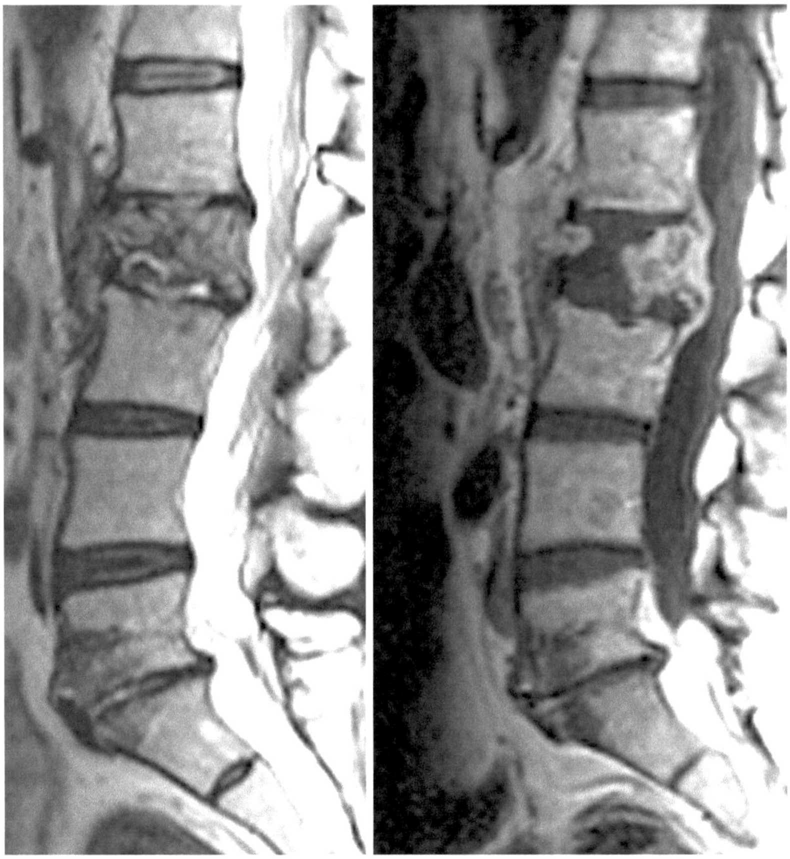

Fig. 31.18 Spinal vertebral osteomyelitis with relative sparing of the disc space; images include T2-w sagittal image (*left*) and a post-contrast T1-w image (*right*). In this instance, the spinal infection has virtually destroyed the L1 vertebral body. There is prominent residual contrast enhancement in the affected vertebral body. There is only minimal edema in the L1–2 disc space and relatively little enhancement. This complex would be consistent with hematogenous seeding of the vascularized vertebral body rather than a primary disc infection with secondary osteomyelitis

concomitant intra-abdominal sepsis), a biopsy should ideally be performed regardless of whether or not blood cultures are positive [174].

Treatment

Targeted antimicrobial therapy, spinal immobilization, and, when necessary, surgical interventions are the mainstays of treatment of vertebral osteomyelitis [149, 150, 152, 157]. About 75% of patients with spinal osteomyelitis can be managed without surgical intervention [149]. Prolonged courses of parental antimicrobials directed by specific culture results and antimicrobial susceptibilities are the rule [152, 157, 184]. Generally, 6 weeks of antimicrobial therapy is recommended [169, 190, 191].

For methicillin-susceptible *S. aureus* (MSSA), high-dose oxacillin (2 g every 4 h) or cefazolin (2 g every 8 h) is recommended. MRSA or coagulase-negative staphylococci can be treated with IV vancomycin (1 g every 12 h) or daptomycin (≥6 mg/kg of body weight once daily). Streptococcal species can be treated with IV penicillin G (five million units every 6 h) or IV ceftriaxone (2 g once daily) depending on susceptibilities. *Enterobacteriaceae* can be treated with ciprofloxacin (750 mg taken orally every 12 h) or IV ceftriaxone (2 g once daily). Infections caused by quinolone-resistant *Enterobacteriaceae* (including extended-spectrum β-lactamase-producing *E. coli*), can be treated effectively with IV meropenem (1–2 g every 8 h). For *P. aeruginosa* infections, cefepime, ceftazidime, or piperacillin/tazobactam every 6 h, may be used, potentially followed by ciprofloxacin (750 mg taken orally every 12 h). Anaerobes can be treated with IV clindamycin (300–600 mg administered intravenously every 6–8 h), IV penicillin G (five million units every 6 h), or IV ceftriaxone (2 g once daily) with metronidazole (500 mg taken orally every 8 h). Tuberculous vertebral osteomyelitis requires an average of 12 months of treatment with a combination of isoniazid, rifampin, ethambutol, and pyrazinamide, depending on regional susceptibility [149, 192]. Treatment of other less common bacterial and fungal causes of vertebral osteomyelitis should be tailored to the individual pathogen and to regional antimicrobial susceptibility profiles. Therapy is guided by clinical response and the ESR/CRP. Continued elevation of inflammatory markers may necessitate more prolonged therapy.

The indications for surgical intervention in spinal osteomyelitis are the presence of a neurological deficit, spinal instability, unresponsiveness to medical therapy, or a non-diagnostic CT-guided biopsy [152, 154]. In addition, surgery is recommended for the drainage of epidural or paraspinal abscesses that often accompany vertebral osteomyelitis [157] The goals of surgery are decompression of the neural elements, correction of spinal deformity, debridement of necrotic tissue, and the promotion of long-term stability [149, 154, 160, 185]. A variety of surgical approaches have been described in the literature, each with its own advantages and disadvantages [149, 154, 185]. The basic principles of surgical intervention include early instrumentation and fusion at the time of the initial operation in order to facilitate ambulation and avoid the complications associated with prolonged bed rest [149, 154, 185].

External Ventricular Drainage

Infectious Considerations

A ventriculostomy is an external ventricular drainage (EVD) device or ventricular catheter that is placed into the cerebral ventricles enabling drainage of CSF externally. It is typically connected by tubing to a CSF collection device that can be elevated or lowered at the bedside to vary the amount of CSF that is drained. EVD devices are an integral aspect of the intensive care management of neurosurgical patients [193–195]. Common indications for their use include management of hydrocephalus, elevated intracranial pressure, or intracranial hemorrhage and the administration of intrathecal medications [193–198]. EVD devices provide diagnostic information and also facilitate therapeutic CSF drainage [199–201]. The most common complication involving the use of EVDs is infection; rates of infection up to 27% have been reported [196, 197, 202–208].

Risk factors for the development of EVD-associated ventriculomeningitis include EVD duration >11 days, frequency of CSF sampling, intraventricular hemorrhage, surgical technique (subcutaneously tunneled EVD, Rickham reservoir with percutaneous CSF drainage), neurosurgical operative procedure, and irrigation or manipulation of the drainage system [197, 203–207]. Conflicting data exist regarding the association between duration of ventricular drainage and the rate of EVD-associated infections [198, 203, 209, 210]. Some clinical series have shown a linear relationship between infection and duration of ventricular drainage [211, 212].

Diagnostic clues for EVD-related ventriculomeningitis may stem from clinical signs, such as fever, meningism, reduced level of consciousness, photophobia, phonophobia, and abnormal laboratory parameters (e.g., reduced CSF glucose, increased CSF protein, CSF pleocytosis, positive CSF culture, or gram's stain) [213]. Erythema and tenderness over the shunt tubing are also indicative of a shunt infection as are peritonitis and abdominal tenderness in patients with ventriculoperitoneal shunts. It should be noted that a negative CSF gram stain does not exclude the presence of infection. Because the results of the CSF leukocyte count may be confounded by intraventricular hemorrhage, Pfausler and colleagues introduced the "cell index" as a new parameter for the diagnosis of EVD-related ventriculomeningitis [214]. They showed that a significant increase of this index is highly indicative of EVD-related ventriculitis in patients with hemorrhagic CSF and that calculation of the "cell index" on a daily basis allows the timely diagnosis and hence initiation of antimicrobial therapy of catheter-related ventriculomeningitis [214]. Coagulase-negative *Staphylococcus* (70%), *S. aureus* (10%), and gram-negative bacteria (15%), including *P. aeruginosa*, *Acinetobacter* spp., *Klebsiella* spp., and *E. coli*, remain the most common microorganisms associated with ventriculomeningitis [213–217].

The role of perioperative and prophylactic antimicrobials in the prevention of EVD-associated infections has been extensively discussed and debated [218–222]. Alleyne and colleagues reviewed over 300 patients who received either daily prophylactic antimicrobials or perioperative antimicrobials alone and found no significant difference in the infection rate between the two groups [218]. Current evidence suggests that antibiotic-impregnated catheters reduce the incidence of shunt infection [219, 222–228]. Other factors thought to be important in preventing infection include perioperative antimicrobial administration prior to skin incision, tunneling of the ventricular catheter, proper surgical skin prep, strict adherence to aseptic technique, use of a closed ventricular drainage system, and meticulously sterile nursing care [203, 204, 211, 218, 229–236]. Antimicrobial-impregnated catheters have been manufactured for a variety of applications and have been shown to be effective in preventing EVD-associated infections [218, 223, 224, 228–232, 237, 238]. Beer and colleagues suggest that the management of EVD-related ventriculitis should involve decisions related to catheter exchange, the type and route of administration (intravenous versus intrathecal) of antimicrobial therapy, based on the type of suspected organism and its resistance pattern, and the duration of antimicrobial therapy [213]. Once the diagnosis is made, broad-spectrum antimicrobials should be administered, followed by diagnostic testing, and targeted antibiotic therapy as soon as antimicrobial susceptibility testing results become available.

Mycobacterium Tuberculosis Infections

Tuberculous Meningitis

Tuberculosis has been known to humankind since antiquity, having been demonstrated by molecular methods in mummies from both the new and the old world dating to 1000–1500 years BCE [239, 240]. Tuberculosis was recognized on clinical grounds in the eighteenth century, and with the isolation of the organism by Robert Koch in 1882, its ability to produce CNS disease was quickly recognized.

Before the HIV pandemic, *M. tuberculosis* infection and disease were already endemic in many economically less-developed countries, though not at pandemic proportions. With the onset of the HIV pandemic, there has been a dramatic, parallel, increase in rates of tuberculosis among HIV-infected patients in many of these countries, especially sub-Saharan Africa, Southeast Asia and, increasingly, the Indian subcontinent. At the end of the first decade of the new millennium, tuberculosis remains the second leading cause of death from an infectious disease worldwide after HIV, despite the availability of highly efficacious treatment for decades. In 2020, there were an estimated ten million cases and 1.5 million deaths attributable to tuberculosis [241]. Indeed, *M. tuberculosis* is one of the most common causes of bloodstream infections in febrile adults who present to emergency rooms in sentinel hospitals in sub-Saharan Africa and Thailand [242–246].

Although comparative rates of *M. tuberculosis* infections are relatively lower among HIV-infected patients in North America and Western Europe, the World Health Organization generally considers *M. tuberculosis* infections a true pandemic that is linked with immunosuppression resulting from HIV infection, although other factors associated with poverty, disasters, and war have also contributed, such as overcrowding, malnutrition, lack of access to healthcare, and poor sanitation [241]. Tuberculosis is the leading cause of death among HIV-infected patients worldwide, and tuberculosis meningitis remains the most rapidly progressive form of the disease.

Treatment of tuberculosis has become challenging since the emergence of tuberculosis resistant to isoniazid and rifampicin—the two most effective first-line drugs. Resistance to both drugs is defined as multidrug-resistant tuberculosis (MDR-TB) [241]. Both MDR-TB and rifampicin-resistant tuberculosis (RR-TB) require treatment with second-line drugs. WHO uses five categories to classify cases of drug-resistant tuberculosis: isoniazid-resistant TB, RR-TB, and MDR-TB (defined above), plus pre-extensively drug-resistant TB (pre-XDR-TB) and XDR-TB [241]. Pre-XDR-TB is tuberculosis that is resistant to rifampicin and any fluoroquinolone (a class of second-line anti-TB drug). XDR-TB is tuberculosis that is resistant to rifampicin, plus any fluoroquinolone, plus at least one of the drugs bedaquiline and linezolid [241]. Emerging resistance has made the management of pulmonary and extrapulmonary tuberculosis, including tuberculous meningitis, more difficult to manage.

Pathogenesis

Tuberculous meningitis can occur as a result of hematogenous seeding of the meninges, reactivation of previously asymptomatic metastatic *M. tuberculosis* foci in the meninges and brain parenchyma, or breakdown of an old tuberculous parameningeal granuloma with rupture into the subarachnoid space. In addition to HIV infection, other predisposing risk factors in adults include alcohol abuse, IV drug abuse, immunosuppression due to steroids and other immunosuppressive therapies, and chronic disorders, such as connective tissue diseases and chronic cardiopulmonary disease.

Pathologically, tuberculous meningitis leads to prodigious inflammation with production of a thick exudate at the base of the brain, particularly involving the optic nerves at the optic chiasm, the pons, and cerebellum. The histologic appearance depends on the stage of the disease. Initially, it consists of polymorphonuclear leukocytes, macrophages, and lymphocytes. After a phase of lymphocytic proliferation, granulomata with caseating centers become a prominent feature (Fig. 31.19). Another feature of tuberculous infection of the meninges is the involvement of the blood vessels traversing the meninges. Small- and medium-sized arteries are most often involved, although capillaries and veins may be similarly affected. The changes include granuloma formation and inflammation of the adventitia, which causes a reactive cellular proliferation of the intima, which in turn may lead to occlusion of the vessel and infarction of the areas supplied by the vessel. Clinically, this vasculitis is frequently found in the distribution of the middle cerebral artery due to its anatomic location at the base of the brain, where the inflammatory response is most intense. This profound inflammatory response with vasculitis causes compression of neural tissues and compromises cerebral blood flow, which can lead to cerebral ischemia, infarction, and edema as well as hydrocephalus.

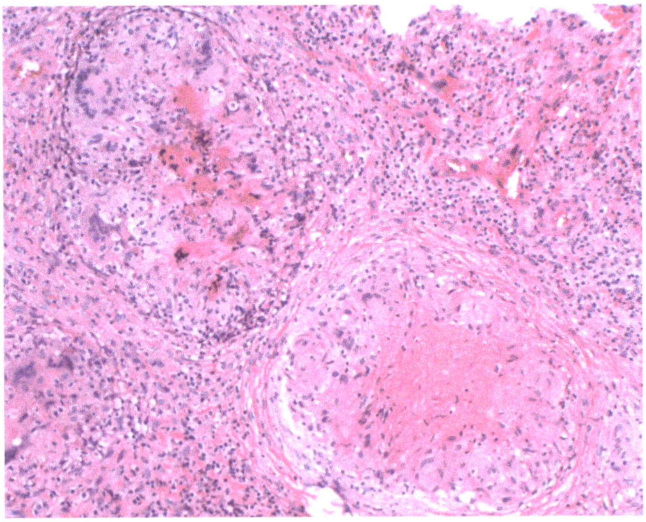

Fig. 31.19 A 40-year-old female with chronic headaches, anosmia, and blurred vision. Biopsy revealed chronic granulomatous meningitis with giant cells and non-caseating and focal caseating (necrotizing) granulomas. Special stains for acid-fast bacilli demonstrated only rare acid-fast organisms (Courtesy of Anthony Yachnis, MD, and Kelly Devers, MD, University of Florida College of Medicine)

Hydrocephalus is one of the most frequent complications of tuberculous meningitis, commonly accompanying symptomatic primary infection in children. Hydrocephalus occurs either by mechanical blockage of the spinal aqueduct or the foramina of Luschka due to the exudate at the base of the brain or to edema of the surrounding brain parenchyma. Hydrocephalus may also be caused by blockage of CSF reabsorption at the base of the brain due to the intense infiltrate. The former mechanism leads to noncommunicating hydrocephalus and the latter mechanism to communicating hydrocephalus.

Clinical Presentation

The classical clinical presentation of tuberculous meningitis in adults is that of fever and headache along with meningismus that becomes progressively more severe over a period of 2–3 weeks. However, the duration of prodromal symptoms can be variable and some patients have reported symptoms for several months before they actually sought medical attention. None of these symptoms or signs is universally present in all patients with tuberculous meningitis. Other frequently observed clinical features include lethargy and behavioral changes in 30–70% of patients, seizures in 10–15%, and cranial nerve palsies in up to 20–30% of adults. Occasionally, abnormal movements such as chorea, hemiballismus, athetosis, myoclonus, and cerebellar signs and symptoms are observed. Localizing neurologic symptoms due to a tuberculoma depends on the size and location of the mass lesion. Strokes due to tuberculous vasculitis described previously usually involve the distribution of the middle cerebral artery and produce symptoms related to that vascular distribution. The most common cranial nerve abnormalities involve the sixth cranial nerve followed by the third, fourth, and seventh but may involve the second, eighth, tenth, eleventh, and twelfth cranial nerves [247]. Coma is present or can develop in up to 30% of adults and children. In some series, as many as 50% of children have a past history of tuberculosis whereas only 8–12% of adults have such a history. Hydrocephalus is a serious and potentially devastating complication that may develop in up to 40% and is associated with a variety of focal neurologic signs, including hemiparesis and blindness.

The differential diagnosis is quite wide and includes bacterial, viral, and fungal infections of the CNS as well as malignancies and noninfectious conditions such as CNS lupus (Table 31.5).

Diagnosis

Routine laboratory tests are not particularly helpful. The single most useful diagnostic procedure is CSF examination. The classic findings of elevated protein, depressed CSF glucose relative to serum, and pleocytosis with a lymphocytic predominance, together with a history of chronic illness over a matter of weeks as opposed to days as in acute bacterial meningitis, is strongly suggestive of a tuberculous or fungal etiology. Staining of CSF smears for acid-fast bacilli has poor sensitivity of about 10–15%. Median CSF protein levels generally range between 100 and 400 mg/dL but may go as high 2 g/dL, although levels of that magnitude usually suggest mechanical blockage of CSF flow. The median white count generally runs between 100 and 200 WBC/mm^3. The CSF glucose is <45 mg/dL in 70–80% of patients. The glucose level tends to become progressively lower and the protein progressively higher as the duration of illness progresses without appropriate therapy; when treatment is successful, the glucose level tends to return towards normal. Although any one of these CSF parameters may be completely normal, it is extremely unusual for all three parameters to be completely normal in a patient with true tuberculous meningitis. If CSF analysis is completely normal and the laboratory reports *M. tuberculosis*, the report should be considered suspect until proven otherwise. Acid-fast smears of CSF are positive in <25% of patients who ultimately have culture-proven tuberculous meningitis, although CSF cultures may ultimately yield *M. tuberculosis* growth in up to 70% of patients.

The ESR varies considerably in series of patients with proven *M. tuberculosis* meningitis, ranging from normal to more than 100 mm/h. Similarly, the syndrome of inappropriate antidiuretic hormone (SIADH), manifest by hyponatremia and hypochloremia, is not uncommon but is by no means diagnostic since the results are confounded by a variety of other events (e.g., vomiting and anorexia) that may accompany *M. tuberculosis* disease.

Chest radiographs are non-diagnostic although 25–50% of adults may show radiographic evidence consistent with current or remote tuberculous infection [248]. In children who develop tuberculous meningitis on the heels of primary tuberculosis infection, chest radiographic evidence of *M. tuberculosis* infection has been observed in 50–80% of cases. Miliary disease was commonly associated with tuberculous meningitis in the pre-antimicrobial era and remains common in HIV-endemic regions of the world; at the present time, though, it remains relatively uncommon in the United States.

Admission tuberculin skin testing as a diagnostic aid for the diagnosis of tuberculous meningitis is of limited utility: the performance of the test varies with age, BCG vaccination and nutritional status, HIV status (HIV-infected patients are often anergic to PPD skin testing), and technique of administration [249–251]. Thus, although skin testing may provide information regarding previous tuberculosis exposure or infection and might be useful in the diagnosis of meningitis in young children, it is not sufficiently sensitivity or specific for routine diagnosis of active *M. tuberculosis* meningitis [249, 252]. Similarly, interferon-gamma release assays (e.g., QuantiFERON-TB Gold or T-SPOT.TB test), which are superior to tuberculin skin testing at diagnosing latent tuberculosis, are neither sufficiently sensitive nor specific for routine diagnosis of *M. tuberculosis* meningitis [253, 254].

Thus, in a patient with a nonspecific history that is suggestive of possible tuberculosis disease but with a CSF profile typical of aseptic meningitis, other causes of aseptic meningitis will have to be considered and ruled out. These alternative causes include cryptococcal and other forms of fungal meningitis, early or partially treated bacterial meningitis, cerebral abscess, and other parameningeal infections, *Listeria* spp. Meningitis, leptospirosis, and syphilis. Noninfective causes that need to be considered in the differential diagnosis include carcinomatous meningitis, including lymphoma, connective tissue diseases, chronic subdural hematoma, and chemical- or drug-induced causes.

Modern radiographic techniques such as CT scan, MRI with gadolinium enhancement, and magnetic resonance angiography (MRA) are extremely sensitive in delineating CNS involvement, readily demonstrating meningeal inflammation and entrapment of cranial nerves in the basilar tuberculous exudate (Figs. 31.5c, d and 31.20) [255]. In addition, MRA can detect characteristic vascular narrowing that accompanies tuberculous meningitis but is less commonly seen with other pathologies. High-field MRA with contrast is more sensitive than conventional MRA in the detection of occlusion of smaller vessels, which are more commonly involved in the pathogenesis of tuberculous meningitis [256].

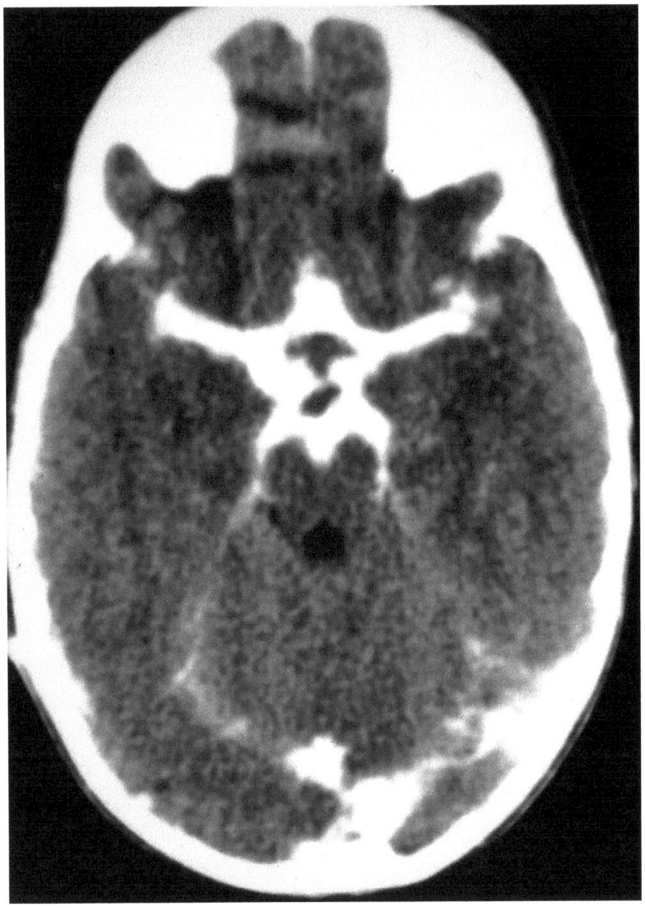

Fig. 31.20 Basilar tuberculous exudate in a patient with tuberculous meningitis

Culture remains the gold standard for laboratory confirmation of tuberculosis and is required for isolating the organism, for drug-susceptibility testing and genotyping and has a sensitivity of about 50–60%. Mycobacteria isolated from cultures are identified using standard biochemical analyses, nucleic acid probes, or 16S rRNA gene sequencing [257]. Real-time PCR assays that rapidly and specifically detect *M. tuberculosis* complex directly from acid-fast, smear-positive specimens and from broth cultures are now routinely conducted in various reference laboratories across the USA and now offer the potential to detect gene mutations responsible for drug resistance within hours of patient specimen collection compared with the average of 2 weeks required for traditional susceptibility testing methods. Real-time PCR assays used in the diagnosis of tuberculous meningitis have reported sensitivities ranging from 25% to 100% and specificities of about 95%. Thus, direct nucleic acid amplification tests should always be performed in conjunction with microscopy and culture, and each test result must be interpreted within the overall clinical setting in which it is used. There is still no *single* diagnostic method that is both sufficiently rapid and sensitive for detecting *M. tuberculosis* infection [258].

Treatment

Treatment of tuberculous meningitis consists of at least three, and usually four, drugs until the susceptibilities are established. Isoniazid (INH), rifampin, ethambutol, and pyrazinamide are the standard, together with pyridoxine at 25–50 mg daily to prevent depletion by INH. Many authors recommend dexamethasone for the first month to improve outcomes. A 2016 Cochrane systematic review and meta-analysis of all relevant published trials concluded that corticosteroids increase survival in HIV-negative patients. Treatment must be continued for at least 12 months. INH is generally used at a dose of 300 mg/day in adults or 10 mg/kg/day in children. The most serious side effect is hepatitis, which ranges from asymptomatic enzyme elevations to fulminant hepatic necrosis. The incidence of hepatotoxicity is higher in persons over 35 years of age, as well as those with other conditions affecting liver function such as alcoholism and viral hepatitis. The dose of rifampin is 600 mg/day and is only infrequently associated with side effects such as a flu-like syndrome and a hypersensitivity reaction with renal, hepatic, and hematologic toxicity. Pyrazinamide is given in a dose of 25 mg/kg/day and has a relatively low incidence of side effects; there is little added toxicity when combined with INH and rifampin. INH, rifampin, ethambutol, and pyrazinamide all have good penetration of the CSF. Ethambutol is generally administered at a dose of 25 mg/kg for the first 1–2 months of treatment with a reduction in dose to approximately 15 mg/kg/day because of the risk of optic neuritis, seen in approximately 25% of patients. The first clue to the development of this complication is loss of red-green vision or diminished visual acuity; ophthalmologic consultation is suggested in these situations. Streptomycin was one of the first drugs found to be active against tuberculosis and is commonly administered in a dose of 20–40 mg/kg/day for children and 1 g/day for adults. Unfortunately, the irreversible ototoxicity is so frequent that it is not advisable to use this agent unless absolutely necessary. Second-line antituberculous drugs such as para-aminosalicylic (PAS), cycloserine, ethionamide, kanamycin, and amikacin should only be used based on treatment failure with primary agents and antimicrobial susceptibility studies. Of these agents, ethionamide and cycloserine penetrate well into the CNS.

Given the time required to definitively diagnose tuberculous meningitis, empiric therapy often must be given while awaiting the results of cultures. A negative test for cryptococcal antigen, absence of encapsulated yeast forms on microscopy of an India ink smear, and no growth of the microorganism within 10–14 days of CSF culture essentially rules out cryptococcal meningitis. In cases where other fungal meningitides cannot be totally ruled out, some patients may have to be placed on empirical therapy with both antituberculous medications and amphotericin B. In patients who show no signs of improvement after the initial phase of treatment, and particularly in situations where the patient is known to have a malignancy, cytological analysis of the CSF should be requested to rule out meningeal carcinomatosis.

Case reports and various studies have demonstrated the immediate effects of steroids in terms of defervescence and clearing of the sensorium, even after a few doses. While there seems to be general agreement that survival from tuberculous meningitis is improved with the use of steroids, survivors often do so with severe sequelae [248]. It is typically recommended to use steroids in all patients with *M. tuberculosis* meningitis, regardless of the severity of the disease at presentation, with a reducing course over 6–8 weeks [61, 62, 249, 259, 260]. The dose of prednisone is 60 mg/day or 1 mg/kg/day, or dexamethasone may also be used at a dose of 8–16 mg/day in divided doses. Steroids are given for 3–6 weeks and then tapered over the ensuing 2–4 weeks. If the results of susceptibility testing implicate multidrug-resistant strains of *M. tuberculosis*, intrathecal therapy might have to be considered [261].

For HIV-infected patients, antituberculous treatment should be initiated promptly and antiretroviral therapy should be delayed for 4 weeks and administered within 8 weeks to limit the development of immune reconstitution inflammatory syndrome [260, 262]. The mortality rate among HIV-infected patients with multidrug-resistant tuberculous meningitis is significantly higher than the comparable rate for meningitis caused by susceptible strains.

Prognosis and Sequelae

Prior to the availability of antituberculous therapy, survival from tuberculous meningitis was exceedingly rare; survival rates currently are 70–80% in the most recent series. Perhaps the most significant prognostic factor for survival is the degree to which the disease has advanced at the time of initial presentation. Other factors correlating with poor response to therapy include age and coexistent miliary disease. The earliest sign of response to therapy in most cases is reduction in peak daily temperatures within the first 1–2 weeks and subjective improvement in fatigue and malaise over the same period. However, early studies pointed out that it was not uncommon for some markers of disease, such as the presence of bacilli in a smear of the CSF or a rise in CSF protein, to occur shortly after the initiation of treatment. In general, the glucose level in the CSF rises with successful treatment while the protein returns to normal more slowly, a process that may take as long as 6 months.

Up to 50% of survivors have a variety of neurologic deficits. As with survival itself, the more seriously ill the patient is upon presentation, the more likely complications or sequelae are to occur. Among children, the most common of these are seizure disorders, ataxia, incoordination, persistent cranial nerve abnormalities, and spastic hemiparesis. Adults are most frequently left with chronic organic brain syndrome, often with cranial nerve palsies, paraplegia, and hemiparesis. Optic atrophy can lead to varying degrees of visual impairment or blindness in both children and adults.

Tuberculoma

Tuberculomas are space-occupying mass lesions within the brain parenchyma ranging in size from <1 mm to >10 cm. The pathogenesis of tuberculomas is similar to that of tuberculous meningitis in that a tuberculous granuloma, seeded during the phase of acquiring the primary infection, breaks down and produces a mass lesion rather than meningitis. Patients may present with fever, headache, focal or generalized seizure, or change in mental status and may manifest signs of proptosis, papilledema, or transient neurologic deficits. Clinical features are related to the anatomic location of the tuberculoma. Generally, patients have a single lesion on presentation. However, autopsy series and sophisticated radiologic studies have shown that in up to 70% of patients, multiple lesions are present. The duration of symptoms prior to presentation is somewhat longer than in tuberculous meningitis, averaging weeks to months with the occasional patient having symptoms for years prior to diagnosis. In fact, 30% of patients with tuberculomas may remain asymptomatic throughout their life. Neuroimaging CT scan and MRI have a 100% diagnostic sensitivity (Fig. 31.21); however, tissue confirmation is essential in order to rule out malignancies or other ring-enhancing, space-occupying lesions, such as pyogenic bacterial abscesses, neurocysticercosis, or toxoplasmosis [118, 249].

Approximately 60% of the specimens from tuberculomas stain positive for acid-fast bacilli on smear, and approximately the same number ultimately grows in culture. Caseating granulomata are invariably seen histologically. Treatment is essentially the same as for tuberculous meningitis, i.e., antituberculous therapy with adjunct corticosteroids if cerebral edema is present, rather than surgery. The utility of adjunct steroids for patients with intracranial tuberculomas without meningitis has not been fully characterized by randomized controlled trials. Steroid therapy can be considered, however, because it mitigates symptoms and reduces the frequency of seizure attacks, tuberculoma size, and perilesional edema [249, 263, 264]. The indications for surgical intervention include the development of hydrocephalus or coalescence of multiple tuberculomas to form a tuberculous cerebral abscess [249, 265].

Spinal Tuberculosis

Spinal tuberculosis is a destructive form of tuberculosis and accounts for approximately half of all cases of musculoskeletal tuberculosis and is more common in children and young adults [266]. Tuberculous spinal meningitis may accompany tuberculous meningitis or may occur as an isolated entity. While tuberculous meningitis is essentially a disease of childhood, tuberculomas and spinal tuberculosis invariably are adult manifestations [264]. The pathogenesis and pathologic findings consist of characteristic exudate surrounding many parts of the spinal cord with symptoms due to compression and vasculitic changes in the arterial supply. Common clinical manifestations include constitutional symptoms (e.g., fever, malaise, weight loss), back pain, spinal tenderness, paraplegia, and spinal deformities [266].

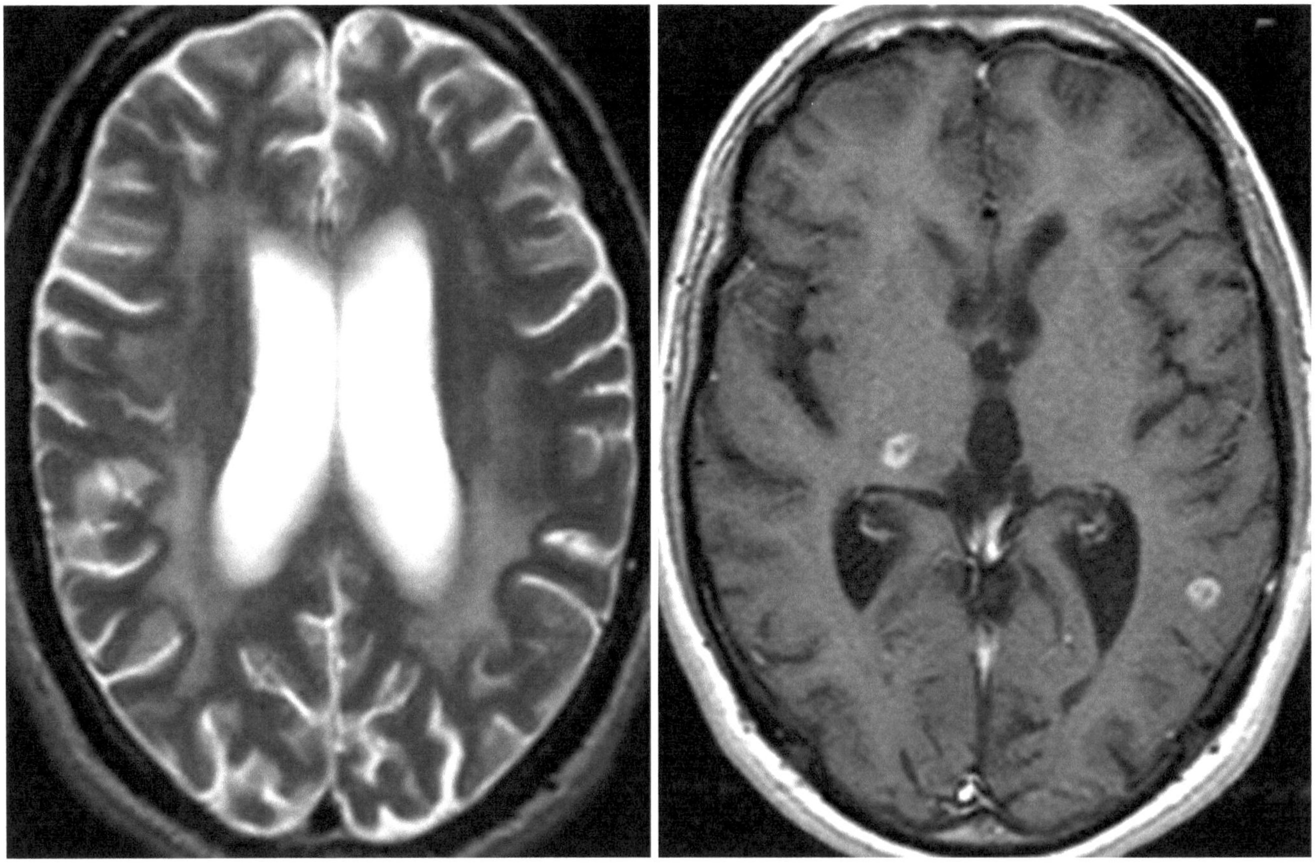

Fig. 31.21 AIDS-related complex and tuberculomas; images include T2-w spine echo (*left*) and post-contrast T1-w sequence (*right*). The T2-w sequence demonstrates features of an AIDS-related complex with global pronounced atrophy and diffuse bilateral loss of myelin within the centrum semiovale. The *right* image demonstrates multicentric brain nodules. Their distribution is consistent with a hematogenous-type of disease dissemination. These nodules were found to be tuberculomas, but evidence of small nodular enhancing lesions has a wide differential diagnosis

Symptoms consistent with transverse myelitis (i.e., paraparesis, loss or disturbance of sensation with a sensory level on the trunk, bowel, and bladder dysfunction) and spinal block, as well as nerve root pain, paresthesia, and motor weakness, may be seen [155].

The thoracic region of the vertebral column is most frequently affected and the formation of a "cold" abscess around the lesion is another characteristic feature [266]. The onset can be sudden or present as a slow ascending paralysis over several months to years. MRI is a more sensitive imaging technique than radiographs and more specific than computed tomography and is generally required for accurate diagnosis of spinal tuberculosis and to rule out intramedullary lesions [249, 266]. Neuroimaging-guided needle biopsy from the affected site in the center of the vertebral body remains the gold standard technique to establish a histopathologic diagnosis and underlying etiology [252, 266]. Antituberculous therapy remains the cornerstone of treatment and essentially is the same as for tuberculous meningitis. Indications for surgical intervention include development of compressive symptoms, large abscess formation, severe kyphosis, an evolving neurological deficit, or lack of response to medical treatment [155, 168, 266].

CNS Infections Caused by Rapidly Growing Mycobacteria

CNS infections associated with rapidly growing mycobacteria are rare. One of the few published reports has implicated *Mycobacterium mucogenicum*, which was isolated in pure culture and detected by PCR sequencing of CSF specimens from two immunocompetent patients who eventually died [267]. *M. mucogenicum* is frequently isolated from tap water or from respiratory specimens and is usually without clinical significance. Other case reports have described CNS infections caused by *Mycobacterium fortuitum*, another rapidly growing mycobacteria found in soil, dust, and water; these infections were all device-associated—a contaminated epidural catheter [268] and manipulation of ventriculoperitoneal shunt [269].

Patients with rapidly growing mycobacterial CNS infection usually present with subacute to chronic meningitis and neutrophilic pleocytosis and usually have a history of trauma or having undergone a neurosurgical procedure or manipulation of a device. CSF smears are often negative for acid-fast organisms but may show gram-positive rods [268–270]. Treatment requires a long course of two or more antimicrobial agents that have the ability to penetrate the blood–brain barrier, with adjunct immunomodulatory therapy with steroids, similar to that used in tuberculous meningitis [268–270].

Fungal CNS Infections

Fungal Meningitis

The most common causes of CNS mycoses include *Cryptococcus* spp. and the dimorphic fungi— *Histoplasma* spp., *Coccidioides* spp., and *Blastomyces* spp. In immunocompromised persons, *Aspergillus* spp., *Candida* spp., and the Mucorales are often implicated. Antifungal therapies that are useful in CNS infections include polyenes (e.g., amphotericin B and its lipid formulations) and azoles (e.g., fluconazole and itraconazole, voriconazole, and posaconazole). Antifungal agents that lack CNS penetration include echinocandins (e.g., caspofungin, micafungin, and anidulafungin). Amphotericin B and flucytosine are used to initiate treatment for CNS yeast infections caused by *Candida* and *Cryptococcus neoformans*. Amphotericin B particularly in lipid formulation and voriconazole are preferred for aspergillus infections.

Cryptococcus Meningitis

Cryptococcus spp. are perhaps the most common fungus implicated in CNS infections. *C. neoformans* has a worldwide distribution and is commonly found in soil that has been contaminated with bird droppings. There are two varieties of *C. neoformans*: *C. neoformans* var. *neoformans* and *C. neoformans* var. gattii. These two species differ in their ecology, distribution in nature, epidemiology, presentation, clinical course, and therapy. *C. neoformans* var. *neoformans* is found worldwide and produces most of the infections in patients in the United States, while *C. neoformans* var. gattii is more commonly found in Southeast Asia, Africa, Australia, and parts of Southern California. The most important determinant of CNS infection caused by *Cryptococcus* spp. is the immune status of the host. This can be most easily demonstrated by the marked increase in the number of cases associated with HIV infection and the fact that as the CD4+ count decreases the incidence of cryptococcal infection increases markedly, particularly at CD4+ counts <200 cells/mm^3. Although a variety of virulence factors have been described in *Cryptococcus* spp. infections, such as the production of the pigment melanin, its thick polysaccharide capsule is probably the most important virulence factor that protects the fungus from phagocytosis by the host.

The initial infection with *Cryptococcus* spp. is due to inhalation and the production of pneumonitis, which is generally asymptomatic even in immunosuppressed patients. Symptomatic patients usually present with fever and cough and a variety of chest radiographic findings, such as nodular, pleural-based lesions, and lobar infiltrates. The initial pneumonia generally clears without treatment, even in immunosuppressed patients. Dissemination from the pneumonitis results in seeding of various organs in the body; the CNS is particularly vulnerable (Fig. 31.22a–c). The organism may remain latent in the lung and at other sites indefinitely. Thus, most patients presenting with cryptococcal meningitis have no evidence of a concurrent pulmonary disease.

C. neoformans is the most common cause of fungal meningitis worldwide. Clinically, the presentation of cryptococcal meningitis is indistinguishable from that seen in chronic meningitis, associated with coccidioidomycosis, histoplasmosis, or tuberculous meningitis. Patients generally describe a history of 1–3 weeks of headache, fever, and stiff neck together with a variety of nonspecific symptoms, such as lethargy, confusion, nausea, vomiting, or rarely, symptoms suggestive of focal neurologic deficits. Patients may develop raised ICP with papilledema (33%), cranial nerve palsies (20%), and seizures; if left untreated, the condition may progress to obtundation and, ultimately, death. Occasionally, total visual loss develops secondary to fungal involvement of the optic tracts, as well as from adhesive arachnoiditis, chorioretinitis, or elevated ICP. Hydrocephalus is a frequent complication even in patients who responded to therapy. Neuroimaging can reveal the extent of CNS involvement: Fig. 31.23 shows *C. neoformans* involvement in the basal ganglia.

The classical method for diagnosis of cryptococcal meningitis is demonstration of the yeast in spinal fluid by India ink stain. Microscopically the India ink particles serve to outline the very large clear polysaccharide capsule surround-

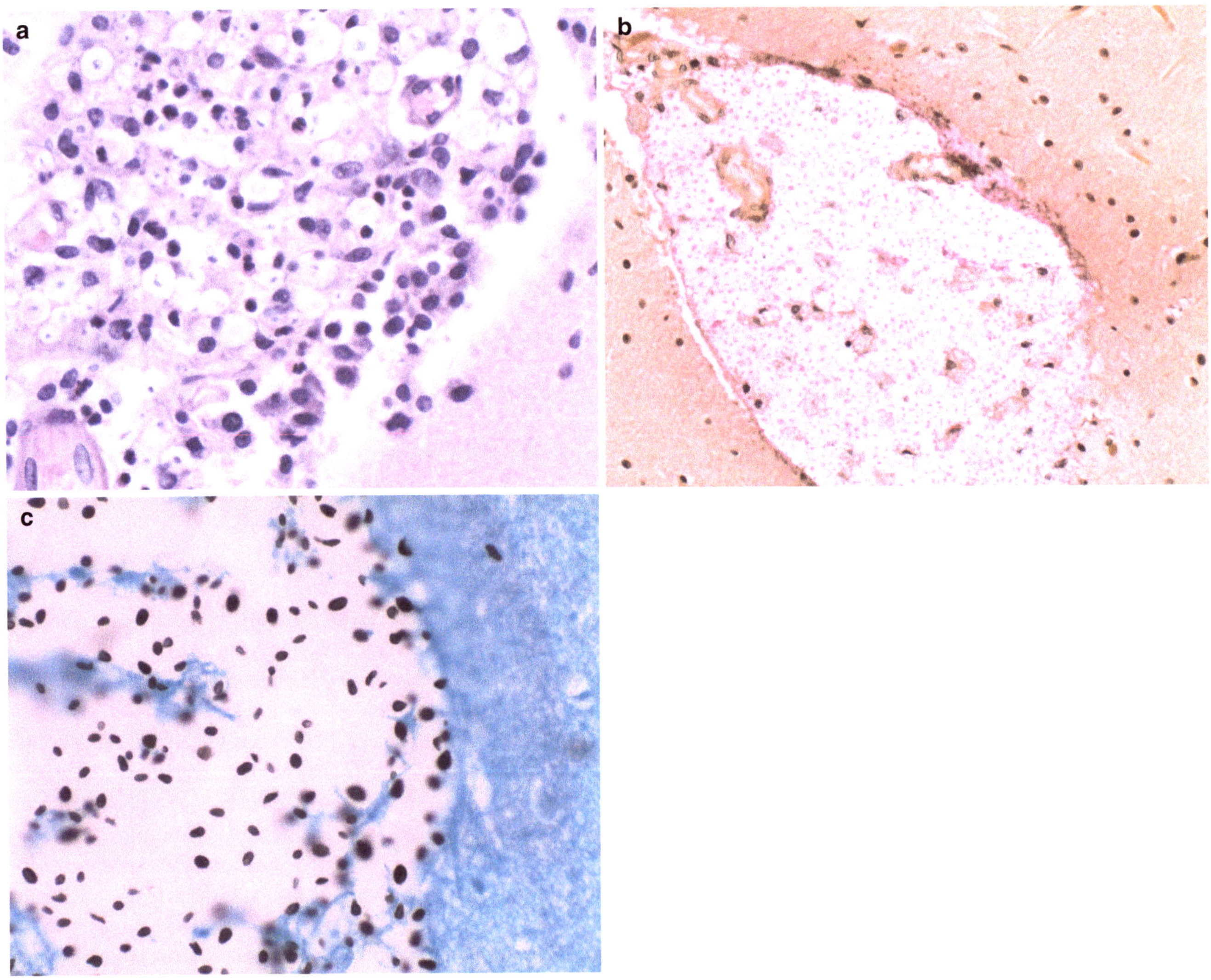

Fig. 31.22 (**a**–**c**) CNS cryptococcosis in a patient with HIV infection. Figure (**a**) shows a distended cerebellar subarachnoid space containing numerous encapsulated *Cryptococcus neoformans* yeast forms with pericapsular clearing (H&E, 40×). Figure (**b**) shows how mucicarmine stains the yeast capsules pink to magenta (Mucicarmine, 20×). Figure (**c**) shows a Gomori methenamine silver (GMS) stain, highlights variably sized yeast forms, with a few yeasts exhibiting "teardrop" budding (GMS, 60×) (All courtesy of Anthony Yachnis, MD, and Kelly Devers, MD, University of Florida College of Medicine)

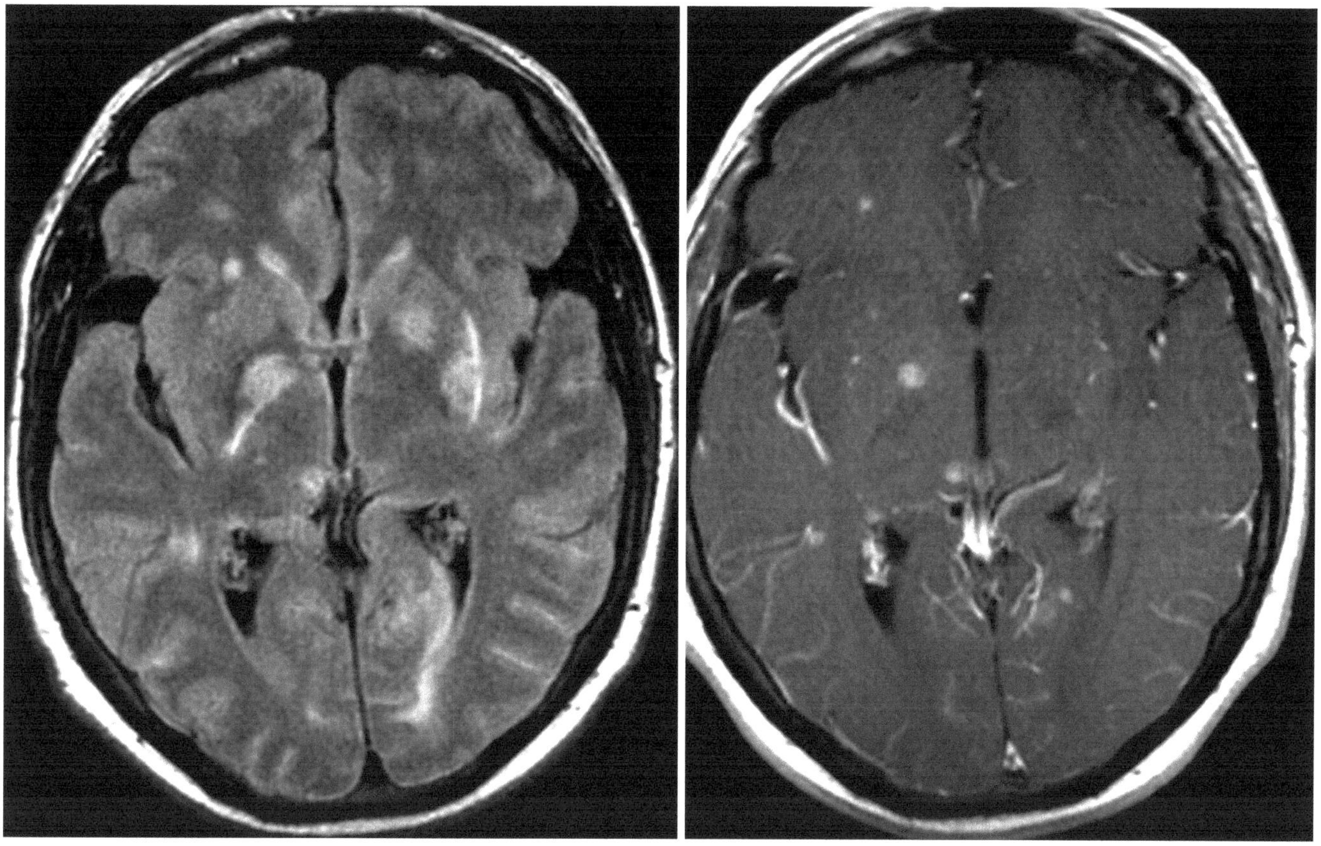

Fig. 31.23 MRI showing *Cryptococcus neoformans* involvement of the basal ganglia

ing the yeast. The test is positive in over 90% of HIV-infected patients but in only 50% of patients with normal immunity. Several latex agglutination tests have been developed that detect the excess polysaccharide capsule produced in the spinal fluid of patients with cryptococcal meningitis. This test is positive in over 95% of patients with the condition. While the test is highly reliable, it is important to recognize that there can be both false-negative and false-positive reactions. For example, HIV-infected patients with overwhelming cryptococcal meningitis may have so much polysaccharide capsule in their CSF that a "prozone" effect occurs, resulting in the finding that undiluted CSF or CSF tested at a 1:2 dilution may appear negative. Generally, upon dilution of the spinal fluid to 1:10 or greater, a positive reaction will be observed. Laboratories must be aware of this prozone effect and physicians who suspect cryptococcal meningitis in HIV-infected patients should alert the laboratory to ensure that this possibility is not overlooked. In addition, cross-reactions with *Trichosporon beigelii* or Capnocytophaga may occasionally produce false-positive latex agglutination tests. The latex agglutination should be confirmed by growth of cryptococci in culture. If a positive cryptococcal antigen titer is found in the CSF from a patient for whom CSF culture did not yield growth of *Cryptococcus* spp., the antigen test cannot be assumed to be false-positive; a large volume (10–20 mL) of CSF should be obtained for repeating the cryptococcal antigen test and reculturing for cryptococcus. The higher the cryptococcal antigen titer, the less likely it is to be a false-positive result. CSF changes in cryptococcal meningitis generally parallel those of chronic tuberculous meningitis and other chronic meningitides (Table 31.2). CSF analysis is typically abnormal as follows: glucose is generally <40 mg/dL, protein is elevated in the large majority of patients, and the white count is usually elevated with a lymphocytic predominance.

Treatment of cryptococcal meningitis depends in part on host susceptibility factors. In patients with no underlying chronic illness or history of HIV infection, IV amphotericin B at a dose of 0.5–0.8 mg/kg/day together with oral flucytosine 37.5 mg/kg every 8 h should be administered until the patient becomes afebrile and culture-negative; generally, this takes approximately 2–6 weeks. Of note, flucytosine may cause severe leukopenia and thrombocytopenia, particularly in patients with impaired renal function, which, in turn, may develop as a result of amphotericin therapy. Therefore, patients need to be monitored carefully for these particular toxic side effects. Some authorities recommend measuring flucytosine levels and adjusting the dose to give a peak of 70–80 mcg/L and a trough of 30–40 mcg/L. However, services for routine measurement of these levels may not be readily available at many hospitals. Alternative therapeutic regimens include various lipid-soluble amphotericin B preparations, which may be used for patients who develop nephrotoxicity. If the patient is intolerant to flucytosine, therapy with amphotericin B at a higher dose of 0.7–1 mg/kg/day for 6–8 weeks may be considered. The initial treatment course is followed by a consolidation course of fluconazole 400–800 mg/day for an additional 2 months. Patients are then transitioned to fluconazole maintenance therapy for at least a year or in some conditions for life.

Histoplasmosis

Histoplasma spp. are dimorphic fungi (i.e., they change their characteristic morphology depending on temperature.) Along with *Coccidioides immitis* and *Blastomyces dermatitidis*, *H. capsulatum* exists as a mold at room temperature (>23 °C) and converts to a yeast form at body temperature of 37 °C. The organism is widely disseminated in nature in the soil and may reach high levels in areas where birds roost and in caves inhabited by large numbers of bats. In vitro, the mold phase is characterized by both macro- and microconidia. The microconidia are small, smooth oval bodies ranging in diameter from 2 to 5 μm and are believed to be the infective phase because their small size enables them to be readily carried down to the terminal bronchioles and alveoli. Although found worldwide, histoplasmosis has a very distinct geographical distribution in the United States. Most cases occur in the Ohio and Mississippi River valleys in the Central Midwestern part of the United States with extension as far eastward as Maryland, Delaware, and some parts of Georgia and Florida. The disease is rarely seen west of Texas, Oklahoma, and Kansas.

Once inhaled, the microconidia are ingested by alveolar macrophages and rapidly undergo conversion to the yeast phase. From the initial pulmonary foci, the yeast rapidly migrates to hilar lymph nodes from which they can disseminate to multiple foci in the body. As is the case with cryptococcus and tuberculosis, an asymptomatic pulmonary infection frequently develops approximately 2–3 weeks after exposure. The development of the cellular immune response limits the spread of the organism and generally clears the initial, early, pulmonary focus, leaving minimal to no calcifications in hilar lymph nodes and lung tissue. The disseminated lesions most commonly manifest through widespread calcific lesions in the spleen and liver after they heal.

Although the vast majority of primary infections in immunologically normal hosts resolve spontaneously, leaving the patient with a positive histoplasma skin test, there are a number of unfavorable outcomes. Dormant infections may reactivate following severe immunosuppression: HIV infection, post transplantation, or after therapy with TNF blockers. Pulmonary disease may go on to produce chronic cavitary histoplasmosis that is radiographically identical to pulmonary tuberculosis. The initial pulmonary infection may result in an acute progressive disseminated infection that characteristically presents with fever, chills, weight loss, hepatosplenomegaly, and pancytopenia from bone marrow involvement. This form of disseminated histoplasmosis most often affects those who are highly immunosuppressed due to AIDS, lymphoma, or iatrogenic therapy.

CNS involvement in this syndrome includes encephalitis, acute meningitis, and encephalopathy. Occasionally, histoplasmomas or mass lesions in the CNS are observed [271–275]. A similar syndrome of disseminated histoplasmosis may also be observed in patients with normal immunity who present with more of a low-grade chronic illness, rather than the acute presentation of disseminated histoplasmosis typically seen in immunosuppressed patients. Symptoms of CNS involvement are secondary to intracranial mass lesions, isolated chronic meningitis with or without other manifestations of disseminated histoplasmosis or meningitis. Some patients may have CNS disease secondary to emboli from histoplasma endocarditis. Wheat and colleagues found that approximately 40% of patients with histoplasma meningitis had chronic meningitis as part of their disseminated disease [273]; 25–30% had isolated chronic meningitis, and the remainder presented with various forms of mass lesions and encephalitis. In general, the duration of symptoms of histoplasma meningitis prior to diagnosis tends to be somewhat longer than the duration of symptoms for cryptococcal or tuberculous meningitis. In Wheat's series, approximately 30% of patients had duration of symptoms <1 month; 44% had symptoms for 2–6 months, and 27% had symptoms lasting >6 months before the diagnosis was made. Patients who present with localizing CNS signs and symptoms should have neuroimaging (CT scans or MRI) to rule out mass lesions. Those with systemic manifestations may have the diagnosis made by culture or biopsy of an enlarged lymph node, liver, or bone marrow. Diagnosis is best made by visualization of yeast in tissue or by culture. CSF findings are typical for chronic fungal and tuberculous meningitis, with 90% of patients having a CSF pleocytosis with lymphocytic predominance (Table 31.2). At least 80% of patients have an elevated CSF protein level and a glucose level <40 mg/dL. CSF white blood cells usually number between 50 and 500 cells/μl and are predominantly mononuclear.

Serologic testing for antibodies to *H. capsulatum* in blood is generally positive in 60–90% of patients with CNS histoplasmosis. The standard assays are the complement fixation test that uses two separate antigens, yeast and mycelial (or histoplasmin), and the immunodiffusion assay [272]. Diagnosis is based on a fourfold rise in antibody titer; a single titer of ≥1:32 is suggestive but not diagnostic. However, in an endemic area, serological tests are often difficult to interpret because patients may have antibodies from prior exposure rather than active infection; likewise, skin testing in an endemic area is probably of no diagnostic value. In the series described by Wheat, CSF cultures were positive in only 26.7% of patients [273].

Treatment

Histoplasmosis involving the CNS is difficult to treat. Amphotericin B given as a lipid formulation should be used for initial therapy in all patients at a dosage of 3–5 mg/kg daily for 3–4 months. Therapy can be assessed with serial weekly or biweekly lumbar punctures for CSF *Histoplasma* antigen levels, white blood cell counts, and complement fixation antibody titers. A rise in the CSF glucose and a fall in the CSF cell count and protein levels would suggest a successful response to treatment. Resolution of abnormal findings can help determine the duration of therapy [272]. Approximately 80% of patients will respond to amphotericin, but at least half of those initial responders will relapse and approximately 20% will die from the disease. Treatment with Amphotericin B should be followed by an oral azole agent for an undetermined period of time. Primary therapy with itraconazole or fluconazole is not useful in the treatment of CNS histoplasmosis—they do not cross the blood–brain barrier particularly well, and failure rates are remarkably high. Kauffman has categorically stated that primary azole therapy of CNS histoplasmosis should be discouraged [272]. Both azoles have been used successfully for secondary treatment following induction therapy with amphotericin B [272]. The dosage suggested for itraconazole is 200 mg twice or thrice daily, and that for fluconazole is 800 mg daily. In HIV-infected patients, suppressive treatment with itraconazole 200 mg orally daily should begin after the initial course of amphotericin.

Coccidioidal Meningitis

Infections with *Coccidioides immitis* have been recognized for over 100 years and were originally believed to be a nearly uniformly fatal. Like the other dimorphic fungi (*Histoplasma capsulatum* and *Blastomyces dermatitidis*), the natural habitat of *C. immitis* is soil. Unlike other dimorphic fungi, *C. immitis* is not distributed worldwide but is limited to the lower Sonoran life zone, found primarily in the desert in the Southwest part of the United States, Mexico, and parts of South and Central America. The characteristics of this particular zone are an arid climate with a yearly rainfall of 5–20 in., hot summers, warm winters, and alkaline soil. In the mold phase of the fungus, which is the form found in soil and other environmental sources, the hyphae fragment into specific structures known as arthrospores which are highly infectious and readily aerosolized when the dust is produced. Thus, on occasion, dust storms have blown infectious spores of *C. immitis* as far north as Sacramento and beyond to produce outbreaks well outside the endemic area of the San Joaquin Valley. Transmission of the organism on fomites as far as the East Coast has been implicated in documented cases. The narrow environmental requirements of this fungus account for its endemic distribution within the United States. Epidemiologic studies of people who migrate into the Central Valley of California suggest that the annual risk of infection is approximately 15%.

Pathogenesis

As is the case with the other dimorphic fungi, the initial route of infection is inhalation with an early focus on infection in lung tissue. The outcome of this infection is highly variable. Approximately one-half to two-thirds of patients demonstrated to be infected with this agent show little or absolutely no initial pulmonary infection. The majority of patients who become symptomatic develop a mild self-limited respiratory infection manifest by fever, cough, malaise, arthralgias, weight loss, and in some patients, a striking clinical syndrome of erythema nodosum and erythema multiforme. The vast majority of these symptomatic cases resolve within 2–4 weeks, occasionally taking up to several months, without treatment. Complications occur in no more than about 10% of all patients with clinically symptomatic primary infections. Occasionally patients will present with fulminant pneumonia and shock-like syndrome, possibly resulting from a particularly high inoculum or perhaps as a result of fungemia and miliary dissemination of the disease. Such a presentation is not uncommon among HIV patients with severe depression of the CD4+ count. Other manifestations include pulmonary nodules, cavities, and chronic lung disease indistinguishable from chronic tuberculosis. The most common site of disseminated lesions is the skin where maculopapular lesions may progress to keratotic and verrucous ulcers with subcutaneous fluctuant abscesses.

The most serious form of disseminated disease following initial pulmonary infection is coccidioidal meningitis which is a result of lymphohematogenous spread from lungs to meninges [276]. Without treatment it is nearly uniformly fatal within 2 years of diagnosis [276–279]. Observational studies suggest about 80% of patients who develop meningitis become symptomatic within 6 months of the initial infection [280]. The signs and symptoms of coccidioidal meningitis are very similar to those of other chronic fungal and tuberculous meningitides. Patients generally present with headache, fever, varying degrees of nuchal rigidity, nausea, vomiting, seizures, and altered mental status [276–280]. Factors that predispose to *C. immitis* dissemination and the development of meningitis include immunosuppression due to HIV infection, diabetes mellitus, alcohol abuse, pregnancy, steroids or other immunosuppressive drugs, and non-Caucasian race [278].

Diagnosis of coccidioidal meningitis is based on analysis of the CSF, which shows typical findings of elevated opening pressure (>25 cm H_2O), elevated leukocyte count with a predominance of lymphocytes, elevated protein, and depressed glucose (Table 31.2). Occasionally, patients may have a significant CSF eosinophilia [281]. Thus, in a patient who presents with a history suggestive of chronic meningitis together with typical CSF findings, a history of travel to or having lived in an endemic area must be carefully sought after. Complications, such as meningitis, may occur as late as 2 years after the initial exposure, which may be exceedingly brief, such as a mere drive through the California's Central Valley [275, 277–280].

Although *C. immitis* grows well on typical fungal media, only about one-third of CSF cultures yield growth of the pathogen [278]. The most reliable method of diagnosis is the detection of complement fixing antibodies in the CSF. Although this testing may be negative in a few patients during the early phase of the disease, they eventually become positive over the ensuing months. In patients with pulmonary disease or extrapulmonary manifestations, biopsy with culture and histopathologic examination of involved tissue may give positive results. The demonstration of a spherule in tissue or a positive culture is diagnostic. MRI scans of the brain invariably are abnormal with evidence of basilar meningitis, hydrocephalus, or cerebral infarcts [278].

Treatment

Fluconazole at 400 mg/day is currently recommended as the treatment of choice for coccidioidal meningitis because the response rate of approximately 70% is very close to that achieved with intrathecal amphotericin B, which was used in the past. In patients who do not respond to the 400 mg/day dose of fluconazole, higher doses may be used. If there is no response to azole therapy, amphotericin B at a dose of 0.1–0.3 mg/kg/day may be given intrathecally, optimally through an Ommaya reservoir. Intravenous amphotericin B has poor CSF penetration and has a limited role in the management of coccidioidal meningitis [278]. Treatment with oral fluconazole must be prolonged for at least 2 years after the spinal fluid becomes completely normal. In patients with HIV infection, therapy is continued for life. It should be noted that the response rate is by no means 100% in either meningitis or disseminated disease and that relapses are not uncommon even in patients who respond initially.

As is the case with other fungi and tuberculosis, patients occasionally present with mass lesions in brain parenchyma caused by *C. immitis*. These lesions often require surgical drainage or excision. In addition, hydrocephalus is relatively common in patients with *C. immitis* meningitis, particularly in children, and must be managed with ventricular shunting. On occasion, *C. immitis* may actually grow in the shunt and cause obstruction. Patients who have a ventricular shunt in place cannot be administered intrathecal amphotericin B in an Ommaya reservoir. Rather, Amphotericin B must be administered intrathecally via intracisternal puncture or lateral neck injection under radiographic guidance. Although intrathecal therapy can be given via the lumbar route, this inevitably leads to varying degrees of potentially severe and debilitating arachnoiditis after several weeks.

Blastomycosis

Blastomycosis is a systemic pyogranulomatous disease caused by *Blastomyces dermatitidis*, another dimorphic fungus that grows as a yeast form at 37 ° C and in a hyphal form at room temperature. *B. dermatitidis* exists in nature in the warm moist soils of wooded areas rich in organic debris, such as decaying vegetation. However, the reports of isolation of the organism in nature have been relatively few and somewhat inconsistent. *B. dermatitidis* occurrence follows the distribution of the Mississippi River and is most commonly reported in states such as Louisiana, Western Alabama, Central Arkansas, Missouri, Kentucky, Western Tennessee, and as far north as Minnesota. Outbreaks have occurred along the St. Lawrence River in Canada and in many parts of North and South Carolina [282].

Pathogenesis

Pulmonary infection occurs by the inhalation of conidia, which convert to the yeast form after deposition in the airways. Pulmonary manifestations vary from asymptomatic to overwhelming multilobar infection with involvement of hilar lymph nodes. From there, dissemination to the skin and other organs may occur via lymphohematogenous spread. Normal host responses generate a characteristic pyogranulomatous reaction. Extrapulmonary involvement in descending order of frequency includes skin (25%), osteoarticular (25%), genitourinary (17%), and CNS (5%) disease [282–286]. CNS disease is more common in immunocompromised patients, for example, 40% of patients with AIDS who have blastomycosis also have CNS involvement as meningitis or mass lesions [282, 287, 288]. Less common metastatic sites include the liver, spleen, and naso–/oro-pharynx. Chronic pulmonary infection resembling tuberculosis or other chronic fungal disease may develop. Dissemination to the skin produces a variety of clinical manifestations, such as chronic verrucous lesions with crusting and purulent drainage, giant keratoacanthoma, and lesions mimicking pyoderma gangrenosum or squamous cell carcinoma. Suppurative granulomatous lesions of the skin and bone may develop and become chronic.

Pathologically, the histological response is that of neutrophils and non-caseating granulomata with epithelioid and giant cells. Because of a vigorous proliferative response, the pseudoepitheliomatous changes seen on skin and mucosal surfaces in response to *B. dermatitidis* may resemble squamous cell carcinoma.

Clinical Manifestations

Most acutely infected patients are asymptomatic or develop a self-limited respiratory illness. The vast majority of patients present with symptoms of pneumonia after an incubation period of 30–45 days. Symptoms are nonspecific, with fever, cough, myalgias, arthralgias, and pleuritic chest pain. Chest examination may reveal lobar or segmental consolidation, including mass lesions mimicking carcinoma with hilar lymphadenopathy. Involvement of the CNS is unusual, with cases generally presenting with meningitis, and rarely as intracranial mass lesion or abscesses that might be solitary or multiple [283, 287, 289].

Clinical involvement of the CNS accounts for 5–10% of extrapulmonary blastomycosis in clinical reviews [286, 290, 291]. Although CNS blastomycosis may develop in patients without evidence of disseminated disease, most reported cases involving the CNS also have evidence of systemic infection. In addition to meningitis, patients with blastomycosis may present with blastomycomas or mass lesions in the CNS more frequently than is seen with other fungal CNS infections [283, 289]. While steroids and immunosuppressive treatment do not predispose to meningitis per se, they may predispose to dissemination of pulmonary blastomycosis and, hence, increase the probability of neurologic involvement.

Diagnosis

Because there is no highly specific serologic or diagnostic skin test material available, the diagnosis rests upon culture of the organism from pulmonary secretions, skin biopsy material, or direct visualization of round, multinucleated yeast forms that produce daughter cells from a single broad-based bud [292]. Histopathologic analysis of tissue specimens stained with methenamine silver or periodic acid-Schiff (PAS) reagents is the standard diagnostic method for extrapulmonary infection [282]. A urinary antigen is available to aid in diagnosis, but it is not particularly specific (79%) and shows cross-reactivity by testing positive (96.3%) in patients with histoplasmosis [293, 294]. Antibody assays by complement fixation or immunodiffusion remain nonspecific and insensitive, and the confirmatory diagnostic test at present remains the growth of the organism in culture [295].

Treatment

Prior to the availability of amphotericin B and itraconazole, the disease was progressive and was associated with mortality rates >60%. Some patients with pulmonary disease have a self-limited infection, but it remains unclear whether the initial primary pulmonary infection should be treated. However, because of the inherent limited ability to predict which cases will disseminate, it is often recommended to treat most cases of pulmonary infection caused by *Blastomyces* spp. In mild to moderate cases of pulmonary disease, the treatment of choice is itraconazole 200 mg once or twice daily for 6–12 months. In moderately severe to severe disseminated blastomycosis, lipid amphotericin B 3–5 mg/kg/day or deoxycholate amphotericin B 0.3–1.0 mg/kg/day for 1–2 weeks should be used followed itraconazole, 200 mg twice daily for 12 months [282]. Mild to moderate disseminated CNS disease should be treated with high-dose lipid amphotericin B 5 mg/kg/day for 1–2 weeks followed itraconazole 200 mg twice daily for 12 months. If the patient is immunosuppressed or is HIV-infected, the recommended therapeutic regimen is lipid amphotericin B 3–5 mg/kg/day or deoxycholate amphotericin B 0.7–1.0 mg/kg/day for 1–2 weeks followed by itraconazole 200 mg twice daily for 12 months; lifelong suppressive therapy may be indicated in some patients, especially if immunosuppression cannot be reversed [282]. In patients with life-threatening disease, the total dose of amphotericin B may have to be increased.

Candida CNS Infections

Candida species are a part of the normal human enteric flora and are the most common microorganism associated with healthcare-associated fungal infections in tertiary care centers in economically developed countries. *Candida* species can cause invasive disease in every major organ system, including the liver, kidney, heart, lungs, spleen, or bone with or without candidemia. In contrast, *Candida* spp. rarely produce CNS disease. Meningitis is uncommon except as a complication of an operation or placement of an in situ ventricular shunt. Neonates and premature infants seem to be at higher risk than adults. Among the various species, *C. albicans* accounts for most of the documented CNS fungal infections, while those caused by non-albicans species (the most encountered are *C. glabrata*, *C. parapsilosis*, *C. tropicalis*, *C. pseudotropicalis*, *C. guilliermondii*, *C. krusei*, or *C. lusitaniae*) are relatively less common; *C. glabrata* is a rare cause of CNS infection. In general, CNS disease caused by *Candida* species occurs as part of disseminated infection in hospitalized patients who have one or more predisposing risk factors, such as prematurity, intravenous hyperalimentation, various intravascular devices and intravenous catheters, treatment with corticosteroids, neutropenia, diabetes, pancreatitis, hemodialysis HIV infection, patients with leukemia, post neurosurgery, broad-spectrum antimicrobial use, or indwelling bladder catheters [296–300].

Four clinicopathologic disease groups of neurocandidiasis have been identified: (1) cerebral microabscesses that cause diffuse encephalopathy. Patients with microabscesses are generally diagnosed with systemic candidiasis before death, and the neurologic involvement is usually only detected at autopsy [298, 300, 301]. (2) *Candida* meningitis occurs together with disseminated microabscesses or alone as chronic meningitis with a dense exudate at the base of the brain and brain stem. Microscopic examination reveals changes consistent with granulomatous meningitis, sometimes with yeasts and hyphae; the onset is usually subacute with fever and headache [300, 302]. A cerebral CT scan might reveal hydrocephalus and CSF culture invariably yields the microorganism. (3) Cerebral macroabscesses are less frequent and may result in seizures and focal neurological signs; diagnosis is based on neuroimaging studies and biopsy [303]. And (4) vasculitis and mycotic aneurysms are recognized vascular complications that often lead to cerebral infarction and subarachnoid hemorrhage if not treated in a timely manner [304]. Thus, depending on the pathophysiology of CNS disease, symptoms can be similar to bacterial meningitis (e.g., fever, headache, neck stiffness, chills, photophobia) or manifest as a subacute infection with headache, low-grade fever, malaise, fatigue, altered mental status, cranial nerve palsies, vomiting, confusion, and lethargy—symptoms that are often seen in patients with cryptococcal and tuberculous meningitis.

The recommended treatment for *Candida* spp. CNS infections is liposomal amphotericin B (5 mg/kg) with or without Flucytosine 25 mg/kg four times/day in patients with normal renal function. This combination is recommended because of in vitro synergism and the excellent CSF concentrations achieved by flucytosine. However, several weeks of therapy are recommended before transitioning to oral azole therapy. Because amphotericin B is associated with renal insufficiency, hypokalemia, hypomagnesemia, hypocalcemia, and hypophosphatemia, patients treated with amphotericin B should have daily monitoring of serum creatinine and electrolytes. The severe side effects of flucytosine include hepatotoxicity and bone-marrow depression that can lead to reduction in hemoglobin, neutrophil, lymphocyte, and platelet counts. In most patients, these side effects are concentration-dependent and often predictable. Critical care monitoring should include weekly lumbar taps for CSF analysis and culture, and daily blood counts and biochemical profiles to monitor electrolytes, renal, and liver function. The optimal length of therapy with amphotericin B alone or in combination with flucytosine has not been studied. However, it follows that one would require clinical improvement in the patient, normalization or improvement in CSF indices, and negative CSF culture before transition to fluconazole 400–800 mg (6–12 mg/kg)/day.

Fluconazole, itraconazole, voriconazole, posaconazole, and isavuconazole demonstrate similar activity against most *Candida* species. However, the choice of agent will depend on the agent's ability to penetrate the CNS. Fluconazole has the greatest penetration into the CSF and is therefore the initial drug of choice for treatment of CNS *Candida* spp. infections. Voriconazole is used for step-down oral therapy in CNS infections caused by *C. krusei* or *C. glabrata*; for the latter microorganism, susceptibility to voriconazole must be confirmed before treatment is initiated. Posaconazole does not achieve therapeutic levels in the CSF and is therefore not recommended for the treatment of CNS *Candida* spp. infections. Flucytosine demonstrates broad antifungal activity against most *Candida* species, except for *C. krusei*. Although echinocandins penetrate brain tissue, their penetration of CSF is substantially lower than azoles.

In summary, IDSA recommends the following:

- Therapy should continue until all signs and symptoms and CSF and radiological abnormalities have resolved.
- Infected CNS devices, including ventriculostomy drains, shunts, stimulators, prosthetic reconstructive devices, and biopolymer wafers that deliver chemotherapy, should be removed if possible.
- For patients in whom a ventricular device cannot be removed, amphotericin B deoxycholate could be administered through the device into the ventricle at a dosage ranging from 0.01 mg to 0.5 mg in 2 mL 5% dextrose in water.

Zygomycetes and Zygomycosis

Zygomycosis is the term used to describe infection caused by any of the zygomycetes—*Absidia*, *Rhizopus*, and *Mucor*. These saprophytic organisms are ubiquitous in the environment, especially soil and commonly found on bread. The genuses *Absidia*, *Rhizopus*, and *Mucor* can invade the CNS by direct extension or from hematogenous spread. Disseminated disease occurring via the hematogenous route may produce CNS mucormycosis resulting in infarction and abscess formation. The Zygomycetes tend to invade the paranasal sinuses or palate with subsequent progression through tissue, nerves, blood vessels, and fascial planes, followed by the vital structures at the base of the brain (Fig. 31.24a, b). In patients with diabetes, this disease typically presents as rhinocerebral mucor (Fig. 31.25). Patients are generally predisposed to this complication if their serum glucose has remained uncontrolled and the patient has been acidotic for at least several weeks. Initial symptoms usually include sinus pain, headache, fever, and nasal stuffiness and discharge, which quickly progresses to facial cellulitis, swelling, proptosis, carotid artery occlusion, cavernous sinus

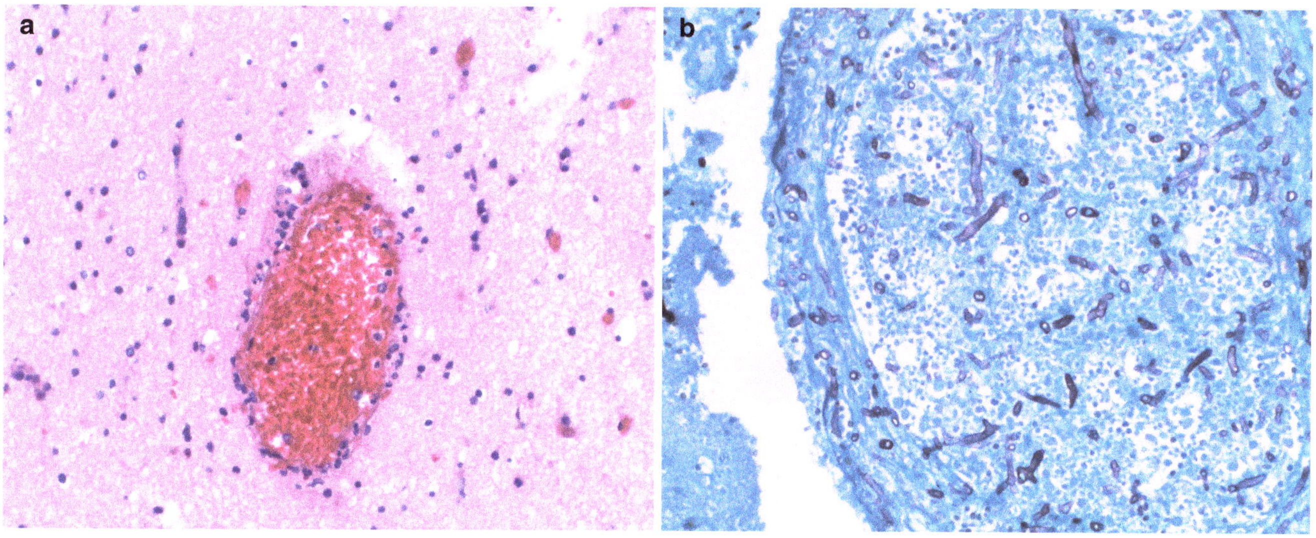

Fig. 31.24 (**a**) A 63-year-old male with disseminated mucor infection. Shows CNS vasculitis with neutrophils invading CNS parenchymal vessels with early vessel wall destruction (H&E, 20×). (**b**) Same patient. Features a Gomori methenamine silver (GMS)-stained specimen demonstrating angioinvasion by fungi with broad aseptate hyphae and right-angle branching (GMS, 20×) (Both courtesy of Anthony Yachnis, MD, and Kelly Devers, MD, University of Florida College of Medicine)

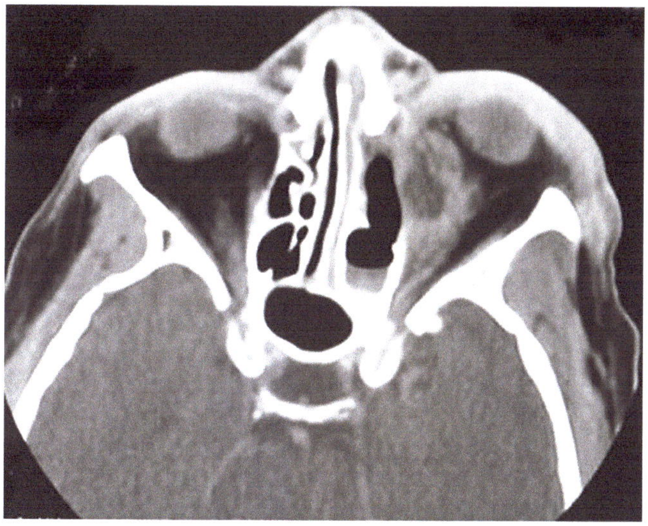

Fig. 31.25 Orbital mucormycosis. Image is a post-contrast axial CT section through the ethmoidal bridge. This case illustrates changes of a left subperiosteal, mesial, orbital abscess. There is little evidence of ethmoid sinusitis. However, it is not uncommon, as in this case, that invasive fungal infections arising either from sinusitis or rhinitis may have only subtle mucosal thickening on imaging, yet still can permeate bone creating soft tissue abscesses in the skull base

thrombosis, CNS infarction due to fungal thrombosis, CNS hemorrhage, abscess, cerebritis, blindness, and airway obstruction caused by head and neck infections. Death ensues if the condition is not treated. Other at-risk populations include persons who have been neutropenic for more than 2–3 weeks as well as those with iron overload, burns, HIV infection and AIDS, blood dyscrasias, transplantation, immunosuppression/on chemotherapy, IV drug abuse, and high-dose steroids. Patients with rhinocerebral mucormycosis may manifest hyperglycemia and metabolic acidosis. Lumbar puncture and CSF analysis often reveal a raised opening pressure, a neutrophilic pleocytosis, normal or slightly elevated protein levels, and low glucose levels. In most cases, however, CSF study findings are normal [305]. Neuroimaging studies help to support the diagnosis of rhinocerebral mucormycosis and to precisely determine the extent of disease. CT scans and MRI reveal soft tissue extent of infection, mucosal thickening, and bony destruction of the sinuses and orbit, presence of cavernous sinus thrombosis, cerebritis, and cerebral edema (Fig. 31.25). Tissue biopsy is necessary to demonstrate the invasive hyphae. The Zygomycetes all appear as ribbon-like nonseptate hyphae in tissue with right- or obtuse-angle branching (Fig. 31.24b). Treatment of the condition is based on three main principles: rapid reversal of underlying predisposing factors, antifungal therapy with amphotericin B, and timely surgical intervention. Treatment includes control of the underlying predisposing condition (e.g., control of diabetic ketoacidosis, hypoxia, and electrolyte abnormalities), IV amphotericin B in a dose of at least 1 mg/kg/day, together with vigorous surgical debridement of all involved tissue. Dexamethasone has been used to treat brain edema. Rhinocerebral mucormycosis carries a prognosis of high morbidity and mortality. Survival depends on the reversibility of underlying risk factors and early surgical intervention [306].

CNS Infections Caused by *Aspergillus* Species

Aspergillus fumigatus and *Aspergillus flavus* can produce CNS disease very similar to that described earlier for mucormycosis. Invasive aspergillosis can occur in patients with preexisting bronchiectasis, chronic bronchitis, asthma, tuberculosis, or in persons who are immunosuppressed (e.g., solid organ transplant recipients). Patients with prolonged and profound neutropenia (< 100 cells/μL) are at high risk for invasive aspergillosis. Colonization with *Aspergillus* spp. can lead to tissue invasion with branching septate hyphae that are best visualized in tissue with silver stains and histologically distinct from other fungi—i.e., *Aspergillus* spp. have frequent septae that branch at 45° angles. Lung invasion can involve blood vessels leading to hematogenous spread. The majority of invasive CNS infections occur in immunosuppressed transplant patients in the hospital who had pulmonary disease that progressed to brain involvement via hematogenous dissemination. Compared with persons with uncontrolled diabetes who are more susceptible to infections caused by mucor, patients with prolonged neutropenia appear to be more susceptible to invasive *Aspergillus* spp. sinus infection with direct extension from the maxillary and ethmoid sinuses with progression to cavernous sinus thrombosis. Voriconazole which has good CNS tissue penetration is usually first-line therapy with surgical debridement of all infected tissue. High-dose amphotericin B may be considered in treatment failure [307].

Opportunistic Infections Associated with HIV Infection

HIV infection predisposes individuals to a variety of opportunistic infections of the brain, including infections caused by *Cryptococcus* spp., *Toxoplasma gondii*, CMV, or the polyomavirus (JC virus) that causes progressive multifocal leukoencephalopathy (PML). In addition, the virus itself is associated with a variety of neuropathologic manifestations.

Toxoplasma Gondii

Toxoplasmic encephalitis is caused by the protozoan *T. gondii*. Disease appears to occur almost exclusively because of reactivation of latent tissue cysts. Primary infection occasionally is associated with acute cerebral or disseminated disease. *T. gondii* causes latent infection in a significant proportion (10–90%) of the world's population but uncommonly causes clinically significant disease [308]. In addition, *T. gondii* infects numerous wild and domestic animals. Human infection generally occurs through the ingestion of raw or undercooked meat that contains cysts, or by the ingestion of food or water contaminated by the oocysts shed in the stool of infected animals. In the United States, the major animal reservoir for this infection is the domestic cat. The life cycle is complex. The sexual phase of the cycle takes place in the cat with formation of oocysts in the mucosal lining of the intestine for approximately 3 weeks after initial infection. During this time, as many as ten million oocysts may be shed daily. Oocysts require 1–5 days to become infectious after being shed by the cat, a process that depends on temperature and availability of oxygen. During intestinal infection, the tachyzoite form of the organism, a 2–4 μm wide by 4–8 μm long crescent-like structure, is produced and disseminates to many different areas in the host. Wide ranges of intermediate hosts ingest the oocysts, which form latent cysts in many tissues, including muscle. In humans, as in many domestic and wild animals, this dissemination is asymptomatic and results in the formation of cysts in brain parenchyma as well as muscle and numerous other organs. Transmission to humans is a result of exposure to excreta from cats, ingestion of undercooked infected meat, or from contaminated water supplies.

Serologic surveys in the United States show that approximately 15% of the general population have been infected with toxoplasmosis at some time in the past [309]. In contrast, the prevalence is much higher in economically underdeveloped countries and in certain parts of Europe where rates may range as high as 75%. Although reactivation of toxoplasmosis in the brain generally leads to local replication with the production of single or multiple abscesses, hematogenous dissemination and infection in the lung and other parts of the body have been documented. The incidence and attributable mortality in Europe and the United States have decreased substantially since the introduction of antiretroviral therapy and the broad use of prophylaxis regimens active against *T. gondii*.

Clinical Manifestations

In humans, primary infection with toxoplasma may, on occasion, produce a mononucleosis-like illness characterized by lymphadenopathy, fever, malaise, liver function abnormalities, and, occasionally, myocarditis. However, in the large majority of cases, primary infection is asymptomatic and only becomes recognized under conditions of extreme immunosuppression, such as occurs when CD4+ counts in HIV-infected individuals fall to levels <100 cells/mm^3, when the cysts break down and initiate symptomatic infection. In immunocompromised patients, reactivation of latent disease can cause life-threatening encephalitis. Patients with toxoplasmic encephalitis generally present with a syndrome of fever, headache and varying degrees of confusion, lethargy, obtundation, focal neurologic signs developing over a period of 1–3 weeks, lymphadenopathy, and splenomegaly. In some patients, the presentation can be abrupt, with seizures or cerebral hemorrhage. Hemiparesis and abnormalities of speech are quite common. Less commonly, brain stem involvement may result in cranial nerve deficits, while dyskinesias such as Parkinsonism, dystonia, tremor, and hemiballismus may also accompany the presenting syndromes. Patients occasionally present with endocrine abnormalities due to involvement of the pituitary axis as well as psychiatric manifestations, such as psychoses and dementia.

Diagnosis

The diagnosis is made by a combination of clinical, imaging, morphological, and serological investigations. In an HIV-infected patient, the finding of single or multiple ring-enhancing lesions by CT or MRI scanning strongly suggests toxoplasma encephalitis (Fig. 31.26a–c). If the patient is also known to be or is found to be, serologically positive for antibodies to toxoplasma, the combination is virtually diagnostic. In patients with a single lesion, the major differential is lymphoma, and a brain biopsy may be required to make a definitive diagnosis. MRI has superior sensitivity when compared with CT scanning and should therefore be used as the initial diagnostic procedure when feasible. Toxoplasmic encephalitis lesions on MRI appear as high-signal abnormalities on T2-weighted studies and have a rim of enhancement surrounding the edema on T1-weighted, contrast-enhanced images. Other imaging techniques, such as PET, radionuclide (e.g., Thallium 201) scanning, and magnetic resonance techniques have been used to evaluate patients with AIDS who have focal CNS lesions and to specifically differentiate between toxoplasmosis and primary CNS lymphoma. Grossly, the acute lesions are hemorrhagic, necrotic, space-occupying lesions with surrounding edema. Histologically, there are cysts, free parasites, necrosis, and vasculitis (Fig. 31.27a, b). These lesions regress with treatment.

Laboratory studies, such as complete blood cell count (CBC), chemistries, and liver function tests, are typically normal. Affected patients may have lymphocytosis. CSF analysis shows nonspecific abnormalities, such as elevated white count and protein levels. Attempts to improve the sensitivity by the detection of toxoplasma oligoclonal antibody bands have been reported but do not add any more diagnostic value than a positive serum antibody test. PCR for toxoplasmosis in CSF has been reported to have a sensitivity of 81% in untreated patients with acute disease; the drawback is that many "in-house" PCR assays suffer from lack of standardization and variable performance according to the laboratory performing the assays [310].

Although a wide variety of antibody tests are available, current commercial ELISA (enzyme-linked immunosorbent assay), IgG, and IgM tests, along with the indirect fluorescent antibody test, are readily available and highly specific. Because the disease in HIV patients is almost always due to reactivation of an old focus, the IgG test should be positive and the IgM test should be negative in these individuals. However, diagnosis based on classical serological testing is often inconclusive as immunodeficient individuals often fail to produce significant titers of specific antibodies [310].

Treatment

Treatment should be instituted empirically for HIV-infected patients with compatible clinical and imaging studies. The standard drug regimens include 6 weeks of therapy with pyrimethamine 200 mg as a loading dose followed by 75–100 mg daily together with either sulfadiazine 1–1.5 g every 6 h or clindamycin 600–1200 mg IV every 6 h. Folinic acid (leucovorin), 10–20 mg/day, is given to reduce bone marrow toxicity. If the patient is intolerant of sulfadiazine or clindamycin, the following may be given in addition to pyrimethamine and folinic acid: clarithromycin 1 g orally every 12 h, atovaquone 700 mg orally every 6 h, azithromycin 1200–1500 mg/day orally, or dapsone 100 mg/day.

A systematic review of therapeutic regimens for the management of toxoplasmic encephalitis in HIV-infected adults concluded that pyrimethamine + sulfadiazine and pyrimethamine + clindamycin were equivalent in effectiveness in the treatment of acute toxoplasmic encephalitis in HIV-infected individuals [310, 311]. The review also found that trimethoprim/sulfamethoxazole, which is cheap and readily available in developing countries, may be suitable first-line therapy for acute toxoplasmic encephalitis in HIV-infected individuals and, in fact, was not found to be inferior compared with pyrimethamine + sulfadiazine [311]. More recent studies indicate that trimethoprim/sulfamethoxazole is indeed an alternative treatment for toxoplasmic encephalitis because it is inexpensive, well-tolerated, and as effective as pyrimethamine-sulfadiazine [312]. Trimethoprim/sulfamethoxazole) may be given 3–5 mg/kg of the trimethoprim component orally or IV every 12 h for 4–6 weeks. Other potential advantages of trimethoprim/sulfamethoxazole include less adverse events, ease of dosing, parenteral formulation, cost, and accessibility [312–314]. Pereira-Chioccola and colleagues recommend that complications, such as expansive brain lesions with a mass effect (e.g., deviation of the middle line structures or imminent risk of cerebral herniation) and cases with diffuse encephalitis should be administered adjunctive corticosteroid therapy. Seizures should be treated with appropriate anticonvulsant agents [313].

Signs of improvement are generally seen in the level of consciousness and in a decrease of fever within 5–7 days, with over 90% generally responding by day 14 [315]. If there is no clinical or radiographic response within 10 days, alternative diagnoses and brain biopsy must be considered. Reactivation of latent infection in the CNS is a common HIV/AIDS-related complication. Thus, current guidelines recommend that patients with toxoplasmic encephalitis should be treated with the initial regimen for 4–6 weeks, depending) upon the degree and rapidity of improvement,

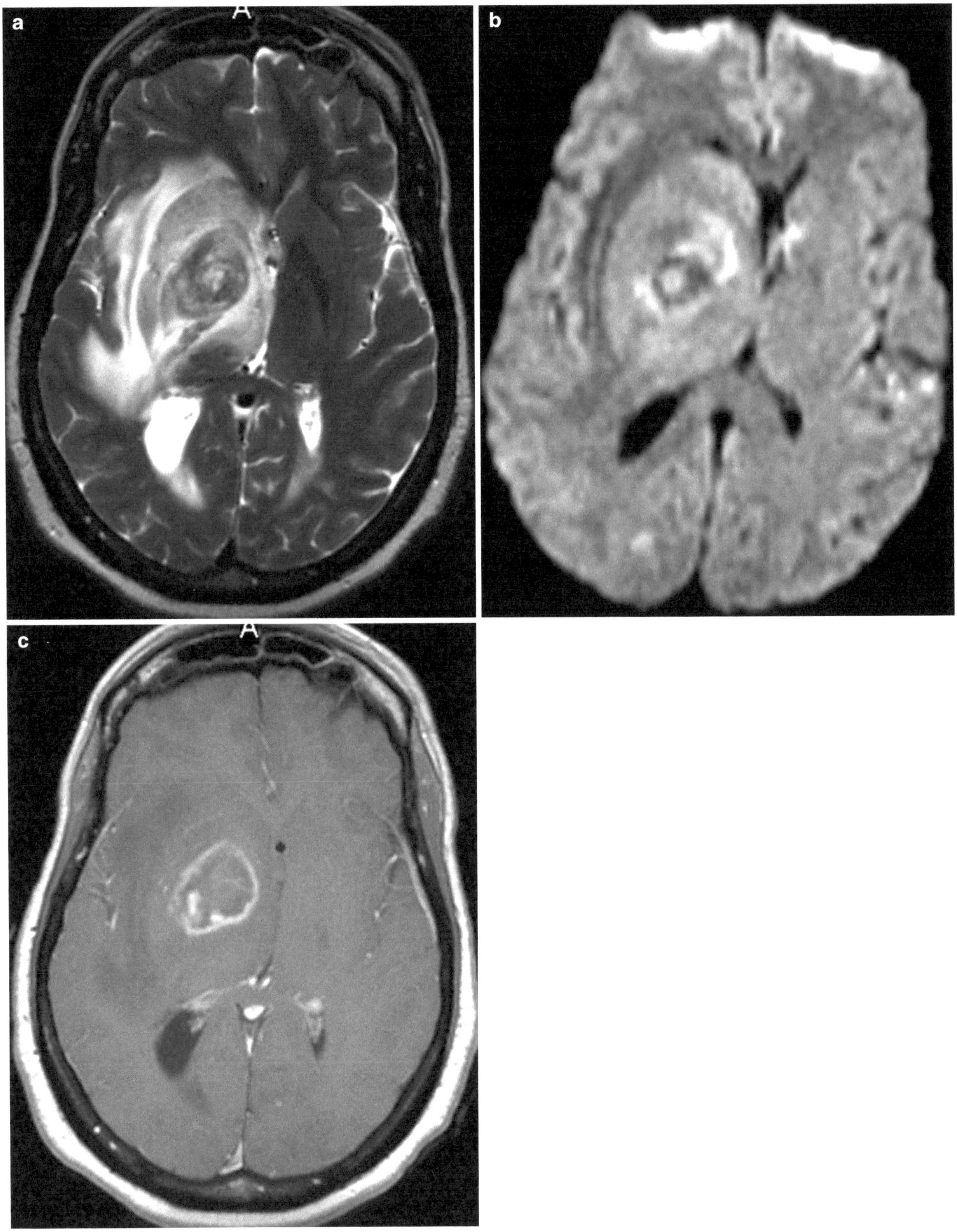

Fig. 31.26 (**a**–**c**) Toxoplasmosis in the right basal ganglia with a T2-w sequence (**a**), a diffusion-weighted image (**b**) and a post gadolinium image (**c**). Toxoplasmosis has a propensity for basal ganglia involvement. It has features that are often very similar to glioblastoma and primary CNS lymphoma and often different from pyogenic abscess. Note in this case that despite the marginal enhancement (similar to pyogenic abscess) the central portion of the abscess forms neither a distinct suppurative cavity nor exhibits water in its center as usually occurs in a pyogenic abscess cavity. In the context of an immunocompromised host, toxoplasmosis should be included as a potential tumefactive entity in the differential of any central nuclear mass

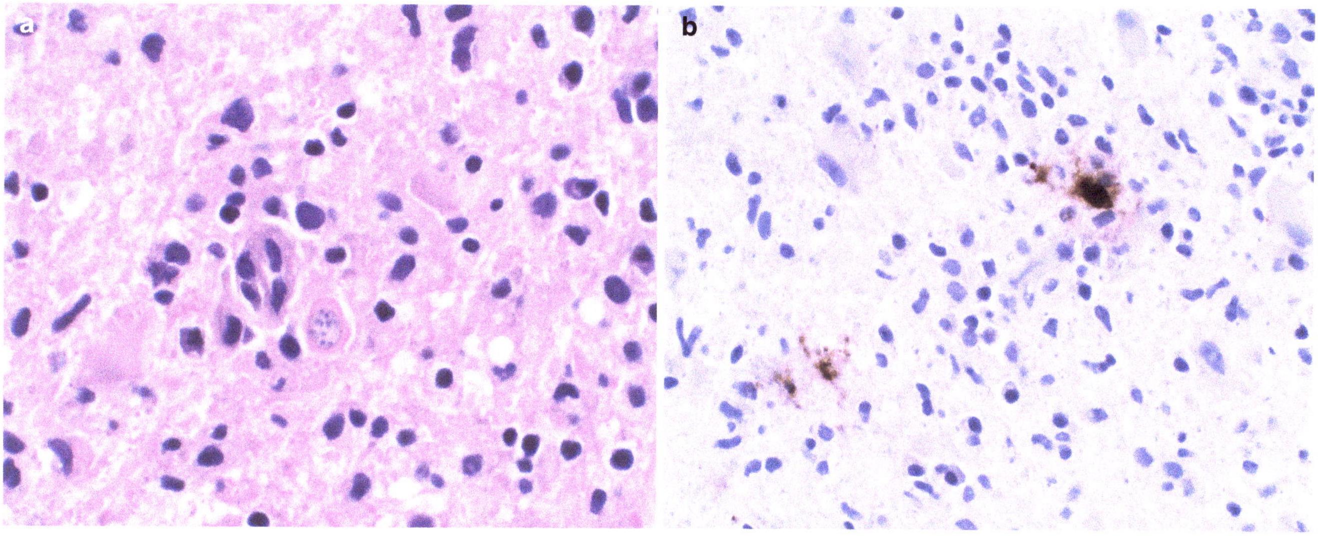

Fig. 31.27 (**a**) CNS toxoplasmosis. This figure features cysts (bradyzoites) of *Toxoplasma gondii* in brain tissue (H&E, 60×). (**b**) Shows an anti-Toxoplasma *gondii* antibody immunohistochemical study that is immunoreactive for both bradyzoites and trophozoites (Both courtesy of Anthony Yachnis, MD, and Kelly Devers, MD, University of Florida College of Medicine)

and then receive lifelong suppression with sulfadiazine 500–1000 mg orally four times daily and with pyrimethamine 25–75 mg and folinic acid 10–20 mg both by mouth daily. Patients on long-term maintenance treatment for cerebral toxoplasmosis have a low risk of subsequently developing *Pneumocystis carinii* pneumonia. This decreased risk is thought to be the result of chronic suppressive treatment with pyrimethamine and sulfonamides [316]. More recent data suggest that discontinuation of maintenance therapy against toxoplasmic encephalitis for individuals infected with HIV/AIDS, who are receiving successful antiretroviral therapy, might be safe and that patients who remain clinically and radiologically free of relapse at 6 months after discontinuation are unlikely to experience a relapse of toxoplasmic encephalitis [317, 318]. However, the overall body of published data in support of a policy that recommends discontinuing secondary prophylaxis remains relatively limited at the present time.

Cytomegalovirus (CMV)

CMV is a DNA herpes virus and is similar to HSV and VZV in its ability to establish latent infection. CMV tends to infect epithelial cells and leukocytes. In HIV-infected adults, serologic evidence of prior CMV infection is present in over 90% of individuals. Serologic surveys in the general adult population show a seroprevalence rate ranging between 50% and 80%, depending upon the socioeconomic status and the particular group studied; the seroprevalence of CMV rises with age. Approximately 10% of all infants born in the United States either have CMV infection at birth or acquire it within the neonatal period. The vast majority of these infections are asymptomatic and result from exposure to reactivated virus that is transmitted transplacentally in seropositive mothers. Subsequently, both children and adults may become infected through exposure to infected urine often from infants in day care; the virus may also be acquired from sexual contact, generally during the late teens and twenties, or by respiratory droplet infection. In non-immunocompromised adults, primary CMV infection is clinically identical to that of infectious mononucleosis and runs a self-limited course of 2–3 weeks characterized by fever, fatigue, malaise, lymphadenopathy, sore throat, and elevated liver enzymes, together with atypical lymphocytes in the blood smear.

In HIV-infected individuals, as long as cell-mediated immunity remains intact, symptomatic reactivation of CMV is not generally seen. However, as the disease progresses and the CD4+ count falls to <50 cells/mm^3, reactivation of CMV becomes more frequent. CMV retinitis is the most common form recognized clinically, and in the pre-ART era, up to 30% of HIV-infected patients showed clinical evidence of CMV retinitis. The diagnosis of CMV retinitis is based on the puffy white retinal infiltrates seen together with retinal hemorrhage. It may or may not be associated with systemic or other manifestations of CMV. Either one or both eyes may be involved at a given time.

There are several forms of CNS involvement with CMV and the pathogenesis appears to follow two different routes: (1) via the ependymal cells in the ventricles and (2) via the blood through capillary endothelial cells. Infection via the ependymal cells and CSF is manifest as necrotizing encephalitis limited to the periventricular areas, with numerous cytomegalic inclusions in and around the lesions. In contrast, infection acquired via hematogenous dissemination results in microglial nodular encephalitis, which is manifest pathologically as glial nodules formed by rod cells, few lymphocytes, and macrophages. Very little tissue damage is associated with these lesions [319]. The microglial nodular disease may involve multiple parts of the brain including the periventricular areas. As with CMV retinitis, these CNS complications occur very late in HIV infection and almost always in patients with CD4+ counts <50 cells/mm^3. In the series reported by Grassi and coworkers, the mean CD4+ count for patients with microglial nodular encephalitis was 21 cells/mm^3, while the average CD4+ count of patients with ventriculoencephalitis was 11 cells/mm^3 [319].

Although there is considerable overlap of symptomatology between these two pathologic conditions, microglial nodular encephalitis is characterized by the onset of acute confusion associated with delirium and psychomotor agitation, whereas the onset of ventriculoencephalitis is insidious and generally characterized by cognitive disturbances, memory deficits, and mental sluggishness. Patients with either type of encephalopathy may complain of headaches and have seizures. CSF examination in these conditions reveals a slightly elevated protein, which tends to be lower in microglial nodular encephalitis, averaging approximately 60 mg/dL as compared with 172 mg/dL in ventriculoencephalitis. Glucose levels are normal and cells are generally, although not always, absent. Although MRI is more sensitive than CT scan in the diagnosis of these conditions, the MRI may be normal or show nonspecific changes [320, 321]. In patients with ventriculoencephalitis, typical MRI findings include a hyperintense ventricular rim on T2-weighted imaging or enhancements with gadolinium. Almost all cases show nonspecific cerebral atrophy. Systemic involvement with CMV is more frequently associated with microglial nodular encephalitis, which may be documented with CMV antigenemia testing or viral culture. Patients with ventriculoencephalitis are more likely to have the clinical syndrome of CMV radiculopathy [319, 321–324]. CMV infection in HIV patients may also involve the spinal cord. A syndrome characterized by ascending weakness of the lower extremities associated with loss of deep tendon reflexes progressing to loss of bowel and bladder control has been described [325]. The syndrome may begin with low back pain with radiation down to the legs or into the groin or anal area, followed over 1–3 weeks by the development of progressive weakness.

Laboratory diagnosis is carried out in several ways: (1) seroconversion, (2) DNA detection in infected tissues using PCR, (3) antigen detection in tissues, (4) cytopathology, (5) isolation of virus from tissue or secretions, or (vi) CMV cytopathology. Pathologically, the CMV radiculopathy is characterized by mononuclear infiltration of the cauda equina and lumbar sacral nerve roots together with CMV inclusions seen in the Schwann's cells and epithelial cells, leading to axonal destruction. Untreated, this condition generally progresses to irreversible paralysis. Analysis of CSF in patients with this syndrome characteristically shows elevation of neutrophils, sometimes as high as 5000 cells/mm^3. Although the CSF protein is only mildly elevated and the glucose generally normal, some patients may have marked hypoglycorrhachia with glucose levels as low as 5–10 mg/dL.

Treatment

Ganciclovir 5 mg/kg IV every 12 h should be given for 14–21 days followed by maintenance with oral or IV doses that must be continued indefinitely to avoid or delay relapses unless CD4+ recovery occurs. Valganciclovir, a prodrug of ganciclovir, possessing excellent oral bioavailability and antiviral activity is effective in both the induction phase and the maintenance phase of CMV retinitis therapy [326, 327]. Ganciclovir blocks CMV replication by inhibiting CMV DNA polymerase. Alternatively, foscarnet 90 mg/kg, adjusted for renal function, can be given IV twice daily for 2–3 weeks. Following induction with ganciclovir or foscarnet, ART therapy can then be given in the hope of sustained improvement in CD4+ count and maintenance of response to therapy. In the pre-ART era, CMV encephalitis responded relatively poorly to ganciclovir, with survival generally in the 3–4-month range. The suppression of HIV replication and elevation in CD4+ cells observed during ART may allow AIDS patients to undergo immune reconstitution. Discontinuation of maintenance CMV therapy for these patients may be considered in these patients [318, 328, 329]. The drawback to withdrawing maintenance therapy is the risk of acquiring sight-threatening inflammatory conditions, including immune recovery uveitis [330, 331]. The treatment of immune recovery uveitis depends on the location of the intraocular inflammation, the severity of the inflammation, and the presence of ocular complications, particularly cystoid macular edema, which results from this inflammation and is a major cause of visual loss in HIV-infected patients. The main symptoms are decreased vision, metamorphopsia, and floaters [331]. More recently, drugs like Leflunomide have proven effective in reducing immune activation in the setting of chronic HIV-1 infection [332].

HIV Encephalopathy and Dementia

HIV is a neurotropic virus that appears to enter the brain via infected macrophages early in the course of infection. HIV infection itself causes CNS complications, including encephalitis and dementia. Encephalopathy usually develops as part of the acute HIV syndrome during the seroconversion phase. Two pathogenic mechanisms are thought to underlie these CNS conditions. In the first mechanism, HIV and its fragments induce damage directly or indirectly through the accumulation of infected or activated macrophage and microglia cells that release neurotoxic mediators including both cellular activation products and viral proteins [333, 334]. The accumulation of these activated macrophage/microglia cells, some of which are infected, release a number of cytokines and small molecule mediators and viral proteins that act on bystander cells. These viral proteins and cellular products have neurotoxic properties and act directly and through induction of astrocyte dysfunction, leading to neuronal injury [334–336]. The second, less predominant, pathogenic mechanism is the ability of HIV to impair neurogenesis [337, 338]. Kaul suggests that both proposed pathogenic mechanisms occur side by side with other host-virus interactions [333].

Pathologically, the most frequent findings in persons with HIV encephalopathy are brain atrophy characterized by sulcal widening and ventricular dilatation together with varying degrees of meningeal fibrosis. The most distinctive histologic feature of this condition is white matter pallor, chiefly seen in a periventricular distribution together with microglial nodules, diffuse astrocytosis, and perivascular mononuclear inflammation. HIV can be readily demonstrated in these nodules by immunohistochemical techniques. HIV-associated dementia is a late phenomenon caused by cortical neuronal loss and abnormalities of the dendritic connections; cerebral atrophy in these patients invariably is confirmed on gross necropsy. Histologically, the brain of a person with HIV encephalitis is characterized by multiple nodules of infected microglia and microglial giant cells in the white matter (Fig. 31.10). These lesions also affect neural function by secreting toxic cytokines.

Clinically, HIV encephalopathy presents with altered mental status characterized by mental slowing frequently accompanied by clinical evidence of subcortical dementia, such as bradykinesia, postural instability, slow and clumsy gait, and altered muscle tone. Radiographically, the most common features are generalized cerebral atrophy together with widespread symmetric hyperintense white matter abnormalities seen on T2 imaging, which generally have a periventricular distribution. Examples are shown in Fig. 31.28. CSF studies are non-diagnostic: the CSF is commonly acellular and a mononuclear pleocytosis is seen in about 25% of patients with cell counts generally <50 cells/mm^3 [339, 340]. CSF protein levels are elevated (usually <200 mg/dL) in 60% of patients, while CSF immunoglobulin G levels are raised in about 80%. Glucose levels in the CSF of HIV-infected patients are usually within normal limits.

HIV may be detected in CSF by a variety of techniques, including PCR, during all the clinical stages of infection, i.e., HIV is present in the CSF in the absence of neurologic abnormalities. Thus, the presence of HIV in the CSF is not diagnostic for HIV encephalopathy and HIV RNA levels in the CSF do not necessarily correlate with the corresponding plasma levels. Neuroimaging studies can support a diagnosis of AIDS dementia complex by revealing cortical atrophy and ventricular enlargement and hyperintense lesions in the periventricular white matter on MRI. ART remains the main mode of medical treatment for HIV encephalopathy and other HIV-related cognitive disorders.

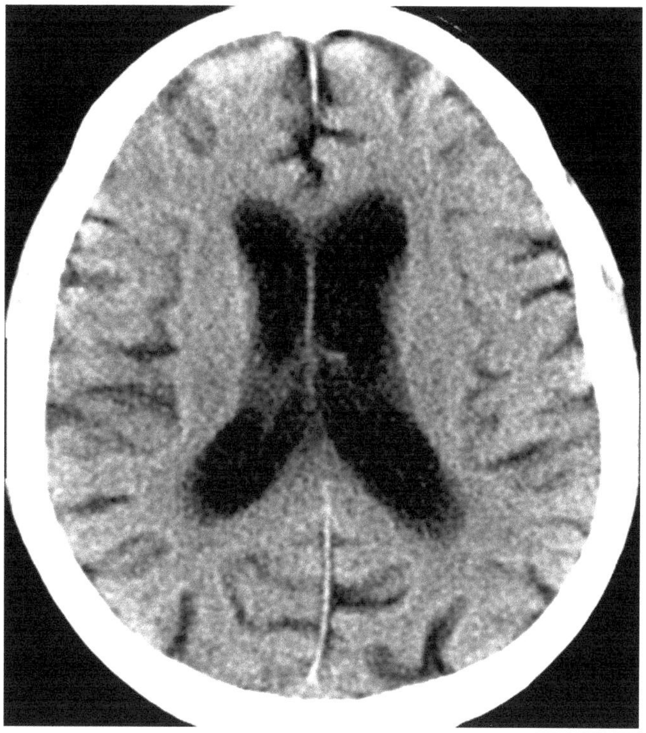

Fig. 31.28 Primary HIV infection of the CNS. Ventriculomegaly and sulcal dilatation (indicating cortical brain atrophy). There is no transependymal fluid to suggest elevated CSF pressure. These findings are indicative of both central and cortical brain atrophy which, in this case, is out of proportion to chronological age. Generalized atrophy is one of the features of primary HIV involvement of brain (Reproduced with permission from Rand et al. [521])

Parasitic Infections of the Central Nervous System

Cerebral Malaria

Despite its eradication from North America and Europe, it is estimated that malaria infects over 2.5 billion people worldwide and causes between one and three million deaths each year. The disease is caused by one of five different *Plasmodium* species: *P. vivax*, *P. ovale*, *P. malariae*, *P. knowlesi*, and *P. falciparum*. Most of the deaths and serious complications of malaria, especially CNS involvement, are caused by *P. falciparum*. Malaria sporozoites are transmitted from the female Anopheles mosquito to the patient at the time the mosquito bites the person for its blood meal.

Sporozoites are carried rapidly to the liver where they multiply in approximately 1 week to become tissue schizonts or the dormant hypnozoites produced by *P. vivax* and *P. ovale*. Infected liver cells then burst, releasing thousands of merozoites, each of which in turn infects red blood cells in the bloodstream. Continued asexual replication in the bloodstream through repeated cycles of maturation and rupture of red cells with release of merozoites eventually results in symptomatic infection. During this process, some of the parasites develop into sexual forms called gametocytes which produce no symptoms themselves, but which may circulate for a prolonged period of time. It is the ingestion of these gametocytes that leads to the sexual reproduction cycle in the Anopheles mosquito resulting in the motile sporozoites which invade the mosquito salivary glands and can be transmitted back to humans at the time of the next feeding.

Malaria is widely distributed in economically less-developed countries, particularly sub-Saharan Africa, Central America and the Caribbean, South America, the Middle East, Far East, and Indonesia. The reader is strongly urged to access the CDC's website for the most up-to-date availability on the distribution and drug resistance among *Plasmodium* spp. on a country-by-country basis.

Pathogenesis

P. falciparum is the cause of the most malignant form of malaria and is associated with almost all serious complications associated with the infection. Cerebral malaria, in particular, is the most prominent and serious of these complications. Attributable mortality remains relatively high (20%) and is often associated with delays in diagnosis and treatment. As *P. falciparum* trophozoites mature in the red blood cells, they induce the formation of small knobs on the surface of the red cell. These knobs bind to adhesion molecules (also known as intercellular adhesion molecule-1) on the microvascular endothelial cells, leading to sequestration. Sequestration is the process whereby erythrocytes containing mature forms of *P. falciparum* adhere to microvascular endothelial cells resulting in marked reduction or disappearance of these cells from the circulation. Sequestration of erythrocytes in small blood vessels and consequent obstruction of microcirculatory flow is a specific property of *P falciparum* and an important mechanism causing coma and death in cerebral malaria. The second important factor in the pathogenesis of cerebral malaria is the increase in cytokine production. In an attempt to control the infection, the host immune system produces a potent proinflammatory response in which cells of the macrophage-monocyte series are induced to release various cytokines, including tumor necrosis factor (TNF)-α, interleukin (IL)-1, IL-6, and IL-8 [341]. However, this response may also induce complications, such as severe anemia, hypoglycemia, and cerebral malaria.

The adhesion molecules are upregulated in malaria as a result of cytokine productions, TNF-α in particular. Furthermore, parasitized erythrocytes tend to adhere to adjacent uninfected cells leading to rosetting. In addition, as the parasite matures inside the erythrocyte, the normally flexible cell becomes more spherical and rigid. Because of the rosetting and increased rigidity of parasitized erythrocytes, the erythrocytes become trapped in the capillaries. The end result of cytoadherence, rosetting, and rigidity is the enhancement of sequestration of *P. falciparum*-parasitized erythrocytes in the cerebral vasculature, stagnation of the cerebral blood flow, and secondary ischemia leading to tissue hypoxia, lactic acidosis, hypoglycemia, and prevention of delivery of nutrients to the tissues. High concentrations of TNF-α can precipitate cerebral malaria by increasing the sequestration of parasitized erythrocytes. Although all tissues potentially can become involved, the brain is the most profoundly affected [342–350].

In the CNS, this process results in delirium, impaired consciousness, convulsions, paralysis, coma, and, ultimately, rapid death if not treated. Systemic manifestations of severe falciparum malaria include anemia, lactic acidosis, hypoglycemia, pulmonary edema, adult respiratory distress syndrome, and disseminated intravascular coagulation. Of note, the pathophysiology of malaria does not include vasculitis or inflammatory cellular infiltration in or around the cerebral vasculature, and most patients have no evidence of cerebral edema. Raised intracranial pressure likely arises from an increase in the overall cerebral blood volume rather than brain swelling arising from cerebral edema and capillary leakage. Coma in malaria is generally not associated with raised intracranial pressure. Clinical features of *P. falciparum* malaria include fever and chills (83%), altered sensorium (48%), jaundice (27%), anemia (75%), cerebral involvement (45%), thrombocytopenia (41%), and renal failure (25%).

The diagnosis should be considered in a person with altered consciousness, fever, and a relevant travel history, which is critically important to elicit, as is the history of whether the patient took or was compliant with prophylaxis for malaria. The location of the travel is particularly critical as *P. falciparum* is typically resistant to chloroquine. Resistance to trimethoprim/sulfamethoxazole, mefloquine, and other agents has been documented in many parts of the world, particularly Southeast Asia and sub-Saharan Africa. Because there is no latent form of *P. falciparum* in the liver, as there is for *P. vivax* and *P. ovale*, cases of *P. falciparum* malaria should become clinically evident within a month after leaving an endemic area.

The laboratory diagnosis of malaria is made from an examination of the blood smear. Although delay is common because of the time needed for their preparation and reading, thick and thin blood smears remain the cornerstone of laboratory diagnosis of malaria in current practice. Despite the availability of rapid diagnostic testing for the detection of malaria based on lateral-flow immunochromatography in which clinicians can detect malaria parasite antigens from finger-prick blood specimens within 10–15 min, microscopic examination of blood smears remains the most cost-effective methodology for diagnosis of malaria, provided the results reach those who need to know in a timely manner.

Rapid diagnostic testing kits based on molecular platforms with high sensitivity and high negative predictive value for *P. falciparum* would be of particular use in acute care settings in regions of low malaria endemicity, where the diagnosis is suspected but lack of laboratory expertise precludes the diagnosis and reading of blood smears. Lastly, rapid diagnostic testing may benefit severely ill patients by confirming or excluding a malaria diagnosis rapidly and facilitating prompt intervention. Rapid test kits for malaria have limitations that preclude replacing microscopy of blood smears any time soon. These limitations include inability to ascertain parasitemia quantitatively or to differentiate between the four plasmodium species.

Treatment

Untreated, cerebral malaria is generally fatal. In cases of severe malaria with CNS involvement, the patient must be treated as though they have falciparum malaria regardless of the preliminary interpretation of the blood smear. According to the CDC, if severe malaria is strongly suspected but a laboratory diagnosis cannot be made at that time, blood should be collected for diagnostic testing as soon as it is available and parenteral antimalarial drugs started empirically. Once the diagnosis is considered likely, IV artesunate should be given. The recommended dose for adults and children who weigh more than 20 kg is 2.4 mg/kg at 0, 12, and 24 h. Patients should have one set of blood smears performed every 12–24 h until a negative result is obtained. If, after the third dose the patient's parasite density is >1%, IV artesunate treatment should be continued until the parasite density is <1% for a maximum of 7 days. After the course of IV artesunate is completed (3 doses) and the parasite density is <1%, and the patient can tolerate oral treatment, a full treatment course with artemether-lumefantrine or atovaquone-proguanil, quinine plus doxycycline or clindamycin or mefloquine is used (CDC) [351].

Parenteral quinidine gluconate is cardiotoxic and can induce hyperinsulinemic hypoglycemia. Thus, a baseline EKG should be obtained before initiating therapy and glucose levels must be monitored closely. Critical care management includes continuous cardiac and blood pressure monitoring with appropriate supportive management of coexisting medical complications often associated with severe malaria: convulsions, renal failure, adult respiratory distress syndrome, disseminated intravascular coagulation, lactic acidosis, hypoglycemia, fluid and electrolyte abnormalities, circulatory collapse, acute renal failure, secondary bacterial infections, and severe anemia.

Intravenous corticosteroids are associated with poor outcomes and are absolutely contraindicated [349]. Brain swelling on CT scan is a common finding in adult patients with cerebral malaria but is not related to coma depth or survival. Mannitol therapy as adjunctive treatment for brain swelling in adult cerebral malaria prolongs coma duration and may be harmful [352]. Results of studies of antipyretics, anticonvulsants (phenobarbitone), anticytokine/anti-inflammatory agents (anti-TNF antibodies, pentoxifylline, dexamethasone), iron chelators, and hyperimmune sera have not proven beneficial in improving patient outcomes [347].

With treatment, almost all patients with CNS malaria recover completely if they survive the acute episode. However, globally, overall mortality in children and adults remains unacceptably high. Approximately 12% of patients with cerebral malaria may have lasting neurologic sequelae, including cortical blindness, tremor, cranial nerve palsies, and sensory and motor deficits, although approximately 50% of these sequelae resolve with time.

Amoebic Meningoencephalitis

A dramatic and almost uniformly fatal primary meningoencephalitis can be seen with infection caused by the free-living amoeba *Naegleria fowleri* and *Acanthamoeba* species. Free-living *N. fowleri* are found widespread in nature, particularly in the upper surface layers of lakes or shallow fresh water in warm climates. Acanthamoeba spp. are usually found in soil and fresh and brackish water. Most cases in the United States, typically children or young adults, occur in the southeastern states. Clinically, patients present with sudden onset of high fever, photophobia, and headaches; progression to obtundation occurs relatively quickly. There is usually a classic history of swimming or waterskiing in warm, freshwater lakes. The amoebae invade the nasal cavity along the blood vessels associated with the olfactory nerves and traverse the cribriform plate to reach the frontal lobes and the surrounding meninges, where they rapidly produce highly necrotizing, purulent, and destructive encephalitis. Because of the olfactory involvement, there may be alterations in smell or taste. Otherwise, nonspecific symptoms such as confusion, irritability, restlessness, and seizures with rapid progression to delirium, stupor, and coma ensue. The CSF is usually bloody, shows a leukocytosis with neutrophil predominance, low glucose levels, and elevated protein. If the diagnosis is strongly suspected, one can examine the unstained CSF with a slide warmer to look for the typical, mobile, amoeboid motion of the trophozoites; gram stain and culture are usually negative. A PCR assay for *Naegleria*,

Acanthamoeba, and *Balamuthia* has been developed by CDC [353, 354].

Frontal lobe involvement is readily seen on MRI but the diagnosis is often delayed because of the rarity of the condition and paucity of immediate diagnostic signs. Only a small number of patients have been reported to have survived and all received amphotericin B, to which the pathogens are susceptible in vitro [355–358]. The optimal treatment regimen is not known for this condition and some authors recommend maximal systemic doses of amphotericin B with intracisternal amphotericin B adjunctive rifampin and doxycycline [359]. Surgical intervention usually involves placement of a reservoir for intrathecal amphotericin B and shunting to alleviate hydrocephalus.

Neurocysticercosis

Neurocysticercosis is the most common helminthic infection of the nervous system, and a leading cause of acquired epilepsy worldwide [360–362]. Cysticercosis is widespread in areas such as Mexico, Central America, South America, Africa, Southeast Asia, India, the Philippines, and Southern Europe. It is also becoming an increasing problem in Europe [360]. Neurocysticercosis in adult patients results from infection of the brain with the larval cysts of the cestode, *Taenia solium*, the pork tapeworm. Human infection occurs by two different mechanisms: [1] ingestion of the eggs leading to embryonation of the eggs and penetration of the intestinal wall with hematogenous transport of cysticerci to many different tissues, primarily muscle and brain, where they encyst and remain potentially infectious for long period of time. Alternatively, ingestion of undercooked pork can result in ingestion of the cysticerci by humans. In the latter instance, the cysticerci mature into the typical tapeworm which attaches to the intestine and may grow to lengths of up to 3 m and live for up to 25 years. During this time, it produces egg-filled segments, called proglottids, which are excreted in the feces. Ingestion of the eggs from these proglottids leads to neurocysticercosis, occasionally even by autoinfection from the patient's own intestinal tapeworm.

Symptomatic neurocysticercosis results from the enlargement of the cysticercal cysts in the brain parenchyma over a period of months to years. In the United States, patients may present with seizures due to neurocysticercosis that was acquired after a visit to an endemic part of the world 30 years previously. The clinical manifestations are nonspecific and varied depending on the number, size, and anatomic location of the cystic lesions. Seizures and headaches are common presenting symptoms. If the cysts block the flow of CSF, symptoms associated with raised ICP, such as headache, nausea, vomiting, changes in vision, dizziness, ataxia, and confusion, may result. When the cysts are located in the meninges, chronic meningitis may occur. An unusual form called "racemes" cysticercosis is caused by the proliferation of cysts at the base of the brain and can result in severe disease, including mental deterioration and death. Intraspinal cysts are common and may produce symptoms of cord compression; severity again depends on location and size of cysts.

The most frequent clinical presentations are seizures (64.8%), symptoms associated with raised intracranial hypertension, and meningism [363]. Radiological studies of the skull show intracranial calcifications suggestive of cysticercosis in up to 50% of patients [363]. Analysis of CSF invariably shows increased pressure, elevated lymphocyte and eosinophil counts, elevated protein levels, and reduced glucose levels. Neurocysticercosis is readily diagnosed by neuroimaging (CT scanning or MRI) studies in which multiple cysts of varying sizes and stages are demonstrated (Fig. 31.29a, b). MRI may show the parasites as well as the changes they induce in the nervous system [362, 364, 365]. Figure 31.29c, d shows the histology of the cyst wall with outer, middle, and inner layers. Serological testing is available with sensitivities as high as 94% in patients with multiple cysts but significantly lower in those with single cysts and calcified lesions [366]. Older cysts are often calcified. PCR assays have the highest sensitivity (95.9%) but variable specificity (80% or 100%) depending on the controls used [366]. Serology is generally available through the CDC or at specific national commercial laboratories. However, the identification of specific antibodies and antigens is currently used only to support the diagnosis because of the limited specificity and sensitivity of current tests.

Treatment

Based on neuroimaging studies, CNS lesions can be classified into active and inactive neurocysticercosis (Fig. 31.29a). Patients with inactive parenchymal neurocysticercosis generally have no evidence of viable or degenerating parasites; the utility of antiparasitic drugs in these patients remains limited. However, these patients are at increased risk of developing seizures, and standard anticonvulsive therapy with phenytoin, phenobarbital, or carbamazepine is indicated. Patients who develop hydrocephalus need to be treated with ventricular peritoneal shunting. Virtually all patients with active neurocysticercosis have seizures, which must be treated with anticonvulsants. The majority of these patients can be treated symptomatically and followed by MRI because the cysticerci typically undergo complete degeneration over a 1- to 2-year period. This process results in either calcified inactive cysticerci that continue to induce seizures thereby requiring continued therapy with anticonvulsants or, in a majority, a normal MRI in which case anticonvulsants may be tapered as long as the patients remain seizure free.

Cysticidal drugs (albendazole and praziquantel) have improved the prognosis of this condition and can be given as praziquantel at doses of 50–100 mg/kg/day for 10–14 days or albendazole 10–15 mg/kg/day for 1–15 days. Albendazole has been superior to praziquantel in trials comparing the efficacy of these drugs [364, 365, 367]. The combination of albendazole and praziquantel has been associated with higher rate of imaging resolution when compared to albendazole alone. Another advantage of albendazole is that it also destroys subarachnoid and ventricular cysts [368, 369]. In some of these cases, particularly in patients with large subarachnoid cysts, higher doses (up to 30 mg/kg/day) or more prolonged, or even repeated, courses of albendazole may be needed. Although these agents kill the cysticerci, some controlled trials have not shown any clinical benefit over symptomatic treatment alone [370–372]. The main adverse side effect of praziquantel is worsening neurologic function, i.e., headaches, dizziness, seizures, and increased ICP probably as a result of an increase in the host inflammatory response and cerebral edema due to the larval death. There is a strong consensus that there is no role for anti-cysticidal drugs in patients with only calcified lesions and those patients with single-enhancing lesions will do well regardless of antiparasitic therapy [373]. Riley and White point out that while antiparasitic therapy is indicated in patients with multiple subarachnoid cysticerci or giant cysticerci they are contraindicated in patients with cerebral edema (cysticercal encephalitis) [373].

Surgery plays an important role in the management of some forms of the disease, particularly hydrocephalus and intraventricular cysts. Standard treatment of ventricular neurocysticercosis has been the surgical removal of cysts that block CSF flow; in patients with ventricular cysticerci, endoscopic removal remains the preferred therapy [373]. Some studies have found fewer shunt failures when such patients are treated with antiparasitic drugs [374–376]. Cysticercosis involving the basilar cisterns is associated with a prominent inflammatory arachnoiditis and can be complicated by both

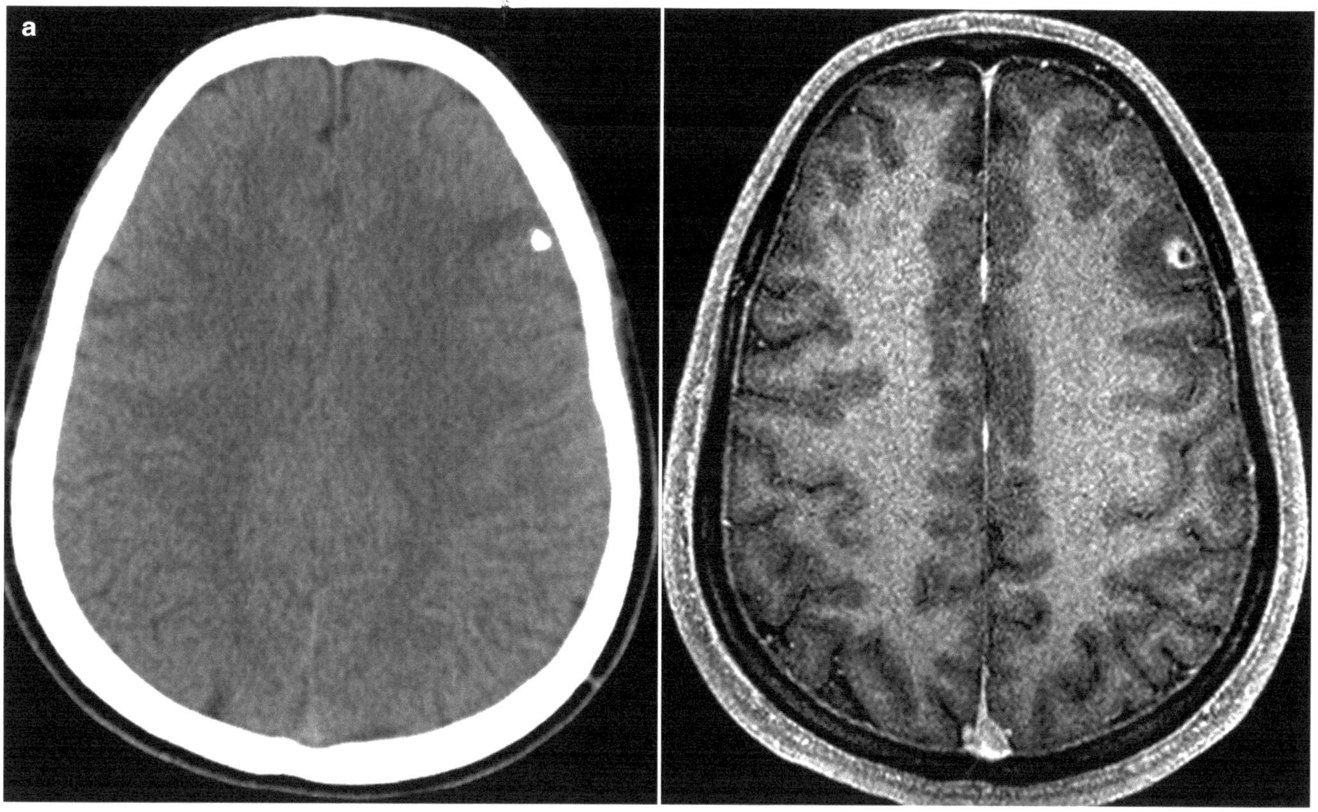

Fig. 31.29 (**a**) Neurocysticercosis. Images include non-contrast CT (*left*) and post-gadolinium-enhanced T1-w MRI (*right*). These images demonstrate the features of chronic neurocysticercosis. The frontal lesion is calcified as evident on the CT. However, it also produces local inflammation evident on the enhanced MR image. This local inflammatory reaction frequently can produce seizure activity. Hence, late-state neurocysticercosis can be a mimic for cortical oligodendroglioma. (**b**) Neurocysticercosis; images include a panorama of the MRI sequences in the mid-convexity level of the brain including pre and post-contrast DT1-w sequences and T2-w spin echo sequences which illustrate typical findings of neurocysticercosis. The findings in this case are those of cystic nodules scattered in brain and the depths of the sulci. The margins of the lesion show reactive hyperemia. Within some of the lesions an organism scolex is evident confirming the basis for the nodules. (**c**) Neurocysticercosis. A 25 year old male from Latin America with a lateral ventricular cyst. The figure shows the cyst wall with outer cuticular layer, middle cellular layer, and inner reticular layer (H&E 20×). (**d**) Features a high-power view of a portion of the scolex (H&E 60×). Courtesy of Anthony Yachnis, MD, and Kelly Devers, MD, University of Florida College of Medicine)

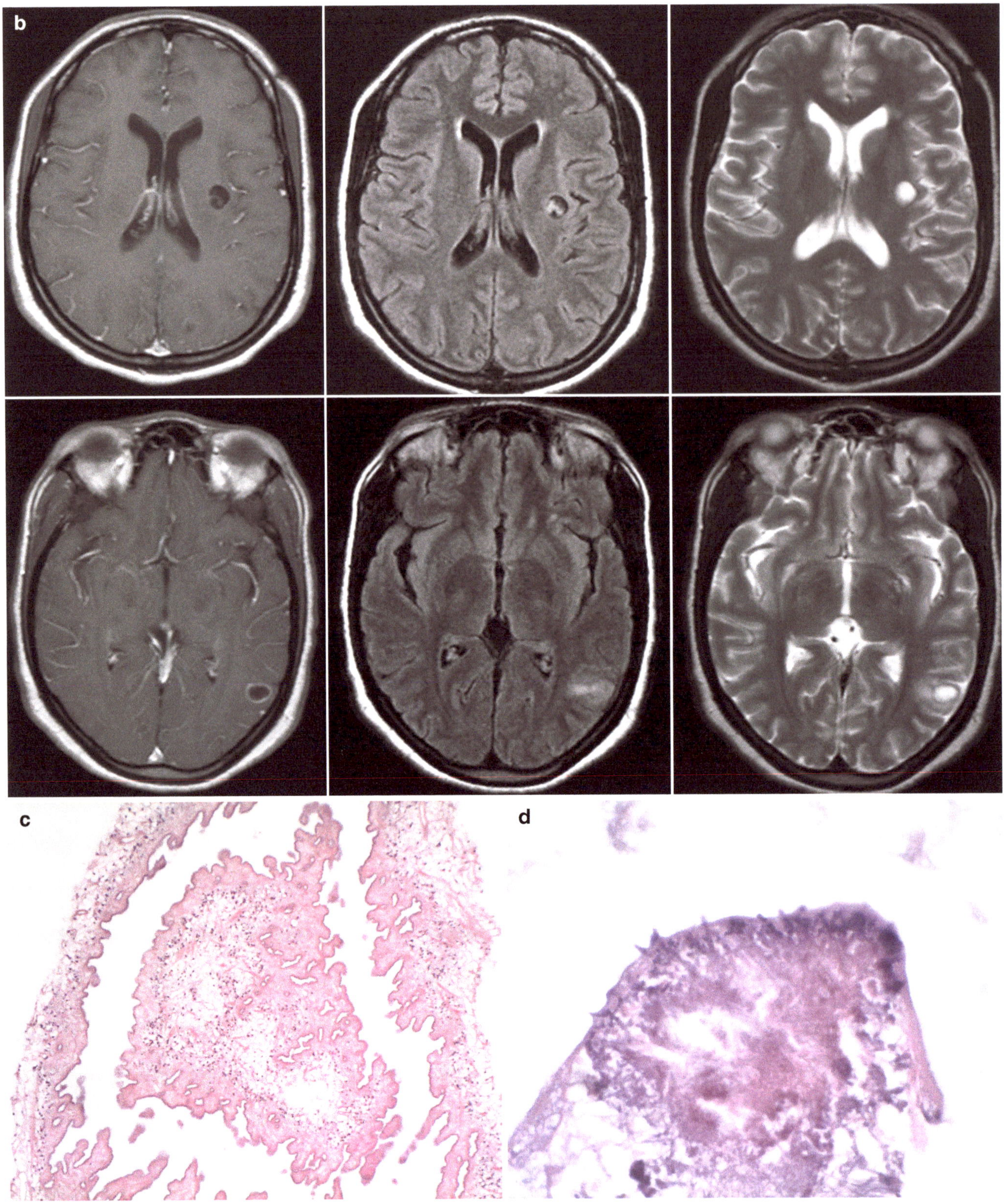

Fig. 31.29 (continued)

vasculitis, resulting in lacunar infarctions, and invasion of the cysticerci into larger vessels, resulting in strokes. Some authors have recommended the addition of corticosteroids together with antiparasitic therapy for the treatment of patients with cisternal cysticercosis as this combination has been shown to be associated with fewer seizures [375–378].

A consensus guideline panel headed by Garcia and coworkers underscored four major tenets of managing neurocysticercosis [379, 380]: (1) individualize therapeutic decisions, including whether to use antiparasitic drugs, based on the number, location, and viability of the parasites within the CNS; (2) actively manage growing cysticerci either with antiparasitic drugs or surgical excision; (3) prioritize the management of intracranial hypertension secondary to neurocysticercosis before considering any other form of therapy; and (4) manage seizures as done for seizures due to other causes of secondary seizures because they are due to an organic focus that has been present for a long time [379].

Echinococcus

Echinococcal disease is caused by tapeworms that commonly infect dogs, cats, wolves, and other carnivores. It is found worldwide but is particularly common in countries surrounding the Mediterranean, parts of East Africa, Russia, and South America. There is very little echinococcal disease in the United States, but it is important to recognize that bears, foxes, and wolves in Canada and Alaska are commonly infected with this parasite. Disease is produced when an egg from an infected animal is ingested and the oncosphere within is activated, penetrates the gut wall, and travels via veins or lymphatics to various tissues in the body where they form hydatid cysts. Up to 80% of cysts occur in the liver and about 10% in the lungs. CNS involvement is uncommon and occurs in only about 2% of cases. At all anatomic sites, cysts may be single or multiple.

Of the four species that infect humans, *Echinococcus granulosus* and *E. multilocularis* account for the vast majority of cases. CNS disease is commonly characterized by slowly enlarging solitary cysts in the brain. Depending on the size and location of the cyst, the patient may remain asymptomatic. However, as the CNS lesion enlarges in size, symptoms may arise from the local effects of the lesion itself or secondary to raised ICP, resulting in headache, nausea and vomiting, seizures, hemiparesis, dysarthria, and cranial nerve palsies. The diagnosis may be suspected from radiographic appearance of the cyst itself seen on CT scanning or MRI. Classic radiographic features include a sharp, spherical border lacking a rim of enhancement or surrounding edema, although a fine rim of peripheral enhancement with perilesional edema may be seen if active inflammation is present. CT is superior for the detection of extrahepatic disease; MRI does not appear to add any diagnostic benefit.

Immunodiagnostic testing is available from CDC; sensitivity of these tests varies from 60% to 90% and they are highly sensitive for liver cysts although less so for cysts in the brain. Thus, a negative test does not absolutely rule out cerebral echinococcal disease. History of travel to or living in an endemic area especially with exposure to sheep also increases the likelihood of the diagnosis of echinococcus. Patients with intracranial hydatid cysts usually present with focal neurological deficit and features of raised intracranial pressure due to interference with CSF flow. The treatment of hydatid cyst is surgical, and the aim of the surgery is to excise the cyst completely and without rupture to prevent recurrence and anaphylactic reaction. Albendazole therapy is given in a daily dose of 10 mg/kg, taken three times for 4 months. It is a broad-spectrum oral antihelminthic agent, which acts by blocking glucose uptake of the larva and adult worm. The glycogen stores are thus depleted thereby decreasing the ATP formation resulting in death of the parasite. Albendazole can decrease the size of large cysts and cause smaller ones to disappear.

Strongyloidiasis

Strongyloides stercoralis is a small nematode with free-living forms found in soil, while parasitic forms (i.e., the adult female) live within intestinal crypts in the duodenum, the jejunal mucosal villi, or in the submucosa; the male does not enter the intestinal mucosa but are passed in stool. Normally, the adult worms bore into the mucosa and produce eggs, which pass out with stool. The eggs deposited by the female may hatch the rhabditiform larvae that enter the lumen of the intestine to be passed out in stool. Eggs released from these organisms normally mature in the soil to produce more rhabditiform larvae. In the environment, these larvae transform into the filariform infective larvae that can directly penetrate intact skin of humans and other mammals. In some patients, the transformation from rhabditiform to the filariform infective larvae can also occur while still in the lower bowel or perianal area, before being passed out in the stool. The filariform larvae burrow through the intestinal wall and perianal skin to reinfect the patient, a phenomenon known as autoinfection. After burrowing through the skin, the filariform larvae enter the lymphatics and, ultimately, the venous system where they are carried to the pulmonary capillaries. Here, they migrate out of the blood vessels into alveoli, up the airways and then down through the esophagus to reach the small bowel. Symptoms include ground itch, urticarial, and pulmonary symptoms. A worm burden in the intestines might lead to a malabsorption syndrome. Chronic strongyloidiasis and autoinfection have been observed in World War II veterans who were in POW camps on the Pacific front up to 30 years after their return to the United States and the United Kingdom.

The most serious consequence of *S. stercoralis* infection occurs as a result of massive autoinfection caused by immunosuppression (e.g., persons on steroid therapy, organ transplant, HTLV-1 coinfection, cancer, or malnutrition) or following treatment of lymphoma, leukemia, or leprosy with corticosteroids or cytotoxic drugs. In this condition, known as the hyperinfection syndrome, the autoinfection cycle escalates to generate massive infection with millions of parasites throughout the whole intestine and hematogenous dissemination of the invasive form of the filariform larvae to all organs, including the liver, lungs, and brain.

As part of this hyperinfection syndrome in immunocompromised patients, CNS involvement may be manifested by headache, altered mentation, meningismus, focal or generalized seizures, or motor weakness. Encephalopathy is common and pyogenic meningitis caused by strongyloides larvae in the meninges can occur. A unique aspect of the hyperinfection syndrome is the likelihood that meningitis and septic shock due to *E. coli* and other gram-negative enteric organisms can occur. These gram-negative infections are thought to be caused by the enteric organisms being carried either on the larvae or within the gut of the larvae as they migrate through the tissues, resulting in bacterial meningitis once the CNS is invaded. Although an eosinophilia is common in strongyloidiasis, it is almost never seen in patients with the hyperinfection syndrome because of existing immunosuppression (usually corticosteroids) and is an indication of poor prognosis: the lower the eosinophil count, the worse the prognosis. The diagnosis can be made by identifying the larvae in stool, duodenal aspirate, or sputum. For massive strongyloidiasis, treatment with thiabendazole 25 mg/kg twice daily for 10 days has been effective. Ivermectin therapy has also proven effective in the treatment of the hyperinfection syndrome.

Toxocariasis

Toxocara canis and *Toxocara cati* are nematodes that infect the intestines of dogs and cats, respectively. As a result of this infection in domestic animals, the eggs of these organisms are distributed widely in the soil to which humans may be exposed. Human infection occurs when eggs are ingested and hatch in the small intestine. Larvae then migrate through the intestinal wall and into various tissues of the body, and most often manifest as visceral larvae migrans (VLM). Symptoms include abdominal pain, hepatomegaly, anorexia, nausea, vomiting, lethargy, behavioral changes, pneumonia, cough, wheezing, lymphadenopathy, or fever. The hallmark of the disease is striking eosinophilia. Older children, adolescents, or young adults may develop unilateral loss of vision; ophthalmoscopy reveals a lesion not unlike a retinoblastoma. When eosinophilia is seen in small children between the ages of 2 and 4, it readily suggests a clinical diagnosis of VLM. Though very uncommon, CNS involvement can manifest as dementia, meningoencephalitis, myelitis, cerebral vasculitis, epilepsy, or optic neuritis [381–384]. CNS involvement in patients with VLM may also present as encephalopathy with seizures. Other manifestations include meningoencephalitis, transverse myelitis, and psychiatric disturbances.

Treatment is diethylcarbamazine 2 mg/kg orally three times daily for 10 days or albendazole 400 mg orally twice a day for 5 days. Steroids are indicated for ocular disease and may be necessary for severe lung, heart, or CNS involvement. The differential diagnosis of parasitic eosinophilic meningitis includes infections caused by *Angiostrongylus cantonensis* and *Gnathostoma* species; meningitis caused by these organisms is caused by their random migration into the CNS.

Syphilis

Syphilis is caused by the spirochete *Treponema pallidum*, belonging to the family Spirochaetaceae. The organisms are thin, tightly coiled bacteria that exhibit a characteristic undulating movement under direct dark-field observation. Syphilis is categorized as early (primary, secondary, and tertiary) or late (late latent, late benign, and late clinical infection). Before penicillin became available, the prevalence of primary and secondary syphilis was high but fell rapidly with the introduction of antimicrobials after the Second World War. Syphilis is transmitted primarily through sexual contact between infected and uninfected persons. Less common modes of transmission include nonsexual contact with infectious lesions, such as breaks in the skin or mucous membranes that come into contact with infectious lesions containing spirochetes, transplacentally from mother to fetus in utero, via transfusion of contaminated blood products, or through laboratory exposures.

Pathogenesis

The initial manifestation is the primary chancre, which begins at the site of inoculation as a painless papule and rapidly ulcerates into a relatively painless and indurated ulcer that is dark-field positive. The primary chancre is frequently associated with regional, nonsuppurative, nontender lymphadenopathy. The chancre generally heals spontaneously within 3–6 weeks. The incubation period from exposure to clinical disease can range anywhere from 3 weeks to 3 months. Spirochetemia occurs at the onset of the primary chancre. For a period of 2–8 weeks following the primary chancre, the treponemes migrate to the lymphatics and gain access to the circulation to cause a systemic illness (the secondary syphilis phase) in approximately 30% of untreated patients. Systemic manifestations of secondary syphilis include fever, malaise, headache, pharyngitis, anorexia, weight loss, and arthralgias. The classic manifestations are maculopapular, papular, or pustular skin lesions, which are distributed over the entire body, including the palms and soles, and patients may develop patchy alopecia. Genital ulcerations, such as condylomata lata and mucous patches, develop in about 20–35% of those with clinically evident secondary syphilis.

During the secondary syphilis phase, between 8 and 40% of affected persons develop some evidence of CNS involvement, including meningitis and cranial nerve involvement. Patients may complain of headache, decreased vision, tinnitus, and vertigo. During the secondary stage, spirochetes can be found in the blood, CNS, and aqueous humor of the eye. However, direct dark-field examination of the CSF in these patients rarely reveals spirochetes. Using rabbit inoculation to test CSF for viable *T. pallidum*, Lukehart and coworkers found that 30% of 40 patients with primary and secondary syphilis had viable treponemes in CSF and that CNS invasion by the spirochete is common in early syphilis and is apparently independent of HIV infection [385].

The clinical manifestations of secondary syphilis resolve spontaneously, without antimicrobial therapy after a period of weeks to several months to enter the latent stage. Patients, however, remain seroreactive. During the secondary syphilis phase, patients generally remain asymptomatic until manifestations of tertiary syphilis appear years later in one-third of untreated patients. Clinically, tertiary syphilis is divided into three general categories: neurosyphilis, cardiovascular syphilis, and gummatous syphilis.

Neurosyphilis

Neurosyphilis is due to damage produced by meningovasculitis and degenerative parenchymal changes in the entire CNS. Since spirochete invasion of the CNS occurs during the primary stage, a small population of patients has continuing CNS involvement. Syphilitic meningitis is an early manifestation, usually occurring within the first 2 years of the primary infection and resulting from small vessel arteritis in the meninges, which accounts for the typical symptoms of headache, nausea, and vomiting seen in approximately 90% of patients. In addition, up to 45% of patients with syphilitic meningitis may have cranial nerve palsies. Seizures have been reported in 17% and fever occurs in <50%. The CSF white count is usually abnormal, but there is only a mild decrease in CSF glucose.

Although there is some overlap of symptomatology, meningovascular syphilis presents with findings of meningitis together with focal neurologic findings due to syphilitic arteritis. The peak incidence of this condition is approximately 7 years after acquisition of syphilis and accounts for approximately 12% of patients with CNS involvement [386 389]. Patients with meningovascular syphilis generally present with a history of several weeks to months of prodromal symptoms and signs, such as headache, vertigo, personality changes, behavioral changes, insomnia or seizures, and stroke-like neurologic deficits, most frequently involving the distribution of vessels in the territory of the middle cerebral artery followed by that of the basilar artery. Thus, while the distribution of strokes in such patients may be similar to that of the patient with atherosclerotic disease, the occlusive symptoms develop gradually over a period of time in meningeal vascular syphilis as opposed to sudden onset in patients with atherosclerotic strokes [389]. In contrast to the findings from the preantibiotic era, neurosyphilis is now most often identified in young patients with HIV coinfection [390, 391].

The majority of neurologic manifestations of tertiary syphilis involve the CNS parenchyma and are classified as parenchymatous neurosyphilis. This category includes two classical syndromes: general paresis and tabes dorsalis. In contrast to the pathogenesis of syphilitic meningitis or meningovascular syphilis, these syndromes result from progressive neuronal destruction with fibrosis and atrophy rather than ischemic damage from vasculitis. General paresis is a chronic progressive meningoencephalitis with a peak incidence 10–20 years after acquisition of syphilis. Patients generally present with gradual deterioration of mental functioning characterized by difficulties in concentration, irritability, and deficits of higher cognitive function. As the condition progresses, these manifestations become more obvious and symptoms may mimic psychiatric disease, including delusions, paranoia, emotional lability, memory loss, or dementia. Difficulties with motor control then develop with a loss of facial muscle and extremity tone, loss of fine motor control, and the development of tremors and dysarthria. Subsequently, patients may have seizures, loss of bowel and bladder control, and paralysis; the pupils become unresponsive to light and painful stimuli and may be constricted and unequal in size (the Argyll Robertson pupil). Untreated, the disease follows a progressive or subacute course over 3–4 years. Pathologically there is diffuse cortical atrophy, dilatation of the ventricles, and neuronal dropout with accompanying gliosis. Spirochetes can be demonstrated in 25–40% of patients with silver stain. The diagnosis is established by a combination of the clinical presentation, positive serology, and elevated CSF white count and protein.

Tabes dorsalis results from progressive neuronal degeneration, especially the dorsal roots and the posterior column of the spinal cord. It has a peak incidence that is generally later than that of paresis, approximately 15–20 years after infection, and the progression of this condition is somewhat slower than that of paresis. The classical early symptomatology is "lightning pains" in the distribution of nerve roots. These pains are described as lancinating, lasting for minutes to hours, and most often involve the lower extremities. Ten percent to 20% of patients with tabes may also present with episodic attacks of abdominal pain. In addition to pain, some patients experience episodic paresthesias. Ultimately, patients experience progressive loss of vibration and proprioceptive sensation, particularly in the lower extremities. As a result, the patients exhibit a characteristic broad-based, shuffling gait and may develop Charcot joints. Muscular atrophy develops in approximately 20% of patients. The Argyll Robertson pupil, in which one or both pupils constrict with accommodation but do not react directly to light, is a characteristic feature of both general paresis and tabes dorsalis. Pathologically there is atrophy of the posterior columns of the spinal cord with inflammatory infiltrates and loss of neurons. In contrast to paresis, it is unusual to be able to stain the spirochete in nerve tissue. The diagnosis is readily made from the characteristic neurologic findings together with positive serology. However, CSF leukocytosis is observed in only 50% of patients, and protein elevation is seen in approximately 53% of patients.

Syphilitic gummas are progressive granulomatous tumor-like lesions primarily involving skin, mucous membranes, and bone but can develop in any organ in the body including the brain. Gummas may arise in almost any part of the CNS but are most often associated with the pia mater and consist of rubbery masses varying in size from several millimeters to centimeters [392, 393]. Localized findings range from small superficial nodules to large radiating lesions. CNS symptoms depend on the anatomic location of the lesions.

Serologic Testing

Laboratory diagnosis of syphilis depends on the stage of the disease and clinical manifestations. Patients with lesions on moist skin or mucous membranes during either primary or secondary syphilis can usually be diagnosed by the demonstration of treponemes on dark-field microscopy. While treponemes can be demonstrated in dry lesions or lymph nodes by biopsy or saline aspiration, the yield is considerably lower. Elevated CSF protein is usually consistent with neurosyphilis. In patients suspected of neurosyphilis who do not have HIV infection and who have a non-reactive CSF-VDRL, a lymphocyte count of more than 5 cells or a protein concentration of 45 mg/dL is usually consistent with a diagnosis of neurosyphilis. Serologic tests for syphilis are generally divided into two different types: nontreponemal and treponemal tests. Nontreponemal tests measure IgG or IgM antibodies directed at cardiolipin, which is released when the treponeme damages cells during an infection. Thus, a positive nontreponemal test is indicative of an active infection, but a confirmatory test with a treponemal test is required to verify that it is indeed a syphilis infection that is causing elevated cardiolipin levels. Currently, a standardized mixture of cardiolipin, cholesterol, and lecithin which has fewer false-positive reactions is used and forms the basis of today's standardized tests. The most common of these are the classic venereal disease research laboratory (VDRL), in which agglutination of the cardiolipin, cholesterol, and lecithin antigen is carried out on a slide using heated serum; the rapid plasma reagin (RPR) card test; the automated reagin test (ART); or the toluidine red unheated test (TRUST). Because of the stringency of the technical requirements for the test, the VDRL is generally performed only on CSF and serum screening tests are generally done with the RPR and its variants. Specific treponemal tests for syphilis include the *T. pallidum* hemagglutination (TPHA) test, the microhemagglutination test with *T. pallidum* antigen, the fluorescent treponemal antibody-absorption test (FTA-abs), the enzyme-linked immunosorbent assay (ELISA), and the hemagglutination treponemal test for syphilis (HATTS).

Nontreponemal tests (RPR and VDRL) rise during primary syphilis and reach their peak in secondary syphilis. They slowly decline with advancing age. It is important to note that the serologic response to syphilis increases gradually over the course of the primary infection, so that when the chancre is first observed no more than 10–20% of patients may be seropositive by any method. However, this will increase with the duration of the chancre during primary infection to approximately 70% for both the treponemal and nontreponemal tests by the time the chancre heals. During secondary syphilis, serologic tests, whether treponemal or nontreponemal, are positive in almost 100% of patients.

Early treatment of the primary infection should render the patient seronegative within a year. Treatment of syphilis during the secondary and latent stages will generally result in a significant fall in the titer of the nontreponemal tests. These tests should display a four-fold decrease within 1 year after treatment, although titers may still remain positive [394].

In general, once the treponemal tests become positive, they remain so for life even if the patient has been successfully treated. Serologic tests can be used to diagnose neurosyphilis during the latent and late latent stages by testing CSF for VDRL antibodies. With the exception of rare false-positive results, possibly resulting from blood contamination, a reactive CSF-VDRL in the absence of substantial contamination of CSF with blood is diagnostic of neurosyphilis.

Although the specificity of the CSF-VDRL in diagnosing likely active neurosyphilis is 100%, the sensitivity is only about 27% and, in early syphilis, is of unknown prognostic significance [395, 396]. The insensitivity of the CSF-VDRL test limits its usefulness as a screening test for neurosyphilis. The CSF-FTA-abs test appears more sensitive for screening CSF but is less specific than the CSF-VDRL test in distinguishing currently active neurosyphilis from past syphilis. These findings imply that clinical judgment remains essential for establishing the diagnosis of active neurosyphilis. Most other tests are both insensitive and nonspecific. Furthermore, one cannot use the more sensitive treponemal antibody tests with CSF to diagnose neurosyphilis as these antibodies cross the blood–brain barrier and are therefore likely to be present in the CSF of all patients who have positive serum treponemal tests for syphilis. Thus, a positive CSF treponemal test does not provide any additional information to that obtained by testing serum alone. For example, in one study the CSF-FTA-abs test was positive in 48 patients of whom only 15 had clinical neurosyphilis [395]. While one can resort to sophisticated methods of CSF analysis, it is generally recommended to treat patients who have reactive serum testing if they have any clinical signs of neurosyphilis. Neuroimaging using CT scanning or MRI can also be used to document CNS gummas or other complications of tertiary syphilis.

Asymptomatic neurosyphilis is defined by the presence of CSF abnormalities consistent with neurosyphilis in persons with serological evidence of syphilis and no neurological symptoms or signs [391]. Also, asymptomatic neurosyphilis can occur in both early and latent stages of syphilis. For example, among a large population with defined latent syphilis and no evidence of symptomatic neurological disease, 13.5% were found to have asymptomatic neurosyphilis [397]. Moreover, patients with latent syphilis and asymptomatic neurosyphilis are more likely to have syphilitic involvement of the skin [397].

Treatment

The preferred treatment for all manifestations of neurosyphilis is intravenous aqueous crystalline penicillin G 12–24 million units/day for 10–14 days. Alternatively, 2.4 million units of procaine penicillin G can be given intramuscularly together with 500 mg/day of probenecid four times a day for 10–14 days. In penicillin-allergic patients, doxycycline 200 mg orally each day for 21 days or ceftriaxone 1 g IM or IV for 14 days has been recommended. However, treatment failures have been documented with ceftriaxone, especially in HIV-infected patients. Patients with syphilitic meningitis or meningovascular syphilis generally respond to treatment with the exception of cases in which the patient has focal cranial nerve abnormalities associated with syphilitic meningitis or larger ischemic defects caused by the arteritis associated with meningovascular syphilis.

For patients with tabes dorsalis or general paresis, improvement approaching cure is relatively uncommon and, in fact, for a majority of patients, disease progression continues despite adequate penicillin treatment [398]. Penicillin remains the drug of choice for all forms of neurosyphilis, but disease progression has been frequently reported following the use of penicillin G benzathine [386]. Thus, documentation of CSF resolution over the months following penicillin therapy is required to confirm curative treatment.

Patients with asymptomatic neurosyphilis appear to respond very well to treatment. In one study, 89% of 454 patients who initially had ≥10 leukocytes/mm^3 of CSF had normalized their cell counts at a 1-year follow-up, as had 69% of those with abnormal protein prior to treatment [399]. Because patients with primary and secondary syphilis are curable with standard treatment of benzathine penicillin G 2.4 million units IM weekly for three weekly doses, the question of proper treatment always arises when an asymptomatic patient is found to have a positive VDRL, RPR, or other screening test for syphilis. The problem is that this regimen does not reliably provide CSF levels in excess of 0.018 μg/mL of CSF in all patients, which is believed to be necessary to kill spirochetes within the CNS [400–402]. The treatment of cerebral gummas is IV penicillin G with neuroimaging follow-up recommended for most patients [403]. Surgery should be reserved for those unresponsive to antibiotics or those with acutely elevated intracranial pressure [403]. All patients found to have serologic evidence of syphilis, assuming that false-positive tests such as those due to pregnancy and other intercurrent illnesses can be ruled out, should have serologic testing for HIV because the ability to eradicate syphilis is considerably lower in HIV-infected patients and re-treatment may be necessary.

Lyme Disease

Lyme disease is due to systemic infection with the microaerophilic spirochete *Borrelia burgdorferi* and the body's immune response to the infection. Lyme disease was first recognized in the United States in the early 1970s when Dr. Allen Steere at Yale University investigated an outbreak of juvenile rheumatoid arthritis in the small towns of Lyme, Old Lyme, and East Haddam, Connecticut. In the initial report, they identified and ascertained 39 children and 12 adults who presented with classic, characteristic, remitting, relapsing oligoarticular arthritis with onset in the summer or early fall. All of these patients lived in rural areas and half of the patients lived on two adjacent country roads. In addition, 13 of these patients had noted an unusual skin lesion an average of 4 months before the onset of the arthritis [404]. Subsequent prospective studies then defined neurologic abnormalities such as Bell's palsy, sensory radiculoneuritis, lymphocytic meningitis, and cardiac conduction abnormalities also associated with Lyme disease. These studies showed that at least a quarter of the patients remembered a tick bite at the site of the initial skin lesion and based on examination of the actual tick from one of these patients, the vector was identified as *Ixodes scapularis* [405, 406]. The agent of Lyme disease was finally isolated by Dr. Willy Burgdorfer from the Rocky Mountain Laboratory in Hamilton, Montana, when he was searching for evidence of Rocky Mountain spotted fever in ticks isolated from New York State. No rickettsiae were found; however, spirochetes were seen in stains of the insect's digestive tract [407, 408].

Pathogenesis

The clinical manifestations fall broadly into three stages: early localized, early disseminated, and chronic disseminated. Approximately 50% of untreated patients progress to disseminated disease. During the first stage, the earliest manifestations of Lyme disease occur at the site of the tick bite beginning as a red macule or papule that may expand to an area 10–15 cm with red outer borders and partial central clearing—the so-called "bull's eye" skin rash. The lesion develops as early as 3 days and as late as 30 days following the initial bite and generally lasts 3–4 weeks. It is most commonly located on the thigh or groin and develops in approximately 80% of patients [409–411]. Following the entry of the spirochete into the patient via the tick bite, dissemination of the spirochete occurs during the development of this initial lesion, and while some patients may develop multiple secondary annular lesions that are similar to the primary site lesion, others may clear the infection without developing symptoms. All patients largely remain seropositive. In the second stage, the organism produces symptoms by direct invasion. Systemic symptoms of fatigue, lethargy, and malaise along with generalized lymphadenopathy, meningismus, encephalopathy, migratory musculoskeletal pain, splenomegaly, sore throat, and cough may develop in varying degrees during this early disseminated phase [410, 411]. For the most part, the systemic manifestations as well as the erythema chronicum migrans lesions themselves usually resolve without treatment in 3–4 weeks. Untreated, however, the Lyme disease spirochete becomes sequestered and persists in various tissues, particularly the CNS, joints, heart, and skin.

In some patients with meningitis, particularly in Europe, where the disease is caused by a different species of spirochete, significant neurologic abnormalities develop, including cranial neuritis which can present as an isolated facial palsy (motor and sensory), radicular mononeuritis multiplex, or myelitis alone or in varying combinations. Although these patients may have some neck stiffness on extreme flexion, typical Kernig's and Brudzinski's signs are not present. Patients may complain of excruciating headaches as well as severe musculoskeletal pain. Early on, examination of the CSF may be normal, but patients may develop a lymphocytic pleocytosis with a normal glucose level.

During this early dissemination stage, cardiac symptoms and signs manifest, usually atrioventricular block with varying degrees of other forms occasionally noted including complete heart block, which rarely persists for more than a week and generally does not require the insertion of a pacemaker [412, 413]. Occasional patients have been described with osteomyelitis, myositis, panniculitis, eosinophilic fasciitis, conjunctivitis, or even deeper involvement of the orbital structures including panophthalmitis and choroid retinitis with exudative retinal detachment or interstitial keratitis.

The third stage of Lyme disease is characterized by arthritis, which develops in about 60% of untreated patients. Symptoms include intermittent attacks of pain particularly involving the large joints (e.g., the knee), in an asymmetric pattern. Attacks of acute arthritis generally last weeks to months followed by periods of remission. Joint fluid counts range from 500 to 100,000 cells/mm^3 with a high percentage of polymorphonuclear leukocytes. Even untreated, this condition resolves gradually over a period of years.

The late manifestations of CNS involvement of Lyme disease generally develop a year or more after the onset of illness and generally do not improve spontaneously. In both North American and European forms of this disease, persistence of the *B. burgdorferi* spirochete has been demonstrated in CSF and in brain parenchyma up to 9 years after the onset of illness [412–416]. The most common neurologic symptoms are speech abnormalities, limb weakness, gait difficulties, ataxia, bladder dysfunction, visual changes, hearing loss, mood changes, sleep disorders, and deteriorating memory and concentration. Symptoms of late progressive Lyme encephalomyelitis may develop either acutely or gradually and then worsen progressively over the ensuing months to years [414, 416–425]. Progression may be gradual or stepwise, characterized by sudden deterioration and only partial improvement between episodes. Headaches, nausea, vomiting, and neck stiffness have been reported but occur less often, while mental deficits such as behavioral changes, poor memory, and concentration are common. More severe changes including confusion, disorientation, dementia, delirium, and somnolence can occur. Symptoms such as apraxia, myoclonus, hemiparesthesia, and visual field abnormalities have been reported. Spinal cord involvement is common and myelitis may present as a progressive paraparesis or quadriparesis that can become very severe. Approximately 45% of patients have cranial nerve palsies; involvement of the optic, facial, oculomotor, and vestibulocochlear cranial nerves have all been reported [413, 418, 426]. Peripheral radiculoneuritis occurs in <10% of patients.

The CSF is abnormal in almost all cases of CNS involvement in Lyme disease. Generally, there is CSF pleocytosis, predominantly monocytic in the range of 100–200 cells/mm^3, although levels as high as 2300 cells/mm^3 have been reported. CSF protein concentrations are usually >50 mg/dL, usually in the range of 100–200 mg/dL, although concentrations levels as high as 1800 mg/dL have been reported; glucose is generally normal to low. Oligoclonal bands specific for *B. burgdorferi* may be present.

EEG and CT abnormalities, including infarcts in the internal capsule, thalamus, lentiform nucleus, hydrocephalus, and cerebral atrophy, have been reported [417, 419, 427–430]. MRI shows additional lesions such as multifocal white matter abnormalities, infarcts, periventricular and sub-insular cavities, as well as atrophy of the pons and medulla [419, 427, 429–432]. MRI imaging in patients with myelitis has shown diffuse or focal signal abnormalities in relevant parts of the spinal cord [419. 433–436].

In contrast to the dramatic and objectively documented neurologic abnormalities and syndromes seen in a small number of patients with Lyme encephalopathy, a certain number of North American patients have reported the development of a less dramatic but nonetheless disabling CNS symptom complex. These patients complain of overwhelming fatigue, accompanied by loss of memory and concentration, and almost always without physical neurologic abnormalities. Psychological testing shows abnormalities or dysfunction in memory, ability to learn or acquire new information, attention span, concentration, problem-solving, perceptual-motor performance, and verbal fluency. Although depression and irritability are frequently reported, general fatigue appears to be the overriding complaint. Many of these patients fit the definition of chronic fatigue syndrome as defined by the CDC. Objective laboratory and radiographic signs of infection are generally absent. CSF pleocytosis is present in <5% of the cases, and CSF protein is elevated in only a minority of patients. Oligoclonal bands for *B. burgdorferi* are absent and patients with these complaints may or may not have antibodies to Lyme disease in the serum. Some of these patients have been reported to have MRI abnormalities, such as focal areas of increased signal in deep cerebral white matter [428, 433–435]. In general, symptoms in these patients do not improve spontaneously. A variable number of persons with this condition apparently do respond to courses of antimicrobial therapy, sometimes for 6 months or more [428, 433–436].

A number of North American patients have developed a mild multifocal polyneuropathy distinct from the meningopolyneuritis of early disseminated Lyme disease as a manifestation of late Lyme disease. Intermittent tingling and paresthesia of the extremities are the most common symptoms, occurring in approximately 50% of patients with this form of late Lyme disease. The onset is generally 8 months to several years after the initial infection. The symptoms are usually distal, may be symmetric or asymmetric, and can involve both arms and legs. About 25% of patients present with carpal tunnel syndrome or develop it at some point. Radicular pain occurs in 25 50% of those with this syndrome; this pain is intermittent, asymmetric, and multifocal, typically radiating from the spine into the limbs or trunk [428, 435, 437–440]. Sensory changes such as mild stocking and glove distal sensory loss, as well as distal asymmetrical or truncal sensory loss also occur [428, 435, 437, 438, 441, 442].

Objective evidence of organic disease is much more common in these patients than in those reporting symptoms of chronic fatigue, with up to 83% of patients having electromyographic abnormalities demonstrable particularly among those with distal paresthesia. In addition, CSF abnormalities, mostly in the form of increased protein concentration and intrathecal antibody synthesis specific for *B. burgdorferi* are found in up to 70% of patients with these symptoms [428, 441]. Treatment with antimicrobials may improve the paresthesia and electrophysiologic conduction abnormalities but may require prolonged regimens from 3 to 7 months [428, 433, 437–439, 441]. Improvement among patients with radicular pain is less frequent and is only seen in about 50%.

The diagnosis of Lyme disease can be made with reasonable assurance by a well-documented history of a tick bite and together with clinical evidence of typical skin lesions (erythema chronicum migrans). However, during this early stage of the disease, only 30–40% of patients will have a serologic test positive for Lyme disease in an acute serum specimen, and only 60–70% of these patients will be positive in the convalescent sera 2–4 weeks later. CDC recommends a two-step approach for serological testing: the first step in the workup of patients with putative Lyme symptoms is to obtain an antibody titer using an ELISA test to screen for the presence of antibodies; the second step is confirmation of positive titers with a Western blot assay; both IgG and IgM antibodies are formed. However, persistence of the IgM antibody alone in the absence of an IgG response after the first month of illness may signal a false-positive reaction. After the first 1–2 months of infection, over 90% of patients will have a specific IgG antibody response to the spirochete. It has been noted that patients treated effectively early in the course of erythema chronicum migrans may never develop a humoral immune response, although cellular immunity may be demonstrated and persist for years.

Treatment

Treatment of early dissemination and localized erythema chronicum migrans consists of doxycycline 100 mg twice a day for 20–30 days or amoxicillin 500 mg three times daily for 20–30 days, with some experts recommending the addition of probenecid 500 mg three times daily to the amoxicillin regimen. Cefuroxime axetil 500 mg orally three times daily for 2–3 weeks has also been recommended as has erythromycin 400 kg/mg/day in four divided doses for 2–4 weeks in children. For patients with arthritis, treatment with doxycycline or amoxicillin is extended to 1–2 months, and intravenous ceftriaxone 2 g a day for 14–30 days is also recommended.

For patients with early or late neurologic abnormalities, ceftriaxone 2 g IV daily for 2–4 weeks is generally recommended. Alternatives include penicillin G 20 million units IV in four divided doses daily for up to 30 days, as well as doxycycline 100 mg orally three times per day for 14–30 days. Treatment failures have been reported for all of these regimens and treatment may need to be repeated.

Cardiac abnormalities are treated as for early infection in those patients with first-degree AV block; IV ceftriaxone or penicillin is used for higher degrees of AV block. In patients with neurologic manifestations of early disseminated Lyme disease, IV therapy with penicillin or ceftriaxone can lead to a mild Herxheimer-like reaction with worsening pain and fever during the first 18–20 h [412, 443]. In general, meningismus, radicular pain, and systemic symptoms improve within days although residual fatigue, arthralgias, and muscular-skeletal pain can persist for some time thereafter. Motor deficits improve more slowly, over 2–3 months, and sometimes never fully recover. CNS abnormalities usually stop progressing and begin to improve slowly, but residual deficits may remain [415, 417–451]. CSF cell counts respond over the course of treatment but may not return to normal for several months, and the protein concentration falls even more slowly and may remain elevated for up to 1 year in some patients. If the patient does not respond by the end of the second week, treatment may be extended for another 2 weeks.

The severe abnormalities of late Lyme disease generally respond well to high-dose penicillin, doxycycline, or ceftriaxone [417, 419, 426, 429, 430, 434, 435, 447, 449–454]. Altogether, 80–90% of patients improve with IV cephalosporins, but recovery is slow and often incomplete, with little change occurring during the treatment itself and only developing over the subsequent weeks after treatment has stopped. At this time, there are no published data that support the routine use of steroid therapy in the management of CNS complications of Lyme disease. Finally, although a controversial issue, there is no convincing data that show prolonged antimicrobial therapy is effective for patients in whom symptoms persist after completing the recommended antimicrobial therapy for acute Lyme disease [455].

Miscellaneous Infections with CNS Complications

Rickettsial Disease

Rickettsiae are small gram-negative, obligate intracellular coccobacilli that are transmitted by tick bites. Rickettsiae grow freely in the cytoplasm of eukaryotic host cells on which they are dependent for nucleotide cofactors and ATP; they do not grow well outside the host cell. They can only be grown in living host cells, such as cell cultures and embryonated eggs. Most rickettsiae have animal reservoirs and are spread by infected arthropod vectors. Infections generally follow the distribution of the main vectors: *Dermacentor andersoni* (the wood tick) is the primary vector in the Western United States; *Dermacentor variabilis* (dog tick) is the principal vector in the Eastern United States. Infections are limited to warmer months.

Following the tick bite, Rickettsiae infects the vascular endothelium lining the small blood vessels causing a vasculitis—the primary pathologic feature of rickettsial infection, particularly RMSF. A combination of endothelial proliferation, necrosis, and perivascular inflammation, predominantly with a mononuclear cell infiltrate, leads to thrombosis and leakage of erythrocytes into surrounding tissues resulting in petechial lesions. Should systemic infection ensue, these vascular lesions occur throughout the body. This is in contrast to the infiltrate of polymorphonuclear leukocytes seen in typical immunocomplex vasculitis.

Rickettsial disease is characterized by fever, headache, rash, myalgias, and myositis. The most important rickettsiosis in the United States is Rocky Mountain spotted fever (RMSF), which is an acute febrile illness caused by *Rickettsia rickettsii*. As the name implies, the disease is seen in the Rocky Mountain States, such as Colorado and Wyoming, but also occurs in the inland parts of North Carolina, Virginia, and other Southeastern States. For RMSF, the incubation period between tick bite and onset of illness is 2–6 days. Fever, headache, rash, mental confusion, and myalgia are the predominant clinical features [456–458]. The rash usually develops on the second or third day of illness, initially on the wrists and ankles followed by spread to the trunk within hours. In contrast with a viral exanthem, the RMSF rash can appear on the palms and soles. About 25% of patients may have encephalitis at presentation with lethargy, confusion, or delirium. This may deteriorate to seizures and coma. As a result of the variability of the vessels involved in the CNS, a wide range of clinical neurologic features are associated with RMSF, including seizures, deafness, facial diplegia, gaze palsies, nystagmus, ataxia, dysphasia, transverse myelitis, neurogenic bladder, hemiplegia, and paraplegia or quadriplegia.

The diagnosis of RMSF is fundamentally a clinical diagnosis and depends on the history of a tick bite together with a compatible systemic illness with or without a rash [458]. The diagnosis of RMSF must be considered in all febrile patients who have known or possible exposure to ticks, especially if they live in or have traveled to endemic regions during warmer months [458]. Because the culture of rickettsiae is difficult, serological testing remains the mainstay of confirming the diagnosis. However, though serologic diagnosis is highly accurate, it is not readily available in most institutions or as a routine service in the acute setting, and therefore treatment must be started empirically; patients with RMSF who received antirickettsial therapy within 5 days of the onset of symptoms are significantly less likely to die than those in whom therapy was delayed [459].

The basic tenet of RMSF management, then, is the commencement of appropriate antimicrobial therapy without delay in conjunction with supportive therapy where indicated, i.e., IV hydration for hypovolemia or circulatory collapse, mechanical ventilatory support especially if the patient has developed ARDS, blood transfusion, and management of DIC. In adults and children, the recommended dose is doxycycline 100 mg per dose administered twice daily (orally or intravenously) for adults or 2.2 mg/kg body weight per dose administered twice daily (orally or intravenously) for children weighing <100 lbs. (45.4 kg) [457]. Previously, for children under the age of 8 years, chloramphenicol was recommended because of the tooth discoloration associated with tetracyclines. However, in 1997, the American Academy of Pediatrics Committee on Infectious Diseases revised its recommendations and identified doxycycline as the drug of choice for treating presumed or confirmed RMSF in children of any age, because of the effectiveness of this antimicrobial in reducing attributable morbidity and potential mortality. Sulfonamides may worsen the disease and are therefore contraindicated.

Most patients show improvement within 2 days but may require up 7–10 days in severe cases. Despite modern therapeutic modalities, the fatality rate of RMSF is still in the range of 5–10% [457]. Even after recovery, CNS abnormalities may persist in a significant number of patients with RMSF, including cognitive defects, impaired fine motor skills, aphasia, and EEG changes. Long-term neurological sequelae include paraparesis; hearing loss; peripheral neuropathy; bladder and bowel incontinence; cerebellar, vestibular, and motor dysfunction; and language disorders [460]. Sexton and colleagues made the point that the mechanism of such abnormalities is rickettsia-induced vasculitis with subsequent infarction of neural tissue and that although early treatment may prevent many such complications, other factors, such as age and race, might be playing a role in the pathogenesis of severe disease [461].

Human Ehrlichiosis

Ehrlichia species are tiny, obligate, leukocyte-associated, gram-negative bacteria that replicate in membrane-bound compartments inside the host white blood cells to cause human disease. *Anaplasma phagocytophilum* causes human granulocytotropic anaplasmosis (HGA), previously known as human granulocytotropic ehrlichiosis (HGE). *A. phagocytophilum* is transmitted by *Ixodes scapularis*, which also transmits the agents that cause Lyme disease and babesiosis. *Ehrlichia chaffeensis*, the cause of human monocytic ehrlichiosis (HME), is transmitted by the Lone Star tick found on the whitetail deer and prefers to invade mononuclear leukocytes (e.g., macrophages). Both diseases are transmitted by deer or dog tick bites; HME is relatively common in the South and Southeast United States, while most cases of human HGA so far have been recorded from the upper Midwest, Northeast, and some parts of the South. HGA is the predominant form of ehrlichiosis in the United States and runs second only to Lyme disease as a tick-borne transmitted infection in the United States. Ehrlichiosis is a seasonal disease with highest rates of occurrence from April to September. DNA studies of the agent that causes HGA show that it is mostly related to *Ehrlichia canis* but probably represents a different subspecies.

Both HGA and HME have incubation periods of about 7 (range 5–14) days after the tick bite. Symptoms of ehrlichiosis include high fever, chills, rigors, malaise, severe headache, myalgias, nausea, and vomiting and may include confusion, disorientation, obtundation, and ataxia in some patients [462]. Presentation may be abrupt or subacute in nature. Compared with RMSF, rashes are relatively uncommon (36% of HME and 2% of HGA) and are characteristically maculopapular with a distribution on the upper and lower limbs, trunk, or face. The petechial rash of RMSF is absent in ehrlichiosis. Patients with HME can develop aseptic meningitis and meningoencephalitis or progress to respiratory and renal insufficiency. Patients may develop hepatosplenomegaly. Although respiratory insufficiency can also occur in HGA, meningoencephalitis is uncommon in this type of human ehrlichiosis.

CSF is frequently normal; other laboratory studies are non-diagnostic or nonspecific; thrombocytopenia is common in both types of ehrlichiosis. Wright stain of a peripheral blood and buffy coat smear might reveal the characteristic intracellular inclusions known as morulae; these inclusions are present in the cytoplasm of neutrophils and monocytes of HGA and HME, respectively. However, presence of morulae in smears is variable. Serologic confirmation of illness is the usual method of diagnosis and is highly accurate but available only from state and other reference laboratories; a fourfold rise of titers is considered diagnostic. The differential diagnosis includes RMSF, Lyme disease, and babesiosis. As with RMSF, treatment with doxycycline (100 mg twice daily) for 14 days or chloramphenicol must be given empirically [457, 462]. Untreated, mortality of all patients with human ehrlichiosis ranges remains significant, ranging from 2% to 10%.

Human Bartonellosis (Cat-Scratch Disease)

Cat-scratch disease is caused by *Bartonella henselae*, a pleomorphic gram-negative bacillus that binds silver and can be identified by Warthin-Starry stains. The condition develops predominantly in persons under the age of 21 years after receiving a scratch from a kitten or feral cat; the organism is transmitted less commonly by cat fleas. The organism proliferates at the site of the injury and, following an incubation period of 3–21 days, one or more papules develop at the site of the bite or scratch. Regional lymphadenitis ensues with enlargement of epitrochlear, axillary, and cervical lymph nodes, along with fever and malaise. In the typical case of cat-scratch disease, a single enlarged, fluctuant lymph node is the most common occurrence; generalized lymphadenopathy is relatively uncommon. About one-third of patients will develop systemic symptoms, such as fever and malaise. Other clinical manifestations include endocarditis and granulomatous or suppurative hepatosplenic and osseous lesions.

B. henselae involvement of the CNS is not uncommon. Patients may actually have a variety of CNS symptoms, including encephalopathy, retinitis, or Parinaud's ocular glandular syndrome (i.e., ocular granuloma or conjunctivitis with preauricular lymphadenopathy). In a large series of 130 seropositive patients with cat-scratch disease, the occurrence of neuroretinitis and encephalopathy was approximately 22% and 15%, respectively.

Bartonella grows slowly on solid and liquid media and, if suspected, the medical microbiology laboratory should be contacted to hold the cultures for an extended period. Histological features of lymph nodes generally are nonspecific, showing features of chronic granulomatous and acute inflammatory changes. Diagnosis can be made serologically using an indirect immunofluorescence assay or enzyme immunosorbent assay to detect *B. henselae* antibodies; PCR assays have proven are more sensitive and specific at detecting *B. henselae*. Although most cases of cat-scratch disease in the normal host are self-limited and resolve over a period of 3–8 weeks, treatment is recommended. A 5-day course of azithromycin is the treatment of choice. Alternatives are clarithromycin, doxycycline, or ciprofloxacin for 10–14 days [463]. In severe cases, including patients with encephalopathy, IV azithromycin or gentamicin plus rifampin is recommended. Although there are reports of the effectiveness of adjunct steroid therapy in the management of patients with cat-scratch encephalitis, no randomized controlled trials have been carried out to determine whether steroids actually improve patient outcomes [464, 465].

Whipple's Disease

Whipple's disease is a slowly progressive systemic disease caused by *Tropheryma whippelii*, a gram-positive rod-shaped bacterium. The disease primarily affects Caucasian men over the age of 40 years. Whipple's disease is relatively uncommon with most reported cases from North America and Western Europe. The typical clinical manifestations are arthralgias (67%), diarrhea (76%), weight loss (92%), abdominal pain (55%), and other features of malabsorption [466]. Less commonly, patients may present with fever, chills, CNS abnormalities, seizures, cardiovascular symptoms, endocarditis, or darkening of the skin. CNS involvement is the most serious complication of Whipple's disease with neurological signs documented in 10–40% of affected patients [466, 467]; damage to the CNS may be irreversible. *T. whippelii* is an unusual bacterium capable of intracellular survival. Left untreated, Whipple's disease is invariably fatal [468]. Although humans are the only known host for *T. whippelii*, a natural source has not been defined. The organism itself is ubiquitous in the environment and has been isolated from the stool of sewage workers suggesting that a possible mode of transmission might be fecal-oral [469]. It appears that the genetic predisposition of the host rather than the genotype of the bacterium is the key risk factor for infection [470, 471].

CNS involvement is one of the more frequent complications of this disease and can, on occasion, occur in the absence of recognized gastrointestinal or systemic involvement. The most frequent neurologic manifestations of Whipple's disease are dementia, decreasing levels of consciousness, progressive supranuclear ophthalmoplegia, myoclonus, and hypothalamic dysfunction. The dementia progresses slowly and is characterized by memory impairment, confusion, personality change, paranoia, emotional instability, and depression [466, 467, 472–478]. An unusual syndrome of synchronized ocular movements and contractions of the jaw, known as oculomasticatory myorhythmia, is sometimes seen and is unique to Whipple's disease [474–476].

The disease is most often diagnosed through upper gastrointestinal endoscopy with biopsy of the small bowel or a mesenteric lymph node. Macroscopically, the duodenal mucosa is pale yellow with dilated villi and ecstatic lymph vessels [466]. Periodic acid-Schiff (PAS) stains will reveal the presence of PAS-positive material (e.g., mucin and carbohydrate) with occasional bacilliform organisms. Pathologic involvement of the brain is most often manifested by chalky, yellowish white, 1–2 mm nodules distributed diffusely throughout the cortical and subcortical gray matter of both the cerebrum and the cerebellum. The most frequently involved sites are the temporal, periventricular, and periaqueductal gray matter as well as the hippocampus, hypothalamus, and basal ganglia. Histologically, the nodules are made up of microglia that stain strongly positive with PAS. Although neuroimaging studies with CT or MRI may reveal cerebral atrophy, ring-enhancing lesions, hydrocephalus, or changes consistent with demyelination, these findings are nonspecific for Whipple's disease.

Although PCR diagnosis of Whipple's disease is possible, healthy carriers can have a positive PCR even if they do not have Whipple's disease. Thus, PCR is better used when there is clinical suspicion of Whipple's disease rather than for screening [466]. Moreover, because of the wide range of conditions in the differential diagnosis of degenerative CNS diseases, tissue biopsy is generally required for diagnosis. For CNS disease, immunohistochemistry testing using specific antibodies is more sensitive than PAS staining by being able to identify *T. whipplei* in tissues, including those with negative PAS staining [466, 479]. CNS involvement, consistent with the characteristic clinical syndromes of Whipple's disease, and occurring in the setting of neuroimaging studies, biopsy-proven systemic Whipple's disease, or PCR are also sufficiently diagnostic [480, 481].

Untreated, Whipple's disease is associated with high mortality rates. And because of the risk of CNS relapse, even while the patient is on oral trimethoprim/sulfamethoxazole, a regimen that includes antimicrobial agents (e.g., a third-generation cephalosporin) that penetrate the CNS is indicated [482, 483]. The initial treatment of CNS involvement in Whipple's disease is ceftriaxone 2 g IV once daily *or* procaine penicillin G 1–two million units IM once daily followed by trimethoprim/sulfamethoxazole one DS tablet twice daily for at least 1 year [466, 471]. Some clinicians continue therapy for 2 years to life. Unfortunately, the overall prognosis of CNS Whipple's disease is poor. With antimicrobial therapy, disease progression can be halted, but significant clinical improvement is limited, relapses are frequent, and established neurological defects are difficult to reverse.

Subacute Sclerosing Panencephalitis (SSPE)

This rare, progressive encephalitis usually occurs 2–10 years after an uncomplicated bout of measles. It occurs most frequently between the ages of 4 and 20 years and has a prolonged clinical course. It is thought to be due to reactivation of latent measles virus with high levels of IgM and IgG in the blood and CSF. Most of the pathologic features of the disease are localized to the CNS and retina. Histological findings include those of subacute meningoencephalitis. Neuronophagia (neuronal degeneration) is common and residual neurons may contain intranuclear or cytoplasmic inclusion bodies. Progressive neurologic disease is characterized by seizures, behavioral abnormalities, and gradual deterioration in intellectual, motor, and autonomic nervous system function. Management of the disease includes medical control of seizures. Although some authors have advocated the use of antiviral and immunomodulatory therapies (e.g., interferon, ribavirin, and Isoprinosine) to slow the progression of the disease and improve life expectancy in patients, the results are conflicting—the condition continues to show relentless progression. The long-term outcome of antiviral treatments remains to be determined. Only 5% of individuals with SSPE undergo spontaneous remission; the remaining 95% invariably die within 5 years of diagnosis [484].

Progressive Multifocal Leukoencephalopathy

Progressive multifocal leukoencephalopathy (PML) is an intractable, severe, usually fatal demyelinating disease that is caused by the JC virus, a small double-stranded, nonenveloped DNA virus, closely related to two other polyomavirus: BK virus and the simian virus SV 40 of monkeys. PML is primarily seen in highly immunosuppressed patients, especially those with AIDS and reticuloendothelial malignancies and in patients on immunosuppressive therapy [485]. In the latter case, the immunomodulatory agent most often implicated in the development of PML is the monoclonal antibody natalizumab [486]. It is believed that under conditions of immunosuppression, replication of JC virus in the CNS increases.

Polyomaviruses are not thought to cause disease in immunocompetent individuals. In the pre-AIDS era, it was recognized that the main risk factor for PML was reduced resistance in persons of any age. The typical clinical features in these patients were impaired vision, motor weakness, and change in mentation, including personality changes [487]. It is estimated that the seroprevalence of the JC virus is 50% in the 20–29 years age group; this rises to about 68% in older persons [488]. Even normal brain tissue from immunocompetent individuals with no evidence of PML or demyelinating lesions has been found to harbor JC virus DNA sequences by PCR methodology, suggesting that the JC virus remains latent in the brain before immunosuppression [489–493]. The JC virus has also been detected in the blood of up to 22% of immunosuppressed patients in the absence of PML [492, 494].

During 1979–1987, deaths related to PML increased fourfold from 1.5/10,000,000 persons in 1979 to 6.1/10,000,000 persons in 1987; this increase was largely attributed to the parallel increase in the incidence of HIV infection in the United States during this period [495]. PML-associated death rates peaked in the mid-1990s and have been decreasing since. For example, death rates decreased from 2.7 deaths per one million persons during 1992–1995 to 0.6 per one million during 2002–2005 [496]. This significant decrease has been attributed to ART which became the standard of care in the United States in 1996 [496]

CNS symptoms associated with PML reflect the anatomic location of pathologic brain lesions. PML characteristically presents with progressive focal neurologic defects, primarily hemiparesis, visual field defects, and cognitive deterioration [491, 496–501]. As the disease progresses, aphasia, ataxia, and cranial nerve defects may occur, ultimately resulting in cortical blindness, quadriparesis, profound dementia, seizures, and coma. The average duration of survival is approximately 4 months, although a subset of 5–10% of patients, including some persons with HIV infection, survive for over a year following diagnosis.

The diagnosis is made from a combination of clinical features with characteristic findings on CT or MRI (Fig. 31.30a, b). The combination of a characteristic clinical picture and typical imaging findings supports a confident presumptive diagnosis of PML [309]. Definitive diagnosis requires brain biopsy and histologic examination, which should demonstrate characteristic cytopathic changes in the oligodendrocytes (Fig. 31.31a, b). These cells typically contain a homogeneous basophilic nuclear inclusion, and virus can be demonstrated by in situ hybridization. Viral damage to the oligodendrocytes, which synthesize and maintain myelin, ultimately leads to widespread, but patchy, multifocal demyelination, surrounded by giant, bizarre astrocytes containing intranuclear inclusions. The pathologic changes generally correlate with the patient's clinical status. Virus particles can be demonstrated in the inclusions by electron microscopy [502].

The CSF is invariably normal in the majority of patients with PML, although slight increases in protein levels and leukocyte counts have been documented for some. JC virus can be detected in the CSF of most patients with PML, whether immunosuppressed or not [490, 503, 504]. In general, however, patients with PML are highly likely to have JC virus DNA in their CSF as compared with normal or immunosuppressed patients without PML. Despite the sensitivity of PCR testing for JC virus, occasional cases of PML have been observed in which no JC virus can be found even in brain tissue at autopsy [505].

Immune reconstitution represents the mainstay of treatment for PML. Thus, for HIV-infected persons with PML, the basis of therapy remains the initiation of antiretroviral therapy for persons who are not on therapy and optimizing the antiretroviral regimen to achieve virologic suppression in patients who are already receiving antiretroviral therapy [309]. With the rapid reversal of immunosuppression followed by immunologic recovery, patients may suffer a paradoxical clinical deterioration termed immune reconstitution inflammatory syndrome (IRIS) [486]. High-dose corticosteroids are often recommended if a clinical and imaging syndrome resembling IRIS develops after immune restoration. The JC virus DNA detection in CSF by nucleic acid amplification techniques and the CD4+ cell count are the most promising prognostic markers; higher levels of CD4+ cell counts are associated with improved survival [499].

A lipid-ester derivative, cidofovir, an agent used in the treatment of CMV infection, does have activity against polyomaviruses in vitro and animal models. However, several large studies, including analytic epidemiologic studies and meta-analyses that included patients from five large studies demonstrated no benefit. Thus, treatment with cidofovir is also not recommended. Initial reports of success with cytosine arabinoside (ara-C) have not been supported by formal clinical trials. Therefore, treatment with cytarabine, too, is not recommended. In summary, there is no effective antiviral therapy for preventing or treating JCV infections or PML. The main basic tenet of management is to preserve immune function and reverse HIV-associated immunosuppression with effective ART. HIV-associated PML is often complicated by clinically significant IRIS that may require administration of corticosteroid therapy. In ART-naive patients who are diagnosed with PML, ART should be started immediately. In patients who are receiving ART but remain viremic because of inadequate adherence or drug resistance, ART should be optimized to achieve HIV suppression [506].

Coronavirus Infection

Human coronaviruses are positive-sense, single-stranded ribonucleic acid (RNA) viruses with a linear, non-segmented viral genome. These viruses are members of the *Coronaviridae* family within the order *Nidovirales*. Amongst all RNA viruses, coronaviruses have the largest genome (~27–32 kb). Coronaviruses cause mainly respiratory and enteric diseases in mammals and birds with varying degrees of severity. Since the first coronavirus was isolated in 1937, and of the 300 strains subsequently identified, only seven cause infections in humans. The first human coronavirus, named HCoV-229E, was isolated during a study of respiratory illness among medical students during the early 1960s. In 1965, two new strains, B814 and HCoV-OC43, were isolated from patients with the common cold [507]. HCoV-229E and HCoVOC43 were the only human coronaviruses followed up during 1965 up through the 1990s largely because they were the only strains that could easily be cultured [507]. Before 2002, only HCoV 229E and HCoV OC43 were known to be circulating in human populations; because they were associated with the common cold and generally associated with mild illness, they were considered relatively harmless.

In November 2002, CDC and WHO reported an investigation of a multicountry outbreak of unexplained severe acute respiratory illness. The illness was named severe acute respiratory syndrome (SARS) and a new coronavirus was identified and named SARS-CoV [508]. This was, officially, the first pandemic of the twenty-first century and first identified in the Guangdong province in South China. A decade later in 2012, another unique human coronavirus that causes a severe respiratory illness, similar to SARS, and renal failure was identified in Saudi Arabia and named Middle East Respiratory

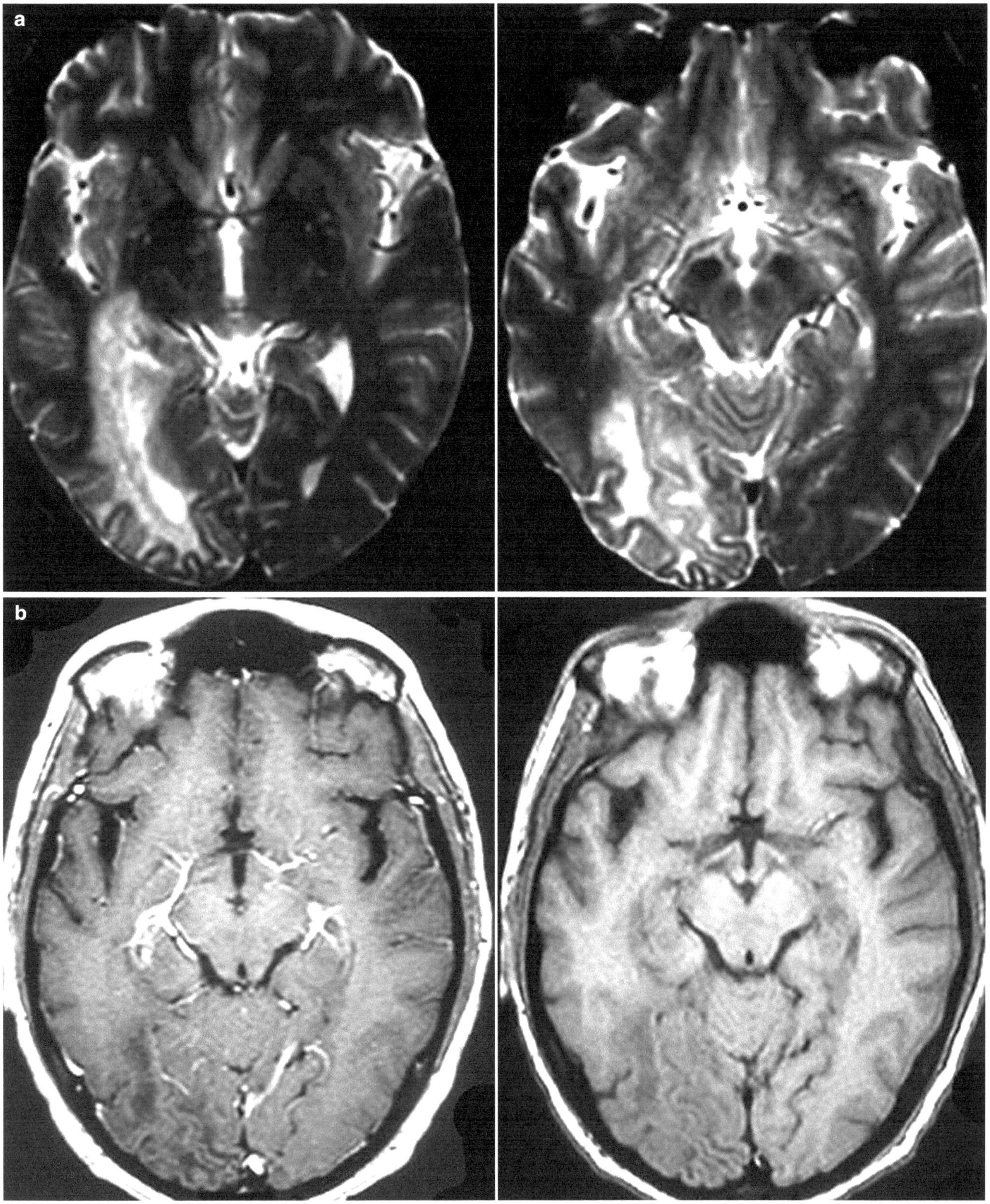

Fig. 31.30 (**a**, **b**) Progressive multifocal leukoencephalopathy (JC virus). Figure (**a**) includes two adjacent T2-w sections. Figure (**b**) includes a post-contrast (*left*) and pre contrast (*right*) images of the same area. These images demonstrate the features of PML with a focal area of abnormality affecting mainly white matter with no appreciable internal contrast enhancement. These findings are nonspecific but in the context of an immune-compromised host, PML is an important consideration. PML can cross the midline through the corpus callosum in which case it simulates both lymphoma and diffusely infiltrating astrocytoma

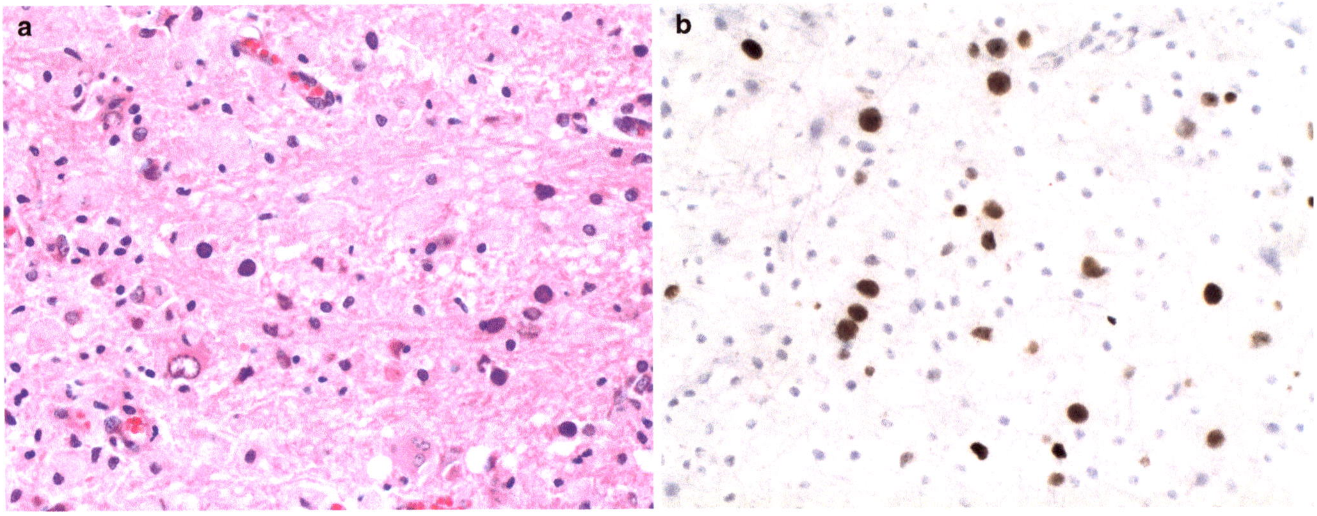

Fig. 31.31 (**a**) Progressive multifocal leukoencephalopathy (JC virus). Numerous foamy macrophages infiltrating CNS white matter and bizarre reactive astrocytes. Scattered oligodendroglia exhibit smudged glassy nuclei (H&E 40×). (**b**) Progressive multifocal leukoencephalopathy (JC virus) Immunohistochemical study for JC virus antibody is immunoreactive in infected glial cells (Both courtesy of Anthony Yachnis, MD, and Kelly Devers, MD, University of Florida College of Medicine)

Syndrome (MERS)-CoV [509]. In December 2019, seven years after the identification of MERS-CoV, a novel human coronavirus that resembles SARS-CoV was isolated from patients suffering from acute pneumonia in the Hubei Province, China. This coronavirus, named SARS-CoV-2, is the seventh coronavirus known to cause infection in humans and causes a syndromic disease (COVID-19), which was declared a pandemic by WHO in 2020 [510].

There is a massive body of literature that describes the various clinical features and presentation of patients with the three pandemic strains of coronavirus. Although primarily an infection of the respiratory system, neurological complications in both the central and peripheral nervous systems are now well-recognized for all three pandemic strains. Neurological sequelae in patients who acquired infection during the first coronavirus pandemic in 2002 and the subsequent MERS outbreak in 2012 are well documented; what emerges from a review the medical literature is that patients with CNS complications generally tend to have severe disease [511, 512].

Neurological complications associated with infection caused by any of the human pandemic coronaviruses (SARS-CoV, MERS-CoV, and SARS-CoV-2) include the following: encephalopathy, encephalitis, and meningitis, acute disseminated encephalomyelitis, seizures, stroke, and neuromuscular disorders (e.g., Guillain-Barre syndrome and polyneuropathy) [511, 512]. During the acute phase of COVID-19 infection, about 36% of cases develop neurological symptoms of which 25% can be attributed to the direct involvement of the central nervous system [513]. Neurological complications of COVID-19 include seizures, cerebrovascular accidents, encephalopathy, cerebral edema, meningitis, cerebral ischemic, loss of smell, myalgia, and Guillain-Barre Syndrome. In a large case series from China, central nervous system symptoms were the main form of neurologic injury in patients with COVID-19. The pathologic mechanism is likely due to direct CNS invasion by SARS-CoV-2, similar to SARS-CoV-1 and the MERS coronavirus. As with other respiratory viruses, SARS-COV-2 can enter the CNS through the hematogenous or retrograde neuronal route; smell impairment is the likely explained by invasion via the latter route.

The neurological complications of COVID-19 are thought to occur through at least four possible pathogenic mechanisms: (a) direct viral encephalitis; (b) systemic inflammation; (c) peripheral organ dysfunction (liver, kidney, lung), and (d) cerebrovascular changes. In most cases, however, it is believed that neurological manifestations of COVID-19 may arise from various combinations of any of the above. Any single factor, or a combination of these mechanisms, puts COVID-19 survivors at risk for developing long-term neurological sequelae by causing a new acute CNS complication or by aggravating a pre-existing neurological disorder [514]. For example, together with endothelial dysfunction, disseminated intravascular coagulation can lead to cerebrovascular ischemia and can exacerbate existing atherosclerotic vascular disease leading to severe ischemic stroke [514]. Patients with severe COVID-19 experience high levels of proinflammatory cytokines and acute respiratory dysfunction and often require assisted ventilation. All these factors likely contribute to cognitive decline. And, while most acute neurological symptoms are ascertained during the acute phase of COVID-19, the epidemiology and clinical characteristics of long-term sequelae in persons with COVID-19 have yet to be fully characterized.

Lymphocyte counts tend to be lower for patients with CNS symptoms than without CNS symptoms [513]. In addition, patients with severe infection tend to have higher D-dimer levels than those with non-severe infection [513]. This may be the reason why patients with severe infections are more likely to develop cerebrovascular disease. This phenomenon may be indicative of immunosuppression in patients with COVID-19 with CNS symptoms [513].

SARS-CoV, MERS-CoV, and SARS-CoV-2 all have neuroinvasive properties. However, it appears that persons with infection caused by SARS-CoV-2 (COVID-19) acquire more neurological complications than those with infection caused by SARS-CoV or MERS-CoV. Moreover, patients with severe COVID-19 infection were more likely to develop cerebrovascular disease, disturbances of consciousness, and skeletal muscle injury [513]. Most neurologic manifestations occur early in the illness and some patients without typical symptoms (fever, cough, anorexia, and diarrhea) may present with only neurologic manifestations as their presenting symptoms [513]. Therefore, for patients with COVID-19, clinicians need to pay close attention to neurologic manifestations, especially for those with severe infections. As pointed out by Mao and colleagues, during the epidemic period of COVID-19, when seeing patients with neurologic manifestations, SARS-CoV-2 infection needs to be included in the differential to avoid delayed diagnosis or misdiagnosis and prevention of transmission [513]. SARS-CoV-2 mainly causes pulmonary disorders; however, current evidence underscores possible neuroinvasion by SARS-CoV-2, as evidenced by isolating SARS-CoV-2 from CSF, SARS-CoV2 discovery in the olfactory system, and various neurologic symptoms in patients with COVID-19 [512]. For patients with central nervous system involvement, the basic tenet of management remains aggressive medical management of COVID-19 pulmonary infection per protocol, supportive care in the critical care setting with mechanical ventilation if deemed necessary, and scrupulous adherence to infection control guidelines. Alternative modes of therapies, such as intranasal drug delivery, in addition to intravenous delivery, as a therapeutic strategy for direct delivery of drugs to the CSF and brain have been discussed but not yet recommended for central nervous system involvement [515]. Masking and immunization, with boosters, remain the mainstays of mitigation.

References

1. Schuchat A, Robinson K, Wenger JD, et al. Bacterial meningitis in the United States in 1995. Active Surveillance Team. N Engl J Med. 1997;337:970–6.
2. Kim KS. Acute bacterial meningitis in infants and children. Lancet Infect Dis. 2010;10:32–42.
3. Mbaeyi SA, Bozio CH, Duffy J, Rubin LG, Hariri S, Stephens DS, et al. Meningococcal vaccination: recommendations of the advisory committee on immunization practices, United States, 2020. MMWR Recomm Rep. 2020;69(9):1–41.
4. Global Burden of Disease Study 2013 Collaborators. Global, regional, and national incidence, prevalence, and years lived with disability for 301 acute and chronic diseases and injuries in 188 countries, 1990–2013: a systematic analysis for the Global Burden of Disease Study 2013. Lancet. 2015;386:743–800.
5. Hsu HE, Shutt KA, Moore MR, et al. Effect of pneumococcal conjugate vaccine on pneumococcal meningitis. N Engl J Med. 2009;360:244–56.
6. Thigpen MC, Whitney CG, Messonnier NE, et al. Bacterial meningitis in the United States, 1998–2007. N Engl J Med. 2011;364:2016–25.
7. Sadarangani M. Protection against invasive infections in children caused by encapsulated bacteria. Front Immunol. 2018;9:2674.
8. Unhanand M, Mustafa MM, McCracken GH Jr, Nelson JD. Gram-negative enteric bacillary meningitis: a twenty-one-year experience. J Pediatr. 1993;122:15–21.
9. Sarff LD, Platt LH, McCracken GH Jr. Cerebrospinal fluid evaluation in neonates: comparison of high-risk infants with and without meningitis. J Pediatr. 1976;88:473–7.
10. Sarff LD, McCracken GH, Schiffer MS, et al. Epidemiology of Escherichia coli K1 in healthy and diseased newborns. Lancet. 1975;1:1099–104.
11. Schiffer MS, Oliveira E, Glode MP, McCracken GH Jr, Sarff LM, Robbins JB. A review: relation between invasiveness and the K1 capsular polysaccharide of Escherichia coli. Pediatr Res. 1976;10:82–7.
12. Nigrovic LE, Kuppermann N, Malley R. Children with bacterial meningitis presenting to the emergency department during the pneumococcal conjugate vaccine era. Acad Emerg Med. 2008;15:522–8.
13. Nigrovic LE, Kuppermann N, Macias CG, et al. Clinical prediction rule for identifying children with cerebrospinal fluid pleocytosis at very low risk of bacterial meningitis. JAMA. 2007;297:52–60.
14. May M, Daley AJ, Donath S, Isaacs D. Early onset neonatal meningitis in Australia and New Zealand, 1992–2002. Arch Dis Child Fetal Neonatal Ed. 2005;90:F324–7.
15. Weisfelt M, van de Beek D, Spanjaard L, de Gans J. Nosocomial bacterial meningitis in adults: a prospective series of 50 cases. J Hosp Infect. 2007;66:71–8.
16. Helbok R, Broessner G, Pfausler B, Schmutzhard E. Chronic meningitis. J Neurol. 2009;256:168–75.
17. Kallstrom H, Blackmer Gill D, Albiger B, Liszewski MK, Atkinson JP, Jonsson AB. Attachment of Neisseria gonorrhoeae to the cellular pilus receptor CD46: identification of domains important for bacterial adherence. Cell Microbiol. 2001;3:133–43.
18. Kallstrom H, Liszewski MK, Atkinson JP, Jonsson AB. Membrane cofactor protein (MCP or CD46) is a cellular pilus receptor for pathogenic Neisseria. Mol Microbiol. 1997;25:639–47.
19. Toleman M, Aho E, Virji M. Expression of pathogen-like Opa adhesins in commensal Neisseria: genetic and functional analysis. Cell Microbiol. 2001;3:33–44.

20. Mulks MH, Plaut AG. IgA protease production as a characteristic distinguishing pathogenic from harmless neisseriaceae. N Engl J Med. 1978;299:973–6.
21. Hill DJ, Griffiths NJ, Borodina E, Virji M. Cellular and molecular biology of Neisseria meningitidis colonization and invasive disease. Clin Sci (Lond). 2010;118:547–64.
22. Rouphael NG, Stephens DS. Neisseria meningitidis: biology, microbiology, and epidemiology. Methods Mol Biol. 2012;799:1–20.
23. Wurzner R, Orren A, Lachmann PJ. Inherited deficiencies of the terminal components of human complement. Immunodefic Rev. 1992;3:123–47.
24. Song JH, Dagan R, Klugman KP, Fritzell B. The relationship between pneumococcal serotypes and antibiotic resistance. Vaccine. 2012;30(17):2728–37.
25. Hausdorff WP, Feikin DR, Klugman KP. Epidemiological differences among pneumococcal serotypes. Lancet Infect Dis. 2005;5:83–93.
26. Pfister HW, Fontana A, Tauber MG, Tomasz A, Scheld WM. Mechanisms of brain injury in bacterial meningitis: workshop summary. Clin Infect Dis. 1994;19:463–79.
27. Pichichero M, Anderson P, Loeb M, Smith D. Do pili play a role in pathogenicity of Haemophilus influenzae type B? Lancet. 1982;2:960–2.
28. Mason EO Jr, Kaplan SL, Wiedermann BL, Norrod EP, Stenback WA. Frequency and properties of naturally occurring adherent piliated strains of Haemophilus influenzae type b. Infect Immun. 1985;49:98–103.
29. Filippidis A, Fountas KN. Nasal lymphatics as a novel invasion and dissemination route of bacterial meningitis. Med Hypotheses. 2009;72:694–7.
30. Mook-Kanamori BB, Geldhoff M, van der Poll T, van de Beek D. Pathogenesis and pathophysiology of pneumococcal meningitis. Clin Microbiol Rev. 2011;24:557–91.
31. Join-Lambert O, Morand PC, Carbonnelle E, et al. Mechanisms of meningeal invasion by a bacterial extracellular pathogen, the example of Neisseria meningitidis. Prog Neurobiol. 2010;91:130–9.
32. Flierl MA, Rittirsch D, Huber-Lang MS, Stahel PF. Pathophysiology of septic encephalopathy—an nsolved puzzle. Crit Care. 2010;14:165.
33. Tunkel AR, Scheld WM. Pathogenesis and pathophysiology of bacterial meningitis. Clin Microbiol Rev. 1993;6:118–36.
34. Durand ML, Calderwood SB, Weber DJ, et al. Acute bacterial meningitis in adults. A review of 493 episodes. N Engl J Med. 1993;328:21–8.
35. Gorse GJ, Thrupp LD, Nudleman KL, Wyle FA, Hawkins B, Cesario TC. Bacterial meningitis in the elderly. Arch Intern Med. 1984;144:1603–7.
36. Verghese A, Gallemore G. Kernig's and Brudzinski's signs revisited. Rev Infect Dis. 1987;9:1187–92.
37. Ward MA, Greenwood TM, Kumar DR, Mazza JJ, Yale SH. Josef Brudzinski and Vladimir Mikhailovich Kernig: signs for diagnosing meningitis. Clin Med Res. 2010;8:13–7.
38. Joffe AR. Lumbar puncture and brain herniation in acute bacterial meningitis: a review. J Intensive Care Med. 2007;22:194–207.
39. Joffe AR. Prognostic factors in adults with bacterial meningitis. N Engl J Med. 2005;352:512–5. author reply 5
40. Oliver WJ, Shope TC, Kuhns LR. Fatal lumbar puncture: fact versus fiction—an approach to a clinical dilemma. Pediatrics. 2003;112:e174–6.
41. Tattevin P, Bruneel F, Regnier B. Cranial CT before lumbar puncture in suspected meningitis. N Engl J Med. 2002;346:1248–51. author reply 51
42. van Crevel H, Hijdra A, de Gans J. Lumbar puncture and the risk of herniation: when should we first perform CT? J Neurol. 2002;249:129–37.
43. Fishman RA. Cerebrospinal fluid in diseases of the nervous system. Philadelphia: WB Saunders Co; 1992.
44. Skipper BJ, Davis LE. Ascertaining hypoglycorrhachia in an acute patient. Am J Emerg Med. 1997;15:378–80.
45. Rand KH, Ulm AJ, Pincus DW. Central nervous system infections. In: Layon AJ, Gabrielli A, Friedman WA, editors. Textbook of neurointensive care. Philadelphia: WB Saunders; 2004.
46. Negrini B, Kelleher KJ, Wald ER. Cerebrospinal fluid findings in aseptic versus bacterial meningitis. Pediatrics. 2000;105:316–9.
47. Feigin RD, Shackelford PG. Value of repeat lumbar puncture in the differential diagnosis of meningitis. N Engl J Med. 1973;289:571–4.
48. Herndon RM, Brumback RA. The cerebrospinal spinal fluid. Boston: Kluwer Academic Publishers; 1989.
49. Neuman MI, Tolford S, Harper MB. Test characteristics and interpretation of cerebrospinal fluid gram stain in children. Pediatr Infect Dis J. 2008;27:309–13.
50. Hayden RT, Frenkel LD. More laboratory testing: greater cost but not necessarily better. Pediatr Infect Dis J. 2000;19:290–2.
51. Mein J, Lum G. CSF bacterial antigen detection tests offer no advantage over Gram's stain in the diagnosis of bacterial meningitis. Pathology. 1999;31:67–9.
52. Gray BM, Simmons DR, Mason H, Barnum S, Volanakis JE. Quantitative levels of C-reactive protein in cerebrospinal fluid in patients with bacterial meningitis and other conditions. J Pediatr. 1986;108:665–70.
53. Skull SA, Leach AJ, Currie BJ. Streptococcus pneumoniae carriage and penicillin/ceftriaxone resistance in hospitalised children in Darwin. Aust NZ J Med. 1996;26:391–5.
54. Jones ME, Draghi DC, Karlowsky JA, Sahm DF, Bradley JS. Prevalence of antimicrobial resistance in bacteria isolated from central nervous system specimens as reported by U.S. hospital laboratories from 2000 to 2002. Ann Clin Microbiol Antimicrob. 2004;3:3.
55. Gouveia EL, Reis JN, Flannery B, et al. Clinical outcome of pneumococcal meningitis during the emergence of penicillin-resistant Streptococcus pneumoniae: an observational study. BMC Infect Dis. 2011;11:323.
56. Lee HY, Wu TL, Su LH, Li HC, Janapatla RP, Chen CL, Chiu CH. Invasive pneumococcal disease caused by ceftriaxone-resistant Streptococcus pneumoniae in Taiwan. J Microbiol Immunol Infect. 2018;51(4):500–9. https://doi.org/10.1016/j.jmii.2016.12.004. Epub 2017 Jun 26. PMID: 28690025
57. Ohga S, Okada K, Ueda K, et al. Cerebrospinal fluid cytokine levels and dexamethasone therapy in bacterial meningitis. J Infect. 1999;39:55–60.
58. Ahmed A, Jafri H, Lutsar I, et al. Pharmacodynamics of vancomycin for the treatment of experimental penicillin- and cephalosporin-resistant pneumococcal meningitis. Antimicrob Agents Chemother. 1999;43:876–81.
59. Lutsar I, Friedland IR, Jafri HS, et al. Factors influencing the anti-inflammatory effect of dexamethasone therapy in experimental pneumococcal meningitis. J Antimicrob Chemother. 2003;52:651–5.
60. McIntyre PB, Berkey CS, King SM, et al. Dexamethasone as adjunctive therapy in bacterial meningitis. A meta-analysis of randomized clinical trials since 1988. JAMA. 1997;278:925–31.
61. Brouwer MC, McIntyre P, Prasad K, van de Beek D. Corticosteroids for acute bacterial meningitis. Cochrane Database Syst Rev. 2015;(9):Art. No.: CD004405. https://doi.org/10.1002/14651858.CD004405.pub5.
62. Griffiths MJ, McGill F, Solomon T. Management of acute meningitis. Clin Med (Lond). 2018;18(2):164–9.
63. Roos KL, Scheld WM. The management of fulminant meningitis in the intensive care unit. Infect Dis Clin N Am. 1989;3:137–54.

64. Roos KL, van de Beek D. Bacterial meningitis. In: Vinken PJ, Bruyn GW, editors. Handbook of clinical neurology, vol. 96. Elsevier; 2010. p. 51–63.
65. Gwer S, Gatakaa H, Mwai L, Idro R, Newton CR. The role for osmotic agents in children with acute encephalopathies: a systematic review. BMC Pediatr. 2010;10:23.
66. Hinson HE, Stein D, Sheth KN. Hypertonic saline and mannitol therapy in critical care neurology. J Intensive Care Med. 2013;28(1):3–11.
67. Liu S, Li L, Luo Z, et al. Superior effect of hypertonic saline over mannitol to attenuate cerebral edema in a rabbit bacterial meningitis model. Crit Care Med. 2011;39:1467–73.
68. Murthy JM. Management of intracranial pressure in tuberculous meningitis. Neurocrit Care. 2005;2:306–12.
69. Qureshi AI, Suarez JI. Use of hypertonic saline solutions in treatment of cerebral edema and intracranial hypertension. Crit Care Med. 2000;28:3301–13.
70. Singhi S, Singhi P, Baranwal AK. Bacterial meningitis in children: critical care needs. Indian J Pediatr. 2001;68:737–47.
71. Czosnyka M, Pickard JD. Monitoring and interpretation of intracranial pressure. J Neurol Neurosurg Psychiatry. 2004;75:813–21.
72. Kumar G, Kalita J, Misra UK. Raised intracranial pressure in acute viral encephalitis. Clin Neurol Neurosurg. 2009;111:399–406.
73. Sala F, Abbruzzese C, Galli D, et al. Intracranial pressure monitoring in pediatric bacterial meningitis: a fancy or useful tool? A case report. Minerva Anestesiol. 2009;75:746–9.
74. Whitney CG, Farley MM, Hadler J, et al. Decline in invasive pneumococcal disease after the introduction of protein-polysaccharide conjugate vaccine. N Engl J Med. 2003;348:1737–46.
75. Pilishvili T, Lexau C, Farley MM, et al. Sustained reductions in invasive pneumococcal disease in the era of conjugate vaccine. J Infect Dis. 2010;201:32–41.
76. Matanock A, Lee G, Gierke R, Kobayashi M, Leidner A, Pilishvili T. Use of 13-valent pneumococcal conjugate vaccine and 23-valent pneumococcal polysaccharide vaccine among adults aged ≥65 years: updated recommendations of the Advisory Committee on Immunization Practices. MMWR Morb Mortal Wkly Rep. 2019;68(46):1069–75.
77. Abedi GR, Watson JT, Nix WA, Oberste MS, Gerber SI. Enterovirus and parechovirus surveillance—United States, 2014–2016. MMWR Morb Mortal Wkly Rep. 2018;67(18):515–8.
78. CDC. Human rabies prevention—United States, 2008: recommendations of the Advisory Committee on Immunization Practices. MMWR Recomm Rep. 2008;57:1–28.
79. Ma X, Monroe BP, Wallace RM, Orciari LA, Gigante CM, Kirby JD, Chipman RB, Fehlner-Gardiner C, Cedillo VG, Petersen BW, Olson V, Bonwitt J. Rabies surveillance in the United States during 2019. J Am Vet Med Assoc. 2021;258(11):1205–20.
80. Sharpe AH, Fields BN. Pathogenesis of viral infections. Basic concepts derived from the reovirus model. N Engl J Med. 1985;312:486–97.
81. Iwasaka T, Kidera Y, Tsugitomi H, Sugimori H. The cellular changes in primary and recurrent infection with herpes simplex virus type 2 in an in vitro model. Acta Cytol. 1987;31:935–40.
82. Esiri MM. Herpes simplex encephalitis. An immunohistological study of the distribution of viral antigen within the brain. J Neurol Sci. 1982;54:209–26.
83. Pleasure SJ, Fischbein NJ. Correlation of clinical and neuroimaging findings in a case of rabies encephalitis. Arch Neurol. 2000;57:1765–9.
84. Peters CJ. Arenaviruses. In: Richman DD, Whitley RJ, Hayden FG, editors. Clinical virology. Washington, DC: American Society of Microbiology Press; 2009. p. 1009–29.
85. Jolles S, Sewell WA, Leighton C. Drug-induced aseptic meningitis: diagnosis and management. Drug Saf. 2000;22:215–26.
86. Dupuis M, Hull R, Wang H, et al. Molecular detection of viral causes of encephalitis and meningitis in New York State. J Med Virol. 2011;83:2172–81.
87. Murphy RF, Caliendo AM. Relative quantity of cerebrospinal fluid herpes simplex virus DNA in adult cases of encephalitis and meningitis. Am J Clin Pathol. 2009;132:687–90.
88. Cinque P, Cleator GM, Weber T, Monteyne P, Sindic CJ, van Loon AM. The role of laboratory investigation in the diagnosis and management of patients with suspected herpes simplex encephalitis: a consensus report. The EU Concerted Action on Virus Meningitis and Encephalitis. J Neurol Neurosurg Psychiatry. 1996;61:339–45.
89. Espy MJ, Uhl JR, Mitchell PS, et al. Diagnosis of herpes simplex virus infections in the clinical laboratory by LightCycler PCR. J Clin Microbiol. 2000;38:795–9.
90. Whitley RJ, Alford CA, Hirsch MS, et al. Vidarabine versus acyclovir therapy in herpes simplex encephalitis. N Engl J Med. 1986;314:144–9.
91. Whitley RJ, Cobbs CG, Alford CA Jr, et al. Diseases that mimic herpes simplex encephalitis. Diagnosis, presentation, and outcome. NIAD Collaborative Antiviral Study Group. JAMA. 1989;262:234–9.
92. CDC. Investigation of rabies infections in organ donor and transplant recipients—Alabama, Arkansas, Oklahoma, and Texas, 2004. MMWR Morb Mortal Wkly Rep. 2004;53:586–9.
93. CDC. Human-to-human transmission of rabies via corneal transplant—Thailand. MMWR Morb Mortal Wkly Rep. 1981;30:473–4.
94. CDC. Human-to-human transmission of rabies by a corneal transplant-Idaho. MMWR. 1979;28:109–11.
95. Houff SA, Burton RC, Wilson RW, et al. Human-to-human transmission of rabies virus by corneal transplant. N Engl J Med. 1979;300:603–4.
96. Jackson AC. Rabies in the critical care unit: diagnostic and therapeutic approaches. Can J Neurol Sci. 2011;38:689–95.
97. Cohen JI, Davenport DS, Stewart JA, Deitchman S, Hilliard JK, Chapman LE. Recommendations for prevention of and therapy for exposure to B virus (cercopithecine herpesvirus 1). Clin Infect Dis. 2002;35:1191–203.
98. Canale DJ. William Macewen and the treatment of brain abscesses: revisited after one hundred years. J Neurosurg. 1996;84:133–42.
99. Nielsen H, Harmsen A, Gyldensted C. Cerebral abscess. A long-term follow-up. Acta Neurol Scand. 1983;67:330–7.
100. Nielsen H, Gyldensted C, Harmsen A. Cerebral abscess. Aetiology and pathogenesis, symptoms, diagnosis and treatment. A review of 200 cases from 1935–1976. Acta Neurol Scand. 1982;65:609–22.
101. Honda H, Warren DK. Central nervous system infections: meningitis and brain abscess. Infect Dis Clin N Am. 2009;23:609–23.
102. Harris PS, Cobbs CG. Cardiac, cerebral, and vascular complications of infective endocarditis. Cardiol Clin. 1996;14:437–50.
103. Muzumdar D, Jhawar S, Goel A. Brain abscess: an overview. Int J Surg. 2011;9:136–44.
104. Le Moal G, Landron C, Grollier G, et al. Characteristics of brain abscess with isolation of anaerobic bacteria. Scand J Infect Dis. 2003;35:318–21.
105. Cunha BA. Central nervous system infections in the compromised host: a diagnostic approach. Infect Dis Clin N Am. 2001;15:567–90.
106. Mathisen GE, Johnson JP. Brain abscess. Clin Infect Dis. 1997;25:763–79. quiz 80–1
107. Mamelak AN, Obana WG, Flaherty JF, Rosenblum ML. Nocardial brain abscess: treatment strategies and factors influencing outcome. Neurosurgery. 1994;35:622–31.
108. Bartzatt R. Tuberculosis infections of the central nervous system. Cent Nerv Syst Agents Med Chem. 2011;11:321–7.

109. Bathla G, Khandelwal G, Maller VG, Gupta A. Manifestations of cerebral tuberculosis. Singapore Med J. 2011;52:124–30. quiz 31
110. Jung A, Korsukewitz C, Kuhlmann T, et al. Intracerebral mass lesion diagnosed as cryptococcoma in a patient with sarcoidosis, a rare opportunistic manifestation induced by immunosuppression with corticosteroids. J Neurol. 2012;259(10):2147–50.
111. Nadkarni T, Goel A. Aspergilloma of the brain: an overview. J Postgrad Med. 2005;51(Suppl. 1):S37–41.
112. Metellus P, Laghmari M, Fuentes S, et al. Successful treatment of a giant isolated cerebral mucormycotic (zygomycotic) abscess using endoscopic debridement: case report and therapeutic considerations. Surg Neurol. 2008;69:510–5. discussion 5
113. Chun CH, Johnson JD, Hofstetter M, Raff MJ, Brain abscess. A study of 45 consecutive cases. Medicine. 1986;65:415–31.
114. Arseni C, Ciurea AV, Cerebellar abscesses. A report on 119 cases. Zentralbl Neurochir. 1982;43:359–70.
115. Turner RC, Dodson SC, Rosen CL. Medical management of cerebellar abscess: a case report and review of the literature. W V Med J. 2011;107:21–3.
116. Kastrup O, Wanke I, Maschke M. Neuroimaging of infections of the central nervous system. Semin Neurol. 2008;28:511–22.
117. Nathoo N, Nadvi SS, Narotam PK, van Dellen JR. Brain abscess: management and outcome analysis of a computed tomography era experience with 973 patients. World Neurosurg. 2011;75:716–26. discussion 612–7
118. Garg RK, Sinha MK. Multiple ring-enhancing lesions of the brain. J Postgrad Med. 2010;56:307–16.
119. Holtas S, Tornquist C, Cronqvist S. Diagnostic difficulties in computed tomography of brain abscesses. J Comput Assist Tomogr. 1982;6:683–8.
120. Nguyen JB, Black BR, Leimkuehler MM, Halder V, Nguyen JV, Ahktar N. Intracranial pyogenic abscess: imaging diagnosis utilizing recent advances in computed tomography and magnetic resonance imaging. Crit Rev Comput Tomogr. 2004;45:181–224.
121. Lai PH, Hsu SS, Ding SW, et al. Proton magnetic resonance spectroscopy and diffusion-weighted imaging in intracranial cystic mass lesions. Surg Neurol. 2007;68(Suppl. 1):S25–36.
122. Lai PH, Hsu SS, Lo YK, Ding SW. Role of diffusion-weighted imaging and proton MR spectroscopy in distinguishing between pyogenic brain abscess and necrotic brain tumor. Acta Neurol Taiwanica. 2004;13:107–13.
123. Desprechins B, Stadnik T, Koerts G, Shabana W, Breucq C, Osteaux M. Use of diffusion-weighted MR imaging in differential diagnosis between intracerebral necrotic tumors and cerebral abscesses. AJNR Am J Neuroradiol. 1999;20:1252–7.
124. Omuro AM, Leite CC, Mokhtari K, Delattre JY. Pitfalls in the diagnosis of brain tumours. Lancet Neurol. 2006;5:937–48.
125. Kang K, Lim I, Roh JK. Positron emission tomographic findings in a tuberculous brain abscess. Ann Nucl Med. 2007;21:303–6.
126. Kosterink JG. Positron emission tomography in the diagnosis and treatment management of tuberculosis. Curr Pharm Des. 2011;17:2875–80.
127. Kumar R, Basu S, Torigian D, Anand V, Zhuang H, Alavi A. Role of modern imaging techniques for diagnosis of infection in the era of 18F-fluorodeoxyglucose positron emission tomography. Clin Microbiol Rev. 2008;21:209–24.
128. Lu CH, Chang WN, Lui CC. Strategies for the management of bacterial brain abscess. J Clin Neurosci. 2006;13:979–85.
129. Mackenzie AR, Laing RB, Smith CC, Kaar GF, Smith FW. Spinal epidural abscess: the importance of early diagnosis and treatment. J Neurol Neurosurg Psychiatry. 1998;65:209–12.
130. Bluman EM, Palumbo MA, Lucas PR. Spinal epidural abscess in adults. J Am Acad Orthop Surg. 2004;12:155–63.
131. Tompkins M, Panuncialman I, Lucas P, Palumbo M. Spinal epidural abscess. J Emerg Med. 2010;39:384–90.
132. Sendi P, Bregenzer T, Zimmerli W. Spinal epidural abscess in clinical practice. QJM. 2008;101:1–12.
133. Martin RJ, Yuan HA. Neurosurgical care of spinal epidural, subdural, and intramedullary abscesses and arachnoiditis. Orthop Clin North Am. 1996;27:125–36.
134. Pradilla G, Ardila GP, Hsu W, Rigamonti D. Epidural abscesses of the CNS. Lancet Neurol. 2009;8:292–300.
135. Soehle M, Wallenfang T. Spinal epidural abscesses: clinical manifestations, prognostic factors, and outcomes. Neurosurgery. 2002;51:79–85. discussion 6–7
136. Curry WT Jr, Hoh BL, Amin-Hanjani S, Eskandar EN. Spinal epidural abscess: clinical presentation, management, and outcome. Surg Neurol. 2005;63:364–71. discussion 71
137. Hlavin ML, Kaminski HJ, Ross JS, Ganz E. Spinal epidural abscess: a ten-year perspective. Neurosurgery. 1990;27:177–84.
138. Nussbaum ES, Rigamonti D, Standiford H, Numaguchi Y, Wolf AL, Robinson WL. Spinal epidural abscess: a report of 40 cases and review. Surg Neurol. 1992;38:225–31.
139. Huang PY, Chen SF, Chang WN, et al. Spinal epidural abscess in adults caused by Staphylococcus aureus: clinical characteristics and prognostic factors. Clin Neurol Neurosurg. 2012;114(6):572–6.
140. Wheeler D, Keiser P, Rigamonti D, Keay S. Medical management of spinal epidural abscesses: case report and review. Clin Infect Dis. 1992;15:22–7.
141. Maslen DR, Jones SR, Crislip MA, Bracis R, Dworkin RJ, Flemming JE. Spinal epidural abscess. Optimizing patient care. Arch Intern Med. 1993;153:1713–21.
142. Khanna RK, Malik GM, Rock JP, Rosenblum ML. Spinal epidural abscess: evaluation of factors influencing outcome. Neurosurgery. 1996;39:958–64.
143. Tang HJ, Lin HJ, Liu YC, Li CM. Spinal epidural abscess—experience with 46 patients and evaluation of prognostic factors. J Infect. 2002;45:76–81.
144. Del Curling JO, Gower DJ, McWhorter JM. Changing concepts in spinal epidural abscess: a report of 29 cases. Neurosurgery. 1990;27:185–92.
145. Davis DP, Salazar A, Chan TC, Vilke GM. Prospective evaluation of a clinical decision guideline to diagnose spinal epidural abscess in patients who present to the emergency department with spine pain. J Neurosurg Spine. 2011;14:765–70.
146. Davis DP, Wold RM, Patel RJ, et al. The clinical presentation and impact of diagnostic delays on emergency department patients with spinal epidural abscess. J Emerg Med. 2004;26:285–91.
147. Reihsaus E, Waldbaur H, Seeling W. Spinal epidural abscess: a meta-analysis of 915 patients. Neurosurg Rev. 2000;23:175–204. discussion 5
148. Obrador GT, Levenson DJ. Spinal epidural abscess in hemodialysis patients: report of three cases and review of the literature. Am J Kidney Dis. 1996;27:75–83.
149. Khan IA, Vaccaro AR, Zlotolow DA. Management of vertebral diskitis and osteomyelitis. Orthopedics. 1999;22:758–65.
150. Strausbaugh LJ. Vertebral osteomyelitis. How to differentiate it from other causes of back and neck pain. Postgrad Med. 1995;97(147–8):51–4.
151. Grammatico L, Baron S, Rusch E, et al. Epidemiology of vertebral osteomyelitis (VO) in France: analysis of hospital-discharge data 2002–2003. Epidemiol Infect. 2008;136:653–60.
152. Zimmerli W. Clinical practice. Vertebral osteomyelitis. N Engl J Med. 2010;362:1022–9.
153. Digby JM, Kersley JB. Pyogenic non-tuberculous spinal infection: an analysis of thirty cases. J Bone Joint Surg Br. 1979;61:47–55.
154. Rezai AR, Woo HH, Errico TJ, Cooper PR. Contemporary management of spinal osteomyelitis. Neurosurgery. 1999;44:1018–25. discussion 25–6

155. Nussbaum ES, Rockswold GL, Bergman TA, Erickson DL, Seljeskog EL. Spinal tuberculosis: a diagnostic and management challenge. J Neurosurg. 1995;83:243–7.
156. Priest DH, Peacock JE Jr. Hematogenous vertebral osteomyelitis due to Staphylococcus aureus in the adult: clinical features and therapeutic outcomes. South Med J. 2005;98:854–62.
157. Sapico FL. Microbiology and antimicrobial therapy of spinal infections. Orthop Clin North Am. 1996;27:9–13.
158. Broner FA, Garland DE, Zigler JE. Spinal infections in the immunocompromised host. Orthop Clin North Am. 1996;27:37–46.
159. Ozuna RM, Delamarter RB. Pyogenic vertebral osteomyelitis and postsurgical disc space infections. Orthop Clin North Am. 1996;27:87–94.
160. Cahill DW, Love LC, Rechtine GR. Pyogenic osteomyelitis of the spine in the elderly. J Neurosurg. 1991;74:878–86.
161. Acosta FL Jr, Chin CT, Quinones-Hinojosa A, Ames CP, Weinstein PR, Chou D. Diagnosis and management of adult pyogenic osteomyelitis of the cervical spine. Neurosurg Focus. 2004;17:E2.
162. Bhavan KP, Marschall J, Olsen MA, Fraser VJ, Wright NM, Warren DK. The epidemiology of hematogenous vertebral osteomyelitis: a cohort study in a tertiary care hospital. BMC Infect Dis. 2010;10:158.
163. Sarria JC, Chutkan NB, Figueroa JE, Hull A. Atypical mycobacterial vertebral osteomyelitis: case report and review. Clin Infect Dis. 1998;26:503–5.
164. Klein JD, Garfin SR. Nutritional status in the patient with spinal infection. Orthop Clin North Am. 1996;27:33–6.
165. Endress C, Guyot DR, Fata J, Salciccioli G. Cervical osteomyelitis due to i.v. heroin use: radiologic findings in 14 patients. AJR Am J Roentgenol. 1990;155:333–5.
166. Lafont A, Olive A, Gelman M, Roca-Burniols J, Cots R, Carbonell J. Candida albicans spondylodiscitis and vertebral osteomyelitis in patients with intravenous heroin drug addiction. Report of 3 new cases. J Rheumatol. 1994;21:953–6.
167. Rahman I, Bhatt H, Chillag S, Duffus W. Mycobacterium chelonae vertebral osteomyelitis. South Med J. 2009;102:1167–9.
168. Colmenero JD, Jimenez-Mejias ME, Sanchez-Lora FJ, et al. Pyogenic, tuberculous, and brucellar vertebral osteomyelitis: a descriptive and comparative study of 219 cases. Ann Rheum Dis. 1997;56:709–15.
169. Livorsi DJ, Daver NG, Atmar RL, Shelburne SA, White AC Jr, Musher DM. Outcomes of treatment for hematogenous Staphylococcus aureus vertebral osteomyelitis in the MRSA ERA. J Infect. 2008;57:128–31.
170. Lora-Tamayo J, Euba G, Narvaez JA, et al. Changing trends in the epidemiology of pyogenic vertebral osteomyelitis: the impact of cases with no microbiologic diagnosis. Semin Arthritis Rheum. 2011;41:247–55.
171. Mylona E, Samarkos M, Kakalou E, Fanourgiakis P, Skoutelis A. Pyogenic vertebral osteomyelitis: a systematic review of clinical characteristics. Semin Arthritis Rheum. 2009;39:10–7.
172. Nolla JM, Ariza J, Gomez-Vaquero C, et al. Spontaneous pyogenic vertebral osteomyelitis in nondrug users. Semin Arthritis Rheum. 2002;31:271–8.
173. Osenbach RK, Hitchon PW, Menezes AH. Diagnosis and management of pyogenic vertebral osteomyelitis in adults. Surg Neurol. 1990;33:266–75.
174. Patzakis MJ, Rao S, Wilkins J, Moore TM, Harvey PJ. Analysis of 61 cases of vertebral osteomyelitis. Clin Orthop Relat Res. 1991;264:178–83.
175. Mete B, Kurt C, Yilmaz MH, et al. Vertebral osteomyelitis: eight years' experience of 100 cases. Rheumatol Int. 2012;32(11):3591–7.
176. Barnes B, Alexander JT, Branch CL Jr. Cervical osteomyelitis: a brief review. Neurosurg Focus. 2004;17:E11.
177. Beluffi G, Bernardo ME, Meloni G, Spinazzola A, Locatelli F. Spinal osteomyelitis due to Aspergillus flavus in a child: a rare complication after haematopoietic stem cell transplantation. Pediatr Radiol. 2008;38:709–12.
178. Chang HM, Yu HH, Yang YH, et al. Successful treatment of Aspergillus flavus spondylodiscitis with epidural abscess in a patient with chronic granulomatous disease. Pediatr Infect Dis J. 2012;31:100–1.
179. Ranjan R, Mishra S, Ranjan S. Aspergillus vertebral osteomyelitis in an immunocompetent person. Neurol India. 2010;58:806–8.
180. Sethi S, Siraj F, Kalra K, Chopra P. Aspergillus vertebral osteomyelitis in immunocompetent patients. Ind J Orthop. 2012;46:246–50.
181. Studemeister A, Stevens DA. Aspergillus vertebral osteomyelitis in immunocompetent hosts: role of triazole antifungal therapy. Clin Infect Dis. 2011;52:e1–6.
182. Tew CW, Han FC, Jureen R, Tey BH. Aspergillus vertebral osteomyelitis and epidural abscess. Singapore Med J. 2009;50:e151–4.
183. Zhu LP, Chen XS, Wu JQ, Yang FF, Weng XH. Aspergillus vertebral osteomyelitis and ureteral obstruction after liver transplantation. Transpl Infect Dis. 2011;13:192–9.
184. An HS, Seldomridge JA. Spinal infections: diagnostic tests and imaging studies. Clin Orthop Relat Res. 2006;444:27–33.
185. Rath SA, Neff U, Schneider O, Richter HP. Neurosurgical management of thoracic and lumbar vertebral osteomyelitis and discitis in adults: a review of 43 consecutive surgically treated patients. Neurosurgery. 1996;38:926–33.
186. Turpin S, Lambert R. Role of scintigraphy in musculoskeletal and spinal infections. Radiol Clin North Am. 2001;39:169–89.
187. Palestro CJ, Love C, Miller TT. Diagnostic imaging tests and microbial infections. Cell Microbiol. 2007;9:2323–33.
188. Palestro CJ, Love C, Miller TT. Infection and musculoskeletal conditions: imaging of musculoskeletal infections. Best Pract Res Clin Rheumatol. 2006;20:1197–218.
189. Vaccaro AR, Shah SH, Schweitzer ME, Rosenfeld JF, Cotler JM. MRI description of vertebral osteomyelitis, neoplasm, and compression fracture. Orthopedics. 1999;22:67–73. quiz 4–5
190. Roblot F, Besnier JM, Juhel L, et al. Optimal duration of antibiotic therapy in vertebral osteomyelitis. Semin Arthritis Rheum. 2007;36:269–77.
191. Hadjipavlou AG, Mader JT, Necessary JT, Muffoletto AJ. Hematogenous pyogenic spinal infections and their surgical management. Spine. 2000;25:1668–79.
192. Perronne C, Saba J, Behloul Z, et al. Pyogenic and tuberculous spondylodiskitis (vertebral osteomyelitis) in 80 adult patients. Clin Infect Dis. 1994;19:746–50.
193. Dey M, Jaffe J, Stadnik A, Awad IA. External ventricular drainage for intraventricular hemorrhage. Curr Neurol Neurosci Rep. 2012;12:24–33.
194. Li LM, Timofeev I, Czosnyka M, Hutchinson PJ. Review article: the surgical approach to the management of increased intracranial pressure after traumatic brain injury. Anesth Analg. 2010;111:736–48.
195. Gigante P, Hwang BY, Appelboom G, Kellner CP, Kellner MA, Connolly ES. External ventricular drainage following aneurysmal subarachnoid haemorrhage. Br J Neurosurg. 2010;24:625–32.
196. The Brain Trauma Foundation. The American Association of Neurological Surgeons. The Joint Section on Neurotrauma and Critical Care. Recommendations for intracranial pressure monitoring technology. J Neurotrauma. 2000;17:497–506.
197. Gutierrez-Gonzalez R, Boto GR, Perez-Zamarron A. Cerebrospinal fluid diversion devices and infection. A comprehensive review. Eur J Clin Microbiol Infect Dis. 2012;31(6):889–97.
198. Ngo QN, Ranger A, Singh RN, Kornecki A, Seabrook JA, Fraser DD. External ventricular drains in pediatric patients. Pediatr Crit Care Med. 2009;10:346–51.

199. Speck V, Staykov D, Huttner HB, Sauer R, Schwab S, Bardutzky J. Lumbar catheter for monitoring of intracranial pressure in patients with post-hemorrhagic communicating hydrocephalus. Neurocrit Care. 2011;14:208–15.
200. Zhong J, Dujovny M, Park HK, Perez E, Perlin AR, Diaz FG. Advances in ICP monitoring techniques. Neurol Res. 2003;25:339–50.
201. Ghajar J. Intracranial pressure monitoring techniques. New Horiz. 1995;3:395–9.
202. Dasic D, Hanna SJ, Bojanic S, Kerr RS. External ventricular drain infection: the effect of a strict protocol on infection rates and a review of the literature. Br J Neurosurg. 2006;20:296–300.
203. Hoefnagel D, Dammers R, Ter Laak-Poort MP, Avezaat CJ. Risk factors for infections related to external ventricular drainage. Acta Neurochir. 2008;150:209–14. discussion 14
204. Kitchen WJ, Singh N, Hulme S, Galea J, Patel HC, King AT. External ventricular drain infection: improved technique can reduce infection rates. Br J Neurosurg. 2011;25:632–5.
205. Kourbeti IS, Jacobs AV, Koslow M, Karabetsos D, Holzman RS. Risk factors associated with postcraniotomy meningitis. Neurosurgery. 2007;60:317–25. discussion 25–6
206. O'Brien D, Stevens NT, Lim CH, et al. Candida infection of the central nervous system following neurosurgery: a 12-year review. Acta Neurochir. 2011;153:1347–50.
207. Schade RP, Schinkel J, Visser LG, Van Dijk JM, Voormolen JH, Kuijper EJ. Bacterial meningitis caused by the use of ventricular or lumbar cerebrospinal fluid catheters. J Neurosurg. 2005;102:229–34.
208. von der Brelie C, Simon A, Groner A, Molitor E, Simon M. Evaluation of an institutional guideline for the treatment of cerebrospinal fluid shunt-associated infections. Acta Neurochir. 2012;154(9):1691–7.
209. Korinek AM, Reina M, Boch AL, Rivera AO, De Bels D, Puybasset L. Prevention of external ventricular drain – related ventriculitis. Acta Neurochir. 2005;147:39–45. discussion 45–6
210. Lo CH, Spelman D, Bailey M, Cooper DJ, Rosenfeld JV, Brecknell JE. External ventricular drain infections are independent of drain duration: an argument against elective revision. J Neurosurg. 2007;106:378–83.
211. Mayhall CG, Archer NH, Lamb VA, et al. Ventriculostomy-related infections. A prospective epidemiologic study. N Engl J Med. 1984;310:553–9.
212. Winfield JA, Rosenthal P, Kanter RK, Casella G. Duration of intracranial pressure monitoring does not predict daily risk of infectious complications. Neurosurgery. 1993;33:424–30. discussion 30–1
213. Beer R, Pfausler B, Schmutzhard E. Management of nosocomial external ventricular drain-related ventriculomeningitis. Neurocrit Care. 2009;10:363–7.
214. Pfausler B, Beer R, Engelhardt K, Kemmler G, Mohsenipour I, Schmutzhard E. Cell index—a new parameter for the early diagnosis of ventriculostomy (external ventricular drainage)-related ventriculitis in patients with intraventricular hemorrhage? Acta Neurochir. 2004;146:477–81.
215. Kim JH, Desai NS, Ricci J, et al. Factors contributing to ventriculostomy infection. World Neurosurg. 2012;77:135–40.
216. Chi H, Chang KY, Chang HC, Chiu NC, Huang FY. Infections associated with indwelling ventriculostomy catheters in a teaching hospital. Int J Infect Dis. 2010;14:e216–9.
217. Stenehjem E, Armstrong WS. Central nervous system device infections. Infect Dis Clin N Am. 2012;26:89–110.
218. Alleyne CH Jr, Hassan M, Zabramski JM. The efficacy and cost of prophylactic and perioprocedural antibiotics in patients with external ventricular drains. Neurosurgery. 2000;47:1124–7. discussion 7–9
219. Ratilal B, Costa J, Sampaio C. Antibiotic prophylaxis for surgical introduction of intracranial ventricular shunts. Cochrane Database Syst Rev. 2006;(3):CD005365.
220. Munch TN, Juhler M. Antibiotic prophylaxis in insertion of intracranial ventricular shunts. A survey of a Cochrane review. Ugeskr Laeger. 2008;170:131–5.
221. Ratilal B, Sampaio C. Prophylactic antibiotics and anticonvulsants in neurosurgery. Adv Tech Stand Neurosurg. 2011;36:139–85.
222. Ratilal B, Costa J, Sampaio C. Antibiotic prophylaxis for surgical introduction of intracranial ventricular shunts: a systematic review. J Neurosurg Pediatr. 2008;1:48–56.
223. Muttaiyah S, Ritchie S, John S, Mee E, Roberts S. Efficacy of antibiotic-impregnated external ventricular drain catheters. J Clin Neurosci. 2010;17:296–8.
224. Abla AA, Zabramski JM, Jahnke HK, Fusco D, Nakaji P. Comparison of two antibiotic-impregnated ventricular catheters: a prospective sequential series trial. Neurosurgery. 2011;68:437–42. discussion 42
225. Eymann R, Chehab S, Strowitzki M, Steudel WI, Kiefer M. Clinical and economic consequences of antibiotic-impregnated cerebrospinal fluid shunt catheters. J Neurosurg Pediatr. 2008;1:444–50.
226. Gutierrez-Gonzalez R, Boto GR. Do antibiotic-impregnated catheters prevent infection in CSF diversion procedures? Review of the literature. J Infect. 2010;61:9–20.
227. Lemcke J, Depner F, Meier U. The impact of silver nanoparticle-coated and antibiotic-impregnated external ventricular drainage catheters on the risk of infections: a clinical comparison of 95 patients. Acta Neurochir Suppl. 2012;114:347–50.
228. Soleman J, Marbacher S, Fandino J, Fathi AR. Is the use of antibiotic-impregnated external ventricular drainage beneficial in the management of iatrogenic ventriculitis? Acta Neurochir. 2012;154:161–4. discussion 4
229. Zingale A, Ippolito S, Pappalardo P, Chibbaro S, Amoroso R. Infections and re-infections in long-term external ventricular drainage. A variation upon a theme. J Neurosurg Sci. 1999;43:125–32. discussion 33
230. Babu MA, Patel R, Marsh WR, Wijdicks EF. Strategies to decrease the risk of ventricular catheter infections: a review of the evidence. Neurocrit Care. 2012;16:194–202.
231. Fichtner J, Guresir E, Seifert V, Raabe A. Efficacy of silver-bearing external ventricular drainage catheters: a retrospective analysis. J Neurosurg. 2010;112:840–6.
232. McCarthy PJ, Patil S, Conrad SA, Scott LK. International and specialty trends in the use of prophylactic antibiotics to prevent infectious complications after insertion of external ventricular drainage devices. Neurocrit Care. 2010;12:220–4.
233. Razmkon A, Bakhtazad A. Maintaining CSF drainage at external ventricular drains may help prevent catheter-related infections. Acta Neurochir. 2009;151:985.
234. Rivero-Garvia M, Marquez-Rivas J, Jimenez-Mejias ME, Neth O, Rueda-Torres AB. Reduction in external ventricular drain infection rate. Impact of a minimal handling protocol and antibiotic-impregnated catheters. Acta Neurochir. 2011;153:647–51.
235. Cummings R. Understanding external ventricular drainage. J Neurosci Nurs. 1992;24:84–7.
236. Narayan RK, Kishore PR, Becker DP, et al. Intracranial pressure: to monitor or not to monitor? A review of our experience with severe head injury. J Neurosurg. 1982;56:650–9.
237. Tamburrini G, Massimi L, Caldarelli M, Di Rocco C. Antibiotic impregnated external ventricular drainage and third ventriculostomy in the management of hydrocephalus associated with posterior cranial fossa tumours. Acta Neurochir. 2008;150:1049–55. discussion 55–6
238. Lopez-Alvarez B, Martin-Laez R, Farinas MC, Paternina-Vidal B, Garcia-Palomo JD, Vazquez-Barquero A. Multidrug-resistant

Acinetobacter baumannii ventriculitis: successful treatment with intraventricular colistin. Acta Neurochir. 2009;151:1465–72.
239. Nerlich AG, Haas CJ, Zink A, Szeimies U, Hagedorn HG. Molecular evidence for tuberculosis in an ancient Egyptian mummy. Lancet. 1997;350:1404.
240. Salo WL, Aufderheide AC, Buikstra J, Holcomb TA. Identification of Mycobacterium tuberculosis DNA in a pre-Columbian Peruvian mummy. Proc Natl Acad Sci U S A. 1994;91:2091–4.
241. WHO. Global tuberculosis report 2021. Geneva: World Health Organization; 2021.
242. Archibald LK, den Dulk MO, Pallangyo KJ, Reller LB. Fatal *Mycobacterium tuberculosis* bloodstream infections in febrile hospitalized adults in Dar es Salaam, Tanzania. Clin Infect Dis. 1998;26:290–6.
243. Archibald LK, McDonald LC, Nwanyanwu O, et al. A hospital-based prevalence survey of bloodstream infections in febrile patients in Malawi: implications for diagnosis and therapy. J Infect Dis. 2000;181:1414–20.
244. Archibald LK, McDonald LC, Rheanpumikankit S, et al. Fever and human immunodeficiency virus infection as sentinels for emerging mycobacterial and fungal bloodstream infections in hospitalized patients greater than ≥15 years old, Bangkok. J Infect Dis. 1999;180:87–92.
245. Bell M, Archibald LK, Nwanyanwu O, et al. Seasonal variation in the etiology of bloodstream infections in a febrile inpatient population in a developing country. Int J Infect Dis. 2001;5:63–9.
246. McDonald LC, Archibald LK, Rheanpumikankit S, et al. Unrecognised Mycobacterium tuberculosis bacteraemia among hospital inpatients in less developed countries. Lancet. 1999;354:1159–63.
247. Kent SJ, Crowe SM, Yung A, Lucas CR, Mijch AM. Tuberculous meningitis: a 30-year review. Clin Infect Dis. 1993;17:987–94.
248. Thwaites GE, Tran TH. Tuberculous meningitis: many questions, too few answers. Lancet Neurol. 2005;4:160–70.
249. Thwaites G, Fisher M, Hemingway C, Scott G, Solomon T, Innes J. British Infection Society guidelines for the diagnosis and treatment of tuberculosis of the central nervous system in adults and children. J Infect. 2009;59:167–87.
250. Joos TJ, Miller WC, Murdoch DM. Tuberculin reactivity in bacille Calmette-Guerin vaccinated populations: a compilation of international data. Int J Tuberc Lung Dis. 2006;10:883–91.
251. Kilpatrick ME, Girgis NI, Tribble D, Farid Z. The value of the tuberculin skin test in patients with tuberculous meningitis. J Egypt Public Health Assoc. 1996;71:1–8.
252. Thwaites GE, Schoeman JF. Update on tuberculosis of the central nervous system: pathogenesis, diagnosis, and treatment. Clin Chest Med. 2009;30:745–54. ix
253. Ferrara G, Losi M, D'Amico R, et al. Use in routine clinical practice of two commercial blood tests for diagnosis of infection with Mycobacterium tuberculosis: a prospective study. Lancet. 2006;367:1328–34.
254. Ferrara G, Losi M, Meacci M, et al. Routine hospital use of a new commercial whole blood interferon-gamma assay for the diagnosis of tuberculosis infection. Am J Respir Crit Care Med. 2005;172:631–5.
255. Foerster BR, Thurnher MM, Malani PN, Petrou M, Carets-Zumelzu F, Sundgren PC. Intracranial infections: clinical and imaging characteristics. Acta Radiol. 2007;48:875–93.
256. Trivedi R, Saksena S, Gupta RK. Magnetic resonance imaging in central nervous system tuberculosis. Indian J Radiol Imaging. 2009;19:256–65.
257. Parsons LM, Somoskovi A, Gutierrez C, et al. Laboratory diagnosis of tuberculosis in resource-poor countries: challenges and opportunities. Clin Microbiol Rev. 2011;24:314–50.
258. Murthy JM. Tuberculous meningitis: the challenges. Neurol India. 2010;58:716–22.
259. Thwaites GE, Nguyen DB, Nguyen HD, et al. Dexamethasone for the treatment of tuberculous meningitis in adolescents and adults. N Engl J Med. 2004;351:1741–51.
260. Marais S, Meintjes G, Pepper DJ, Dodd LE, Schutz C, Ismail Z, Wilkinson KA, Wilkinson RJ. Frequency, severity, and prediction of tuberculous meningitis immune reconstitution inflammatory syndrome. Clin Infect Dis. 2013;56(3):450–60.
261. Berning SE, Cherry TA, Iseman MD. Novel treatment of meningitis caused by multidrug-resistant Mycobacterium tuberculosis with intrathecal levofloxacin and amikacin: case report. Clin Infect Dis. 2001;32:643–6.
262. Garg RK, Sinha MK. Tuberculous meningitis in patients infected with human immunodeficiency virus. J Neurol. 2011;258:3–13.
263. Afghani B, Lieberman JM. Paradoxical enlargement or development of intracranial tuberculomas during therapy: case report and review. Clin Infect Dis. 1994;19:1092–9.
264. Galimi R. Extrapulmonary tuberculosis: tuberculous meningitis new developments. Eur Rev Med Pharmacol Sci. 2011;15:365–86.
265. Hall WA, Truwit CL. The surgical management of infections involving the cerebrum. Neurosurgery. 2008;62(Suppl. 2):519–30. discussion 30–1
266. Garg RK, Somvanshi DS. Spinal tuberculosis: a review. J Spinal Cord Med. 2011;34:440–54.
267. Adekambi T, Foucault C, La Scola B, Drancourt M. Report of two fatal cases of *Mycobacterium mucogenicum* central nervous system infection in immunocompetent patients. J Clin Microbiol. 2006;44:837–40.
268. Madaras-Kelly KJ, DeMasters TA, Stevens DL. *Mycobacterium fortuitum* meningitis associated with an epidural catheter: case report and a review of the literature. Pharmacotherapy. 1999;19:661–6.
269. Midani S, Rathore MH. *Mycobacterium fortuitum* infection of ventriculoperitoneal shunt. South Med J. 1999;92:705–7.
270. Talati NJ, Rouphael N, Kuppalli K, Franco-Paredes C. Spectrum of CNS disease caused by rapidly growing mycobacteria. Lancet Infect Dis. 2008;8:390–8.
271. Bradsher RW. Histoplasmosis and blastomycosis. Clin Infect Dis. 1996;22(Suppl. 2):S102–11.
272. Kauffman CA. Histoplasmosis: a clinical and laboratory update. Clin Microbiol Rev. 2007;20:115–32.
273. Wheat LJ, Batteiger BE, Sathapatayavongs B. *Histoplasma capsulatum* infections of the central nervous system. A clinical review. Medicine. 1990;69:244–60.
274. Gottfredsson M, Perfect JR. Fungal meningitis. Semin Neurol. 2000;20:307–22.
275. Chakrabarti A. Epidemiology of central nervous system mycoses. Neurol India. 2007;55:191–7.
276. Williams PL. Coccidioidal meningitis. Ann N Y Acad Sci. 2007;1111:377–84.
277. Johnson RH, Einstein HE. Coccidioidal meningitis. Clin Infect Dis. 2006;42:103–7.
278. Mathisen G, Shelub A, Truong J, Wigen C. Coccidioidal meningitis: clinical presentation and management in the fluconazole era. Medicine. 2010;89:251–84.
279. Bouza E, Dreyer JS, Hewitt WL, Meyer RD. Coccidioidal meningitis. An analysis of thirty-one cases and review of the literature. Medicine. 1981;60:139–72.
280. Vincent T, Galgiani JN, Huppert M, Salkin D. The natural history of coccidioidal meningitis: VA-Armed Forces cooperative studies, 1955–1958. Clin Infect Dis. 1993;16:247–54.
281. Ragland AS, Arsura E, Ismail Y, Johnson R. Eosinophilic pleocytosis in coccidioidal meningitis: frequency and significance. Am J Med. 1993;95:254–7.
282. Chapman SW, Dismukes WE, Proia LA, et al. Clinical practice guidelines for the management of blastomycosis: 2008 update

by the Infectious Diseases Society of America. Clin Infect Dis. 2008;46:1801–12.
283. Bariola JR, Perry P, Pappas PG, et al. Blastomycosis of the central nervous system: a multicenter review of diagnosis and treatment in the modern era. Clin Infect Dis. 2010;50:797–804.
284. Borgia SM, Fuller JD, Sarabia A, El-Helou P. Cerebral blastomycosis: a case series incorporating voriconazole in the treatment regimen. Med Mycol. 2006;44:659–64.
285. Chowfin A, Tight R, Mitchell S. Recurrent blastomycosis of the central nervous system: case report and review. Clin Infect Dis. 2000;30:969–71.
286. Gonyea EF. The spectrum of primary blastomycotic meningitis: a review of central nervous system blastomycosis. Ann Neurol. 1978;3:26–39.
287. Bakleh M, Aksamit AJ, Tleyjeh IM, Marshall WF. Successful treatment of cerebral blastomycosis with voriconazole. Clin Infect Dis. 2005;40:e69–71.
288. Pappas PG, Pottage JC, Powderly WG, et al. Blastomycosis in patients with the acquired immunodeficiency syndrome. Ann Intern Med. 1992;116:847–53.
289. Chander B, Deb P, Sarkar C, Garg A, Mehta VS, Sharma MC. Cerebral blastomycosis: a case report. Indian J Pathol Microbiol. 2007;50:821–4.
290. Bradsher RW, Chapman SW, Pappas PG. Blastomycosis. Infect Dis Clin N Am. 2003;17:21–40. vii
291. Pappas PG. Blastomycosis. Semin Respir Crit Care Med. 2004;25:113–21.
292. Saccente M, Woods GL. Clinical and laboratory update on blastomycosis. Clin Microbiol Rev. 2010;23:367–81.
293. Durkin M, Witt J, Lemonte A, Wheat B, Connolly P. Antigen assay with the potential to aid in diagnosis of blastomycosis. J Clin Microbiol. 2004;42:4873–5.
294. Smith JA, Kauffman CA. Blastomycosis. Proc Am Thorac Soc. 2010;7:173–80.
295. Martynowicz MA, Prakash UB. Pulmonary blastomycosis: an appraisal of diagnostic techniques. Chest. 2002;121:768–73.
296. Casado JL, Quereda C, Corral I. Candidal meningitis in HIV-infected patients. AIDS Patient Care STDs. 1998;12:681–6.
297. Goldani LZ, Santos RP. Candida tropicalis as an emerging pathogen in Candida meningitis: case report and review. Braz J Infect Dis. 2010;14:631–3.
298. Montero A, Romero J, Vargas JA, et al. Candida infection of cerebrospinal fluid shunt devices: report of two cases and review of the literature. Acta Neurochir. 2000;142:67–74.
299. Rodriguez-Arrondo F, Aguirrebengoa K, De Arce A, et al. Candidal meningitis in HIV-infected patients: treatment with fluconazole. Scand J Infect Dis. 1998;30:417–8.
300. Sanchez-Portocarrero J, Perez-Cecilia E, Corral O, Romero-Vivas J, Picazo JJ. The central nervous system and infection by Candida species. Diagn Microbiol Infect Dis. 2000;37:169–79.
301. Parker JC Jr, McCloskey JJ, Lee RS. Human cerebral candidosis—a postmortem evaluation of 19 patients. Hum Pathol. 1981;12:23–8.
302. Bayer AS, Edwards JE Jr, Seidel JS, Guze LB. Candida meningitis. Report of seven cases and review of the english literature. Medicine. 1976;55:477–86.
303. Black JT. Cerebral candidiasis: case report of brain abscess secondary to Candida albicans, and review of literature. J Neurol Neurosurg Psychiatry. 1970;33:864–70.
304. Lipton SA, Hickey WF, Morris JH, Loscalzo J. Candidal infection in the central nervous system. Am J Med. 1984;76:101–8.
305. Bengel D, Susa M, Schreiber H, Ludolph AC, Tumani H. Early diagnosis of rhinocerebral mucormycosis by cerebrospinal fluid analysis and determination of 16s rRNA gene sequence. Eur J Neurol. 2007;14:1067–70.
306. Mallis A, Mastronikolis SN, Naxakis SS, Papadas AT. Rhinocerebral mucormycosis: an update. Eur Rev Med Pharmacol Sci. 2010;14:987–92.
307. Schwartz S, Thiel E. Cerebral aspergillosis: tissue penetration is the key. Med Mycol. 2009;47(Suppl. 1):S387–93.
308. Montoya JG, Liesenfeld O. Toxoplasmosis. Lancet. 2004;363:1965–76.
309. Kaplan JE, Benson C, Holmes KH, Brooks JT, Pau A, Masur H. Guidelines for prevention and treatment of opportunistic infections in HIV-infected adults and adolescents: recommendations from CDC, the National Institutes of Health, and the HIV Medicine Association of the Infectious Diseases Society of America. MMWR Recomm Rep. 2009;58:1–207. quiz CE1–4
310. Contini C. Clinical and diagnostic management of toxoplasmosis in the immunocompromised patient. Parassitologia. 2008;50:45–50.
311. Dedicoat M, Livesley N. Management of toxoplasmic encephalitis in HIV-infected adults—a review. S Afr Med J. 2008;98:31–2.
312. Beraud G, Pierre-Francois S, Foltzer A, et al. Cotrimoxazole for treatment of cerebral toxoplasmosis: an observational cohort study during 1994–2006. Am J Trop Med Hyg. 2009;80:583–7.
313. Pereira-Chioccola VL, Vidal JE, Su C. Toxoplasma gondii infection and cerebral toxoplasmosis in HIV-infected patients. Future Microbiol. 2009;4:1363–79.
314. Portegies P, Solod L, Cinque P, et al. Guidelines for the diagnosis and management of neurological complications of HIV infection. Eur J Neurol. 2004;11:297–304.
315. Luft BJ, Hafner R, Korzun AH, et al. Toxoplasmic encephalitis in patients with the acquired immunodeficiency syndrome. Members of the ACTG 077p/ANRS 009 Study Team. N Engl J Med. 1993;329:995–1000.
316. Heald A, Flepp M, Chave JP, et al. Treatment for cerebral toxoplasmosis protects against Pneumocystis carinii pneumonia in patients with AIDS. The Swiss HIV Cohort Study. Ann Intern Med. 1991;115:760–3.
317. Bertschy S, Opravil M, Cavassini M, et al. Discontinuation of maintenance therapy against toxoplasma encephalitis in AIDS patients with sustained response to anti-retroviral therapy. Clin Microbiol Infect. 2006;12:666–71.
318. Soriano V, Dona C, Rodriguez-Rosado R, Barreiro P, Gonzalez-Lahoz J. Discontinuation of secondary prophylaxis for opportunistic infections in HIV-infected patients receiving highly active antiretroviral therapy. AIDS. 2000;14:383–6.
319. Grassi MP, Clerici F, Perin C, et al. Microglial nodular encephalitis and ventriculoencephalitis due to cytomegalovirus infection in patients with AIDS: two distinct clinical patterns. Clin Infect Dis. 1998;27:504–8.
320. Clifford DB, Arribas JR, Storch GA, Tourtellote W, Wippold FJ. Magnetic resonance brain imaging lacks sensitivity for AIDS associated cytomegalovirus encephalitis. J Neurovirol. 1996;2:397–403.
321. Arribas JR, Storch GA, Clifford DB, Tselis AC. Cytomegalovirus encephalitis. Ann Intern Med. 1996;125:577–87.
322. Anders HJ, Goebel FD. Neurological manifestations of cytomegalovirus infection in the acquired immunodeficiency syndrome. Int J STD AIDS. 1999;10:151–9. quiz 60–1
323. Cinque P, Cleator GM, Weber T, et al. Diagnosis and clinical management of neurological disorders caused by cytomegalovirus in AIDS patients. European Union Concerted Action on Virus Meningitis and Encephalitis. J Neurovirol. 1998;4:120–32.
324. Silva CA, Oliveira AC, Vilas-Boas L, Fink MC, Pannuti CS, Vidal JE. Neurologic cytomegalovirus complications in patients with AIDS: retrospective review of 13 cases and review of the literature. Rev Inst Med Trop São Paulo. 2010;52:305–10.

325. Eidelberg D, Sotrel A, Vogel H, Walker P, Kleefield J, Crumpacker CS 3rd. Progressive polyradiculopathy in acquired immune deficiency syndrome. Neurology. 1986;36:912–6.
326. Kurup A, Torriani FJ. Therapy and prevention of cytomegalovirus retinitis. Curr Infect Dis Rep. 2001;3:371–7.
327. Spector SA, McKinley GF, Lalezari JP, et al. Oral ganciclovir for the prevention of cytomegalovirus disease in persons with AIDS. Roche Cooperative Oral Ganciclovir Study Group. N Engl J Med. 1996;334:1491–7.
328. Waib LF, Bonon SH, Salles AC, et al. Withdrawal of maintenance therapy for cytomegalovirus retinitis in AIDS patients exhibiting immunological response to HAART. Rev Inst Med Trop São Paulo. 2007;49:215–9.
329. Macdonald JC, Torriani FJ, Morse LS, Karavellas MP, Reed JB, Freeman WR. Lack of reactivation of cytomegalovirus (CMV) retinitis after stopping CMV maintenance therapy in AIDS patients with sustained elevations in CD4 T cells in response to highly active antiretroviral therapy. J Infect Dis. 1998;177:1182–7.
330. Wohl DA, Kendall MA, Owens S, et al. The safety of discontinuation of maintenance therapy for cytomegalovirus (CMV) retinitis and incidence of immune recovery uveitis following potent antiretroviral therapy. HIV Clin Trials. 2005;6:136–46.
331. Urban B, Bakunowicz-Łazarczyk A, Michalczuk M. Immune recovery uveitis: pathogenesis, clinical symptoms, and treatment. Mediat Inflamm. 2014;2014:971417.
332. Read SW, DeGrezia M, Ciccone EJ, DerSimonian R, Higgins J, Adelsberger JW, et al. The effect of leflunomide on cycling and activation of T-cells in HIV-1-infected participants. PLoS One. 2010;5(8):e11937.
333. Kaul M. HIV-1 associated dementia: update on pathological mechanisms and therapeutic approaches. Curr Opin Neurol. 2009;22:315–20.
334. Yadav A, Collman RG. CNS inflammation and macrophage/microglial biology associated with HIV-1 infection. J Neuroimmune Pharmacol. 2009;4:430–47.
335. Giulian D, Vaca K, Noonan CA. Secretion of neurotoxins by mononuclear phagocytes infected with HIV-1. Science. 1990;250:1593–6.
336. Giulian D, Wendt E, Vaca K, Noonan CA. The envelope glycoprotein of human immunodeficiency virus type 1 stimulates release of neurotoxins from monocytes. Proc Natl Acad Sci USA. 1993;90:2769–73.
337. Krathwohl MD, Kaiser JL. HIV-1 promotes quiescence in human neural progenitor cells. J Infect Dis. 2004;190:216–26.
338. Okamoto S, Kang YJ, Brechtel CW, et al. HIV/gp120 decreases adult neural progenitor cell proliferation via checkpoint kinase-mediated cell-cycle withdrawal and G1 arrest. Cell Stem Cell. 2007;1:230–6.
339. Nogales-Gaete J, Syndulko K, Tourtellotte WW. Cerebrospinal fluid (CSF) analyses in HIV-1 primary neurological disease. Ital J Neurol Sci. 1992;13:667–83.
340. Navia BA, Jordan BD, Price RW. The AIDS dementia complex: I. Clinical features. Ann Neurol. 1986;19:517–24.
341. Freitas do Rosario AP, Langhorne J. T cell-derived IL-10 and its impact on the regulation of host responses during malaria. Int J Parasitol. 2012;42(6):549–55.
342. Garg RK. Cerebral malaria. J Assoc Physicians India. 2000;48:1004–13.
343. Higgins SJ, Kain KC, Liles WC. Immunopathogenesis of falciparum malaria: implications for adjunctive therapy in the management of severe and cerebral malaria. Expert Rev Anti-Infect Ther 2011;9:803–19.
344. Mackintosh CL, Beeson JG, Marsh K. Clinical features and pathogenesis of severe malaria. Trends Parasitol. 2004;20:597–603.
345. Medana IM, Day NP, Sachanonta N, et al. Coma in fatal adult human malaria is not caused by cerebral oedema. Malar J. 2011;10:267.
346. Ponsford MJ, Medana IM, Prapansilp P, et al. Sequestration and microvascular congestion are associated with coma in human cerebral malaria. J Infect Dis. 2012;205:663–71.
347. Warrell DA. Management of severe malaria. Parassitologia. 1999;41:287–94.
348. Warrell DA, Looareesuwan S, Phillips RE, et al. Function of the blood-cerebrospinal fluid barrier in human cerebral malaria: rejection of the permeability hypothesis. Am J Trop Med Hyg. 1986;35:882–9.
349. Warrell DA, Looareesuwan S, Warrell MJ, et al. Dexamethasone proves deleterious in cerebral malaria. A double-blind trial in 100 comatose patients. N Engl J Med. 1982;306:313–9.
350. Warrell DA, White NJ, Warrell MJ. Dexamethasone deleterious in cerebral malaria. Br Med J (Clin Res Ed). 1982;285:1652.
351. Dondorp AM, Fanello CI, Hendriksen IC, et al. Artesunate versus quinine in the treatment of severe falciparum malaria in African children (AQUAMAT): an open-label, randomised trial. Lancet. 2010;376:1647–57.
352. Mohanty S, Mishra SK, Patnaik R, et al. Brain swelling and mannitol therapy in adult cerebral malaria: a randomized trial. Clin Infect Dis. 2011;53:349–55.
353. Qvarnstrom Y, James C, Xayavong M, et al. Comparison of real-time PCR protocols for differential laboratory diagnosis of amebiasis. J Clin Microbiol. 2005;43:5491–7.
354. Qvarnstrom Y, Visvesvara GS, Sriram R, da Silva AJ. Multiplex real-time PCR assay for simultaneous detection of *Acanthamoeba* spp., *Balamuthia mandrillaris*, and *Naegleria fowleri*. J Clin Microbiol. 2006;44:3589–95.
355. Seidel JS, Harmatz P, Visvesvara GS, Cohen A, Edwards J, Turner J. Successful treatment of primary amebic meningoencephalitis. N Engl J Med. 1982;306:346–8.
356. CDC. Primary amebic meningoencephalitis—Arizona, Florida, and Texas, 2007. MMWR Morb Mortal Wkly Rep. 2008;57:573–7.
357. Lopez C, Budge P, Chen J, et al. Primary amebic meningoencephalitis: a case report and literature review. Pediatr Emerg Care. 2012;28:272–6.
358. Soltow SM, Brenner GM. Synergistic activities of azithromycin and amphotericin B against Naegleria fowleri in vitro and in a mouse model of primary amebic meningoencephalitis. Antimicrob Agents Chemother. 2007;51:23–7.
359. Visvesvara GS. Amebic meningoencephalitides and keratitis: challenges in diagnosis and treatment. Curr Opin Infect Dis. 2010;23:590–4.
360. Del Brutto OH. Neurocysticercosis in Western Europe: a re-emerging disease? Acta Neurol Belg. 2012;112(4):335–43.
361. Del Brutto OH. Neurocysticercosis among international travelers to disease-endemic areas. J Travel Med. 2012;19:112–7.
362. Del Brutto OH. Neurocysticercosis: a review. ScientificWorldJournal. 2012;2012:159821.
363. Takayanagui OM, Jardim E. Clinical aspects of neurocysticercosis: analysis of 500 cases. Arq Neuropsiquiatr. 1983;41:50–63.
364. Sotelo J, Del Brutto OH. Review of neurocysticercosis. Neurosurg Focus. 2002;12:e1.
365. Sotelo J, Del Brutto OH. Brain cysticercosis. Arch Med Res. 2000;31:3–14.
366. Michelet L, Fleury A, Sciutto E, et al. Human neurocysticercosis: comparison of different diagnostic tests using cerebrospinal fluid. J Clin Microbiol. 2011;49:195–200.
367. Sotelo J, del Brutto OH, Penagos P, et al. Comparison of therapeutic regimen of anticysticercal drugs for parenchymal brain cysticercosis. J Neurol. 1990;237:69–72.

368. Del Brutto OH. Albendazole therapy for subarachnoid cysticerci: clinical and neuroimaging analysis of 17 patients. J Neurol Neurosurg Psychiatry. 1997;62:659–61.
369. Takayanagui OM, Jardim E. Therapy for neurocysticercosis. Comparison between albendazole and praziquantel. Arch Neurol. 1992;49:290–4.
370. Padma MV, Behari M, Misra NK, Ahuja GK. Albendazole in neurocysticercosis. Natl Med J India. 1995;8:255–8.
371. Carpio A, Santillan F, Leon P, Flores C, Hauser WA. Is the course of neurocysticercosis modified by treatment with antihelminthic agents? Arch Intern Med. 1995;155:1982–8.
372. Padma MV, Behari M, Misra NK, Ahuja GK. Albendazole in single CT ring lesions in epilepsy. Neurology. 1994;44:1344–6.
373. Riley T, White AC Jr. Management of neurocysticercosis. CNS Drugs. 2003;17:577–91.
374. Shandera WX, White AC Jr, Chen JC, Diaz P, Armstrong R. Neurocysticercosis in Houston, Texas. A report of 112 cases. Medicine. 1994;73:37–52.
375. White AC, Garcia HH. Recent developments in the epidemiology, diagnosis, treatment, and prevention of neurocysticercosis. Curr Infect Dis Rep. 1999;1:434–40.
376. White AC Jr. Neurocysticercosis: a major cause of neurological disease worldwide. Clin Infect Dis. 1997;24:101–13. quiz 14–5
377. Jimenez-Vazquez OH, Nagore N. Cisternal neurocysticercosis. Br J Neurosurg. 2008;22:774–5.
378. Sotelo J. Clinical manifestations, diagnosis, and treatment of neurocysticercosis. Curr Neurol Neurosci Rep. 2011;11:529–35.
379. Garcia HH, Evans CA, Nash TE, et al. Current consensus guidelines for treatment of neurocysticercosis. Clin Microbiol Rev. 2002;15:747–56.
380. Garcia HH, Del Brutto OH, Nash TE, White AC Jr, Tsang VC, Gilman RH. New concepts in the diagnosis and management of neurocysticercosis (Taenia solium). Am J Trop Med Hyg. 2005;72:3–9.
381. Sommer C, Ringelstein EB, Biniek R, Glockner WM. Adult Toxocara canis encephalitis. J Neurol Neurosurg Psychiatry. 1994;57:229–31.
382. Moreira-Silva SF, Rodrigues MG, Pimenta JL, Gomes CP, Freire LH, Pereira FE. Toxocariasis of the central nervous system: with report of two cases. Rev Soc Bras Med Trop. 2004;37:169–74.
383. Maiga Y, Wiertlewski S, Desal H, Marjolet M, Damier P. Presentation of cerebral toxocariasis with mental confusion in an adult: case report and review of the literature. Bull Soc Pathol Exot. 2007;100:101–4.
384. Finsterer J, Auer H. Neurotoxocarosis. Rev Inst Med Trop São Paulo. 2007;49:279–87.
385. Lukehart SA, Hook EW 3rd, Baker-Zander SA, Collier AC, Critchlow CW, Handsfield HH. Invasion of the central nervous system by Treponema pallidum: implications for diagnosis and treatment. Ann Intern Med. 1988;109:855–62.
386. Simon RP. Neurosyphilis. Arch Neurol. 1985;42:606–13.
387. Hotson JR. Modern neurosyphilis: a partially treated chronic meningitis. West J Med. 1981;135:191–200.
388. Hooshmand H, Escobar MR, Kopf SW. Neurosyphilis. A study of 241 patients. JAMA. 1972;219:726–9.
389. Holmes MD, Brant-Zawadzki MM, Simon RP. Clinical features of meningovascular syphilis. Neurology. 1984;34:553–6.
390. Flood JM, Weinstock HS, Guroy ME, Bayne L, Simon RP, Bolan G. Neurosyphilis during the AIDS epidemic, San Francisco, 1985–1992. J Infect Dis. 1998;177:931–40.
391. Ghanem KG. Review: neurosyphilis: a historical perspective and review. CNS Neurosci Ther. 2010;16:e157–68.
392. Weinert LS, Scheffel RS, Zoratto G, et al. Cerebral syphilitic gumma in HIV-infected patients: case report and review. Int J STD AIDS. 2008;19:62–4.
393. Horowitz HW, Valsamis MP, Wicher V, et al. Brief report: cerebral syphilitic gumma confirmed by the polymerase chain reaction in a man with human immunodeficiency virus infection. N Engl J Med. 1994;331:1488–91.
394. Seña AC, Wolff M, Behets F, Martin DH, Leone P, Langley C, et al. Rate of decline in nontreponemal antibody titers and seroreversion after treatment of early syphilis. Sex Transm Dis. 2017;44(1):6–10.
395. Davis LE, Schmitt JW. Clinical significance of cerebrospinal fluid tests for neurosyphilis. Ann Neurol. 1989;25:50–5.
396. Workowski KA, Berman S. Sexually transmitted diseases treatment guidelines, 2010. MMWR Recomm Rep. 2010;59:1–110.
397. Moore JE. Asymptomatic neurosyphilis V: a comparison of early and late asymptomatic neurosyphilis. Arch Dermatol Syphilol. 1928;18:99–108.
398. Wilner E, Brody JA. Prognosis of general paresis after treatment. Lancet. 1968;2:1370–1.
399. Curtis AC, Cutler JC, Gammon G, et al. Penicillin treatment of asymptomatic central nervous system syphilis. I. Probability of progression to symptomatic neurosyphilis. AMA. Arch Dermatol. 1956;74:355–66.
400. Dunlop EM, Al-Egaily SS, Houang ET. Penicillin levels in blood and CSF achieved by treatment of syphilis. JAMA. 1979;241:2538–40.
401. Mohr JA, Griffiths W, Jackson R, Saadah H, Bird P, Riddle J. Neurosyphilis and penicillin levels in cerebrospinal fluid. JAMA. 1976;236:2208–9.
402. Schoth PE, Wolters EC. Penicillin concentrations in serum and CSF during high-dose intravenous treatment for neurosyphilis. Neurology. 1987;37:1214–6.
403. Fargen KM, Alvernia JE, Lin CS, Melgar M. Cerebral syphilitic gummata: a case presentation and analysis of 156 reported cases. Neurosurgery. 2009;64:568–75. discussion 75–6
404. Steere AC, Malawista SE, Snydman DR, et al. Lyme arthritis: an epidemic of oligoarticular arthritis in children and adults in three connecticut communities. Arthritis Rheum. 1977;20:7–17.
405. Steere AC, Malawista SE, Hardin JA, Ruddy S, Askenase W, Andiman WA. Erythema chronicum migrans and Lyme arthritis. The enlarging clinical spectrum. Ann Intern Med. 1977;86:685–98.
406. Wallis RC, Brown SE, Kloter KO, Main AJ Jr. Erythema chronicum migrans and lyme arthritis: field study of ticks. Am J Epidemiol. 1978;108:322–7.
407. Burgdorfer W. Discovery of the Lyme disease spirochete and its relation to tick vectors. Yale J Biol Med. 1984;57:515–20.
408. Burgdorfer W. The enlarging spectrum of tick-borne spirochetoses: R. R. Parker Memorial Address. Rev Infect Dis. 1986;8:932–40.
409. Steere AC, Broderick TF, Malawista SE. Erythema chronicum migrans and Lyme arthritis: epidemiologic evidence for a tick vector. Am J Epidemiol. 1978;108:312–21.
410. Steere AC, Bartenhagen NH, Craft JE, et al. Clinical manifestations of Lyme disease. Zentralbl Bakteriol Mikrobiol Hyg A. 1986;263:201–5.
411. Steere AC, Bartenhagen NH, Craft JE, et al. The early clinical manifestations of Lyme disease. Ann Intern Med. 1983;99:76–82.
412. Steere AC. Lyme disease. N Engl J Med. 1989;321:586–96.
413. Yoshinari NH, Steere AC, Cossermelli W. A review of Lyme disease. Rev Assoc Med Bras. 1989;35:34–8.
414. Keller TL, Halperin JJ, Whitman M. PCR detection of Borrelia burgdorferi DNA in cerebrospinal fluid of Lyme neuroborreliosis patients. Neurology. 1992;42:32–42.
415. Preac-Mursic V, Weber K, Pfister HW, et al. Survival of Borrelia burgdorferi in antibiotically treated patients with Lyme borreliosis. Infection. 1989;17:355–9.
416. Shadick NA, Phillips CB, Logigian EL, et al. The long-term clinical outcomes of Lyme disease. A population-based retrospective cohort study. Ann Intern Med. 1994;121:560–7.

417. Ackermann R, Rehse-Kupper B, Gollmer E, Schmidt R. Chronic neurologic manifestations of erythema migrans borreliosis. Ann N Y Acad Sci. 1988;539:16–23.
418. Hanny PE, Hauselmann HJ. Lyme disease from the neurologist's viewpoint. Schweiz Med Wochenschr. 1987;117:901–15.
419. Kohler J, Kern U, Kasper J, Rhese-Kupper B, Thoden U. Chronic central nervous system involvement in Lyme borreliosis. Neurology. 1988;38:863–7.
420. Kuntzer T, Bogousslavsky J, Miklossy J, Steck AJ, Janzer R, Regli F. Borrelia rhombencephalomyelopathy. Arch Neurol. 1991;48:832–6.
421. Meurers B, Kohlhepp W, Gold R, Rohrbach E, Mertens HG. Histopathological findings in the central and peripheral nervous systems in neuroborreliosis. A report of three cases. J Neurol. 1990;237:113–6.
422. Mokry M, Flaschka G, Kleinert G, Kleinert R, Fazekas F, Kopp W. Chronic Lyme disease with an expansive granulomatous lesion in the cerebellopontine angle. Neurosurgery. 1990;27:446–51.
423. Pachner AR. Borrelia burgdorferi in the nervous system: the new "great imitator". Ann N Y Acad Sci. 1988;539:56–64.
424. Rafto SE, Milton WJ, Galetta SL, Grossman RI. Biopsy-confirmed CNS Lyme disease: MR appearance at 1.5 T. AJNR Am J Neuroradiol. 1990;11:482–4.
425. Crisp D, Ashby P. Lyme radiculoneuritis treated with intravenous immunoglobulin. Neurology. 1996;46:1174–5.
426. O'Connell S. Lyme borreliosis: current issues in diagnosis and management. Curr Opin Infect Dis. 2010;23:231–5.
427. Mertens HG, Martin R, Kohlhepp W. Clinical and neuroimmunological findings in chronic Borrelia burgdorferi radiculomyelitis (Lyme disease). J Neuroimmunol. 1988;20:309–14.
428. Logigian EL, Kaplan RF, Steere AC. Chronic neurologic manifestations of Lyme disease. N Engl J Med. 1990;323:1438–44.
429. Reik L Jr. Stroke due to Lyme disease. Neurology. 1993;43:2705–7.
430. Weder B, Wiedersheim P, Matter L, Steck A, Otto F. Chronic progressive neurological involvement in Borrelia burgdorferi infection. J Neurol. 1987;234:40–3.
431. Agarwal R, Sze G. Neuro-lyme disease: MR imaging findings. Radiology. 2009;253:167–73.
432. Hildenbrand P, Craven DE, Jones R, Nemeskal P. Lyme neuroborreliosis: manifestations of a rapidly emerging zoonosis. AJNR Am J Neuroradiol. 2009;30:1079–87.
433. Halperin JJ, Luft BJ, Anand AK, et al. Lyme neuroborreliosis: central nervous system manifestations. Neurology. 1989;39:753–9.
434. Halperin JJ. Nervous system lyme disease: diagnosis and treatment. Rev Neurol Dis. 2009;6:4–12.
435. Halperin JJ. Nervous system Lyme disease. J R Coll Physicians Edinb. 2010;40:248–55.
436. Halperin JJ. Central nervous system Lyme disease. Curr Neurol Neurosci Rep. 2005;5:446–52.
437. Halperin JJ, Pass HL, Anand AK, Luft BJ, Volkman DJ, Dattwyler RJ. Nervous system abnormalities in Lyme disease. Ann N Y Acad Sci. 1988;539:24–34.
438. Halperin J, Luft BJ, Volkman DJ, Dattwyler RJ. Lyme neuroborreliosis. Peripheral nervous system manifestations. Brain. 1990;113(Pt 4):1207–21.
439. Halperin JJ. Neuroborreliosis: central nervous system involvement. Semin Neurol. 1997;17:19–24.
440. Halperin JJ. Neuroborreliosis (nervous system Lyme disease). Curr Treat Options Neurol. 1999;1:139–46.
441. Logigian EL, Steere AC. Clinical and electrophysiologic findings in chronic neuropathy of Lyme disease. Neurology. 1992;42:303–11.
442. Halperin JJ. North American Lyme neuroborreliosis. Scand J Infect Dis Suppl. 1991;77:74–80.
443. Steere AC, Pachner AR, Malawista SE. Neurologic abnormalities of Lyme disease: successful treatment with high-dose intravenous penicillin. Ann Intern Med. 1983;99:767–72.
444. Kohler J, Kasper J, Kern U, Thoden U, Rehse-Kupper B. Borrelia encephalomyelitis. Lancet. 1986;2:35.
445. Agosta F, Rocca MA, Benedetti B, Capra R, Cordioli C, Filippi M. MR imaging assessment of brain and cervical cord damage in patients with neuroborreliosis. AJNR Am J Neuroradiol. 2006;27:892–4.
446. Bigi S, Aebi C, Nauer C, Bigler S, Steinlin M. Acute transverse myelitis in Lyme neuroborreliosis. Infection. 2010;38:413–6.
447. Chang BL, Shih CM, Ro LS, et al. Acute neuroborreliosis with involvement of the central nervous system. J Neurol Sci. 2010;295:10–5.
448. Kalish RA, Kaplan RF, Taylor E, Jones-Woodward L, Workman K, Steere AC. Evaluation of study patients with Lyme disease, 10-20-year follow-up. J Infect Dis. 2001;183:453–60.
449. Pfister HW, Preac-Mursic V, Wilske B, Einhaupl KM. Cefotaxime vs penicillin G for acute neurologic manifestations in Lyme borreliosis. A prospective randomized study. Arch Neurol. 1989;46:1190–4.
450. Pfister HW, Preac-Mursic V, Wilske B, Schielke E, Sorgel F, Einhaupl KM. Randomized comparison of ceftriaxone and cefotaxime in Lyme neuroborreliosis. J Infect Dis. 1991;163:311–8.
451. Pfister HW, Rupprecht TA. Clinical aspects of neuroborreliosis and post-Lyme disease syndrome in adult patients. Int J Med Microbiol. 2006;296(Suppl 40):11–6.
452. Halperin JJ. Diagnosis and treatment of the neuromuscular manifestations of lyme disease. Curr Treat Options Neurol. 2007;9:93–100.
453. Logigian EL, Kaplan RF, Steere AC. Successful treatment of Lyme encephalopathy with intravenous ceftriaxone. J Infect Dis. 1999;180:377–83.
454. Halperin JJ, Shapiro ED, Logigian E, et al. Practice parameter: treatment of nervous system Lyme disease (an evidence-based review): report of the Quality Standards Subcommittee of the American Academy of Neurology. Neurology. 2007;69:91–102.
455. Klempner MS, Hu LT, Evans J, et al. Two controlled trials of antibiotic treatment in patients with persistent symptoms and a history of Lyme disease. N Engl J Med. 2001;345:85–92.
456. Sexton DJ, Kaye KS. Rocky mountain spotted fever. Med Clin North Am. 2002;86:351–60. vii–viii
457. Chapman AS, Bakken JS, Folk SM, et al. Diagnosis and management of tickborne rickettsial diseases: Rocky Mountain spotted fever, ehrlichioses, and anaplasmosis – United States: a practical guide for physicians and other health-care and public health professionals. MMWR Recomm Rep. 2006;55:1–27.
458. Chen LF, Sexton DJ. What's new in Rocky Mountain spotted fever? Infect Dis Clin N Am. 2008;22:415–32. vii–viii
459. Kirkland KB, Wilkinson WE, Sexton DJ. Therapeutic delay and mortality in cases of Rocky Mountain spotted fever. Clin Infect Dis. 1995;20:1118–21.
460. Archibald LK, Sexton DJ. Long-term sequelae of Rocky Mountain spotted fever. Clin Infect Dis. 1995;20:1122–5.
461. Sexton DJ, Kirkland KB. Rickettsial infections and the central nervous system. Clin Infect Dis. 1998;26:247–8.
462. Ismail N, Bloch KC, McBride JW. Human ehrlichiosis and anaplasmosis. Clin Lab Med. 2010;30:261–92.
463. Windsor JJ. Cat-scratch disease: epidemiology, aetiology and treatment. Br J Biomed Sci. 2001;58:101–10.
464. Weston KD, Tran T, Kimmel KN, Maria BL. Possible role of high-dose corticosteroids in the treatment of cat-scratch disease encephalopathy. J Child Neurol. 2001;16:762–3.
465. Genizi J, Kasis I, Schif A, Shahar E. Effect of high-dose methylprednisolone on brainstem encephalopathy and basal gan-

glia impairment complicating cat scratch disease. Brain Dev. 2007;29:377–9.
466. Schneider T, Moos V, Loddenkemper C, Marth T, Fenollar F, Raoult D. Whipple's disease: new aspects of pathogenesis and treatment. Lancet Infect Dis. 2008;8:179–90.
467. Slowik A, Szczudlik A. Whipple's disease—a rare cause of neurological symptoms and disorders. Neurol Neurochir Pol. 2002;36:959–70.
468. Relman DA, Schmidt TM, MacDermott RP, Falkow S. Identification of the uncultured bacillus of Whipple's disease. N Engl J Med. 1992;327:293–301.
469. Schoniger-Hekele M, Petermann D, Weber B, Muller C. Tropheryma whipplei in the environment: survey of sewage plant influxes and sewage plant workers. Appl Environ Microbiol. 2007;73:2033–5.
470. Moos V, Loddenkemper C, Schneider T. Tropheryma whipplei infection. Colonization, self-limiting infection and Whipple's disease. Pathologe. 2011;32:362–70.
471. Moos V, Schneider T. Changing paradigms in Whipple's disease and infection with *Tropheryma whipplei*. Eur J Clin Microbiol Infect Dis. 2011;30:1151–8.
472. Abreu P, Azevedo E, Lobo L, Moura CS, Pontes C. Whipple disease and central nervous system. Acta Medica Port. 2005;18:199–208.
473. Bermejo P, Burgos A. Whipple's disease and central nervous system. Med Clin (Barc). 2006;127:379–85.
474. Durand DV, Lecomte C, Cathebras P, Rousset H, Godeau P. Whipple disease: clinical review of 52 cases. The SNFMI Research Group on Whipple Disease. Medicine. 1997;76(3):170–84.
475. Louis ED. Whipple disease. Curr Neurol Neurosci Rep. 2003;3:470–5.
476. Louis ED, Lynch T, Kaufmann P, Fahn S, Odel J. Diagnostic guidelines in central nervous system Whipple's disease. Ann Neurol. 1996;40:561–8.
477. Scheld WM. Whipple disease of the central nervous system. J Infect Dis. 2003;188:797–800.
478. Vital Durand D, Gerard A, Rousset H. Neurological manifestations of Whipple disease. Rev Neurol. 2002;158:988–92.
479. Baisden BL, Lepidi H, Raoult D, Argani P, Yardley JH, Dumler JS. Diagnosis of Whipple disease by immunohistochemical analysis: a sensitive and specific method for the detection of Tropheryma whipplei (the Whipple bacillus) in paraffin-embedded tissue. Am J Clin Pathol. 2002;118:742–8.
480. Gerard A, Sarrot-Reynauld F, Liozon E, et al. Neurologic presentation of Whipple disease: report of 12 cases and review of the literature. Medicine. 2002;81:443–57.
481. Panegyres PK, Edis R, Beaman M, Fallon M. Primary Whipple's disease of the brain: characterization of the clinical syndrome and molecular diagnosis. QJM. 2006;99:609–23.
482. Schnider PJ, Reisinger EC, Berger T, Krejs GJ, Auff E. Treatment guidelines in central nervous system Whipple's disease. Ann Neurol. 1997;41:561–2.
483. Schnider PJ, Reisinger EC, Gerschlager W, et al. Long-term follow-up in cerebral Whipple's disease. Eur J Gastroenterol Hepatol. 1996;8:899–903.
484. Gutierrez J, Issacson RS, Koppel BS. Subacute sclerosing panencephalitis: an update. Dev Med Child Neurol. 2010;52:901–7.
485. Weissert R. Progressive multifocal leukoencephalopathy. J Neuroimmunol. 2011;231:73–7.
486. Fox R. Advances in the management of PML: focus on natalizumab. Cleve Clin J Med. 2011;78(Suppl. 2):S33–7.
487. Brooks BR, Walker DL. Progressive multifocal leukoencephalopathy. Neurol Clin. 1984;2:299–313.
488. Egli A, Infanti L, Dumoulin A, et al. Prevalence of polyomavirus BK and JC infection and replication in 400 healthy blood donors. J Infect Dis. 2009;199:837–46.
489. White FA 3rd, Ishaq M, Stoner GL, Frisque RJ. JC virus DNA is present in many human brain samples from patients without progressive multifocal leukoencephalopathy. J Virol. 1992;66:5726–34.
490. Vago L, Cinque P, Sala E, et al. JCV-DNA and BKV-DNA in the CNS tissue and CSF of AIDS patients and normal subjects. Study of 41 cases and review of the literature. J Acquir Immune Defic Syndr. 1996;12:139–46.
491. Quinlivan EB, Norris M, Bouldin TW, et al. Subclinical central nervous system infection with JC virus in patients with AIDS. J Infect Dis. 1992;166:80–5.
492. Koralnik IJ, Boden D, Mai VX, Lord CI, Letvin NL. JC virus DNA load in patients with and without progressive multifocal leukoencephalopathy. Neurology. 1999;52:253–60.
493. Ferrante P, Caldarelli-Stefano R, Omodeo-Zorini E, Vago L, Boldorini R, Costanzi G. PCR detection of JC virus DNA in brain tissue from patients with and without progressive multifocal leukoencephalopathy. J Med Virol. 1995;47:219–25.
494. Dubois V, Dutronc H, Lafon ME, et al. Latency and reactivation of JC virus in peripheral blood of human immunodeficiency virus type 1-infected patients. J Clin Microbiol. 1997;35:2288–92.
495. Holman RC, Janssen RS, Buehler JW, Zelasky MT, Hooper WC. Epidemiology of progressive multifocal leukoencephalopathy in the United States: analysis of national mortality and AIDS surveillance data. Neurology. 1991;41:1733–6.
496. Christensen KL, Holman RC, Hammett TA, Belay ED, Schonberger LB. Progressive multifocal leukoencephalopathy deaths in the USA, 1979–2005. Neuroepidemiology. 2010;35:178–84.
497. Amend KL, Turnbull B, Foskett N, Napalkov P, Kurth T, Seeger J. Incidence of progressive multifocal leukoencephalopathy in patients without HIV. Neurology. 2010;75:1326–32.
498. Focosi D, Marco T, Kast RE, Maggi F, Ceccherini-Nelli L, Petrini M. Progressive multifocal leukoencephalopathy: what's new? Neuroscientist. 2010;16:308–23.
499. Hernandez B, Dronda F, Moreno S. Treatment options for AIDS patients with progressive multifocal leukoencephalopathy. Expert Opin Pharmacother. 2009;10:403–16.
500. Lima MA, Bernal-Cano F, Clifford DB, Gandhi RT, Koralnik IJ. Clinical outcome of long-term survivors of progressive multifocal leukoencephalopathy. J Neurol Neurosurg Psychiatry. 2010;81:1288–91.
501. Tavazzi E, White MK, Khalili K. Progressive multifocal leukoencephalopathy: clinical and molecular aspects. Rev Med Virol. 2012;22:18–32.
502. Silverman L, Rubinstein LJ. Electron microscopic observations on a case of progressive multifocal leukoencephalopathy. Acta Neuropathol. 1965;5:215–24.
503. McGuire D, Barhite S, Hollander H, Miles M. JC virus DNA in cerebrospinal fluid of human immunodeficiency virus-infected patients: predictive value for progressive multifocal leukoencephalopathy. Ann Neurol. 1995;37:395–9.
504. Hammarin AL, Bogdanovic G, Svedhem V, Pirskanen R, Morfeldt L, Grandien M. Analysis of PCR as a tool for detection of JC virus DNA in cerebrospinal fluid for diagnosis of progressive multifocal leukoencephalopathy. J Clin Microbiol. 1996;34:2929–32.
505. Dorries K, Arendt G, Eggers C, Roggendorf W, Dorries R. Nucleic acid detection as a diagnostic tool in polyomavirus JC induced progressive multifocal leukoencephalopathy. J Med Virol. 1998;54:196–203.

506. Masur H, Brooks JT, Benson CA, Holmes KK, Pau AK, Kaplan JE. Prevention and treatment of opportunistic infections in HIV-infected adults and adolescents: Updated Guidelines from the Centers for Disease Control and Prevention, National Institutes of Health, and HIV Medicine Association of the Infectious Diseases Society of America. Clin Infect Dis. 2014;58(9):1308–11.
507. Mulabbi EN, Tweyongyere R, Byarugaba DK. The history of the emergence and transmission of human coronaviruses. Onderstepoort J Vet Res. 2021;88(1):e1–8.
508. Tsang K, Zhong NS. SARS: pharmacotherapy. Respirology. 2003;8(s1):S25–30.
509. Widagdo W, Okba NMA, Stalin Raj V, Haagmans BL. MERS-coronavirus: From discovery to intervention. One Health (Amsterdam, Netherlands). 2017;3:11–6.
510. Zhu N, Zhang D, Wang W, Li X, Yang B, Song J, et al. A novel coronavirus from patients with pneumonia in China, 2019. N Engl J Med. 2020;382(8):727–33.
511. Alshebri MS, Alshouimi RA, Alhumidi HA, Alshaya AI. Neurological complications of SARS-CoV, MERS-CoV, and COVID-19. SN Comp Clin Med. 2020;2(11):2037–47.
512. Wan D, Du T, Hong W, Chen L, Que H, Lu S, et al. Neurological complications and infection mechanism of SARS-COV-2. Signal Transduct Target Ther. 2021;6(1):406.
513. Mao L, Jin H, Wang M, Hu Y, Chen S, He Q, et al. Neurologic manifestations of hospitalized patients with coronavirus disease 2019 in Wuhan, China. JAMA Neurol. 2020;77(6):683–90.
514. Heneka MT, Golenbock D, Latz E, Morgan D, Brown R. Immediate and long-term consequences of COVID-19 infections for the development of neurological disease. Alzheimers Res Ther. 2020;12(1):69.
515. Siddiqui R, Khan NA. Proposed intranasal route for drug administration in the management of central nervous system manifestations of COVID-19. ACS Chem Neurosci. 2020;11(11):1523–4.
516. Carpenter RR, Petersdorf RG. The clinical spectrum of bacterial meningitis. Am J Med. 1962;33:262–75.

Status Epilepticus

32

Katherine Schwartz, Katharine R. Colton, and Thomas P. Bleck

Contents

Abstract

Status epilepticus is a neurological emergency requiring prompt recognition and management. This term describes a range of etiologies united by continuous or frequent seizures, diagnosed either clinically or electrographically. The morbidity and mortality of status epilepticus are clearly time dependent, necessitating urgent intervention. Refractory and super-refractory status epilepticus describe seizures that persist after appropriate therapy with antiseizure medications; treatment of these etiologies remains controversial and is best managed in a critical care environment.

K. Schwartz (✉)
Department of Neurology, Rosalind Franklin University of Medicine and Science, North Chicago, IL, USA
e-mail: katherine.schwartz@aah.org

K. R. Colton
Department of Neurology, Duke University School of Medicine, Durham, NC, USA

T. P. Bleck
Department of Neurology, Northwestern University Feinberg School of Medicine, Chicago, IL, USA

Introduction

Status epilepticus (SE) is a neurologic emergency commonly encountered in the intensive care unit (ICU). While the definition of SE has evolved over time, it can be broadly described as a prolonged seizure or repeated seizures without interim return to neurologic baseline. SE is associated with high morbidity and mortality, although there is wide heterogeneity between studies with mortality rates ranging from 7% to 39% in adults and < 5% in children [1–3]. A recent meta-analysis showed disappointingly little improvement in mortality over time, despite a trend toward more aggressive

E. Mahanna Gabrielli et al. (eds.), *Textbook of Neurointensive Care: Volume 1*, https://doi.org/10.1007/978-3-031-62220-5_32

protocols for treatment of SE [4]. SE is generally dichotomized into convulsive (associated with rhythmic jerking of the extremities and mental status impairment) or nonconvulsive, although there is crossover between these groups; generalized convulsive SE accounts for 45–74% of cases [1]. SE can be further classified by underlying etiology, duration, and treatment responsiveness.

Definitions

Since its early recognition as a dire complication of epilepsy, the definition of SE has evolved. In the WHO Dictionary of Epilepsy published in 1973, and mirroring the classification set out by the International League Against Epilepsy (ILAE) in 1970 and 1981, the French neurologist Henri Gastaut described SE as "a condition characterized by an epileptic seizure that is sufficiently prolonged or repeated at sufficiently brief intervals so as to produce an unvarying and enduring epileptic condition" [5]. This definition proved valuable but imprecise. A seminal study later showed irreversible neuronal injury due to excitotoxicity after 82 min of seizure activity in baboons [6], giving a pathophysiologic basis for defining SE as seizure duration of 60, and later 30 min. In 1999, Lowenstein and colleagues urged that the definition of SE be changed to 5 min in order to terminate seizures before such damage would occur [7]. The Neurocritical Care Society recommendations followed this suggestion, using 5 or more minutes of continuous seizure activity or recurrent seizures without a return to baseline, losing some specificity in favor of earlier and more aggressive treatment of prolonged seizure activity. The ILAE has proposed an operational definition, stating that SE is "a condition resulting either from the failure of the mechanisms responsible for seizure termination or from the initiation of mechanisms, which lead to abnormally prolonged seizures (after time point t1). It is a condition, which can have long-term consequences (after time-point t2), including neuronal death, neuronal injury, and alteration of neuronal networks depending on the type and duration of seizures" [8].

The ILAE's definition of SE gives us two operational dimensions—both the length of seizure that should be considered abnormally prolonged (t1) and the seizure duration with which there is increased risk of permanent neuronal damage (t2). These domains likely vary significantly between different forms of SE [convulsive versus non-convulsive (NCSE), focal, or absence]. Once defined, t1 identifies a reasonable time point at which to initiate treatment, and t2 determines how aggressively therapy should be escalated in order to reduce the risk of long-term damage.

Current recommendations from the ILAE are to define t1 and t2 in convulsive SE as 5 and 30 min, respectively [9]. Data from populations with refractory epilepsy undergoing continuous EEG monitoring showed that most convulsive seizures self-abort within 5 min [1, 8]. Studies in the pediatric general population suggest two populations of patients, one with relatively brief seizures (<5 min) and one predisposed to prolonged seizures. One study showed a threshold of 7 min as the time above which seizures were likely to be prolonged [10]. Taken with others, these studies form the background from which the ILAE Task Force made the consensus recommendation to initiate treatment of convulsive seizures at 5 min. T2 was defined in the same publication at 30 min, in line with previous definitions of SE [8]. These thresholds are yet undefined in focal or absence SE. Further, the likelihood of damage is dependent on the location of the epileptic focus, the intensity of the status, the age of the patient, and other factors [8].

As acknowledged above, the ILAE has created a framework within which different subtypes of SE can be delineated. SE with prominent motor symptoms includes convulsive SE as characterized by prominent motor symptoms and impairment of consciousness, either sustained or interrupted. Myoclonic, focal motor (including epilepsia partialis continua (EPC)), and tonic status are all characterized by prominent abnormal muscular contractions. NCSE is primarily divided into patients with or without coma. NCSE without coma includes absence status and focal status without motor symptoms—potentially involving language (aphasic status) or persistent sensory phenomena (visual, auditory, gustatory, or other experiential symptoms) [8].

Refractory SE is continuous seizure activity not adequately controlled by first- or second-line antiseizure medications (ASMs). Per guidelines published by the Neurocritical Care Society (NCS), these are appropriate doses of a benzodiazepine followed by an acceptable ASM. A third category of super-refractory SE does not have a single definition but generally refers to SE not controlled by third-line agents [11] or seizures persisting longer than 24 h after an anesthetic agent is given [12].

Etiology

Underlying etiology remains the most important prognostic factor for mortality in SE. Per the ILAE, the etiology of SE can be divided into unknown/cryptogenic or known/symptomatic, which is further broken down into acute symptomatic, remote symptomatic, and progressive symptomatic based on time course (see Table 32.1). Common underlying causes in adults include acute trauma, tumors, vascular disorders, alcohol withdrawal, and low antiseizure medication (ASM) levels (often due to missed doses). Children are more likely to suffer cryptogenic SE or from remote symptomatic causes [3].

Table 32.1 Etiologies of status epilepticus

	Causes of status epilepticus
Cryptogenic/ unknown	Undiscovered causes
Remote symptomatic	Prior insults, such as stroke or traumatic brain injury, genetic predisposition (e.g. Dravet syndrome)
Acute symptomatic	Stroke, traumatic brain injury, central nervous system infection, electrolyte imbalance, hypoxia, febrile illness, alcohol withdrawal, tumor, antiseizure medication noncompliance
Progressive	Brain tumors, progressive myoclonic epilepsies, dementia

Just over half of first episodes of SE occur in patients without a previous diagnosis of epilepsy [13]. Acute symptomatic etiologies (stroke, anoxic/hypoxic injury, and drug overdose) are more common and associated with higher morbidity and mortality than chronic etiologies [14], with underlying stroke as the most common acute etiology and anoxic injury associated with the highest mortality [1]. Chronic epilepsy with low antiseizure medication levels is the most common cause of SE among chronic or acute causes and is associated with a relatively low mortality [1].

Refractory SE appears to have similar underlying etiologies to SE, although several studies have shown it to be more commonly associated with encephalitis [15, 16], particularly of viral origin [17]. Multiple studies showed super refractory SE (SRSE) to be more commonly associated with encephalitis [15, 16, 18, 19]. In the past 15 years, the term new-onset refractory status epilepticus (NORSE) has been used to describe patients with prolonged, refractory status epilepticus without an easily identifiable etiology. In the largest retrospective analysis of NORSE cases (n = 130), half were cryptogenic and the other half included paraneoplastic and non-paraneoplastic autoimmune disease causes. Of the half with an identified cause, 37% were paraneoplastic diseases and 40% were non-paraneoplastic autoimmune diseases. Anti-NMDA receptor encephalitis was the most common cause and infectious causes comprised 16% [20].

Classification

Status epilepticus is classified based on whether the seizure is generalized (involving the entire cortex in both hemispheres) or focal (involving a portion of cortex). While generalized seizures are accompanied by impaired awareness, focal seizures may be associated with either preserved or impaired awareness. Some focal seizures evolve into generalized seizures, and these are named "focal to bilateral tonic-clonic seizures" and then classified based on the first prominent sign or symptom (motor or nonmotor). If the onset is unknown, then the seizure is named as such [21]. Epilepsia partialis continua (EPC) is a subset of focal aware motor status epilepticus (previously known as simple focal motor status) in which the patient has frequent repetitive muscle jerks that are not usually rhythmic and continue over prolonged periods of time (1 h to multiple years). EPC has many causes, which can be local or systemic, including stroke, non-ketotic hyperglycemia, Rassmussen encephalitis, Russian tick-borne spring-summer encephalitis, and mitochondrial diseases [22].

Pathophysiology

While the underlying pathophysiology of SE is multifactorial and not thoroughly understood, it can be simply stated as a failure of native mechanisms to stop seizure activity. This can result from both excessive neuronal excitation or from a loss of inhibition, allowing a single seizure to progress into SE, with its attendant self-reinforcing mechanisms. Multiple observations that prolonged (e.g. >30 min) seizures become much harder to terminate suggest a dynamic pathophysiology.

The earliest physiologic changes (within seconds) include the sequelae of protein phosphorylation, neurotransmitter release, ion channel opening and closing, and receptor desensitization [23]. Within minutes, cellular internalization of inhibitory GABA receptors and an increase in excitatory NMDA receptors potentiate abnormal excitatory activity [23]. Synaptic inhibitory receptors can become encapsulated in endosomes, or previously stored excitatory receptors can be mobilized to the synaptic membrane. Over minutes to hours, changes including alterations in excitatory (substance P) and inhibitory (neuropeptide Y) neuropeptide expression can work maladaptively to maintain a hyperexcitable state. Long-term changes in gene expression over hours to weeks after seizures can contribute to the development of epilepsy.

Changes in receptor presence on the synaptic membrane likely contribute to the well-documented progressive pharmacoresistance to benzodiazepines seen in SE. An in vivo study of an SE model in rats showed a ten-fold increase in the dose of diazepam required to halt seizures after 45 min of seizures compared to after 10 min. This effect appears to be related to GABA receptor modulation [24]. Better understanding of these mechanisms has justified aggressive clinical management guidelines in an attempt to avoid maladaptive physiologic changes.

As seizure activity continues, neurologic injury and mortality increase. Meldrum's seminal study on convulsive SE in baboons showed neuronal injury and death [25], and the animals developed systemic hypotension, hypoxia, and hyperthermia, all of which are particularly deleterious to vulnerable neurons. Later, animal models identified multiple underlying mechanisms. Mitochondrial dysfunction, apoptosis, overproduction of reactive oxygen species, and intracellular calcium accumulation have all been posited as potential mechanisms for neuronal death during and after SE. Neuron-specific enolase, a nonspecific marker of brain injury, was shown to be elevated in all major subtypes of SE [26] and has been proposed as a biomarker of ongoing seizure activity and neuronal damage [27].

Diagnosis

Since initiation of therapy for SE is emergent, convulsive SE is a clinical diagnosis, although electroencephalography (EEG) monitoring is useful to guide treatment and to detect ongoing seizure activity. High clinical suspicion is often necessary to detect NCSE in patients with unexplained or fluctuating mental status, and clinicians should consider extended EEG monitoring early in the evaluation of these often-undifferentiated patients.

Electroencephalography

EEG plays a critical role in the diagnosis and ongoing management of SE. While convulsive SE is a clinical diagnosis, NCSE can present with a nonspecific encephalopathy and can be diagnosed only with EEG monitoring.

In 2013, the American Clinical Neurophysiology Society (ACNS) published standardized terminology of patterns commonly seen in ICU EEG recordings in order to facilitate communication and research involving such patterns. These patterns include periodic discharges, rhythmic delta activity, and spike and wave or sharp and wave activity and are defined in Table 32.2. In 2021, the ACNS updated those guidelines and included definitions for seizures and status epilepticus that are shown in Table 32.3 [28].

In convulsive SE, the EEG can be obscured by muscle artifact but can show continuous, generalized spike and wave morphology. By the same ACNS guidelines as above, a time-locked clinical correlate with a repetitive EEG pattern—for instance, stereotypic periodic discharges at a lower frequency—can also be classified as SE. Clinical correlates can be subtle, including facial twitching or eye deviation.

Table 32.2 Standard EEG pattern terminology

	Definition
Periodic discharges	Repetition of a waveform with relatively uniform morphology and duration with an interdischarge interval between consecutive waveforms and recurrence of the waveform at nearly regular intervals
Rhythmic delta activity	Repetition of a waveform with relatively uniform morphology and duration and without an interval between consecutive waveforms, occurring at ≤4 Hz
Spike-and-wave or sharp-and-wave	Polyspike, spike, or sharp wave followed by a slow wave in a regularly repeating and alternating pattern, with a consistent relationship between the spike (or polyspike or sharp) component and the slow wave and no interval between one spike-wave complex and the next

Table 32.3 Definitions of seizures and status epilepticus

	Seizure	Status epilepticus
Electrographic	(a) Epileptiform discharges averaging >2.5 Hz and lasting ≥10 s or (b) any pattern with definite evolution and lasting ≥10 s	(a) Electrographic seizure lasting ≥10 continuous minutes or (b) Electrographic seizures for ≥20% of any 60-min period of recording
Electroclinical	(a) the presence of a clinical correlate time locked to an EEG pattern or (b) EEG and clinical improvement after ASM administration[a]	(a) Electroclinical seizure ≥10 min, for a total duration of ≥20% of any 60-min period or (b) ≥ 5 min of bilateral tonic-clonic activity

[a]Electroclinical seizures need not meet requirements of an electrographic seizure

Imaging

Multiple imaging modalities are employed in the evaluation and management of SE, including computed tomography (CT), magnetic resonance imaging (MRI), positron emission tomography (PET) scan, and single-photon emission CT (SPECT). Initial work-up for the etiology SE often includes a head CT to evaluate for mass lesion, stroke or intracranial hemorrhage, evidence of infection, anoxic injury, or other structural abnormalities. Consequences of SE that may be observed on CT scans include edema, loss of gray-white matter differentiation, and enhancement of the gyri . MRI imaging can show signal abnormalities resembling those seen in acute stroke, although typically in not in major vascular distributions. These can include restricted diffusion and T2 hyperintensity. These changes are commonly found in the cortex and hippocampi, although can be present in many structures including the basal ganglia, thalami, corpus callosum, and leptomeninges (with abnormal enhancement), as can be seen in image 32.1. Epilepsy-specific MRI protocols include sequences chosen to assess for underlying causative structural abnormalities including hippocampal sclerosis, cortical developmental abnormalities, and calcified lesions.

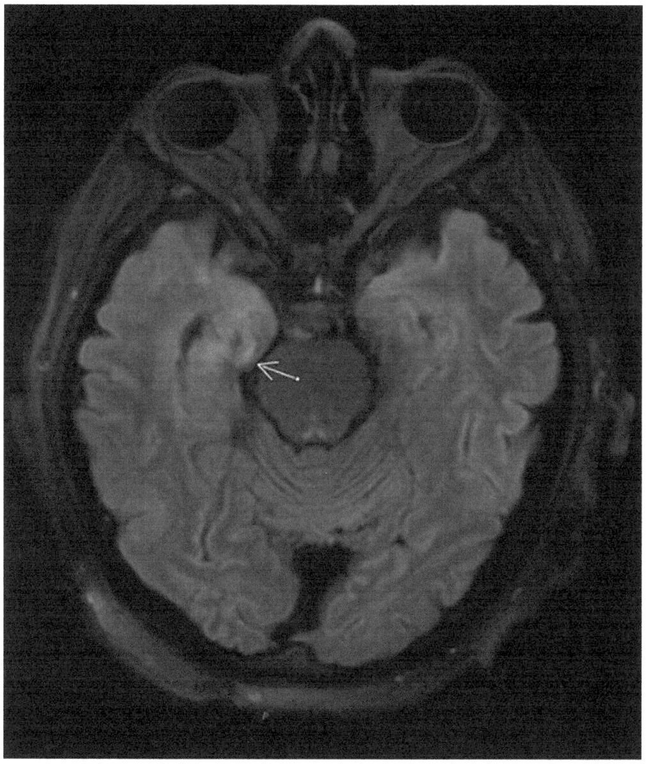

Image 32.1 An axial FLAIR sequence MRI image from a 50-year-old woman who had a prolonged seizure in the setting of hyponatremia demonstrates hyperintensity in the right hippocampus (arrow)

Treatment

Generalized convulsive status epilepticus is a medical emergency. Initial critical care begins with managing the patient's airway, either noninvasively (with options including nasal/oral airways, head positioning, supplemental oxygen), or invasively with endotracheal intubation. Many patients maintain oxygenation if supported with noninvasive means, but if intubation is required, short-acting paralytics are preferred to allow for continued assessment of ongoing clinical seizure activity. Vital signs should be continuously monitored and supported appropriately, including with fluid resuscitation or vasopressors as needed. Intravenous (IV) access should be obtained, although initial ASMs (weight-dosed benzodiazepines, generally) can be given via the intramuscular route. The RAMPART study [29] showed that intra-muscular (IM) midazolam was noninferior to IV lorazepam in equivalent doses when administered in the prehospital setting to terminate SE. In the hospital setting, IV administration is typically preferred. Abnormalities in blood glucose (more commonly hypoglycemia) should be ruled out or treated immediately, and if dextrose is needed, then thiamine should first be administered to prevent precipitous thiamine deficiency (although dextrose should never be delayed if thiamine is not readily available) [1, 28, 30]. Laboratory tests should be sent promptly and include a basic chemistry panel, a complete blood count, and ASM levels (if appropriate).

Emergent Initial Therapy

Benzodiazepines (typically lorazepam in the inpatient setting) are generally accepted as the emergent initial ASM therapy. The seminal Veterans Affairs Status Epilepticus Cooperative Study Group in 1998 showed superior efficacy of lorazepam over phenytoin as an initial abortive agent for GSE [31]. Alldredge and colleagues later published the first rigorous prehospital evaluation of the efficacy and safety of benzodiazepine use in SE and showed superiority of lorazepam and diazepam to placebo in terminating SE [32]. Despite concerns for respiratory depression with benzodiazepine administration, this study showed lower rates of respiratory compromise with the treatment groups, likely due to shorter duration of seizures. As mentioned above, the RAMPART trial later showed noninferiority of IM midazolam to IV lorazepam in prehospital seizure abortion [29]. The study design does not permit conclusion that midazolam is more effective, as the group difference may have been related to route or timing of administration.

Urgent Control Therapy

Patients presenting with SE should receive urgent second-line control therapy with an accepted ASM following administration of a short-acting benzodiazepine (first-line therapy) unless a rapidly correctable cause (i.e. hypoglycemia) is identified and addressed. This serves the dual purpose of treating the patient who has failed initial therapy and establishing therapeutic ASM levels if SE has resolved. The ESETT trial, published in 2020, compared effectiveness of three agents in terminating established SE (in patients that have failed to respond to initial benzodiazepine dosing). Patients were randomized to receive weight-based dosing of levetiracetam (60 mg/kg, maximum dose 4.5 g), fosphenytoin (20 mg/kg, maximum dose 1.5 g), or valproic acid (40 mg/kg, maximum dose 3 g). There were no significant differences in the primary outcome (absence of clinically apparent seizures and improving responsiveness at 60 min) or secondary outcomes (ICU admission or safety outcomes), and the trial was stopped early after meeting predetermined futility criteria [33]. The study found no difference in the primary efficacy outcome between the different drugs in pediatric, adult, or older adults (aged >65 years).

Other agents studied for use in urgent control in SE include phenytoin, phenobarbital, lacosamide, and infusion of midazolam [34]. Since the publication of ESETT, the use of levetiracetam as a second-line agent has been increasing due to tolerability and relatively few drug–drug interactions. In the ESETT trial, leveteracitam was administered as a 15 min infusion, but several recent studies have suggested more rapid infusion or IV push dosing is safe [35, 36]. In patients chronically established on a different commonly used medication, it is reasonable to provide an IV bolus of that medication to ensure a therapeutic level and to administer another medication to establish seizure control. It can be expected that each subsequent agent is less likely to control SE.

Treatment of Refractory SE and Super-Refractory SE

Once seizures persist beyond 60 min with adequate treatment of a benzodiazepine (first-line therapy) and an appropriate parenteral ASM (second-line therapy), a patient is in RSE [3]. A substantial minority of patients in SE will progress to RSE (published studies report progression rates of 23–43%) [1, 2, 15, 16, 37]. SE that persists despite the addition of an anesthetic agent is termed super-refractory SE (SRSE). Additional treatment might include repeat bolus dosing of the second-line ASM, additional agents, or the initiation of a continuous ASM at anesthetic dosing. These are insufficient data to guide choice of therapy or an optimal therapeutic target (extent of seizure suppression) for treatment of RSE. One study showed improved functional outcome after a treatment was targeted toward electrographic seizure suppression, rather than an isoelectric background or burst suppression [38].

When convulsive SE lasts for >30 min, the patient should be intubated and mechanically ventilated, a continuous anesthetic agent should be started, and the patient should be admitted or transferred to an ICU with continuous EEG capabilities. Once started, these agents are typically not weaned before 24–48 h, but there has been no definitive trial to guide this timing. Commonly used agents include propofol, midazolam, pentobarbital, and ketamine. Pentobarbital, midazolam, and propofol are GABA agonists, whereas ketamine and propofol are NMDA antagonists. They are all hepatically metabolized. Choice of agent is again made on a case-by-case basis, taking into account underlying etiology, patient characteristics, drug interactions, and hemodynamic stability.

Propofol is commonly used in the ICU population and is often readily available. It is a highly lipophilic phenol derivative unrelated to any other anesthetic agents. A loading dose of 1–2 mg/kg is given and can be repeated up to a total dose of 10 mg/kg, after which a continuous infusion is started. Propofol titration may be limited by dose-dependent hypotension that frequently necessitates volume resuscitation or vasopressor use. At higher doses and with prolonged use (in adults), propofol can be associated with the propofol-related infusion syndrome (PRIS), a constellation of hemodynamic collapse, severe metabolic acidosis, renal failure, hypertriglyceridemia, and rhabdomyolysis. PRIS is more common in children, leading many to avoid or minimize the use of propofol in pediatric SE.

Midazolam is a rapid-acting benzodiazepine preferred over lorazepam infusion due to concern with propylene glycol toxicity associated with the latter at the high doses required for SE treatment. It is initiated with bolus dosing of 0.2 mg/kg that can be repeated and followed by an infusion of up to 3 mg/kg/h. It is less likely to cause hemodynamic instability than a barbiturate or propofol but may cause hypotension at high doses. It is commonly associated with tachyphylaxis, which would require rapid dose escalation. When infused for days, its metabolism slows and its half-life lengthens beyond the initial 1–4 h.

Pentobarbital (or thiopental, outside of the US) has a long history of use in SE, and there is older data to suggest less treatment failure with pentobarbital compared to midazolam or propofol [39]. Pentobarbital is administered with loading dosing of 5 mg/kg, with additional boluses and a continuous infusion of 1–5 mg/kg/h. Hypotension requiring vasopressor use is nearly universal, and patients are at high risk of associated complications including ileus, pneumonia, and hepatotoxicity. The very long half-life of pentobarbital predisposes patients to prolonged sedation (extremely delayed emergence). Pentobarbital, or intermittent dosing of phenobarbital, is commonly used as a salvage therapy in patients with recurrent seizures during an anesthetic wean.

Ketamine is an NMDA antagonist that has gained traction in the literature as a viable agent for cessation of RSE, although it has yet to be studied in a prospective trial. As SE progresses, receptor trafficking results in internalization of synaptic GABA receptors and upregulation of NMDA receptors. A retrospective study published in 2020 examined seizure burden in the 24 h after initiation of ketamine for SRSE; authors found that 63% of patients had complete seizure cessation within 24 h, and another 18% showed at least 50% reduction in total seizure burden [40]. Its use was associated with reduced vasopressor requirements in the days following initiation, and no effect was seen on cerebral blood flow, cerebral perfusion pressure, or intracranial pressure. Ketamine can be loaded at a dose of 2 mg/kg (similar to a dissociative or intubating dose) followed by an infusion of approximately 1.5–10 mg/kg/h and is ideally titrated to an EEG endpoint.

Other adjunctive medications can be added as needed with the goal of electrographic seizure suppression. Lacosamide, perampanel, clobazam, topiramate, and brivaracetam have all been studied and found to have varying degrees of efficacy in RSE/SRSE.

Alternative therapies can and should be considered in patients with SRSE. In SE with an underlying autoimmune etiology, immunomodulatory therapy has been attempted with varying success. Plasma exchange, IV immunoglobulin, and steroids can all be considered after infection is excluded. Neurosurgical consultation can be considered if a seizure focus can be identified and is amenable to surgical resection. The ketogenic diet is a logistically challenging but medically promising intervention extrapolated from pediatric literature. Therapeutic hypothermia has been attempted as a treatment for RSE/SRSE, although a well-powered trial in 2016 showed no improvement in outcome at 90 days in patients treated with standard care or standard care plus hypothermia for 24 h. Some centers will use inhaled anesthetics in patients who have persistent electrographic seizures despite parenteral anesthetic administration, although evidence to support his approach is lacking.

Treatment of Focal Motor and Nonconvulsive SE

The optimal treatment of non-convulsive status epilepticus is less well defined owing to a paucity of data, but some important considerations are worth highlighting. Unlike generalized convulsive status epilepticus, most forms of non-convulsive status epilepticus are not associated with life-threatening systemic dysfunction and are therefore perceived as less of a medical emergency. The initial treatment of non-convulsive status epilepticus, including focal status epilepticus with dyscognitive features (previously known as complex partial status epilepticus), focal status epilepticus without dyscognitive features (previously known as simple partial status epilepticus), and absence status epilepticus, is similar to generalized convulsive status epilepticus and begins with benzodiazepines. If seizure activity persists, a repeat dose of benzodiazepines should be considered, followed by an ASM. For most forms of non-convulsive status epilepticus that persist after treatment with benzodiazepines and an antiseizure medication, additional trials of antiseizure medications are often preferred rather than early escalation to anesthetics.

Epilepsia partialis continua (EPC) is another subset of status epilepticus that has some additional considerations. Treatment should take into account the etiology of the seizures. However, in general, EPC tends to be drug resistant. Epilepsy surgery is often indicated in Rasmussen encephalitis [22].

References

1. Betjemann JP, Lowenstein DH. Status epilepticus in adults. Lancet Neurol. 2015;14:615–24.
2. Novy J, Logroscino G, Rossetti AO. Refractory status epilepticus: a prospective observational study. Epilepsia. 2010;51(2):251–6.
3. Seinfeld S, Goodkin HP, Shinnar S. Status epilepticus. Cold Spring Harbor Perspective in Medicine. 2016;6:1–12.
4. Neligan A, Noyce AJ, Gosavi TD, Shorvon SD, Köhler S, Walker MC. Change in mortality of generalized convulsive status epilepticus in high-income countries over time: a systematic review and meta-analysis. JAMA Neurol. 2019;76(8):897–905. https://doi.org/10.1001/jamaneurol.2019.1268.
5. Gastaut H. Epileptic seizure. Developmental Medicine and Child Neurology. 1973;15(5):688–9.
6. Meldrum BS, Horton RW. Physiology of status epilepticus in primates. Arch Neurol. 1973;28(1):1–9.
7. Lowenstein DH, Bleck T, Macdonald RL. It's time to revise the definition of status epilepticus. Epilepsia. 1999;40:120–2.
8. Trinka E, Cock H, Hesdorffer D, et al. A definition and classification of status epilepticus–report of the ILAE task force on classification of status epilepticus. Epilepsia. 2015;56(10):1515–23.
9. Cock HR, Coles LD, Elm J, et al. Lessons from the established status epilepticus treatment trial. Epilepsy Behav. 2020;101(pt B):106296.
10. Shinnar S, Berg AT, Moshe SL, Sinnar R. How long do new-onset seizures in children last. Ann Neurol. 2001;49(5):659–64.
11. Reznik ME, Berger K, Claassen J. Comparison of intravenous anesthetic agents for the treatment of refractory status epilepticus. J Clin Med. 2016;5(5):E54. https://doi.org/10.3390/jcm5050054
12. Kantanen AM, Reinikainen M, Parviainen I, et al. Incidence and mortality of super-refractory status epilepticus in adults. Epilepsy Behav. 2015;49:131–4. https://doi.org/10.1016/j.yebeh.2015.04.065.

13. Hesdorffer DC, Logroscino G, Cascino G, Annegers JF, Hauser WA. Incidence of status epilepticus in Rochester, Minnesota, 1965–1984. Neurology. 1998;50:735–41.
14. Coeytaux A, Jallon P, Galobardes B, Morabia A. Incidence of status epilepticus in French-speaking Switzerland: (EPISTAR). Neurology. 2000;55:693–7.
15. Holtkamp M, Othman J, Buchheim K, Meierkord H. Predictors of refractory status epilepticus treater in a neurological intensive care unit. J Neurol Neurosurg Psychiatry. 2005a;76(4):534–9.
16. Holtkamp M, Othman J, Buchheim K, et al. A "malignant" variant of status epilepticus. Arch Neurol. 2005b;62(9):1428–31. https://doi.org/10.1001/archneur.62.9.1428.
17. Vooturi S, Jayalakshmi S, Sahu S, Mohandas S. Prognosis and predictors of outcome of refractory generalized convulsive status epilepticus in adults treated in neurointensive care unit. Clin Neurol Neurosurg. 2014;126:7–10. https://doi.org/10.1016/j.clineuro.2014.07.038.
18. Jayalakshmi S, Ruikar D, Vooturi S, et al. Determinants and predictors of outcome in super refractory status epilepticus—a developing country perspective. Epilepsy Res. 2014;108(9):1609–17. https://doi.org/10.1016/j.eplepsyres.2014.08.010.
19. Tian L, Li Y, Xue X, et al. Super-refractory status epilepticus in West China. Acta Neurol Scand. 2015;132(1):1–6. https://doi.org/10.1111/ane.12336.
20. Gaspard N, Foreman BP, Alvarez V, et al. New onset refractory status epilepticus. Neurology. 2015;85(18):1604–13.
21. Fisher RS, Cross JH, D'Souza C, et al. Instruction manual for the ILAE 2017 operational classification of seizure types. Epilepsia. 2017;58(4):531–42.
22. Mameniskiene R, Wolf P. Epilepsia partialis continua: a review. Seizure. 2017;44:74–80.
23. Chen JW, Wasterlain CG. Status epilepticus: pathophysiology and management in adults. Lancet Neurol. 2006;5(3):246–56.
24. Kapur J, Macdonald RL. Rapid seizure-induced reduction of benzodiazepine and Zn2+ sensitivity of hippocampal dentate granule cell GABAA receptors. Journal of Neuroscience. 1997;17(19):7532–40.
25. Meldrum BS, Vigouroux RA, Brierley JB. Systemic factors and epileptic brain damage. Prolonged seizures in paralyzed, artificially ventilated baboons. Arch Neurol. 1973;29(2):82–7.
26. DeGiorgio CM, Heck CN, Rabinowicz AL, Gott PS, Smith T, Correale J. Serum neuron-specific enolase in the major subtypes of status epilepticus. Neurology. 1999;52(4):746–9. https://doi.org/10.1212/wnl.52.4.746.
27. Hanin A, Demeret S, Denis JA, Nguyen-Michel VH, Rohaut B, Marois C, Imbert-Bismut F, Bonnefont-Rousselot D, Levy P, Navarro V, Lambrecq V. Serum neuron-specific enolase: a new tool for seizure risk monitoring after status epilepticus. Eur J Neurol. 2021;29(3):883–9. https://doi.org/10.1111/ene.15154.
28. Hirsch LJ, Fong MWK, Leitinger M, et al. American clinical neurophysiology society's standardized critical care EEG terminology: 2021 version. J Clin Neurophysiol. 2021;38(1):1–29.
29. Silbergleit R, Lowenstein D, Durkalski V, et al. RAMPART (rapid anticonvulsant medication prior to arrival trial): a double-blind randomized clinical trial of the efficacy of intramuscular midazolam versus intravenous lorazepam in the prehospital treatment of status epilepticus by paramedics. Epilepsia. 2011;52(suppl. 8):45–57.
30. Working Group on Status Epilepticus. Treatment of convulsive status epilepticus: recommendations of the epilepsy foundation of America's working group on status epilepticus. JAMA. 1993;21370:854–9.
31. Treiman DM, Meyers PD, Walton NY, et al. A comparison of four treatments for generalized convulsive status epilepticus. NEJM. 1998;339:792–8.
32. Alldredge BK, Gelb AM, et al. A comparison of lorazepam, diazepam, and placebo for the treatment of out-of- hospital status epilepticus. N Engl J Med. 2001;345(9):631–7.
33. Chamberlain JM, Kapur J, Shinnar S, et al. Efficacy of levetiracetam, fosphenytoin, and valproate for established status epilepticus by age group (ESETT): a double-blind, responsive-adaptive, randomized controlled trial. Lancet. 2020;395:1217–24.
34. Yasiry Z, Shorvon SD. The relative effectiveness of five antiepileptic drugs in treatment of benzodiazepine-resistant convulsive status epilepticus: a meta-analysis of published studies. Seizure. 2014;23(3):167–74. https://doi.org/10.1016/j.seizure.2013.12.007.
35. Haller JT, Bonnin S, Radosevich J. Rapid administration of undiluted intravenous levetiracetam. Epilepsia. 2021 Aug;62(8):1865–70. https://doi.org/10.1111/epi.16961.
36. Morgan O, Medenwald B. Safety and tolerability of rapid administration undiluted Levetiracetam. Neurocrit Care. 2020 Feb;32(1):131–4. https://doi.org/10.1007/s12028-019-00708-5.
37. Mayer SA, Claassen J, Lokin J, et al. Refractory status epilepticus: frequency, risk factors, and impact on outcome. Arch Neurol. 2002;59:205–10.
38. Hocker SE, Britton JW, Mandrekar JN. Predictors of outcome in refractory status epilepticus. JAMA Neurol. 2013;70(1):72–7.
39. Claassen J, Hirsch LJ, Emerson RJ, Mayer SA. Treatment of refractory status epilepticus with pentobarbital, propofol, or midazolam: a systematic review. Epilepsia. 2002;43(2):146–53.
40. Alkhachroum A, Der-Nigoghossian CA, Mathews E, Massad N, Letchinger R, Doyle K, Chiu WT, Kromm J, Rubinos C, Velazquez A, Roh D, Agarwal S, Park S, Connolly ES, Claassen J. Ketamine to treat super-refractory status epilepticus. Neurology. 2020;95(16):e2286–94.

Neuromuscular Disorders

33

Starane Shepherd, Ryan Jones, Uttara Koul, and Caitlin Radnis

Contents

S. Shepherd (✉)
Department of Neurology, Piedmont Atlanta Hospital, Atlanta, GA, USA

R. Jones
Department of Neurosurgery, Lenox Hill Hospital, New York, NY, USA

U. Koul · C. Radnis
Department of Neurology, Rush University Medical Center, Chicago, IL, USA

E. Mahanna Gabrielli et al. (eds.), *Textbook of Neurointensive Care: Volume 1*, https://doi.org/10.1007/978-3-031-62220-5_33

Abstract

Neuromuscular diseases, as an admitting diagnosis, can present with life-threatening symptoms requiring admission to the intensive care unit (ICU). This chapter provides an overview of the main neuromuscular diseases that may be seen in the ICU. The discussion includes an examination of the epidemiology, pathophysiology, clinical presentation, diagnostic evaluation, and management of each disease. A thorough understanding of these conditions is essential for the neurologist and critical care clinician in order to diagnose, treat, and manage patients effectively and minimize complications. Herein, we provide a comprehensive resource, highlighting the key aspects of each disease and providing the latest evidence-based recommendations for their management in the ICU setting.

Introduction

As critical care clinicians, a portion of our patients will present with various forms of neuromuscular disease, ranging from autoimmune-mediated disorders such as myasthenia gravis to toxin-mediated conditions like botulism.

Understanding these complex disorders, their diagnosis, and appropriate treatment can be the key to improving patient outcomes and reducing morbidity and mortality in the intensive care unit (ICU).

In this chapter, we will delve into the intricacies of six specific neuromuscular diseases: Myasthenia gravis, Guillain-Barré syndrome, Lambert-Eaton myasthenic syndrome, ALS, ICU-acquired weakness, and botulism. We will examine the pathophysiology, clinical presentation, diagnostic approach, and management strategies of these conditions that may present in the ICU.

Myasthenia Gravis

Myasthenia gravis (MG) is an autoimmune disease caused by antibodies that interfere with neurotransmission at the motor end plate. While a thorough discussion of the incidence of these antibodies is beyond the scope of this chapter, in short, the most common antibodies associated with MG are those targeting the acetylcholine receptor (AChR), muscle-specific kinase (MuSK), and low-density lipoprotein receptor-related protein 4 (LRP-4). Seronegative MG is a known clinical entity and is thought to be the result of currently undiscovered autoantibodies.

Clinical presentation of MG can vary, but includes proximal limb weakness, diplopia, ptosis, dysarthria, dysphagia, inability to maintain a sustained upgaze, palatal and bulbar weakness resulting in a weak cough and dysphonia, and neck extensor and flexor weakness. The differential diagnoses in patients with new onset of neuromuscular failure includes Lambert-Eaton Myasthenic Syndrome, Guillain-Barre syndrome, and tick paralysis, among others [1]. In patients with known MG, it can be difficult to differentiate between exacerbation of symptoms due to MG versus a cholinergic crisis, precipitated by the patient's maintenance medication (pyridostigmine). However, cholinergic crises are rare and are more likely to occur as a result of organophosphate poisoning.

Many medications are known to worsen MG, some of which include magnesium sulfate or citrate, beta-blockers, calcium channel blockers, aminoglycosides, fluoroquinolones, and iodinated contrast agents [1]. Other drugs are known to cause de novo MG or MG-like symptoms, such as immune checkpoint inhibitors, D-penicillamine, and statins [2].

A myasthenic crisis (MC) is defined as a MG exacerbation severe enough to compromise respiratory status. Within 2 years of diagnosis, 15–20% of patients with MG will develop a life-threatening crisis [3–7]. The mortality rate has fallen from 62% in the early 1960s to 4–10% due to improved ICU management and therapies such as intravenous immunoglobulins (IVIg) and plasmapheresis (PE) [6, 8, 9]. Symptoms suggestive of an impending myasthenic crisis include paradoxical breathing pattern and staccato speech (inability to speak full sentences with one breath) [8] and are the result of worsening bulbar, diaphragmatic, and accessory breathing muscle weakness. The risk of developing a myasthenic crisis is greater in patients exhibiting oropharyngeal weakness [1, 6, 10].

Causes of MC can be unknown at the time of presentation, but can be preceded by infection (e.g., nonspecific upper respiratory infection, pneumonia, sepsis), pregnancy, and postoperative status [1].

Immediate Management

As with all patients, the primary survey is of utmost importance in patients admitted to the neurocritical care unit for MC, with particular attention to airway compromise. Oxygen saturation can be normal as hypoxemia is typically a late presentation of MC, after tachypnea and hypercarbia. The most significant contributors to airway compromise in those with neuromuscular respiratory failure are inspiratory and expiratory muscle weakness and airway compromise [11–14]. An assessment of the patient's neck muscle weakness, extensor more than flexor, and bulbar function is a helpful surrogate measure of diaphragmatic muscle weakness, and the ability to maintain airway patency, respectively. Single breath count test has been shown to have significant correlation with forced vital capacity, negative inspiratory force, and neck flexor strength [15].

If the decision is made to intubate, the neuromuscular blocking agent should be chosen with great consideration. Succinylcholine requires approximately 2.5 times standard dosing, while non-depolarizing agents will have prolonged duration in patients with myasthenia [16, 17]. Prolonged need for intubation and mechanical ventilation is not uncommon and can lead to further complications. One multicenter retrospective study yielded a mean duration of mechanical ventilation of 12 days [18].

Long-Term Clinical Course

First-line therapies for MC are IVIg (0.4 g/kg/day given over 5 days or less) and PE, usually for a total of five exchanges. These therapies are equally effective in the treatment of myasthenic crisis/relapse, but PE is more rapid in its effect than IVIg [19]. Although PE has been shown to be more rapid in onset, it carries the inherent risks of placing a hemodialysis central venous catheter, hemodynamic instability, and increased risk of infection. Risks of IVIg include allergic reaction, thrombotic events, and hypervolemia in patients predisposed to fluid overload.

It is important to identify the appropriate situation to continue pyridostigmine or other cholinomimetics as they may exacerbate bronchial secretions, further worsening an already tenuous clinical status of a patient in crisis. As such, it is usually standard to discontinue this medication until clinical improvement has been achieved [19]. It is often restarted at a dose of 30 mg orally every 3–4 h [1, 20].

Initiation of corticosteroids while the patient is clinically improving might seem counterintuitive, as there can be transient worsening of symptoms during the first 2 weeks of steroid initiation [21, 22]. However, this effect is thought to be counteracted in those currently receiving IVIg or PE and best initiated while the patient is already under close monitoring. Corticosteroids may take 2–4 months to take effect, and as such, early initiation may also reduce the likelihood of another crisis [19].

Early initiation of rituximab, particularly in anti-MuSK myasthenia gravis patients, should be considered in patients showing no improvement (i.e., inability to be weaned from the ventilator) after administration of immunotherapy. It should be noted that rituximab is contraindicated in pregnancy and can greatly increase risk of infection [19, 22, 23]. A promising novel treatment is eculizumab, a C5 complement inhibitor, studied in AChR-positive patients in the REGAIN trial. Though it did not demonstrate significant differences in the primary endpoint of disability, it did show benefit on quality of life for 52 weeks [24–26].

Endotracheal extubation failure is common and has been shown to lead to prolonged mechanical ventilation, ICU, and hospital length of stay and a higher incidence of ventilator-associated pneumonia [18, 27–29]. Early tracheostomy placement after less than 10 days of mechanical ventilation has been shown to lead to a significant decrease in duration of mechanical ventilation, ICU, and hospital length of stays. However, in one study, those who received early tracheostomy placement had a higher number of comorbidities [7]. If the decision is made to commit a patient to early tracheostomy placement, it is helpful to identify factors that might predict the need for prolonged ventilation such as age or degree of respiratory muscle weakness [6, 30]. A study by Seneviratne et al. showed that the strongest predictor of extubation failure is atelectasis [28].

There are no guidelines on the decision as to when or how to extubate. If able to tolerate minimal sedation, it is the authors' experience that patients with MC are able to follow commands for a reliable focused neurological exam. An improvement in bulbar and neck muscle strength should accompany the patient's improvement in respiratory status, and if not, extubation failure is more likely to occur [15]. Extubation is often preceded by a spontaneous breathing trial with minimal ventilatory settings. However, a systematic literature review yielded no eligible studies that compared weaning protocols, whether it be with pressure support, T-piece, or various modes of mechanical ventilation [11].

Near Misses

A significant number of patients (15–20%) with newly diagnosed MG will develop a life-threatening crisis [3–7]. Those who have MC as their initial presentation can be a particular challenge, as diagnosis can be confused with other neurological diseases. A careful history should be obtained with attention to certain details, including preceding illness, personal or family history of concurrent autoimmune disease, and episodes of unexplained muscle fatigue, particularly in the latter half of the day.

Key Monitoring

Trending pulmonary tests initially every 2 h may be useful. A forced vital capacity (FVC) of <10–20 mL/kg and maximal inspiratory pressure (MIP) < 20–30 cm H_2O are concerning. However, the patient's clinical status should supersede these objective values as they were derived from studies in patients with Guillain Barre Syndrome, not MG [30–33]. Because the value of bedside pulmonary function tests has not been well elucidated, the clinician should have a low threshold to initiate non-invasive ventilation with BiPAP prior to the onset of hypercarbia [27, 34]. A retrospective cohort study found that 14 out of 24 patients with MC initially treated with BiPAP avoided intubation [31, 35]. Another study by Rabinstein and Wijdicks found similar results in 7 of 11 patients treated with BiPAP [31, 36]. Hypercarbia with a $PaCO_2$ > 45 and 50, predicted failure of NIV in each study, respectively.

Take Home Message

Myasthenic crisis (MC) is defined as a MG exacerbation severe enough that the patient's respiratory status is compromised. A significant fraction of those with newly diagnosed MG will suffer from a MC within 2 years of their initial diagnosis. Of utmost importance is monitoring the patient's airway and respiratory strength, which should be done with examination of bulbar function, looking for signs of accessory respiratory muscle use, and assessing neck flexor and extensor strength. Monitoring PFTs should not supersede clinical assessment as there may be waxing and waning symptoms throughout the day. A trial of NIPPV may help avoid the need for intubation, particularly if the patient is not already hypercarbic. For acute treatment, IVIg or PE may be used, but it is generally accepted that PE is faster in time to recovery. Initiation of corticosteroids and pyridostigmine is reasonable when the patient is clinically improving, as the beneficial effects of IVIg and PE will eventually wane over the following weeks. Extubation failure is common, and limited data indicate that early tracheostomy may be of some benefit. Finally, there is a fair amount of ongoing clinical and basic science research aimed at predicting the need for intubation, establishing parameters for extubation, discovery of associated diseases and new therapeutic targets.

Guillain-Barre Syndrome

Guillain-Barré syndrome (GBS) is an acute, monophasic polyradiculoneuropathy that is immune mediated and typically manifests as ascending paralysis and areflexia [37]. Early diagnosis is critical, as it is the second most common cause of rapidly progressive neuromuscular respiratory failure seen in the ICU; accounting for just under 15% of these cases after myasthenia gravis. Annual incidence of GBS is 0.81–1.89 cases (median, 1.11) per 100,000 persons worldwide. GBS has a mortality of roughly 2.6–2.8% in the ICU environment and 10% are left with severe disability [24, 37].

GBS is a consequence of immune mediated destruction of myelin with or without secondary axonal injury involving T cell and macrophage infiltrates [38].

Several antecedent infections are implicated. The most notable is *Campylobacter jejuni*. Significant molecular mimicry exists between the glycan present on lipo-oligosaccharides of this bacteria and the neuronal membrane gangliosides GM1 and GD1a, which are implicated in acute motor axonal neuropathy (AMAN), a variant of GBS [37].

Other infections that can be responsible include Epstein-Barr virus, Cytomegalovirus (anti-GM2), *Mycoplasma pneumoniae*, Influenza A, *Haemophilus influenzae*, severe acute respiratory syndrome coronavirus 2 (SARS-CoV-2), Zika virus, and very rarely HIV [37]. The antigens from these infectious agents cause an early humoral and a later cell-mediated attack on myelin [39]. The specific neuronal membrane ganglioside GQ1b (found in ocular motor nerves and in the brainstem) is the target in the Miller Fisher variant of GBS. Major surgery can also trigger GBS, although the mechanism remains unclear.

Clinical Presentation

Almost two-thirds of GBS cases have a prodromal upper respiratory tract or gastrointestinal tract infection in the 4 weeks before symptom onset. Poorly characterized crampy pain and paresthesias in buttocks, thighs, and back are often described by patients; however, objective sensation is preserved. This is followed by acute to subacute onset, rapidly progressive ascending paralysis. This often starts in the proximal legs and ultimately can progress to involve the arms, diaphragm, and cranial nerves. Facial and bulbar weakness happens in about half the patients and may sometimes present before limb weakness, confusing the clinical picture and raising incorrect suspicion for myasthenia gravis or botulism [38, 39]. Weakness peaks in about 3 weeks and should not progress beyond 4 weeks. Additional progression beyond 4 weeks should raise concern for an alternative diagnosis, such as chronic inflammatory demyelinating polyradiculoneuropathy (CIDP). Hyporeflexia or areflexia is characteristic in GBS and CIDP.

Dysautonomia in GBS is very common and indicates more severe involvement of the peripheral nervous system. This can take the form of fixed tachycardia (most common), orthostasis, hypertension (fixed or labile), abnormal sweating, ileus, incontinence, urinary retention, and diarrhea [39]. One study of 187 patients found at least 38% patients with at least one manifestation of dysautonomia. Quadriparesis, bulbar and neck flexor weakness, and mechanical ventilation were associated with dysautonomia. Mortality was 6% in patients with autonomic dysfunction versus 2% in the entire cohort ($P = 0.02$) [40]. Fatal arrhythmias (ventricular tachyarrhythmias, heart block, and asystole) are well illustrated in numerous case reports and necessitate the need for early recognition and potential cardiac pacing in the ICU [41, 42].

Early/Immediate Management

When establishing a diagnosis in a suspected patient, the following diagnostic criteria (Table 33.1) enlisted by NINDS can be helpful [43]:

The diagnosis of GBS is primarily clinical. Supportive studies include CSF analysis showing albuminocytological dissociation, nerve conduction studies and EMG, and antibody testing. Delayed F responses may be the first sign on EMG; however, it may be normal in the hyperacute phase. Spinal imaging should be done in the setting of hyperacute onset of symptoms, a definite sensory level, or hyperreflexia, or when the weakness is asymmetric. MRI of the spine with gadolinium can be helpful to view enhancement of the nerve roots, but is nonspecific [37].

Table 33.1 Diagnosis of GBS

Features required for diagnosis:-
Progressive bilateral weakness of arms and legs
Absent or decreased tendon reflexes in affected limbs
Features that strongly support diagnosis:-
Progresses from days to 4 weeks (usually <2 weeks)
Relative symmetry of symptoms and signs
Sensory symptoms are relatively mild
Cranial nerve involvement, especially bilateral facial palsy
Autonomic dysfunction
Muscular or radicular back or limb pain
Increased protein level in CSF; normal protein levels do not rule out the diagnosis
Electrodiagnostic features of motor or sensorimotor neuropathy
Features that cast doubt on diagnosis:-
Increased numbers of mononuclear or polymorphonuclear cells in CSF
Marked persistent asymmetry of weakness
Bladder or bowel dysfunction at onset or persistent during disease course
Severe respiratory dysfunction with limited limb weakness at onset
Sensory signs with limited weakness at onset
Fever at onset
Nadir <24 h
Sharp sensory level indicating spinal cord injury
Hyperreflexia or clonus
Extensor plantar responses
Abdominal pain
Slow progression with limited weakness without respiratory involvement
Alteration of consciousness

Key Monitoring

Once a diagnosis has been made, treatment is initiated in a timely manner. A substantial number of these patients develop neuromuscular respiratory failure [24]. Predictors for ICU admission and need for mechanical ventilation include:

1. Exam based: inability to cough, inability to stand, inability to lift the elbows or head.
2. Dysautonomia.
3. Shorter time to peak of illness (rapid progressor): < 7 days.
4. Impending respiratory failure:
   (a) Forced vital capacity (FVC) < 20 mL/kg.
   (b) Decrease in baseline vital capacity by 30%.
   (c) Maximum inspiratory pressure (MIP) < 30 cm H_2O.
   (d) Maximum expiratory pressure (MEP) < 40 cm H_2O.

This is often referred to as the 20/30/40 rule [24].

Treatment Pearls

GBS patients may have hypercarbia and hypoxemia late so oxygen saturation monitoring is not often helpful. Some may exhibit a paradoxical breathing pattern. GBS patients should be intubated rather than treated with noninvasive ventilation, as the respiratory failure is unlikely to reverse quickly. Noninvasive ventilation also poses a high risk for aspiration if they have bulbar weakness [44].

Therapeutic Modalities

Currently, IVIg (intravenous immunoglobulin) and PE (plasma exchange) are used to treat up to 92% of GBS patients in the United States [45]. PE was the first proven immunotherapy for GBS, followed by IVIg. Both treatments, when administered to non-ambulatory patients, are proven to be effective at reducing the length of time patients require mechanical ventilation and also lead to faster recovery [37]. However, little evidence supports their use in patients with mild GBS.

Long Term Clinical Course

Some physicians have tried a second round of IVIG in cases that continue to deteriorate or experience fluctuations of symptoms after the initial dose. However, this has not been corroborated in treatment trials and is not a standard of care. Also, combination therapy, such as plasma exchange followed by IVIg, is not known to be more effective than monotherapy [37]. There is no role for corticosteroids.

Poor prognostic factors for recovery include axonal variant, old age, rapid onset of weakness, dysautonomia, prolonged mechanical ventilation, and insufficient rehabilitation after discharge.

Goals-of-care discussions should be initiated discussing the potential need for early tracheostomy in patients with severe weakness. This may be a short-term measure until recovery over weeks to months. Some predictors of prolonged mechanical ventilation include the inability to lift the arms at 1 week and evidence of axonal degeneration, as seen in AMAN [44].

Near Misses

Table 33.2 demonstrates alternate diagnoses that should be ruled out.

Table 33.2 Alternative diagnoses of neuromuscular weakness to consider in acute neuromuscular weakness

Central nervous system pathologies: 1. Brainstem infection or inflammation (sarcoidosis, Sjogrens, neuromyelitis optica or myelin oligodendrocyte glycoprotein antibody-associated disorder, Bickerstaff encephalitis) 2. Brainstem ischemia or compression 3. Acute transverse myelitis 4. Leptomeningeal carcinomatosis in the base of the brain
Anterior horn cell pathologies: 1. Acute flaccid paraparesis (as a result of polio, enterovirus D68 or A71, West Nile virus, Japanese encephalitis virus, or rabies virus)
Nerve root pathologies: 1. Polyradiculopathy from infections (Lyme disease, cytomegalovirus, HIV, Epstein–Barr virus or varicella zoster virus) 2. Compression (cauda equina) 3. Leptomeningeal spread to nerve roots from malignancies, neurolymphomatosis
Peripheral nerve pathologies: 1. CIDP 2. Vitamin B1, B12, E, and copper deficiencies 3. Toxins (drugs, alcohol, vitamin B6, lead, thallium, arsenic, organophosphate, ethylene glycol, diethylene glycol, methanol, or N-hexane) 4. Critical illness neuropathy 5. Vasculitis 6. Amyotrophy
Neuromuscular junction pathologies: 1. Myasthenia gravis 2. Lambert–Eaton syndrome 3. Toxic (botulinum, snake venom, tetanus, and tick paralysis) 4. Organophosphate poisoning
Muscle pathologies: 1. Critical illness myopathy 2. Hypokalemic/hyperkalemic periodic paralysis, hypothyroidism 3. Rhabdomyolysis 4. Inflammatory myositis 5. Drug related myopathy (chloroquine, statins, etc.)
Conversion disorder/malingering

Complications of Plasmapheresis and IVIg

The main complications of plasmapheresis include increased risk of infections, coagulopathy, and fluid overload.

Regarding IVIG, renal failure, fluid overload, TRALI, allergic reactions—most ominously anaphylaxis (in individuals with selective IgA deficiency)—are the main potential complications. Headache with IVIg due to aseptic meningitis can also occur [39].

A Comment on SARS-CoV-2 and GBS

Several cases of Guillain–Barré syndrome (GBS) resulting from SARS-CoV-2 infection have been reported. The most notable study is a systematic review which included 73 patients that developed GBS after COVID-19 [46]. It is postulated that GBS occurs in COVID-19 patients due to the same immune-mediated pathogenetic mechanisms.

The clinical variants and electrophysiological subtypes resemble those of classic GBS, with a higher prevalence of the classic sensorimotor form and the acute inflammatory demyelinating polyneuropathy. Cerebrospinal fluid (CSF) albumin-cytological dissociation was present in most cases, and more than 70% of patients showed a good prognosis after treatment with intravenous immunoglobulin. A handful of GBS cases have also been described after the administration of adenovirus vector vaccines, specifically the J&J/Janssen COVID-19 vaccine.

A study by Patone et al., which followed neurological outcomes and complications in the 28 days following a COVID-19 infection, established that, although there may be an increased risk of GBS in those who received COVID-19 vaccines, the risk of these complications is greater following a positive SARS-CoV-2 test [47].

Amyotrophic Lateral Sclerosis

Amyotrophic lateral sclerosis (ALS) is an idiopathic, progressive, and universally fatal disease affecting the motor system; incidence varies by region and ancestral origin [48]. In Europe, the incidence is 2.16 per 100,000 person-years [49]. Men are affected more frequently than women and onset is typically in the fifth to seventh decade of life. The majority of cases are sporadic, but a small proportion—5–15%—are familial [48]. The presentation of ALS is heterogenous, but the two main subtypes are limb-onset, characterized by early extremity weakness, and bulbar onset, characterized by early speech and swallowing difficulties. Typical signs and symptoms include muscle weakness, atrophy, fasciculations, cramps, hyperreflexia, as well as dysarthria, dysphagia, bulbar/pseudobulbar signs, and dyspnea [50]. The pathophysiologic mechanisms of motor neuron degeneration in ALS are suspected to be multifactorial and discussion of the current leading theories is beyond the scope of this chapter.

Early/Immediate Managment

Acute respiratory failure is the most common cause for hospital admission in patients with ALS [51]. While establishing adequate ventilation is the primary concern, there are special considerations when treating patients with ALS. Difficulty weaning from the ventilator after endotracheal intubation is common and the prospect of tracheostomy is controversial among both patients and providers [52, 53]. Noninvasive ventilation along with cough assist devices may be helpful in avoiding intubation when treating acute respiratory failure in patients with motor neuron disease and should be considered when appropriate [54].

After ensuring adequate ventilation, one should consider the cause of acute decompensation. Patients with ALS are at increased risk of multiple pulmonary complications including aspiration pneumonitis and pneumonia. In addition to primary hypoventilation due to loss of phrenic nerve function, as bulbar muscle coordination declines, airway clearance is impaired, and aspiration risk increases. Furthermore, ineffective cough can lead to atelectasis and mucus plugging [51, 53, 55]. Additionally, ALS patients, in particular those with spinal onset, are at higher risk for deep vein thrombosis and subsequent pulmonary embolism [56]. Determining the underlying cause of the acute decompensation promptly is essential to guide treatment.

Long-Term Clinical Course

In the context of chronic respiratory failure, noninvasive ventilation (NIV) can prolong survival and improve quality of life in patients with ALS [57]. Current guidelines dictate that an FCV less than 50% of predicted warrants consideration of NIV as respiratory failure may be imminent [55]. In both the acute and long-term care setting, management of respiratory secretions poses challenges. Mechanical insufflation–exsufflation may provide helpful cough assistance [58]. Sialorrhea is commonly managed initially with anti-cholinergics [59], but the strongest evidence exists for treatment with Botulinum toxin injection [60].

Malnutrition, dehydration, and weight loss are common, and there is evidence to support PEG placement for stabilization of body weight [61]. Benefits of enteral nutrition must be weighed against risk of the procedure, particularly in patients with FVC less than 50% of predicted [59], as the risk of complications increases.

Near Misses

On occasion, respiratory failure may be the initial presenting symptom of previously undiagnosed ALS [62]. Motor neuron disease should be considered in patients presenting with unexplained neuromuscular respiratory failure.

If intubation is required, the use of succinylcholine should be avoided as it can cause life-threatening hyperkalemia in patients with chronic denervation [63].

Key Radiologic Features

Both structural and functional neuroimaging have been studied in ALS, but currently these have little diagnostic role [64]. EMG changes remain central to the diagnosis of ALS. EMG testing in conjunction with the physical exam demonstrates lower motor neuron dysfunction. Evidence of active and chronic denervation are necessary for the diagnosis and fasciculation potentials are supportive. Conversely nerve conduction studies are typically normal to near normal [65].

Key Monitoring

Pulmonary function testing, nocturnal oximetry, sniff nasal inspiratory testing, mean inspiratory pressures (MIP), and forced vital capacity (FVC) are used to monitor disease progression and need for noninvasive ventilation in the outpatient setting [61, 66]. Current guidelines dictate that an MIP of less than 60 cm H_2O or an FVC of <50% of predicted should warrant consideration for noninvasive ventilation. Invasive ventilation should be considered if PaO_2 is <90 mm Hg or $PaCO_2$ is >50 mm Hg despite optimal noninvasive ventilation [61].

Take Home Message

ALS is an idiopathic progressive disease in which respiratory failure is ubiquitous. Typically, patients present to the ICU with a known diagnosis of ALS but, occasionally, the diagnosis will be made in the ICU setting [62]. Management in the acute setting should focus on ensuring adequate ventilation. Given the progressive nature of the disease, early goals of care/End of Life conversations should be undertaken, as once intubated, liberation from the ventilator may not be possible.

Intensive Care Unit Acquired Weakness

ICU-acquired weakness (ICU-AW) is a severe motor and sensory polyneuropathy that was first described in critically ill patients by Bolton and colleagues [67]. Typical present ing symptoms include generalized weakness, diminished deep tendon reflexes, and difficulty with ventilator weaning [67, 68]. There are two broad categories of ICU-AW: critical illness myopathy and critical illness neuropathy. There is frequent overlap between the two entities with patients demonstrating features of both neuropathy and myopathy [69].

The pathophysiology of ICU-AW is thought to be complex and multifactorial. There is evidence that dysfunction of the microcirculation as well as biochemical changes within nerve and muscle cells induced by critical illness and muscle inactivity contribute to development of neuromuscular weakness [70]. ICU-AW is more prevalent in female patients, the elderly and those with greater severity of illness [71]. Systemic inflammation, neuromuscular blockade, poor glycemic control, and immobility have also been noted to increase the risk of ICU-AW [72].

Diagnosis of ICU-AW requires formal muscle strength testing, most commonly with the Medical Research Council Score (MRC) which grades muscle strength from 0 to 5 [71–73]. An MRC total score of <48 is consistent with the diagnosis [71, 74]. Electrophysiologic testing may be helpful in some patients.

Immediate/Early Managment

Management of ICU-AW begins with prevention. Strict glycemic control with the use of insulin has been associated with lower risk of ICU-AW, decreased duration of mechanical ventilation, and improved long-term outcomes [75–77]. However, this must be balanced with the risk of hypoglycemia, which has been associated with increased mortality in critically ill patients [78, 79]. Blood glucose goals should be carefully followed accordingly.

The extent to which medications may contribute to ICU-AW is somewhat fraught. The use of corticosteroids was previously suspected to contribute to the development of ICU-AW, but newer evidence argues against a correlation [77]. The use of neuromuscular blocking agents (NMBAs) has been associated with increased risk of ICU-AW in certain populations [80]. However, in patients with acute respiratory distress syndrome (ARDS) the use of NMBAs does not consistently portend worse neuromuscular outcomes and, *per* current guidelines, the benefit of NMBAs in this population outweighs the risk [80, 81].

There is evidence for early mobility as a protective factor against ICU-AW [77]. Patients who undergo early physical and occupational therapy during sedation holidays have better functional status on discharge and fewer ventilator dependent days [82].

Long-Term Clinical Course

Many patients experience prolonged neuromuscular recovery after surviving critical illness. One study found evidence of persistent motor and sensory deficits in more than half of patients who were 5 years removed from their initial illness. Electrophysiologic evidence of neuromuscular dysfunction also persisted for many years [83].

Near Misses

Features including pain, autonomic instability, and facial weakness are atypical for ICU-AW and should prompt investigation into alternative causes of neuromuscular weakness. Laboratory studies including creatinine kinase are typically normal in ICU-AW, and severe derangements can suggest an alternative diagnosis [70].

Diagnostic Testing

If ICU-AW is present, EMG will demonstrate a severe axonal polyneuropathy [67] with reduced compound muscle action potential (CMAP) amplitude and normal to minimally reduced nerve conduction [70]. If myopathy is present, there will also be reduced muscle excitability on direct stimulation and increased CMAP duration. In critical illness polyneuropathy, there will also be reduced compound sensory nerve action potential (SNAP) amplitude [70].

Take Home Message
ICU-AW is a complication of critical illness characterized by generalized weakness, decreased deep tendon reflexes, and difficulty weaning from the ventilator. Once identified, the treatment for ICU-AW is supportive care. Measures including glucose control and early mobility should be implemented to prevent the development of ICU-AW in critically ill patients.

Lambert-Eaton Myasthenic Syndrome

Lambert–Eaton myasthenic syndrome (LEMS) is a presynaptic neuromuscular disease, in which antibodies are directly against the presynaptic P/Q type voltage-gated calcium channel, resulting in characteristic weakness and autonomic dysfunction. In the majority of LEMS patients, antibodies are targeted against the alpha 1A subunit of the P/Q type voltage-gated calcium channel. These calcium channels are present in autonomic synapses and within the cerebellum [84].

LEMS is a rare disease, with an annual incidence nearly 10 times less than that of MG. Due to it being a rare disease, having overlapping clinical features with MG, and nonspecific symptoms, LEMS is often misdiagnosed as MG, diagnosed late, or even discovered incidentally in patients who experience prolonged paralysis following neuromuscular blockade during surgery and other procedures [85–87].

Immediate Management

Clinical presentation often involves weakness of the proximal lower and upper and lower limbs, with a significant proportion of patients exhibiting autonomic dysfunction, leg weakness, blurry vision, dry mouth, constipation, and orthostasis [88, 89]. Autonomic dysfunction is reported in 96% of patients [90]. Of cranial muscle involvement, ptosis and diplopia are the most common manifestations, although oropharyngeal symptoms have been reported [84].

Weakness typically spreads proximally to distally and caudally to cranially, though involvement of the bulbar muscles is typically less severe than that in MG [85]. A presenting symptom of ocular weakness virtually excludes LEMS [91]. Pain and elevated creatine kinase are rare in LEMS and if present should prompt workup for an alternative etiology [92]. Diaphragmatic and respiratory muscle weakness can occur although these are uncommon [93–97]. Finally, LEMS has been reported as an adverse event in those receiving immune checkpoint inhibitor therapy [84].

The detection of P/Q type voltage-gated calcium channel antibodies is highly sensitive and specific for the diagnosis of LEMS, though low titers have been found in controls and in patients with cancer and amyotrophic lateral sclerosis. Furthermore, about 10–15% of LEMS patients are seronegative for these antibodies [84].

EMG facilitates diagnosis through the triad of low CMAP amplitude, a decremental (10%) CMAP response to low-frequency repetitive stimulation (2–5 Hz) and an incremental (100%) CMAP response to high frequency repetitive stimulation (20–50 Hz) or facilitation after a brief muscle contraction. It is important to note that MG also exhibits a decremental response to low-frequency repetitive stimulation [85]. Single fiber EMG has increased sensitivity for LEMS, but does not differentiate between LEMS and myasthenia gravis [85].

3,4-Diaminopyridine (3,4-DAP) at a starting dose of 15–30 mg daily in adults, with a max daily dose of 80 mg, is first-line therapy. Significant albeit rare adverse events associated with 3,4-diaminopyridine are seizures and Q-T prolongation. More frequently, oral and digital paresthesias, nausea, and diarrhea are seen [84]. 3,4-DAP is a potassium channel blocker that prolongs the action potential at the neuromuscular junction, resulting in more calcium entering the nerve terminal and increased neurotransmitter release [98].

When symptoms are disabling, immunotherapy should be instituted, typically consisting of prednisone alone or in combination with azathioprine. If refractory, IVIg or plasmapheresis in parallel with 3,4-diaminopyridine are reasonable [84, 85].

Long-Term Clinical Course

Survival is shorter in patients with squamous cell lung cancer (SCLC) LEMS as compared to LEMS where no malignancy is found [84]. Interestingly, patients with SCLC-LEMS exhibit a longer median length of survival than those with SCLC without neurological symptoms (17.3 months vs. 10 months) [84, 99].

Near Misses

Approximately 50% of LEMS patients have a primary autoimmune disorder, and 50–60% of patients with LEMS have an associated cancer [90, 100]; in 90% of cases, that cancer is small-cell lung cancer (SCLC-LEMS). Nontumor LEMS (NT-LEMS) is associated with other autoimmune diseases, such as rheumatoid arthritis, pernicious anemia, and Sjogren syndrome [85].

Once LEMS has been diagnosed, aggressive screening for SCLC should ensue, which should include CT of the chest and, if negative, a PET scan. SOX1 antibodies are a specific marker for SCLC-LEMS with a sensitivity and specificity of 67% and 95%, respectively [90, 100].

Key Monitoring

The Dutch-English LEMS Tumor Association Prediction (DELTA-P) was developed to assist with deciding how long oncologic screening should be repeated if the first turns out negative. It consists of assigning scores for dysarthria, dysphagia, neck weakness, erectile dysfunction, weight loss, tobacco use, age of onset, and Karnofski performance status [85, 92, 101].

Take Home Message

LEMS is a rare presynaptic neuromuscular disease often misdiagnosed as myasthenia gravis. Presenting symptoms often involve weakness of the proximal upper and lower limbs, spreading distally and caudally to cranially. Autonomic nervous system involvement (blurry vision, dry mouth, constipation, and orthostasis) is common. Bulbar muscle weakness is typically less severe than that in myasthenia gravis, and respiratory muscle weakness is uncommon. Detection of P/Q type volta-gated calcium channel antibodies are highly sensitive and specific for the diagnosis of LEMS; EMG can only facilitate diagnosis. 3,4-Diaminopyridine is the mainstay of treatment, but care must be taken as it can lower seizure threshold and cause a prolonged QT interval. Severe symp toms can be treated with IVIg or plasma exchange with or without immunomodulators. LEMS has a strong association with SCLC and various autoimmune disorders.

Botulism

Botulinum neurotoxin is the most powerful toxin known to humankind, being discovered in 1897 during an outbreak of food poisoning by Belgian microbiologist van Ermengem [102]. Some authors estimate 1 gram of aerosolized botulinum toxin could kill over 1.5 million people [103].

Botulism is a disease caused by the neurotoxin produced by the bacterium *Clostridium botulinum*, which is commonly found in soil. Other types of *Clostridium* bacteria can also cause botulism. The toxin can survive food preservation and grow in low-acid, low-solute, and anaerobic conditions. It is internalized via receptor-mediated endocytosis, where it then prevents presynaptic release of acetylcholine by binding irreversibly to the presynaptic nerve endings of peripheral and cranial nerves [102]. The large size of the toxin prevents it from crossing the blood–brain barrier and affecting the central nervous system [104].

Foodborne botulism can be caused by low-acid home-canned or processed foods, baked potatoes in foil, garlic in oil, and sauteed onions with butter or cheese sauce. The incidence of wound botulism from black tar heroin use has also increased [102].

Botulinum neurotoxin causes four clinical illnesses in humans: foodborne botulism, wound botulism, adult infectious, and infant botulism. From 1973 through 1996, 724 cases of foodborne botulism, and 103 cases of wound botulism were reported to the Centers for Disease Control and Prevention [102].

Botulinum neurotoxin type A causes about half of foodborne, wound, and infant botulism and is more severe and deadly than types B and E. Type A is common West of the Mississippi River, while type B is common East of the Mississippi [102]. Type F botulinum is rare but progresses quickly and also has an earlier recovery [104].

Immediate Management

Initial symptoms of foodborne botulism may include nausea, vomiting, abdominal pain, or diarrhea, but constipation usually develops after neurological symptoms have manifested. Initial neurological symptoms may involve dysphonia, dysarthria, dysphagia, and muscle weakness, followed by symmetric descending paralysis involving the respiratory muscles. The onset in foodborne botulism usually occurs 18–36 h after exposure. Wound botulism manifests similarly to foodborne botulism, but has a longer incubation period of about 1–2 weeks [102].

Confirmatory tests for botulism include detecting the neurotoxin in serum, stool, gastric fluid, or food, or finding the bacterium in stool or wound culture. The gold standard for identifying botulinum neurotoxin is the mouse bioassay, available at specialized public health labs and the CDC's National Botulism Laboratory. Other methods include PCR and mass spectrometry [104]. Electromyography can differentiate botulism from other neuromuscular disorders, but results are nonspecific.

Botulinum antitoxin should be administered quickly, as lab confirmation may take several days. Each vial of antitoxin, can neutralize 100 times more circulating toxin than ever measured by the CDC, and contains antibodies to types A to G. It is licensed for adults and children and is available through the CDC's 24-h service. Administering antitoxin within 24–48 h of symptom onset decreases mortality, ICU treatment, and hospitalization. Antitoxin cannot reverse existing paralysis. It rarely causes anaphylaxis (less than 2%), and skin testing is no longer recommended. Antimicrobials do not help in botulism treatment and wound botulism should be treated with debridement [104].

Long-Term Clinical Course

Ventilatory support is commonly needed for 2–8 weeks, and clinical recovery may take months, correlating with the formation of new presynaptic end plates and neuromuscular junctions. If left untreated, botulism has a mortality rate of 40–50% [105, 106]. Due to the advent of mechanical ventilation, the mortality rate of foodborne botulism has drastically decreased to 5–10% [102].

Key Monitoring

Due to the lack of clinical data available on respiratory monitoring in patients with botulism, incorporation of data from other neuromuscular disease (such as Guillain-Barre syndrome), as is done with myasthenia gravis, is reasonable. Spirometry with vital capacity (FVC) under 20 mL/kg, maximum inspiratory pressure (MIP) under 30 cm H_2O, and maximum expiratory pressure under 40 cm H_2O should be concerning, but not taken as independent indicators for need for mechanical ventilation. End tidal CO_2 monitoring and frequent monitoring for bulbar dysfunction are also reasonable [104].

Take Home Message

Botulinum neurotoxin is a highly potent and dangerous substance, and patients presenting with symptoms of botulism require immediate assessment and consideration for treatment with botulinum antitoxin. The only FDA-approved identification of the toxin is done through a mouse bioassay, and patients may require intubation and a long period of hospitalization for recovery, which can take months.

Conclusion

Although this chapter covers a number of key neuromuscular diseases a clinician may encounter in the ICU, there are many others that are beyond the scope of this book. This chapter provided a comprehensive review of the clinical presentation and management strategies for several neuromuscular diseases, including myasthenia gravis, Lambert–Eaton myasthenic syndrome, and ICU acquired weakness among others. Early recognition of these conditions along with prompt diagnosis are essential so that optimal patient outcomes can be achieved.

References

1. Lacomis D. Myasthenic crisis. Neurocrit Care. 2005;3(3):189–94.
2. Sheikh S, Alvi U, Soliven B, Rezania K. Drugs that induce or cause deterioration of myasthenia gravis: an update. J Clin Med. 2021;10(7):1537. https://doi.org/10.3390/jcm10071537.
3. Phillips LH. The epidemiology of myasthenia gravis. Ann N Y Acad Sci. 2003;998:407–12.
4. Fink M. Treatment of the critically ill patient with myasthenia gravis. In: Ropper AH, editor. Neurological and neurosurgical intensive care. 3rd ed. Raven Press; 1993. p. 351–62.
5. Alshekhlee A, Miles JD, Katirji B, Preston DC, Kaminski HJ. Incidence and mortality rates of myasthenia gravis and myasthenic crisis in US hospitals. Neurol Int. 2009;72(18):1548–54.
6. Thomas CE, Mayer SA, Gungor Y, Swarup R, Webster EA, Chang I, Brannagan TH, Fink ME, Rowland LP. Myasthenic crisis: clinical features, mortality, complications, and risk factors for prolonged intubation. Neurol Int. 1997;48(5):1253–60.
7. Angstwurm K, Vidal A, Stetefeld H, Dohmen C, Mergenthaler P, Kohler S, Schonenberger S, Bosel J, Neumann U, Lee DH, Gerner ST, Huttner HB, Thieme A, Dunkel J, Roth C, Schneider H, Schimmel E, Reichmann H, Fuhrer H, Berger B, Kleiter I, Schneider-Gold C, Alberty A, Zinke J, Schalke B, Steinbrecher A, Meisel A, Neumann B. Early tracheostomy is associated with shorter ventilation time and duration of ICU stay in patients with myasthenic crisis-a multicenter analysis. J Intensive Care Med. 2020;25:885066620967646.
8. Lizarraga AA, Lizarraga KJ, Benatar M. Getting rid of weakness in the ICU: an updated approach to the acute management of myasthenia gravis and guillain-Barre syndrome. Semin Neurol. 2016;36(6):615–24.
9. Cohen MS, Younger D. Aspects of the natural history of myasthenia gravis: crisis and death. Ann N Y Acad Sci. 1981;377:670–7.
10. Oosterhuis HJ. Observations of the natural history of myasthenia gravis and the effect of thymectomy. Ann N Y Acad Sci. 1981;377:678–90.
11. Bernardes Neto SCG, Torres-Castro R, Lima I, Resqueti VR, Fregonezi GAF. Weaning from mechanical ventilation in people with neuromuscular disease: a systematic review. BMJ Open. 2021;11(9):e047449.
12. Benditt JO, Boitano LJ. Pulmonary issues in patients with chronic neuromuscular disease. Am J Respir Crit Care Med. 2013;187(10):1046 55.
13. Racca F, Vianello A, Mongini T, Ruggeri P, Versaci A, Vita GL, Vita G. Practical approach to respiratory emergencies in neurological diseases. Neurol Sci. 2020;41(3):497–508.
14. Vassilakopoulos T, Petrof BJ. Ventilator-induced diaphragmatic dysfunction. Am J Respir Crit Care Med. 2004;169(3):336–41.
15. Elsheikh B, Arnold WD, Gharibshahi S, Reynolds J, Freimer M, Kissel JT. Correlation of single-breath count test and neck flexor muscle strength with spirometry in myasthenia gravis. Muscle Nerve. 2016;53(1):134–6.
16. Rajajee V, Riggs B, Seder DB. Emergency neurological life support: airway, ventilation, and sedation. Neurocrit Care. 2017;27(Suppl 1):4–28.
17. Abel M, Eisenkraft JB. Anesthetic implications of myasthenia gravis. Mt Sinai J Med. 2002;69(1-2):31–7.
18. Neumann B, Angstwurm K, Mergenthaler P, Kohler S, Schonenberger S, Bosel J, Neumann U, Vidal A, Huttner HB, Gerner ST, Thieme A, Steinbrecher A, Dunkel J, Roth C, Schneider H, Schimmel E, Fuhrer H, Fahrendorf C, Alberty A, Zinke J, Meisel A, Dohmen C, Stetefeld HR. German Myasthenic crisis study group. Myasthenic crisis demanding mechanical ventilation: a multicenter analysis of 250 cases. Neurol Int. 2020;94(3):e299–313.
19. Farrugia ME, Goodfellow JA. A practical approach to managing patients with myasthenia gravis-opinions and a review of the literature. Front Neurol. 2020;11:604.
20. Rezania K, Goldenberg FD, White S. Neuromuscular disorders and acute respiratory failure: diagnosis and management. Neurol Clin. 2012;30(1):161.
21. Kanai T, Uzawa A, Kawaguchi N, Oda F, Ozawa Y, Himuro K, Kuwabara S. Predictive score for oral corticosteroid-induced initial worsening of seropositive generalized myasthenia gravis. J Neurol Sci. 2019;396:8–11.
22. Narayanaswami P, Sanders DB, Wolfe G, Benatar M, Cea G, Evoli A, Gilhus NE, Illa I, Kuntz NL, Massey J, Melms A, Murai H, Nicolle M, Palace J, Richman D, Verschuuren J. International consensus guidance for management of myasthenia gravis: 2020 update. Neurol Int. 2021 January 19;96(3):114–22.
23. Hamel J, Ciafaloni E. An update: myasthenia gravis and pregnancy. Neurol Clin. 2018;36(2):355–65.
24. Patel A, Lynch F, Shepherd SA. Newer immunotherapies for the treatment of acute neuromuscular disease in the critical care unit. Curr Treat Options Neurol. 2020;22(3):7–8.
25. Dhillon S. Eculizumab: a review in generalized myasthenia gravis. Drugs. 2018;78(3):367–76.
26. Howard JF, Utsugisawa K, Benatar M, Murai H, Barohn RJ, Illa I, Jacob S, Vissing J, Burns TM, Kissel JT, Muppidi S, Nowak RJ, O'Brien F, Wang JJ, Mantegazza R, REGAIN Study Group. Safety and efficacy of eculizumab in anti-acetylcholine receptor antibody-positive refractory generalised myasthenia gravis (REGAIN): a phase 3, randomised, double-blind, placebo-controlled, multicentre study. Lancet Neurol. 2017;16(12):976–86.
27. Rabinstein AA, Mueller-Kronast N. Risk of extubation failure in patients with myasthenic crisis. Neurocrit Care. 2005;3(3):213–5.
28. Seneviratne J, Mandrekar J, Wijdicks EF, Rabinstein AA. Predictors of extubation failure in myasthenic crisis. Arch Neurol. 2008;65(7):929–33.
29. Wu JY, Kuo PH, Fan PC, Wu HD, Shih FY, Yang PC. The role of non-invasive ventilation and factors predicting extubation outcome in myasthenic crisis. Neurocrit Care. 2009;10(1):35–42.
30. Mehta S. Neuromuscular disease causing acute respiratory failure. Respir Care. 2006;51(9):1016–3.
31. Roper J, Fleming ME, Long B, Koyfman A. Myasthenia gravis and crisis: evaluation and management in the emergency department. J Emerg Med. 2017;53(6):843–53.
32. Lawn ND, Fletcher DD, Henderson RD, Wolter TD, Wijdicks EF. Anticipating mechanical ventilation in guillain-Barre syndrome. Arch Neurol. 2001;58(6):893–8.
33. Sharshar T, Chevret S, Bourdain F, Raphael JC. French cooperative group on plasma exchange in Guillain-Barre syndrome. Early predictors of mechanical ventilation in guillain-Barre syndrome. Crit Care Med. 2003;31(1):278–83.

34. Rabinstein AA. Noninvasive ventilation for neuromuscular respiratory failure: when to use and when to avoid. Curr Opin Crit Care. 2016;22(2):94–9.
35. Seneviratne J, Mandrekar J, Wijdicks EF, Rabinstein AA. Noninvasive ventilation in myasthenic crisis. Arch Neurol. 2008;65(1):54–8.
36. Rabinstein A, Wijdicks EF. BiPAP in acute respiratory failure due to myasthenic crisis may prevent intubation. Neurol Int. 2002;59(10):1647–9.
37. Birch TB. Neuromuscular disorders in the intensive care unit. Continuum (Minneapolis, Minn). 2021;27(5):1344–64; https://search.proquest.com/docview/2580691582.
38. Shang P, Zhu M, Baker M, Feng J, Zhou C, Zhang HL. Mechanical ventilation in guillain-Barre syndrome. Expert Rev Clin Immunol. 2020;16(11):1053–64.
39. Salardini A, Triggs WJ. Neuromuscular Disorders in the ICU. In: Textbook of Neurointensive Care. London: Springer London; 2013. p. 777–98; http://link.springer.com/10.1007/978-1-4471-5226-2_38. https://doi.org/10.1007/978-1-4471-5226-2_38.
40. Chakraborty T, Kramer CL, Wijdicks EFM, Rabinstein AA. Dysautonomia in Guillain–Barré syndrome: Prevalence, clinical spectrum, and outcomes. Neurocritical Care. 2020;32(1):113–20. https://doi.org/10.1007/s12028-019-00781-w.
41. Fryman E, Saleem S, Singh A. Guillain-Barre syndrome induced dysautonomia resulting in cardiac arrest. Cureus. 2020;12(12):e12149.
42. Abbas Z, Sardar Z. Use of pacemaker in GBS dysautonomia. BMJ Case Rep. 2021;14(10):e242464. https://doi.org/10.1136/bcr-242464.
43. Dimachkie MM, Barohn RJ. Guillain-barré syndrome and variants. Neurol Clin. 2013;31(2):491–510; https://pubmed.ncbi.nlm.nih.gov/23642721. https://www.ncbi.nlm.nih.gov/pmc/articles/PMC3939842/.
44. Melone M, Heming N, Meng P, Mompoint D, Aboab J, Clair B, Salomon J, Sharshar T, Orlikowski D, Chevret S, Annane D. Early mechanical ventilation in patients with guillain-barré syndrome at high risk of respiratory failure: a randomized trial. Ann Intensive Care. 2020;10(1):128. https://doi.org/10.1186/s13613-020-00742-z.
45. Verboon C, Doets AY, Galassi G, Davidson A, Waheed W, Péréon Y, Shahrizaila N, Kusunoki S, Lehmann HC, Harbo T, Monges S, Van den Bergh P, Willison HJ, Cornblath DR, Jacobs BC, on behalf of the, IGOS Consortium. Current treatment practice of guillain-barré syndrome. Neurology. 2019;93(1):e59; http://n.neurology.org/content/93/1/e59.abstract.
46. Abu-Rumeileh S, Abdelhak A, Foschi M, Tumani H, Otto M. Guillain–Barré syndrome spectrum associated with COVID-19: An up-to-date systematic review of 73 cases. J Neurol. 2020;268(4):1133–70; https://link.springer.com/article/10.1007/s00415-020-10124-x.
47. Patone M, Handunnetthi L, Saatci D, Pan J, Katikireddi SV, Razvi S, Hunt D, Mei XW, Dixon S, Zaccardi F, Khunti K, Watkinson P, Coupland CAC, Doidge J, Harrison DA, Ravanan R, Sheikh A, Robertson C, Hippisley-Cox J. Neurological complications after first dose of COVID-19 vaccines and SARS-CoV-2 infection. Nat Med. 2021;27(12):2144–53.
48. Kiernan MC, Vucic S, Cheah BC, Turner MR, Eisen A, Hardiman O, Burrell JR, Zoing MC. Amyotrophic lateral sclerosis. Lancet. 2011;377(9769):942–55.
49. Logroscino G, Traynor BJ, Hardiman O, Chió A, Mitchell D, Swingler RJ, Millul A, Benn E, Beghi E. Incidence of amyotrophic lateral sclerosis in europe. J Neurol Neurosurg Psychiatry. 2010;81(4):385–90.
50. Ringel SP, Murphy JR, Alderson MK, Bryan W, England JD, Miller RG, Petajan JH, Smith SA, Roelofs RI, Ziter F, Lee MY, Brinkmann JR, Almada A, Gappmaier E, Graves J, Herbelin L, Mendoza M, Mylar D, Smith P, Yu P. The natural history of amyotrophic lateral sclerosis. Neurology. 1993;43(7):1316–22.
51. Lechtzin N, Wiener CM, Clawson L, Chaudhry V, Diette GB. Hospitalization in amyotrophic lateral sclerosis: causes, costs, and outcomes. Neurology. 2001;56(6):753–7.
52. Bradley MD, Orrell RW, Clarke J, Davidson AC, Williams AJ, Kullmann M, Hirsch N. Outcome of ventilatory support for acute respiratory failure in motor neurone disease. BMJ. 2002;72:752. https://doi.org/10.1136/jnnp.72.6.752.
53. Niedermeyer S, Murn M, Choi PJ. Respiratory failure in amyotrophic lateral sclerosis. Chest. 2019;155(2):401–8. https://doi.org/10.1016/j.chest.2018.06.035.
54. Servera E, Sancho J, Zafra MJ, Catalá A, Vergara P, Marín J. Alternatives to endotracheal intubation for patients with neuromuscular diseases. Am J Phys Med Rehabil. 2005;84(11):851–7; https://www.ncbi.nlm.nih.gov/pubmed/16244522.
55. Lechtzin N, Rothstein J, Clawson L, Diette GB, Wiener CM. Amyotrophic lateral sclerosis: Evaluation and treatment of respiratory impairment. Amyotroph Lateral Scler Other Motor Neuron Disord. 2002;3(1):5–13. https://doi.org/10.1080/146608202317576480.
56. Gil J, Funalot B, Verschueren A, Danel-Brunaud V, Camu W, Vandenberghe N, Desnuelle C, Guy N, Camdessanche JP, Cintas P, Carluer L, Pittion S, Nicolas G, Corcia P, Fleury MC, Maugras C, Besson G, Le Masson G, Couratier P. Causes of death amongst french patients with amyotrophic lateral sclerosis: a prospective study. Eur J Neurol. 2008;15(11):1245–51.
57. Bourke SC, Tomlinson M, Williams TL, Bullock RE, Shaw PJ, Gibson GJ. Effects of non-invasive ventilation on survival and quality of life in patients with amyotrophic lateral sclerosis: a randomised controlled trial. Lancet Neurol. 2006;5(2):140–7.
58. Mustfa N, Aiello M, Lyall RA, Nikoletou D, Olivieri D, Leigh PN, Davidson AC, Polkey MI, Moxham J. Cough augmentation in amyotrophic lateral sclerosis. Neurology. 2003;61(9):1285–7.
59. Miller RG, Jackson CE, Kasarskis EJ, England JD, Forshew D, Johnston W, Kalra S, Katz JS, Mitsumoto H, Rosenfeld J, Shoesmith C, Strong MJ, Woolley SC. Practice parameter update: the care of the patient with amyotrophic lateral sclerosis: multidisciplinary care, symptom management, and cognitive/behavioral impairment (an evidence-based review): report of the quality standards subcommittee of the american. Neurology. 2009;73(15):1227–33.
60. Jackson CE, Gronseth G, Rosenfeld J, Barohn RJ, Dubinsky R, Simpson CB, Mcvey A, Kittrell PP, King R, Herbelin L, Griggs R, Tawil R, Jackson C, Kissel JT, Pandya S, Downing K, Rose M, McDermott M. Randomized double-blind study of botulinum toxin type B for sialorrhea in ALS patients. Muscle Nerve. 2009;39(2):137–43.
61. Miller RG, Jackson CE, Kasarskis EJ, England JD, Forshew D, Johnston W, Kalra S, Katz JS, Mitsumoto H, Rosenfeld J, Shoesmith C, Strong MJ, Woolley SC. Practice parameter update: the care of the patient with amyotrophic lateral sclerosis: drug, nutritional, and respiratory therapies (an evidence-based review): report of the quality standards subcommittee of the american academy of neurology. Neurology. 2009;73(15):1218–26.
62. Serrano MC, Rabinstein AA. Causes and outcomes of acute neuromuscular respiratory failure. Arch Neurol. 2010;67(9):1089–94.
63. Cooperman LH. Succinylcholine-induced hyperkalemia in neuromuscular disease. JAMA. 1970;213(11):1867–71.
64. Chiò A, Pagani M, Agosta F, Calvo A, Cistaro A, Filippi M. Neuroimaging in amyotrophic lateral sclerosis: Insights into structural and functional changes. 2014;13(12):1228–40. https://doi.org/10.1016/S1474-4422(14)70167-X.
65. Brooks BR, Miller RG, Swash M, Munsat TL. El Escorial revisited: revised criteria for the diagnosis of amyotrophic lateral sclerosis. Amyotroph Lateral Scler. 2000;1(5):293–9.

66. Morgan RK, McNally S, Alexander M, Conroy R, Hardiman O, Costello RW. Use of sniff nasal-inspiratory force to predict survival in amyotrophic lateral sclerosis. Am J Respir Crit Care Med. 2005;171(3):269–74.
67. Bolton CF, Gilbert JJ, Hahn AF, Sibbald WJ. Polyneuropathy in critically ill patients. J Neurol Neurosurg Psychiatry. 1984;47(11):1223–31.
68. De Jonghe B, Bastuji-Garin S, Sharshar T, Outin H, Brochard L. Does ICU-acquired paresis lengthen weaning from mechanical ventilation? Intensive Care Med. 2004;30(6):1117–21.
69. Bednarik J, Lukas Z, Vondracek P. Critical illness polyneuromyopathy: the electrophysiological components of a complex entity. Intensive Care Med. 2003;29(9):1505–14.
70. Kress JP, Hall JB. ICU-acquired weakness and recovery from critical illness. N Engl J Med. 2014;370(17):1626–35.
71. Vanhorebeek I, Latronico N, Van den Berghe G. ICU-acquired weakness. Intensive Care Med. 2020;46(4):637–53. https://doi.org/10.1007/s00134-020-05944-4.
72. Schweickert WD, Hall J. ICU-acquired weakness. Chest. 2007;131(5):1541–9.
73. Medical Research Council. Aids to the examination of the peripheral nervous system. HM Stationery Office; 1976.
74. Stevens RD, Marshall SA, Cornblath DR, Hoke A, Needham DM, de Jonghe B, Ali NA, Sharshar T. A framework for diagnosing and classifying intensive care unit-acquired weakness. Crit Care Med. 2009;37(10):S299–308; https://journals.lww.com/ccmjournal/Fulltext/2009/10001/A_framework_for_diagnosing_and_classifying.3.aspx.
75. Van den Berghe G, Wouters P, Weekers F, Verwaest C, Bruyninckx F, Schetz M, Vlasselaers D, Ferdinande P, Lauwers P, Bouillon R. Intensive insulin therapy in critically ill patients. N Engl J Med. 2001;345(19):1359–67. https://doi.org/10.1056/NEJMoa011300.
76. Van den Berghe G, Schoonheydt K, Becx P, Bruyninckx F, Wouters PJ. Insulin therapy protects the central and peripheral nervous system of intensive care patients. Neurol Int. 2005;64(8):1348; http://n.neurology.org/content/64/8/1348.abstract.
77. Hermans G, De Jonghe B, Bruyninckx F, Van den Berghe G. Interventions for preventing critical illness polyneuropathy and critical illness myopathy. Cochrane Database Syst Rev. 2014;1:1283. https://doi.org/10.1002/14651858.CD006832.pub3.
78. Bagshaw SM, Bellomo R, Jacka MJ, Egi M, Hart GK, George C, the ANZICS CORE, Management Committee. The impact of early hypoglycemia and blood glucose variability on outcome in critical illness. Critical Care. 2009;13(3):R91. https://doi.org/10.1186/cc7921.
79. NICE-SUGAR Study Investigators, Finfer S, Chittock DR, et al. Intensive versus conventional glucose control in critically ill patients. N Engl J Med. 2009;360(13):1283–97. https://doi.org/10.1056/NEJMoa0810625.
80. Murray MJ, DeBlock H, Erstad B, Gray A, Jacobi J, Jordan C, McGee W, McManus C, Meade M, Nix S, Patterson A, Sands MK, Pino R, Tescher A, Arbour R, Rochwerg B, Murray CF, Mehta S. Clinical practice guidelines for sustained neuromuscular blockade in the adult critically ill patient. Crit Care Med. 2016;44(11):179. https://doi.org/10.1093/ajhp/59.2.179.
81. De Jonghe B, Sharshar T, Lefaucheur JP, Authier FJ, Durand-Zaleski I, Boussarsar M, Cerf C, Renaud E, Mesrati F, Carlet J, Raphaël JC, Outin H, Bastuji-Garin S. Groupe de Réflexion et d'Etude des Neuromyopathies en Réanimation. Paresis acquired in the intensive care unit: a prospective multicenter study. JAMA. 2002;288(22):2859–67.
82. Schweickert WD, Pohlman MC, Pohlman AS, Nigos C, Pawlik AJ, Esbrook CL, Spears L, Miller M, Franczyk M, Deprizio D, Schmidt GA, Bowman A, Barr R, McCallister KE, Hall JB, Kress JP. Early physical and occupational therapy in mechanically ventilated, critically ill patients: a randomised controlled trial. Lancet. 2009;373(9678):1874–82.
83. Fletcher SN, Kennedy DD, Ghosh IR, Misra VP, Kiff K, Coakley JH, Hinds CJ. Persistent neuromuscular and neurophysiologic abnormalities in long-term survivors of prolonged critical illness*. Crit Care Med. 2003;31(4):1012; https://journals.lww.com/ccmjournal/Fulltext/2003/04000/Persistent_neuromuscular_and_neurophysiologic.3.aspx.
84. Giannoccaro MP, Avoni P, Liguori R. Presynaptic paraneoplastic disorders of the neuromuscular junction: an update. Brain Sci. 2021;11(8):1035. https://doi.org/10.3390/brainsci11081035.
85. Evoli A, Liguori R, Romani A, Mantegazza R, Di Muzio A, Giometto B, Pegoraro E, Rodolico C, Vigliani MC, Italian Working Group on Myasthenic Syndromes. Italian recommendations for lambert-Eaton myasthenic syndrome (LEMS) management. Neurol Sci. 2014;35(4):515–20.
86. Juel VC, Sanders DB. The Lambert–Eaton myasthenicsyndrome. In: Engel AG, editor. Myasthenia gravis and myasthenic disorders. 2nd ed. Oxford: Oxford University Press; 2012. p. 156–69.
87. Sanders DB, Guptill JT. Myasthenia gravis and lambert-eaton myasthenic syndrome. Continuum (Minneap Minn). 2014;20(5 Peripheral Nervous System Disorders):1413–25.
88. Wirtz PW, Smallegange TM, Wintzen AR, Verschuuren JJ. Differences in clinical features between the lambert-Eaton myasthenic syndrome with and without cancer: an analysis of 227 published cases. Clin Neurol Neurosurg. 2002;104(4):359–63.
89. Kesner VG, Oh SJ, Dimachkie MM, Barohn RJ. Lambert-Eaton myasthenic syndrome. Neurol Clin. 2018;36(2):379–94.
90. Huang K, Luo YB, Yang H. Autoimmune channelopathies at neuromuscular junction. Front Neurol. 2019;10:516.
91. Wirtz PW, Sotodeh M, Nijnuis M, Van Doorn PA, Van Engelen BG, Hintzen RQ, De Kort PL, Kuks JB, Twijnstra A, De Visser M, Visser LH, Wokke JH, Wintzen AR, Verschuuren JJ. Difference in distribution of muscle weakness between myasthenia gravis and the lambert-Eaton myasthenic syndrome. J Neurol Neurosurg Psychiatry. 2002;73(6):766–8.
92. Titulaer MJ, Lang B, Verschuuren JJ. Lambert-Eaton myasthenic syndrome: from clinical characteristics to therapeutic strategies. Lancet Neurol. 2011;10(12):1098–107.
93. Wilcox PG, Morrison NJ, Anzarut AR, Pardy RL. Lambert-Eaton myasthenic syndrome involving the diaphragm. Chest. 1988;93(3):604–6.
94. Mantegazza R, Meisel A, Sieb JP, Le Masson G, Desnuelle C, Essing M. The european LEMS registry: baseline demographics and treatment approaches. Neurol Ther. 2015;4(2):105–24.
95. Nicolle MW, Stewart DJ, Remtulla H, Chen R, Bolton CF. Lambert-Eaton myasthenic syndrome presenting with severe respiratory failure. Muscle Nerve. 1996;19(10):1328–33.
96. Nicolle MW. Myasthenia gravis and lambert-eaton myasthenic syndrome. Continuum (Minneap Minn). 2016;22(6, Muscle and Neuromuscular Junction Disorders):1978–2005.
97. Smith AG, Wald J. Acute ventilatory failure in lambert-Eaton myasthenic syndrome and its response to 3,4-diaminopyridine. Neurol Int. 1996;46(4):1143–5.
98. Argov Z. Management of myasthenic conditions: nonimmune issues. Curr Opin Neurol. 2009;22(5):493–7.
99. Maddison P, Gozzard P, Grainge MJ, Lang B. Long-term survival in paraneoplastic lambert-Eaton myasthenic syndrome. Neurol Int. 2017;88(14):1334–9.
100. O'Neill JH, Murray NM, Newsom-Davis J. The lambert-Eaton myasthenic syndrome. A review of 50 cases. Brain. 1988;111(Pt 3):577–96.
101. Timmermann C. 'Just give me the best quality of life questionnaire': the karnofsky scale and the history of quality of life measurements in cancer trials. Chronic Illn. 2013;9(3):179–90.

102. Shapiro RL, Hatheway C, Swerdlow DL. Botulism in the United States: a clinical and epidemiologic review. Ann Intern Med. 1998;129(3):221–8.
103. Chalk CH, Benstead TJ, Pound JD, Keezer MR. Medical treatment for botulism. Cochrane Database Syst Rev. 2019;4:CD008123.
104. Rao AK, Sobel J, Chatham-Stephens K, Luquez C. Clinical guidelines for diagnosis and treatment of botulism, 2021. MMWR Recomm Rep. 2021;70(2):1–30.
105. Chatham-Stephens K, Fleck-Derderian S, Johnson SD, Sobel J, Rao AK, Meaney-Delman D. Clinical features of foodborne and wound botulism: a systematic review of the literature, 1932-2015. Clin Infect Dis. 2017;66(suppl_1):S11–6.
106. Dembek ZF, Smith LA, Rusnak JM. Botulism: cause, effects, diagnosis, clinical and laboratory identification, and treatment modalities. Disaster Med Public Health Prep. 2007;1(2):122–34.

Cardiac Implications of Neurological Disease

34

Cesare Iani, Ennio Montinaro, Novella Bonaffini, Loreta Quaranta, Alessandra Cinque, and Achille Gaspardone

Contents

Abstract

For a long time, empirical observation and popular wisdom have suggested a close link between neurological disease and cardiac complications, yet only in recent years have new technical approaches allowed a more detailed insight into the mechanisms underlying such connection. Both acute and chronic brain diseases may have relevant impacts on the heart eliciting arrhythmias and myocardial ischemia, which might have catastrophic consequences.

C. Iani (✉) · E. Montinaro · N. Bonaffini · L. Quaranta
Department of Neurology and Stroke Unit, Ospedale S. Eugenio-ASL RMC, Rome, Italy
e-mail: loreta.quaranta@aslroma2.it

A. Cinque · A. Gaspardone (✉)
Division of Cardiology, Department of Medicine, Ospedale S. Eugenio-ASL RMC, Rome, Italy
e-mail: alessandra.cinque@aslroma2.it

Introduction

This chapter will illustrate the most frequent acute and chronic neurological diseases in which clinically relevant cardiac complications manifest [1].

The physiological basis of the complex and intriguing relationship between heart and brain under physiological conditions will be discussed in the first section. After that,

E. Mahanna Gabrielli et al. (eds.), *Textbook of Neurointensive Care: Volume 1*, https://doi.org/10.1007/978-3-031-62220-5_34

we will focus on cerebrovascular accidents, traumatic brain and spinal cord injury, epilepsy, immune-mediated polyradiculoneuropathies, and myasthenia gravis, which represent the most frequent categories for acute neurocardiac complications. In the second part of this chapter, recent additions to our knowledge on dysautonomia and myocardial denervation observed in neurological degenerative disease will be illustrated. A summarizing table of cardiac implications of neurological diseases is presented below (Table 34.1).

A better understanding of the intimate connections between brain and heart is the basis for more effective prevention of cardiac complications in patients with neurological disease and customized therapeutical interventions for neurological disorders.

Table 34.1 Cardiac implications of neurological diseases

Neurological diseases	Temporal profile: acute/chronic	Neuroanatomic involvement:CNS/PNS/ANS Plaque/muscle	Cardiac manifestations	Diagnostic tools
Cerebrovascular disorders				
Ischemic stroke	Acute/chronic	CNS	Arrhythmias, myocardial infarct	EKG, Holter-EKG-loop recovery arteriography
Hemorrhagic stroke	Acute/chronic	CNS	Takotsubo-like syndrome	Echocardiography transthoracic (TTE)
Subarachnoid hemorrhage (SAH)	Acute/chronic	CNS	Sudden death	Echocardiography transesophageal (TEE)
PRES (posterior reversible encephalopathy syndrome)	Acute	CNS	Myocardial Ischemia	Coronary arteriography/ventriculography
			Takotsubo-like syndrome	MRI-CT-cardiac
				Cardiac SPECT-I ^{123}MIBG
				Cardiac PET
Traumatic injury				
Brain trauma	Acute/chronic	CNS	Arrhythmias, sudden death, dysautonomia	EKG, Holter-EKG
Spinal cord injury	Acute/chronic	CNS/PNS	Arrhythmias, sudden death, dysautonomia	TTE-TEE
Immune-mediated injury				
Acute polyradiculoneuropathy (GBS)	Acute	PNS	Arrhythmias, dysautonomia	EKG, Holter-EKG, TTE-TEE
			Takotsubo-like syndrome	
Myasthenia gravis crisis	Acute	PNS/muscle, plaque	Arrhythmias, Takotsubo-like syndrome	EKG, Holter-EKG, TTE-TEE
Polymyositis	Acute/chronic	Muscle	Arrhythmias	EKG, Holter-EKG
Epilepsy				
Epileptic status	Acute	CNS	Arrhythmias, sudden death	EKG, Holter-EKG, loop recording
			Takotsubo-like syndrome	TTE-TEE
				EEG-polysomnography
SUDEP (Sudden Unexpected Death in Epilepsy)	Acute/chronic		Sudden death	
Degenerative diseases				
Synucleinopathies				
Parkinson's disease	Chronic	CNS, ANS	Dysautonomia	SPECT I ^{123}-MIBG
Multiple-system atrophy				PET- ^{18}FD
Lewy body dementia				EKG, Holter-EKG, loop recording
PAF (pure autonomic failure)				Tilt test
Tauopathies				
Alzheimer disease	Chronic	CNS, ANS?	Dysautonomia	SPECT I ^{123}-MIBG
Progressive supranuclear palsy				PET- ^{18}FD
Frontotemporal dementia				EKG, Holter-EKG, loop recording

(continued)

Table 34.1 (continued)

Neurological diseases	Temporal profile: acute/chronic	Neuroanatomic involvement:CNS/PNS/ANS Plaque/muscle	Cardiac manifestations	Diagnostic tools
Miscellanea				
Neurocardiogenic syncope (vasovagal, carotid sinus syndrome, situational)	Acute	CNS, ANS	Dysautonomia	EKG, Holter-EKG, loop recording
				Tilt test
Neurogenic orthostatic hypotension (hereditary amyloidosis, hereditary sensory and autonomic neuropathy (HSAN type III), immune-mediated autonomic neuropathy)	Chronic	PNS, ANS	Dysautonomia	EKG, Holter-EKG, loop recording
				Tilt test
				Genetic test, serum autoantibodies
Channelopathies	Chronic	CNS, PNS	QT prolongation, ventricular arrhythmias, sudden death	EKG, Holter-EKG, loop recording
				Genetic test

CNS central nervous system, *PNS* peripheral nervous system, *musc* muscle, *ANS* autonomic nervous system

The Brain and the Heart

Folk wisdom and literature anticipate what science only much later can confirm. Conditions referred to as "heartache," "broken heart," and sudden deaths occurring shortly after losing one's beloved or stressful emotions have been attributed to a close connection between heart and brain. The heart and brain have a close and bidirectional interaction. Interestingly, there is no definite concept for mind or heart in Chinese traditional medicine. Instead, it embraces both and could be translated as a unique word: heart-mind [2].

Physiologically, the brain may be considered one of the first vascular stations of the circulatory system after its origin in the heart. On the other hand, a vast network of selective innervation links brain structures to the heart, which is deeply permeated by a tiny neural network (intrinsic cardiac nerve) (Fig. 34.1a, b).

Sudden cardiac death—the "voodoo death" [3]—precipitated by psychological stress represents an extreme example of the interaction of brain activation with cardiac activity. During earthquakes, people without any evidence of coronary artery disease or cardiomyopathy died suddenly without explanation [4]. There is such a thing as being "scared to death." In recent years, scientific evolution has allowed a more factual investigation of the mechanisms implied in such phenomena. Many studies have focused on a condition known as "myocardial stunning" or "Takotsubo cardiomyopathy," where emotions and stress lead to heart dysfunction. Indeed, it is well known that strong emotions and mental stress can precipitate cardiac dysrhythmias and sudden death in patients with heart disease.

To date, many cerebral areas are recognized as being involved in brain–heart regulation. We are still unsure if a discrete cerebral area influences cardiac activity or whether a more complex network interaction resulting from stimulation/inhibition processes is responsible for the final effect. Further, we are unsure whether conditioning activity—as in an ischemic cardiac insult—can modulate the heart's internal cellular environment and later predispose the same subject to cerebro-mediated cardiac insult [5].

The anatomy and physiology of the neurocardiac axis suggest an interaction between the central nervous system (CNS), autonomic nervous system (ANS), and the heart. This interaction has been studied for the last four decades. Animal models or human pathologic conditions, with or without pharmacological interventions, electrocardiography (ECG), electroencephalography (EEG), and evoked potential recordings, hormones level, plasma and urine levels of catecholamines have been employed to investigate the neurocardiac axis.

Recently, functional magnetic resonance imaging (fMRI) and positron emission tomography (PET) have allowed us to define a more complex neurocardiac network. Drawing on the anatomy and physiology studies of the last century, which identified autonomic cerebral control centers in the brainstem and hypothalamus, neuroimaging has expanded our knowledge from a static concept of central effectors to a more dynamic interaction of anatomical structures [6, 7].

Early scientific works identified the hypothalamus, brainstem, and spinal cord as the autonomic effectors of cardiocirculatory activity. Cortical areas such as the anterior cingulate cortex, insular cortex, amygdaloid nucleus, basal ganglia, and their connections with the brainstem and spinal cord

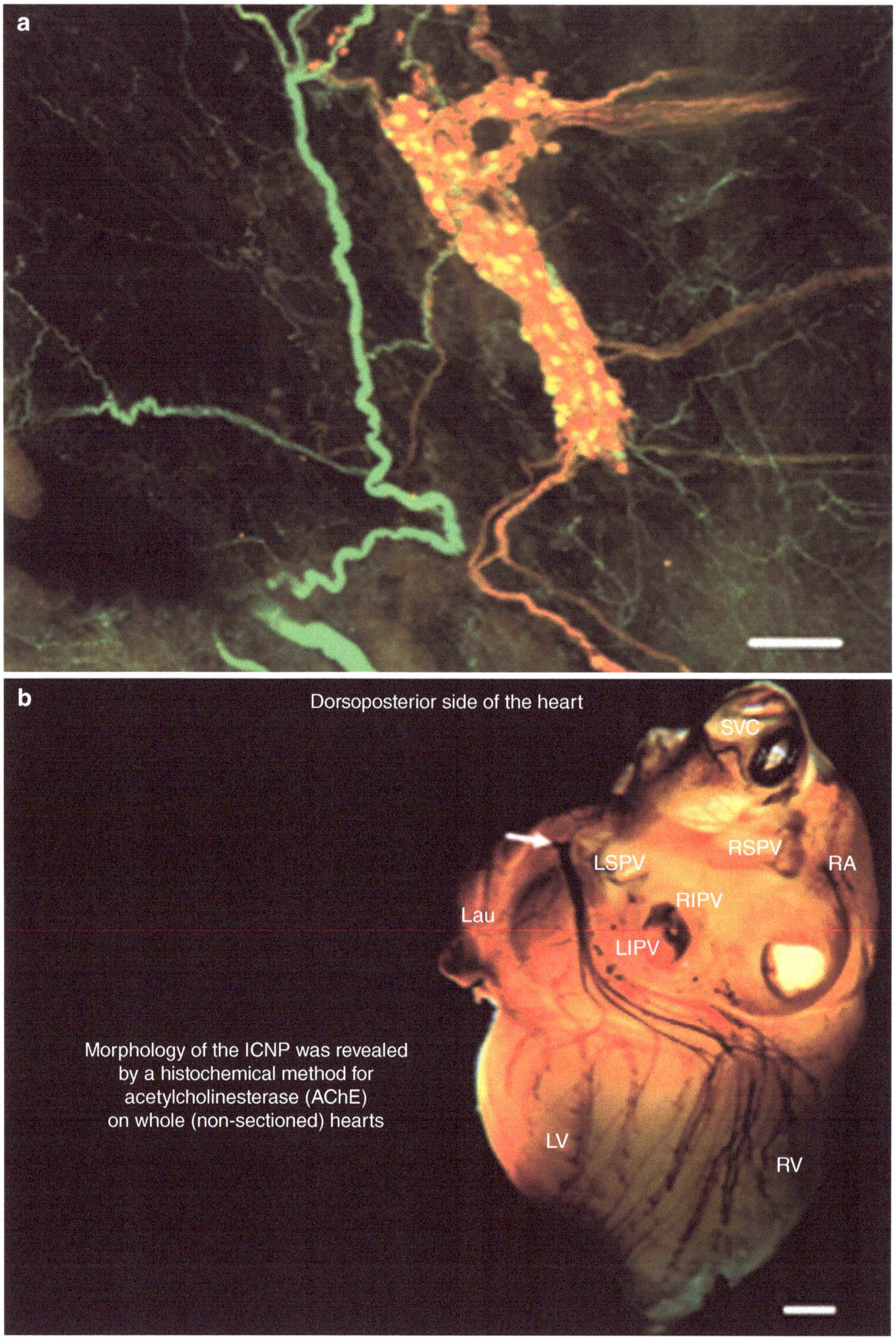

Fig. 34.1 (**a**, **b**) Intrinsic cardiac nervous system. (**a**) Microphotograph of left mouse atrium preparation demonstrating simultaneous staining of choline acetyltransferase (ChAT-positive in *red*) and tyrosine hydroxylase (TH-positive in *green*) as different nerve pathways. (**b**) Photomicrograph of the dorsoposterior side of the 1-month-old canine heart illustrates the location, course, and extent (capacity) of the left dorsal neural ganglionated plexus revealed on the total heart employing histochemical staining for acetylcholinesterase. Note the high concentration of epicardial ganglionated nerves inside the Marshall ligament on the left atrium that massively proceed forward of the coronary sinus and to ventricular coronary blood vessels. Epicardial ganglia are seen as dark differently sized spots along the stained nerves. The *arrow* points to the site where the extrinsic cardiac nerves are reflected onto the heart and subsequently course epicardially as the left dorsal ganglionated nerve subplexus. *ICV* orifice of the inferior vena cava, *Lau* left auricle, *LIPV* root of the left inferior pulmonary vein, *LSPV* root of the left superior pulmonary vein, *LV* left ventricle, *RA* right atrium, *RIPV* root of the right inferior pulmonary vein, *RSPV* root of the right superior pulmonary vein, *RV* right ventricle, *SVC* root of the superior vena cava. Scale bar 2 mm (Figures from Professor Dainius Pauza with permission of BMJ Publishing Group Ltd. from Taggart et al. [1])

situated below these structures have now been recognized as the anatomic link connecting emotions and cardiac activity [8–10] (Figs. 34.2 and 34.3).

Some authors have focused on stress as a critical factor in cerebral–cardiac interactions. Toivonen investigated arousal effects on the ambulatory ECG of 30 healthy physicians without known heart diseases. Recordings were compared just before and during emergency calls [12]. An inversion of the T wave was seen in 67% of subjects, and asymptomatic ST depression was recorded in 33%, suggesting that arousal can significantly affect ventricular repolarization even in normal hearts, presumably through sympathetic stimulation [13].

Cardiac dysrhythmia can therefore be linked to psychological stress and is associated with abnormal activation of

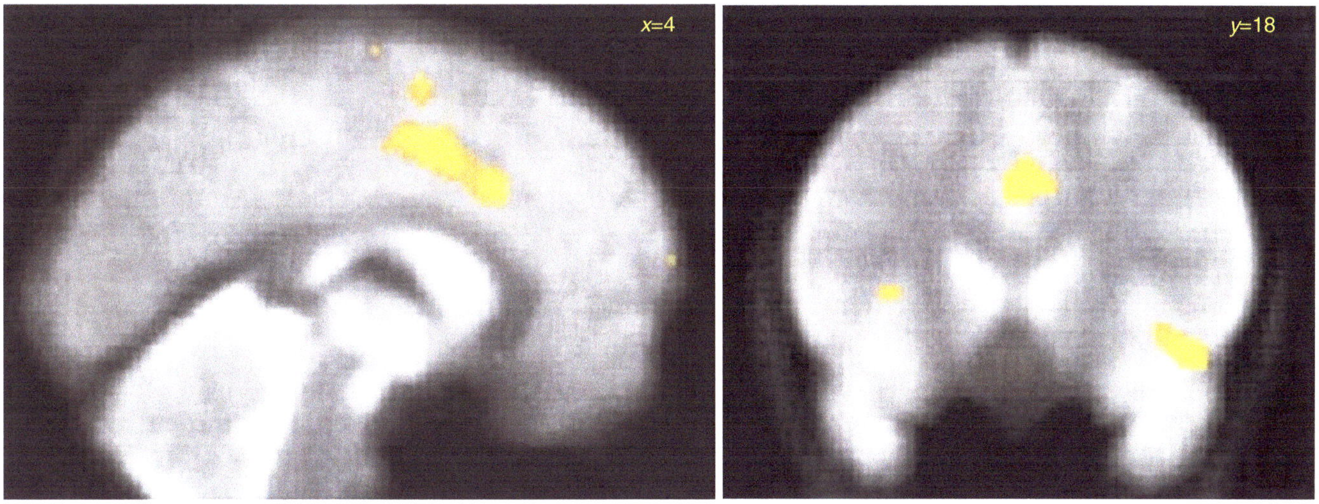

Fig. 34.2 Brain activity is associated with sympathetic cardiac control. Significant changes in regional brain activity associated with increasing low-frequency (LF, sympathetic) power derived from frequency analysis of beat interval (from ECG). Numbers illustrate laterality (mm) in normal space. This *t* contrast (a method to statistically extrapolate signals of sympathetic activity), resulting from multiple regression *t*-tests statistical analysis of specific signals, represents an activity that is uniquely related to sympathetic influences on heart rate (Reprinted with permission of Oxford University Press in part from Critchley et al. [11])

some cerebral areas, which leads to abnormal efferent autonomic drive to the heart. On the other hand, cerebral dysrhythmia of the autonomic centers may be amplified by afferent feedback from dysfunctional cardiac activity [6]. Moreover, a heartbeat-evoked potential (HEP), an index of afferent cardiac signals, has been described through EEG recording and is supposed to reflect individual differences in interoceptive sensitivity or the awareness of one's heartbeats. Patients subjected to stressors and studied by co-recorded EEG–fMRI techniques can express different functional responses of the myocardium through cardio-cortical feedback of cardiac function during stress [6, 14].

Cardiac stress-induced dysrhythmias can also result from repolarization inhomogeneity, induced by cardiac autonomic drive [15]. Other clues on the potential role of mental stress in predisposing to dysrhythmias derive from studies in patients without coronary disease with implantable cardiac defibrillators. In these patients, ventricular tachycardia was observed when subjected to difficult mental arithmetic tasks [16].

Research conducted on late-stage Parkinson's disease or dystonia patients treated with deep brain stimulation (DBS) has shown that specific electrical activity in the studied areas can affect cardiovascular functions, thus confirming a dynamic heart–brain interaction [17]. An object of further research is the possibility of therapeutically controlling heart activity through stimulation of specific brain areas [18].

Psychological stress triggering cardiac alterations is the key feature of a novel clinical entity known as transient left ventricular apical ballooning (TLVAB) or Takotsubo-like cardiomyopathy. The name Takotsubo is a Japanese term referring to the distinctive ballooning appearance of the mid and apical left ventricle on an angiogram, resembling an octopus cap. The apical ballooning syndrome is characterized by sudden onset of chest pain and ECG alterations such as ST-segment elevation, diffuse T-wave inversions, and abnormal QS-wave development. Echocardiography or left ventriculography of these patients shows wall motion abnormalities involving the lower anterior wall and apex. These abnormalities are associated with a slight increase in myocardial enzymes in patients without significant coronary artery lesions.

Nonetheless, the clinical presentation mimics acute myocardial infarction, its onset often preceded by emotional or psychological stress and characterized by highly rapid resolution. Takotsubo cardiomyopathy was first described in 1991 in Japanese literature with a dramatic female predominance. Initially considered a geographical or ethnic disorder, it is now described worldwide [19–21] (Fig. 34.4a–c). The pathophysiology of TLVAB is unknown, but most authors attribute TLVAB to a sudden surge of sympathetic activity in the CNS, resulting in high catecholamine levels in the blood and high levels of norepinephrine released directly into the myocardium [23]. In a study conducted by Wittstein, reversible TLVAB was investigated in 19 previously healthy patients admitted to the coronary care unit for chest pain or symptomatic heart failure precipitated by acute emotional stress. Plasma levels of catecholamines, metabolites, and neuropeptides were measured on day one and throughout the patients' hospital stay and compared with a sample of patients with myocardial infarction [20]. On the first hospital days, plasma levels of catecholamines among patients with stress cardiomyopathy were 2–3 times the values of patients with myocardial infarction and 7–34 times normal values.

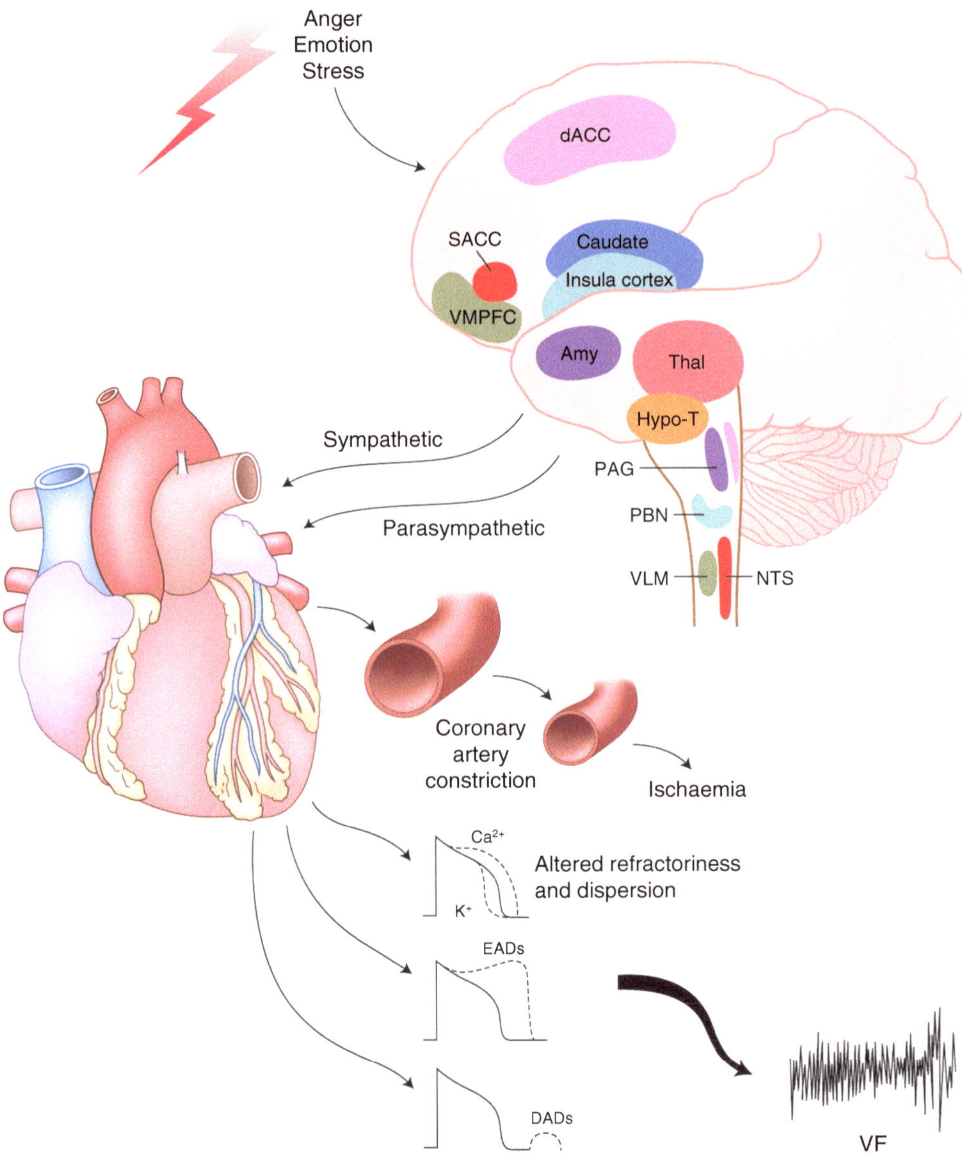

Fig. 34.3 Schematic view of brain autonomic nerves and the heart as an interactive system. Brain and brainstem regions are shown to interact with processing mental stress and emotion and with autonomic nerves and reflexes and the heart. Autonomically mediated effects modulate epicardial coronary artery and microvascular tone and thus myocardial perfusion. Both sympathetic and parasympathetic neural inputs to the heart influence a number of electrophysiological parameters, the result of which includes altered action potential duration and refractoriness and the generation of early and delayed after-depolarizations. *AMY* amygdala, *dACC* dorsal anterior cingulate cortex, *DAD* delayed after-depolarization, *EAD* early after-depolarization, *HYPO-T*, hypothalamus, *NTS* nucleus tractus solitarius, *PAG* periaqueductal gray, *PBN* parabrachial nucleus, *THAL* thalamus, *VF* ventricular fibrillation, *VLM* ventrolateral medulla, *VMPFC* ventromedial prefrontal cortex (Reprinted with permission of BMJ Publishing Group Ltd. from Taggart et al. [1])

These results led the authors to conclude that exaggerated sympathetic stimulation is probably the central cause of stress cardiomyopathy.

There are three suggested hypotheses to explain the pathophysiology of this event. One is a coronary arterial spasm, despite the absence of ST-segment elevation and a significant increase in cardiac enzymes. An alternative hypothesis is a sympathetically mediated microcirculatory dysfunction. The third possible mechanism of catecholamine-mediated myocardial stunning is direct myocyte injury. The histological correlate of the latter is called contraction band necrosis. It is a unique form of myocyte injury characterized by hypercontracted sarcomeres, dense eosinophilic transverse bands, and an interstitial mononuclear inflammatory response different from the polymorphonuclear inflammation seen in infarction. Contraction band necrosis (CBN) has been described in clinical states of catecholamine excess such as pheochromocytoma and SAH. It is also seen in the postmortem examination of people who died under terrifying circumstances, such as a fatal asthma attack or violent assault; this is consistent with the hypothesis of damage related to elevated levels of catecholamines [24, 25].

In stress-related myocardial stunning, contractile abnormalities are limited to the apex and midportion of the left ventricle, with relative sparing of the basal segments.

These findings are probably due to a greater density of sympathetic nerves at the base of the heart than at the apex with enhanced responsiveness of the apical myocardium to sympathetic stimulation.

An alternative explanation has been attributed to a base to apex perfusion gradient, resulting in regional differences in myocardial blood flow in the setting of catecholamine-mediated

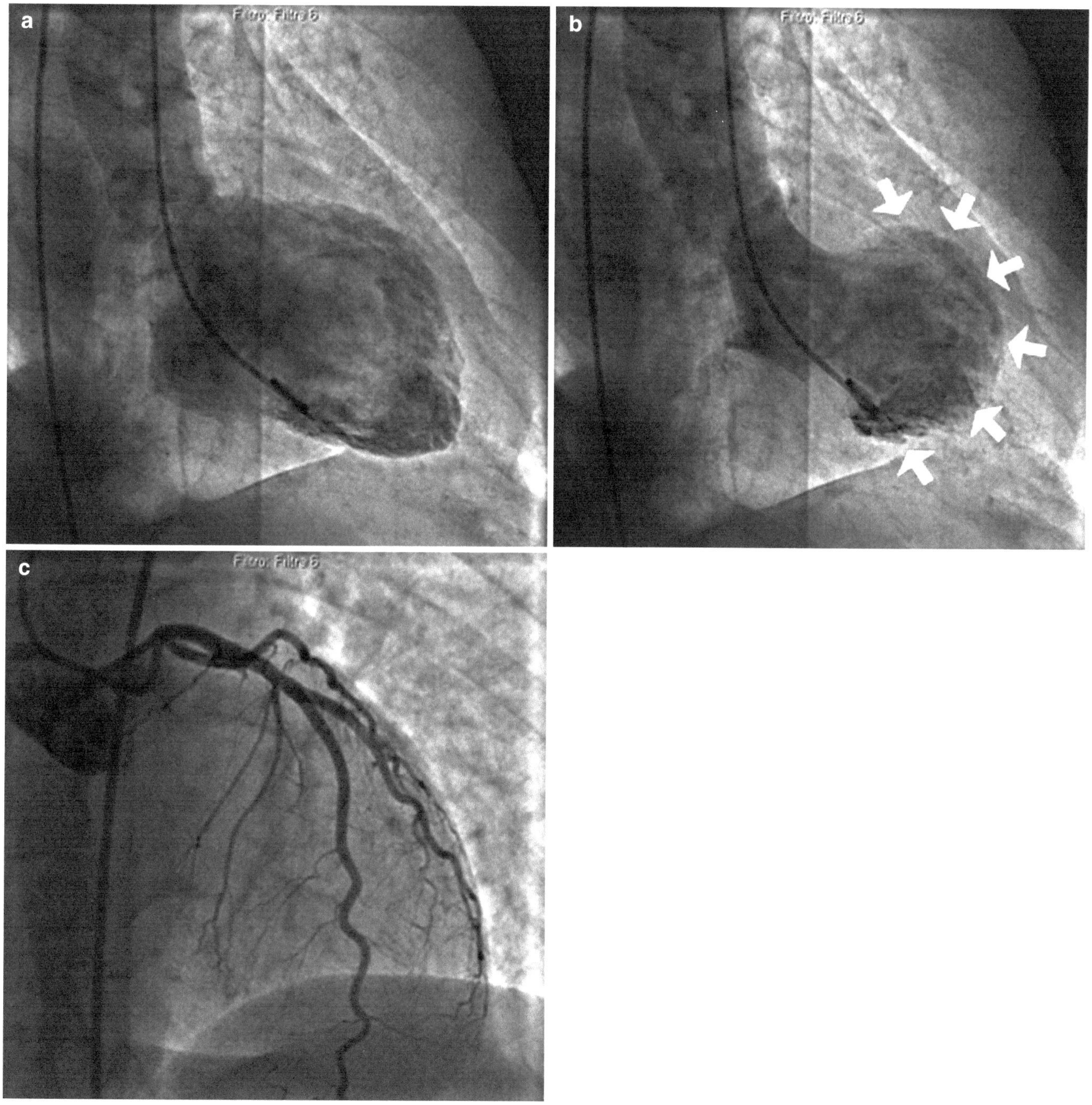

Fig. 34.4 (**a–c**) Left ventriculography in a young female patient with a Takotsubo syndrome occurring after an emotional stress. During diastole, left ventricle appears moderately enlarged (**a**). During systole, a large hypo-akinetic area involving the anterolateral, apical, and distal inferior segments of the left ventricle can be observed (**b**, *white arrows*). Left ventricular dysfunction occurs in the absence of epicardial left coronary artery abnormalities (**c**). Reprinted from Radfar et al. [22]

epicardial or microvascular vasoconstriction. The female propensity of the condition is possibly related to a different hormonal environment through mechanisms that remain to be identified [20].

The autonomic nervous system is likely a critical link between brain activity and the heart in the genesis of dysrhythmias. Functional neuroimaging and advances in molecular cardiology have added essential details in comprehending the precise mechanisms by which brain activity influences cardiac electrophysiology [1]. Focal stimulation of selected brain regions can produce changes in heart rate, blood pressure, ECG, and rhythm. In rats, stimulation of the left insular cortex may induce QT-segment prolongation, ST-segment depression, a decrease in heart rate, heart block, and asystole, suggesting the importance of hemispheric laterality in cardiac autonomic regulation [26]. In a related manner, in patients undergoing surgery for epilepsy, stimulation of the left insula induces bradycardia and a decrease in blood pressure, while stimulation of the opposite side increases both heart rate and BP.

Studies conducted in recent years with fMRI have added precious evidence to the analysis of the circuitry involved in stress-induced dysrhythmias. A specific group of cortical and subcortical brain regions (such as the anterior cingulated cortex, insular cortex, amygdala, basal ganglia) plays key roles in autonomic balance. The lack of sympathetic and parasympathetic activities balance could be responsible for stress-induced arrhythmogenesis and sudden cardiac death [9, 15, 27]. Given its characteristics, Takotsubo syndrome (TTS) has provided a model for investigating the neurocardiac axis. Several studies have engaged advanced brain imaging techniques to confirm the hypothesized pathogenetic mechanisms. A recent retrospective imaging study conducted on patients undergoing clinically indicated 18F-FDG-PET/CT imaging, who later developed TTS, showed an increased activity (seen as increased uptake of FDG on PET CT imaging)in the amygdala in PTS with subsequent TTS compared to controls [22]. Therefore, the amygdala has a pivotal role in the stress-induced phenomenon [28]. Resting-state fMRI in 15 TTS patients showed hypoconnectivity of central brain regions and the limbic system, under the influence of the autonomic nervous system.

A longitudinal PET/CT study by Tawakol et al. showed that increased amygdala activity was also associated with acute cardiovascular disease and increase inflammatory mediators [29], linking inflammation to cardiovascular disease [30]. Common features to all functional imaging studies cited are the evidence that sympathetic system activation plays a detrimental role on the cardiovascular system, with the amygdala playing a crucial part (Fig. 34.4d [29]).

Finally, case reports of typical Takotsubo have been described in neurological conditions such as SAH, during which a catecholamine surge has been demonstrated, Myasthenia gravis and, most recently, also during Sars-Cov2 infection [31].

Neurological Disease and the Heart

Cerebrovascular disease—the third leading cause of mortality in the world and first in western countries—is linking to neurological diseases. Data from both North American and European databases suggest that 25–30% of ischemic strokes are of cardioembolic origin. Around 25–80% of ischemic or hemorrhagic strokes induce cardiac complications such as acute myocardial ischemia, rhythm disturbances, myocardial stunning, and sudden death [32–38].

During the first 10 min post traumatic brain injury (TBI), cerebral hypoxia and stress-related catecholamine surge lead to a synergistic injury effect. In spinal cord injury (SCI), the heart lacks cardio-accelerated spinal control. Besides neurovascular and TBI/SCI influence on cardiac activity, other complex pathologic processes can affect heart function. For example, an immune-mediated dysautonomic failure can be observed during acute demyelinating polyradiculopathy or Guillain-Barré syndrome (GBS). Epilepsy can be complicated by sudden death, and, finally, cardiac failure can follow neurodegenerative processes such as Parkinson's disease.

Subarachnoid Hemorrhage

Subjects affected by SAH have a prevalence of cardiac injury ranging from 17% to 40%. The alterations described in patients affected by SAH are elevated cardiac troponin I levels (cTnI), QTc prolongation, ST-segment depression or elevation, T-wave changes, and dysrhythmias. Subarachnoid aneurysmal rupture causes a catecholamine surge in cardiac nerve endings, resulting in subendocardial myocyte damage known as contraction band necrosis (CBN) [39]. Cardiac injury is relevant in such patients. It has been observed that elevated cTnI is associated with an increased risk of cardiopulmonary complications, delayed cerebral ischemia, and death or poor functional outcome at discharge [40]. Moreover, myocardial damage seems to be worse as SAH severity increases; alterations in QTc persist in a consistent percentage of patients on follow-up ECG performed 5–12 days after the acute event. Finally, regional wall motion abnormalities (RWMA) have been found to be more frequent in SAH patients and may fail to normalize on follow-up echocardiography [40].

To better define the pathophysiology of left ventricular (LV) systolic dysfunction observed in SAH, Banki and colleagues designed a study to simultaneously evaluate myocardial sympathetic innervation and myocardial perfusion (both by scintigraphic imaging), and LV systolic function in SAH patients. The LV systolic dysfunction was associated with normal myocardial perfusion, but abnormal sympathetic innervation, suggesting an association between functional myocardial sympathetic denervation and cardiac injury. These findings support the hypothesis that excessive release of catecholamines from myocardial sympathetic nerves after SAH results in cardiac dysfunction; this may be considered a form of neurocardiogenic injury [41] (Fig. 34.5a). Genetic polymorphisms, which modulate the catecholamine sensitivity of the adrenoceptors, are associated with an increased risk of cardiac injury and dysfunction after SAH. Patients with particular types of polymorphism showed a 10- to 15-fold increase in the odds ratio of developing myocardial injury and LV dysfunction [44]. An increase in plasma B-type natriuretic peptide (BNP) is also common in SAH patients. High BNP levels were significantly associated with

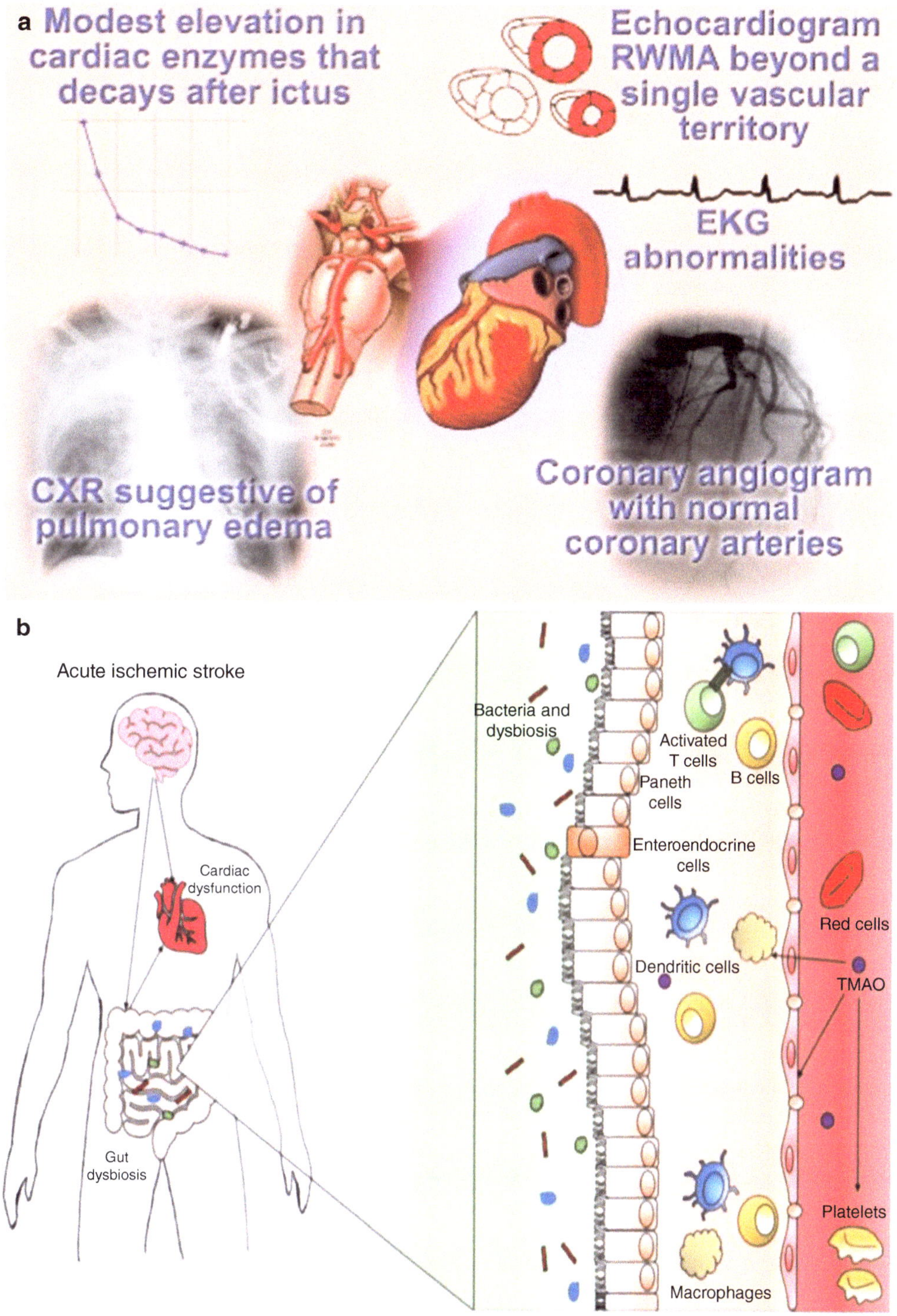

Fig. 34.5 (**a**) Cardiac manifestations during acute SAH (Reprinted with kind permission of Springer Science + Business Media from Lee et al. [42]). (**b**) Gut dysbiosis causes increased gut-blood barrier permeability and possible atherosclerosis and thrombosis through enhancement of the inflammatory response and platelet hyperactivation and thrombosis. Reprinted from Battaglini et al. [43] (**c**) Activation of different brain areas during stroke followed by specific cardiovascular complications. Depending on the extent of subsequent brain damage, stroke triggers different central regulatory regions, thus activating corresponding pathways that depend on the injured area. Therefore, post-stroke cardiac dysfunctions may be referred to specific brain areas. Right sides stroke is usually associated with more cardiac complications than left-sides stroke. *Qtc* corrected QT interval. Reprinted from Battaglini et al. [43]

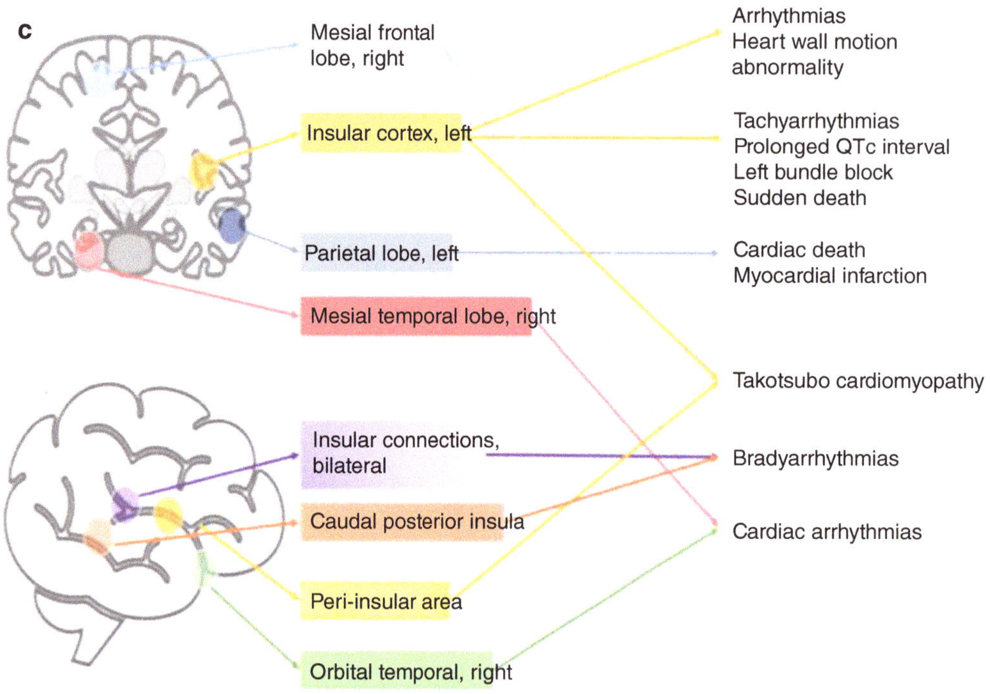

Fig. 34.5 (continued)

inpatient mortality, thus yielding additional evidence of cardiac injury and dysfunction occurring during SAH [45].

The pathogenesis of SAH-induced cardiac dysfunction can be explained by the following theories: (1) multivessel coronary artery spasm causing ischemia, (2) microvascular dysfunction, and (3) catecholamine toxicity. The first two hypotheses are not well supported by clinical evidence. The rare cases in which coronary angiograms of SAH patients were performed have demonstrated normal coronary arteries even in presence of ongoing S-T segment elevation. No alteration in myocardial perfusion of SAH patients has been documented supporting the microvascular dysfunction hypothesis [41, 42] should be the most likely explanation for SAH-induced myocardial injury.

Clinical evidence of the "catecholamine hypothesis" is supported by an increase in plasma norepinephrine within 48 h of symptom onset from SAH, persisting in the first week [46]. Pathologic myocardial changes described in patients with SAH are specific forms of myocyte injury characterized by hypercontracted sarcomeres, dense eosinophilic transverse bands, and an interstitial mononuclear inflammatory response [20, 47]. Similar histological changes have been reported in conditions such as Takotsubo cardiomyopathy, pheochromocytoma, status epilepticus, and assault victims who were found dead without clear explanation [20, 48]. A common feature between SAH-induced myocardial damage and stress-related cardiac dysfunction is a massive sympathetic discharge [9, 20, 42, 46].

Ischemic Stroke

Incidence of cardiovascular complication after acute ischemic stroke (AIS) is significant, with a 3% risk for myocardial infarction and one-third of AIS having >50% coronary artery stenosis despite no prior history of cardiovascular disease [49]. The autonomic function is impaired in 24% of stroke patients and linked to a worse outcome [50]. Almost 30% of patients show impaired ventricular ejection fraction, and systolic dysfunction develops in 13–29% of patients. EKG abnormalities are present up to 85% of AIS in the first 24 h, both in telemetry [51] and at baseline EKG [43, 52].

The wide spectrum of cardiac abnormalities observed in AIS includes sudden death, bradycardia, ectopic supraventricular or ventricular beats, supraventricular paroxysmal tachycardia, flutter, or atrial fibrillation; QT-segment prolongation; ischemic damage; left ventricular wall motion dysfunction; and cerebrogenic pulmonary edema.

Since the first clinical reports of case series in the late 1960s, clinicians have noticed the close interaction between neurological insults and cardiac activity [35, 53]. Norris and colleagues collected prospective data on 312 consecutive patients with either ischemic or hemorrhagic stroke, or transient ischemic attack (TIA), observing a 50% incidence of cardiac dysrhythmias after brain insult. These dysrhythmias were seen primarily with hemispheric involvement rather than with brainstem involvement. The investigators observed elevated plasma levels of the myocardial fraction of creatinine phosphokinase (CK-MB), suggesting clinically undetected myocardial lesions during acute neurological illness. Pathologic studies have revealed diffuse myocardial damage characterized by micro-islands of necrosis and subendocardial hemorrhages in stroke patients [35]. Acute cerebrovascular diseases are, therefore, a well-recognized cause of cardiac derangement. Ischemic stroke represents an excellent model to investigate neurocardiac influences through anatomic correlations of brain lesions [13].

The insular region was identified as the anatomical site linked most closely to cerebrogenic cardiac dysfunction after ischemic stroke. Stimulation of the right anterior insular cortex, in preoperative patients undergoing epilepsy surgery, generates sympathetic-derived cardiovascular responses, while left insular stimulation results in parasympathetic effects [54]. In a murine model of middle cerebral artery (MCA) stroke, occlusion of the MCA resulted in increased pulse and arterial pressure, increased plasma catecholamines, and subendocardial damage. In a feline model of the same injury, only the involvement of the insula resulted in significant increases in plasma catecholamines, suggesting an abnormal sympathetic stimulation [55, 56].

The insula is a deep cortical region located inside the Sylvian fissure at the intersection of frontal-parietal and temporal lobes in the opercular region, formed by about six cortical gyri and subdivided by a central sulcus into an anterior and posterior insular cortex. Embryologically, the insular cortex overlies the cerebral site where the telencephalon (which gives origin to the whole cortex) and the diencephalon (from which the thalamus and hypothalamus originate) are fused developmentally [57]. Ultrastructurally, the insula belongs to the paralimbic cortex. It is connected with the frontal cortex (opercular, premotor, and medial areas), temporal cortex (auditory cortex, polar and superior temporal cortex), parietal cortex (primary and secondary sensory areas), and limbic structures (amygdala, entorhinal cortex, and olfactory cortex) [58]. The insula is also connected to the basal ganglia and thalamus through the underlying claustrum and striatum [59]. The insula represents an important somatosensory/interoceptive and vestibular cortical processing area [60]. Its arterial supply emanates from the MCA—primarily the MCA-2 segment—whose origins are at the apex of the insula itself but also, to a lesser extent, from the M1 and M3 segments [61]. Over the past 10–15 years, the insular cortex has been identified as a key region in the genesis of cerebral-cardiac complications, resulting from its extensive autonomic and limbic connections. The right insula has generally been identified as the center for sympathetic autonomic modulation, whereas the left has a role in parasympathetic control [33]. In clinical studies, insular infarcts strongly correlate with sympathetic activation (high norepinephrine plasma concentration), and nighttime blood pressure increases [62]. Other recent clinical work with newer MRI techniques underscored the importance of right insula involvement for cerebrogenic cardiac effect, finding a solid correlation with raised plasma levels of cardiac troponin T (cTnT) [63]. In 208 ischemic stroke patients, reduced heart rate variability (HRV), a marker of cardiac autonomic derangement, and increased 1-year mortality were noted among patients with right insular lesions [64]. Other relatively small clinical studies supported the view of a right insular stroke lesion prevalence in patients with dysautonomic imbalance [51, 65]. An increased 1-year probability of adverse cardiac outcomes in patients without coronary artery disease has been noted when the left insula is involved in an ischemic stroke [66]. Lateralization of the injury does not appear to affect cardiovascular outcome [67]. There may be a different mechanism for the effect of acute and chronic cerebral ischemia, attributable to a reorganization of neuronal circuitry and rebalancing of parasympathetic and sympathetic nervous system activity. Long-term activation of the autonomic nervous system after an acute stroke event has been noted, with increased levels of norepinephrine and nighttime blood pressure. This combination represents an independent risk for future cardiovascular and cerebrovascular events [33].

Cerebrogenic cardiac abnormalities are mainly due to the direct toxic effect of raised catecholamine plasma levels on the myocardium. Secondly, catecholamine autoxidation may cause damage via the generation of free radicals. Moreover, there may be sympathetic-mediated coronary vasoconstriction [66]. Contraction band necrosis (CBN) is common in these patients, resulting from an intense sympathetic nervous system activation [63] peripheral adrenal medullary [3]. In a prospective study including 5817 AIS patients, 23 met the diagnostic criteria for Takotsubo-like myocardial dysfunction (TMD). Stroke patients with TMD had a higher inflammatory marker level and lower triglyceride level. Ischemic lesions were frequently located in the anterior circulation, with specific dominant regions being the insula and peri-insular areas [68]. The mechanisms affecting the stroke-heart crosstalk involve the hypothalamic-pituitary-adrenal axis (HPA), immune and inflammatory responses, and potentially gut dysbiosis [69]. Gut dysbiosis causes increased gut–blood barrier permeability and possible atherosclerosis and thrombosis by enhancing the inflammatory response and platelet hyperactivation and thrombosis [43] (Fig. 34.5b, c).

Many patients suffering from ischemic stroke have preexisting heart disease. About 20% of stroke patients have non-symptomatic CAD [70]. The presence of CAD, or any other overt cardiomyopathy, can alter the feedback between cardiac function and cerebral structures, determining an abnormal output to the heart. Neurological disease often uncovers an underlying cardiac condition.

An autopsy study reviewed 803 consecutive patients having died secondary to stroke or other neurological disorders, without a clear history of CAD [71]. Coronary artery stenosis greater than 50% was noted in 72% and 38% of subjects, respectively. Further, 40.8% had evidence of previous myocardial infarct, of which about 66% were clinically silent.

Comparing pre-and post-stroke ECGs, Lavy found new cardiac dysrhythmias in 39% of patients without a cardiac history [72]. In a similar study, Goldstein compared ECGs obtained within 24 h of stroke onset with those obtained 4 months earlier in 53 patients with stroke and controls. Thirty-two percent of stroke patients had new QT-segment prolongation, compared to just 2% of controls. T-wave inversion and U waves were present in 15% of stroke patients but none of the controls. New-onset cardiac dysrhythmias, of which atrial fibrillation (AF) was the most frequent, were noted in 25% of stroke patients but only 3% of controls [73].

Other studies evaluated dysrhythmia in ischemic stroke patients with ECG-Holter monitoring. Ventricular dysrhythmias after stroke, varied from 25% to 75%, but no statistical correlation with cardiac comorbidities or preexistent conditions was noted [35, 74, 75]. Atrial fibrillation (AF) is a common finding in ECG stroke studies [76]. About 20–25% of ischemic strokes occur related to AF [77]. In about 25% of older adults with AF, the dysrhythmia is intermittent and termed paroxysmal atrial fibrillation (PAF); AF and PAF share essentially the same odds of developing ischemic stroke [78].

Thirty-six percent of stroke survivors have a cryptogenic stroke, 19% of which have been of cardioembolic origin. These patients are at high risk of stroke recurrence and benefit from a preemptive diagnosis [79]. One consecutive series reported a 4.9% rate of previously unknown AF at stroke presentation [80], while Holter monitoring in post-stroke patients has yielded a detection range for AF/PAF of 3.8–6.1% [81]. Heart rate variability (HRV) studies have found impaired cardiovascular autonomic function expressed through lower parasympathetic tone and a tendency for right-sided strokes to present increased sympathetic cardiac activity, an increased risk for cardiac dysrhythmias [82].

Acute myocardial infarct (MI) is another potential complication of ischemic stroke [71]. While somewhat challenging to recognize due to a nonspecific cTnI elevation during the acute phase of stroke, it is a significant prognostic factor for in-hospital death or non-fatal cardiac event [83].

In a retrospective 6-year case series of 1357 patients, an overall 0.9% post-stroke MI (12 patients) rate was observed, usually occurring during the initial ten days. Half of these patients were noted to have an acute DWI lesion in the insular region on MRI. In 8 of the 12 patients, the cardiac event occurred as a painless infarction only recognized by cardiac monitoring [84].

Takotsubo-like wall motion abnormalities or myocardial stunning may follow acute stroke; this process is due to massive catecholamine release secondary to a stress response. A recent study examined 569 consecutive patients within 24 h of stroke onset and found seven female-gendered patients developing Takotsubo cardiomyopathy, with the dysfunction extending to 12 days [85].

Prosser and colleagues retrospectively analyzed the natural history in 846 acute stroke patients enrolled in a neuroprotective drug (lubeluzole) trial. The 3-month mortality was 21.3%, with cardiac etiology being the second most frequent cause, accounting for 19.4% of deaths, and peaking around day 14. Severe but non-fatal cardiac events occurred in 161/846 (19%) stroke patients, 80% of whom had a previous history of ischemic heart disease or chronic heart failure. Mortality was more frequent (46%) in patients suffering from at least one cardiac adverse event, most of which occurred during the first three days post-stroke [86]. Early cardiac mortality in stroke patients has been reported at about 6% in several studies [87, 88]. The annual cardiac mortality after stroke (5–10%) represents the single most common cause of death in long-term follow-up of ischemic stroke patients [89]. Kaplan and coworkers reported in a prospective population-based cohort study of stroke in adults 65 years of age and older [90], that over a median follow-up of 3.2 years, 57% of patients died, 22% suffered from a recurrence of ischemic stroke, while up to 17.4% showed signs of ischemic coronary disease.

In summary, monitoring cardiac function during the acute phase of ischemic stroke is essential for appropriate monitoring and planning therapeutic interventions aiming to decrease mortality from acute coronary artery diseases and dysrhythmias [91].

Intracerebral Hemorrhage

Spontaneous intracerebral hemorrhage (ICH) accounts for 15% of cerebrovascular accidents with higher 30-day mortality (30–52%) than ischemic stroke. Cardiac derangement could account for a significant proportion of early mortality in this subset of patients.

While there are data from investigations on the cardiac effects of ischemic stroke and subarachnoid hemorrhage, few studies have addressed cardiac abnormalities after ICH. In the acute phase of ICH, a murine study has shown a direct link between ICH and cardiomyocyte intracellular calcium metabolism dysregulation [92]. QTc-segment prolongation, ST-T segment morphologic changes, sinus bradycardia, and inverted T waves were the most frequently observed ECG abnormalities [38]. In a case series of 100 cerebrovascular accidents, 12 patients with ICH had ECG changes [53]. In another retrospective series [35], 47% of 30 patients with ICH had cardiac dysrhythmias with ventricular ectopic beats, the most common rhythm disturbance.

Another two studies use troponin levels as a marker of cardiac insult in ICH patients. At the Mayo Clinic, in a series of 110 patients [93], 64% had ECG abnormalities, whereas a positive TnT was detected only in about 20% of subjects. Hays and colleagues studied a population of 729 ICH patients [94]. While 18% showed an increased TnT level, 1.2% died from cardiac causes.

PRES and Cardiac Abnormalities

Posterior reversible encephalopathy syndrome (PRES) is a recent clinical entity characterized by transient neurological features and neuroimaging findings following a hypertensive crisis. PRES can lead to a reversible stunned myocardium. PRES has been associated with TTS in 10 patients. In a retrospective study of 224 patients with TTS, PRES was found in 2.7% of them. The link between the two conditions remains an object of speculation, yet suggesting careful cardiac monitoring in all these patients, in the acute phase [95–98].

Traumatic Brain Injury

Traumatic brain injury (TBI), a common condition in clinical practice, is frequently complicated by cardiac abnormalities, depending mainly on its severity. Blunt TBI consists of different types of cerebral lesions, which vary, on a severity scale, from focal to diffuse axonal injury (DAI). Severe TBI is usually accompanied by cerebral edema and elevation of intracranial pressure (ICP), which compromises cerebral perfusion pressure (CPP) and may result in cerebral ischemia [99].

TBI produces ECG abnormalities in up to 40% of patients, the gravity of which depends on the initial Glasgow Coma Scale (GCS) score and the presence of cardiac comorbidity. There is a general agreement that autonomic instability is the leading mechanism underlying cardiac pathophysiology [100–102], in general manifesting as a paroxysmal autonomic nervous system overactivity [100–104].

The clinical picture includes autonomic dysregulation signs, blood pressure, and cardiac rhythm abnormalities, elevated body temperature and diaphoresis, and muscle dystonia with a hypercatabolic state. Cardiac abnormalities include rhythm alteration with increased and decreased heart rate, ST-segment depression, and abnormal ventricular wall motion.

It is speculated that the dysautonomia following TBI results from "disconnection" of upper brainstem structures, causing a release of excitatory activity, or "diencephalic seizures." The lack of inhibitory drive from diencephalic-mesencephalic centers increases neurological stimuli through the spinal cord, originating in paroxysmal autonomic overactivity [101]. Indeed, non-painful stimuli, e.g., muscle stretching, skin touching, and loud noise or emotional inputs, can trigger autonomic paroxysms. TBI patients can present with dysautonomia and dissociation of sympathetic-parasympathetic heart rate variability (HRV) balance up to 1 year after the event [105], thus the rationale to administer gabapentin or baclofen as helpful medications in head-injured patients.

Premature atrial contraction and prolonged QTc interval have been observed in children undergoing therapeutic hypothermia [106, 107]. Therapy with beta-blockers may reduce the mortality of TBI patients, albeit data on functional outcomes are still missing [108]. Ongoing trials aim to clarify the issue of the use of beta-blockers in TBI based on the high sensitive troponin T status [109].

Spinal Cord Injury

Traumatic spinal cord injury (SCI) often involves a younger population, with about 80% male prevalence. A bimodal median age of 32 years and 74 years of age for older victims has been observed, with a mortality rate of between 1% and 3% and about 25% and 39%, respectively [110]. A significant degree of disability follows severe SCI, which leads to about 50% complete or partial tetraplegia and 40% complete or partial paraplegia [111]. Interruption of medullary pathways determines acute sensorimotor deficits and autonomic derangements, which depend upon the lesion level. Recent data have highlighted how cardiovascular disturbances are the second leading cause of death in the acute—as well as in the chronic—stages of SCI after respiratory failure [112, 113].

Sympathetic intermediolateral nuclei in the lateral medulla extend from the level of T1 through the L2 segment of the spinal cord, giving rise to preganglionic sympathetic neurons, which synapse with postganglionic neurons in the paravertebral sympathetic chain or in perivisceral ganglia structures. At the T1–T6 level, postganglionic sympathetic fibers, known as the cardiac sympathetic chain, are directed to the heart and related vessels. The basic mechanism of cardiovascular derangement in the SCI patient is interruption of descending autonomic control pathways, and suppression of sympathetic outflow resulting in unbalanced vagal nerve-mediated parasympathetic activity. Compared with controls, the analysis of heart rate variability (HRV) in acute SCI patients showed marked alteration in low frequencies. In contrast, high frequencies variabilities were comparable to controls, indicating a lack of sympathetic and parasympathetic tone in SCI [114]. Sympathetic activity raises pulse rate and blood pressure. Parasympathetic activity via the right vagal nerve predisposes to brady dysrhythmias and, through the left vagal nerve, to atrioventricular block.

Heart disease accounts for about 30% of SCI patients' acute and long-term death rates. The period of peak mortality is within 6 weeks of injury. Older patients are more affected for reasons not yet completely understood [112, 115, 116]. In long-term patients, the most frequent causes of death related to the circulatory system occur at a median of 55 months post-SCI. Causes were, in decreasing order of frequency, heart failure, atrial fibrillation, atherosclerosis, and ischemic heart disease, ventricular tachycardia, abdominal aneurysm rupture, cerebrovascular disease, cardiac arrest, cardiomyopathy, and "ill-defined heart disease" [110, 116].

In the acute stage of SCI, the sudden lack of sympathetic drive exposes the patients to bradycardia, hypotension, and hypothermia. This neurogenic shock must not be confused with hypovolemic shock, where hypotension occurs with tachycardia; unfortunately, the two situations may coexist and are difficult to separate. Cardiac dysrhythmias are linked to the SCI level and hence severity; the more cranial the lesion, the more severe the dysrhythmia. In the acute setting and for the first 4–6 weeks post-injury, the risk of dysrhythmias is particularly high [116]. The most common dysrhythmia is ventricular bradycardia which may progress to asystole/cardiac arrest. The response to vagolytic agents such as atropine or glycopyrrolate might be insufficient to sustain cardiac output. Isoproterenol and methylxanthines have been used for refractory cases while a temporary pacemaker is inserted. In the chronic phase, brady dysrhythmias are more frequent in high cervical lesions and sometimes require permanent pacemaker implantation.

Although less frequent, tachydysrhythmias are represented by paroxysmal supraventricular tachycardia (PSVT), sinus tachycardia, and atrial flutter or fibrillation. Not infrequently seen are ST-segment elevation and other abnormalities such as premature atrial contractions (PACs), intraventricular conduction delay (IVCD), and bundle branch block (BBB). Nonetheless, brady dysrhythmias represent the most frequent (64–77%) rhythm disturbances seen in cervical spine injuries.

Autonomic dysreflexia, rare in the acute phase of SCI, usually is seen after the first month of injury and mainly in patients with T6 or higher-level lesions. It is due to the reorganization of an imbalanced sympathetic system. In particular, the aberrant sprouting of peptidergic fibers below the cord lesion may amplify disinhibited sympathetic spinal neurons and responsiveness of peripheral alpha-adrenoceptors. Autonomic dysreflexia is characterized by sudden episodes of arterial hypertension, with systolic blood pressure values up to 300 mmHg, accompanied by reflex bradycardia and other signs of sympathetic hyperreactivity. The disorder is usually triggered by noxious stimuli such as endotracheal suctioning, bladder emptying, or bowel stimulation. The episodes may recur three to four times a day and may precipitate post-event tachydysrhythmias or acute coronary syndrome in predisposed patients. Finally, one may see cardiovascular deconditioning, with resultant upregulation of nitric oxide synthase and increased plasma nitric oxide levels, both of which contribute to prolonged hypotension [110, 116, 117].

Therapeutic interventions are limited and are directed toward sustaining blood pressure in case of neurogenic shock, controlling hypertensive emergencies with appropriate drugs, and preventing inappropriate stimuli, which may precipitate autonomic dysreflexia.

A recent analysis of a large cohort of SCI survivors, with a variety of injury levels and severities, has shown an increased incidence of AF in these patients, with long-term autonomic dysregulation being a significant risk factor [118]. Abnormal lipid profile, with an increase in total cholesterol and low-density lipoprotein cholesterol (LDL-cholesterol) occurs in chronic SCI leading to a high risk of developing coronary heart disease and systemic atherosclerosis. The reason for the lipid profile alteration has been indicated as possibly linked to a combination of inappropriate diet, adrenergic dysfunction, and lack of physical activity [119].

Guillain-Barrè Syndrome and Peripheral Neuropathies

Autonomic dysfunction is a well-recognized manifestation of Guillain-Barrè syndrome (GBS) and has been reported more commonly in the acute demyelinating subtype of the disease [120]. Dysautonomia is considered a distinctive feature of GBS and part of differential diagnosis with chronic inflammatory demyelinating polyneuropathy (CIDP) [121]. Different degrees of autonomic nervous system involvement have been reported and can be seen in up to 70% of patients with GBS.

Autonomic dysfunction manifests as increased heart rate and labile hypertension associated with elevated plasma noradrenaline concentrations. The diseased peripheral nerves' impairment of catecholamine uptake is responsible for plasma catecholamine elevation [122]. Cardiovascular abnormalities attributed to autonomic neuropathy in GBS patients take different forms. Rhythm abnormalities range from sustained sinus tachycardia—the most commonly observed feature and usually not requiring treatment—to brady dysrhythmias, reported in 50% of patients; a small percentage of these cases present with potentially serious events necessitating administration of vagolytic agents or pacemaker placement [123, 124]. Blood pressure variability has been attributed to impaired baroreceptor reflex and altered catecholamine levels, causing postural hypotension alternated to hypertensive episodes [122].

A wide spectrum of electrocardiographic changes, such as QT-segment prolongation, giant T waves, ST-T segment changes, and atrioventricular blocks, have all been described in patients with GBS, suggesting myocardial involvement

[122]. On postmortem evaluation, a fatal case of intractable cardiac dysrhythmias was reported that showed signs of severe myocarditis [125].

Anecdotal reports of reversible left ventricular dysfunction during GBS match the characteristics described in stunned neurogenic myocardium (i.e., rapid onset and resolution of symptoms, ECG changes accompanied by mildly elevated cardiac enzymes, severe left ventricular systolic dysfunction, and segmental wall motion abnormalities) [126, 127].

Cardiac autonomic neuropathy (CAN) is the least recognized and understood complication of peripheral neuropathy. CAN is a common complication of diabetic neuropathy, with 20–34% of all diabetic patients being affected. Symptoms vary from paroxysmal tachycardia, postural hypotension, exercise intolerance, silent myocardial ischemia, and infarction to major cardiovascular events such as myocardial infarction and heart failure. QT interval prolongation indicates an imbalance between right and left sympathetic innervation. Prolongation of QT interval may increase the risk of dysrhythmia and sudden death. Peripheral neuropathies are the most common neurological complication in HIV/AIDS, with a prevalence of CAN described in up to 70%. Manifestations of CAN are seen both in HIV-positive and AIDS patients ranging from bradycardia to prolongation of QT interval [128].

Recent interest has been focusing on Transthyretin (TTR) amyloidosis, especially due to the availability of disease-modifying therapies [129, 130]. TTR amyloidosis is a systemic disorder caused by the deposition of aggregated fibrils of a misfolded mutated plasma protein for thyroxin and vitamin A (TTR). TTR amyloid fibrils accumulate in various organs and tissues, causing progressive dysfunction. Peripheral nerves are frequently involved with TTR amyloidosis, presenting as a progressive axonal sensory autonomic and motor neuropathy (familial amyloid polyneuropathy TTR -FAP, also known as FAP or ATTR-PN). Cardiac involvement is due to infiltrative cardiomyopathy (familial amyloid cardiomyopathy). Disease prevalence varies across individuals and geographic locations. Amyloid deposition, regardless of the amyloid deposit's substance, has a direct effect on cardiac function and indirect cardiovascular downfall. Dysrhythmias include bundle branch block, atrioventricular and sinoatrial block, and autonomic dysfunction [128, 131].

Myasthenia Gravis

Myasthenia gravis (MG) is an autoimmune disorder leading to fluctuating muscle weakness and fatigability. Circulating antibodies bind acetylcholine receptors at the postsynaptic neuromuscular junction. ICU admission of patients affected by myasthenia is mainly related to respiratory failure. Bronchopneumonia from aspiration is a common autopsy finding in patients with myasthenia gravis [132]. Patients with myasthenia gravis may also develop MG-related heart disease in a minority of cases, mainly when a thymoma is present. Symptoms of myocardial involvement are mainly dysrhythmias. Microscopic study of symptomatic patients has shown signs of focal myocarditis [133]. Myocarditis is a much more rare complication of MG [134]. Overall, 12% of MG patients may experience various clinical signs of cardiac disease. Generally, patients with late-onset (50 years of age) or thymoma associated MG are the highest risk group for cardiovascular events [135–137].

Recent case reports have described the association of Takotsubo syndrome with myasthenic crisis. MG crisis itself or plasmapheresis treatments played to treat it may have a causative role in the development of TLVAB [138].

Myasthenic and multiple sclerosis patients have increased numbers of plasma T-helper 1 and T-helper 7 cells and proinflammatory cytokines such as interleukin(IL)-1, IL-6, IL-17, interferon-gamma, and tumor necrosis factor alfa (TNFα) [139, 140].

Autonomic and immune systems are linked by a feedback mechanism.

An immunomodulating loop was identified between the vagal nerve (VN) and the immune system as a cholinergic anti-inflammatory pathway. Therefore, the modulation of vagal activity may result in beneficial therapeutic effects in both MG and MS [141–143].

A recent study has assessed cardiac autonomic responses to an orthostatic test in 23 Myasthenia Gravis (MG) patients. A shift of autonomic nervous system balance toward sympathetic predominance in the MG group was recognized, with an impaired baroreflex mechanism [135, 144].

Cardiac involvement in MG has been reported and ranged from asymptomatic ECG findings through conduction abnormalities to heart failure and sudden death [145–147].

Abnormal baroreceptor reflex may also be the result of impaired synaptic transmission in autonomic ganglia through a cross-reactivity of muscular anti-AChR Ab with ganglionic AChR [148–151].

In summary, the cardiac autonomic function of patients with MG is frequent and often misdiagnosed. Coronary artery disease may be present as a comorbidity. However, it may not be easily excluded because of patients' exercise intolerance [135–137].

Dermatomyositis and Polymyositis

Polymyositis and dermatomyositis are chronic inflammatory muscle diseases clinically characterized by muscle weakness due to inflammatory cell infiltration in skeletal muscle. Extramuscular involvement is common, such as skin inflammation, interstitial lung disease, arthritis, gastrointestinal involvement, and Raynaud's phenomenon. Myositis is a systemic inflammatory connective tissue disease. Annual incidence per 100,000 population is approximately 0.5 [152].

The frequency of heart involvement in patients with myositis varies between 6% and 75% [153]. Cardiac involvement as a cause of death in polymyositis is present in 10–20% of cases, and congestive heart failure between 3% and 45% of cases [154]. Subclinical cardiac involvement is much more common than overtly manifest heart disease. ECG changes are the most commonly observed alterations and include atrial and ventricular dysrhythmias, atrioventricular block, BBB, prolongation of P-R intervals, nonspecific ST-T wave changes, and abnormal Q waves [155].

Histopathological studies have documented mononuclear inflammatory cell infiltrates in the endomysium and perivascular areas [156]. Coronary artery vasculitis, intimal proliferation, medial sclerosis, and microvascular disease are potential causes of clinical symptoms such as dysrhythmias and angina pectoris [154]. Echocardiographic studies show left ventricular diastolic dysfunction as the most common alteration. Gadolinium-DTPA-enhanced MRI, which can detect myocardial inflammation, and endomyocardial biopsy have also been used to assess myocardial involvement. However, troponin I remains the most used and specific laboratory test to detect myocardial involvement [154].

Epilepsy

Seizures are associated with an increased risk of dysrhythmias. Various heart rhythm alterations occur during (ictal) or after (postictal) seizures. Sinus tachycardia is the most common ictal pattern [157]. The most frequent clinically relevant arrhythmia is ictal asystole, assumed to be self-limiting. It may cause falls and injuries due to seizure-induced syncope [158]. Ictal asystole, bradycardia, and AV block predominantly occur in people with temporal lobe epilepsy. Postictal asystole is less common, associated with convulsive rather than focal (temporal lobe) seizures, and with a higher fatality rate [159].

Cardiac asystole induced by epileptic seizures is a rare complication (Fig. 34.6a). Five patients developed temporary asystole self-resolving in a recent retrospective study of

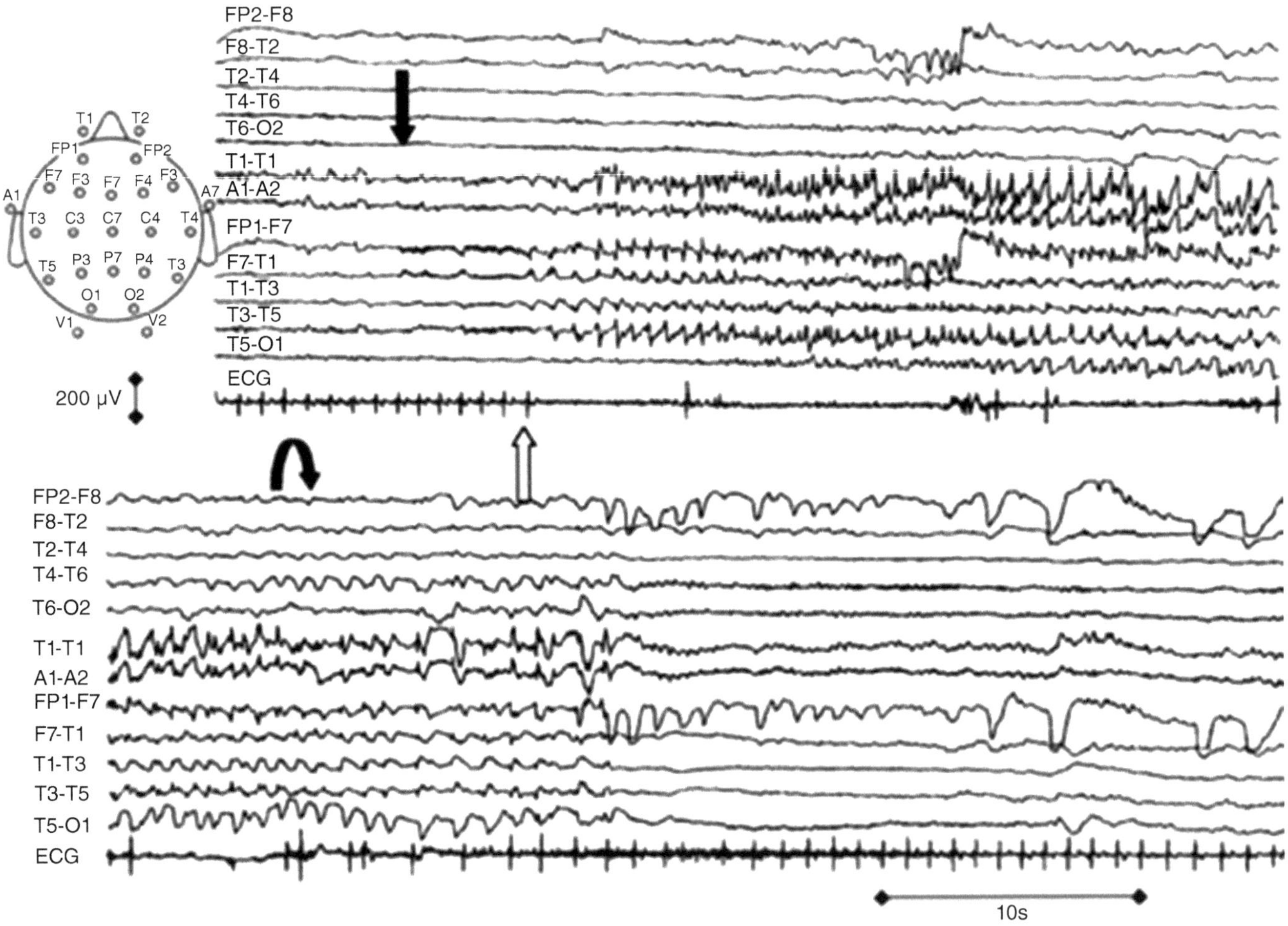

Fig. 34.6 (**a**, **b**) Conceptual framework of the link between chronic epilepsy and development of an "epileptic heart" due to cardiotoxic effects of catecholamines, repeated hypoxemia, with increased cardiac electrical instability manifest as TWA, a repeating ABAB beat-to-beat pattern in the ST-segment and T wave of the EKG. (Reprinted from Verrier RL et al. [160])

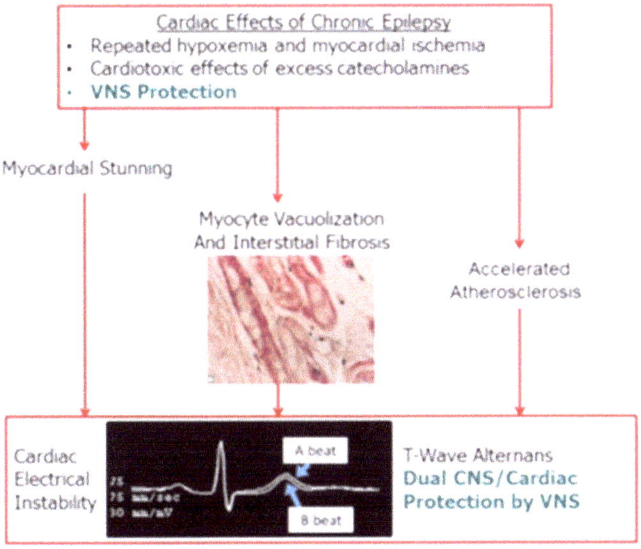

Fig. 34.6 (continued)

1244 patients undergoing long-term video-EEG monitoring [161].

The precise mechanism of ictal asystole is unknown. It may result from epileptic activity directly stimulating the central autonomic networks. Alternatively, seizure-induced catecholamine may evoke a vasovagal response causing cardiac conduction inhibition and vasodilation [162].

Many genes that potentially link epilepsy to cardiac dysrhythmias have been identified; genes implicated in ion channel disorders (channelopathies) play a significant role.

Patients can develop transient myocardial ischemia during seizures, which lowers the threshold for dysrhythmias. Epileptic individuals are also more likely to present structural and functional cardiac abnormalities, a sedentary lifestyle, obesity, and antiepileptic drugs (AEDs) altering lipid metabolisms, such as carbamazepine and phenytoin [162].

Status epilepticus (SE) [160] is a dramatic complication of epilepsy and a medical emergency carrying a mortality rate up to 30%. Anoxia followed by cardiac arrest accounts for the highest mortality in older patients with SE; other complications affecting mortality are stroke, metabolic alterations, drug overdose, tumors, and trauma [163].

Interestingly, 90% of SE-induced mortality does not occur during the seizures, or even within the initial 24 h of the events, but within the 30 days following seizure activity, even if metabolic variables are controlled [164–166].

Two different patterns in hemodynamic instability precede death [167] a gradual decline in blood pressure and heart rate that correlates with myocardial injury in the post mortem examinations, and sudden death with autopsy studies showing no evidence of cardiac damage [163]. A murine study evaluated myocardial damage, consistent with activation of the sympathetic nervous system and induced cardiac myofilament damage [168]. The cardiorespiratory effects of seizure activity are probably due to a seizure-induced excitation of the rostral brain areas projecting to the autonomic centers in the brainstem [168].

Seizure activity could cause repetitive myocardial injury with a catecholamine-mediated mechanism, leading to the concept of the "epileptic heart" (Fig. 34.6b), resulting in myocardial fibrosis, accelerated atherosclerosis, systolic and diastolic dysfunction, severe dysrhythmias [160, 169], and Takotsubo cardiomyopathy [170–172]. ECG monitoring for all patients admitted to the hospital for epilepsy is recommended [172].

Patients affected by epilepsy are at increased risk of a sudden death condition termed sudden unexpected death in epilepsy (SUDEP). The death may be witnessed or unwitnessed and may occur with or without evidence of a seizure. The autopsy is always negative for toxicology [173]. SUDEP ranges from 0.35 to 2.7 per 1000 person-years; SUDEP accounts for up to 17% of all deaths in patients with epilepsy [174, 175]. Risk factors for SUDEP include a history of epilepsy and, in particular, refractory generalized tonic-clonic seizures (GTCS). Nocturnal GTCS and living alone are associated with markedly increased risk of SUDEP. Among comorbid diseases, a previous diagnosis of substance abuse or alcohol dependence is associated with an increased risk of SUDEP [176]. Interestingly, polytherapy with antiepileptic drugs and frequent dose changes appear associated with SUDEP, independent of seizure frequency [174]. The current consensus is that SUDEP is primarily a "seizure-related" event, but the mechanisms underlying cardiac arrest are still unclear. A frequent finding of pulmonary edema in SUDEP patients at autopsy or in animal models may link the death to hypoxia from neurogenic pulmonary edema [175, 177]. Epilepsy surgery and vagal nerve stimulation techniques reduce the risk of SUDEP [178].

Genetic predisposition contributes to SUDEP: (a) sodium and potassium ion channels subunits were the most frequently reported genetic variants discovered by molecular autopsy [179, 180].

Degenerative Neurological Diseases and the Heart

The critical feature of cardiovascular dysfunction in Parkinson's disease (PD) and other basal ganglia disorders is dysautonomia [181, 182]. Studies of autonomic dysfunction in such diseases provide new insights into their pathophysiological mechanism and potential for therapies.

For example, orthostatic hypotension (OH) and postprandial hypotension are well-recognized examples of cardiac autonomic dysfunctions in Parkinsonian syndromes, probably due to lack not only in dopamine neurotransmission but also in noradrenergic mediated neurotransmission. Other dysautonomic disturbances, such as urinary incontinence, constipation, heat/cold intolerance, sweating, and salivary gland dysfunction, have been noted.

Common clinical manifestations underlie common cellular abnormalities. Parkinson's disease (PD), Lewy body dementia (LBD), multiple-system atrophy (MSA), and pure autonomic failure (PAF) share the name of synucleinopathies where α-synuclein, a cytosolic protein, pathologically accumulates, leading to progressive cellular degeneration. Strong genetic correlation has been observed in familial forms of PD with synuclein gene mutation or triplication [183]. Cognitive and motor disturbances, such as progressive supranuclear palsy (PSP), cortico-basal ganglionic degeneration (CBD), frontotemporal dementia (FTD), and Alzheimer's disease (AD), share a cellular level of deposits of hyperphosphorylated tau protein. This group of degenerative abnormalities is often grouped as tauopathies.

Synucleinopathies

Parkinson's Disease (PD), Multiple-System Atrophy (MSA), and Lewy Body Dementia (LBD)

Synucleinopathies share the presence of Lewy body deposits into neurons, a hallmark of cell degeneration. In PD and LBD, there is postganglionic autonomic structure damage involving the heart and paravertebral sympathetic ganglia. In MSA, there is predominant involvement of spinal and brainstem structures [184] (Fig. 34.7).

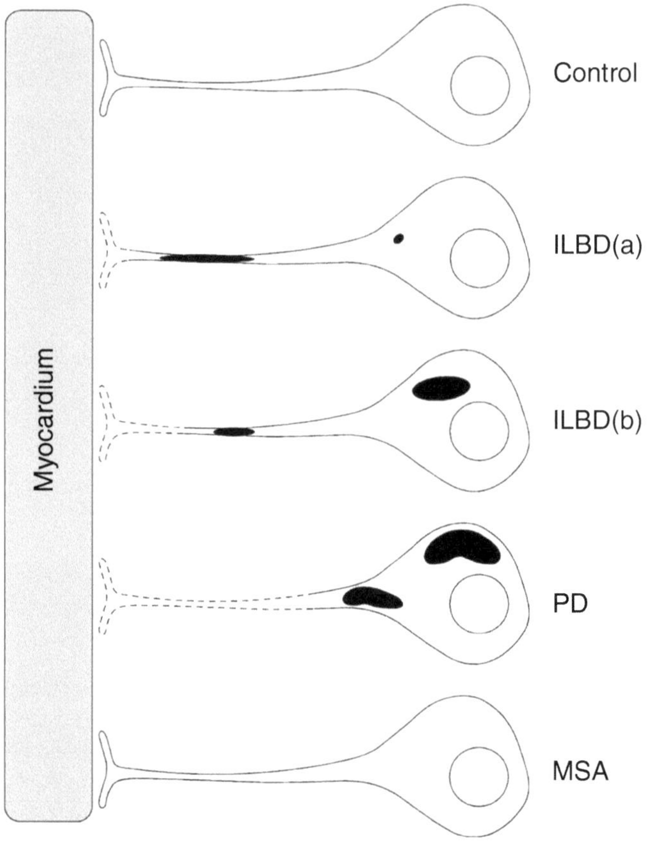

Fig. 34.7 Schematic illustration of the degenerative process of the cardiac sympathetic nervous system. In ILBD(a) α-synuclein aggregates accumulate in the distal axons and sparse α-synuclein aggregates in the paravertebral sympathetic ganglia. *Black shading* indicates α-synuclein aggregates. The *line* indicates the outline of TH-ir axons or their mother neurons. The *dotted line* indicates degeneration of TH-ir axons. *ILBD(a)* ILBD with preserved TH-ir axons, *ILBD(b)* ILBD with decreased TH-ir axons (Reprinted with permission of Oxford University Press from Orimo et al. [184])

Cell loss or Lewy body formation is present in the locus coeruleus of PD patients, which is the primary source of norepinephrine in the brain. The dorsal motor nucleus of the vagal nerve also shows cell loss or Lewy bodies in PD patients [185, 186]. There is still unclarity as to the precise mechanisms of these disorders [183], and the peripheral versus central origin of OH in PD remains a debated topic.

Newer imaging techniques have confirmed "in vivo" pathologic findings. Goldstein and colleagues found, in PD, a significantly low myocardial concentration of 6[^{18}F]fluoro-dopamine with positron emission tomographic (PET) scanning and low plasma concentrations of norepinephrine and its metabolites. This finding is evidence of postganglionic cardiac noradrenergic denervation, and it is seen in the early stages of the disease, labeled as "sympathetic cardio-neuropathy." Patients with MSA and autonomic failure (Shy-Drager syndrome) have increased 6[^{18}F]fluoro-dopamine cardiac concentrations and slightly increased norepinephrine spillover (Fig. 34.8).

Many authors have demonstrated a reduction in cardiac innervation in PD patients with or without clinical evidence of dysautonomia, even in the early stages of the disease [187–193]. Sudden falls in blood pressure vary from 40% to 60%, depending upon the clinical phase of the disease [181, 182].

The arterial baroreflex is the primary neurocirculatory reflex implicated in OH. Distortion of stretch-sensitive cells in large artery walls and in the heart causes increased vagal outflow to the heart, resulting in bradycardia and, with decreased sympathetic outflow to the cardiovascular system, vasodilation [185]. The site, or sites, of the central neural lesions that produce baroreflex failure in PD are largely unknown.

Baroreflex failure involving both vagal and sympathetic circuits is associated with sympathetic denervation [185], and often abnormal patterns of HRV are recorded during polysomnography [192, 194].

A recent cross-sectional study including 50 PD patients and matched controls showed that PD patients had a higher incidence of left ventricular hypertrophy, diastolic dysfunction, and heart failure [195].

Knowledge of cardiac and autonomic derangement is beneficial in degenerative disease for differential clinical diagnostic determination and therapy. Antipsychotic drugs

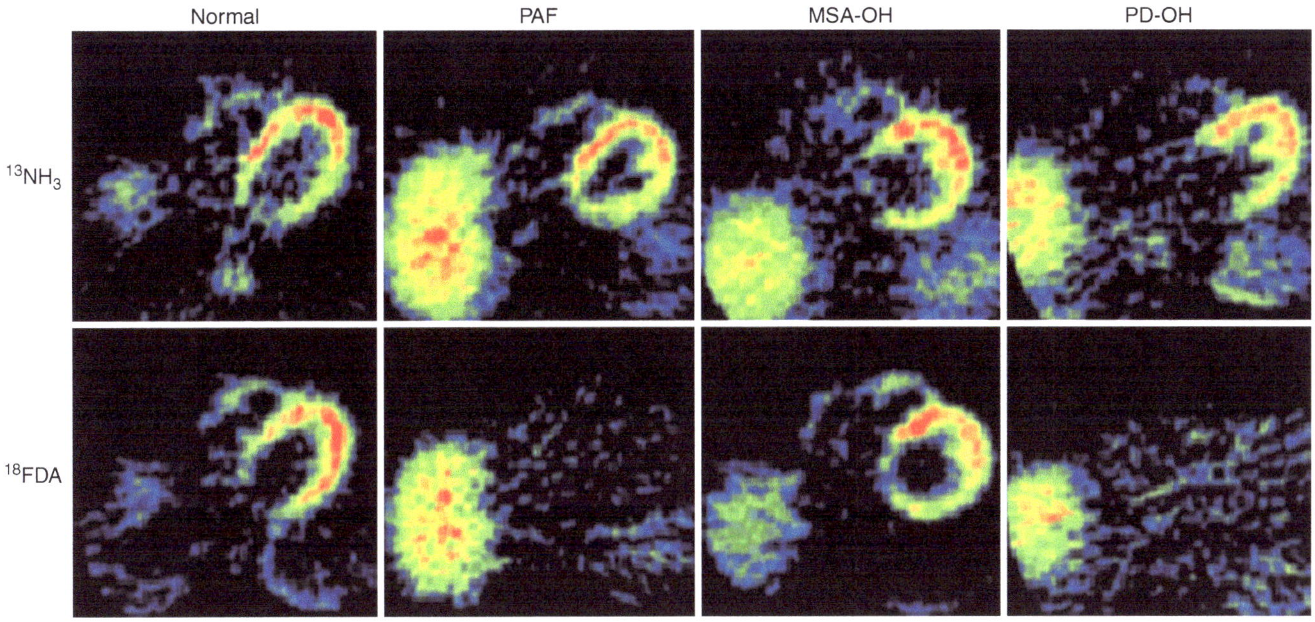

Fig. 34.8 Cardiac PET scans in a control subject and in patients with pure autonomic failure (*PAF*), multiple-system atrophy with orthostatic hypotension (*MSA-OH*), and PD with orthostatic hypotension (*PD-OH*). *Top*: nitrogen-13-labeled ammonia ($^{13}NH_3$) perfusion scans. *Bottom*: ^{18}F-dopa 3 (^{18}FDA) sympathoneural scans in each patient. Note absence of cardiac ^{18}F-dopa imaging in PAF and PD-OH and normal radioactivity in MSA-OH (Reprinted with permission of Elsevier from Goldstein [185])

for behavioral disturbance control in these patients, for example, may further prolong the QTc, putting the patient at risk for dysrhythmias.

L-Dopa therapy in PD patients contributes to OH with its vasodilatory effect. Moreover, selegiline, amantadine, and dopamine agonists, common therapeutic tools, may potentiate OH in PD and MSA patients [193, 196]. On the contrary, fludrocortisone and midodrine to counteract OH may exacerbate hypertension. Calcium antagonists and nitrates may be safer drugs to treat hypertension [182, 185], since orthostatic hypotension can exacerbate cognitive decline [197].

Tauopathies

Alzheimer Disease (AD), Progressive Supranuclear Palsy (PSP), Cortico-Basal Degeneration (CBD), and Frontotemporal Dementia (FTD)

Clinical AD is associated with a wide range of dysautonomic phenomena, such as increased pupillary dilation, altered skin conductivity, blunted autonomic response to noxious stimuli, diminished HRV, depressed baroreflex sensitivity, and orthostasis. Among the brain regions implicated in autonomic control, the insula has been widely investigated as a potential cause of autonomic dysfunction.

The insula appears to be involved in the degenerative process of AD very early in the disorder's course. Autopsies have noted that as many as 40% of non-demented elderly may have AD pathology sufficiently advanced to affect the insular cortex.

Recent experimental evidence has shown that neurodegenerative diseases may have a cardiovascular involvement due to the direct deposition of beta-amyloid or Tau proteins in peripheral organs [198] (Fig. 34.9).

Many cardiac and noncardiac "age-related" changes may actually be secondary to AD. Twenty-four-hour ECG recordings of subjects older than 80 have shown frequent unexplained tachy or brady dysrhythmias and increased QTc [199]. Myocardial scintigraphy with meta-iodobenzylguanidine (MIBG) imaging distinguishes AD from LBD, since a marked reduction of MIBG uptake is present in most patients with LBD but not in AD [200].

Cankar et al., studying 31 patients affected by Huntington's disease (HD) confirmed a traceable gene mutation, with nonspecific changes in ECG variables that may represent initial signs of cardiomyopathy [201].

Other tauopathies like Friedreich's Ataxia (FA) show an autosomal recessive tract of neuro and cardio degenerative disorder, with cardiomyopathy as the cause of death in 66% of patients.

Muscular Dystrophies

Muscular dystrophies (MD) are a group of hereditary muscle diseases in which a defect in muscle proteins leads to muscle cell death, with consequent progressive muscle weakness

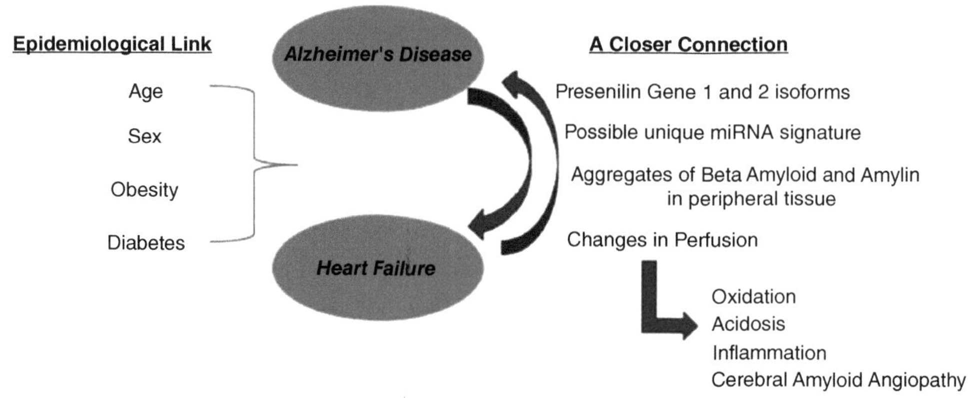

Fig. 34.9 Overall schematic summary of the new findings on the head to heart connection in Alzheimer disease bringing attention to either a more systemic profile or a metastatic condition. This closer connection has some main tenants: (1) A shared genetic profile with presenilin 1 (PSEN1) and PSEN2 isoforms; (2) Discovery of aggregations of Aβ (β-amyloid) and amylin in peripheral tissue and their proteotoxic effects. Tublin et al. [198]

and wasting. The most common, and also the most severe, form of MD is Duchenne's type (DMD), an X-linked, very early-age onset, early dependency, and short life expectancy MD. Mortality in DMD patients is primarily related to cardiac and/or respiratory muscle failure. It is estimated that approximately 75% of patients with DMD die of respiratory failure and 20% die from heart failure. Cardiac involvement in DMD is characterized by cardiac muscle degeneration with fibrous tissue replacement and fatty infiltration, typically occurring late in the course of the disease [202]. Many studies have attempted to detect early myocardial damage, or to correlate left ventricular dysfunction with skeletal muscle or lung function tests, but have failed to find any useful relationship [63]. More recent studies have used MRI to evaluate heart involvement and have noted that T2 relaxation times of cardiac muscle in DMD patients free of cardiac complaints were decreased in comparison to healthy volunteers [203]. Another more recent MRI study has investigated myocardial inflammation in DMD as a precipitating factor for heart failure, documenting myocardial fibrosis in 6 of 20 patients, and evidence of active myocarditis on histological analysis in four of the six patients with fibrosis. Considering that abnormal dystrophin has also been identified as a potential susceptibility gene product for viral infection of the myocardium and that dystrophin deficiency seems to potentiate the unfavorable course of enterovirus-induced cardiomyopathy, inflammatory aspects of myocardial dysfunction in DMD could be an important object of future interest [203].

Miscellanea

Neuro-mediated cardiocirculatory syndromes include syncope, neurogenic orthostatic hypotension syndromes, and channelopathies. Neurocardiogenic syncope is a relatively frequent condition characterized by acute failure of the autonomic nervous system to maintain blood pressure when a subject changes posture. Carotid sinus syndrome and situational syncope, which might occur after vagal stimulation with urination, defecation, or coughing, are other well-known conditions of this category. Vagal syncope tends to occur more frequently in adolescents. It may be elicited by visual, olfactory, or situational stimuli—such as closed, crowded, hot, or smoky environments. For idiopathic vagal reactions, there is no specific treatment. The patient must be informed to avoid vagal stimuli, recognize prodromal symptoms such as decreased heart rate, sweating, yawning, or nausea with epigastric heaviness, and manage syncopal episodes (lying down with legs uplifted). Drinking water and salting food can prevent vagal syncope in predisposed patients.

Neurogenic orthostatic hypotension is more than one condition that operates through a common mechanism of reduced baroreflex responsiveness, decreased cardiac compliance, and attenuation of the vestibulo sympathetic reflex. It is characterized by a reduction of at least 20 mmHg of systolic blood pressure or 10 mmHg of diastolic blood pressure during the first 3 min of standing after being in a supine position for a prolonged period. Primary causes of neurogenic orthostatic hypotension can be degenerative, such as hereditary amyloidosis, hereditary sensory and autonomic neuropathy (HSAN type III), and immune-mediated autonomic neuropathy [204, 205].

Channelopathies (ion channel disease) represent the most common cause of sudden arrhythmic death syndrome (SADS). This heterogeneous disease group includes Brugada syndrome, early repolarization syndrome, long QT syndrome, catecholaminergic polymorphic ventricular tachycardia, short QT syndrome, progressive cardiac conduction defect, and inherited atrial fibrillation. Common features of ion channel diseases are a structurally normal heart, a genetic basis, and predisposition to fatal dysrhythmias. Occasionally, they may have neurologic-associated clinical manifestations, including epilepsy and familial hemiplegic migraine. Various genetic mutations have been identified, and the chance of a positive genetic test varies from 20% to 70%. A history of sudden death is present in up to 30% of patients' families.

Patent Fossa Ovalis Associated Neurological Syndromes

Patent fossa ovalis (PFO) is an anatomical communication between the right and left atrium. It is caused by the failed closure of the oval fossa that normally occurs after birth with the fusion of septum primum and septum secundum. About 25% of the healthy population has a PFO. The PFO, allowing paradoxical embolization of thrombotic material from the venous district to the systemic arterial system, contributes to the pathogenesis of cerebral ischemic syndromes.

PFO prevalence is significantly higher in patients with cryptogenic stroke or transient ischemic attack, reaching 40–56% in patients younger than 55 years [206–209].

Contrast transthoracic echocardiography and transesophageal echocardiography are the diagnostic techniques to define PFO anatomy and stratify the risk of paradoxical embolization [210, 211].

The existence of other risk factors for stroke (first of all atrial fibrillation) does not exclude the role of PFO [212, 213].

A paradoxical embolism (RoPE) score integrates with clinical judgment to define the causal role of PFO in cryptogenic stroke. The score includes younger age, cortical location of the stroke, diabetes, hypertension, smoking, and a prior stroke or TIA [214].

PFO has been associated with other medical and neurological conditions, such as migraine and decompression sickness in divers [215, 216].

The underlying association with migraine is currently a matter of investigation in various clinical trials. Beyond the role of paradoxical cerebral embolisms, another potential cause is the release of active metabolites from platelet activated by shear stress during the passage of blood through the PFO [217]. Retrospective case-controlled epidemiological studies support the association between PFO and DCS. A recent meta-analysis of patients with decompression sickness showed an odds ratio (increased risk) of 5.63 if a PFO was present [218].

Transcatheter closure of the interatrial communication in patients with PFO is indicated to prevent systemic thrombo embolism [214, 219]. PFO closure for intractable migraine has been considered only in clinical trials [218].

Percutaneous PFO closure is feasible with several implantable devices based on an umbrella-like design [220]. Recently, percutaneous suture-mediated PFO closure has been introduced in clinical practice [221, 222], showing a favorable efficacy and safety profile in most PFO cases [223, 224].

References

1. Taggart P, Critchley H, Lambiase PD. Heart-brain interactions in cardiac arrhythmia. Heart. 2011;97(9):698–708.
2. Schwartz B. The world of thought in ancient China. Cambridge: Harvard University Press; 1985.
3. Samuels MA. 'Voodoo' death revisited: the modern lessons of neurocardiology. Cleve Clin J Med. 2007;74(Suppl. 1):S8–16.
4. Leor J, Poole WK, Kloner RA. Sudden cardiac death triggered by an earthquake. N Engl J Med. 1996;334(7):413–9.
5. Hua F, et al. c-Fos expression in rat brain stem and spinal cord in response to activation of cardiac ischemia-sensitive afferent neurons and electrostimulatory modulation. Am J Physiol Heart Circ Physiol. 2004;287:H2728–38.
6. Gray MA, Taggart P, Sutton PM, Groves D, Holdright DR, Bradbury D, Brull D, Critchley HD. A cortical potential reflecting cardiac function. Proc Natl Acad Sci USA. 2007;104(16):6818–23.
7. Hagemann D, Waldstein SR, Thayer JF. Central and autonomic nervous system integration in emotion. Brain Cogn. 2003;52(1):79–87.
8. Natelson BH. Neurocardiology. An interdisciplinary area for the 80s. Arch Neurol. 1985;42(2):178–84. Review
9. Davis AM, Natelson BH. Brain-heart interactions. The neurocardiology of arrhythmia and sudden cardiac death. Tex Heart Inst J. 1993;20(3):158–69. Review
10. Benarroch E. Chapter 4. In: Robertson D, et al., editors. Primer on autonomic nervous system. 2nd ed. Philadelphia: Elsevier; 2004.
11. Critchley HD, Mathias CJ, Oliver J, et al. Human cingulated cortex and autonomic control: converging neuroimaging and clinical evidence. Brain. 2003;126:213–2152.
12. Toivonen L, Helenius K, Viitasalo M. Electrocardiographic repolarization during stress from awakening on alarm call. J Am Coll Cardiol. 1997;30:774–9.
13. Oppenheimer S. Cerebrogenic cardiac arrhythmias: cortical lateralization and clinical significance. Clin Auton Res. 2006;16:6–11.
14. Critchley HD, Wiens S, Rotshtein P, Ohman A, Dolan RJ. Neural systems supporting interoceptive awareness. Nat Neurosci. 2004;7(2):189–95.
15. Critchley HD, Taggart P, Sutton PM, Holdright DR, Batchvarov V, Hnatkova K, Malik M, Dolan RJ. Mental stress and sudden cardiac death: asymmetric midbrain activity as a linking mechanism. Brain. 2005;128(Pt 1):75–85.
16. Lampert R, Jain D, Burg MM, Batsford WP, McPherson CA. Destabilizing effects of mental stress on ventricular arrhythmias in patients with implantable cardioverter-defibrillators. Circulation. 2000;101(2):158–64.
17. Green AL, Paterson DJ. Identification of neurocircuitry controlling cardiovascular function in humans using functional neurosurgery: implications for exercise control. Exp Physiol. 2008;93(9):1022–8.
18. Green AL, Wang S, Owen SL, Paterson DJ, Xie K, Liu X, Bain PG, Stein JF, Aziz TZ. Functional Neurosurgery Resident Award: controlling the cardiovascular system with deep brain stimulation. Clin Neurosurg. 2006;53:316–23.
19. Dote K, Sato KT, et al. Myocardial stunning due to simultaneous multi vessel coronary spasms: a review of 5 cases. J Cardiol. 1991;21:203–14.

20. Wittstein I, Thiemann DR, et al. Neurohumoral features of myocardial stunning due to sudden emotional stress. N Engl J Med. 2005;352:539–48.
21. Sharkey S, Lesser J, et al. Acute and reversible cardiomyopathy provoked by stress in women from the United States. Circulation. 2005;111:472–9.
22. Radfar A, Abohashem S, Osborne MT, et al. Stress-associated neurobiological activity associates with the risk for and timing of subsequent Takotsubo syndrome. Eur Heart J. 2021;42(19):1898–908. https://doi.org/10.1093/eurheartj/ehab029.
23. Hessel E. The brain and the heart. Anesth Analg. 2006;103(3):522–6.
24. Desmet W, Dynamic LV. Obstruction in apical ballooning syndrome: the chicken or the egg? Eur J Echocardiogr. 2006;7:1–3.
25. Merli E, Sutcliffe S, et al. TakoTako-Tsubo cardiomyopathy: new insights into the possible underlying pathophysiology. Eur J Echocardiogr. 2006;7:53.
26. Oppenheimer SM, Wilson JX, et al. Insular cortex stimulation produces lethal cardiac arrhythmias: a mechanism of sudden death? Brain Res. 1991;550:115–21.
27. Critchley HD, Corfield DR, et al. Cerebral correlates of autonomic cardiovascular arousal: a functional neuroimaging investigation in humans. J Physiol. 2000;523:259–70.
28. Templin C, Hänggi J, Klein C, et al. Altered limbic and autonomic processing supports brain-heart axis in Takotsubo syndrome. Eur Heart J. 2019;40(15):1183–7. https://doi.org/10.1093/eurheartj/ehz068.
29. Tawakol A, Ishai A, Takx RA, et al. Relation between resting amygdalar activity and cardiovascular events: a longitudinal and cohort study. Lancet. 2017;389(10071):834–45. https://doi.org/10.1016/S0140-6736(16)31714-7.
30. Hinterdobler J, Schott S, Jin H, et al. Acute mental stress drives vascular inflammation and promotes plaque destabilization in mouse atherosclerosis. Eur Heart J. 2021:ehab371. https://doi.org/10.1093/eurheartj/ehab371. Published online July 19, 2021
31. Meyer P, Degrauwe S, Van Delden C, Ghadri JR, Templin C. Typical takotsubo syndrome triggered by SARS-CoV-2 infection. Eur Heart J. 2020;41(19):1860. https://doi.org/10.1093/eurheartj/ehaa306.
32. Kolominsky-Rabas PL, Weber M, et al. Epidemiology of ischemic stroke subtypes according to TOAST criteria: incidence, recurrence, and long-term survival in ischemic stroke subtypes: a population-based study. Stroke. 2001;32:2735–40.
33. Rincon F, Dhamoon M, et al. Stroke location and association with fatal cardiac outcomes. Northern Manhattan Study (NOMAS). Stroke. 2008;39:2425–51.
34. Grau AJ, Weimar C, et al. Risk factors, outcome, and treatment in subtypes of ischemic stroke: the German stroke data bank. Stroke. 2001;32(11):2559–66.
35. Norris JW, Froggatt GM, Hachinski VC. Cardiac arrhythmias in acute stroke. Stroke. 1978;9(4):392–6.
36. Cheung RTF, Hachinski W. The insula and cerebrogenic sudden death. Arch Neurol. 2000;57:1685–8.
37. Touzé E, Varenne O, et al. Risk of myocardial infarction and vascular death after transient ischemic attack and ischemic stroke: a systematic review and meta-analysis. Stroke. 2005;36(12):2748–55. Review
38. van Bree MD, Roos YB, et al. Prevalence and characterization of ECG abnormalities after intracerebral hemorrhage. Neurocrit Care. 2010;12(1):50–5.
39. Hravanak M, Frangiskakis M, et al. Elevated cardiac troponin I and relationship to persistence of electrocardiographic and echocardiographic abnormalities after aneurysmal subarachnoid hemorrhage. Stroke. 2009;40:3478–84.
40. Naidech AN, Kreiter KT, et al. Cardiac troponin elevation, cardiovascular morbidity and outcome after subarachnoid hemorrhage. Circulation. 2005;112:2851–6.
41. Banki N, Kopelnik A, et al. Acute neurocardiogenic injury after subarachnoid hemorrhage. Circulation. 2005;112:3314–9.
42. Lee V, Oh JK, et al. Mechanisms in neurogenic stress cardiomyopathy after aneurismal subarachnoid hemorrhage. Neurocrit Care. 2006;05:243–9.
43. Battaglini D, Robba C, Lopes da Silva A, et al. Brain–heart interaction after acute ischemic stroke. Crit Care. 2020;24(1):163. https://doi.org/10.1186/s13054-020-02885-8.
44. Zaroff JG, Pawlikoska L, et al. Adrenoceptor polymorphisms and the risk of cardiac injury and dysfunction after subarachnoid hemorrhage. Stroke. 2006;37:1680–5.
45. Tung PP, Olmsted E, et al. Plasma B-type natriuretic peptide levels are associated with early cardiac dysfunction after subarachnoid hemorrhage. Stroke. 2005;36:1567–71.
46. Naredi S, Lambert G, et al. Increased sympathetic nervous activity in patients with non-traumatic subarachnoid hemorrhage. Stroke. 2000;31:901–6.
47. Manno EM, Pfeifer EA, et al. Cardiac pathology in patients with status epilepticus. Neurocrit Care. 2005;2:231.
48. Cebelin MS, Hirsch CS. Human stress cardiomyopathy. Myocardial lesions in victims of homicidal assaults without internal injuries. Hum Pathol. 1980;11:123–32.
49. Gunnoo T, Hasan N, Khan MS, Slark J, Bentley P, Sharma P. Quantifying the risk of heart disease following acute ischaemic stroke: a meta-analysis of over 50,000 participants. BMJ Open. 2016;6(1):e009535. https://doi.org/10.1136/bmjopen-2015-009535.
50. Xiong L, Tian G, Leung H, et al. Autonomic dysfunction predicts clinical outcomes after acute ischemic stroke: a prospective observational study. Stroke. 2018;49(1):215–8. https://doi.org/10.1161/STROKEAHA.117.019312.
51. Christensen H, Boysen G, Christensen AF, Johannesen HH. Insular lesions, ECG abnormalities, and outcome in acute stroke. J Neurol Neurosurg Psychiatry. 2005;76(2):269–71.
52. Adeoye AM, Ogah OS, Ovbiagele B, et al. Prevalence and prognostic features of ECG abnormalities in acute stroke: findings from the SIREN study Among Africans. Glob Heart. 2017;12(2):99. https://doi.org/10.1016/j.gheart.2017.01.002.
53. Dimant J, Grob D. Electrocardiographic changes and myocardial damage in patients with acute cerebrovascular accidents. Stroke. 1977;8(4):448–55.
54. Oppenheimer SM, Gelb A, Girvin JP, Hachinski VC. Cardiovascular effects of human insular cortex stimulation. Neurology. 1992;42(9):1727–32.
55. Cechetto DF, Wilson JX, Smith KE, Wolski D, Silver MD, Hachinski VC. Autonomic and myocardial changes in middle cerebral artery occlusion: stroke models in the rat. Brain Res. 1989;502(2):296–305.
56. Hachinski VC, Smith KE, Silver MD, Gibson CJ, Ciriello J. Acute myocardial and plasma catecholamine changes in experimental stroke. Stroke. 1986;17(3):387–90.
57. Nolte J. The human brain. 4th ed. St. Louis: Mosby; 1999.
58. Cereda C, Ghika J, Maeder P, Bogousslavsky J. Strokes restricted to the insular cortex. Neurology. 2002;59(12):1950–5.
59. Augustine JR. Circuitry and functional aspects of the insular lobe in primates including humans. Brain Res Brain Res Rev. 1996;22(3):229–44. Review
60. Critchley HD. The human cortex responds to an interoceptive challenge. Proc Natl Acad Sci USA. 2004;101(17):6333–4.
61. Türe U, Yasargil MG, Al-Mefty O, Yasargil DCH. Arteries of insula. J Neurosurg. 2000;92:676–87.

62. Sander D, Winbeck K, Klingelhöfer J, Etgen T, Conrad B. Prognostic relevance of pathological sympathetic activation after acute thromboembolic stroke. Neurology. 2001;57(5): 833–8.
63. Ay H, Koroshetz WJ, et al. Neuroanatomic correlates of stroke-related myocardial injury. Neurology. 2006;66:1325–9.
64. Colivicchi F, Bassi A, Santini M, Caltagirone C. Prognostic implications of right-sided insular damage, cardiac autonomic derangement, and arrhythmias after acute ischemic stroke. Stroke. 2005;36(8):1710–5.
65. Tokgosoglu SL, Batur MK, et al. Effects of stroke localization on cardiac autonomic balance and sudden death. Stroke. 1999;30:1307–11.
66. Laowattana S, Zeger SL, Lima JA, Goodman SN, Wittstein IS, Oppenheimer SM. Left insular stroke is associated with adverse cardiac outcome. Neurology. 2006;66(4):477–83.
67. Fink JN, Frampton CM, Lyden P, Lees KR. Virtual international stroke trials archive investigators. Does hemispheric lateralization influence functional and cardiovascular outcomes after stroke? An analysis of placebo-treated patients from prospective acute stroke trials. Stroke. 2008;39(12):3335–40.
68. Jung JM, Kim JG, Kim JB, et al. Takotsubo-like myocardial dysfunction in ischemic stroke: a hospital-based registry and systematic literature review. Stroke. 2016;47(11):2729–36. https://doi.org/10.1161/STROKEAHA.116.014304.
69. Stanley D, Mason LJ, Mackin KE, et al. Translocation and dissemination of commensal bacteria in post-stroke infection. Nat Med. 2016;22(11):1277–84. https://doi.org/10.1038/nm.4194.
70. Urbinati S, Di Pasquale G, Andreoli A, Lusa AM, Ruffini M, Lanzino G, Pinelli G. Frequency and prognostic significance of silent coronary artery disease in patients with cerebral ischemia undergoing carotid endarterectomy. Am J Cardiol. 1992;69(14):1166–70.
71. Gongora-Rivera F, Labreuche J, Jaramillo A, Steg PG, Hauw JJ, Amarenco P. Autopsy prevalence of coronary atherosclerosis in patients with fatal stroke. Stroke. 2007;38(4):1203–10.
72. Lavy S, Yaar I, Melamed E, Stern S. The effect of acute stroke on cardiac functions as observed in an intensive stroke care unit. Stroke. 1974;5(6):775–80.
73. Goldstein D. The electrocardiogram in stroke: relationship to pathophysiological type and comparison with prior tracings. Stroke. 1979;10:253–9.
74. Rem JA, Hachinski VC, Boughner DR, Barnett HJ. Value of cardiac monitoring and echocardiography in TIA and stroke patients. Stroke. 1985;16(6):950–6.
75. Orlandi G, Fanucchi S, Strata G, Pataleo L, Landucci Pellegrini L, Prontera C, Martini A, Murri L. Transient autonomic nervous system dysfunction during hyperacute stroke. Acta Neurol Scand. 2000;102(5):317–21.
76. Lin HJ, Wolf PA, Benjamin EJ, Belanger AJ, D'Agostino RB. Newly diagnosed atrial fibrillation and acute stroke. The Framingham Study. Stroke. 1995;26(9):1527–30.
77. Hart RG. Atrial fibrillation and stroke prevention. N Engl J Med. 2003;349(11):1015–6.
78. Hart RG, Pearce LA, Rothbart RM, McAnulty JH, Asinger RW, Halperin JL. Stroke with intermittent atrial fibrillation: incidence and predictors during aspirin therapy. Stroke Prevention in Atrial Fibrillation Investigators. J Am Coll Cardiol. 2000;35(1): 183–7.
79. Tayal AH, Tian M, Kelly KM, Jones SC, Wright DG, Singh D, Jarouse J, Brillman J, Murali S, Gupta R. Atrial fibrillation detected by mobile cardiac outpatient telemetry in cryptogenic TIA or stroke. Neurology. 2008;71(21):1696–701.
80. Paciaroni M, Agnelli G, Caso V, Venti M, Milia P, Silvestrelli G, Parnetti L, Biagini S. Atrial fibrillation in patients with first-ever stroke: frequency, antithrombotic treatment before the event and effect on clinical outcome. J Thromb Haemost. 2005;3(6):1218–23.
81. Liao J, Khalid Z, Scallan C, Morillo C, O'Donnell M. Noninvasive cardiac monitoring for detecting paroxysmal atrial fibrillation or flutter after acute ischemic stroke: a systematic review. Stroke. 2007;38(11):2935–40.
82. Dütsch M, Burger M, Dörfler C, Schwab S, Hilz MJ. Cardiovascular autonomic function in poststroke patients. Neurology. 2007;69(24):2249–55.
83. Di Angelantonio E, Fiorelli M, Toni D, Sacchetti ML, Lorenzano S, Falcou A, Ciarla MV, Suppa M, Bonanni L, Bertazzoni G, Aguglia F, Argentino C. Prognostic significance of admission levels of troponin I in patients with acute ischemic stroke. J Neurol Neurosurg Psychiatry. 2005;76(1):76–81.
84. Lee SJ, Lee KS, Kim YI, An JY, Kim W, Kim JS. Clinical features of patients with a myocardial infarction during acute management of an ischemic stroke. Neurocrit Care. 2008;9(3):332–7.
85. Yoshimura S, Toyoda K, Ohara T, Nagasawa H, Ohtani N, Kuwashiro T, Naritomi H, Minematsu K. Takotsubo cardiomyopathy in acute ischemic stroke. Ann Neurol. 2008;64(5):547–54.
86. Prosser J, MacGregor L, Lees KR, Diener HC, Hacke W, Davis S, VISTA Investigators. Predictors of early cardiac morbidity and mortality after schemic stroke. Stroke. 2007;38(8):2295–302.
87. Silver FL, Norris JW, Lewis AJ, Hachinski VC. Early mortality following stroke: a prospective review. Stroke. 1984;15(3):492–6.
88. Algra A, Gates PC, Fox AJ, Hachinski V, Barnett HJ, North American Symptomatic Carotid Endarterectomy Trial Group. Side of brain infarction and long-term risk of sudden death in patients with symptomatic carotid disease. Stroke. 2003;34(12):2871–5.
89. North American Symptomatic Carotid Endarterectomy Trial Collaborators. Beneficial effect of carotid endarterectomy in symptomatic patients with high-grade carotid stenosis. N Engl J Med. 1991;325(7):445–53.
90. Kaplan RC, Tirschwell DL, Longstreth WT Jr, Manolio TA, Heckbert SR, Lefkowitz D, El-Saed A, Psaty BM. Vascular events, mortality, and preventive therapy following ischemic stroke in the elderly. Neurology. 2005;65(6):835–42.
91. Adams HP Jr, del Zoppo G, Alberts MJ, Bhatt DL, Brass L, Furlan A, Grubb RL, Higashida RT, Jauch EC, Kidwell C, Lyden PD, Morgenstern LB, Qureshi AI, Rosenwasser RH, Scott PA, Wijdicks EF, American Heart Association, American Stroke Association Stroke Council, Clinical Cardiology Council, Cardiovascular Radiology and Intervention Council, Atherosclerotic Peripheral Vascular Disease and Quality of Care Outcomes in Research Interdisciplinary Working Groups. Guidelines for the early management of adults with ischemic stroke: a guideline from the American Heart Association/American Stroke Association Stroke Council, Clinical Cardiology Council, Cardiovascular Radiology and Intervention Council, and the Atherosclerotic Peripheral Vascular Disease and Quality of Care Outcomes in Research Interdisciplinary Working Groups: the American Academy of Neurology affirms the value of this guideline as an educational tool for neurologists. Stroke. 2007;38(5):1655–711. Stroke. 2007; 38(9):e96
92. Fang CX, Wu S, Ren J. Intracerebral hemorrhage elicits aberration in cardiomyocyte contractile function and intracellular Ca2+ transients. Stroke. 2006;37(7):1875–82.
93. Maramattom BV, Manno EM, Fulgham JR, Jaffe AS, Wijdicks EF. Clinical importance of cardiac troponin release and cardiac abnormalities in patients with supratentorial cerebral hemorrhages. Mayo Clin Proc. 2006;81(2):192–6.
94. Hays A, Diringer MN. Elevated troponin levels are associated with higher mortality following intracerebral hemorrhage. Neurology. 2006;66(9):1330–4.

95. Banuelos PA, Temes R, Lee VH. Neurogenic stunned myocardium associated with reversible posterior leukoencephalopathy syndrome. Neurocrit Care. 2008;9(1):108–11.
96. Papanikolaou J, Tsirantonaki M, Koukoulitsios G, Papageorgiou D, Mandila C, Karakitsos D, Karabinis A. Reversible posterior leukoencephalopathy syndrome and takotsubo cardiomyopathy: the role of echocardiographic monitoring in the ICU. Hell J Cardiol. 2009;50(5):436–8.
97. Finsterer J, Wahbi K. CNS disease triggering Takotsubo stress cardiomyopathy. Int J Cardiol. 2014;177(2):322–9. https://doi.org/10.1016/j.ijcard.2014.08.101.
98. Grimaldi S, Doche E, Rey C, et al. Association of posterior reversible encephalopathy syndrome and transient apical ballooning syndrome (Takotsubo): first case report of a man and review of the literature. Case Rep Neurol. 2017;9(2):173–8. https://doi.org/10.1159/000474933.
99. Layon J, Friedman WA, Gabrielli A, editors. Textbook of neurointensive care. Philadelphia: WB Saunders; 2003. Chapter 8
100. Blackman JA, Patrick PD, Buck ML, Rust RS Jr. Paroxysmal autonomic instability with dystonia after brain injury. Arch Neurol. 2004;61(3):321–8. Review
101. Baguley IJ, Heriseanu RE, Cameron ID, Nott MT, Slewa-Younan S. A critical review of the pathophysiology of dysautonomia following traumatic brain injury. Neurocrit Care. 2008;8(2):293–300. Review
102. Singleton RH, Adelson PD. Chapter 3: Diffuse axonal injury and dysautonomia. In: Bhardwa JA, Ellegala DB, Kirsch JR, editors. Acute brain and spinal cord injury: evolving paradigms and management. New York: Informa Healthcare; 2008.
103. Boeve BF, Wijdicks EF, Benarroch EE, Schmidt KD. Paroxysmal sympathetic storms ("diencephalic seizures") after severe diffuse axonal head injury. Mayo Clin Proc. 1998;73(2):148–52.
104. Kishner S, et al. Post head injury autonomic complications; 2008. http://emedicine.medscape.com/article/325994-overview#showall.
105. Baguley IJ, Heriseanu RE, Felmingham KL, Cameron ID. Dysautonomia and heart rate variability following severe traumatic brain injury. Brain Inj. 2006;20(4):437–44. (Abstract)
106. Bourdages M, et al. Cardiac arrhythmias associated with severe traumatic brain injury and hypothermia therapy. Pediatr Crit Care Med. 2010;11(3):439–41.
107. Bourdages M, Bigras JL, Farrell CA, Hutchison JS, Lacroix J, Canadian Critical Care Trials Group. Cardiac arrhythmias associated with severe traumatic brain injury and hypothermia therapy. Pediatr Crit Care Med. 2010;11(3):408–14.
108. Alali AS, Mukherjee K, McCredie VA, et al. Beta-blockers and Traumatic Brain Injury: a systematic review, meta-analysis, and Eastern Association for the Surgery of Trauma Guideline. Ann Surg. 2017;266(6):952–61. https://doi.org/10.1097/SLA.0000000000002286.
109. El-Menyar A, Goyal A, Latifi R, Al-Thani H, Frishman W. Brain-heart interactions in traumatic brain injury. Cardiol Rev. 2017;25(6):279–88. https://doi.org/10.1097/CRD.0000000000000167.
110. Furlan JC, Fehlings MG. Cardiovascular complications after acute spinal cord injury: pathophysiology, diagnosis, and management. Neurosurg Focus. 2008;25(5):E13. Review
111. Rowland JW, Hawryluk GW, Kwon B, Fehlings MG. Current status of acute spinal cord injury pathophysiology and emerging therapies: promise on the horizon. Neurosurg Focus. 2008;25(5):E2. Review
112. Garshick E, Kelley A, Cohen SA, Garrison A, Tun CG, Gagnon D, Brown R. A prospective assessment of mortality in chronic spinal cord injury. Spinal Cord. 2005;43(7):408–16.
113. Stein DM, Menaker J, McQuillan K, Handley C, Aarabi B, Scalea TM. Risk factors for organ dysfunction and failure in patients with acute traumatic cervical spinal cord injury. Neurocrit Care. 2010;13(1):29–39.
114. Bunten DC, Warner AL, Brunnemann SR, Segal JL. Heart rate variability is altered following spinal cord injury. Clin Auton Res. 1998;8(6):329–34.
115. Furlan JC, Fehlings MG. The impact of age on mortality, impairment, and disability among adults with acute traumatic spinal cord injury. J Neurotrauma. 2009;26(10):1707–17.
116. Grigorean VT, Sandu AM, Popescu M, Iacobini MA, Stoian R, Neascu C, Strambu V, Popa F. Cardiac dysfunctions following spinal cord injury. J Med Life. 2009;2(2):133–45. Review
117. Mathias CJ. Chapter 81: Autonomic disturbances in spinal cord injuries. In: Robertson D, editor. Primer on the autonomic nervous system. 2nd ed. Philadelphia: Elsevier; 2004.
118. Manogue M, Hirsh DS, Lloyd M. Cardiac electrophysiology of patients with spinal cord injury. Heart Rhythm. 2017;14(6):920–7. https://doi.org/10.1016/j.hrthm.2017.02.015.
119. Popa C, Popa F, Grigorean VT, et al. Vascular dysfunctions following spinal cord injury. J Med Life. 2010;3(3):275–85.
120. Asahina M, Kuwabara S, et al. Autonomic function in demyelinating and axonal subtypes of Guillain Barrè syndrome. Acta Neurol Scand. 2002;105(1):44–50.
121. Dionne A, Nicolle MW, Hahn AF. Clinical and electrophysiological parameters distinguishing acute-onset chronic inflammatory demyelinating polyneuropathy from acute inflammatory demyelinating polyneuropathy. Muscle Nerve. 2010;41:202–7.
122. Mukerji S, Aloka F, et al. Cardiovascular complications of the Guillain-Barrè syndrome. Am J Cardiol. 2009;104:1452–5.
123. Pfeiffer G, Schiller H, et al. Indicators of dysautonomia in sever Guillain Barrè syndrome. J Neurol. 1999;246:1015–22.
124. Greenland P, Griggs RC. Arrhythmic complications in the Guillain Barrè syndrome. Arch Intern Med. 1980;40:1053–5.
125. Hodson AK, Hurwitz BJ, et al. Dysautonomia in Guillain-Barrè syndrome with dorsal root ganglioneuropathy, wallerian degeneration and fatal myocarditis. Ann Neurol. 1984;15(1):88–95.
126. Finkelstein JS, Melek BH. Guillain-Barrè syndrome as a cause of reversible cardiomyopathy. Tex Heart Inst J. 2006;33:57–9.
127. Iga K, Himura Y, et al. Reversible left ventricular dysfunction associated with Guillain Barrè syndrome-an expression of catecholamine cardiotoxicity? Jpn Circ J. 1995;59:236–40.
128. Burakgazi AZ, AlMahameed S. Cardiac involvement in peripheral neuropathies. J Clin Neuromusc Dis. 2016;17(3):120–8. https://doi.org/10.1097/CND.0000000000000106.
129. Maurer MS, Schwartz JH, Gundapaneni B, et al. Tafamidis treatment for patients with transthyretin amyloid cardiomyopathy. N Engl J Med. 2018;379(11):1007–16. https://doi.org/10.1056/NEJMoa1805689.
130. Adams D, Gonzalez-Duarte A, O'Riordan WD, et al. Patisiran, an RNAi therapeutic, for hereditary transthyretin amyloidosis. N Engl J Med. 2018;379(1):11–21. https://doi.org/10.1056/NEJMoa1716153.
131. Ando Y, Coelho T, Berk JL, et al. Guideline of transthyretin-related hereditary amyloidosis for clinicians. Orphanet J Rare Dis. 2013;8(1):31. https://doi.org/10.1186/1750-1172-8-31.
132. Gibson TC. The heart in myasthenia gravis. Am Heart J. 1975;90(3):389–96.
133. Hofstad H, Ohm OJ, Mork SJ, Aarli JA. Heart disease in myasthenia gravis. Acta Neurol Scand. 1984;70(3):176–84.
134. Suzuki S, Utsugisawa K, et al. Autoimmune targets of heart and skeletal muscles in myasthenia gravis. Arch Neurol. 2009;66(11):1334–8.
135. Rzepinski L, et al. Cardiac autonomic dysfunction in myasthenia gravis and relapsing–remitting multiple sclerosis. J Clin Med. 2021;10(2173):1–15.

136. Shivamurthya P, Parkerb MW. Cardiac manifestations of myasthenia gravis: a systematic review. IJC Metab Endocr. 2014;5:3–6.
137. Romi F, Skeie GO, Gilhus NE, Aarli JA. Striational antibodies in myasthenia gravis: reactivity and possible clinical significance. Arch Neurol. 2005;62:442–6.
138. Beydoun SR, Wang JT, et al. Emotional stress as a trigger of myasthenic crisis and concomitant takotsubo cardiomyopathy: a case report. J Med Case Rep. 2010;4:393.
139. Danikowski KM, Jayaraman S, Prabhakar BS. Regulatory T cells in multiple sclerosis and myasthenia gravis. J Neuroinflamm. 2017;14:117.
140. Kataria H, Hart CG, Alizadeh A, Cossoy M, Kaushik DK, Bernstein CN, Marrie RA, Yong VW, Karimi-Abdolrezaee S. Neuregulin-1 beta 1 is implicated in pathogenesis of multiple sclerosis. Brain. 2021;12:162–85.
141. Uzawa A, Kanai T, Kawaguchi N, Oda F, Himuro K, Kuwabara S. Changes in inflammatory cytokine networks in myasthenia gravis. Sci Rep. 2016;6:25886.
142. Benarroch EE. Autonomic nervous system and neuroimmune interactions. New insights and clinical implications. Neurology. 2019;92:377–85.
143. Borovikova LV, Ivanova S, Zhang M, Yang H, Botchkina GI, Watkins LR, Wang H, Abumrad N, Eaton JW, Tracey KJ. Vagus nerve stimulation attenuates the systemic inflammatory response to endotoxin. Nature. 2000;405:458–62.
144. Grassi G, Serravalle G, Mancia G. Sympathetic activation in cardiovascular disease: evidence, clinical impact and therapeutic implications. Eur J Clin Investig. 2015;45:1367–75.
145. Kato T, Hirose S, Kumagai S, Ozaki A, Matsumoto S, Inoko M. Electrocardiography as the first step for the further examination of cardiac involvement in myasthenia gravis. Biomed Res Int. 2016;2016:1–4.
146. Tsugawa J, Tsuboi Y, Inoue H, Suzuki S, Yamada T. Recurrent syncope due to sick sinus syndrome in a patient with myasthenia gravis associated with thymoma. Rinsho Shinkeigaku. 2011;51:32–4.
147. Calin C, Savu O, Dumitru D, Ghiorghiu I, Calin A, Capraru C, et al. Cardiac involvement in myasthenia gravis—is there a specific pattern? Rom J Intern Med. 2009;47:179–89.
148. Owe FJ, Davidson ES, Eide GE. Left ventricular long axis function in myasthenia gravis. J Neurol. 2008;255:1777–84.
149. Benjamin RN, Aaron S, Sivadasan A, Devasahayam S, Sebastin A, Alexander M. The spectrum of autonomic dysfunction in myasthenic crisis. Ann Indian Acad Neurol. 2018;21:42–8.
150. Kocabas ZU, Kizilay F, Basarici I, Uysal H. Evaluation of cardiac autonomic functions in myasthenia gravis. Neurol Res. 2018;40(5):405–12.
151. Vernino S, Hopkins S, Wang Z. Autonomic ganglia, acetylcholine receptor antibodies, and autoimmune ganglionopathy. Auton Neurosci. 2009;146:3–7.
152. Bradley WG. Polymyositis: an overdiagnosed entity. Neurology. 2004;63(2):402.
153. Gottdiener JS, Sherber HS, et al. Cardiac manifestations in polymyositis. Am J Cardiol. 1978;41(7):1141–9.
154. Lundberg IE. The heart in dermatomyositis and polymyositis. Rheumatology. 2006;45:iv18–21.
155. Stern R, Godbold JH, et al. ECG abnormalities in polymyositis. Arch Intern Med. 1984;144:2185–9.
156. Haupt HM, Hutschins GM, et al. The heart and cardiac conduction system in polymyositis-dermatomyositis: a clinicopathologic study of 16 autopsied patients. Am J Cardiol. 1982;50:998–1006.
157. Sevcencu C, Struijk JJ. Autonomic alterations and cardiac changes in epilepsy. Epilepsia. 2010;51(5):725–37.
158. Moseley BD, Ghearing GR, Munger TM, Britton JW. The treatment of ictal asystole with cardiac pacing. Epilepsia. 2011;52(4):e16–9.
159. van der Lende M, Surges R, Sander JW, Thijs RD. Cardiac arrhythmias during or after epileptic seizures. J Neurol Neurosurg Psychiatry. 2016;87(1):69–74.
160. Verrier RL, Pang TD, Nearing BD, Schachter SC. The epileptic heart: concept and clinical evidence. Epilepsy Behav. 2020;105:106946.
161. Rocamora R, Kurthen M, et al. Cardiac asystole in epilepsy: clinical and neurophysiologic features. Epilepsia. 2003;44(2):179–85.
162. Shmuely S, van der Lende M, Lamberts RJ, Sander IW, Thijs RD. The heart of epilepsy: current views and future concepts. Seizure. 2017;44:176–83.
163. Boggs JG. Mortality associated with status epilepticus. Epilepsy Curr. 2004;4(1):25–7.
164. Nevander G, Ingvar M, et al. Status epilepticus in well-oxygenated rats causes neuronal necrosis. Ann Neurol. 1985;18:281–90.
165. De Lorenzo RJ, Towne AR, et al. Status epilepticus in children, adults and the elderly. Epilepsia. 1992;33(suppl 4):S15–25.
166. Towne AR, Pellock JM, et al. Determinants of mortality in status epilepticus. Epilepsia. 1994;35:27–34.
167. Boggs JG, Maramarou A, et al. Hemodynamic monitoring prior to and at the time of death in status epilepticus. Epilepsy Res. 1998;31(3):199–209.
168. Metcalf C, Poelzing S, et al. Status epilepticus induces cardiac myofilament damage and increased susceptibility to arrhythmias in rats. Am J Physiol Heart Circ Physiol. 2009;297:H2120–7.
169. Fialho GL, Wolf P, Walz R, Lin K. Epilepsy and ultrastructural heart changes: the role of catecholaminergic toxicity and myocardial fibrosis. What can we learn from cardiology? Seizure. 2019;71:105–9.
170. Lemke DM, Hussain SI, et al. Tako-tsubo cardiomyopathy associated with seizures. Neurocrit Care. 2008;9:112–7.
171. Legriel S, Bruneel F, et al. Recurrent takotsubo cardiomyopathy triggered by convulsive status epilepticus. Neurocrit Care. 2008;9:118–21.
172. Shimutzu M, Kagawa A, et al. Neurogenic stunned myocardium associated with status epilepticus and postictal catecholamine surge. Intern Med. 2007;47:269–73.
173. Nashef L. Sudden unexpected death in epilepsy: terminology and definitions. Epilepsia. 1997;38(Suppl. 11):S6–8.
174. Tomson T, Walczak T, et al. Sudden unexpected death in epilepsy: a review of incidence and risk factors. Epilepsia. 2005;46(Suppl. 11):54–61.
175. Jehi L, Najm IM. Sudden unexpected death in epilepsy: impact, mechanisms and prevention. Cleve Clin J Med. 2008;75(Suppl. 2):s66–70.
176. Sveinsson O, Andersson T, Mattsson P, Carlsson S, Tomson T. Clinical risk factors in SUDEP A nationwide population-based case-control study. Neurology. 2020;94:e419–29.
177. Ryvlin P, So EL, Gordon CM, Hesdorffer DC, Sperling MR, Devinsky O, Bunker MT, Olin B, Friedman D. Long-term surveillance of SUDEP in drug-resistant epilepsy patients treated with VNS therapy. Epilepsia. 2018;59(3):562–72.
178. Li R, Buchanan GF. Scurrying to understand sudden expected death in epilepsy: insights from animal models. Epilepsy Curr. 2019;19:390–6.
179. Chahal CAA, Salloum MN, Alahdab F, Gottwald JA, Tester DJ, Anwer LA, So EL, Murad MH, St Louis EK, Ackerman MJ, Somers VK. Systematic review of the genetics of sudden unexpected death in epilepsy: potential overlap with sudden cardiac death and arrhythmia-related genes. J Am Heart Assoc. 2020;9:e012264.
180. Costagliola G, Orsini A, Coll M, Ramon Brugada R, Pasquale Parisi P, Pasquale SP. The brain–heart interaction in epilepsy: implications for diagnosis, therapy, and SUDEP prevention. Ann Clin Transl Neurol. 2021;8(7):1557–68.

181. Goldstein DS. Cardiac denervation in patients with Parkinson disease. Cleve Clin J Med. 2007;74(Suppl. 1):S91–4.
182. Walter BL. Cardiovascular autonomic dysfunction in patients with movement disorders. Cleve Clin J Med. 2008;75(Suppl. 2): S54–8.
183. Goldstein DS. Neuroscience and heart-brain medicine: the year in review. Cleve Clin J Med. 2010;77(Suppl. 3):S34–9.
184. Orimo S, Uchihara T, Nakamura A, Mori F, Kakita A, Wakabayashi K, Takohashi H. Axonal alpha-synuclein aggregates herald centripetal degeneration of cardiac sympathetic nerve in Parkinson's disease. Brain. 2008;131(Pt3):642–50.
185. Goldstein D. Dysautonomia in Parkinson's disease: neurocardiological abnormalities. Lancet Neurol. 2003;2:669–76.
186. Post S, Papetropulos KK. Chapter 5C. In: Halliday G, Barker R, Rowe D, editors. Non dopamine lesions in Parkinson diseases. Cambridge: Oxford Press; 2010.
187. Orimo S, Ozawa E, Nakade S, Sugimoto T, Mizusawa H. (123)I-metaiodobenzylguanidine myocardial scintigraphy in Parkinson's disease. J Neurol Neurosurg Psychiatry. 1999;67(2):189–94.
188. Yoshita M, Taki J, Yamada M. A clinical role for [(123)I]MIBG myocardial scintigraphy in the distinction between dementia of the Alzheimer's-type and dementia with Lewy bodies. J Neurol Neurosurg Psychiatry. 2001;71(5):583–8.
189. Nagayama H, Hamamoto M, Ueda M, Nagashima J, Katayama Y. Reliability of MIBG myocardial scintigraphy in the diagnosis of Parkinson's disease. J Neurol Neurosurg Psychiatry. 2005;76(2):249–51.
190. Marquié Sayagués M, Da Silva AL, Molina-Porcel L, Alcolea Rodríguez D, Sala Matavera I, Sánchez-Saudinós MB, Camacho Martí V, Estorch Cabrera M, Blesa González R, Blesa González R, Gómez-Isla T, Gómez-Isla T, Lleó Bisa A, Lleó BA. (123)I-MIBG myocardial scintigraphy in the diagnosis of Lewy body dementia. Neurologia. 2010;25(7):414.
191. Camacho V, Marquié M, Lleó A, Alvés L, Artigas C, Flotats A, Duch J, Blesa R, Gómez-Isla T, Carrió I, Estorch M. Cardiac sympathetic impairment parallels nigrostriatal degeneration in probable dementia with Lewy bodies. Q J Nucl Med Mol Imaging. 2011;55(4):476–83.
192. Valappil RA, Black JE, Broderick MJ, Carrillo O, Frenette E, Sullivan SS, Goldman SM, Tanner CM, Langston JW. Exploring the electrocardiogram as a potential tool to screen for premotor Parkinson's disease. Mov Disord. 2010;25(14): 2296–303.
193. Goldstein DS, Eldadah BA, Holmes C, Pechnik S, Moak J, Saleem A, Sharabi Y. Neurocirculatory abnormalities in Parkinson disease with orthostatic hypotension: independence from levodopa treatment. Hypertension. 2005;46(6):1333–9.
194. Iranzo A, Molinuevo JL, Santamaría J, Serradell M, Martí MJ, Valldeoriola F, Tolosa E. Rapid-eye-movement sleep behavior disorder as an early marker for a neurodegenerative disorder: a descriptive study. Lancet Neurol. 2006;5(7):572–7.
195. Piqueras-Flores J, López-García A, Moreno-Reig Á, et al. Structural and functional alterations of the heart in Parkinson's disease. Neurol Res. 2018;40(1):53–61. https://doi.org/10.1080/01616412.2017.1390933.
196. Wenning GK, Colosimo C, Geser F, Poewe W. Multiple system atrophy. Lancet Neurol. 2004;3(2):93–103. Erratum in: Lancet Neurol. 2004;3(3):137
197. Espay AJ, LeWitt PA, Hauser RA, Merola A, Masellis M, Lang AE. Neurogenic orthostatic hypotension and supine hypertension in Parkinson's disease and related synucleinopathies: prioritisation of treatment targets. Lancet Neurol. 2016;15(9):954–66. https://doi.org/10.1016/S1474-4422(16)30079-5.
198. Tublin JM, Adelstein JM, del Monte F, Combs CK, Wold LE. Getting to the heart of Alzheimer disease. Circ Res. 2019;124(1): 142–9. https://doi.org/10.1161/CIRCRESAHA.118.313563.
199. Royall DR. Insular Alzheimer disease pathology and the psychometric correlates of mortality. Cleve Clin J Med. 2008;75(Suppl. 2):S97–9.
200. Nakajima K, Yoshita M, et al. Ionidne-123-MIBG sympathetic imaging in Lewy-body diseases and related movement disorders. Q J Nucl Med Mol Imaging. 2008;52:378–87.
201. Cankar K, Melik Z, Kobal J, Starc V. Evidence of cardiac electrical remodeling in patients with Huntington disease. Brain Behav. 2018;8(8):e01077. https://doi.org/10.1002/brb3.1077.
202. Sasaki K, Sakata K, et al. Sequential changes in cardiac structure and function in patients with Duchenne-type muscular dystrophy: a two-dimensional echocardiographic study. Am Heart J. 1998;135:937–44.
203. Mavrogeni S, Tzelepis G, et al. Cardiac and sternocleidomastoid muscle involvement in Duchenne muscular dystrophy an MRI study. Chest. 2005;127:143–8.
204. Grubb BP. Clinical practice. Neurocardiogenic syncope. N Engl J Med. 2005;352(10):1004–10.
205. Freeman R. Clinical practice. Neurogenic orthostatic hypotension. N Engl J Med. 2008;358(6):615–24.
206. Webster M, Chancellor A, Smith H, Swift D, Sharpe D, Bass N, Glasgow G. Patent foramen ovale in young stroke patients. Lancet. 1988;2:11–2.
207. Overell JR, Bone I, Lees KR. Interatrial septal abnormalities and stroke: a meta-analysis of case control studies. Neurology. 2000;55:1172–9.
208. Handke M, Harloff A, Bode C, Geibel A. Patent foramen ovale and cryptogenic stroke: a matter of age? Semin Thromb Hemost. 2009;35:505–14.
209. Gaspardone A, Iani C, Papa MG. Percutaneous closure of patent foramen ovale: a wise approach. Ital Cardiol. 2008;9(9):593–602.
210. Pepi M, Evangelista A, Nihoyannopoulos P, Flachskampf FA, Athanassopoulos G, Colonna P, Habib G, Ringelstein EB, Sicari R, Zamorano JL, Sitges M, Caso P, European Association of Echocardiography. Recommendations for echocardiography use in the diagnosis and management of cardiac sources of embolism: European Association of Echocardiography (EAE). Eur J Echocardiogr. 2010;11:461–76.
211. Pristipino C, Anzola GP, Ballerini L, Bartorelli A, Cecconi M, Chessa M, Donti A, Gaspardone A, Neri G, Onorato E, Palareti G, Rakar S, Rigatelli G, Santoro G, Toni D, Ussia GP, Violini R. Management of patients with patent foramen ovale and cryptogenic stroke: a collaborative, multidisciplinary, position paper. Catheter Cardiovasc Interv. 2013;82:1–14.
212. Gaspardone A, Sgueglia GA. Cryptogenic stroke over 60 years of age: should patent foramen ovale be closed? Eur Heart J Suppl. 2020;22(Suppl. E):E82–6.
213. Mazzucco S, Li L, Binney L, Rothwell PM, Oxford Vascular Study Phenotyped Cohort. Prevalence of patent foramen ovale in cryptogenic transient ischaemic attack and non-disabling stroke at older ages: a population-based study, systematic review, and meta-analysis. Lancet Neurol. 2018;17:609–17.
214. Pristipino C, Sievert H, D'Ascenzo F, Louis Mas J, Meier B, Scacciatella P, Hildick-Smith D, Gaita F, Toni D, Kyrle P, Thomson J, Derumeaux G, Onorato E, Sibbing D, Germonpré P, Berti S, Chessa M, Bedogni F, Dudek D, Hornung M, Zamorano J, Evidence Synthesis Team, Eapci Scientific Documents and Initiatives Committee, International Experts. European position paper on the management of patients with patent foramen ovale. General approach and left circulation thromboembolism. Eur Heart J. 2019;40(38):3182–95.

215. Kahya Eren N, Bülbül NG, Yakar Tülüce S, Nazlı C, Beckmann Y. To be or not to be patent: the relationship between migraine and patent foramen ovale. Headache. 2015;55:934–42.
216. Kanwar SM, Noheria A, DeSimone CV, Rabinstein AA, Asirvatham SJ. Coincidental impact of transcatheter patent foramen ovale closure on migraine with and without aura—a comprehensive meta-analysis. Clin Trials Regul Sci Cardiol. 2016;15:7–13.
217. Zeller JA, Frahm K, Baron R, Stingele R, Deuschl G. Platelet-leukocyte interaction and platelet activation in migraine: a link to ischemic stroke? J Neurol Neurosurg Psychiatry. 2004;75:984–7.
218. Pristipino C, Germonpré P, Toni D, Sievert H, Meier B, D'Ascenzo F, Berti S, Onorato EM, Bedogni F, Mas JL, Scacciatella P, Hildick-Smith D, Gaita F, Kyrle PA, Thomson J, Derumeaux G, Sibbing D, Chessa M, Hornung M, Zamorano J, Dudek D, Evidence Synthesis Team, D'Ascenzo F, Omedè P, Ballocca F, Barbero U, Giordana F, Gili S, Iannaccone M, International Experts, Akagi T, Anzola G, Carroll J, Dalvi B, Angelis C, Junbo G, Kasner SE, Michel-Behnke I, Musumeci G, Søndergaard L, Tarantini G, Biondi-Zoccai GGL. European position paper on the management of patients with patent foramen ovale. Part II: Decompression sickness, migraine, arterial deoxygenation syndromes and select high-risk clinical conditions. Eur Heart J. 2021;42(16):1545–53.
219. Lee PH, Song JK, Kim JS, Heo R, Lee S, Kim DH, Song JM, Kang DH, Kwon SU, Kang DW, Lee D, Kwon HS, Yun SC, Sun BJ, Park JH, Lee JH, Jeong HS, Song HJ, Kim J, Park SJ. Cryptogenic stroke and high-risk patent foramen ovale: the DEFENSE-PFO trial. J Am Coll Cardiol. 2018;71:2335–42.
220. Kent DM, Dahabreh IJ, Ruthazer R, Furlan AJ, Reisman M, Carroll JD, Saver JL, Smalling RW, Jüni P, Mattle HP, Meier B, Thaler DE. Device closure of patent foramen ovale after stroke: pooled analysis of completed randomized trials. J Am Coll Cardiol. 2016;67(8):907–17.
221. Gaspardone A, De Marco F, Sgueglia GA, De Santis A, Iamele M, D'Ascoli E, Tusa M, Corciu A, Mullen M, Nobles A, Carminati M, Bedogni F. Novel percutaneous suture-mediated patent foramen ovale closure technique: early results of the NobleStitch EL Italian Registry. EuroIntervention. 2018;14(3):e272–9.
222. Gaspardone A, Sgueglia GA, De Santis A, D'Ascoli E, Iamele M, Piccioni F, Giannico B, D'Errico F, Gioffrè G, Summaria F, Gaspardone C, Versaci F. Predictors of residual right-to-left shunt after percutaneous suture-mediated patent fossa ovalis closure. JACC Cardiovasc Interv. 2020;13(18):2112–20.
223. Gaspardone A, De Santis A, Giannico MB, Sgueglia GA. Modified percutaneous suture-mediated patent fossa ovalis closure for prevention of cerebral ischemic events. Catheter Cardiovasc Inter. 2020;96(3):638–42.
224. Gaspardone A, Cinque A, Beggio E, D'Ascoli E, Piccioni F, Iamele M, Sgueglia GA, Gaspardone C, Versaci F. Percutaneous suture-mediated Patent Fossa Ovalis (PFO) closure: two-year clinical follow-up. Minerva Cardiol Angiol. 2021.
225. Lim ECH, Lim S-H, Wilder-Smith E. Brain seizes, heart ceases: a case of ictal asystole. J Neurol Neurosurg Psychiatry. 2000;69:557–9.
226. Handara G, Hetsch FJA, Jüttner R, Schick A, Haupt C, Rathjen FG, Kröger S. The role of agrin, Lrp4 and MuSK during dendritic arborization and synaptogenesis in cultured embryonic CNS neurons. Dev Biol. 2019;445:54–67.
227. Trinka E, Cock H, Hesdorffer D, Rossetti AO, Scheffer IE, Shinnar S, Shorvon S, Lowenstein DH. A definition and classification of status epilepticus—report of the ILAE Task Force on Classification of Status Epilepticus. Epilepsia. 2015;56(10):1515–23.

Endocrine Issues in Neurocritical Care

35

Micah T. Long, Eric R. Leiendecker, John T. Dollerschell, Arthur Tokarcyzk, and Douglas B. Coursin

Contents

M. T. Long (✉)
Division of Critical Care Anesthesiology, Departments of Anesthesiology, Internal Medicine & Emergency Medicine, University of Wisconsin Hospitals & Clinics, Madison, WI, USA
e-mail: mtlong@wisc.edu

E. R. Leiendecker
Divisions of Cardiothoracic and Critical Care Anesthesiology, Department of Anesthesiology, Emory University, Atlanta, GA, USA
e-mail: eric.richard.leiendecker@emory.edu

J. T. Dollerschell
Division of Cardiothoracic and Critical Care Anesthesiology, Department of Anesthesiology, University of Wisconsin Hospitals & Clinics, Madison, WI, USA
e-mail: dollerschell@wisc.edu

A. Tokarcyzk
Department of Anesthesiology, University of Chicago, NorthShore University Health Systems, Evanston, IL, USA

D. B. Coursin
Emeritus of Anesthesiology and Medicine, University of Wisconsin School of Medicine and Public Health, Madison, WI, USA

Department of Anesthesiology, University of Minnesota Medical School, Minneapolis, MN, USA
e-mail: dcoursin@wisc.edu

E. Mahanna Gabrielli et al. (eds.), *Textbook of Neurointensive Care: Volume 1*, https://doi.org/10.1007/978-3-031-62220-5_35

Abstract

The endocrine system is integral to maintain organ system function and homeostasis in humans. Critical illness causes dysregulation of the endocrine system and may disrupt hormonal balance. Neurologically injured patients are at particular risk to develop various endocrinopathies specific to their individual insults and comorbidities. Hormonal imbalances seen in the neurocritically ill can vary temporally as part of the acute, subacute, and chronic phases of critical illness. Emerging therapies continue to be investigated in order to reverse the deleterious effects of acute and chronic hormonal dysregulation. Neurointensivists should be aware of the various endocrinopathies that are present or may evolve in their patients, as well as the associated ICU polypharmacy that may cause endocrine dysfunction. Expeditious recognition of these issues and timely intervention may limit morbidity and enhance outcomes.

Introduction

The endocrine system is vital to physiologic homeostasis and includes a variety of glands that secrete hormones into the bloodstream, which then modulate end organs to regulate metabolism, growth, mood, development, tissue integrity, and cardiovascular and immune function in humans. The endocrine system exhibits numerous similarities to the nervous system, and these systems are intimately interrelated. The term "neuroendocrine" infers that hormones are similar to neurotransmitters, and certainly both rely on signaling and function of stimulus–response interactions. Typical neuroendocrine hormones are produced by the hypothalamus and stored in axons in the brain. Uniquely, however, hormones are secreted in the bloodstream and often act by stimulating or suppressing distant target cells. The endocrine and nervous systems do closely interact. For example, the sympathetic and parasympathetic nervous systems, along with neurotransmitters like dopamine, serotonin, endorphins, and encephalins can promote or suppress hormonal secretion. Hormone release is also closely modulated by nervous system-derived stimuli (e.g., tactile, auditory or olfactory). It is imperative to understand the close interactions between these two systems—the endocrine and nervous systems—in order to identify and manage abnormalities that may occur in both systems.

Neurologic injury causes a marked physiologic stress response that results in endocrine abnormalities. The most common endocrinopathy in the neurointensive care unit (NICU) patient is dysglycemia, defined as hypo- or hyperglycemia, or labile glucose levels termed glycemic variability [1]. All have potentially deleterious impact on the injured brain. Glucose monitoring technology has changed drastically in the last decade and glycemic goals in the critically ill have similarly evolved [2].

In addition to dysglycemia, other endocrine abnormalities are seen frequently with specific neurologic pathologies. These include traumatic brain injury (TBI), stroke, subarachnoid hemorrhage (SAH), intracranial hemorrhage (ICH), meningitis and encephalitis, endocrine secreting tumors, and progressive neurologic diseases. Brain death also causes a host of endocrine aberrancies.

This chapter will review the physiology and pathophysiology of the hypothalamic–pituitary axis and the neuroendocrine stress response during critical illness. Endocrinopathies encountered in the NICU will then be reviewed, including those related to premorbid endocrinopathies such as diabetes or thyroid abnormalities, and those that develop secondary to neurologic insults. We also explore endocrinopathies that can induce mental status changes, drug-induced endocrine disorders, and, finally, the endocrinopathy of brain death.

Anatomy and Physiology of the Hypothalamic–Pituitary Axis (HPA)

The hypothalamus and pituitary gland are closely integrated and responsible for the majority of endocrine function. The hypothalamus, a part of the diencephalon located below the thalamus, is responsible for releasing neuropeptides into the hypophyseal tract. These activate or inhibit responses from both the posterior and anterior pituitary glands. The pituitary gland consists of two portions, the anterior adenohypophysis and the posterior neurohypophysis. Uniquely, the posterior pituitary is not separate from the hypothalamus, but consists of a bundle of axons and nerve endings of nerves beginning in the hypothalamus [3, 4]. Figure 35.1 depicts the anatomy of both the anterior and posterior pituitary glands, while Table 35.1 lists specific glands, their respective hormones, and predominant actions [4].

The endocrine activity of the hypothalamus is provided by two types of neurosecretory cells. First are the magnocellular neurons, located in the paraventricular and supraoptic nuclei of the hypothalamus. These produce oxytocin and arginine vasopressin (AVP), hormones that are then released from the posterior pituitary gland. AVP primarily targets the collecting ducts of the kidney, increasing aquaporin density and, thus, free water reabsorption, as well as smooth muscle cells in the arteries, causing vasoconstriction. Oxytocin acts on the uterus and mammary epithelial cells and is responsible for uterine contraction and milk release [3, 5].

Second, the parvocellular neurons release both inhibitory and releasing neurohormones that interact with the anterior pituitary gland. These include corticotropin-releasing

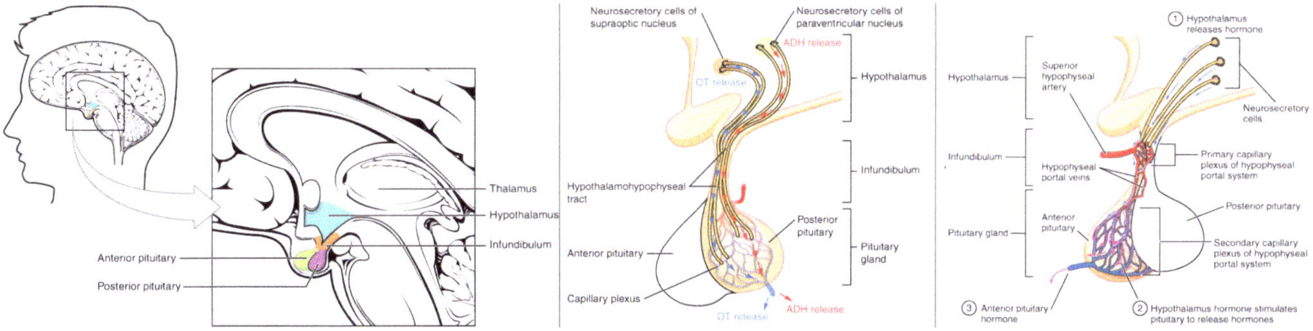

Fig. 35.1 Anatomy of the anterior and posterior pituitary glands. Reproduced, with permission from Biga et al. [4]

Table 35.1 Endocrine glands and action of the primary hormones

Gland	Hormone	Action
Posterior pituitary	Oxytocin	Uterine smooth muscle contraction, milk expulsion (mammary glands)
	Antidiuretic hormone (ADH)	Vasoconstriction Increases renal water reabsorption
Anterior pituitary	Thyroid-stimulating hormone (TSH)	Stimulates release of T3 and T4 by thyroid gland
	Adrenocorticotropic hormone (ACTH)	Involved in synthesis of glucocorticoids and mineralocorticoids and androgens, redistributes body energy in response to stress/starvation
	Prolactin	Growth of breasts Lactogenesis
	Luteinizing hormone (LH)	Promotes testosterone secretion and spermatogenesis in men Promotes ovulation and estrogen release in females
	Follicle-stimulating hormone (FH)	Spermatogenesis in men Promotes follicular growth/egg development in women
Thyroid gland	Thyroxine and triidothyronine	Augments metabolic rate Temperature regulation Increases O_2 consumption
Adrenal cortex	Mineralocorticoids	Increases sodium/water renal reabsorption facilitates renal potassium excretion
	Glucocorticoids	Increases blood glucose level Suppresses inflammation Modulates vascular homeostasis
	Androgens	Precursor to testosterone Secondary sexual characteristic development
Gland	Hormone	Action
Pancreatic islet cells	Insulin	Reduces serum glucose Drives glucose into cells Stimulates protein synthesis and storage of glycogen and fat
	Glucagon	Increases serum glucose Increases lipolysis Enhances hepatic glucose production and glycogenolysis
	Somatostatin	Inhibits release of insulin, glucagon, and some GI hormones
Ovary	Estrogen	Promotes growth/development of female sex organs
	Progesterone	Stimulates development/differentiation of sex organs

hormone (CRH), luteinizing hormone-releasing hormone (LHRH), somatostatin (SS), dopamine (DA), thyroid releasing hormone (TRH), and growth hormone-releasing hormone (GHRH). An intricate capillary system allows for the transport of these neurohormones from the hypothalamus to the anterior pituitary gland. In addition, venous connections between the anterior and posterior glands allow for neuropeptides to crossover (Fig. 35.1) [3–5].

While the posterior pituitary gland releases only two primary hormones, the anterior pituitary gland releases several hormones to organs throughout the body including growth hormone (GH), adrenocorticotropic hormone (ACTH), thyroid-stimulating hormone (TSH), luteinizing hormone (LH), follicle-stimulating hormone (FSH), and prolactin (PRL).

Growth hormone is primarily an anabolic peptide that participates in the growth of muscle and bone. Somatostatin inhibits its release, while GHRH allows for its secretion. ACTH is released in response to physical and emotional stress/starvation and targets the adrenal gland, promoting the production of adrenocortical hormones (glucocorticoids, mineralocorticoids, and androgens) [6]. It also acts on melanocytes to cause skin coloration. These hormones may contribute to hyperglycemia as well as suppression of the inflammatory response to both beneficial and harmful ends. Thyroid-stimulating hormone result in the release of triiodothyronine (T3) and thyroxine (T4) by the thyroid gland, which then suppress further TRH and TSH release. These hormones are integral to metabolism, growth, and development [5].

The anterior pituitary gland also produces sex hormones including LH, FSH, and PRL. Luteinizing hormone stimulates androgen production in both men and women. In men, FSH combined with testosterone aids in sperm production, whereas in women FSH promotes aromatization of androgens to estrogens. Prolactin is released in a diurnal fashion and is a stress hormone with immune-supporting capabilities as evidenced by the presence of PRL receptors on human B and T lymphocytes [5].

Pathophysiology of the HPA

Indirect or direct injury to the central nervous system (CNS) can have profound effects on the integrity of the endocrine system and cause inadequate release, production, or inhibition of hormones or the response to them. Hypopituitarism is a common endpoint from a myriad of conditions and, broadly, can result from either pituitary or hypothalamic dysfunction. It has been associated with excess deaths with a mortality ratio between 1.44 and 2.44 compared to age- and sex-matched controls [7, 8]. While the incidence (12–42 new cases per million per year) and prevalence (300–455 per million) are rare, hypopituitarism is likely underestimated, particularly in neurocritical care patients [9].

Etiology

There are multiple causes of hypopituitarism with some more frequently encountered in the NICU. Etiologies of hypopituitarism can be divided into several broad categories, shown in Table 35.2 [10]. Brain injury and ischemia may account for upward of 70% of cases of hypopituitarism [9, 10]. Clinical features depend on the magnitude and type of hormone deficiency; the diagnosis is likely underreported and underrecognized due to nonspecific findings like fatigue, hypotension, cold intolerance, or infertility. Special consideration of hypopituitarism is recommended for those patients with severe TBI, severe SAH, basilar skull fractures, diffuse axonal injury, increased intracranial pressure, and those who have a prolonged length of stay in the NICU [11]. Note that the amount of intracerebral blood and/or cerebral edema has been associated with an increased risk for hypopituitarism [11].

Table 35.2 Categories of hypopituitarism. Etiologies of hypopituitarism (right) can be divided into several broad categories (left) [10]

Congenital	Can cause multiple or isolated hormonal deficits
Tumors	Both functioning pituitary adenomas and nonfunctioning pituitary and peripituitary tumors
Infiltrative	Sarcoidosis, histiocytosis X, lymphocytic hypophysitis, and primary hemochromatosis
Infectious	Specific infections include tuberculosis, syphilis, mycoses, and meningitis, but hypopituitarism may also occur in broad conditions like septic shock
Ischemic	Pituitary apoplexy or Sheehan syndrome
Cellular injury and anatomic	Traumatic brain injury, cerebral edema, aneurysms, subarachnoid hemorrhage, irradiation, or interruption of the hypothalamohypophyseal portal blood supply (e.g., secondary to trauma)
Drug-induced	Antineoplastic agents and immune checkpoint inhibitors, or ribavirin

Symptomatology and Diagnosis

Clinical features of hypopituitarism depend on the underlying pathology, rapidity of onset, and severity. Compression lesions that are responsible for producing hypopituitarism usually cause visual abnormalities and headache due to proximity to the optic nerves. Less commonly, cerebrospinal rhinorrhea, temporal lobe epilepsy, or changes in personality can be seen with space-occupying lesions that also induce hypopituitarism [9].

Pituitary tumors can cause symptoms by affecting the HPA function with excessive production, reduced production from mass effect, or interference of delivery of hypothalamic hormones. Patients with PRL-secreting adenomas, for example, often present with hypogonadism because high levels of PRL inhibit FSH and LH. A patient with a GH-secreting tumor, alternatively, may develop both acromegaly and hypogonadism, due to a combination of symptoms associated with hormone excess and deficiency. Mixed symptomatology makes accurate and timely diagnoses very challenging and a combination of medical history, examination including visual field assessments, laboratory work, and imaging may be required [9]. Finally, magnetic resonance imaging (MRI) should be obtained, although computerized tomography (CT) with contrast may be an adequate alternative if the former is unobtainable or contraindicated [9, 12].

Basal serum hormonal measurements often include TSH, thyroxine (free T4), FSH, LH, estradiol, testosterone, PRL, insulin-like growth factor 1, and a 9:00 A.M. cortisol [13]. More advanced testing is required to assess GH secretion and ACTH-adrenal axis-related problems. Table 35.3 depicts the clinical features and testing for several core hormonal deficiencies. Other laboratory assessments can help delineate rare causes of hypopituitarism, such as serum and cerebro-

Table 35.3 Clinical features and tests for hypopituitarism

Hormone deficiency	Symptomatology	Testing
TSH	Fatigue, apathy, cold intolerance, weight gain, dry skin, psychomotor retardation, constipation	Decreased serum free/total T4 + inappropriately normal or low TSH
ACTH	Fatigue, weakness, anorexia, weight loss, nausea, vomiting, hypoglycemia, hemodynamic compromise	Basal 9 am cortisol <100 nmol/ or > 400–500 nmol/L Requires provocative test: Insulin tolerance test (ITT): Cortisol level > 500 nmol/L with normal ACTH
GH	Decreased muscle mass, strength, energy Increased central adiposity Impaired thermogenesis Decreased sweating	ITT (gold standard): Severe deficiency when peak GH response <3 μg/L Alternative tests: GHRH + arginine test Glucagon stimulation test
ADH	Polyuria, polydipsia, nocturia	Diabetes insipidus: Large urine volumes >3 L/day or low osmolality <300 mOsmol/kg 8-h water deprivation test with administration of desmopressin
Prolactin	Inability to breast feed	Prolactin levels
Gonadotropins	*Men:* decrease muscle mass, erythopoiesis, energy, and vitality; erectile dysfunction, soft testes *Females*: dyspareunia, breast atrophy, amenorrea, or oligomenorrhea *Both sexes:* infertility, loss of libido, hot flashes	Low serum testosterone with normal or low gonadotropin levels in men and low estradiol levels in premenopausal women without appropriate increased gonadotropins Post-menopausal women: absence of normal increase in gonadotropins

spinal fluid angiotensin converting enzyme levels (elevated in sarcoidosis), serum ferritin (elevated in hemochromatosis), and serum human chorionic gonadotropin (elevated in germ cell tumors) [9].

Management

Management of hypopituitarism focuses on replacement of deficient hormones, reducing hormone excess when applicable, and treating the underlying etiology in a directed manner. Prolactinomas, for example, are usually medically treated with dopamine agonists, whereas GH-producing adenomas are typically resected because of high surgical cure rates [9]. Surgical resection is also preferred for most compressing lesions, although an in-depth discussion of the management of all hormone deficiencies is beyond the scope of this chapter.

Recent clinical practice guidelines set by the Endocrine Society recommend hormonal replacement to approximate normal physiologic pattern as much as possible [13]. For instance, GH deficiency is typically managed with a nighttime subcutaneous dose of GH [9]. Exogenous replacement of GH may improve bone and mineral density, exercise capabilities, strength, and limit hyperlipidemia [9] and excess mortality [8]. Patients with ACTH deficiency, meanwhile, require exogenous basal hydrocortisone replacement and supplemental doses to prevent life-threatening adrenal insufficiency during windows of physiologic stress. An 8-h serum daytime cortisol curve can be obtained to diagnose over- or undertreatment [6, 9]. Unlike ACTH deficiency, treatment of TSH deficiency with L-thyroxine is primarily assessed clinically, though free T4 levels may also be beneficial [13]. Overtreatment may result in tachydysrhythmias including atrial fibrillation, weakness, weight loss, and hyperactivity and even vertebral fractures on occasion [14].

Gonadotropin deficiency requires specific sex hormone replacement. Testosterone replacement in men given by the intramuscular, buccal, transdermal patch or gel route can have beneficial effects on body composition, behavior, and sexual function [9, 13]. Testosterone levels and resolving symptomatology gauge the success of therapy. In women, estrogen replacement can mitigate bone density loss, fatigue, hot flashes and other symptoms of deficiency. Replacement therapy is monitored by assessment of symptom amelioration and side effect assessment, rather than by estrogen levels [13, 15].

Neuroendocrine Stress Response in Critical Illness

Dysglycemia in the Neurointensive Care Unit

There is a worldwide epidemic of diabetes mellitus (DM). Most recent epidemiology suggests that approximately 15% of adult Americans have DM, with approximately 3.4% being unaware that they have the disease [16]. Chronic hyperglycemia seen in DM causes both micro- and macrovascular complications that impact the brain. Diabetes doubles the risk of stroke [17] and may be associated with worse outcomes after stroke [18]. Diabetes also likely increases the risk of cognitive dysfunction [19] and dementia, which are closely interwoven with the incidence of hypoglycemia [20, 21].

Acute dysglycemia also occurs frequently in critically ill patients and likely impacts outcomes. Dysglycemia may include hyperglycemia, either absolute or relative to baseline glycemia, hypoglycemia that can be absolute or relative, spontaneous or treatment-induced, and labile glucose, termed glycemic variability [22]. In the critically ill, hyperglycemia can cause mitochondrial damage, oxidative stress, endothelial dysfunction, inflammation, and more. It has been associated with morbidity, like acute kidney injury, liver dysfunction, infection, and mortality in a broad array of critical illness states [23]. Historically, concerns about hyperglycemia-induced infectious complications and insulin-resistance-induced negative outcomes drove glycemic goals in the critically ill toward "physiologic," or "tight" ranges, from previously targeted renal-threshold glycemic control (e.g., 80–110 mg/dL from <200–220 mg/dL) [24]. Broad, less-specific application of aggressive control of hyperglycemia, however, was found to be less beneficial and in fact harmful compared to the evolved and now broadly adopted "intermediate" control of glucose (varied guidelines exist, typically targeting 130–180 mg/dL) [25]. This may be related to treatment-induced hypoglycemia [26], hypokalemia, or glycemic variability [27].

The brain has high metabolic activity, limited glucose reserves, and does not tolerate inadequate energy delivery. Hypoglycemia, therefore, is particularly detrimental to neuronal survival and overall outcome after brain injury [28]. In the NICU, subarachnoid hemorrhage, TBI, or stroke may result in changes in the brain and blood brain barrier (BBB) that alter normal glucose availability to neurons. Injured brain tissue and the surrounding penumbra develop abnormal glucose transport through the damaged BBB. Therefore, measured arterial or venous glucose may not reflect glucose levels within the injured brain. Supporting this, certain states such as TBI and aneurysmal hemorrhage have displayed markers of hypoglycemic stress in states of systemic plasma euglycemia (80–110 mg/dL) [29], making glycemic goals particularly challenging to determine, and risky to achieve. Altered glucose transport may be a result of up- and down-regulation of neuronal cell glucose transporter (GLUT) proteins. Upregulation of GLUT3, in severe TBI, may contribute to the glucose uptake, and downregulation of GLUT1 at the BBB, in severe TBI, decreases cerebral glucose availability even in the face of systemic euglycemia [28–31]. These aberrancies can cause regional hypoglycemia with resultant energy production failure, cellular distress, and injury.

The evolving use of brain microdialysis allows detection of glucose levels at the site of injury and in the future may guide therapeutic measures to adjust the supply of glucose delivery to the injured brain [28, 29]. The Krebs cycle is the predominant glucose-mediated method to generate cellular energy. The Krebs cycle is oxygen dependent, therefore during states of ischemia energy production shifts to anaerobic pathways, which require NAD^+, produced from NADH by converting pyruvate to lactate. This causes an increase in lactate and decrease in pyruvate leading to an increased lactate/pyruvate ratio (LPR). Microdialysis enables repetitive sampling of the neuronal extracellular fluid via a microcatheter to determine the LPR, as well as other metabolic markers of energy failure such as glycerol and glutamate [29]. In states of anaerobic metabolism, the LPR should increase prior to the onset of ICP changes or clinical symptoms of cerebral distress; an LPR greater than 25 is considered an early warning sign of cerebral energy failure [29, 32, 33].

Hyperglycemia in ischemic brain tissue is also detrimental, promoting anaerobic glycolysis that results in local intracellular metabolic and lactic acidosis and, in turn, intracellular hypercalcemia that yields glutamate and free fatty acid accumulation and resultant injury. Hyperglycemia also impacts the endothelium and may disrupt small vasculature flow through vasospasm and increased viscosity. Finally, hyperglycemia can produce an increased inflammatory milieu and general oxidative stress [34].

Further, glucose variability develops commonly in critically ill patients. The greater the degree of glucose variability, even at the same average glucose, the greater the morbidity and mortality [27, 35]. Evolving work suggests that glucose variability induces ischemia-reperfusion phenomena and oxidative stress which, in the brain, can be particularly deleterious [36].

Knowing the above, the appropriate glucose target range in the neurocritically ill remains elusive and a "one-size fits all approach" may not be optimal for the individual patient. Patients with poorly controlled diabetes, for instance, may benefit from higher glucose goals than a patient without diabetes [2]. Adding complexity, temporal differences may exist. The patient with TBI, for instance, may benefit from higher glucose acutely and lower glucose after the first week [37]. Nonetheless, prospective trials in the NICU, including work in TBI, SAH, stroke, and after neurosurgery, have compared "tight" glucose control (generally with glucose goals of ~80–120 mg/dL) with conventional goals. Crucially, these studies did not reveal a benefit in mortality or neurologic outcomes with tighter goals, only a higher incidence of hypoglycemia [2], unless the conventional glucose target was severely elevated and not consistent with current guidelines (e.g. >200 mg/dL) [28]. Current recommendations, therefore, support intermediate glucose goals in the neurocritically ill, generally 130–180 mg/dL, to maximize benefit and mitigate risk.

Hormonal Changes During the Acute Phase of Critical Illness

Critical illness is associated with dysregulation of the hypothalamic–pituitary axis, occurring differently in the acute, sub-acute, and chronic phases of critical illness (Fig. 35.2 and Table 35.4) [38, 39]. The acute neuroendocrine changes associated with critical illness involve the adrenal, somatotropic, thyroid, and gonadal/lactotropic axes.

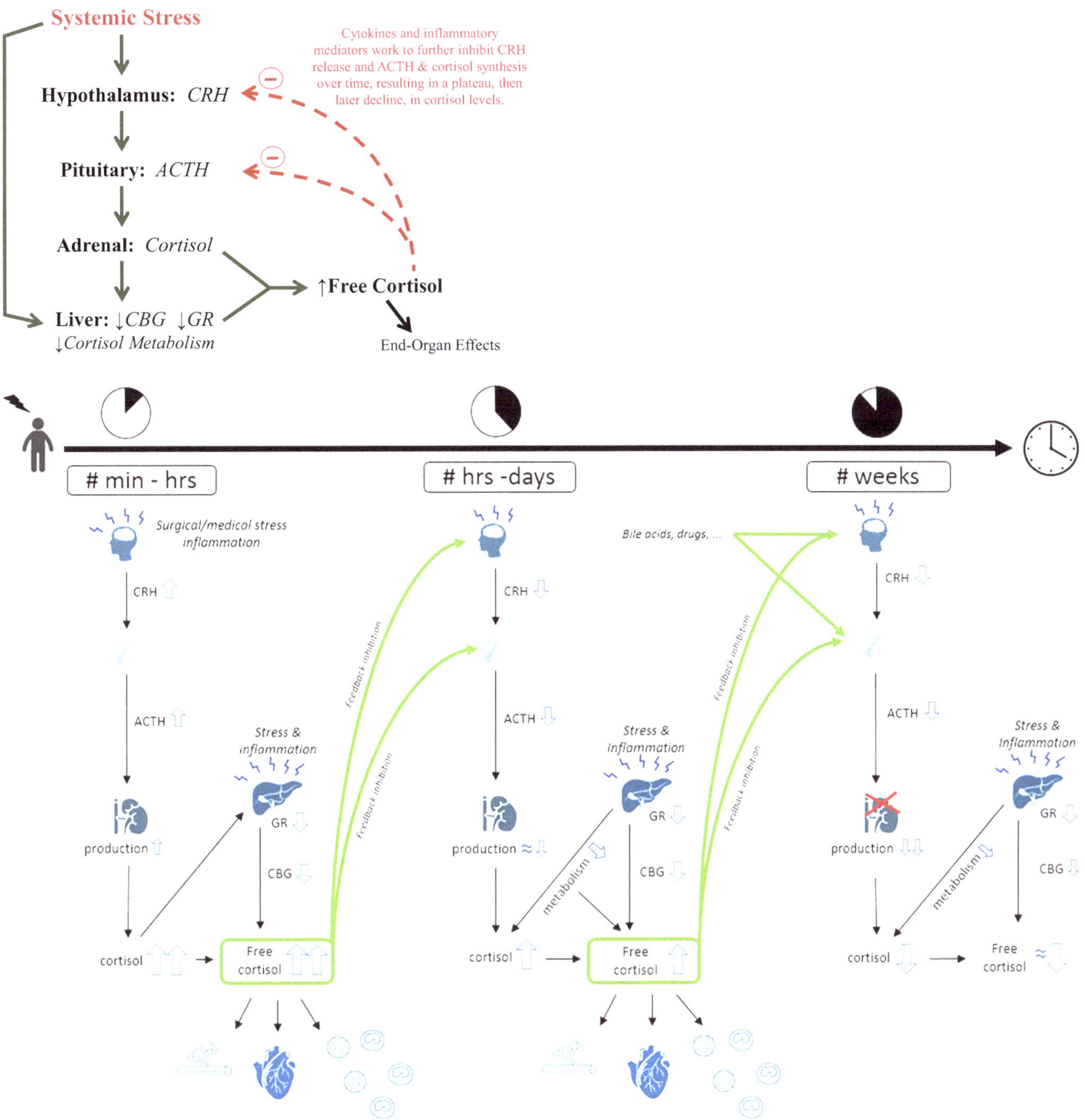

Figs. 35.2 and 35.3 Hormonal and adrenocortical impact of critical illness. Acute medical or surgical stress and/or inflammation results in an immediate hormonal cascade that causes a spike in both total and free cortisol (acute phase). The liver participates by decreasing cortisol-binding globulin acutely and by decreasing cortisol metabolism over time (subacute and chronic). Free cortisol results in important end-organ effects including effects on the cardiovascular system, metabolism, and immune system. Free cortisol causes progressive feedback inhibition, limiting its production at the hypothalamus and anterior pituitary and resulting in a post-peak plateau of free and total cortisol levels (subacute phase) and eventual chronic-phase normalization of levels. Meanwhile, however, reductions in cortisol metabolism can be longstanding. *ACTH* adrenocorticotropic hormone, *CBG* cortisol-binding globulin, *CRH* cortisol-releasing hormone, *GR* glucocorticoid receptor

The adrenal axis plays an integral role in the body's response to critical illness. Under normal circumstances, healthy individuals secrete cortisol in a diurnal pattern, and cortisol provides negative feedback on both CRH and ACTH release. In acute illness, a change in this control has been attributed to the hypoperfusion and inflammatory damage to the pituitary gland, thereby leading to reduced CRH and Argentine vasopressin (AVP) release [40]. Concurrently, the

Table 35.4 Hormonal changes during the acute and chronic phases of critical illness

Hormone	Acute phase	Prolonged phase
Somatotropic axis		
Pulsatile GH release	+	–
GHBP	–	+
IGF-1	–	--
ALS	–	--
AGFBP-3	–	--
Thyroid axis		
Pulsatile TSH release	+/=	–
T4	+/=	–
T3	–	--
rT3	+	+/=
Gonadal & lactotropic axis		
Pulsatile LH release	+/=	–
Testosterone	–	--
Pulsatile prolactin release	+	–
Adrenal axis		
ACTH	+	–
Cortisol	++	+/=/–

Modified and with permission, from Vanhorebeek and Van den Berghe [43]
+ Increased
= Unchanged
– Decreased

diurnal pattern of cortisol release disappears. Cortisol levels may remain elevated, reflecting increased production and decreased metabolism, along with a reduced level of cortisol-binding globulin (Fig. 35.2) [38, 41]. While higher levels of cortisol may reflect a greater stressor, low levels may reflect an inadequate response to stress. Acute stress-induced hypercortisolism is vital to protect critically ill patients from hyperinflammation, hemodynamic instability, and malnourishment with cellular injury failure during the high metabolic state of critical illness [39]. This rise in cortisol serves to tamp down the activity of proinflammatory T cells, facilitate catabolism, and ensure an adequate supply of substrate for metabolism and energy formation. However, persistent hypercortisolism may be a significant negative prognosticator, especially among patients with septic shock [42].

Production of proinflammatory cytokines due to stress-induced injury increases abruptly during the acute phase of critical illness. This increase in cytokines causes downregulation of GH receptors, especially in the muscle and liver, causing significant GH resistance [43]. While GH release sharply escalates, there is a decrease in effector protein levels of insulin-like growth factor-1 (IGF-1) and GH-dependent IGF-binding proteins (IGFBPs). This reduction of circulating IGF-1, which typically inhibits GH release, is thus partly responsible for the increased GH secretion [44]. From a teleologic viewpoint, inhibition of anabolism via a reduction in functional GH may ensure the body maintains necessary energy substrates [43, 45].

Thyroid hormones are integral to the regulation of metabolism. During the early phase of critical illness, plasma levels of T3 are reduced and reverse triiodothyronine (rT3), an isomer of T3, levels are increased due to the increased conversion of T4 [46]. This is now commonly referred to as non-thyroidal illness syndrome (NTIS) and is part of the adaptation to acute illness and not an intrinsic thyroid disorder. During most acute illnesses, TSH and T4 transiently rise and then return to normal levels (except in severe illness where T4 levels may be low). While TSH normalizes, low levels of T3 persist. The persistence of low T3 is referred to as the "low T3 syndrome." Decreased levels of T3 during the first day of critical illness may indicate the severity of illness and may be somewhat prognostic: survivors have been found to have higher nadir levels of T3 than non-survivors [47]. The acute reduction in T3 levels may enact the protective processes seen during starvation that reduce energy expenditure and maintain energy delivery to organs [46].

The gonadal and lactotropic axes are also affected during the acute phase of critical illness. Despite increased levels of LH, testosterone levels are reduced during acute injury [6, 43], which may reduce anabolism, thereby conserving energy and diverting energy expenditures to the most vital organ systems [6, 43]. Unlike testosterone, PRL levels are elevated during acute critical illness. This process may be directed by cytokines, oxytocin, and/or vasoactive intestinal peptide and may enhance immunity and mitigate infection. Finally, estradiol levels in the acute phase of critical illness may be elevated, maintained, or decreased [6, 43]. The impact of these changes is unclear.

Hormonal Changes During the Chronic Phase of Critical Illness

The transition to the chronic phase of critical illness is marked by hormonal adaptation. While cortisol levels remain elevated in the chronically critically ill, cortisol-binding globulin returns to near normal levels during this phase of chronic illness (Figs. 35.2 and 35.3) [41, 43]. This hypercortisolism may be responsible for an increased risk of infection.

The GH resistance seen in acute illness is somewhat reversed in the chronic state, and evidence suggests that GH-secretagogues can increase IGF-1 and IGFBP levels during the chronic phase of critical illness. Thus, GH resistance is partially corrected, particularly when nutrition is restored [44]. In addition to a reduction in somatostatin activity, a deficiency originating from the hypothalamus or inactivity of endogenous GHRP-like GH secretagogues is a likely contributor of hyposomatotropism [6]. There is also a lack of pulsatile GH release, which may help explain the development of the protein wasting syndrome encountered during chronic critical illness [45]. There are some observational studies suggesting that the GH axis is more suppressed in men than women, though it remains unclear if this suppression explains the poorer outcomes associated with endocrinologic abnormalities in men versus women [45].

Pulsatile TSH secretion is markedly reduced during prolonged critical illness and replaced with a constant low level secretion, resulting in reduced serum T3 and T4 [46]. There is a reduced TRH gene expression in prolonged critical illness, which results in reduced TRH-induced stimulation of TSH, and subsequently results in reduced serum T3 and T4 [48]. This reduction of gene expression of TRH seen in studies of chronically sick patients who subsequently died likely accounts for the primary mechanism of reduced TSH levels [46].

In addition to reduced thyroid hormone production, thyroid hormone metabolism is altered due to a reduction in the type 1 deiodinase enzyme, which converts T4–T3. This contributes to the aforementioned low T3 syndrome. This metabolism is also impacted by the interrelationship between the thyroid and somatotropin axes, a relationship exemplified by the combination of TRH with growth hormone-releasing peptide-2 (GHRP-2) which facilitates increases in serum levels of TSH, T4, and T3 [46]. With a predominance of TRH reduction, as opposed to an increase in GHRP-2, low levels of TSH, T4, and T3 coupled with higher rT3 are encountered, which may be prognostic in chronically critically ill patients [46, 49]. In fact, the addition of the free T3 level to the APACHE-2 score has been shown to significantly increase the score's ability to predict outcomes [49]. The mechanism for this negative prognosis has yet to be elucidated however.

Similar to the thyroid axis, the gonadal and lactotropic axes are also profoundly depressed during chronic critical illness. Serum levels of testosterone become nearly undetectable due to suppressed LH release [43]. This likely contributes to muscle weakness; there is evidence that supplementation can aid in rehabilitation of these patients [50]. Meanwhile, while total estradiol concentrations are low, free estradiol levels are relatively maintained due to a reduction in sex hormone-binding globulin [43]. Finally, prolactin secretion is reduced to a greater degree during chronic critical illness versus the acute phase [43]. Reduced PRL secretion may contribute to an increased risk of infection or other morbidities. Drugs such as dopamine may further suppress PRL secretion and contribute to further immunosuppression [43, 51].

Endocrine Issues in Specific Neuropathology

Stroke

Cerebrovascular accidents (CVA) are a leading cause of morbidity and mortality. Most (80–85%) CVAs are thrombotic or embolic events that disrupt cerebral blood flow and cause ischemic damage to affected brain. The remaining 15–20% of CVAs are hemorrhagic strokes evenly divided between intracerebral hemorrhage (ICH), usually due to uncontrolled hypertension, and SAH [52, 53]; each have associated neuroendocrine pathology.

Subarachnoid Hemorrhage

Subarachnoid hemorrhages (SAH) can arise from trauma, arteriovascular malformations, illicit drug use (e.g. cocaine or amphetamines), vasculitides, and bleeding diatheses. The most common cause of SAH is due to ruptured saccular aneurysms (aSAH) from weakened cerebral arterial vasculature [53]. Risk factors for aneurysms include smoking, hypertension, moderate to heavy alcohol use, a family history of aneurysms, and genetic diseases such as autosomal dominant polycystic kidney disease, glucocorticoid-remediable aldosteronism, or Ehlers–Danlos syndrome. Additionally, over-the-counter sympathomimetic drugs, estrogen deficiency, antithrombic therapy, and statin use have been associated with aneurysm development [53, 54].

Most SAHs occur in adults between 40 and 60 years of age. Approximately 10% of patients with SAH die before reaching the hospital. Over 60% of the remaining SAH patients have high morbidity and disability [53]. Mortality of treated patients is approximately 50% in the first 30 days. The high mortality and morbidity associated with a SAH are due to complications that occur in the 15 days after the aneurysm is surgically or angiographically managed. The most dreaded complications of a SAH are bleeding and vasospasm [53, 55].

Subarachnoid hemorrhage is a risk factor for neuroendocrine dysfunction, both acutely and in long-term survivors. The most common endocrine abnormality following SAH is hypopituitarism with GH and CRF deficiency. One study of 60 patients with spontaneous SAH found that 56.9% of patients developed at least one anterior pituitary hormone deficiency within 72 h of insult. Gonadotropin and GH secretion failure were the most prominent at 33.3% and 22.0%, respectively. Meanwhile, ACTH and TSH deficiencies were less frequent at 7.1% and 1.8%, respectively [56].

Ischemic Stroke

Endocrine dysfunction can occur in all types of CVAs, in both the acute and chronic phases of the disease process. Pituitary and hypothalamic strokes, although rare, cause the greatest dysfunction. In these cases, panhypopituitarism is common with minimal recovery [57]. Elevated levels of endothelin-1, AVP, and cortisol in acute stroke patients may be implicated in exacerbating neurologic deficits and contributing to worse outcomes. Lastly, leptin secretion is frequently abnormal during and after stroke, which may lead to the poor nutritional status [58].

Traumatic Brain Injury and Adrenal Insufficiency

Persistent hypopituitarism after TBI approaches 12%. GH is the most common hormone lost, followed by ACTH [59]. The neurocritical care patient in shock usually presents with hypotension refractory to vasopressors and volume resuscitation. Laboratory findings consistent with adrenal insufficiency include hypoglycemia, hyponatremia, hyperkalemia, azotemia, hypercalcemia, and eosinophilia. High-dose methylprednisolone treatment in TBI has been shown to be detrimental to outcomes; however, treatment with low-dose glucocorticoid supplementation for hemodynamically unstable patients may be necessary in the first few days [60].

Chronic hypopituitarism requiring hormone replacement occurs in 20% of TBI patients. Mild hormonal deficits occur in approximately 30% of patients after mild, moderate, or severe TBI. These data suggest the importance of long-term follow-up testing for hormonal deficiencies in patients recovering from TBI [59]. Importantly, recent studies show that this may occur after smaller repeated brain injuries, such as in repeated concussions seen with aggressive sports activity [61].

Progressive Neurologic Disease: Guillain Barré Syndrome

The term Guillain–Barré syndrome (GBS) or Landry-Guillain Barré Syndrome is an eponym used to describe a spectrum of peripheral sensorimotor, inflammatory polyneuropathies that are the most common causes of acute, flaccid paralysis with an incidence of 1–2 per 100,000 [62, 63]. Guillain, Barré, and Strohl described this syndrome in 1916, and it was traditionally viewed as an acute inflammatory demyelinating polyradiculoneuropathy (AIDP). The onset of GBS is commonly preceded by a viral illness or infectious process within 6 weeks in 2/3 of patients [64]. The six pathogens most commonly associated with the development of GBS are *Campylobacter jejuni*, Epstein-Barr virus, Cytomegalovirus, Hepatitis E, Mycoplasma pneumonia, and Zika virus; it has also been associated with surgery, immunization, Hodgkin disease, and systemic lupus erythematosus [62].

Patients with GBS typically present with weakness and paresthesias located in the fingers or toes, which progresses proximally into the limbs within days. Weakness is typically "ascending" and may include the arms, trunk and respiratory muscles and the facial or pharyngeal muscles. Pain can be pronounced and typically peaks alongside of muscle weakness within the first 1–3 weeks, then persists for several weeks prior to a slow resolution over months. Autonomic dysfunction is common and may affect 50% of all patients suffering from GBS [65]. The severity of dysautonomia varies and can include sympathetic or parasympathetic nervous system hyperactivity or deficiency with dysrhythmias, hypertension, ileus, and/or incontinence. Less severe GBS forms may present with only mild weakness, but the duration may extend for several months [63].

The diagnostic work up of GBS/AIDP is based on clinical history and physical examination and may include analysis of cerebral spinal fluid (CSF), electrophysiologic studies, a complete blood count (CBC), an electrolyte panel, and more. CSF analysis typically reveals elevated protein in the absence of pleocytosis, termed albumino-cytological dissociation. CSF abnormalities may be delayed and not appear for up to 1 week after onset. Electrophysiolgic studies reveal slowed nerve conduction velocity or even blockage of conduction, while evaluation of axonal variants will reveal low amplitudes and normal velocities [62]. The CBC is usually unchanged, while serum electrolytes may demonstrate hyponatremia from SIADH [62, 63].

The management of patients with GBS will involve the evaluation of respiratory function, the need for intubation, anticipation and treatment of autonomic dysfunction, and consideration for specific treatment. The standard treatment for progressive GBS is either IVIG administration or plasma pheresis/exchange therapy (PLEX). Although pheresis/exchange was formerly the gold standard for treatment, IVIG has been demonstrated as being at least as effective with improved ease of administration [63, 66]. Plasmapheresis is recommended in patients with severe symptoms, including inability to walk, respiratory failure or distress, or bulbar muscle weakness. Other immunotherapies such as use of the monoclonal antibody, eculizumab, to modulate C-5 complement activation, remain under investigation [66].

Patients with progressive weakness will require close respiratory monitoring and pulmonary clearance, with the need for intubation determined by the ability to protect the airway, adequacy of self-management of secretions, and the risk of hypoventilation. Factors that may be associated with the need for mechanical ventilation include rapid onset (<7 days from symptom onset to admission), inability to lift the head, and a vital capacity <1–1.5 L or a rapid drop in vital capacity [67]. Clinicians should evaluate patient respiratory muscle strength and pulmonary function prior to weaning these patients from the ventilator. Duration of intubation is variable, although tracheostomy may be required in a small percentage of patients [62, 63]. Typical ICU care should be performed on patients with GBS including prophylaxis for deep vein thrombosis, nutritional support, monitoring for pressure sores, and provision of appropriate pain relief.

Endocrine Abnormalities and Guillain Barré Syndrome

GBS has been associated with numerous endocrine disturbances, specifically Hashimoto thyroiditis, elevated serum cortisol, and the syndrome of inappropriate antidiuretic hormone secretion (SIADH) or diabetes insipidus (DI). There are no specific associations between GBS and abnormalities of the somatotropic or gonadal axis.

Albeit rare, GBS has been associated with other autoimmune disorders, including Hashimoto thyroiditis (HT) [68]. HT is an autoimmune disorder characterized by antibodies against thyroid peroxidase and thyroglobulin resulting in antibody-mediated destruction of the thyroid gland follicles. This eventually results in hypothyroidism due to depletion of the thyroid gland follicles. The mechanism of association is incompletely understood but may be due to a common autoimmune antibody against thyroid tissue and ganglioside/neuronal cells [68, 69].

Stress-induced hypercortisolism may be the straightforward mechanism by which GBS patients are observed to have elevated cortisol levels, though this is not yet clear and may be related to cytokine induction of steroidogenesis [70]. Elevated cortisol levels at presentation can be predictive of need for mechanical ventilation and development of dysautonomia [70]. Accordingly, corticotrophin and corticosteroids were initially considered for therapy, though later analyses refuted any benefit [71]. Therefore, specific treatment for hypercortisolism may not be necessary, as levels appear to quickly improve with resolution of the underlying illness.

Disturbances in AVP may also be seen in patients with GBS [72]. Diabetes insipidus (DI) is rarely seen in GBS and results from insufficient levels of or response to AVP and may lead to hypernatremia and hypovolemia. Contrarily, SIADH occurs frequently in patients with GBS with an incidence between 11.8% and 48% [72, 73]. Symptoms of moderate hyponatremia (serum sodium <130 mEq/L) include confusion, mental status changes, cramping, and weakness, whereas more severe hyponatremia (Na <115 mEq/L) may result in seizures or coma. The mechanism for SIADH development in GBS is poorly understood and likely multifactorial. It may not be directly due to excessive secretion of AVP [73]. SIADH may develop at any point in the course of GBS, even after treatment initiation. This, however, also suggests that pseudohyponatremia due to IVIG therapy-induced increased serum viscosity may be an additional cause of hyponatremia in GBS [72–74]. SIADH is often secondary to an underlying process, and reversal of the cause yields resolution of SIADH. With mild to moderate hyponatremia (Na >120 mEq/L), appropriate therapy may be limited to fluid restriction, treatment of the underlying causative disorder and watchful waiting. Worsening or symptomatic hyponatremia, however, may be treated with hypertonic saline or a vasopressin receptor antagonist such as conivaptan or tolvaptan. When symptomatic, hyponatremia should be corrected deliberately with exceeding caution and close monitoring. The rate of correction should be limited to 10–12 mEq/L per 24 h, or 0.5 mEq/L per hour, as an excessively rapid correction may result in osmotic demyelination syndrome [75].

Without recognizing that acute rapid development of SIADH can occur in conjunction with GBS, clinicians may fail to make a timely diagnosis of GBS, particularly as weakness may be attributed to hyponatremia. Specific risks for SIADH in GBS include the need for mechanical ventilation and bulbar weakness. Critically, SIADH in GBS has been associated with higher mortality [72, 73]. The intensivist must remain vigilant for changes in sodium alongside of GBS.

Endocrine Abnormalities in Meningitis/Encephalitis

Central nervous system (CNS) infections such as meningitis and encephalitis can be associated with endocrine abnormalities both independently and in conjunction with critical illness. Both infectious meningitis and encephalitis carry significant risk of morbidity and mortality, dependent on the causative organism, particularly if diagnosis and/or therapy are delayed [76]. The clinical presentation, diagnosis, and management of both nosocomial and community-acquired CNS infections are reviewed in Chap. 31.

Several pathogens that cause meningitis and encephalitis may cause endocrine abnormalities, noting that these may also be incidentally discovered in patients with primary intracranial masses or hormone-secreting tumors who also develop CNS infection. In at-risk patients, infections directly attack the pituitary and yield hypopituitarism. These include patients with pituitary abscesses, tuberculous meningitis or brain abscesses, and neurosyphilis [77]. Fungal infections due to aspergillus, nocardia, or *Candida albicans*, viral infections due to Herpes simplex, varicella, enterovirus, and others, including tick borne viruses, and parasitic infections due to *Toxoplasma gondii* may result in hypophysitis [77]. Specific endocrine derangements associated with CNS infections remain poorly studied, though existing literature suggests that over 30% of patients with CNS infections may have acute pituitary abnormalities along with infection [77–79].

Uniquely, imaging including brain CT or MRI does not yield consistent abnormalities of the hypothalamus or pituitary gland in patients with these abnormalities, though occasionally enhancing tissue or nodular lesions are revealed [80]. These changes may endure, with chronic pituitary sequelae observed in over 30% of patients 12 months after initial illness [78]. Specifically, GH deficiency frequently complicates acute meningitis and can last years [79, 80].

Thyroid hormone abnormalities can also be seen in patients with CNS infections. In patients with acute meningitis that are not critically ill, low T3 syndrome has been demonstrated in a significant portion of patients on admission [78]. Fortunately, low T3 syndrome typically resolves and does not appear to lead to chronic thyroid hormone deficiency [78]. Abnormal TSH and free T4 levels are not readily demonstrated in patients with meningitis, suggesting a primary lack of consistent pituitary or thyroid gland dysfunction in meningitis [78, 79, 81].

Deficiencies in sex hormones secondary to abnormal pituitary function are also observed in patients with meningitis. While these gonadotropic derangements are seen in the acute phase of meningitis, gonadotropic dysfunction appears to resolve over time or result in only mild deficiency [81].

Adrenal insufficiency has received significant attention in the setting of critical illness, as discussed above. After resolution of meningitis, however, 21–25% of patients suffer from ACTH deficiency [78, 80]. This may be due to decreased CRH from the hypothalamus [81].

The reversibility of endocrine abnormalities due to CNS infection depends on the underlying endocrine abnormality, concomitant control and treatment of the underlying infection, and chance. Some endocrine sequelae, such as low T3, are self-limited and should not require treatment except in extreme circumstances with persistent symptoms [46]. Gonadotropin deficiencies observed in patients with CNS infections may be treated with administration and monitoring of testosterone in men and estradiol and progesterone in women. CNS infection-associated ACTH deficiency may be treated initially with hydrocortisone, transitioning to longer-acting steroids for chronic administration. These patients are prone to Addisonian crisis or adrenal insufficiency with stress and steroid dosing should be increased during periods of physiologic stress.

Endocrine Response in CNS and Endocrine-Secreting Tumors

Pituitary Tumors

Pituitary tumors are common, occurring in as many as 20% of the general population [82]. They are typically classified by size, either as microadenomas if less than 1 cm and macroadenomas if greater than 1 cm, though size may not correlate to secretory function. Macroadenomas are drastically less common, with an incidence of 0.16–0.2% in the general population [82]. Pituitary adenomas can also be differentiated by their hormonal secretory activity (i.e., PRL-secreting tumors causing hyperprolactinemia, GH-secreting tumors causing acromegaly or gigantism, ACTH-secreting tumors causing Cushing syndrome, and TSH-secreting tumors causing hyperthyroidism) [82]. The treatment of choice for symptomatic tumors is surgical resection, with the exception of PRL-secreting tumors [82]. The intensivist will primarily encounter the patient with a pituitary adenoma postoperatively. Rarely, however, a pituitary adenoma may hemorrhage or necrose, leading to pituitary apoplexy. This results in a sudden increase in sellar pressure and pituitary impairment that may require immediate supportive therapy, hormone replacement, and surgical evaluation [83].

The physiology, symptomatology, and management of a pituitary adenoma depend on its classification. A significant proportion of pituitary adenomas are hormonally active, with PRL-secreting adenomas being the most common, accounting for 15% of brain tumors and 40–45% of pituitary tumors [82]. More aggressive forms of PRL-secreting tumors are typically associated with multiple endocrine neoplasia-1 (MEN-1) syndrome [84]. Other active adenomas include GH and ACTH adenomas, followed by less common LH/FSH and TSH adenomas [82]. Overall, prolactinomas occur far more often in females (10:1), though after 50 years of age this sex differential is, in fact, eliminated. Men more typically have macroadenomas and aggressive disease [82]. Patients can present with amenorrhea, infertility, galactorrhea, hypogonadism, impotence, gynecomastia, or osteoporosis.

Evaluation of patients with PRL-secreting tumors includes a morning serum PRL level coupled with TSH and thyroid hormone levels, IGF-1 levels, serum electrolytes, and a pregnancy test [82]. Though most prolactinomas present as microadenomas, all symptomatic patients and those with macroadenomas should have visual acuity assessed. The goal of treatment is to normalize prolactinoma levels, with first-line therapy consisting of dopamine agonists such as bromocriptine or cabergoline, with the latter being preferred due to heightened selectiveness toward dopamine receptors in the pituitary. Cabergoline typically offers therapeutic success, normalizing prolactin levels in over 95% of patients and decreasing tumor size in most; therapy is generally long term. Endoscopic trans-sphenoidal surgery is reserved for patients unresponsive to, or intolerant of, dopamine agonist therapy, which can infrequently cause cardiac valvular disease and impulse control disorders. If needed, radiation may be required for surgical failure [82].

GH-secreting somatotropinomas are the next most common hormonally active pituitary adenoma. Most present as macroadenomas with slow growth rates thus yielding a many-years delay in diagnosis [82]. Adults can present with acromegaly, tachycardia, hypertension, left ventricular hypertrophy, dysrhythmias, obstructive sleep apnea (OSA), airway obstruction, insulin resistance, diabetes, polyneuropathy, and myalgias. Hypopituitarism, hyperthyroidism, and and hyperprolactinemia may also be seen in patients with GH-secreting tumors [85]. An evaluation of these patients consists of an oral glucose tolerance test, serum IGF-1, thyroid hormone, PRL levels, and serum electrolytes [85]. An MRI can be used to detect a pituitary source of acromegaly; tumor size often correlates with GH elevation [12, 85]. A thorough cardiorespiratory evaluation prior to surgery is essential due to an increased incidence of atherosclerosis, hypertension, dysrhythmias, and OSA. Patients over 40 years of age should undergo colonoscopy due to increased incidence of colorectal neoplasms with acromegaly [86].

The goal of therapy is to normalize both GH and IGF-1 levels and to reduce the size of the tumor. Surgical therapy is the first-line treatment for GH-secreting adenomas, though presurgical medical therapy and primary medical therapy is on the rise [87]. Medical therapy consists of somatostatin receptor ligands such as octreotride, lanreotide, and the second-generation drug pasireotide [82, 86]. These primarily inhibit hormonal secretion of GH, which then secondarily reduces IGF-1; successful biochemical reductions in GH and IGF-1 are seen in approximately 50% of patients [82, 86]. Note that pasireotide may cause hyperglycemia in many patients and warrants close follow-up. Patients that do not achieve success or who are intolerant of these therapies are treated with pegvisomant, a GH-receptor antagonist, which can also be used in combination with somatostatin receptor ligands [87]. Other evolving therapeutics including octreotride, CRN00808, newer somatostatin receptor ligands and antisense synthetic oligonucleotides, which inhibit GH receptor mRNA translation [82].

Patients with ACTH-secreting tumors can initially present with Cushing syndrome from high levels of circulating glucocorticoids, with signs and symptoms including headaches, central obesity, cutaneous thinning and purple striae, acne, thinning of the hair, muscle weakness, hypertension, osteopenia, oligomenorrhea, amenorrhea, depression, anxiety, decreased libido, and impotence. Cardiovascular, metabolic, and infectious complications drive morbidity and mortality from the disease, which occurs more often in women [82]. Cushing disease is typically due to pituitary microadenomas, which may or may not be seen on MRI [82].

Initial evaluation of patients with ACTH-secreting adenomas should include a CBC and serum electrolytes. A 24-h urine cortisol will be significantly elevated in Cushing syndrome, and when coupled with an elevated ACTH level, a pituitary ACTH-secreting adenoma is strongly suggested, although ectopic foci still occur frequently. A high-dose dexamethasone suppression or CRH test may be performed to further delineate the source of the hormonal abnormality.

Treatment for Cushing disease is primarily surgical, though 20–40% patients are not cured with surgery, and relapse is common [82, 87]. The somatostatin receptor ligand pasireotide can decrease ACTH release and decrease the size of these tumors. This therapy is frequently complicated by significant hyperglycemia [82]. Cabergoline, temozolomide, roscovitine, and gefitinib may be evolving therapeutic options and all act via unique pathways.

Control of excessive cortisol production is typically reserved for patients that do not achieve normal cortisol levels after surgery and/or radiation, or for patients who are unable to undergo surgery or radiation. Ketoconazole can control excessive cortisol levels in these patients by inhibiting steroid synthesis. It may rarely cause severe hepatic injury, including failure, particularly at high doses, and has other concerning side effects [82]. Therefore, serum cortisol levels should be monitored closely, and dosage titrated accordingly. Metyrapone and mitotane are also able to inhibit steroid synthesis, and finally, if excessive cortisol secretion results in persistent symptomatic Cushing syndrome despite medical therapy, bilateral adrenalectomy can be considered. Afterward, these patients may develop Nelson syndrome, hyperpigmentation due to persistent ACTH elevation [82].

Luteinizing hormone and FSH-secreting adenomas do not typically present with defining symptomatology and hypersecretion of gonadotropins occurs only in a minority of patients [82]. Instead, presenting symptoms of a gonadotropic pituitary adenoma are frequently due to mass effect and may include visual changes, hypopituitarism, or headaches. Signs of hypogonadism may be present, such as loss of libido, low testosterone, impotence, infertility, oligomenorrhea, or amenorrhea. Evaluation should include broad assessment of hormonal levels including serum LH, FSH, PRL, testosterone, estradiol, TSH, thyroid hormone, ACTH, cortisol, and IGF-1. Surgery is the first line of therapy for gonadotropin-secreting adenomas, with radiation therapy as an option for recurrent or unresectable tumors. Medical therapy with dopamine agonists or somatostatin analogs has not been successful [87].

Finally, TSH-secreting neoplasms are rare and typically present with signs and symptoms of hyperthyroidism. Evaluation includes contrast-enhanced MRI, CBC, electrolytes, and hormonal levels including TSH, free T_3 and T_4, PRL, and GH. Thyroid ultrasound may detect a goiter or nodules due to chronic stimulation. Management of TSH-secreting adenomas is primarily surgical. Somatostatin analogs such as octreotride have been used to some benefit [87].

Perioperative Management of Pituitary Adenomas

The neurointensivist will most commonly encounter patients with pituitary adenomas in the postoperative period. Postoperative complications can include intracranial bleeding, wound infection or meningitis, vision changes, CSF leakage, airway obstruction, obtundation, epistaxis, electrolyte disturbances, and delirium. Endocrine complications that are observed in the postoperative period include DI, SIADH, adrenal insufficiency, and hyper- and hypoglycemia.

Diabetes insipidus is the most common endocrine abnormality after resection of pituitary tumors and is frequently short lived [88, 89]. Patients typically present with thirst and polyuria, up to 3–6 L daily with mild AVP deficiency and up to 18 L per day in severe cases, with measured urine osmolality less than serum osmolality. The diagnosis of DI can be made when serum sodium is above 145 mEq/L, and urine osmolality is below 200 mOsm/kg. If patients are not closely monitored, volume depletion, hypernatremia, and hyperosmolality can develop and result in hemodynamic instability and mental status changes [75]. The mechanism of AVP deficiency is likely due to injury to the posterior pituitary gland or neurohypophyseal system from surgical manipulation [73]. For mild AVP deficiency—polyuria of less than 6 L per day—patients with DI should be able to maintain adequate oral intake. If polyuria worsens or continues, AVP replacement therapy should be provided. Desmopressin (DDAVP), a synthetic analog of AVP, is currently used due to its rapid onset and ease of use. Diligent monitoring of urine output and sodium levels is critical to avoid free water retention and hyponatremia from overtreatment [75].

In contrast, the syndrome of inappropriate antidiuretic hormone secretion (SIADH) is caused by excessive AVP secretion and results in fluid retention and hyponatremia. This may be due to primary secretion of AVP or secondary to hypocortisolism or hypothyroidism [73]. Laboratory evaluation reveals hyponatremia and concentrated urine with urine sodium greater than 20 mEq/L and osmolality greater than 300 mOsm/kg; serum uric acid will be decreased. If the patient exhibits signs of severe hypothyroidism, such as cold intolerance, muscle weakness, thinning hair, or bradycardia, thyroid hormone levels should be assessed. Hypocortisolism, alternatively, is suggested by hypotension and, when present, evaluation of serum cortisol and/or a cosyntropin stimulation test is indicated. Treatment of SIADH is based on the severity of hyponatremia. For mild to moderate hyponatremia (Na >120 mEq/L), appropriate therapy may be limited to treatment of the underlying causative disorder and fluid restriction. If the patient becomes symptomatic or sodium worsens, hypertonic saline or a vasopressin receptor antagonist such as conivaptan or tolvaptan can be utilized. Crucially, osmotic demyelination syndrome can result from over-rapid correction of hyponatremia and a maximal rate of sodium rise under 0.5 mMol/L/h to a maximum of 8 mMol/L/day is advised [73, 75].

Patients with pituitary adenomas may develop new hypopituitarism after surgery. Low serum cortisol levels or refractory hypotension of unclear etiology should prompt immediate glucocorticoid replacement therapy. Dexamethasone may be considered initially, since hydrocortisone can interfere with interpretation of the cosyntropin stimulation test. Dexamethasone, however, has limited mineralocorticoid activity and timely conversion to hydrocortisone and in some patients oral fludricortisone is warranted.

Patients with GH-secreting tumors may develop fluid retention and edema through renal sodium retention [90]. Postoperatively, then, the expected decline in GH can result in mobilization of fluid as early as the first postoperative day.

Finally, postoperative management of patients after surgery for PRL- and TSH-secreting tumors is typically uncomplicated. For PRL-secreting adenomas, a serum PRL level is measured on the first or second postoperative day to assess surgical cure, and for TSH-secreting tumors, a serum TSH-level is checked. Diligent monitoring for hypo- or hyperthyroidism should continue longitudinally, noting that acute hypothyroidism is unlikely due to the long half-life of thyroxine.

Craniopharyngiomas

Craniopharyngiomas are sellar or parasellar epithelial tumors that occur along the path of the craniopharyngeal duct, with two histologic subtypes: adamantinomatous and papillary. In children, the adamantinomatous subtype occurs nearly exclusively, whereas adults more often suffer from papillary craniopharyngiomas [91]. These tumors are generally benign and usually only locally invasive, though malignant forms can occur or complicate surgery by seeding [91, 92]. These rare tumors have an incidence of 0.14 cases per 100,000 person-years and account for approximately 0.7% of primary intracranial tumors in adults and 2.5–3.4% in children. There is a bimodal incidence that peaks at 5–14 and 50–74 years of age [91, 93].

Initial symptoms are dependent on the location and size of the craniopharyngioma and may include headache in 50%, visual changes in over 60%, lost or depressed consciousness, nausea and/or vomiting [93]. These can be grouped into specific symptomatology syndromes including high intracranial pressure/chiasmal (most frequent), hypothalamic and pituitary, and the infundibulo-tuberal syndromes [91]. Up to 87% of patients present with hormonal deficiencies which are frequently in combination and may include GH, TSH, or ACTH deficiency, hypogonadism, or diabetes insipidus. These cause broad and varied symptomatology that can include growth failure or sexual development aberrancies, amenorrhea, polyuria and polydipsia, hypotension and orthostasis, weight gain or weight loss, and fatigue [94, 95]. Broad hormonal assessment should be performed. Supplementation of adrenal and thyroid hormones and monitoring of sodium concentrations may be necessary.

There is significant variability in the management and treatment of craniopharyngiomas due to variability in location and presentation [91, 92]. Preoperatively, a CSF shunt may be required for intracranial hypertension. Surgical management is challenging as craniopharyngiomas occur near important neurovascular structures and are particularly adherent; they carry an approximate 50% rate of recurrence [91, 92]. Nonetheless, in general, surgical resection is performed followed by external beam radiation [91]. Although overall survivorship is high, most patients have persistent sequelae [91, 92].

Postoperative complications may include CSF leak, new neurologic deficits, meningitis, and new hormonal abnormalities [91, 92]. Hormonal aberrancies must be managed, including both preoperative and new postoperative deficiencies with the exception of therapy for GH deficiency or hypogonadism, which is typically deferred in the acute perioperative period [96]. First, DI may occur due to a primary deficiency of AVP, and urine output may be profound with resultant hypovolemia and hypernatremia. As above, DDAVP may be required. Note that patients with DI may have a heightened risk for thrombotic events, thus institution of pharmacologic thromboprophylaxis is encouraged once feasible and safe [73, 75]. Postoperative hypocortisolism and adrenal crisis may also occur. As above, dexamethasone may be initially used, then transitioned to hydrocortisone after the cosyntropin stimulation test. Further Addisonian crises may occur and prophylaxis with additional steroids during periods of physiologic stress is frequently indicated.

Thyroid replenishment should be continued if the patient was on therapy preoperatively. Intravenous levothyroxine at a reduced dose (50–70% of oral dose) can be initiated when oral intake is not possible. Postoperative levels of thyroid hormones should be followed.

Meningiomas

Meningiomas are some of the most common primary intracranial tumors and originate from arachnoid cap cells near the arachnoid villi [97]. They account for 20% of all intracranial tumors and are typically discovered in middle to late adult life, due to symptoms generally related to the size and location of the mass. Meningiomas occur more often in females and African Americans and are more commonly benign than malignant [98].

The presence of sex hormone receptors on meningiomas may have prognostic implications, and manipulation of estrogen or progesterone levels could theoretically alter the risk of developing meningiomas. Gender differences in meningioma incidence may be due to the presence of estrogen and progesterone receptors on these tumors [97, 98]. Thus, estrogen and progesterone levels may alter disease risk. Premenopausal women have been shown to have higher rates of meningioma formation compared to post-menopausal women or those on hormone replacement therapy (HRT), though the risk was not modified by the use of oral contraception [97, 99]. More recently though, there has been a nationwide study from Denmark reporting an association between HRT and the development of meningiomas with an OR approaching 2.2 for those on prolonged combined estrogen/progesterone therapy [99]. This hypothesis is substantiated by looking at women on an estrogen receptor blocker, tamoxifen, who have been shown to have a 36% lower rate of meningioma formation [100]. Meningiomas may also express additional cell surface hormone receptors (i.e., androgen, glucocorticoid, somatostatin, PRL, IGF-1, IGF-2, thyroid hormone, and GHRH). Although the importance of these is not well delineated, GH and IGF-1 may be involved in meningioma occurrence and growth.

Meningiomas are typically surgically managed, with or without adjunctive radiation therapy. In a minority of cases, the meningioma recurs or is only partially resected. In these cases, or when patients are not candidates for surgery or radiation, chemotherapy and hormonal therapy are considered. Hormonal therapy has focused on targeting progesterone activity, since estrogen receptors are only present in 8 to 40% of meningiomas. Unfortunately, work with tamoxifen and mifepristone has not yielded benefit [101]. Other chemotherapeutic and directed therapies are actively being assessed [101].

Hormonal Therapy for Critical Illness

Hormone replacement therapy during critical illness is controversial [6, 102]. It is challenging for clinicians to determine which neuroendocrine response to illness is helpful or harmful, and in what phase of illness therapy would benefit. As mentioned previously, the acute illness phase is marked by energy conservation, while the chronic phase is signified by catabolism, weakness, and prolonged recovery. Targeted interventions that slow or reverse the deterioration that occurs in the chronic phase may be advantageous to human survival.

Full stress-dose replacement glucocorticoids, typically at 200–300 mg of hydrocortisone daily, are used frequently in the critically ill with severe sepsis and septic shock, refractory shock, critical illness-related corticosteroid insufficiency (CIRCI), or in ARDS, though the optimal dose and timing remain unclear [103–107]. It is unclear if certain subgroups stand to gain more with, or are at higher potential risk from, steroid therapy, and results have varied between severity and type of critical illness (e.g., respiratory versus abdominal sepsis, ARDS, or surgical patients). Nonetheless, steroidal therapy may reduce inflammation and hypercortisolism, maintain vascular tone and the endothelial barrier, and improve sensitivity to catecholamines [102]. Steroids, however, are not without risks, which include persistent weakness or myopathy, delirium, and immune suppression. In general, for the patient with refractory septic shock, it is rationale to consider stress dose steroids after shock develops, with approximately 200 mg of hydrocortisone equivalents with a recommended duration of 5–7 days and without needed dose tapering/weaning [106]. Note that "more" is not better; supraphysiologic dosing is rarely utilized in the modern era.

Hormonal therapy attempting to reduce catabolism or increase anabolism has been trialed in the critically ill. Growth hormone and insulin-like growth factor-1 (IGF-1) derangements yield altered metabolism and likely contribute to catabolism, weakness, and delayed recovery from critical illness [6]. Notably, while GH has anabolic effects, it also may also promote edema formation, cause insulin resistance, and alter immune system activity. Unfortunately, GH therapy in the critically ill was associated with a markedly elevated mortality in the critically ill [6]. Though the reason for this outcome is unclear and debated, only selective groups of critically ill patients should now be considered for GH therapy, including patients with burns, select pediatric patients, and, possibly, large trauma [90]. Ongoing work is evaluating ghrelin, a GH receptor ligand, IGF-1, and other hypothalamic-releasing hormone combinations (e.g., growth hormone-releasing peptide-2) to improve outcomes in the critically ill patients [6, 90].

Testosterone and other similar androgens may also beneficially alter the anabolism–catabolism relationship in the critically ill. While the early native deficiency of testosterone may be an adaptation to benefit the overall energy conservation and redirection needs of early shock states, testosterone, and analogs may improve functional recovery and attenuate muscle loss and catabolism in the post-shock state [6, 50]. Testosterone has been utilized in COPD, HIV muscle-wasting, and heart failure, and oxandrolone—an oral testosterone analog—use is an area of active interest and study, though limited data exist in the general critically ill population [50]. Both adult and pediatric burn patients, who suffer from immense catabolism, have benefited from the use of oxandrolone; however, with studies showing improved muscle and bone outcomes, wound healing, weight gain, and even mortality [50].

Thyroid hormones play an integral role in the regulation of metabolism, impacting protein synthesis, lipolysis, and more, and sepsis yields a fall in T3 and increased rT3, with varying TSH and T4 aberrancies [46]. The pattern of low T3, high rT3, and normal TSH has been termed low T3 syndrome, or nonthyroidal illness syndrome (NTIS; formerly euthyroid sick syndrome). In this setting, diagnosing hypothyroidism is challenging due to inflammation, cytokine expression, disease course, and co-administered agents like steroids or anticonvulsants. To date, no definitive benefit for supplemental therapy with thyroid hormones or TSH, however, otherwise exists [6, 46, 48]. The use of hypothalamic-releasing hormones and other hormonal combinations remains a focus of ongoing study [6].

Altered Mental Status and Endocrine Abnormalities

Altered mental status may occur as the presenting symptom of an endocrine abnormality. Derangements in thyroid hormones, glucose, and endogenous cortisol levels account for most of the endocrine-related mental status changes that occur in the NICU [108].

Hyper or hypothyroidism has a prevalence of 2% of adults. Changes in mental status may occur in approximately 50% of patients suffering from thyroid dysfunction [46]. This may be due to the role of the thyroid axis in metabolism and its relationship with neurotransmission. Patients with hyperthyroidism may present with fatigue, anxiety, or emotional lability. The nonspecific symptoms may lead to the underdiagnosis of hyperthyroidism in the NICU. Hypothyroidism is also associated with mental status changes. A decrease in cerebral blood flow, glucose utilization, and a desensitization of neuroreceptors are primarily responsible for the presenting symptomatology. Weakness, depression, and even coma are all symptoms. Due to the nonspecific nature, thyroid indices may be measured during the initial workup of the patient with altered mental status [46, 108].

Both hyper- and hypoglycemia can cause profound mental status changes. Lethargy, weakness, confusion, fatigue, emotional lability, seizures, and even coma are all associated with dysglycemia, particularly with hypoglycemia. These symptoms usually mark impending neurologic injury without prompt reversal in the glucose abnormality. It is imperative that glucose is checked in anyone who has developed acute mental status changes in the NICU. In patients who are intubated and sedated, symptoms of autonomic system activation (tachycardia, sweating, tremors, and hypertension) may be blunted or misinterpreted; the clinician must maintain a high clinical suspicion for glucose aberrancies.

Adrenal dysfunction may also present in patients with altered mental status. Approximately 20% of patients with Cushing syndrome can present with psychosis that may be difficult to distinguish from schizophrenia [108]. Cushing syndrome and Addison disease can also present as severe depression.

Drug-Induced Endocrine Abnormalities in the NICU

Critically ill patients are at particular risk of iatrogenic medication errors, polypharmacy, and drug-induced endocrine disorders. Many drugs used in the NICU may cause endocrine abnormalities (Table 35.5) [51].

Table 35.5 Drug-induced endocrine disorders in the ICU[51]

Hormone	Drugs	Proposed mechanism
CRH and ACTH	Glucorticoids, opioids, and benzodiazepines	Negative feedback suppression
Cortisol	Phenobarbital	Induces cortisol metabolism
	Phenytoin	Same
	Rifampin	Same
	Etomidate	Inhibits cortisol production
	Azole antifungals	Chronic use inhibits cortisol synthesis
	Opioids	Decreases cortisol secretion Decreases free fraction cortisol
TSH	Dobutamine	Decrease TSH concentration
	Dopamine	Same
	Corticosteroids	Direct inhibition of TSH release
Thyroid hormone	Phenobarbital	Increase clearance of thyroxine
	Phenytoin	Same
	Rifampin	Same
	Carbamazepine	Same
	Amiodarone	Increases thyroid hormone synthesis Inhibits type I 5-deiodinase
	Iodinated contrast dye	Increases thyroid hormone through iodine administration
	Heparin	Increases free fraction of thyroid hormone
	Furosemide	Increase free fraction by displacement from protein-binding sites
	Lithium	Decreases thyroid hormone secretion
	Atypical antipsychotics	Unknown—decreases free and total T4
Insulin	ACE inhibitors	Hypoglycemia—increases peripheral insulin sensitivity
	Fluoroquinolones	Hypoglycemia—promotes insulin secretion
	Pentamidine	Hypoglycemia—increases insulin secretion
	Sulfonylureas	Same
	Salicylates	Hypoglycemia—Increase insulin secretion, glucose utilization, decreases gluconeogensis
	Glucocorticoids	Hyperglycemia—increases gluconeogenesis, decreases insulin secretion, increases insulin resistance
	Pentamidine	Hyperglycemia—impair insulin release
	Calcineurin inhibitors	Hyperglycemia—decreases insulin production and release
	Vasopressors (epinephrine)	Hyperglycemia—promotes glycogenolysis, gluconeogenesis
	Atypical antipsychotics	Unknown

Drug-Induced Adrenal Abnormalities

Drug-induced adrenal insufficiency may occur due to commonly administered therapies in the critically ill. First, recent or active glucocorticoid use is pervasive in the critically ill and is discussed above. New hypotension after steroid cessation or during steroid tapering should prompt consideration for stress-dose replenishment.

Analgosedation regimens may also suppress the adrenal axis [109]. Benzodiazepines, for example, can result in a dose-dependent reduction in serum cortisol levels, and opioids can reduce cortisol secretion and increase levels of cortisol-binding globulin, reducing free cortisol [109]. Critically ill patients may be especially susceptible to the adrenal suppressive effects of these agents. Etomidate, typically only used for intubation induction, also predictably suppresses the adrenal axis by inhibiting 11β-hydroxylase, decreasing cortisol synthesis. This was found to cause mortality when used as a continuous infusion for sedation in the ICU. Evidence now points to problems with even single-dose etomidate in the critically ill, particularly in patients that are more severely ill [110]. Thus, caution and restraint should be deployed with its use and alternatives such as ketamine should be considered.

Commonly used antiepileptics may also cause adrenal insufficiency. Phenytoin and phenobarbital, for instance, induce the CYP-450 system and may increase metabolism of cortisol [51]. This may exacerbate adrenal insufficiency in critically ill patients with existing adrenal dysfunction and reduce the effect of exogenous steroids or cause adrenal insufficiency in patients on chronic steroid therapy. Phenytoin may also facilitate an increase in the urinary excretion of 6β-hydroxycortisol: cortisol within 1 week of initiation. This may yield adrenal suppression in patients with TBI, though the frequency of this is unclear [51].

Antifungal agents ("the azoles") have also been implicated in causing adrenal suppression. These medications inhibit CYP-450 enzymes integral to endogenous steroid metabolism. The most potent inhibitor appears to be ketoconazole. Mixed results are available regarding the steroid inhibitory effect of both fluconazole and iatroconazole [51]. Those patients who are on both exogenous steroid replacement and azole-antifungals are more susceptible to steroid-induced adverse effects due to the azole agents' inhibition of the CYP-450 metabolism of steroids.

Drug-Induced Thyroid Hormone Abnormalities

Amiodarone, lithium, and dopamine all impact the thyroid axis [51]. Amiodarone is a common antidysrhythmic agent utilized for both ventricular and supraventricular dysrhythmias. Amiodarone is very similar in structure to thyroxine and is composed of approximately 40% iodine. The iodine moiety may contribute to hyperthyroidism due to "amiodarone-induced thyrotoxicosis (AIT). AIT may be seen several weeks after drug initiation and can present as late as several months after cessation due to amiodarone's long half-life. Two types exist: AIT Type 1 is most commonly seen in patients with established thyroid disease such as Grave disease and is due to increased thyroid hormone synthesis from the iodine load of amiodarone. AIT Type 2, meanwhile, is an injurious thyroiditis that causes release of already synthesized thyroid hormones into the circulation. These can be difficult to distinguish and frequently occur in combination [111]. Amiodarone-induced thyrotoxicosis has been associated with nearly a threefold increased risk of stroke, myocardial infarction, and mortality. Treatment includes the institution of antithyroid agents, methimazole, and/or propylthiouracil. Concomitant steroid therapy is also recommended, particularly for AIT Type 2 and when the etiology is unclear [111, 112].

Amiodarone is also associated with the development of hypothyroidism, though rarely in the acute setting and more often following months of treatment [112]. The mechanism remains unclear but may be due to abnormalities in iodine organification and thyroid hormone production. Fortunately for patients, this type of hypothyroidism is symptomatically mild and readily treated with levothyroxine [112].

Dopamine, a neuroendocrine mediator and vasoactive catecholamine hormone with dose-dependent chronotropy, inotropy, and vasoconstriction, can decrease TSH and thyroxine production [51]. This effect may occur within 24 h of administration and is usually reversed after 24 h of discontinuing dopamine. Lithium, primarily used in patients with bipolar disease, also inhibits thyroid function by reducing thyroxine release and thyroid hormone synthesis. This is more common among chronic users of lithium and rarely causes myxedema coma [113].

Other notable drugs that may cause thyroid hormone abnormalities include phenobarbital, phenytoin, and carbamazepine, via increased thyroid hormone metabolism; heparins, which increase the free fraction of thyroid hormone; iodinated contrast dye, which causes increased thyroid hormone synthesis; and furosemide, which displaces protein-bound T4 and thereby increases both T3 and T4 [51].

Drug-Induced Glucose Abnormalities

A myriad of drugs can cause glucose aberrancies; this review will focus on agents common to the ICU. Hypoglycemia is particularly injurious to the brain and several agents warrant review. First, antihyperglycemic agents for diabetes may cause hypoglycemia. Sulfonylureas, especially older drug generations, may be associated with severe hypoglycemia in patients with sulfonylurea overdose and in those who receive concomitant drugs that inhibit the CYP2C9 enzyme system [114]. Octreotide may reverse the hypoglycemic effect, but these drugs are not easily reversible due to their long duration of action [114]. Other antihyperglycemics including glucagon-like peptide-1 (GLP-1) receptor agonists, dipeptidyl peptide-4 (DDP-4) inhibitors, and thiazolidinediones can cause hypoglycemia, though this only occurs rarely with metformin, a common agent used in diabetes management.

Most crucially, the ubiquitous use of insulin to meet glycemic goals can cause iatrogenic hypoglycemia. A myriad of approaches minimize this risk, including the use of standardized hospital or web-based algorithms, frequent monitoring, and the use of new monitoring technology, and more. Importantly, hypoglycemia causes patient harm whether it is treatment-induced or spontaneous [26].

Other drugs may cause hypoglycemia, such as fluoroquinolone antibiotics, which stimulate pancreatic insulin production [51]. Both levofloxacin and gatifloxacin are associated with the most frequent reports of hypoglycemia, while ciprofloxacin is a notable exception [115]. Risk factors for fluoroquinolone-induced hypoglycemia include renal failure, sepsis, and simultaneous hypoglycemic agent administration [51]. ACE inhibitor use may also lead to hypoglycemia by increasing peripheral insulin sensitivity, though this is poorly validated in the critically ill [51].

The sodium-glucose cotransporter-2 (SGLT-2) inhibitors, such as canagliflozin, dapagliflozin, and empagliflozin, are newer agents used in the management of diabetes. These drugs decrease renal tubular glucose reabsorption and thus improve plasma glucose independent of insulin. They are only rarely associated with hypoglycemia. They can, however, cause euglycemic diabetic ketoacidosis, a unique phenomenon that can occur in stress states and underfeeding, both common in the ICU. This can occur 1–3 days after drug cessation and is frequently missed due to euglycemia and thus a lack of a prompt to check for ketones. It is managed similarly to diabetic ketoacidosis [116].

Alternatively, drugs and polypharmacy contribute significantly to hyperglycemia in the critically ill. Glucocorticoids are often administered to NICU patients to reduce brain swelling and/or inflammation, such as in patients with bacterial meningitis, brain tumors, to treat autoimmune diseases such as lupus cerebritis, and for non-neurologic indications such as for ARDS, severe sepsis and/or shock, chronic obstructive pulmonary disease, or asthma exacerbations. Glucocorticoids induce hyperglycemia by promoting gluconeogenesis, insulin resistance, and by decreasing pancreatic insulin secretion [117].

Drugs typically administered to transplant or immune suppressed patients may also cause hyperglycemia. The calcineurin inhibitors, cyclosporine and tacrolimus, can cause post-transplant diabetes, likely via reduced insulin synthesis and release [118]. This phenomenon usually occurs early in the transplant course [118]. Pentamidine, an anti-pneumocystis agent, has a biphasic effect on glucose levels with an initial increase in insulin secretion, risking hypoglycemia, that progresses to hyperglycemia due to pancreatic β-cell destruction that occurs with chronic use [51].

Epinephrine, through its profound β_2-adrenergic activation, has the most prominent hyperglycemic effect among adrenergic agents, though all beta-agonists, including inhaled therapies such as albuterol, activate glycogenolysis, hepatic gluconeogenesis, and stimulate the release of glucagon and cortisol [119]. Finally, second-generation antipsychotics, particularly clozapine and olanzapine, can cause significant hyperglycemia, even inducing life-threatening diabetic ketoacidosis or hyperglycemic, hyperosmolar, and nonketoic coma [120].

The Endocrinopathy of Brain Death

Hormonal changes occur after brain death and are secondary to both posterior and anterior pituitary dysfunction [121]. Diabetes insipidus due to posterior pituitary dysfunction, for instance, occurs in 80% of brain-dead organ donors, requiring aggressive treatment to maintain organ viability. The anterior pituitary gland may also become dysfunctional upon brain death, yielding abnormalities in thyroid and adrenal function. In addition, dysglycemia is common [122]. The etiology of thyroid abnormalities after brain death is unclear. One study involving 22 brain-dead donors demonstrated that the majority displayed reductions in TSH, free T4, and T3 [122]. Other studies suggest, instead, that nonthyroidal illness syndrome (NTIS) is more likely than is TSH deficiency [122]. An expedient decrease in T3 as a result of reduced secretion of TSH by the anterior pituitary can also be seen in brain-dead patients and may result in lower blood pressure. Therefore, both T3 and T4 infusions have been trialed to improve graft survival and success [123–125].

Note that T4 is generally considered as a cheaper alternative to T3 and relies on conversion to T3, which can take several hours and is compromised by conversion to rT3, which may yield lesser benefit. The most robust evidence supporting its use is derived from an analysis of the UNOS database [126]. Analyses of this database suggest that utilizing triple hormonal therapy (thyroid replacement, cortisol, and insulin) improves survival of heart grafts and reduces the overall odds of death [123–125].

Brain-dead patients also exhibit decreased cortisol levels, with adrenal insufficiency occurring in approximately 50% of brain-dead organ donors [127]. This may be due to reduced CRF or ACTH secretion from the anterior pituitary. The combination of reduced cortisol and T3 may contribute to hemodynamic instability, and thus, steroids are frequently administered or considered for brain-dead organ donors [127].

Recent practice suggests that there is a benefit to a combination of hormone replacement. Specifically, methylprednisolone (15 mg/kg bolus), triiodothyronine (4 mcg bolus followed by infusion of 3 mcg/h), and arginine vasopressin (1 U bolus followed by 0.5–4 mU/kg/h) administration to brain-dead organ donors has been associated with an increased rate of successful organ donations [128]. This combination may also reduce the odds of organ recipient death within 30 days by 46% [128]. Beneficial effects may also be seen in brain-dead organ donors who receive corticosteroids alone or with T3/T4 [128]. In addition to the hemodynamic effects of corticosteroids, they may also reduce cytokine release, which may improve graft survival.

Hyperglycemia is also commonly seen in brain-dead organ donors and occurs due to insulin resistance and decreased insulin secretion [127]. This can result in impaired glucose uptake with cellular starvation and dependence on anaerobic metabolism, yielding stress and acidemia. High doses of intravenous insulin, matched to co-infused dextrose, are sometimes administered to brain-dead organ donors in order to minimize severe hyperglycemia-induced hypovolemia and hypoperfusion [127].

Summary

The endocrine system is a complex organ system that produces and secretes hormones that travel broadly through the body and play a crucial role in homeostasis, immune function, catabolism, anabolism, and in our response to stress, which include cardiovascular function. During critical illness, certain hormones mitigate the catabolic response and others exacerbate it. Clinicians should be aware of hormonal changes that occur during the acute, subacute, and chronic phases of critical illness and be aware of potential hormonal therapies that may impact outcomes.

Dysglycemia occurs frequently as part of the stress response of critical illness, including neurologic injuries that also alter glucose transport in the brain. Newer monitoring techniques such as cerebral microdialysis catheters may aid clinicians in minimizing CNS glucose derangements that cause cellular energy before overt symptoms develop. Simply put, avoiding hypo- and hyperglycemia is a priority for neurointensive care patients.

Several pathological responses to neurologic insult have been discussed in this chapter relating to their impact on homeostasis in the endocrine system. The somatotropic, thyroid, gonadal, lactotropic, and adrenal axes are frequently dysfunctional during neurocritical illness. Changes in the hormonal milieu are underrecognized and underreported due to heterogeneous etiologies and concurrent pathologies. Intensivists should be cognizant of these changes and the potential resultant endocrinopathies and their deleterious effect in order to alter management and enhance outcomes.

PEARLS

1. The endocrine system is vital to maintaining homeostasis in humans, but dysregulation of various hormonally mediated functions are common during critical illness. In particular, in NICU patients, the hypothalamic–pituitary hormone axis is universally impacted, Depending on the underlying brain insult, this may significantly compromise outcomes.
2. Neurologic patients are at particular risk for various endocrinopathies depending on their original neurologic insult, associated comorbidities, and evolution of their ICU course.
3. Hormonal abnormalities vary depending on the acute or chronic phase of critical illness.
4. Dysglycemia in the neurocritically ill is common, and glucose transport is altered in the injured brain. Optimal glucose measurement and management remains open to debate, but an intermediate goal (130–180 mg/dL) is recommended in the NICU.
5. New therapeutic hormonal interventions continue to be investigated in critically ill patients in an attempt to curb and/or reverse the catabolic state seen in the chronic phase of critical illness.
6. Recognition of endocrine dysfunction during Guillain–Barre syndrome is important in the overall management of this syndrome and may prompt earlier diagnosis.
7. Meningitis and encephalitis can cause derangements in hormonal homeostasis. Failure to recognize these abnormalities may result in worse patient outcomes.
8. Pituitary adenomas, craniopharyngiomas, and meningiomas all cause specific perioperative endocrine abnormalities that warrant monitoring and sometimes directed therapy.
9. Physicians should recognize medications used commonly in the NICU that are associated with endocrine abnormalities: glucocorticoids, antihyperglycemics, dopamine, phenytoin, phenobarbital, fluoroquinolones, lithium, ACE inhibitors, vasopressors, benzodiazepines, and opioids, among others.
10. The polypharmacy seen in the ICU can result in drug-induced endocrine disorders.

References

1. Smith FG, Sheehy AM, Vincent J-L, Coursin DB. Critical illness-induced dysglycaemia: diabetes and beyond. Crit Care. 2010;14(6):327.
2. Krinsley JS, Chase JG, Gunst J, et al. Continuous glucose monitoring in the ICU: clinical considerations and consensus. Crit Care. 2017;21(1):197.
3. Amar AP, Weiss MH. Pituitary anatomy and physiology. Neurosurg Clin N Am. 2003;14(1):11–23. v
4. Biga LM, Dawson S, Harwell A, et al. Anatomy & physiology. Covrallis, OR: OpenStax, Oregon State University; 2019. https://open.oregonstate.education/aandp/chapter/17-3-the-pituitary-gland-and-hypothalamus/. Accessed December 7, 2021
5. Dorton AM. The pituitary gland: embryology, physiology, and pathophysiology. Neonatal Netw. 2000;19(2):9–17.
6. Téblick A, Langouche L, Van den Berghe G. Endocrine interventions in the intensive care unit. Handb Clin Neurol. 2021;182:417–31.
7. Jasim S, Alahdab F, Ahmed AT, et al. Mortality in adults with hypopituitarism: a systematic review and meta-analysis. Endocrine. 2017;56(1):33–42.
8. Pappachan JM, Raskauskiene D, Kutty VR, Clayton RN. Excess mortality associated with hypopituitarism in adults: a meta-analysis of observational studies. J Clin Endocrinol Metab. 2015;100(4):1405–11.
9. Ascoli P, Cavagnini F. Hypopituitarism. Pituitary. 2006;9(4):335–42.
10. Prodam F, Caputo M, Mele C, Marzullo P, Aimaretti G. Insights into non-classic and emerging causes of hypopituitarism. Nat Rev Endocrinol. 2021;17(2):114–29.
11. Schneider HJ, Kreitschmann-Andermahr I, Ghigo E, Stalla GK, Agha A. Hypothalamopituitary dysfunction following traumatic brain injury and aneurysmal subarachnoid hemorrhage: a systematic review. JAMA. 2007;298(12):1429–38.
12. Kirsch CFE. Imaging of Sella and Parasellar region. Neuroimaging Clin N Am. 2021;31(4):541–52.
13. Fleseriu M, Hashim IA, Karavitaki N, et al. Hormonal replacement in hypopituitarism in adults: an endocrine society clinical practice guideline. J Clin Endocrinol Metab. 2016;101(11):3888–921.
14. Mazziotti G, Mormando M, Cristiano A, et al. Association between l-thyroxine treatment, GH deficiency, and radiological vertebral fractures in patients with adult-onset hypopituitarism. Eur J Endocrinol. 2014;170(6):893–9.
15. Pitkin J, Rees MC, Gray S, et al. Management of premature menopause. Menopause Int. 2007;13(1):44–5.
16. Wang L, Li X, Wang Z, et al. Trends in prevalence of diabetes and control of risk factors in diabetes among US Adults, 1999–2018. JAMA. 2021;326(8):1–13.
17. Hill MD. Stroke and diabetes mellitus. Handb Clin Neurol. 2014;126:167–74.
18. Lau LH, Lew J, Borschmann K, Thijs V, Ekinci EI. Prevalence of diabetes and its effects on stroke outcomes: a meta-analysis and literature review. J Diab Investig. 2019;10(3):780–92.
19. McCrimmon RJ, Ryan CM, Frier BM. Diabetes and cognitive dysfunction. Lancet. 2012;379(9833):2291–9.
20. Meneilly GS, Tessier DM. Diabetes, dementia and hypoglycemia. Can J Diabetes. 2016;40(1):73–6.
21. van Sloten TT, Sedaghat S, Carnethon MR, Launer LJ, Stehouwer CDA. Cerebral microvascular complications of type 2 diabetes:

stroke, cognitive dysfunction, and depression. Lancet Diabetes Endocrinol. 2020;8(4):325–36.
22. Lheureux O, Prevedello D, Preiser JC. Update on glucose in critical care. Nutrition. 2019;59:14–20.
23. Gunst J, Van den Berghe G. Blood glucose control in the ICU: don't throw out the baby with the bathwater! Intensive Care Med. 2016;42(9):1478–81.
24. van den Berghe G, Wouters P, Weekers F, et al. Intensive insulin therapy in critically ill patients. N Engl J Med. 2001;345(19):1359–67.
25. Finfer S, Chittock DR, Su SY, et al. Intensive versus conventional glucose control in critically ill patients. N Engl J Med. 2009;360(13):1283–97.
26. Finfer S, Liu B, Chittock DR, et al. Hypoglycemia and risk of death in critically ill patients. N Engl J Med. 2012;367(12):1108–18.
27. Egi M, Bellomo R, Stachowski E, French CJ, Hart G. Variability of blood glucose concentration and short-term mortality in critically ill patients. Anesthesiology. 2006;105(2):244–52.
28. Kramer AH, Roberts DJ, Zygun DA. Optimal glycemic control in neurocritical care patients: a systematic review and meta-analysis. Crit Care. 2012;16(5):R203.
29. Kurtz P, Rocha EEM. Nutrition therapy, glucose control, and brain metabolism in traumatic brain injury: a multimodal monitoring approach. Front Neurosci. 2020;14:190.
30. Vespa P, Boonyaputthikul R, McArthur DL, et al. Intensive insulin therapy reduces microdialysis glucose values without altering glucose utilization or improving the lactate/pyruvate ratio after traumatic brain injury. Crit Care Med. 2006;34(3):850–6.
31. Vespa P, McArthur DL, Stein N, et al. Tight glycemic control increases metabolic distress in traumatic brain injury: a randomized controlled within-subjects trial. Crit Care Med. 2012;40(6):1923–9.
32. Timofeev I, Carpenter KL, Nortje J, et al. Cerebral extracellular chemistry and outcome following traumatic brain injury: a microdialysis study of 223 patients. Brain. 2011;134(Pt 2):484–94.
33. Plummer MP, Notkina N, Timofeev I, Hutchinson PJ, Finnis ME, Gupta AK. Cerebral metabolic effects of strict versus conventional glycaemic targets following severe traumatic brain injury. Crit Care. 2018;22(1):16.
34. Shi J, Dong B, Mao Y, et al. Review: Traumatic brain injury and hyperglycemia, a potentially modifiable risk factor. Oncotarget. 2016;7(43):71052–61.
35. Bellaver P, Schaeffer AF, Dullius DP, Viana MV, Leitão CB, Rech TH. Association of multiple glycemic parameters at intensive care unit admission with mortality and clinical outcomes in critically ill patients. Sci Rep. 2019;9(1):18498.
36. Watt C, Sanchez-Rangel E, Hwang JJ. Glycemic variability and CNS inflammation: reviewing the connection. Nutrients. 2020;12(12):3906.
37. Meier R, Béchir M, Ludwig S, et al. Differential temporal profile of lowered blood glucose levels (3.5–6.5 mmol/L versus 5–8 mmol/L) in patients with severe traumatic brain injury. Crit Care. 2008;12(4):R98.
38. Téblick A, Peeters B, Langouche L, Van den Berghe G. Adrenal function and dysfunction in critically ill patients. Nat Rev Endocrinol. 2019;15(7):417–27.
39. Langouche L, Van den Berghe G. Hypothalamic-pituitary hormones during critical illness: a dynamic neuroendocrine response. Handb Clin Neurol. 2014;124:115–26.
40. Peeters B, Meersseman P, Vander Perre S, et al. ACTH and cortisol responses to CRH in acute, subacute, and prolonged critical illness: a randomized, double-blind, placebo-controlled, crossover cohort study. Intensive Care Med. 2018;44(12):2048–58.
41. Boonen E, Vervenne H, Meersseman P, et al. Reduced cortisol metabolism during critical illness. N Engl J Med. 2013;368(16):1477–88.
42. Annane D, Sébille V, Troché G, Raphaël JC, Gajdos P, Bellissant E. A 3-level prognostic classification in septic shock based on cortisol levels and cortisol response to corticotropin. JAMA. 2000;283(8):1038–45.
43. Vanhorebeek I, Van den Berghe G. The neuroendocrine response to critical illness is a dynamic process. Crit Care Clin. 2006;22(1):1–15.
44. Van den Berghe G. On the neuroendocrinopathy of critical illness. Perspectives for feeding and novel treatments. Am J Respir Crit Care Med. 2016;194(11):1337–48.
45. Taylor BE, Buchman TG. Is there a role for growth hormone therapy in refractory critical illness? Curr Opin Crit Care. 2008;14(4):438–44.
46. Maiden MJ, Torpy DJ. Thyroid hormones in critical illness. Crit Care Clin. 2019;35(2):375–88.
47. Peeters RP, Wouters PJ, van Toor H, Kaptein E, Visser TJ, Van den Berghe G. Serum 3,3′,5′-triiodothyronine (rT3) and 3,5,3′-triiodothyronine/rT3 are prognostic markers in critically ill patients and are associated with postmortem tissue deiodinase activities. J Clin Endocrinol Metab. 2005;90(8):4559–65.
48. Fliers E, Boelen A. An update on non-thyroidal illness syndrome. J Endocrinol Investig. 2021;44(8):1597–607.
49. Wang F, Pan W, Wang H, Wang S, Pan S, Ge J. Relationship between thyroid function and ICU mortality: a prospective observation study. Crit Care. 2012;16(1):R11.
50. Wischmeyer PE, Suman OE, Kozar R, Wolf SE, Molinger J, Pastva AM. Role of anabolic testosterone agents and structured exercise to promote recovery in ICU survivors. Curr Opin Crit Care. 2020;26(5):508–15.
51. Thomas Z, Bandali F, McCowen K, Malhotra A. Drug-induced endocrine disorders in the intensive care unit. Crit Care Med. 2010;38(Suppl. 6):S219–30.
52. Powers WJ. Acute ischemic stroke. N Engl J Med. 2020;383(3):252–60.
53. Lawton MT, Vates GE. Subarachnoid hemorrhage. N Engl J Med. 2017;377(3):257–66.
54. Greving JP, Wermer MJ, Brown RD Jr, et al. Development of the PHASES score for prediction of risk of rupture of intracranial aneurysms: a pooled analysis of six prospective cohort studies. Lancet Neurol. 2014;13(1):59–66.
55. Kale SP, Edgell RC, Alshekhlee A, et al. Age-associated vasospasm in aneurysmal subarachnoid hemorrhage. J Stroke Cerebrovasc Dis. 2013;22(1):22–7.
56. Franceschini R, Tenconi GL, Zoppoli F, Barreca T. Endocrine abnormalities and outcome of ischaemic stroke. Biomed Pharmacother. 2001;55(8):458–65.
57. Boehncke S, Ackermann H, Badenhoop K, Sitzer M. Pituitary function and IGF-I levels following ischemic stroke. Cerebrovasc Dis. 2011;31(2):163–9.
58. Menon B, Krishnan R. Role of leptin in acute ischemic stroke. J Neurosci Rural Pract. 2018;9(3):376–80.
59. Bavisetty S, Bavisetty S, McArthur DL, et al. Chronic hypopituitarism after traumatic brain injury: risk assessment and relationship to outcome. Neurosurgery. 2008;62(5):1080–93. discussion 1093–1084
60. Roberts I, Yates D, Sandercock P, et al. Effect of intravenous corticosteroids on death within 14 days in 10008 adults with clinically significant head injury (MRC CRASH trial): randomised placebo-controlled trial. Lancet. 2004;364(9442): 1321–8.
61. Ives JC, Alderman M, Stred SE. Hypopituitarism after multiple concussions: a retrospective case study in an adolescent male. J Athl Train. 2007;42(3):431–9.
62. Leonhard SE, Mandarakas MR, Gondim FAA, et al. Diagnosis and management of Guillain-Barré syndrome in ten steps. Nat Rev Neurol. 2019;15(11):671–83.

63. Shahrizaila N, Lehmann HC, Kuwabara S. Guillain-Barré syndrome. Lancet. 2021;397(10280):1214–28.
64. Doets AY, Verboon C, van den Berg B, et al. Regional variation of Guillain-Barré syndrome. Brain. 2018;141(10):2866–77.
65. Zaeem Z, Siddiqi ZA, Zochodne DW. Autonomic involvement in Guillain-Barré syndrome: an update. Clin Auton Res. 2019;29(3):289–99.
66. Lin J, Gao Q, Xiao K, Tian D, Hu W, Han Z. Efficacy of therapies in the treatment of Guillain-Barre syndrome: a network meta-analysis. Medicine (Baltimore). 2021;100(41):e27351.
67. Sharshar T, Chevret S, Bourdain F, Raphaël JC. Early predictors of mechanical ventilation in Guillain-Barré syndrome. Crit Care Med. 2003;31(1):278–83.
68. Tu Y, Gong X, Zeng G, Zhuo W, Li Z, Yu X. Differences in thyroid function and autoantibodies in the development of Guillain-Barré syndrome vs. chronic inflammatory demyelinating polyradiculoneuropathy. Front Neurol. 2020;11:1018.
69. Toudou Daouda M, Obenda NS, Maazou L, et al. Guillain-Barre syndrome and Hashimoto's thyroiditis. QJM. 2016;109(8):547–8.
70. Strauss J, Aboab J, Rottmann M, et al. Plasma cortisol levels in Guillain-Barré syndrome. Crit Care Med. 2009;37(8):2436–40.
71. Hughes RA, Brassington R, Gunn AA, van Doorn PA. Corticosteroids for Guillain-Barré syndrome. Cochrane Database Syst Rev. 2016;10(10):Cd001446.
72. Rumalla K, Reddy AY, Letchuman V, Mittal MK. Hyponatremia in Guillain-Barré syndrome. J Clin Neuromuscul Dis. 2017;18(4):207–17.
73. Cui H, He G, Yang S, et al. Inappropriate antidiuretic hormone secretion and cerebral salt-wasting syndromes in neurological patients. Front Neurosci. 2019;13:1170.
74. Steinberger BA, Ford SM, Coleman TA. Intravenous immunoglobulin therapy results in post-infusional hyperproteinemia, increased serum viscosity, and pseudohyponatremia. Am J Hematol. 2003;73(2):97–100.
75. Sterns RH. Disorders of plasma sodium--causes, consequences, and correction. N Engl J Med. 2015;372(1):55–65.
76. Bystritsky RJ, Chow FC. Infectious meningitis and encephalitis. Neurol Clin. 2022;40(1):77–91.
77. Pekic S, Popovic V. Diagnosis of endocrine disease: expanding the cause of hypopituitarism. Eur J Endocrinol. 2017;176(6):R269–r282.
78. Tsiakalos A, Xynos ID, Sipsas NV, Kaltsas G. Pituitary insufficiency after infectious meningitis: a prospective study. J Clin Endocrinol Metab. 2010;95(7):3277–81.
79. Beatrice AM, Selvan C, Mukhopadhyay S. Pituitary dysfunction in infective brain diseases. Indian J Endocrinol Metab. 2013;17(Suppl. 3):S608–11.
80. Tanriverdi F, De Bellis A, Teksahin H, et al. Prospective investigation of pituitary functions in patients with acute infectious meningitis: is acute meningitis induced pituitary dysfunction associated with autoimmunity? Pituitary. 2012;15(4):579–88.
81. Schaefer S, Boegershausen N, Meyer S, Ivan D, Schepelmann K, Kann PH. Hypothalamic-pituitary insufficiency following infectious diseases of the central nervous system. Eur J Endocrinol. 2008;158(1):3–9.
82. Gheorghiu ML, Negreanu F, Fleseriu M. Updates in the medical treatment of pituitary adenomas. Horm Metab Res. 2020;52(1):8–24.
83. Briet C, Salenave S, Chanson P. Pituitary apoplexy. Endocrinol Metab Clin N Am. 2015;44(1):199–209.
84. Cohen-Cohen S, Brown DA, Himes BT, et al. Pituitary adenomas in the setting of multiple endocrine neoplasia type 1: a single-institution experience. J Neurosurg. 2020;134(3):1132–8.
85. Vilar L, Vilar CF, Lyra R, Lyra R, Naves LA. Acromegaly: clinical features at diagnosis. Pituitary. 2017;20(1):22–32.
86. Melmed S, Bronstein MD, Chanson P, et al. A consensus statement on acromegaly therapeutic outcomes. Nat Rev Endocrinol. 2018;14(9):552–61.
87. Mehta GU, Lonser RR. Management of hormone-secreting pituitary adenomas. Neuro-Oncology. 2017;19(6):762–73.
88. Blumberg DL, Sklar CA, Wisoff J, David R. Abnormalities of water metabolism in children and adolescents following craniotomy for a brain tumor. Childs Nerv Syst. 1994;10(8):505–8.
89. Snyder MH, Asuzu DT, Shaver DE, Vance ML, Jane JA. Routine postoperative fluid restriction to prevent syndrome of inappropriate antidiuretic hormone secretion after transsphenoidal resection of pituitary adenoma. J Neurosurg. 2021;136(2):405–12.
90. Elijah IE, Branski LK, Finnerty CC, Herndon DN. The GH/IGF-1 system in critical illness. Best Pract Res Clin Endocrinol Metab. 2011;25(5):759–67.
91. Henderson F Jr, Schwartz TH. Update on management of craniopharyngiomas. J Neuro-Oncol. 2022:1–12.
92. Kiliç M, Can SM, Özdemir B, Tanik C. Management of craniopharyngioma. J Craniofac Surg. 2019;30(2):e178–83.
93. Müller HL, Merchant TE, Warmuth-Metz M, Martinez-Barbera JP, Puget S. Craniopharyngioma. Nat Rev Dis Primers. 2019;5(1):75.
94. Feng Y, Ni M, Wang YG, Zhong LY. Comparison of neuroendocrine dysfunction in patients with adamantinomatous and papillary craniopharyngiomas. Exp Ther Med. 2019;17(1):51–6.
95. Manuylova E, Calvi LM, Vates GE, Hastings C, Shafiq I. Morning serum cortisol level after transphenoidal surgery for pituitary adenoma predicts hypothalamic-pituitary-adrenal function despite intraoperative dexamethasone use. Endocr Pract. 2015;21(8):897–902.
96. Thompson CJ, Costello RW, Crowley RK. Management of hypothalamic disease in patients with craniopharyngioma. Clin Endocrinol. 2019;90(4):506–16.
97. Wiemels J, Wrensch M, Claus EB. Epidemiology and etiology of meningioma. J Neuro-Oncol. 2010;99(3):307–14.
98. Buerki RA, Horbinski CM, Kruser T, Horowitz PM, James CD, Lukas RV. An overview of meningiomas. Future Oncol. 2018;14(21):2161–77.
99. Andersen L, Friis S, Hallas J, Ravn P, Schrøder HD, Gaist D. Hormone replacement therapy increases the risk of cranial meningioma. Eur J Cancer. 2013;49(15):3303–10.
100. Sun LM, Lin CL, Sun S, Hsu CY, Shae Z, Kao CH. Long-term use of tamoxifen is associated with a decreased subsequent meningioma risk in patients with breast cancer: a nationwide population-based cohort study. Front Pharmacol. 2019;10:674.
101. Kim L. A narrative review of targeted therapies in meningioma. Chin Clin Oncol. 2020;9(6):76.
102. Wasyluk W, Wasyluk M, Zwolak A. Sepsis as a pan-endocrine illness-endocrine disorders in septic patients. J Clin Med. 2021;10(10):2075.
103. Venkatesh B, Cohen J. Hydrocortisone in vasodilatory shock. Crit Care Clin. 2019;35(2):263–75.
104. Venkatesh B, Finfer S, Cohen J, et al. Adjunctive glucocorticoid therapy in patients with septic shock. N Engl J Med. 2018;378(9):797–808.
105. Suffredini AF. A role for hydrocortisone therapy in septic shock? N Engl J Med. 2018;378(9):860–1.
106. Qadir N, Chang SY. Pharmacologic treatments for acute respiratory distress syndrome. Crit Care Clin. 2021;37(4):877–93.
107. Villar J, Ferrando C, Martínez D, et al. Dexamethasone treatment for the acute respiratory distress syndrome: a multicentre, randomised controlled trial. Lancet Respir Med. 2020;8(3):267–76.
108. Park E, Abraham MK. Altered mental status and endocrine diseases. Emerg Med Clin North Am. 2014;32(2):367–78.
109. Carli F, Mistraletti G. Metabolic and endocrine effects of sedative agents. Minerva Anestesiol. 2006;72(6):395–9.

110. Albert SG, Sitaula S. Etomidate, adrenal insufficiency and mortality associated with severity of illness: a meta-analysis. J Intensive Care Med. 2021;36(10):1124–9.
111. Tsang W, Houlden RL. Amiodarone-induced thyrotoxicosis: a review. Can J Cardiol. 2009;25(7):421–4.
112. Narayana SK, Woods DR, Boos CJ. Management of amiodarone-related thyroid problems. Ther Adv Endocrinol Metab. 2011;2(3):115–26.
113. Gitlin M. Lithium side effects and toxicity: prevalence and management strategies. Int J Bipolar Disord. 2016;4(1):27.
114. Carr R, Zed PJ. Octreotide for sulfonylurea-induced hypoglycemia following overdose. Ann Pharmacother. 2002;36(11):1727–32.
115. Singh M, Jacob JJ, Kapoor R, Abraham J. Fatal hypoglycemia with levofloxacin use in an elderly patient in the post-operative period. Langenbeck's Arch Surg. 2008;393(2):235–8.
116. Hsia DS, Grove O, Cefalu WT. An update on sodium-glucose co-transporter-2 inhibitors for the treatment of diabetes mellitus. Curr Opin Endocrinol Diab Obes. 2017;24(1):73–9.
117. Clore JN, Thurby-Hay L. Glucocorticoid-induced hyperglycemia. Endocr Pract. 2009;15(5):469–74.
118. Chowdhury TA. Post-transplant diabetes mellitus. Clin Med (Lond). 2019;19(5):392–5.
119. Barth E, Albuszies G, Baumgart K, et al. Glucose metabolism and catecholamines. Crit Care Med. 2007;35(Suppl. 9):S508–18.
120. Zhang Y, Liu Y, Su Y, et al. The metabolic side effects of 12 antipsychotic drugs used for the treatment of schizophrenia on glucose: a network meta-analysis. BMC Psychiatry. 2017;17(1):373.
121. Smith M. Physiologic changes during brain stem death--lessons for management of the organ donor. J Heart Lung Transplant. 2004;23(Suppl. 9):S217–22.
122. Sazontseva IE, Kozlov IA, Moisuc YG, Ermolenko AE, Afonin VV, Ilnitskiy VV. Hormonal response to brain death. Transplant Proc. 1991;23(5):2467.
123. Anwar A, Lee JM. Medical management of brain-dead organ donors. Acute Crit Care. 2019;34(1):14–29.
124. Turco LM, Glorsky SL, Winfield RD. Hormone replacement therapy in brain-dead organ donors: a comprehensive review with an emphasis on traumatic brain injury. J Trauma Acute Care Surg. 2019;86(4):702–9.
125. Hahnenkamp K, Böhler K, Wolters H, Wiebe K, Schneider D, Schmidt HH. Organ-protective intensive care in organ donors. Dtsch Arztebl Int. 2016;113(33-34):552–8.
126. Rosendale JD, Kauffman HM, McBride MA, et al. Hormonal resuscitation yields more transplanted hearts, with improved early function. Transplantation. 2003;75(8):1336–41.
127. Howlett TA, Keogh AM, Perry L, Touzel R, Rees LH. Anterior and posterior pituitary function in brain-stem-dead donors. A possible role for hormonal replacement therapy. Transplantation. 1989;47(5):828–34.
128. Rosengard BR, Feng S, Alfrey EJ, et al. Report of the crystal city meeting to maximize the use of organs recovered from the cadaver donor. Am J Transplant. 2002;2(8):701–11.

Cardiac Arrest and Post-Arrest Management

36

Benjamin S. Abella

Contents

Abstract

Cardiac arrest is an exquisitely time-sensitive critical illness that strikes over 400,000 people each year in the United States. Initial treatment is based on the "chain of survival," a paradigm described by the American Heart Association that includes prompt recognition of cardiac arrest, early delivery of cardiopulmonary resuscitation, use of defibrillation when appropriate, followed by advanced care in the hospital for those who attain return of spontaneous circulation (ROSC). Hospital-based care for patients with ROSC includes the use of careful neurologic monitoring including electroencephalography, hemodynamic support to maintain adequate brain perfusion, careful oxygen titration, and the use of targeted temperature management (TTM), either to a cooled state such as 33 °C or at a very minimum to a strict avoidance of fever (i.e., TTM technology employed to maintain strict normothermia). The goal of hospital-based critical care for post-arrest patients is to minimize the risk of crippling neurologic injury, which can occur as a component of post-cardiac arrest syndrome, an overlapping set of pathophysiologic processes that are activated in the first few days following resuscitation. This chapter will review current understandings of TTM, neurologic monitoring, and related topics pertaining to post-arrest care.

B. S. Abella (✉)
Department of Emergency Medicine, University of Pennsylvania, Philadelphia, PA, USA
e-mail: benjamin.abella@pennmedicine.upenn.edu

Introduction

Cardiac arrest remains a massive public health burden and challenge to clinical care around the world. Defined as the abrupt cessation of cardiac output leading rapidly to the loss of global organ perfusion, cardiac arrest afflicts over 400,000

E. Mahanna Gabrielli et al. (eds.), *Textbook of Neurointensive Care: Volume 1*, https://doi.org/10.1007/978-3-031-62220-5_36

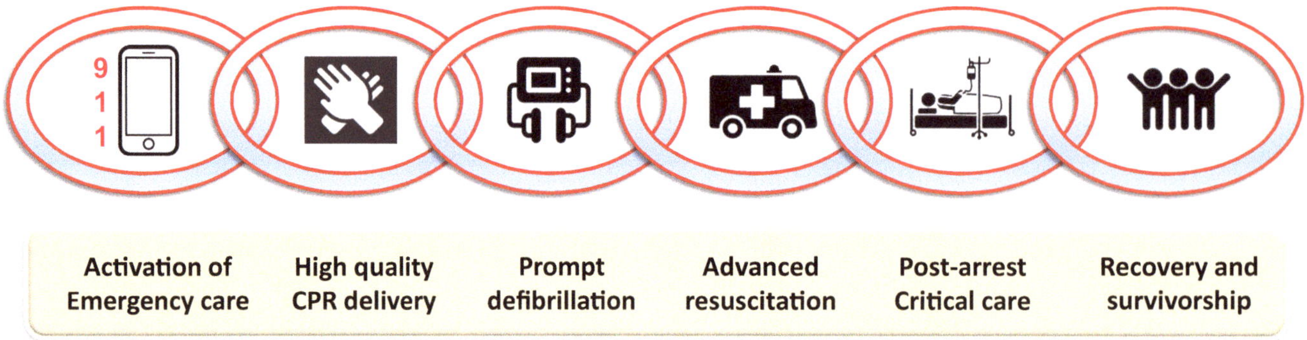

Fig. 36.1 The "chain of survival" paradigm for cardiac arrest and post-arrest care. The original conception of the chain had four links. In current form, two additional links have been added in the AHA guidelines, highlighting the importance of both post-arrest care and recovery after critical illness

people in the United States each year, with an overall survival to hospital discharge rate of 10–15% in many US communities [1, 2]. Cardiac arrest can occur in the home or public setting, both together termed out-of-hospital cardiac arrest (OHCA), or within the hospital, known as in-hospital cardiac arrest (IHCA). Swift recognition of cardiac arrest is essential, followed by initial treatment as outlined in a framework known as the "chain of survival" (Fig. 36.1) [3]. Initial treatment of cardiac arrest consists of the delivery of cardiopulmonary resuscitation (CPR) and, when appropriate, the use of automated external defibrillators (AEDs). The treatment of cardiac arrest is exquisitely time sensitive. For every minute, a cardiac arrest victim remains untreated, the probability of survival falls by 10–15% [4]. Thus, prompt prehospital care for OHCA victims is essential, including involvement from both lay bystanders and prehospital care providers, including personnel from emergency medical services (EMS) agencies.

Initial survival from cardiac arrest, known as return of spontaneous circulation (ROSC), is followed by complex critical illness that carries significant morbidity and mortality [5, 6]. Among cardiac arrest survivors, long-term neurologic disabilities are common, related to ischemia-reperfusion injury of brain tissue that evolves during post-arrest care in the hospital. These disabilities are highly variable. They range from mild deficits such as modestly impaired fine motor coordination, to severe injuries such as long-term vegetative state [7]. However, some survivors exhibit full neurologic recovery and return to normal activities of daily living, serving as evidence that intact survival is possible after cardiac arrest.

Chapter Goals

In the following discussion, readers will:

- Understand the role of initial evaluation of the post-arrest patient in the Emergency Department
- Be able to appreciate the role of targeted temperature management during critical care
- Appreciate the data pertaining to different goal temperatures during post-arrest care
- Understand the role of cardiac evaluation and in particular coronary angiography
- Learn about key pitfalls and challenges that can arise during post-arrest care

Prehospital Care

Much of the post-arrest care and outcome trajectory is determined by the quality of immediate care received for patients with OHCA. For prognostication and treatment purposes, it is therefore crucial for inhospital providers to ascertain key variables pertaining to initial arrest (e.g., pre-arrest symptoms, initial rhythm) and the care provided before hospital arrival (e.g., provision of bystander CPR and/or defibrillation), both by lay providers and EMS professionals (see Table 36.1). Given the confusion that often surrounds initial OHCA recognition and care, it may not be possible to obtain reliable information but the attempt to do so is important. For example, survival from OHCA is 2–3x higher among patients receiving bystander CPR than those who do not receive it [8]. In another example, patients with initial ventricular fibrillation with subsequent coronary angiography that reveals no evidence of atherosclerosis often require the placement of implantable cardiac defibrillators (ICDs) [9].

Bystander CPR is generally comprised of chest compressions interposed with rescue breaths, given in a 30:2 sequence (30 compressions, followed by 2 breaths). The American Heart Association (AHA) guidelines for CPR have suggested an alternative form of CPR is acceptable for initial bystander response and may indeed generate equivalent outcomes, in which "hands only" CPR is performed [10], without the delivery of rescue breaths. Studies have shown that the quality of CPR delivery is directly linked to survival. [11–13] Appropriate compression rate (100–120 compression per minute) and depth (2–2.4 inches), minimization of pauses in CPR, and

Table 36.1 Key prehospital variables in cardiac arrest care. It is important for providers to obtain data on these variables, when possible, from bystanders, family members, and Emergency Medical Services providers

Prehospital arrest variable	Response categories
Pre-arrest symptoms	Chest pain Shortness of breath Leg pain or swelling
Witnessed arrest status	Yes or no
Bystander CPR delivery	Yes or no
Initial rhythm	Ventricular fibrillation Ventricular tachycardia Pulseless electrical activity Asystole
Defibrillation attempt	Automated external defibrillator Manual monitor/defibrillator
Shocks delivered	Number of shocks
EMS CPR method	Manual CPR Mechanical CPR

adequate recoil (complete removal of hand pressure on the chest between compressions) are all aspects of high-quality CPR. For readers interested in the topic of CPR provision, an excellent summary of the data surrounding delivery of CPR has been generated by an AHA expert consensus group [14].

Use of automated external defibrillators (AEDs) has grown substantially over recent decades and has represented a crucial improvement in the care of OHCA [15]. Available in public settings such as airports, train stations, and health clubs, AEDs are designed for untrained users, often providing both audio and/or visual instructions at the point of care. For patients with initial ventricular fibrillation and/or ventricular tachycardia as causes of arrest, defibrillation is essential. EMS professional may use either AEDs or manual monitor/defibrillators to provide this function. Standard energies delivered by these devices vary by manufacturer; 200 J is a commonly delivered energy in a typical “biphasic waveform” defibrillator. EMS providers with advanced cardiovascular life support (ACLS) training may also intubate the OHCA victim and provide pharmacologic adjuncts such as intravenous epinephrine. The role of epinephrine in cardiac arrest resuscitation has come under intense study in recent years, with the growing consensus that while the drug may increase initial rates of ROSC, it may also contribute to worsened reperfusion injury of the brain and in some cases worse neurologic outcomes [16, 17].

Essential Management Priorities

Post-Arrest Care: Early Phase (0–6 h Post Arrest)

Initial care for resuscitated OHCA victims is based in the Emergency Department (ED). ED providers have a number of key tasks following ROSC, including hemodynamic stabilization, placement of adequate intravenous access (often via central venous catheters and arterial lines), and establishment of a definitive airway. Often in parallel to these actions, the early acquisition of an electrocardiogram (ECG) within 15–30 min of ED arrival is crucial to determine whether the cause of arrest was due to underlying ST-segment myocardial infarction (STEMI) [18]. OHCA patients with STEMI require immediate cardiac catheterization and percutaneous coronary intervention; patients without STEMI may require cardiac evaluation during subsequent hospital care but randomized trials have supported the notion that this may occur in delayed fashion without negative impact on patient outcomes in most cases [19, 20]. While serum troponin should be tested as well as ECG, troponin levels should be interpreted with caution, myocardial infarction leading to immediate cardiac arrest may yield initially normal troponin levels, and prolonged CPR may lead to elevated troponin even without underlying myocardial infarction.

Within the first few hours following ROSC, ED providers should also obtain non-contrast brain computed tomography, to rule out traumatic hemorrhage such as subdural hematoma that might have occurred during the initial collapse of the victim. Use of initial brain imaging to provide prognostic information, however, is controversial [21]. Early findings of cerebral edema or diffuse axonal injury have insufficient predictive value in many cases. Other initial neurologic assessment tools, such as serum biomarkers of neuronal injury [22–24] (nerve specific enolase or glial fibrillary acidic protein, for example) and initial quantitative pupillometry [25], may have prognostic value but are still subjects of intense research efforts.

Ventilator management during the early phase should rest on the principle of avoiding arterial hyperoxia. A number of clinical studies have suggested that hyperoxia contributes to post-arrest inflammatory changes, free radical generation, and worsened outomes [26, 27]. As a practical matter, FiO_2 should be reduced every few hours if oxygen saturation remains >92%, with a goal $FiO_2 = 0.6$ or less.

During ED and initial ICU-based care of the post-arrest patient, a careful search for the underlying cause of arrest should be conducted. Such potential causes not only include myocardial infarction but also include a broad array of other etiologies, including pulmonary embolism, drug overdose, metabolic derangements (e.g., hyperkalemia in a patient with renal failure, or marked acidosis in a patient with Type I diabetes mellitus), and significant hemorrhage (e.g., from gastrointestinal bleeding). An illustrative list of underlying causes of arrest is shown in Table 36.2. Immediate testing post-arrest may include chest computed tomography to evaluate for PE, serum or urine drug testing to evaluate for opioids or other pharmacologic agents, and blood testing such as complete blood count and blood gas analysis. It is important to test initial serum lactate; although lactate elevations post-arrest are common and nonspecific, they often provide a

Table 36.2 Differential diagnosis of cardiac arrest. During and after resuscitation, it is important for providers to seek for underlying treatable causes of arrest

Category	Arrest etiologies
Cardiac	Myocardial infarction[a] Arrythmia from genetic Channelopathy Arrythmia from myocardial scar[a] Medication induced long QT Severe aortic stenosis Aortic dissection
Pulmonary	Pulmonary embolism[a] Status asthmaticus Tension pneumothorax Opioid overdose respiratory arrest[a]
Metabolic	Hyperkalemia Acidemia (e.g., diabetic ketoacidosis hypoglycemia)
Neurologic	Cerebrovascular accident Subarachnoid hemorrhage Seizure-related sudden death
Situational	Environmental hypothermia Asphyxia (e.g., drowning or hanging)

[a] Most common causes

clue regarding duration of arrest. Serial lactate measurements (e.g., every 6–8 h) will allow the assessment of lactate clearance over the first 24 h, which has been strongly associated with arrest outcomes [28, 29].

Another crucial action during the early phase of care is the initiation of targeted temperature management (TTM) for appropriate patients, or at a minimum, using TTM technology to institute strict normothermia/fever avoidance. Strong evidence has suggested that neurogenic fever is common after arrest resuscitation and is associated with worse outcomes [30–32]. Other studies have suggested that implementation of TTM is time sensitive, with improved outcomes associated with shorter "door-to-TTM initiation time" [33]. A realistic goal is to begin TTM within 4 h of arrival and preferably within 2 h. Details regarding TTM will be described below.

ED-based disposition planning for post-arrest patients is highly variable. That is, whether patients are dispositioned to the medical ICU, cardiac ICU, or neurologic ICU depends on local hospital resources and expertise. Given that post-arrest care is often centered on brain assessment and neurologic support, disposition to the neurologic ICU is ideal, with medical or cardiac critical care consultants engaged as needed.

Post-Arrest Care: ICU Phase—TTM

After ICU admission, the use of TTM is a key principle of post-arrest patient management. Three randomized trials and many observational studies have demonstrated that lowering core body temperature to 33 °C following arrest leads to improved neurologic outcomes (Table 36.3) [34–39]. These studies are supported by a body of laboratory science [40–42] that provides convincing mechanistic underpinning for TTM, showing that TTM lessens cerebral edema, markers of post-arrest inflammation, and other injury processes that are part of what is known as the post-cardiac arrest syndrome (PCAS) [6], a constellation of overlapping pathophysiologic changes that occur over the first few days follow ROSC.

Table 36.3 Brief description of the 5 major post-arrest TTM dosing trials in adults. Three trials showed improved outcome with a TTM 33 °C target, and three trials were neutral. It is important to note that no published RCT has demonstrated a worse outcome with a TTM 33 °C target temperature

Trial	Setting	Patients	Comparison groups	Outcomes
HACA (2002) [34]	OHCA	Adults, shockable arrest	32-34 °C vs. normothermia	32-34 °C better neurologic outcomes RR 1.4 (95% CI 1.08–1.81)
Bernard (2002) [35]	OHCA	Adults, shockable arrest	33 °C vs. normothermia	33 °C better neurologic outcomes OR 5.25 (95% CI 1.47–18.76
Nielsen (2013) [43]	OHCA	Adults, presumed cardiac cause	33 °C vs. 36 °C	No difference in outcomes HR 1.06, 95% CI 0.89–1.28
Lascarrou (2019) [36]	OHCA, IHCA	Adults, nonshockable arrest	33 °C vs. 37 °C	33 °C better neurologic outcomes 4.5% difference, 95% CI 0.1–8.9%
Dankiewiz (2021) [44]	OHCA	Adults, presumed cardiac cause	33 °C vs. <37.8 °C	No difference in outcomes HR 1.00; 95% CI, 0.92 to 1.09

Two randomized trials from Europe, known as the TTM1 and TTM2 trials, have called into question the appropriate goal temperature of post-arrest TTM [43, 44]. The TTM1 trial revealed equivalent outcomes when managing patients at 33 °C vs. 36 °C; the more recent TTM2 trial showed equivalent outcomes at 33 °C vs. "therapeutic normothermia" (aggressive maintanance <37.8 °C). This has led to a global debate about the appropriate "dose" of TTM following arrest resuscitation.

However, a question has been raised about generalizability of these studies to the broader array of post-arrest patients, as the overwhelming majority of patients in these trials had both witnessed arrest and provision of bystander CPR, and both trial cohorts exhibited a low prevalence of post-arrest shock states. These observations suggest that on balance patients enrolled in these trials may have sustained more modest neuronal injuries, for which aggressive TTM may not be required. Indeed, three recent observational studies have suggested that TTM to 33 °C shows benefit for patients with more significant evidence of injury (e.g., based on electroencephalographic [EEG] findings of moderate encephalopathy in one study and based on clinical evidence of end-organ injury in another) [45–47]. In these studies, less injured patients had similar outcomes when managed at 36 °C, consistent with the TTM1 and TTM2 trial results. Taken together, these findings suggest that the future of TTM therapy should involve specific patient-tailored approaches, employing physiologic markers of injury severity. This remains an active area of intensive research. However, as a practical matter, many hospitals have retained 33 °C as the default TTM target based on the balance of data inclusive of three positive RCTs and the newer studies showing a benefit of 33 °C for more injured patients. For patients who fit the TTM1 or TTM2 criteria (witnessed arrest, provision of bystander CPR, and no evidence of shock), a goal temperature of 36 °C or even normothermia may be considered.

Post-Arrest Care: ICU Phase—Cardiac Management

During critical care of the post-arrest patient, it is important to obtain echocardiographic assessment serially (e.g., daily for the first 3–5 days) for a number of reasons. First, assessment of regional wall motion abnormalities may be the key data to support myocardial ischemia as a cause of the arrest and may prompt coronary intervention. Second, myocardial stunning is common in the first 24–48 h follow resuscitation [48], during which systolic ejection fraction may fall precipitously but recover over subsequent days. Initial hemodynamic instability may be due to a variety of causes, but one etiology is this myocardial stunning phenomenon. Studies have suggested that the addition of dobutamine may be helpful to mitigate stunning [49].

The role of cardiac catheterization in non-STEMI post-arrest patients remains controversial, as two European trials have suggested that survival outcomes were equivalent when angiography was performed early or in delayed fashion [19, 20]. That said, patient selection is crucial [50], and recent evidence suggests that the presence of chest pain before arrest onset may enrich for patients with underlying cardiac ischemia who would benefit from coronary evaluation [51]. It is reasonable that most post-arrest patients receive cardiology consultation in the critical care setting, to advise regarding echocardiography findings and to consider the timing, or necessity, of coronary angiography. In addition, this consultation is important as some patients may be appropriate candidates for ICD placement as a long-term secondary prevention measure [52]. This consultation may not be required for post-arrest patients with clear causes of arrest that are not cardiac in nature (e.g., drug overdose, drowning, and status asthmaticus).

Throughout critical care of the post-arrest patient, it is essential to maintain adequate hemodynamic support. AHA guidelines recommend targeting a mean arterial pressure (MAP) > 65 mm Hg, based on observational data from several clinical studies [53, 54]. Maintaining a high MAP is essential for brain perfusion, given that many post-arrest patients have increased intracranial pressure. Hypotension during the first several days of post-arrest care is to be avoided whenever possible.

Post-Arrest Care: ICU Phase—Prognostication and Neurologic Management

Neurologic assessment of patients following arrest represents a rapidly evolving field, with the increased introduction of multimodal brain monitoring including microdialysis and other techniques to assess brain perfusion and physiology [55, 56]. At a minimum, patients following arrest should receive EEG monitoring, ideally continuously. This allows for the identification of malignant EEG patterns that might auger poor prognosis [57, 58]. For example, a number of studies have suggested that suppression patterns on EEG (defined as EEG background activity below 10 μV) have nearly 100% specificity for poor neurologic outcome at 24 h post-arrest. EEG burst suppression patterns, in which suppression is interposed with "burst" periods of electrical activity, are also associated with poor prognosis but with somewhat lessened specificity [57]. Yet another common EEG pattern, known as periodic lateralized epileptiform discharges (PLEDs), is a hallmark of intermittent electrical seizure activity that may benefit from treatment.

EEG can also identify electrical evidence of seizure activity, found in up to 20% of comatose post-arrest patients [58]. Seizures typically occur early, often within 8–24 h following ROSC, and can lead to secondary brain injuries through such mechanisms as glutamate excitotoxicity and increased metabolic rate. No specific pharmacologic anticonvulsant agents have been shown superior to others for post-arrest seizure management, although generally benzodiazepines and phenytoin are used only with great caution due to the potential for hypotension, which should be avoided given the possibility of elevated intracranial pressure in many patients following resuscitation. Whether post-arrest patients should receive prophylactic treatment with anticonvulsants is unknown, representing a key knowledge gap in post-arrest care.

For centers that have capabilities for multimodal monitoring, such an approach should be considered for all post-arrest patients; evidence is growing that such approaches yield additional insights into post-arrest cerebral physiology that might change care approaches or offer additional value for prognostication [59].

Neuroprognostication following cardiac arrest resuscitation remains an enormous challenge for the ICU practitioner. Available tools in addition to EEG include the use of somatosensory evoked potentials (SSEPs), with strong evidence that an absent N20 response 72 h following arrest is a poor prognostic indicator [60]. The use of magnetic resonance imaging (MRI) in the post-arrest time frame from days 3–7 post-arrest may also provide key information regarding likely irreversible neurologic injuries [61, 62]. Clinical bedside examination is, unfortunately, a very poor prognostic tool, as many patients remain comatose with poor or absent brain stem reflexes for several days following arrest and yet may still make a full recovery. A major hazard of ICU care is the early and inappropriate withdrawal of care following arrest based on clinical examination [63]. The AHA strongly recommends avoidance of early withdrawal based on clinical assessment, for at least 3 days following arrest, and likely longer if TTM is employed. [64] Observational work has suggested that many patients do not exhibit volitional motor movements (more precisely, a Glasgow motor score of 6) until days 4–7 post arrest, and many of these patients attain a good neurologic outcome (Fig. 36.2) [65].

A crucial knowledge gap in the field remains the identification of early markers that reliably auger a very poor prognosis, to guide decisions regarding ICU care and TTM use. Serum biomarkers might theoretically be an ideal tool for this, but data are mixed for all markers assessed to date. The most promising of these, neurofilament light chain (NFL), demonstrated a receiver-operator characteristic area under the curve of 0.94 for poor prognosis, meaning that some patients had good prognosis despite markedly elevated NFL. [66] Whether combinations of markers or markers plus clinical factors, could be arranged into a prognostic scoring system, remain to be determined.

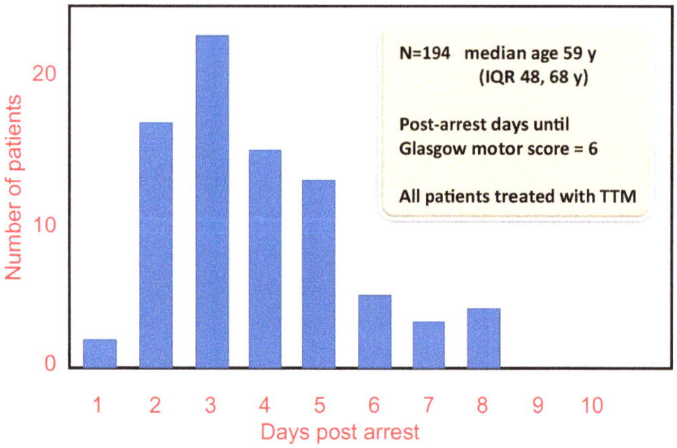

Fig. 36.2 Timeline of post-arrest awakening, adapted from Grossestreuer et al. [65] TTM, targeted temperature management. The vertical bars represent the number of patients to achieve purposeful motor function on a specific post-arrest day during the index hospitalization

Post-Arrest Care: ICU Phase—Family Management

The critical care practitioner must not only manage the post-arrest patient, but the family members of the victim. Unlike many critically ill patients who are in the ICU following progression of chronic illnesses, it must be appreciated that most OHCA patients had a high functional level immediately before cardiac arrest, thus their arrest represents an abrupt and catastrophic change in clinical status. Family members are therefore confronted with dramatic changes in their loved one's status, at breathtaking speed. First, they are informed their otherwise "healthy" family member died and may not survive resuscitation. Then, they are informed that their loved one is critically ill and requires sophisticated care in the critical care setting with a significant change of brain injury. It is, therefore, often the case that family members become overwhelmed during the first few days of care. It is incumbent on the critical care team to advise and promote family members self-care, calling upon resources such as other family members, chaplains, or friends to support them during the subacute phase of patient management.

Given that many patients remain unresponsive for days following resuscitation (through a combination of PCAS brain injury and sedative treatment), it is important to stress to families that information about recovery and prognostication may not be forthcoming for several days at a minimum. It is useful to set expectations for potentially poor outcomes but to advise against hasty decision making. Many resuscitation care experts summarize post-arrest care to families with the phrase "post-arrest recovery is a marathon, not a sprint"—such simple metaphors capture the need for families to pace themselves regarding expectations and the need to take breaks from care, to sleep and to eat. This is especially important to help critical care practitioners during the later days of critical care (often days 4–8) when weighty decisions must be discussed with family members, potentially regarding withdrawal of care, or long-term care planning with potential tracheostomy, and other issues.

Post-Arrest Care: ICU Discharge and Long-Term Management

For patients who recover substantial neurologic function and are transferred to the ward setting, a number of key items need to be addressed by practitioners. Some patients who had initial shockable arrest rhythms may benefit from ICD placement; for those who do, but are not yet clinically well enough to undergo the procedure, the use of bridging devices such as wearable defibrillation vests may be considered. [67] Most patients will require physical therapy and occupational therapy evaluation and may require placement in acute rehabilitation following hospitalization, to address motor deficits and/or overall debility following prolonged hospitalization [68].

Follow-up planning for post-arrest patients should include continued ambulatory care via both cardiology and neurology practitioners. Referral to brain injury specialists may be appropriate for ongoing granular neurocognitive assessments and management of neurologic deficits. Patients may be referred to national support groups for cardiac arrest survivors, including the Sudden Cardiac Arrest Foundation. A number of cardiac arrest survivors have spoken publicly about their experiences, and such internet resources may be helpful for families and survivors [69, 70].

Selected Challenges During Post-Arrest Care: Avoid These Near Misses

Challenges During TTM Administration

While the adverse effects of TTM are relatively modest, a few of these effects warrant mention to prepare care teams. During TTM targeted to 33 °C, hypokalemia may occur due to "cold diuresis," in which whole body cooling provokes a diuretic effect on glomerular function [71]. Serial evaluation of serum electrolytes, every 6–8 h, will allow for repletion to take place as needed. While cooled to 33 °C, many patients become bradycardic, to heart rates as low as 30–40 per minute. It is important for practitioners to resist the urge to administer atropine or employ electrical pacing, as in the great majority of cases this bradycardia is well tolerated. Provided that the patient maintains adequate mean arterial pressure and urine output, the bradycardia may remain untreated, as it will resolve upon restoration of a euthermic state. Finally and perhaps most importantly, when rewarming from 33 °C, practitioners should be aware that venodilation as a response to warming may lead to hypotension. It is crucial that patients receive adequate intravenous fluids during post-arrest care so that this hypotension can be minimized. Inadequate fluid resuscitation, combined with rewarming hypotension, can lead to significant organ impacts on already injured brain tissue.

Challenges During Early Post-Arrest Care

Ischemia from cardiac arrest on occasion leads to organ impacts that can manifest insidiously over the first 24–72 h post-arrest. An important variant of this phenomenon is bowel ischemia that can be provoked by the arrest and resuscitation. Practitioners should remain vigilant, as sedated and intubated patients are challenging to clinically assess for this problem. Blood per rectum during the first few days of critical care and an unexplained rising serum lactate post-arrest are worrisome findings that warrant consideration of bowel ischemia. Another important clinical problem is secondary infection during post-arrest care. Ventilator-associated pneumonia, often provoked from aspiration during arrest and resuscitation, is common in post-arrest patients; however, the use of TTM prevents the manifestation of fever. Therefore, practitioners should have a low threshold to initiate antimicrobial therapy in the context of a rising white blood cell count or the appearance of infiltrate on chest radiography.

Challenges During Post-ICU Care

An important pitfall can reside in the consideration of post-arrest ICD placement. It is essential that care providers obtain cardiac rhythm data from AEDs or monitor/defibrillators from initial prehospital resuscitation care, whenever possible, as it is standard of care to place ICDs for patients with shockable arrest rhythms and no evidence of coronary disease on subsequent cardiac catheterization. A dangerous miss resides in the failure to recognize an initial shockable rhythm, followed by the discharge home of a patient without an ICD who then remains unprotected from a second lethal arrhythmic event. A second pitfall in evaluating post-arrest patients on the ward is the need for a secondary trauma evaluation. Given that many post-arrest patients collapsed from standing, followed by receiving chest compressions known to sometimes cause rib fractures, it is important to perform and document a thorough musculoskeletal examination once patients are awake and responsive. Secondary discovery of wrist or hand fractures, subtle rib fractures, dental injuries, and other bone findings is not unheard of following initial post-arrest care. These should be documented and potentially addressed before hospital discharge.

Conclusions

Cardiac arrest and post-arrest management remain highly challenging clinical scenarios for hospital-based providers. In many cases, cardiac arrest outcomes are dependent on neurologic injuries, and therefore, post-arrest care is centered supportive care for the brain. Following initial CPR and electrical defibrillation, hospital-based management includes such modalities as TTM, coronary angiography, EEG monitoring, and hemodynamic support. While survival remains poor, and many survivors experience some degree of neurologic impairment, an increasing number of patients worldwide have recovered from cardiac arrest and enjoyed a return to normal activities, demonstrating that survival is indeed possible. High-quality post-arrest management, including the modalities listed above in addition to the avoidance of early withdrawal of care, should be codified in hospital-based protocols and reviewed on a regular basis as part of quality assurance efforts. In this fashion, more cardiac arrest victims can be restored to health over coming years.

References

1. Virani SS, Alonso A, Aparicio HJ, et al. Heart disease and stroke statistics—2021 update: a report from the American Heart Association. Circulation. 2021;143:e254–743.
2. Engdahl J, Holmberg M, Karlson BW, et al. The epidemiology of out-of-hospital "sudden" cardiac arrest. Resuscitation. 2002;52:235.
3. Merchant RM, Topjian AA, Panchal AR, et al. Part 1: executive summary: 2020 American Heart Association guidelines for cardiopulmonary resuscitation and emergency cardiovascular care. Circulation. 2020;142:S337–57.
4. Valenzuela T, Roe D, Cretin S, et al. Estimating effectiveness of cardiac arrest interventions: a logistic regression survival model. Circulation. 1997;96:3308–13.
5. Neumar RW, Nolan JP, Adrie C, et al. Post-cardiac arrest syndrome: epidemiology, pathophysiology, treatment, and prognostication. Circulation. 2008;118(23):2452–83.
6. Jozwiak M, Bougouin W, Geri G, et al. Post-resuscitation shock: recent advances in pathophysiology and treatment. Ann Intensive Care. 2020;10(1):170.
7. Perez CA, Samudra N, Aiyagari V. Cognitive and functional consequence of cardiac arrest. Curr Neurol Neurosci Rep. 2016;16(8):70.
8. Hasselqvist-Ax I, Riva G, Herlitz J, et al. Early cardiopulmonary resuscitation in out-of-hospital cardiac arrest. N Engl J Med. 2015;372(24):2307–15.
9. Suryanarayana P, Garza HK, Klewer J, et al. Electrophysiologic considerations after sudden cardiac arrest. Curr Cardiol Rev. 2018;14(2):102–8.
10. Nagao K. Chest compression-only cardiocerebral resuscitation. Curr Opin Crit Care. 2009;15(3):189–97.
11. Edelson DP, Litzinger B, Arora V, et al. Improving in-hospital cardiac arrest process and outcomes with performance debriefing. Arch Intern Med. 2008;168(10):1063–9.
12. Bobrow BJ, Vadeboncoeur TF, Stolz U, et al. The influence of scenario-based training and real-time audiovisual feedback on out-of-hospital cardiopulmonary resuscitation quality and survival from out-of-hospital cardiac arrest. Ann Emerg Med. 2013;62(1):47–56. e1.
13. Vaillancourt C, Petersen A, Meier EN, et al. The impact of increased chest compression fraction on survival for out-of-hospital cardiac arrest patients with a non-shockable initial rhythm. Resuscitation. 2020 Sep;154:93–100.
14. Meaney PA, Bobrow BJ, Mancini ME, et al. Cardiopulmonary resuscitation quality: improving cardiac resuscitation outcomes both inside and outside the hospital: a consensus statement from the American Heart Association. Circulation. 2013;128(4):417–35.
15. Delhomme C, Njeim M, Varlet E, et al. Automated external defibrillator use in out-of-hospital cardiac arrest: current limitations and solutions. Arch Cardiovasc Dis. 2019;112(3):217–22.
16. Finn J, Jacobs I, Williams TA, et al. Adrenaline and vasopressin for cardiac arrest. Cochrane Database Syst Rev. 2019;1(1):CD003179.
17. Perkins GD, Ji C, Deakin CD, et al. A randomized trial of epinephrine in out-of-hospital cardiac arrest. N Engl J Med. 2018;379(8):711–21.
18. Baldi E, Schnaubelt S, Caputo ML, et al. Association of Timing of electrocardiogram acquisition after return of spontaneous circulation with coronary angiography findings in patients with out-of-hospital cardiac arrest. JAMA Netw Open. 2021;4(1): e2032875.
19. Lemkes JS, Janssens GN, van der Hoeven NW, et al. Coronary angiography after cardiac arrest without ST-segment elevation. N Engl J Med. 2019;380(15):1397–407.
20. Desch S, Freund A, Akin I, et al. Angiography after out-of-hospital cardiac arrest without ST-segment elevation. N Engl J Med. 2021;385(27):2544–53.
21. Elmer J, Liu C, Pease M, et al. Deep learning of early brain imaging to predict post-arrest electroencephalography. Resuscitation. 2022;172:17–23.
22. Moseby-Knappe M, Mattsson-Carlgren N, Stammet P, et al. Serum markers of brain injury can predict good neurological outcome after out-of-hospital cardiac arrest. Intensive Care Med. 2021;47(9):984–94.
23. Chung-Esaki HM, Mui G, Mlynash M, et al. The neuron specific enolase (NSE) ratio offers benefits over absolute value thresholds in post-cardiac arrest coma prognosis. J Clin Neurosci. 2018;57:99–104.
24. Hoiland RL, Rikhraj KJK, Thiara S, et al. Neurologic prognostication after cardiac arrest using brain biomarkers: a systematic review and meta-analysis. JAMA Neurol. 2022;79(4):390–8.
25. Oddo M, Sandroni C, Citerio G, et al. Quantitative versus standard pupillary light reflex for early prognostication in comatose cardiac arrest patients: an international prospective multicenter double-blinded study. Intensive Care Med. 2018;44(12):2102–11.
26. Roberts BW, Kilgannon JH, Hunter BR, et al. Association between early Hyperoxia exposure after resuscitation from cardiac arrest and neurological disability: prospective multicenter protocol-directed cohort study. Circulation. 2018;137(20):2114–24.
27. Okuma Y, Becker LB, Hayashida K, et al. Effects of post-resuscitation normoxic therapy on oxygen-sensitive oxidative stress in a rat model of cardiac arrest. J Am Heart Assoc. 2021;10(7):e018773.
28. Donnino MW, Miller J, Goyal N, et al. Effective lactate clearance is associated with improved outcome in post-cardiac arrest patients. Resuscitation. 2007;75(2):229–34.
29. Williams TA, Martin R, Celenza A, et al. Use of serum lactate levels to predict survival for patients with out-of-hospital cardiac arrest: a cohort study. Emerg Med Australas. 2016 Apr;28(2):171–8.
30. Leary M, Grossestreuer AV, Iannacone S, et al. Pyrexia and neurologic outcomes after therapeutic hypothermia for cardiac arrest. Resuscitation. 2013;84(8):1056–61.
31. Gebhardt K, Guyette FX, Doshi AA, et al. Prevalence and effect of fever on outcome following resuscitation from cardiac arrest. Resuscitation. 2013;84(8):1062–7.
32. Grossestreuer AV, Gaieski DF, Donnino MW, et al. Magnitude of temperature elevation is associated with neurologic and survival outcomes in resuscitated cardiac arrest patients with postrewarming pyrexia. J Crit Care. 2017;38:78–83.
33. Stanger D, Kawano T, Malhi N, et al. Door-to-targeted temperature management initiation time and outcomes in out-of-hospital cardiac arrest: insights from the continuous chest compressions trial. J Am Heart Assoc. 2019;8(9):e012001.
34. The Hypothermia After Cardiac Arrest Study Group. Mild therapeutic hypothermia to improve the neurologic outcome after cardiac arrest. N Engl J Med. 2002;346:549.
35. Bernard SA, Gray TW, Buist MD, et al. Treatment of comatose survivors of out-of-hospital cardiac arrest with induced hypothermia. N Engl J Med. 2002;346:557.

36. Lascarrou JB, Merdji H, Le Gouge A, et al. Targeted temperature Management for Cardiac Arrest with nonshockable rhythm. N Engl J Med. 2019;381(24):2327–37.
37. Walker AC, Johnson NJ. Targeted temperature management and Postcardiac arrest care. Emerg Med Clin North Am. 2019;37(3):381–93.
38. Gaieski DF, Band RA, Abella BS, et al. Early goal-directed hemodynamic optimization combined with therapeutic hypothermia in comatose survivors of out-of-hospital cardiac arrest. Resuscitation. 2009;80(4):418–24.
39. DeLia D, Wang HE, Kutzin J, et al. Prehospital transportation to therapeutic hypothermia centers and survival from out-of-hospital cardiac arrest. BMC Health Serv Res. 2015;15:533.
40. Kim T, Paine MG, Meng H, et al. Combined intra- and post-cardiac arrest hypothermic-targeted temperature management in a rat model of asphyxial cardiac arrest improves survival and neurologic outcome compared to either strategy alone. Resuscitation. 2016;107:94–101.
41. Li J, Li C, Yuan W, et al. Targeted temperature management suppresses hypoxia-inducible factor-1α and vascular endothelial growth factor expression in a pig model of cardiac arrest. Neurocrit Care. 2021;35(2):379–88.
42. Che D, Li L, Kopil CM, et al. Impact of therapeutic hypothermia onset and duration on survival, neurologic function, and neurodegeneration after cardiac arrest. Crit Care Med. 2011;39(6):1423–30.
43. Nielsen N, Wetterslev J, Cronberg T, et al. Targeted temperature management at 33°C versus 36°C after cardiac arrest. N Engl J Med. 2013;369(23):2197–206.
44. Dankiewicz J, Cronberg T, Lilja G, et al. Hypothermia versus Normothermia after out-of-hospital cardiac arrest. N Engl J Med. 2021;384(24):2283–94.
45. Callaway CW, Coppler PJ, Faro J, et al. Association of Initial Illness Severity and Outcomes after Cardiac Arrest with Targeted Temperature Management at 36 °C or 33 °C. JAMA Netw Open. 2020;3(7):e208215.
46. Nishikimi M, Ogura T, Nishida K, et al. Outcome related to level of targeted temperature Management in Postcardiac Arrest Syndrome of low, moderate, and high severities: a Nationwide multicenter prospective registry. Crit Care Med. 2021;49(8):e741–50.
47. Nutma S, Tjepkema-Cloostermans MC, Ruijter BJ, et al. Effects of targeted temperature management at 33 °C vs. 36 °C on comatose patients after cardiac arrest stratified by the severity of encephalopathy. Resuscitation. 2022;173:147–53.
48. Chalkias A, Xanthos T. Pathophysiology and pathogenesis of post-resuscitation myocardial stunning. Heart Fail Rev. 2012;17(1):117–28.
49. Vasquez A, Kern KB, Hilwig RW, et al. Optimal dosing of dobutamine for treating post-resuscitation left ventricular dysfunction. Resuscitation. 2004;61(2):199–207.
50. Abella BS, Gaieski DF. Coronary angiography after cardiac arrest - the right timing or the right patients? N Engl J Med. 2019;380(15):1474–5.
51. Helfer DR, Helber AR, Ferko AR, et al. Clinical factors associated with significant coronary lesions following out-of-hospital cardiac arrest. Acad Emerg Med. 2022;29(4):456–64.
52. Aro AL, Chugh SS. Prevention of sudden cardiac death in children and young adults. Prog Pediatr Cardiol. 2017;45:37–42.
53. Ai HB, Jiang EL, Yu JH, et al. Mean arterial pressure is associated with the neurological function in patients who survived after cardiopulmonary resuscitation: a retrospective cohort study. Clin Cardiol. 2020;43(11):1286–93.
54. Beylin ME, Perman SM, Abella BS, et al. Higher mean arterial pressure with or without vasoactive agents is associated with increased survival and better neurological outcomes in comatose survivors of cardiac arrest. Intensive Care Med. 2013;39(11):1981–8.
55. Beekman R, Maciel CB, Balu R, et al. Neuromonitoring after cardiac arrest: can twenty-first century medicine personalize post cardiac arrest care? Neurol Clin. 2021 May;39(2):273–92.
56. Balu R, Rajagopalan S, Baghshomali S, et al. Cerebrovascular pressure reactivity and intracranial pressure are associated with neurologic outcome after hypoxic-ischemic brain injury. Resuscitation. 2021;164:114–21.
57. Faro J, Coppler PJ, Dezfulian C, et al. Differential association of subtypes of epileptiform activity with outcome after cardiac arrest. Resuscitation. 2019;136:138–45.
58. Wiley SL, Razavi B, Krishnamohan P, et al. Quantitative EEG metrics differ between outcome groups and change over the first 72 h in comatose cardiac arrest patients. Neurocrit Care. 2018;28(1): 51–9.
59. Mayasi Y, Geocadin RG. Updates on the Management of Neurologic Complications of post-cardiac arrest resuscitation. Semin Neurol. 2021;41(4):388–97.
60. Youn CS, Park KN, Kim SH, et al. External validation of the 2020 ERC/ESICM prognostication strategy algorithm after cardiac arrest. Crit Care. 2022;26(1):95.
61. Greer DM, Wu O. Neuroimaging in cardiac arrest prognostication. Semin Neurol. 2017;37(1):66–74.
62. Lopez Soto C, Dragoi L, Heyn CC, et al. Imaging for Neuroprognostication after cardiac arrest: systematic review and meta-analysis. Neurocrit Care. 2020;32(1):206–16.
63. Grossestreuer AV, Gaieski DF, Abella BS, et al. Factors associated with post-arrest withdrawal of life-sustaining therapy. Resuscitation. 2017;110:114–9.
64. Geocadin RG, Callaway CW, Fink EL, et al. Standards for studies of neurological prognostication in comatose survivors of cardiac arrest: a scientific statement from the American Heart Association. Circulation. 2019;140(9):e517–42.
65. Grossestreuer AV, Abella BS, Leary M, et al. Time to awakening and neurologic outcome in therapeutic hypothermia-treated cardiac arrest patients. Resuscitation. 2013;84(12):1741–6.
66. Moseby-Knappe M, Mattsson N, Nielsen N, et al. Serum Neurofilament light chain for prognosis of outcome after cardiac arrest. JAMA Neurol. 2019;76(1):64–71.
67. Cheung CC, Olgin JE, Lee BK. Wearable cardioverter-defibrillators: a review of evidence and indications. Trends Cardiovasc Med. 2021;31(3):196–201.
68. Lilja G, Nielsen N, Bro-Jeppesen J, et al. Return to work and participation in society after out-of-hospital cardiac arrest. Circ Cardiovasc Qual Outcomes. 2018;11(1):e003566.
69. https://www.hmpgloballearningnetwork.com/site/emsworld/article/1224743/five-questions-dr-glaucomflecken-surviving-cardiac-arrest, Accessed 30 May 2022.
70. https://www.theguardian.com/football/2012/mar/25/muamba-collapse-minute-by-minute, Accessed 30 May 2022.
71. Raper JD, Wang HE. Urine output changes during Postcardiac arrest therapeutic hypothermia. Ther Hypothermia Temp Manag. 2013;3(4):173–7.

Neurologic Prognostication in Neurocritical Care

37

Henry Chang, Vishank A. Shah, and Romergryko G. Geocadin

Contents

H. Chang · V. A. Shah · R. G. Geocadin (✉)
Johns Hopkins University School of Medicine,
Baltimore, MD, USA
e-mail: rgeocad1@jhmi.edu

E. Mahanna Gabrielli et al. (eds.), *Textbook of Neurointensive Care: Volume 1*, https://doi.org/10.1007/978-3-031-62220-5_37

Abstract

Neurological prognostication is an indispensable component of neurointensive care with significant ramifications—not just for patients with regard to survival and functional outcomes, or for families and caregivers, but also for the scientific advancement for a particular neurologic pathology. Accurate, reliable, and objective determination of prognosis after acute brain injury requires a multifaceted approach and consideration of all aspects of the patient's condition, including the pathophysiology of the specific acute neurologic injury, its clinical course, pertinent neurologic clinical assessment, neuroimaging information, neurophysiologic data, blood/CSF-based biomarkers, and importantly the timing of these parameters in relation to the injury and subsequent interventions. Despite some advances, there is a growing realization that existing neuro-prognostic markers have serious limitations that may impact both patient care and clinical research after life-threatening neurologic injury. In particular, the majority of prognostication models are confounded by self-fulfilling prophecies created by the bias of early care limitations and do not take into account the influence of post-hospitalization events such as treatment response and exposure to factors causing secondary neurologic injury. Additionally, patient and caregiver perspectives regarding what constitutes an acceptable level of disability is often not incorporated into prognostication methods. This chapter will present the state of the science vis-à-vis the prevailing practices in neurologic prognostication in common acute life-threatening neurologic illnesses and highlight these important limitations and their impact on patient care.

Clinical Significance of Neurologic Prognostication

Neurologic prognostication has far-reaching consequences on patient survival and recovery, as well as on the scientific advancement of medical research. Survival after neurologic injury is often a direct consequence of neurologic prognostication. Outcomes predicted by physicians inform exceedingly consequential decisions regarding continuation of medical care versus withdrawal of life-sustaining therapies (WLST) that inevitably lead to demise of the patient. Up to 80% of the deaths in the neurointensive care unit occur due to WLST [1]. Inclusion of WLST in prognostication models negates the effect of other variables, implying that the most important prognostic variable for survival and recovery may be the degree of medical support received based on the estimated neurologic prognosis [2].

Acute neurologic injuries often lead to significant disability in the early phase, although if given adequate time, good functional outcome may occur in a large proportion of patients. For example, among traumatic brain injury (TBI) patients with impaired consciousness at discharge, 80% regained consciousness and approximately 40% regained partial functional independence [3]. Likewise, the median modified Rankin score (mRS) at days 30–90 after intracerebral hemorrhage (ICH) is reported to be 4–5 [4, 5], but >40% of such severely disabled ICH survivors may recover to a good functional outcomes by 1-year [6, 7]. In propensity-score matched analyses of more than 4000 out-of-hospital cardiac arrest patients, 17% of the patients that died due to early WLST could have achieved a favorable functional outcome [8]. On the other hand, maximizing therapy among patients with a poor likelihood of recovery may lead to significant socioeconomic burden for caregivers, healthcare systems, and society. Thus, accurate and unbiased neurologic prognostication is necessary to help identify patients with potential to make significant functional recovery and provide them with necessary time to permit recovery, while at the same time avoiding futile and often invasive care in those who will not recover to a functional status acceptable to them.

Finally, neurologic prognostication has a significant impact on the interpretation of mortality and functional outcomes in clinical trials. Neurologic prognostication is invariably performed early in the course of the injury even though clinical trials often assess primary outcomes at 90 days and beyond. Thus, early pessimistic neurologic prognostication may result in WLST decisions in the first few days after brain injury leading to early deaths, causing a significant impact on the interpretation of the effect of the study intervention on mortality. Unfortunately, mortality in clinical trials is often not differentiated between deaths as a consequence of the neurologic injury (i.e., brain death), somatic death (e.g., intractable hypotension), and WLST. There is a need to delineate these factors and to allow more time for the intervention to take effect and influence recovery prior to WLST in clinical trials, in order to accurate assess the true course of the brain injury and subsequent interventions.

Self-Fulfilling Prophecy in Prognostication

Numerous factors impact the interpretation and execution of existing prognostication literature and warrant discussion up front. A careful review of neurologic prognostication studies across multiple acute neurologic injuries demonstrates the lack of scientific rigor and standardization which is not in line with other clinical interventional trials in which it is expected that study design is prospectively defined, confounders are minimized, and well-validated outcome metrics are employed. The majority of studies assessing prognostic markers are retrospective, do not blind the treating physicians to the prognostic marker under study, may incorporate that prognostic marker in WLST-decision making, and may not collect blinded outcomes [9, 10]. By far, the most important limitation is the strong influence of mortality due to a WLST decision—which is itself influenced by certain prognostic markers—on the analysis of outcomes in the cohorts used to evaluate these same prognostic markers [9].When treating physicians use the prognostic markers under study to make decisions regarding WLST and then include the very same patients in the cohorts to test the predictive accuracy of the prognostic markers, this creates a confirmation bias termed the self-fulfilling prophecy. The self-fulfilling prophecy often leads to overestimation of poor prognosis and falsely elevates positive predictive values for markers of poor prognosis. This practice can have a profound impact on patient care, survival, and functional outcomes. Understanding these limitations is thus key to interpreting existing prognostication models in acute neurologic injury. Considering that clinical trial outcomes are largely driven by survival, limitations in biased neurologic prognostication are a major hindrance to scientific advancement.

Neurologic Prognostication in Specific Disease States

In this section, we will discuss prognostication literature and its limitations in commonly encountered neurocritical care conditions that have the most literature and guidance on prognostication, including hypoxic–ischemic brain injury, intracerebral hemorrhage, acute ischemic stroke, subarachnoid hemorrhage, and traumatic brain injury.

Hypoxic–Ischemic Brain Injury

Background

Most studies concerning neurologic prognostication are dedicated to hypoxic–ischemic brain injury in survivors of cardiac arrest, which is a global cerebral ischemic event. Greater than 180,000 people experience an out-of-hospital cardiac arrest per year in the United States, of which approximately 11% survive to hospital discharge. Another 200,000 experience an in-hospital cardiac arrest, which has better survivorship: up to 25% [11]. Approximately 80% of cardiac arrest survivors are comatose in the acute phase [9], but the true anatomic burden of brain injury that determines the potential for future neurologic recovery is widely heterogenous, depending on the type of cardiac arrest, clinical setting of its occurrence, time-to-CPR initiation, duration of CPR, quality of CPR, intra- and post-resuscitation care, underlying comorbid conditions, premorbid cerebral reserve, and patient demographics [12, 13]. Up to a third of comatose survivors may regain consciousness [9] (with notably 35% having delayed awakening from coma [>48 h after stopping sedation]), and more than 70% of these patients have the potential for an eventual good functional recovery [14]. Thus, neurologic prognostication is of utmost importance, as it drives important patient care decisions that influence survival and functional recovery, and it serves as a major purpose for the involvement of neurologists and neurointensivists in post-cardiac arrest care. There has been a steady increase in long-term survival and neurologic recovery after cardiac arrest likely driven by standardization of post-cardiac arrest care and—more importantly—by limiting early WLST [15], highlighting the significance of accurate prognostication on cardiac arrest survivorship.

Pre-Requisites to Neurologic Prognostication in Cardiac Arrest Survivors

Prior to neurologic prognostication, all external and potentially reversible factors that may affect the patient's neurological examination and other ancillary tests need to be excluded [16]. This is often not straightforward, especially in the intensive care unit (ICU) setting. Metabolic abnormalities such as electrolyte and acid–base disturbances, sepsis, and multiorgan failure can be severe and profoundly affect the patient's neurological status. Also, many of the medications frequently used in the ICU with sedating effects can linger for a significant period of time even after being discontinued. Such factors limit interpretation of early neurologic prognostication during the acute phase.

Targeted temperature management (TTM) to normothermia or hypothermia is currently utilized in the acute period after cardiac arrest due its association with improved clinical outcomes in comatose survivors in multiple clinical trials [17–19]. While the patient is being cooled, neurologic prognostication cannot be reliably performed. Hypothermia itself can impair consciousness and delay awakening [20], and metabolic consequences of hypothermia—such as delayed clearance of sedatives and paralytics, and slowed body metabolism—may also confound interpretation of the clinical examination and ancillary tests [21]. Seizures are another important consideration, as patients with nonconvulsive status epilepticus may initially exhibit impaired consciousness, but once treated may demonstrate neurological recovery [22, 23].

Perhaps the most essential factor to consider is time. Even after mitigation of all other apparent confounders, if performed too soon, neurologic prognostication is unreliable and may be overly pessimistic. Current guidelines (the American Heart Association [22, 23]and the European Society of Intensive Care Medicine guidelines [24, 25]) generally recommend waiting at least 72 h after sedation has been halted and the patient has been rewarmed to normothermia before performing neurologic prognostication. Moreover, a recent American Heart Association (AHA) consensus statement recommends waiting for 7 days [16] to account for the subset of patients known as "late awakeners," in whom neurological recovery may be substantial but significantly delayed [26]. A 2022 study in post CA survivors where WLST was not a factor showed that median time for post-CA survivors to regain consciousness and have a favorable outcome was 12 days [27].

Clinical Assessment

Consciousness

The neurologic prognostication examination begins with evaluation of consciousness; that is, the patient's level of arousal and awareness. Consciousness is a complex process that involves a network of connections between the brainstem (in particular, the pons and midbrain), thalami, and cortical structures. Ultimately, the goal of neurologic prognostication is to predict awakening from a comatose state and the likelihood of meaningful functional recovery. The most commonly used measures of consciousness are the Glasgow Coma Scale (GCS) and the Full Outline of UnResponsiveness (FOUR) score. An initial assessment is often used to make decisions regarding post-resuscitation care including therapeutic hypothermia, but early assessments may not have prognostic value. Serial assessments over time, after elimination of confounders such as sedation, are more valuable than a single measurement [28].

Brainstem Reflexes

Absence of bilateral pupillary light reflex, 72 h after return of spontaneous circulation (ROSC) and after rewarming to normothermia in those treated with TTM, is highly specific for poor neurological recovery, with a false positive rate (FPR) of <5% and specificity of 98% [24, 25] [29]. However, pupillary response assessment is a qualitative method with concerns for inter-observer reliability. Quantitative pupillometry offers a more reliable tool for detecting the presence or absence of the pupillary response using the neurological pupil index (NPi). NPi less than 2 is shown to have a 100% positive predictive value, with a 0% FPR. Early pupillometry (within the first 72 h) is as specific at predicting poor outcome as a delayed (after 72 h) standard pupillary light reflex [30–32]. An important caveat is that in most studies assessing qualitative and quantitative pupillometry, clinicians providing patient care and outcome assessors were not blinded to the prognostic indicator. Thus, it is possible that these measurements may have influenced clinical decision making and led to a higher mortality due to WLST, which would result in artificially low false-positive rates due to this confirmation bias. However, Oddo et al. did blind clinicians and outcome assessors to pupillometry data and did not include pupillometry in their algorithm for cardiac arrest prognostication, and their study still demonstrated that quantitative pupillometry with an NPi of <2 had a 100% positive predictive value for an unfavorable outcome [32].

Similarly, bilaterally absent corneal reflex 72 h after ROSC also indicates poor outcome with high specificity, though lower than pupillary reflex—particularly in post-TTM patients (specificity 96%, FPR 4%)—given the vulnerability of the corneal reflex to residual effects of sedation and paralytics [29, 33].

It is again important to highlight that in most of the studies assessing brainstem reflexes and motor responses as prognostic indicators, WLST occurred at high rates, with up to 60–80% of the deaths in these cohorts being related to WLST [9]. This suggests a profound influence of a self-fulfilling prophecy, which limits the validity of the low false positive rates and high predictive values of these tests.

Motor Responses

A fully intact motor exam consists of voluntary cortical initiation of movement, transmission of this signal through the thalamus and brainstem into the spinal cord, and on to the target muscle group. Disruption of this pathway results in abnormal findings which are usually graded by the motor subscale of the Glasgow Coma Scale. A GCS motor subscore of 1–2 (corresponding to absent motor response or abnormal extensor posturing) has a sensitivity of 77% for poor neurological outcome, making this a reasonable screening method to identify patients who should undergo neurologic prognostication. However, this finding has a high false positive rate of 10–15% for predicting a poor neurological outcome, so it should not be used on its own to make withdrawal of care decisions [24, 25, 33].

Post-anoxic status myoclonus—defined as continuous and generalized myoclonus lasting at least 30 min in comatose survivors of cardiac arrest [24, 25, 29]—seems to be an extremely reliable predictor of poor neurological outcome when present within the first 72 h [29]. In particular, concurrent electroencephalogram (EEG) demonstrating a burst-suppression pattern with time-locked high amplitude polyspikes was associated with a 100% positive predictive value for poor outcome [34]. However, there are reports of patients with myoclonic status epilepticus recovering with a good outcome, so it is recommended to be used in conjunction with other modalities.

Neuroimaging Markers

Non-contrast CT scan of the brain may show diffuse cerebral edema and loss of gray-white differentiation at the cortex and deep nuclei. The gray-white ratio (GWR) can be quantified using the value of the Hounsfield units which measures the densities at specified gray and white matter locations (basal ganglia, centrum semiovale, and high convexity). A GWR on CT scans performed within first 24 h after ROSC, between 1.16 and 1.22 predicted poor neurological outcome with 0% false-positive rate in some studies, while in other studies it only predicted hospital mortality. This variability may be due to lack of standardized methods to calculate GWR [29].

MRI is more sensitive for neurological injury than CT scan but typically presents more logistic challenges, limiting its applicability. The most useful MRI sequences for neurologic prognostication are diffusion weighted imaging, apparent diffusion coefficient (ADC), and T2 sequences, which do not require gadolinium contrast [35–37]. The appearance of widespread abnormalities in the cortex and deep nuclei on these sequences is highly predictive for a poor neurological outcome, but the sensitivity and specificity of these findings vary between different studies. Additionally, the timing of MRI remains controversial; most guidelines currently recommend that the MRI be performed at least 48 h after ROSC [24, 25, 29]. Given variability in data and lack of availability of expertise at all centers, neuroimaging markers should be used only in conjunction with other modalities [24, 25, 29].

Neurophysiologic Markers

Electroencephalogram

A number of EEG patterns have been described in the setting of anoxic brain injury. For neurologic prognostication, an EEG demonstrating a "malignant" pattern—global suppression iso-electric (<10uV for >99% of the recording) or burst suppression with identical spikes (<10uV for 50–99% of the recording)—is predictive of a poor neurological outcome [29]. On the other hand, an EEG with normal-appearing background activity and reactivity (e.g., to command) is predictive of a good neurological recovery [38]. Out of a cohort of 104 unresponsive patients 4 days after brain injury (of which 33% were cardiac arrest survivors), 15% of the patients had brain activation to verbal commands detected by machine learning algorithms before they had motor activation to verbal commands. 44% of such patients had a good functional outcome versus only 14% of those that did not demonstrate such cognitive motor dissociation [39]. Similarly, in a cohort of 94 comatose cardiac arrest survivors undergoing therapeutic hypothermia, semiautomated quantification of EEG responses to auditory discrimination was able to predict awakening with a predictive value of 93% [40].

Since EEG patterns evolve over the first few days, recommendations are to wait at least 24–72 h before making neurologic prognostication judgments. As highlighted previously, EEG prognostic markers for cardiac arrest may also be partly influenced by a confirmation bias, since most studies did not blind the clinicians making WLST decisions to EEG findings [10]. The persistence of malignant patterns over time is of more value than a single reading, so continuous EEG monitoring is recommended. Detecting seizures and status epilepticus are also important as these may be treatable causes of unresponsiveness after cardiac arrest. Finally, it is also important to keep in mind that medications and metabolic disturbances can significantly alter the EEG and affect its reliability [24, 25].

Somatosensory Evoked Potentials (SSEP)

SSEPs are most commonly performed by electrical stimulation of the median nerve at the wrist, creating a signal which is transmitted through the brachial plexus, high spinal cord, brainstem, and thalamus to the somatosensory cortex, where the N20 response (named for the Negative waveform deflection seen after 20 ms) is measured. While SSEPs are less affected by sedation and are most reliable when the patient is paralyzed or sedated, they are affected by peripheral structural lesions (e.g. neuropathy or root avulsion) or other metabolic abnormalities (e.g., electrolyte derangement or hypothermia) that compromise nerve conduction. When performed 72 h after brain injury, bilaterally absent cortical N20 signals is a very reliable predictor of poor neurological outcome, with a false-positive rate of 0.4–1% [24, 25, 29]. A low-voltage N20 response (eg <0.65 uV) may also predict poor neurological outcome [41, 42]. The presence of an N20 response does not necessarily predict a favorable outcome; however, a retrospective study demonstrated that a 12- and 24-h N20 amplitude of 3 uV, when coupled with a benign EEG rhythm, had a 91% sensitivity for favorable functional outcome [43]. These findings need further prospective validation but serve to highlight the significant dearth of prognostic markers of good functional recovery and overemphasis on identifying patients with an unfavorable outcome in existing literature.

Serological Biomarkers

The benefit of serological biomarkers is that they are unaffected by sedation; however, limitations include the need to identify a specific and reliable threshold for prognostication judgments, effect of hypothermia on levels, and possibility of contamination from extracerebral sources [29]. Neuro-specific enolase (NSE) is an enzyme found in neurons and neuroendocrine cells that is released after neuronal injury. Serum levels of NSE typically decrease after 24 h in patients with a good outcome, whereas they peak at 48–72 h in patients with a poor outcome [44]. NSE thresholds associated with poor neurological outcome were >61 ng/mL at 24 h, >46 ng/mL at 48 h, and 35 ng/mL at 72 h after ROSC [45]. Current guidelines recommend serial assessments to ensure that these results are reproducible [24, 25, 29]. While NSE has been extensively studied and demonstrates high reliability in several neurologic prognostication trials, its use remains somewhat limited due to lack of standardization between different laboratories and lack of specific thresholds in updated guidelines as compared to original American Academy of Neurology (AAN) guidelines [46].

Other serological markers of significance include S100B (released by glial cells), tau levels (released due to axonal injury), and microRNAs. However, these markers have not yet been widely adopted and are not included in guidelines for neurologic prognostication.

Future Directions

As neurological prognostication after cardiac arrest remains an area of active ongoing research, practices are likely to continue rapidly evolving in the near future. Advancements in important areas such as expected time to neurological recovery, incorporation of newer technologies into guidelines, and eliminating WLST biases from studies are likely to have a significant impact on neurologic prognostication guidelines in upcoming years (Fig. 37.1).

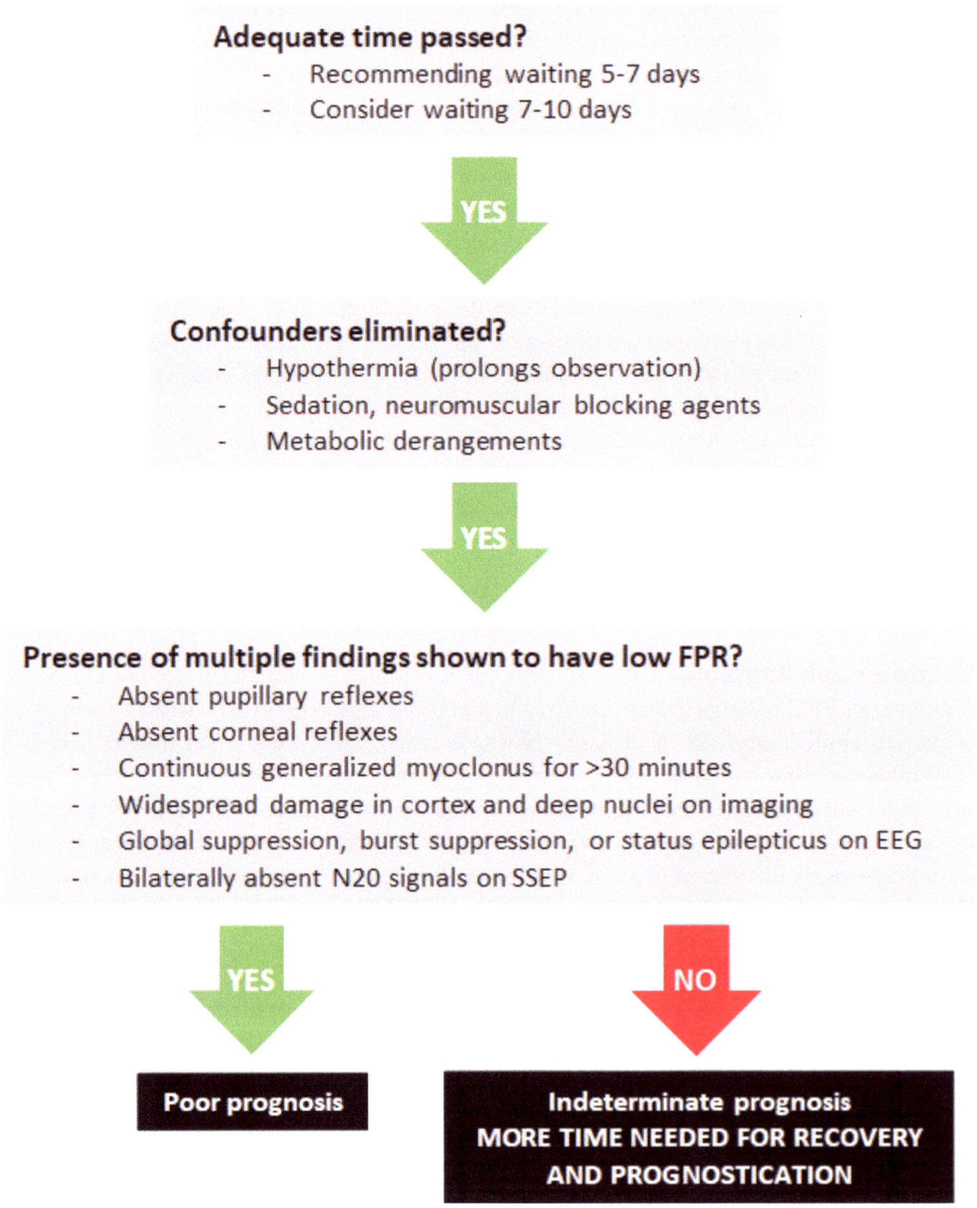

Fig. 37.1 Stepwise approach to neurologic prognostication after hypoxic/ischemic injury

Intracerebral Hemorrhage (ICH)

Background

Intracerebral hemorrhage is the second most common form of acute cerebrovascular injury—comprising 20% of all strokes worldwide [47]—yet is associated with the highest mortality of all stroke types, with limited to no therapeutic interventions that improve functional outcomes. ICH incidence is reported to be 43 per 100,000 person-years, with a steady increase in ICH incidence among patients greater than 75 years in age due to an increase in anticoagulant use [48]. In addition to high mortality, ICH has a high morbidity, particularly in the early months, with an average of 4 years lived with disability, 6 years of life lost, and ten disability adjusted life-years, creating a significant burden on healthcare systems and society [49]. The median mRS in the first months after ICH is reported to be 4 to 5 [4, 5]. There are limited data on future recovery in ICH patients, but a meta-analysis revealed that a range of 12–39% of ICH survivors eventually gained functional independence in the long-term [50]. Importantly, collective statistics for recovery after ICH may be significantly underestimated, given that early WLST is the single most important predictor of mortality in ICH [2, 51]. These factors serve to emphasize the importance of accurate neurologic prognostication, not only for care of the patient with ICH but also for patient selection in clinical trials and development of therapeutic interventions. Commonly measured outcomes in ICH include 30-day mortality, 30, 90, and 180-day mRS, and Glasgow outcome scales (GOS).

Clinical Assessment

By far, the most commonly used prognostication models in ICH are a composite of baseline clinical and radiological severity and are summarized in Table 37.1. It is important to note the survival estimates assigned to these scores describe population averages rather than truly predict prognosis. The ICH score was the first widely adopted tool to predict outcomes in patients with ICH, incorporating the GCS, ICH volume, presence of intraventricular hemorrhage (IVH), infratentorial location, and age [55]. Originally designed to estimate 30-day mortality, the ICH score has been validated to predict 12-month functional outcomes [64]. However, these cohorts were significantly influenced by death due to WLST (20–30%) raising concerns for a confirmation bias widely known as the self-fulfilling prophecy. After excluding patients with early care limitations, the ICH score had significantly lower predictive accuracy for mortality and functional outcomes among maximally treated ICH patients [58, 65].

Alternatives to the ICH score include the FUNC score, which incorporates baseline functional status into the ICH score, and the Essen score, which incorporates the National Institute of Health Stroke Scale (NIHSS); both predict 3-month functional outcomes [56, 57]. The max-ICH score was developed to account for WLST by excluding those that died due to WLST [58]. However, none of the models have gained widespread acceptance in clinical practice and subjective clinician judgment seems to outperform the traditional ICH prognostication models for predicting 3 month outcomes [66].

These existing ICH prognostication models do not incorporate the use of systemic anticoagulation which is a strong predictor of poor outcomes in patients with ICH. Additionally, they only include admission characteristics without accounting for factors such as temporal evolution of the hemorrhage and the impact of treatment interventions and hospital events on survival and recovery. In a recent analysis of clinical trials data, outcome prognostication models incorporating first 30-day hospital complications, procedures, and resolution of ICH and IVH on delayed imaging had significantly improved predictive accuracy with an 11% increase in area-under-curve in ROC analysis, compared to models that used traditional admission ICH and IVH severity characteristics alone [7]. Thus, current AHA guidelines recommend against early WLST (defined as before the second full day of hospitalization) based on an estimate of poor prognosis using admission characteristics [67].

Neuroimaging Markers

In addition to the well-known significance of initial ICH volume, presence of IVH and location of intracerebral hemorrhage, several other radiological factors impact outcomes after ICH but are not traditionally incorporated in ICH prognostication models. Hematoma expansion occurs in 13–32% of ICH patients and is an independent predictor of poor mRS at 90-days [68]. IVH volume has higher prognostic value than the presence of IVH alone, particularly at higher IVH severity [69]. Several IVH grading scales are available to quantify IVH severity and have demonstrated significant associations with functional outcomes [69–73]. Other factors that may also impact outcomes in ICH patients with IVH include hydrocephalus [74] and IVH expansion [75]. The presence of a "spot sign" on CT angiograms, indicating active extravasation of blood, or the "black hole sign," indicating heterogenous density of blood and ongoing hemorrhage, is also associated with poor neurologic outcome [76]. Finally, significant reduction in hematoma volumes is also associated with improved functional outcomes [77]. Other radiologic markers of poor neurologic outcome after ICH may include premorbid leukoariosis [78], peak perihematomal edema [79], and acute ischemic lesions after ICH [80]. In summary, delaying prognostication until after treatment may provide an opportunity to incorporate radiological evolution of hemorrhage, responses to therapy, and secondary neurological injury. Incorporating these factors improves accuracy of prognostication, minimize false positive prediction of poor outcome, and most importantly provide an opportunity for neurological recovery in patients that would have otherwise succumbed to early WLST based on prognostication using only admission characteristics [7].

Serologic and Neurophysiologic Biomarkers

In a recent systematic review of 36 studies, 50 discrete serologic prognostic biomarkers of ICH were identified in the literature [81]. Serologic prognostic markers in ICH include inflammatory, oxidative, and neuron/astrocyte specific biomarkers. The most commonly studied biomarkers include S100 calcium-binding protein B (S100B), white blood cell count, neutrophil/lymphocyte ratio, and copectin [81]. S100B and glial fibrillary astrocyte protein (GFAP), markers of astrocyte degeneration, as well as vascular endothelial growth factor (VEGF), had the highest predictive accuracy (receiver operative curve areas >0.950 for predicting functional outcome) [81]. Limitations of these studies include lack of external cross-validation in independent datasets, lack of blinded assessment of outcomes, and limited reporting of the impact of WLST. Neurophysiologic markers are less well studied in ICH. In one retrospective study of >100 ICH patients undergoing continuous EEG monitoring, 30% developed seizures, which were associated with hematoma expansion. Periodic discharges were independent predictors of poor neurologic outcome after adjusting for baseline ICH severity [82]. Currently, serologic and EEG markers have not been validated for prognostication in ICH.

Future Directions

Medical and surgical treatments of ICH, including timely reduction of ICH and IVH volumes with minimally invasive approaches, treatment of perihematomal edema, prevention of cerebral ischemic injury after ICH, continue to be active areas of research. As such, it will become even more necessary to incorporate responses to ICH treatment, evolution of hemorrhage, and secondary neurological injury as part of neurologic prognostication after ICH [7]. Using only admission characteristics for prognostication and for decisions regarding WLST must be strongly discouraged. Proteomics, while demonstrating promise for ICH prognostication with excellent predictive accuracy, still has several limitations as discussed above which need to be addressed in future studies, including prospective external validation, multivariable analyses incorporating well known predictors of ICH outcome, blinded assessment of outcomes, and exclusion of patients with early WLST.

Ischemic Stroke

Background

Ischemic stroke is infarcted tissue from a sudden reduction or cessation of blood flow to an area of the brain, most frequently due to vascular or cardiac disease. While mortality rates have declined significantly (overall decrease of 13.6% from 2007 to 2017), [83] long-term functional impairment remains common and often debilitating, with >30% of stroke survivors reporting activity and participation limitations after 4 years [84]. Reliable neurologic prognostication after ischemic strokes can be challenging due to the highly heterogenous nature of stroke presentations. Many factors seem to profoundly impact patient outcomes—stroke characteristics (e.g. infarct size, location, and etiology), patient demographics, and comorbidities, which vary considerably between populations and studies. Additionally, significant evolution of acute stroke therapies, including intravenous thrombolysis, standardization of stroke care, and the rapid evolution of endovascular therapy with constantly evolving therapeutic windows using advanced imaging selection, have substantially influenced outcomes over the past several decades. These factors likely all contribute to the poor reliability of clinical judgment alone in predicting death or disability at discharge and 30-day mortality [85].

Clinical Assessment

Many different objective risk scores for ischemic strokes have been developed which seem to outperform clinician judgment, but there has been limited acceptance in clinical practice [86, 87].

Table 37.1 lists several such scores—ASTRAL, DRAGON, PLAN, and iSCORE—as a representative sample of externally validated measures, but several other scores have also been proposed [88]. Common variables used for these scores include baseline NIHSS score, baseline functional status, imaging findings, age, cardiac comorbidities, and serum glucose level. Commonly measured outcomes include mortality and mRS at 30 days, 90 days, and 1 year after stroke.

Serological and Neurophysiological Biomarkers

At present, no serological biomarkers have been validated for prognostication in acute ischemic stroke. Various biomarkers of neuronal injury (such as matrix metalloproteinase 9 and S100B) and inflammation (including TNF-α, IL-6, and

Table 37.1 Existing prediction models in different acute neurological diseases

Disease state	Prediction model	Outcome	Performance	Externally validated
Ischemic stroke	ASTRAL score [52]	mRS ≥3 at 90 days	ROC AUC 0.85	Yes
	DRAGON score [53]	mRS ≤2 at 90 days in IV-thrombolysis patients	ROC AUC 0.80	Yes
	PLAN score [54]	mRS ≥5 at 30 days and at 1 year	ROC AUC 0.86	Yes
	iSCORE [54]	mRS ≥3 at 30 days and at 1 year	ROC AUC 0.83	Yes
ICH	ICH score [55]	30 day mortality	ROC AUC 0.80	Yes
	FUNC score [56]	GOS ≥4 at 90-days		Yes
	ESSEN score [57]	BI 100 at 100 days		Yes
	Max-ICH score [58]	mRS ≥4 at 3 months and at 1 year	ROC AUC 0.81	Yes
SAH	Hunt & Hess Scale [59]	Mortality, GOS	–	Yes
	WFNS scale	Mortality, GOS	–	Yes
	SAFIRE Score [60]	mRS ≥4 at 2 months	ROC AUC 0.82	Yes
	FRESH Score [61]	mRS ≥4 at 1 year	ROC AUC 0.85	Yes
TBI	IMPACT score [62]	GOS ≤3 at 6 months	ROC AUC 0.80	Yes
	CRASH score [63]	Death at 14 days, GOS ≤3 at 6 months	ROC AUC 0.90	Yes

BI barthel index, *GOS* glasgow outcome scale, *mRS* modified Rankin scale, *ROC AUC* receiver-operating characteristic area under the curve

glutamate) seem to be correlated with outcomes [89, 90], but this area remains under investigation and should not be used for clinical prognostication.

While a clear association between clinical seizures (excluding status epilepticus) and outcomes has not been well established the utility of electroencephalography after stroke has been a topic of growing interest. EEG findings such as decreased alpha activity, increased delta-alpha ratio, and lateralized periodic discharges (LPDs) have been correlated with outcomes such as mRS, NIHSS, and Montreal Cognitive Assessment (MoCA) scores [91, 92]. However, EEG has not yet been fully validated in the clinical setting for prognostication after stroke.

Malignant Infarcts and Decompressive Hemicraniectomy

A special consideration is the patient with an acute malignant MCA stroke, generally defined as high NIHSS with imaging showing an infarct size >50% of the MCA territory. These patients are at high risk for developing massive cerebral edema and transtentorial herniation causing brain death, and have a mortality rate of 70–80% [93, 94]. A pooled analysis of three trials—HAMLET, DESTINY, and DECIMAL—demonstrated that decompressive hemicraniectomy reduced this mortality rate to 22% [94]. However, the proportion of patients with mRS 4 at 1-year increased as well, indicating that most of these additional survivors remain unable to care for themselves independently. Although this is traditionally not deemed an acceptable outcome among treating physicians, survivors reported an acceptable quality of life and 80% of the patients and their families reported that despite knowing their current outcome, they would have agreed to decompressive surgery [95]. Such studies highlight the immense value of placing ordinal functional outcome scales, such as mRS, into the right context with respect to patient preferences, beliefs, and personal acceptability.

Future Directions

Given the relatively recent advent of endovascular treatment for acute ischemic strokes, and the substantial impact it has had on stroke outcomes, it becomes more important for prognostication models to account for the degree of revascularization along with other more traditional neurologic prognostic characteristics.

Traumatic Brain Injury (TBI)

Background

TBI is a broad umbrella term for any brain injury caused by an external force and encompasses a wide range of etiologies, presentations, and intracranial pathologies. Mortality is high in moderate and severe TBI patients (patients with loss of consciousness >30 min, amnesia >24 h, GCS <13, ICH, cerebral contusion, penetrating skull injury, brainstem injury, or subarachnoid hemorrhage)—40.3% at 6 months in adults 16–65 years, and 50.0% in the elderly >65 years [96]. In one study of 86 TBI survivors at 8 years, 19.8% remained severely disabled, 46.5% remained moderately disabled, and 33.7% had a good recovery (using the Extended Glasgow Outcome Scale), and the majority reported cognitive impairment [97]. Development of neurologic prognostication markers has been difficult due to the heterogeneity of TBI. That said, it is of substantial clinical importance especially when considering that TBI tends to disproportionately affect young, otherwise healthy individuals compared to other neurological diseases. https://www.liebertpub.com/doi/full/10.1089/neu.2014.3742

Clinical Assessment

The IMPACT score (Table 37.1) was created using a dataset consisting of 8509 patients with moderate and severe TBI from eleven studies [62]. It predicts the likelihood of an unfavorable outcome (death, vegetative state, or severe disability) at 6 months, using age, GCS motor sub-score, and pupillary light reflex. Expanded versions of this score (called the CT and CT + laboratory scores) also incorporate hypoxia, hypotension, CT findings, presence of traumatic SAH or EDH, glucose, and hemoglobin, though addition of these additional variables does not clearly improve the accuracy of prognostication [62, 98].

The CRASH score (Table 37.1) was created using the CRASH trial dataset which consists of 10,008 patients who sustained mild, moderate, and severe TBI [63]. It predicts the likelihood of death at 14 days and unfavorable outcome (death, vegetative state, or severe disability) at 6 months incorporating the IMPACT score but recognizing the significance of any major extracranial injury on survival and outcomes after TBI. Both these scores have been externally validated using several different cohorts of TBI patients; however, these scores do not demonstrate enough reliability to use if neurologic prognostication may affect withdrawal of care decisions.

Neuroimaging Markers

CT findings in TBI include edema and multicompartmental hemorrhages causing midline shift and/or compression of basal cisterns. Two scales incorporating these findings are the Marshall system and the newer Rotterdam score [99]; their ability to provide reliable prognostic value is yet to be confirmed. MRI has the additional capability to detect more subtle changes, particularly white matter structural damage using standard DWI and T2 sequences [100], and more advanced techniques such as diffusion tensor imaging [100] and proton spectroscopy [101]. However, the ability to perform reliable neurologic prognostication using MRI has not yet been established.

Serologic and Neurophysiologic Biomarkers

Elevated serum levels of NSE, S100BB, and GFAP have been shown to be associated with poor outcomes in TBI [102, 103]. Elevated tau protein in both serum and CSF and serum tau protein have also been shown to be correlated with poor neurological outcomes [104, 105]. However, the clinical utility of these biomarkers remains under investigation, and they have not yet been sufficiently validated for use in clinical practice.

While EEG monitoring is frequently utilized in TBI patients, studies have failed to show a clear association between electrographic seizures and mortality [106]. Other EEG patterns, including poor background reactivity, absent sleep patterns, interhemispheric asymmetries, and decreased alpha activity, have been shown to be correlated with poor neurological outcomes [106].

Future Directions

Neurologic prognostication scores in TBI have yet to be validated for clinical use, especially for decisions about WLST. Given the high stakes involved, there is significant interest in developing technological advances in imaging and biomarkers to improve neurologic prognostication in the future.

Aneurysmal Subarachnoid Hemorrhage (SAH)

Background

Aneurysmal SAH, which is defined as bleeding in the subarachnoid space from rupture of an intracranial arterial aneurysm, accounts for 5% of all stroke types, but is associated with the highest pre-hospital mortality and most significant loss of productivity among all stroke-types [107]. The annual worldwide incidence of SAH is 7.9 per 100,000 person-years, with a declining trend in incidence overall, likely related to improved management of risk factors such as hypertension and smoking, as well as early detection and treatment of aneurysms [107]. However, SAH continues to be associated with significant mortality, with a reported case-fatality rate ranging from 31–41% [108], although there is an overall decline in mortality after SAH over past several decades [109, 110]. Regardless, survivors have significant disability, and given that >50% of SAH patients are less than 55 years of age, SAH contributes to 27% of all stroke-related years of life lost before age 65 [107, 111]. Many SAH patients present to the hospital with little early disability (median GCS 13) [112], but suffer multiple hospital complications such as hydrocephalus, early brain injury, elevated intracranial pressure, aneurysmal re-bleeding, seizures and most importantly delayed cerebral ischemia, all of which contribute to significant accumulation of secondary brain injury and increased morbidity. Thus, neurologic prognostication in SAH is often difficult, given significant heterogeneity in baseline injury, neurological and medical complications, significant variability in patient care, and limited understanding of the pathophysiology. However, as in other critical neurologic illnesses, prognostication is an essential part of the clinical care of SAH patients and can have significant influence on patient selection and interpretation in clinical trials and on designing therapeutic interventions that impact factors influencing prognosis.

Clinical and Neuroimaging Assessment

The classic prognostication models in aneurysmal SAH such as Hunt and Hess or World Federation of Neurological Surgeons scale (WFNS) incorporate a combination of physical symptoms, focal neurological deficits, and/or level of alertness such as the GCS (Table 37.1). In the original studies, 100% of Hunt Hess grade V and 70% of grade IV patients died [59]. For decades, this prognostic information was historically used to withhold surgical interventions in high grade patients. Updated outcome information in the last decade has shown that up to 40% of poor grade SAH patients can survive with favorable outcome and moderate functional independence [113]. This is largely due to improvement in aneurysmal repair techniques that have significantly improved survival (number needed to treated [NNT] = 2) and favorable functional outcomes (NNT = 3) in SAH patients [59, 112], Newer outcome models combine classic SAH grading scales with neuroimaging grading of SAH severity to improve predictive accuracy (SAFIRE score; Table 37.1) [60]. Other factors that contribute to long-term outcomes include critical illness score (APACHE score) upon admission, aneurysmal rebleeding, and age, which are incorporated in the FRESH (Table 37.1) score, demonstrating high predictive accuracy (area under curve: 0.90) [61].

Neuroimaging Markers

The most important factor that determines SAH outcome is the amount of blood in the subarachnoid space and ventricles, which determines the risk of delayed cerebral ischemia. This is graded by the modified Fisher scale (ranging from 0 to 4), which has a linear correlation with risk of delayed cerebral ischemia after SAH, and is also shown to predict poor functional outcomes after SAH [114, 115]. Other imaging factors associated with poor outcome after SAH include presence of intraparenchymal hematoma, posterior circulation aneurysm, larger aneurysmal size, and development of new cerebral infarction on delayed imaging [116].

Serologic and Neurophysiologic Biomarkers

Several serological prognostic markers in SAH have been studied. In a systematic review of 55 studies, the predominant biomarkers studied in SAH included neuron and astrocyte specific markers, inflammatory markers, molecular adhesion markers, and markers of systemic injury such as cardiac troponins [117]. The most commonly studied marker with excellent predictive accuracy for short- and long-term SAH outcomes is S100-B—a marker of astrocyte degeneration—in both blood and cerebrospinal fluid [117]. Among inflammatory markers, elevated interleukins (IL-1, IL-6, IL-8, and TNF-alpha) are associated with unfavorable outcome at 3–12 months after SAH [117], and elevated CRP is associated with development of delayed cerebral ischemia [117]. Most of these studies have small sample sizes (<100 patients), are not externally validated, and do not include standardized outcome measures or assess outcomes in a blinded fashion, which limits their interpretation. Among neurophysiologic markers, presence of seizures or nonconvulsive status epilepticus in patients with SAH is known to be associated with poor neurological outcome [118]. Additionally, quantitative analysis of continuous EEG data can predict delayed cerebral ischemia in real time, a complication known to be the primary cause of increased morbidity after SAH [119].

Future Directions

Advancement of our understanding of the pathophysiology in SAH complications is currently an area of active research. As our understanding of these processes improves, we can expect to be able to better predict and treat feared complications such as delayed cerebral ischemia, which can impact outcomes after SAH. Current studies also focus on improving our understanding and prediction of the trajectories of patient-centered outcomes, such as cognitive function, quality of life, and mood/pain disorders, among others, which are important to SAH survivors.

Prevailing Challenges in Neurologic Prognostication

Clinical Course and Outcomes

When communicating neurological prognosis in clinical practice, it is important to recognize the somewhat arbitrary dichotomy between good and poor neurological outcomes, which is commonly used in neurologic prognostication guidelines and studies. In fact, the term "poor neurological outcome" is a moving target and has been variably defined in the literature as a cerebral performance categories (CPC) score of 4 to 5, CPC score of 3 to 5, modified Rankin Scale (mRS) score of 5 to 6, mRS score of 4 to 6, among others. Furthermore, these measures, while useful for broadly categorizing population outcomes, lack the meaningful granularity which can be critical for individual patient cases. Patients, families, and clinicians are sure to have very different perspectives regarding what particular neurological deficits qualify as comprising a poor versus good outcome. Most prognostication studies have largely focused on graded functional outcomes, but other measures may be more meaningful to survivors and their families, including quality of life, cognitive recovery, ability to return to work, behavior, mood, and pain control, among others. Complicating this picture further is the evolution of neurological function over time [120]. Trajectories of recovery over time are not yet well-defined and studies have measured outcomes at heterogeneous time points varying from hospital discharge all the way through 1-year and beyond. Prognostication of outcomes at early time points can often overestimate poor neurological outcome due to the influence of multiple acute confounders (e.g., hospital complications) and failure to consider the benefits of neuro-rehabilitation. Very few studies have prospectively and longitudinally assessed recovery over longer periods of time, and such studies are often affected by selection biases created by WLST.

Other limitations in prognostication models include an overemphasis on prognostication upon admission without incorporation of treatment interventions and hospital complications. In clinical practice, neurologists most often make the determination of prognosis at the end of the acute treatment phase, at which point multiple other factors may be more predictive of outcome than admission characteristics. Thus, it is prudent to consider inclusion of such factors in outcome prediction. Moreover, accounting for the ever-changing landscape of treatment interventions in acute brain injury and their profound relevance to patient outcomes, constant re-assessment of prognostication data is necessary as outcomes are likely to change over time with improved care, as noted in SAH and cardiac arrest survivors with the advent of aneurysm treatment and targeted temperature management [59].

Self-Fulfilling Prophecy

The enormously important concept of the "self-fulfilling prophecy," introduced earlier in this chapter, occurs when clinicians have a pessimistic expectation of a poor neurological outcome which then influences family discussions and treatment plans, ultimately leading to WLST and therefore assuring a poor outcome (i.e. death). This bias has the potential to skew any nonblinded study to produce a greater proportion of poor outcomes, particularly when one considers that the mortality rate in severe neurological injury is largely driven by voluntary withdrawal of life support [121, 122]. The overall results from this study then further feed into clinicians' pessimistic bias, creating a positive-feedback loop and propagating the self-fulfilling prophecy of predicting (and assuring) poor outcomes. Examples of this bias have been discussed extensively in earlier sections.

Culture and Communication

Often the most challenging aspect of neurologic prognostication is navigating family dynamics and discussions. Family members, coming from a range of educational backgrounds and personal experiences, are asked to make exceedingly difficult decisions during a period of high emotional stress based on information and data that is often of unclear certainty. It is of utmost importance to communicate clearly and compassionately when discussing results with family members and to be aware of the different values held by families when discussing continued medical care. Significant discordance exists between surrogate decision-makers and physicians, particularly with respect to differences in beliefs and understanding [123]. This discordance may be due to overemphasis of predicting mortality and poor outcome rather than recovery and good outcome. Poor outcome models may help with patient selection in clinical trials and alleviate futile care, but often they do not have significant utility when answering important questions for patients and their families in daily clinical practice, leading to significant uncertainty among decision-makers. However, disclosing this prognostic uncertainty may be more acceptable to surrogate decision-makers/families and patients than physicians believe [124]. Acknowledging such uncertainty in prognosis, pursuing early aggressive treatment, and avoiding WLST within the first 72 h are some strategies suggested for navigating goals of care discussions and communicating prognosis with patients and families [125] (Fig. 37.2).

Future Directions

Significant innovation in the field of neurologic prognostication is underway with the advent of artificial intelligence (AI) and machine learning, advanced neuroimaging modalities, and proteomics. These technological developments have the ability to improve the accuracy of prognostication and eliminate biases created by provider preferences and beliefs if properly designed and executed. Automated

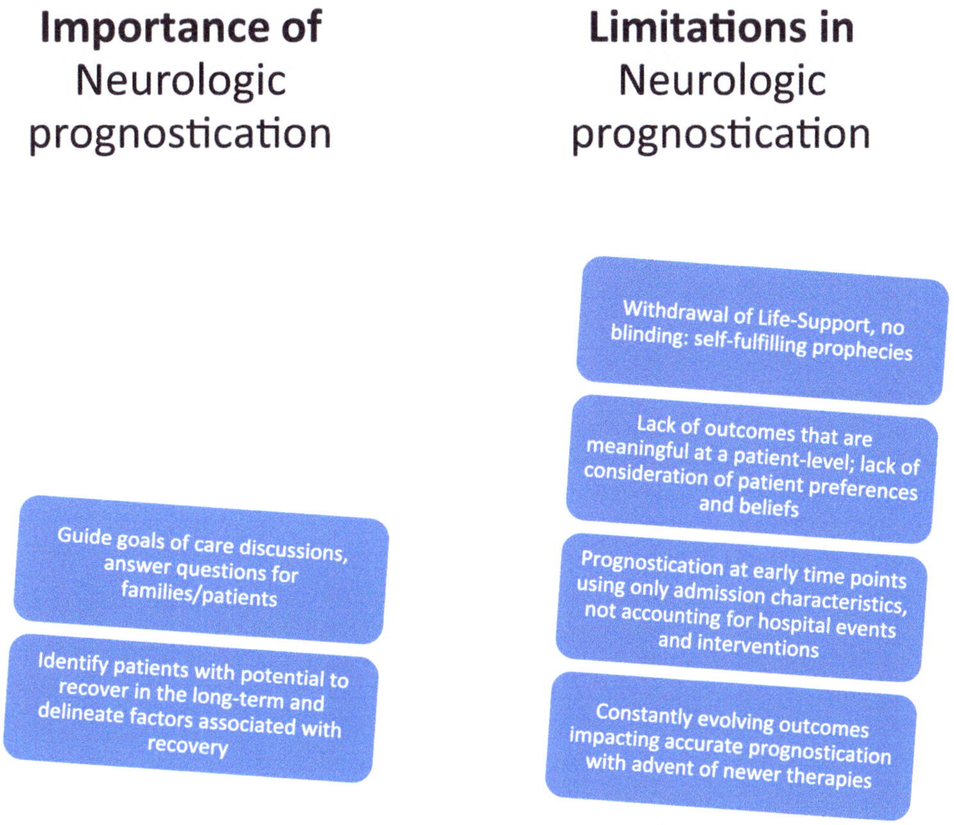

Fig. 37.2 Weighing the importance of neurologic prognostication against the existing limitations in neurologic prognostication practices

machine-learning models have been shown to demonstrate significantly improved prediction accuracy over traditional logistic regression for survival and functional outcomes in cardiac arrest [126], intracerebral hemorrhage [127], subarachnoid hemorrhage [128], and traumatic brain injury [129]. Additionally, machine learning can identify individual phenotypes of patients that account for the variability in response to therapies and outcomes [130]. These machine learning techniques can be applied to neuroimaging, EEG, and other physiologic data to identify novel predictors of recovery. For example, EEG reactivity and covert consciousness may be detected with such machine-learning algorithms before overt clinical motor recovery [39, 131]. Machine learning-based techniques can be applied to identify white matter hyperintensities and intrinsic functional connectivity associated with outcome and functional recovery in brain injury patients [132, 133]. As this field matures, careful attention will be required to ensure the quality of data used for machine learning is held to rigorous standards prior to widespread clinical adoption [16].

Advanced neuroimaging techniques such as MR-based diffusion tensor imaging, functional MRI, convolutional neural networks, and AI-based morphometric/volumetric analysis and connectomes have great promise in more precise and personalized outcome prognostication [134]. Ascending arousal network connectivity identified by high angular resolution diffusion imaging may also have significance in predicting arousal from a comatose state [135]. Personalized connectome mapping may have applicability in predicting arousal and designing therapies for arousal that target-specific neural networks [136].

Proteomics, the study of proteins expressed by an organism, permits the identification of novel biomarkers that may have prognostic significance. In cardiac arrest survivors, poor neurological outcome was predicted by novel biomarkers involved in well-known pathophysiologic pathways for secondary brain injury (such as alpha-enolase and 14-3-3 protein), with better accuracy than standard models [137]. Similarly, fluid and CSF proteomic profiling studies in severe TBI patients identified multiple neuroinflammatory markers that were associated with long-term outcomes. Going forward, it will become increasingly important to consider that biomarker levels that are physiologically correlated with the degree of nonspecific brain tissue injury may be less predictive of functional outcome than biomarker levels which are correlated with injury to specific regions of the brain, such as the brainstem or other highly eloquent regions.

In addition to improving accuracy of prognostication, another area of much needed research is individualizing prognostic communications based on individual patient preferences [138]. In addition, standardizing prognostic communications with the help of decision aids may help improve the discordance between physicians and surrogates [139, 140].

The implications of neurologic prognostication are immense, and improving the accuracy and reliability of prognostication as well as its communication can by itself impart survival benefit, improve neurological outcomes, and advance medical science research. While neurologic prognostication must be based on rigorous science, it is important to acknowledge that the "art" in neurologic prognostication may in fact be heavily based on biases. It is imperative to acknowledge the limitations in our practices and pivot to objective and multifaceted methods, including complete knowledge of the full extent of the natural history of the disease and injury, study of an amalgamation of properly validated predictors, AI-based algorithms, advanced neuroimaging, proteomics, individual patient preferences, and empathetic communications in accordance with the standards of medical ethics.

References

1. Stachulski F, Siegerink B, Bosel J. Dying in the neurointensive care unit after withdrawal of life-sustaining therapy: associations of advance directives and health-care proxies with timing and treatment intensity. J Intensive Care Med. 2021;36(4):451–8. https://doi.org/10.1177/0885066620906795.
2. Becker KJ, Baxter AB, Cohen WA, et al. Withdrawal of support in intracerebral hemorrhage may lead to self-fulfilling prophecies. Neurology. 2001;56(6):766–72. https://doi.org/10.1212/wnl.56.6.766.
3. Kowalski RG, Hammond FM, Weintraub AH, et al. Recovery of consciousness and functional outcome in moderate and severe traumatic brain injury. JAMA Neurol. 2021;78(5):548–57. https://doi.org/10.1001/jamaneurol.2021.0084.
4. Sreekrishnan A, Leasure AC, Shi FD, et al. Functional improvement among intracerebral hemorrhage (ICH) survivors up to 12 months post-injury. Neurocrit Care. 2017;27(3):326–33. https://doi.org/10.1007/s12028-017-0425-4.
5. Oie LR, Madsbu MA, Solheim O, et al. Functional outcome and survival following spontaneous intracerebral hemorrhage: A retrospective population-based study. Brain Behav. 2018;8(10):e01113. https://doi.org/10.1002/brb3.1113.
6. Shah V, McBee N, Yenokyan G, et al. The one year fate of day 30 poor outcome survivors of large intracerebral and intraventricular hemorrhage. Int J Stroke. 2020;15(1_Suppl):47.
7. Shah VA, Thompson RE, Yenokyan G, et al. One-year outcome trajectories and factors associated with functional recovery among survivors of intracerebral and intraventricular hemorrhage with initial severe disability. Arch Neurol (Chicago). 2022;79(9):856–68. https://doi.org/10.1001/jamaneurol.2022.1991.
8. Elmer J, Torres C, Aufderheide TP, et al. Association of early withdrawal of life-sustaining therapy for perceived neurological prognosis with mortality after cardiac arrest. Resuscitation. 2016;102:127–35. https://doi.org/10.1016/j.resuscitation.2016.01.016.
9. Kalanuria AA, Geocadin RG. Early prognostication in acute brain damage: where is the evidence? Curr Opin Crit Care. 2013;19(2):113–22. https://doi.org/10.1097/MCC.0b013e32835eba56.
10. Bronder J, Cho S, Geocadin R, Ritzl E. Revisiting EEG as part of the multidisciplinary approach to post-cardiac arrest care and prognostication: A review. Resusc Plus. 2022;9:100189.
11. Sawyer KN, Camp-Rogers TR, Kotini-Shah P, et al. Sudden cardiac arrest survivorship: A scientific statement from the american heart association. Circulation. 2020;141(12):e654–85. https://doi.org/10.1161/CIR.0000000000000747.
12. Fernando SM, Tran A, Cheng W, et al. Pre-arrest and intra-arrest prognostic factors associated with survival after in-hospital cardiac arrest: systematic review and meta-analysis. BMJ. 2019;367:l6373. https://doi.org/10.1136/bmj.l6373.
13. Xue JK, Leng QY, Gao YZ, et al. Factors influencing outcomes after cardiopulmonary resuscitation in emergency department. World J Emerg Med. 2013;4(3):183–9. https://doi.org/10.5847/wjem.j.1920-8642.2013.03.005.
14. Rey A, Rossetti A, Miroz J, Eckert P, Oddo M. Late awakening in survivors of postanoxic coma:Early neurophysiologic predictors and associationwith ICU and long-term neurologic recovery. Crit Care Med. 2019;47:85–92.
15. Elmer J, ea. Long-term survival benefit from treatment at a specialty center after cardiac arrest. Resuscitation. 2016;108:48–53.
16. Geocadin RG, Callaway CW, Fink EL, et al. Standards for studies of neurological prognostication in comatose survivors of cardiac arrest: A scientific statement from the american heart association. Circulation. 2019;140(9):e517–42. https://doi.org/10.1161/CIR.0000000000000702.
17. Rasmussen TP, Bullis TC, Girotra S. Targeted temperature management for treatment of cardiac arrest. Curr Treat Options Cardiovasc Med. 2020;22(11):39. https://doi.org/10.1007/s11936-020-00846-6.
18. Lascarrou JB, Merdji H, Le Gouge A, et al. Targeted temperature management for cardiac arrest with nonshockable rhythm. N Engl J Med. 2019;381(24):2327–37. https://doi.org/10.1056/NEJMoa1906661.
19. Donnino MW, Andersen LW, Berg KM, et al. Temperature management after cardiac arrest: an advisory statement by the advanced life support task force of the international liaison committee on resuscitation and the american heart association emergency cardiovascular care committee and the council on cardiopulmonary, critical care, perioperative and resuscitation. Resuscitation. 2016;98:97–104. https://doi.org/10.1016/j.resuscitation.2015.09.396.
20. Ponz I, Lopez-de-Sa E, Armada E, et al. Influence of the temperature on the moment of awakening in patients treated with therapeutic hypothermia after cardiac arrest. Resuscitation. 2016;103:32–6. https://doi.org/10.1016/j.resuscitation.2016.03.017.
21. Shah V, Geocadin R. Therapeutic hypothermia in neurocritical care. In: Nelson SE, Nyquist PA, editors. *Neurointensive care unit: Clinical practice and organization*. Cham: Humana; 2020. p. 57–72.
22. Cronberg T. Should postanoxic status epilepticus be treated agressively? Yes! J Clin Neurophysiol. 2015;32(6):449–51. https://doi.org/10.1097/WNP.0000000000000020.
23. Dragancea I, Backman S, Westhall E, Rundgren M, Friberg H, Cronberg T. Outcome following postanoxic status epilepticus in patients with targeted temperature management after cardiac

arrest. Epilepsy Behav. 2015;49:173–7. https://doi.org/10.1016/j.yebeh.2015.04.043.
24. Callaway CW, Donnino MW, Fink EL, et al. Part 8: post-cardiac arrest care: 2015 american heart association guidelines update for cardiopulmonary resuscitation and emergency cardiovascular care. Circulation. 2015;132(18 Suppl 2):465. https://doi.org/10.1161/CIR.0000000000000262.
25. Nolan JP, Sandroni C, Bottiger BW, et al. European resuscitation council and european society of intensive care medicine guidelines 2021: post-resuscitation care. Resuscitation. 2021;161:220–69. https://doi.org/10.1007/s00134-021-06368-4.
26. Paul M, Bougouin W, Geri G, et al. Delayed awakening after cardiac arrest: prevalence and risk factors in the parisian registry. Intensive Care Med. 2016;42(7):1128–36. https://doi.org/10.1007/s00134-016-4349-9.
27. Tsai M, Chen W, Chen W, et al. Should we prolong the observation period for neurological recovery after cardiac arrest? Crit Care Med. 2022;50(3):389–97. https://doi.org/10.1097/CCM.0000000000005264.
28. Schefold JC, Storm C, Kruger A, Ploner CJ, Hasper D. The Glasgow coma score is a predictor of good outcome in cardiac arrest patients treated with therapeutic hypothermia. Resuscitation. 2009;80(6):658–61. https://doi.org/10.1016/j.resuscitation.2009.03.006.
29. Sandroni C, D'Arrigo S, Nolan JP. Prognostication after cardiac arrest. Crit Care. 2018;22(1):150–7. https://doi.org/10.1186/s13054-018-2060-7.
30. Riker RR, Sawyer ME, Fischman VG, et al. Neurological pupil index and pupillary light reflex by pupillometry predict outcome early after cardiac arrest. Neurocrit Care. 2020;32(1):152–61. https://doi.org/10.1007/s12028-019-00717-4.
31. Wang CH, Wu CY, Liu CC, et al. Neuroprognostic accuracy of quantitative versus standard pupillary light reflex for adult post-cardiac arrest patients: A systematic review and meta-analysis. Crit Care Med. 2021;49(10):1790–9. https://doi.org/10.1097/CCM.0000000000005045.
32. Oddo M, Sandroni C, Citerio G, et al. Quantitative versus standard pupillary light reflex for early prognostication in comatose cardiac arrest patients: an international prospective multicenter double-blinded study. Intensive Care Med. 2018;44(12):2102–11. https://doi.org/10.1007/s00134-018-5448-6.
33. Golan E, Barrett K, Alali AS, et al. Predicting neurologic outcome after targeted temperature management for cardiac arrest: systematic review and meta-analysis. Crit Care Med. 2014;42(8):1919–30. https://doi.org/10.1097/CCM.0000000000000335.
34. Elmer J, Rittenberger JC, Faro J, et al. Clinically distinct electroencephalographic phenotypes of early myoclonus after cardiac arrest. Ann Neurol. 2016;80(2):175–84. https://doi.org/10.1002/ana.24697.
35. Jeon CH, Park JS, Lee JH, et al. Comparison of brain computed tomography and diffusion-weighted magnetic resonance imaging to predict early neurologic outcome before target temperature management comatose cardiac arrest survivors. Resuscitation. 2017;118:21–6. https://doi.org/10.1016/j.resuscitation.2017.06.021.
36. Wijman CA, Mlynash M, Caulfield AF, et al. Prognostic value of brain diffusion-weighted imaging after cardiac arrest. Ann Neurol. 2009;65(4):394–402. https://doi.org/10.1002/ana.21632.
37. Choi SP, Park KN, Park HK, et al. Diffusion-weighted magnetic resonance imaging for predicting the clinical outcome of comatose survivors after cardiac arrest: A cohort study. Crit Care. 2010;14(1):R17. https://doi.org/10.1186/cc8874.
38. Muhlhofer W, Szaflarski JP. Prognostic value of EEG in patients after cardiac arrest-an updated review. Curr Neurol Neurosci Rep. 2018;18(4):16. https://doi.org/10.1007/s11910-018-0826-6.
39. Claassen J, Doyle K, Matory A, et al. Detection of brain activation in unresponsive patients with acute brain injury. N Engl J Med. 2019;380(26):2497–505. https://doi.org/10.1056/NEJMoa1812757.
40. Tzovara A, Rossetti AO, Juan E, et al. Prediction of awakening from hypothermic postanoxic coma based on auditory discrimination. Ann Neurol. 2016;79(5):748–57. https://doi.org/10.1002/ana.24622.
41. Endisch C, Storm C, Ploner CJ, Leithner C. Amplitudes of SSEP and outcome in cardiac arrest survivors: A prospective cohort study. Neurology. 2015;85(20):1752–60. https://doi.org/10.1212/WNL.0000000000002123.
42. Carrai R, Scarpino M, Lolli F, et al. Early-SEPs' amplitude reduction is reliable for poor-outcome prediction after cardiac arrest? Acta Neurol Scand. 2019;139(2):158–65. https://doi.org/10.1111/ane.13030.
43. Scarpino M, et al. SSEP amplitude accurately predicts both good and poor neurological outcome early after cardiac arrest; a post-hoc analysis of the ProNeCA multicentre study. Resuscitation. 2021;163:162–71.
44. Streitberger KJ, Leithner C, Wattenberg M, et al. Neuron-specific enolase predicts poor outcome after cardiac arrest and targeted temperature management: A multicenter study on 1,053 patients. Crit Care Med. 2017;45(7):1145–51. https://doi.org/10.1097/CCM.0000000000002335.
45. Stammet P, Collignon O, Hassager C, et al. Neuron-specific enolase as a predictor of death or poor neurological outcome after out-of-hospital cardiac arrest and targeted temperature management at 33 degrees C and 36 degrees C. J Am Coll Cardiol. 2015;65(19):2104–14. https://doi.org/10.1016/j.jacc.2015.03.538.
46. Wijdicks EF, Hijdra A, Young GB, Bassetti CL, Wiebe S. Quality standards Subcommittee of the American Academy of neurology. Practice parameter: prediction of outcome in comatose survivors after cardiopulmonary resuscitation (an evidence-based review): report of the quality standards subcommittee of the american academy of neurology. Neurology. 2006;67(2):203–10. https://doi.org/10.1212/01.wnl.0000227183.21314.cd.
47. Feigin VL, Lawes CM, Bennett DA, Barker-Collo SL, Parag V. Worldwide stroke incidence and early case fatality reported in 56 population-based studies: A systematic review. Lancet Neurol. 2009;8(4):355–69. https://doi.org/10.1016/S1474-4422(09)70025-0.
48. Lioutas VA, Beiser AS, Aparicio HJ, et al. Assessment of incidence and risk factors of intracerebral hemorrhage among participants in the Framingham heart study between 1948 and 2016. JAMA Neurol. 2020;77(10):1252–60. https://doi.org/10.1001/jamaneurol.2020.1512.
49. Haupenthal D, Kuramatsu JB, Volbers B, et al. Disability-adjusted life-years associated with intracerebral hemorrhage and secondary injury. JAMA Netw Open. 2021;4(7):e2115859. https://doi.org/10.1001/jamanetworkopen.2021.15859.
50. van Asch C, Luitse M, Rinkel G, van der Tweel I, Algra A, Klijn CJM. Incidence, case fatality, and functional outcome ofintracerebral haemorrhage over time, according to age, sex,and ethnic origin: A systematic review and meta-analysis. Lancet Neurol. 2010;9:167–76.
51. Zahuranec DB, Brown DL, Lisabeth LD, et al. Early care limitations independently predict mortality after intracerebral hemorrhage. Neurology. 2007;68(20):1651–7.
52. Ntaios G, Faouzi M, Ferrari J, Lang W, Vemmos K, Michel P. An integer-based score to predict functional outcome in acute ischemic stroke: the ASTRAL score. Neurology. 2012;78(24):1916–22. https://doi.org/10.1212/WNL.0b013e318259e221.
53. Strbian D, Meretoja A, Ahlhelm FJ, et al. Predicting outcome of IV thrombolysis-treated ischemic stroke patients: the DRAGON

score. Neurology. 2012;78(6):427–32. https://doi.org/10.1212/WNL.0b013e318245d2a9.
54. Saposnik G, Kapral MK, Liu Y, et al. IScore: A risk score to predict death early after hospitalization for an acute ischemic stroke. Circulation. 2011;123(7):739–49. https://doi.org/10.1161/CIRCULATIONAHA.110.983353.
55. Hemphill JC 3rd, Bonovich DC, Besmertis L, Manley GT, Johnston SC. The ICH score: A simple, reliable grading scale for intracerebral hemorrhage. Stroke. 2001;32(4):891–7.
56. Rost NS, Smith EE, Chang Y, et al. Prediction of functional outcome in patients with primary intracerebral hemorrhage: the FUNC score. Stroke. 2008;39(8):2304–9. https://doi.org/10.1161/STROKEAHA.107.512202.
57. Weimar C, Benemann J, Diener HC. German stroke study collaboration. Development and validation of the Essen intracerebral haemorrhage score. J Neurol Neurosurg Psychiatry. 2006;77(5):601–5. https://doi.org/10.1136/jnnp.2005.081117.
58. Sembill JA, Gerner ST, Volbers B, et al. Severity assessment in maximally treated ICH patients: The max-ICH score. Neurology. 2017;89(5):423–31. https://doi.org/10.1212/WNL.0000000000004174.
59. Konczalla J, Seifert V, Beck J, et al. Outcome after hunt and hess grade V subarachnoid hemorrhage: A comparison of pre-coiling era (1980-1995) versus post-ISAT era (2005-2014). J Neurosurg. 2018;128(1):100–10. https://doi.org/10.3171/2016.8.JNS161075.
60. van Donkelaar CE, Bakker NA, Birks J, et al. Prediction of outcome after aneurysmal subarachnoid hemorrhage. Stroke. 2019;50(4):837–44. https://doi.org/10.1161/STROKEAHA.118.023902.
61. Witsch J, Frey HP, Patel S, et al. Prognostication of long-term outcomes after subarachnoid hemorrhage: the FRESH score. Ann Neurol. 2016;80(1):46–58. https://doi.org/10.1002/ana.24675.
62. Marmarou A, Lu J, Butcher I, et al. IMPACT database of traumatic brain injury: design and description. J Neurotrauma. 2007;24(2):239–50. https://doi.org/10.1089/neu.2006.0036.
63. MRC CRASH Trial Collaborators, Perel P, Arango M, et al. Predicting outcome after traumatic brain injury: practical prognostic models based on large cohort of international patients. BMJ. 2008;336(7641):425–9. https://doi.org/10.1136/bmj.39461.643438.25.
64. Hemphill JC 3rd, Farrant M, Neill TA Jr. Prospective validation of the ICH score for 12-month functional outcome. Neurology. 2009;73(14):1088–94. https://doi.org/10.1212/WNL.0b013e3181b8b332.
65. McCracken DJ, Lovasik BP, McCracken CE, et al. The intracerebral hemorrhage score: A self-fulfilling prophecy? Neurosurgery. 2019;84(3):741–8. https://doi.org/10.1093/neuros/nyy193.
66. Hwang DY, Dell CA, Sparks MJ, et al. Clinician judgment vs formal scales for predicting intracerebral hemorrhage outcomes. Neurology. 2016;86(2):126–33. https://doi.org/10.1212/WNL.0000000000002266.
67. Hemphill JC 3rd, Greenberg SM, Anderson CS, et al. Guidelines for the management of spontaneous intracerebral hemorrhage: A guideline for healthcare professionals from the american heart association/american stroke association. Stroke. 2015;46(7):2032–60. https://doi.org/10.1161/STR.0000000000000069.
68. Dowlatshahi D, Demchuk AM, Flaherty ML, et al. Defining hematoma expansion in intracerebral hemorrhage: relationship with patient outcomes. Neurology. 2011;76(14):1238–44. https://doi.org/10.1212/WNL.0b013e3182143317.
69. Trifan G, Arshi B, Testai FD. Intraventricular hemorrhage severity as a predictor of outcome in intracerebral hemorrhage. Front Neurol. 2019;10:217. https://doi.org/10.3389/fneur.2019.00217.
70. Hallevi H, Dar NS, Barreto AD, et al. The IVH score: A novel tool for estimating intraventricular hemorrhage volume: Clinical and research implications. Crit Care Med. 2009;37(3):969–74, e1. https://doi.org/10.1097/CCM.0b013e318198683a.
71. Morgan TC, Dawson J, Spengler D, et al. The modified graeb score: an enhanced tool for intraventricular hemorrhage measurement and prediction of functional outcome. Stroke. 2013;44(3):635–41. https://doi.org/10.1161/STROKEAHA.112.670653.
72. Hansen BM, Morgan TC, Betz JF, et al. Intraventricular extension of supratentorial intracerebral hemorrhage: The modified graeb scale improves outcome prediction in lund stroke register. Neuroepidemiology. 2016;46(1):43–50. https://doi.org/10.1159/000442575.
73. Graeb DA, Robertson WD, Lapointe JS, Nugent RA, Harrison PB. Computed tomographic diagnosis of intraventricular hemorrhage. Etiology and prognosis. Radiology. 1982;143(1):91–6. https://doi.org/10.1148/radiology.143.1.6977795.
74. Bhattathiri PS, Gregson B, Prasad KS, Mendelow AD, Investigators STICH. Intraventricular hemorrhage and hydrocephalus after spontaneous intracerebral hemorrhage: results from the STICH trial. Acta Neurochir Suppl. 2006;96:65–8.
75. Roh DJ, Asonye IS, Carvalho Poyraz F, et al. Intraventricular hemorrhage expansion in the CLEAR III trial: A post hoc exploratory analysis. Stroke. 2022;53:1847. https://doi.org/10.1161/STROKEAHA.121.037438.
76. Sporns P, Kemmling A, Schwake M, et al. Triage of 5 noncontrast computed tomography markers and spot sign for outcome prediction after intracerebral hemorrhage. Stroke. 2018;49(10):2317–22. https://doi.org/10.1161/STROKEAHA.118.021625.
77. Polster SP, et al. Intracerebral hemorrhage volume reduction and timing of intervention versus functional benefit and survival in the MISTIE III and STICH trials. Neurosurgery. 2021;88(5):961–70.
78. Caprio FZ, Maas MB, Rosenberg NF, et al. Leukoaraiosis on magnetic resonance imaging correlates with worse outcomes after spontaneous intracerebral hemorrhage. Stroke. 2013;44(3):642–6. https://doi.org/10.1161/STROKEAHA.112.676890.
79. Ironside N, Chen C, Ding D, Mayer S, Connolly E. Perihematomal edema after spontaneous intracerebral hemorrhage. Stroke (1970). 2019;50(6):1626–33. https://doi.org/10.1161/STROKEAHA.119.024965.
80. Murthy SB, Cho SM, Gupta A, et al. A pooled analysis of diffusion-weighted imaging lesions in patients with acute intracerebral hemorrhage. JAMA Neurol. 2020;77(11):1390–7.
81. Troiani Z, Ascanio L, Rossitto CP, et al. Prognostic utility of serum biomarkers in intracerebral hemorrhage: A systematic review. Neurorehabil Neural Repair. 2021;35(11):946–59.
82. Claassen J, Jette N, Mayer SA, et al. Electrographic seizures and periodic discharges after intracerebral hemorrhage. Neurology. 2007;69(13):1356–65. https://doi.org/10.1212/01.wnl.0000281664.02615.6c.
83. Virani S, Alonso A, Benjamin E, et al. Heart disease and stroke statistics—2020 update: A report from the american heart association. Circulation (New York, N.Y.). 2020;141(9):e139–51. https://doi.org/10.1161/CIR.0000000000000757.
84. Winstein C, Stein J, Arena R, et al. Guidelines for adult stroke rehabilitation and recovery: A guideline for healthcare professionals from the american heart association/american stroke association. Stroke. 2016;47(6):e98–e169. https://doi.org/10.1161/STR.0000000000000098.
85. Saposnik G, Cote R, Mamdani M, et al. JURaSSiC: Accuracy of clinician vs. risk score prediction of ischemic stroke outcomes. Neurology. 2013;81(5):448–55. https://doi.org/10.1212/WNL.0b013e31829d874e.
86. Matsumoto K, Nohara Y, Soejima H, Yonehara T, Nakashima N, Kamouchi M. Stroke prognostic scores and data-driven prediction of clinical outcomes after acute ischemic stroke.

Stroke. 2020;51(5):1477–83. https://doi.org/10.1161/STROKEAHA.119.027300.
87. Drozdowska BA, Singh S, Quinn TJ. Thinking about the future: A review of prognostic scales used in acute stroke. Front Neurol. 2019;10:274. https://doi.org/10.3389/fneur.2019.00274.
88. Gao M, Wang J, Saposnik G. The art and science of stroke outcome prognostication. Stroke (1970). 2020;51(5):1358–60. https://doi.org/10.1161/STROKEAHA.120.028980.
89. Jickling GC, Sharp FR. Blood biomarkers of ischemic stroke. Neurotherapeutics. 2011;8(3):349–60. https://doi.org/10.1007/s13311-011-0050-4.
90. Saenger AK, Christenson RH. Stroke biomarkers: Progress and challenges for diagnosis, prognosis, differentiation, and treatment. Clin chemistry (Baltimore, Md.). 2010;56(1):21–33. https://doi.org/10.1373/clinchem.2009.133801.
91. Doerrfuss JI, Kilic T, Ahmadi M, Holtkamp M, Weber JE. Quantitative and qualitative EEG as a prediction tool for outcome and complications in acute stroke patients. Clin EEG Neurosci. 2020;51(2):121–9.
92. Bentes C, Peralta AR, Viana P, et al. Quantitative EEG and functional outcome following acute ischemic stroke. Clin Neurophysiol. 2018;129(8):1680–7. https://doi.org/10.1016/j.clinph.2018.05.021.
93. Hacke W, Schwab S, Horn M, Spranger M, De Georgia M, von Kummer R. 'Malignant' middle cerebral artery territory infarction: clinical course and prognostic signs. Arch Neurol. 1996;53(4):309–15. https://doi.org/10.1001/archneur.1996.00550040037012.
94. Vahedi K, Hofmeijer J, Juettler E, et al. Early decompressive surgery in malignant infarction of the middle cerebral artery: A pooled analysis of three randomised controlled trials. Lancet Neurol. 2007;6(3):215–22. https://doi.org/10.1016/S1474-4422(07)70036-4.
95. Woertgen C, Erban P, Rothoerl RD, Bein T, Horn M, Brawanski A. Quality of life after decompressive craniectomy in patients suffering from supratentorial brain ischemia. Acta Neurochir. 2004;146(7):691–5. https://doi.org/10.1007/s00701-004-0280-x.
96. Flaada JT, Leibson CL, Mandrekar JN, et al. Relative risk of mortality after traumatic brain injury: A population-based study of the role of age and injury severity. J Neurotrauma. 2007;24(3):435–45. https://doi.org/10.1089/neu.2006.0119.
97. Ruet A, Bayen E, Jourdan C, et al. A detailed overview of long-term outcomes in severe traumatic brain injury eight years post-injury. Front Neurol. 2019;10:120. https://doi.org/10.3389/fneur.2019.00120.
98. Dijkland SA, Foks KA, Polinder S, et al. Prognosis in moderate and severe traumatic brain injury: A systematic review of contemporary models and validation studies. J Neurotrauma. 2020;37(1):1–13. https://doi.org/10.1089/neu.2019.6401.
99. Maas AI, Hukkelhoven CW, Marshall LF, Steyerberg EW. Prediction of outcome in traumatic brain injury with computed tomographic characteristics: A comparison between the computed tomographic classification and combinations of computed tomographic predictors. Neurosurgery. 2005;57(6):1173–82. https://doi.org/10.1227/01.neu.0000186013.63046.6b.
100. Richter S, Winzeck S, Kornaropoulos EN, et al. Neuroanatomical substrates and symptoms associated with magnetic resonance imaging of patients with mild traumatic brain injury. JAMA Netw Open. 2021;4(3):e210994. https://doi.org/10.1001/jamanetworkopen.2021.0994.
101. Garnett MR, Blamire AM, Corkill RG, Cadoux-Hudson TA, Rajagopalan B, Styles P. Early proton magnetic resonance spectroscopy in normal-appearing brain correlates with outcome in patients following traumatic brain injury. Brain. 2000;123(Pt 10):2046–54. https://doi.org/10.1093/brain/123.10.2046.
102. Chabok SY, Moghadam AD, Saneei Z, Amlashi FG, Leili EK, Amiri ZM. Neuron-specific enolase and S100BB as outcome predictors in severe diffuse axonal injury. J Trauma Acute Care Surg. 2012;72(6):1654–7. https://doi.org/10.1097/TA.0b013e318246887e.
103. Vos PE, Lamers KJB, Heniks JCM, et al. Glial and neuronal proteins in serum predict outcome after severe traumatic brain injury. Neurology. 2004;62(8):1303–10. https://doi.org/10.1212/01.WNL.0000120550.00643.DC.
104. Liliang P, Liang C, Weng H, et al. T proteins in serum predict outcome after severe traumatic brain injury. J Surg Res. 2010;160(2):302–7. https://doi.org/10.1016/j.jss.2008.12.022.
105. Öst M, Nylen K, Csajbok L, et al. Initial CSF total tau correlates with 1-year outcome in patients with traumatic brain injury. Neurology. 2006;67(9):1600–4. https://doi.org/10.1212/01.wnl.0000242732.06714.0f.
106. Wallace BE, Wagner AK, Wagner EP, McDeavitt JT. A history and review of quantitative electroencephalography in traumatic brain injury. J Head Trauma Rehabil. 2001;16(2):165–90. https://doi.org/10.1097/00001199-200104000-00006.
107. Etminan N, Chang H, Hackenberg K, et al. Worldwide incidence of aneurysmal subarachnoid hemorrhage according to region, time period, blood pressure, and smoking prevalence in the population: A systematic review and meta-analysis. JAMA Neurol. 2019;76(5):588–97. https://doi.org/10.1001/jamaneurol.2019.0006.
108. Mahlamäki K, Rautalin I, Korja M. Case fatality rates of subarachnoid hemorrhage are decreasing with substantial between-country variation: A systematic review of population-based studies between 1980 and 2020. Neuroepidemiology. 2022;56:402–12. https://doi.org/10.1159/000526983.
109. Nieuwkamp DJ, Setz LE, Algra A, Linn FH, de Rooij NK, Rinkel GJ. Changes in case fatality of aneurysmal subarachnoid haemorrhage over time, according to age, sex, and region: A meta-analysis. Lancet Neurol. 2009;8(7):635–42. https://doi.org/10.1016/S1474-4422(09)70126-7.
110. Lovelock CE, GJE R, Rothwell PM. Time trends in outcome of subarachnoid hemorrhage: population-based study and systematic review. Neurology. 2010;74(19):1494–501. https://doi.org/10.1212/WNL.0b013e3181dd42b3.
111. Al-Khindi T, Macdonald RL, Schweizer TA. Cognitive and functional outcome after aneurysmal subarachnoid hemorrhage. Stroke (1970). 2010;41(8):e519–36. https://doi.org/10.1161/STROKEAHA.110.581975.
112. Bae I, Chun H, Choi K, Yi H. Modified Glasgow coma scale for predicting outcome after subarachnoid hemorrhage surgery. Medicine (Baltimore). 2021;100(19):e25815. https://doi.org/10.1097/MD.0000000000025815.
113. Chou SH. Subarachnoid hemorrhage. Continuum (Minneap Minn). 2021;27(5):1201–45. https://doi.org/10.1212/CON.0000000000001052.
114. Frontera JA, Claassen J, Harnof S, et al. Prediction of symptomatic vasospasm after subarachnoid hemorrhage : the modified fisher scale. Neurosurgery. 2006;59(1):21–7.
115. Kramer AH, Hehir M, Nathan B, et al. A comparison of 3 radiographic scales for the prediction of delayed ischemia and prognosis following subarachnoid hemorrhage. J Neurosurg. 2008;109(2):199–207. https://doi.org/10.3171/JNS/2008/109/8/0199.
116. Rosengart AJ, Schultheiss KE, Tolentino J, Macdonald RL. Prognostic factors for outcome in patients with aneurysmal subarachnoid hemorrhage. Stroke. 2007;38(8):2315–21. https://doi.org/10.1161/STROKEAHA.107.484360.
117. Hong CM, Tosun C, Kurland DB, Gerzanich V, Schreibman D, Simard JM. Biomarkers as outcome predictors in subarachnoid

hemorrhage - a systematic review. Biomarkers. 2014;19(2):95–108. https://doi.org/10.3109/1354750X.2014.881418.

118. De Marchis G, Pugin D, Meyers E, et al. Seizure burden in subarachnoid hemorrhage associated with functional and cognitive outcome. Neurology. 2016;86(3):253–60. https://doi.org/10.1212/WNL.0000000000002281.

119. Rosenthal ES, Biswal S, Zafar SF, et al. Continuous electroencephalography predicts delayed cerebral ischemia after subarachnoid hemorrhage: A prospective study of diagnostic accuracy. Ann Neurol. 2018;83(5):958–69. https://doi.org/10.1002/ana.25232.

120. Tong JT, Eyngorn I, Mlynash M, Albers GW, Hirsch KG. Functional neurologic outcomes change over the first 6 months after cardiac arrest. Crit Care Med. 2016;44(12):e1202–7. https://doi.org/10.1097/CCM.0000000000001963.

121. Dragancea I, Wise MP, Al-Subaie N, et al. Protocol-driven neurological prognostication and withdrawal of life-sustaining therapy after cardiac arrest and targeted temperature management. Resuscitation. 2017;117:50–7. https://doi.org/10.1016/j.resuscitation.2017.05.014.

122. Dragancea I, Rundgren M, Englund E, Friberg H, Cronberg T. The influence of induced hypothermia and delayed prognostication on the mode of death after cardiac arrest. Resuscitation. 2013;84(3):337–42. https://doi.org/10.1016/j.resuscitation.2012.09.015.

123. Kiker WA, Rutz Voumard R, Andrews LIB, et al. Assessment of discordance between physicians and family members regarding prognosis in patients with severe acute brain injury. JAMA Netw Open. 2021;4(10):e2128991. https://doi.org/10.1001/jamanetworkopen.2021.28991.

124. Jones K, Quinn T, Mazor KM, Muehlschlegel S. Prognostic uncertainty in critically ill patients with traumatic brain injury: A multicenter qualitative study. Neurocrit Care. 2021;35(2):311–21. https://doi.org/10.1007/s12028-021-01230-3.

125. Graham M. Burying our mistakes: dealing with prognostic uncertainty after severe brain injury. Bioethics. 2020;34(6):612–9. https://doi.org/10.1111/bioe.12737.

126. Johnsson J, Bjornsson O, Andersson P, et al. Artificial neural networks improve early outcome prediction and risk classification in out-of-hospital cardiac arrest patients admitted to intensive care. Crit Care. 2020;24(1):474–1. https://doi.org/10.1186/s13054-020-03103-1.

127. Wang HL, Hsu WY, Lee MH, et al. Automatic machine-learning-based outcome prediction in patients with primary intracerebral hemorrhage. Front Neurol. 2019;10:910. https://doi.org/10.3389/fneur.2019.00910.

128. Savarraj JPJ, Hergenroeder GW, Zhu L, et al. Machine learning to predict delayed cerebral ischemia and outcomes in subarachnoid hemorrhage. Neurology. 2021;96(4):e553–62. https://doi.org/10.1212/WNL.0000000000011211.

129. Abujaber A, Fadlalla A, Gammoh D, Abdelrahman H, Mollazehi M, El-Menyar A. Prediction of in-hospital mortality in patients on mechanical ventilation post traumatic brain injury: machine learning approach. BMC Med Inform Decis Mak. 2020;20(1):336-z. https://doi.org/10.1186/s12911-020-01363-z.

130. Elmer J, Coppler PJ, May TL, et al. Unsupervised learning of early post-arrest brain injury phenotypes. Resuscitation. 2020;153:154–60. https://doi.org/10.1016/j.resuscitation.2020.05.051.

131. Amorim E, van der Stoel M, Nagaraj SB, et al. Quantitative EEG reactivity and machine learning for prognostication in hypoxic-ischemic brain injury. Clin Neurophysiol. 2019;130(10):1908–16. https://doi.org/10.1016/j.clinph.2019.07.014.

132. Wu X, Zou Q, Hu J, et al. Intrinsic functional connectivity patterns predict consciousness level and recovery outcome in acquired brain injury. J Neurosci. 2015;35(37):12932–46. https://doi.org/10.1523/JNEUROSCI.0415-15.2015.

133. Stone JR, Wilde EA, Taylor BA, et al. Supervised learning technique for the automated identification of white matter hyperintensities in traumatic brain injury. Brain Inj. 2016;30(12):1458–68. https://doi.org/10.1080/02699052.2016.1222080.

134. Irimia A, Wang B, Aylward SR, et al. Neuroimaging of structural pathology and connectomics in traumatic brain injury: toward personalized outcome prediction. Neuroimage Clin. 2012;1(1):1–17. https://doi.org/10.1016/j.nicl.2012.08.002.

135. Snider SB, Bodien YG, Frau-Pascual A, Bianciardi M, Foulkes AS, Edlow BL. Ascending arousal network connectivity during recovery from traumatic coma. Neuroimage Clin. 2020;28:102503. https://doi.org/10.1016/j.nicl.2020.102503.

136. Edlow BL, Barra ME, Zhou DW, et al. Personalized connectome mapping to guide targeted therapy and promote recovery of consciousness in the intensive care unit. Neurocrit Care. 2020;33(2):364–75. https://doi.org/10.1007/s12028-020-01062-7.

137. Distelmaier K, Muqaku B, Wurm R, et al. Proteomics-enriched prediction model for poor neurologic outcome in cardiac arrest survivors. Crit Care Med. 2020;48(2):167–75. https://doi.org/10.1097/CCM.0000000000004105.

138. Wendler D. A call for a patient preference predictor. Crit Care Med. 2021;49(6):877–80. https://doi.org/10.1097/CCM.0000000000004949.

139. Goostrey KJ, Lee C, Jones K, et al. Adapting a traumatic brain injury goals-of-care decision aid for critically ill patients to intracerebral hemorrhage and hemispheric acute ischemic stroke. Crit Care Explor. 2021;3(3):e0357. https://doi.org/10.1097/CCE.0000000000000357.

140. Muehlschlegel S, Hwang DY, Flahive J, et al. Goals-of-care decision aid for critically ill patients with TBI: development and feasibility testing. Neurology. 2020;95(2):e179–93. https://doi.org/10.1212/WNL.0000000000009770.

Brain Death

38

Ariane Lewis, Matthew P. Kirschen, and David M. Greer

Contents

Abstract

Clinicians who work in neurointensive care units must be familiar with brain death/death by neurologic criteria (BD/DNC). To declare BD/DNC, a patient must be in a permanent coma due to a known etiology, have brainstem areflexia, and be unable to breathe spontaneously in the setting of a hypercarbic acidemic challenge. The presence of confounders must be excluded, and the standardized examination must be performed accurately to prevent false-positive determinations of death. It is imperative that clinicians involved in BD/DNC evaluations be adept at communicating with families/legally authorize representatives about BD/DNC. The goals of this chapter are (1) Examine the etiologies for BD/DNC; (2) review techniques for successful communication with families/LARs about BD/DNC; (3) identify the prerequisites to perform an evaluation for BD/DNC; (4) review performance of a clinical evaluation for BD/DNC; (5) summarize the assessment for apnea; and (6) examine the indications for, and interpretation of, ancillary testing.

Supplementary Information The online version contains supplementary material available at https://doi.org/10.1007/978-3-031-62220-5_38.

A. Lewis
Departments of Neurology and Neurosurgery, NYU Langone Medical Center, New York, NY, USA

M. P. Kirschen
Departments of Anesthesiology and Critical Care Medicine, Neurology, and Pediatrics, The Children's Hospital of Philadelphia, Philadelphia, PA, USA

D. M. Greer (✉)
Department of Neurology, Boston University Chobanian and Avedisian School of Medicine and Boston Medical Center, Boston, MA, USA
e-mail: dgreer@bu.edu

Introduction

The end of life was identified following an evaluation for brain death/death by neurologic criteria (BD/DNC) for 2% of hospitalized patients who died in the United States from 2012 to 2016 [1]. During that time, the incidence increased from 34.47 cases/100,000 discharges in 2012 to 43.19 cases/100,000 discharges in 2016. BD/DNC occurred at a younger age than in-hospital death by cardiopulmonary criteria (48 ± 1 years vs. 70 ± 19 years, $p < 0.0001$). Accordingly, BD/DNC is more common in pediatric intensive care units (PICUs), comprising 7% of deaths from 2012

E. Mahanna Gabrielli et al. (eds.), *Textbook of Neurointensive Care: Volume 1*, https://doi.org/10.1007/978-3-031-62220-5_38

to 2016 in a PICU in Saudi Arabia and 21% of deaths in PICUs in the United States from 2012 to 2017 [2, 3]. There is a linear association between PICU size and number of annual cases of BD/DNC [3].

The goals of this chapter are (1) Examine the etiologies for BD/DNC; (2) review the techniques to communicate with a family/legally-authorized representative (LAR) about BD/DNC; (3) identify the prerequisites to perform an evaluation for BD/DNC; (4) review performance of a clinical evaluation for BD/DNC; (5) summarize the assessment for apnea; and (6) examine the indications for, and interpretation of, ancillary testing.

Key Clinical Questions

The chapter will answer the following questions:

1. What are the standards for performance of an evaluation for BD/DNC?
2. When should an evaluation for BD/DNC be performed?
3. What are the components of an evaluation for BD/DNC?
4. How do you perform apnea testing for patients on extracorporeal membrane oxygenation?
5. When should ancillary testing be performed?
6. What is the time of death?

Prehospital

Most patients who are evaluated for BD/DNC are neurologically normal prior to an event that results in sudden and catastrophic brain injury, but a review of pediatric deaths in the United States found that 15% of patients had a preexisting neurologic disability, and 0.5% were comatose or vegetative [3]. BD/DNC most commonly occurs following admission for a primary disorder of the central nervous system, but it can result from brain injury due to non-neurologic diseases including disorders of the respiratory system, circulatory system, hepatobiliary system, toxic effects of drugs, and trauma [1]. In pediatric patients, the primary causes of BD/DNC include hypoxic–ischemic injury after cardiac arrest, shock and/or respiratory failure without cardiac arrest, and traumatic brain injury [3]. Compared to in-hospital death due to cardiopulmonary criteria, the incidence of BD/DNC is higher among men (56.5% vs. 51.5% for women, $p < 0.0001$) [1]. The incidence of BD/DNC is also higher among Blacks in the United States (38.1 cases/100,000 Black people vs. 15.4 cases/100,000 White people, $p < 0.0001$) [1]. Among pediatric patients, male sex and Black race were also risk factors for progression to BD/DNC, compared with death by cardiopulmonary criteria ($p = 0.02$ and $p < 0.001$, respectively) [3]. Other factors associated with BD/DNC included age 2–12 years old (as compared with <2-years-old or ≥ 13-years-old; $p < 0.001$), trauma ($p < 0.001$) and higher Pediatric Index of Mortality score ($p < 0.001$) [3]. However, female sex was a risk factor for progression to BD/DNC compared with death due to cardiopulmonary criteria or survival amongst patients with hypoxic–ischemic injury after out-of-hospital cardiac arrest on univariate analysis ($p = 0.012$); other risk factors included nonshockable rhythm ($p < 0.001$), neurological cause of arrest ($p < 0.001$), and lower Glasgow Coma Scale score 24 hours post-arrest ($p < 0.001$) [4].

In the prehospital setting, severe catastrophic brain injury that may progress to BD/DNC may be suspected. However, this determination cannot be made until neuroimaging and a detailed neurologic examination are performed and confounding conditions/mimics of BD/DNC are ruled out. Prehospital management should be targeted toward a patient's known or suspected primary pathology as described elsewhere throughout this book. Patients with the inability to protect their airway and/or lack of spontaneous breathing should be intubated, and appropriate interventions, based on the known or suspected primary pathology, should be performed in an attempt to mitigate brain injury.

Essential Management Priorities

Early: Immediate/First 24 hours

Patients whose history and examination suggest a catastrophic brain injury should have emergent imaging with head computed tomography (CT). The initial management should be based on the etiology of their injury, but should be restricted to interventions that are clinically indicated. The World Brain Death Project (WBDP), an international consensus statement on the evaluation for BD/DNC, advised against performance of interventions to decrease intracranial pressure (e.g., mannitol, hypertonic saline, external ventricular drain placement, and hemicraniectomy) simply for the purpose of determining whether the injury is irreversible if they are not judged to be clinically indicated [5].

The concept of BD/DNC should be introduced to a patient's family/LAR as soon as it is apparent the patient has sustained a severe brain injury and has the potential to progress to BD/DNC [5, 6]. Although consent is not required to perform a BD/DNC evaluation, reasonable efforts should always be made to notify a patient's family/LAR about the potential for progression to BD/DNC and the intent to perform an evaluation [5, 7]. The patient's family/LAR should be invited to observe the evaluation, and told that the goal of the evaluation is to look for any sign of life. This conversation should address the fact that BD/DNC occurs in the setting of devastating irreparable damage to the brain, permanently preventing integration with the other organs, necessitating machines to provide organ support. Further, it must be noted that BD/DNC is the legal equivalent to death by cardiopulmonary criteria. Communication about BD/DNC must be empathetic, clear, and transparent. For the most part, the general public does not know about BD/DNC or harbors misconceptions about BD/DNC, believing it to be equivalent to a coma, a state from which recovery is possible. It can be beneficial to incorporate a social worker, palliative care specialist, or chaplain in discussions about BD/DNC to provide support for the family/LAR [8].

Long-Term Clinical Course

The duration of time between admission and progression to BD/DNC can vary, but it is typically shorter than the time between admission and death by cardiopulmonary criteria (median of 3 days (interquartile range (IQR) 2–4) vs. 5 days (IQR 1–15) in pediatric patients, $p < 0.001$, and mean of 4 days ± 8 vs. 8 ± 13 in all patients, $p < 0.0001$) [1, 3]. The amount of time between admission and evaluation for BD/DNC must be determined on a case-by-case basis to exclude the potential for reversibility of the patient's condition without doubt, but in the case of hypoxic–ischemic brain injury, the WBDP advises waiting at least 24 h after resuscitation, and longer after treatment with targeted temperature management [5]. Before commencing an evaluation for BD/DNC, there must be an identified etiology for the patient's neurologic condition that would cause permanent coma, brainstem areflexia, and inability to breathe spontaneously.

Because there are inconsistencies in policies regarding the prerequisites, examination, apnea testing and use of ancillary testing for the determination of BD/DNC around the world, the WBDP, published in 2020, was created to provide international expert guidance on the minimum clinical standards for BD/DNC) (see Supplementary Data 38.1 and 38.2 flow diagrams sections 1–4 and checklist) [5, 9]. In the United States, the current accepted medical standards on BD/DNC were published in 2023 jointly by the American Academy of Neurology (AAN), the Society of Critical Care Medicine (SCCM), the American Academy of Pediatrics (AAP) and the Child Neurology Society [10]. The WBDP suggests one clinical examination and one apnea test is the minimum requirement for BD/DNC determination in adults [5], but the AAN/SCCM/AAP/CNS guidelines recommend two examinations to reduce the possibility of false positives due to diagnostic error, and mandate that 2 examinations and 2 apnea tests be performed in children.

The prerequisites for a BD/DNC evaluation necessitate exclusion of confounding or reversible conditions that could lead to a false positive determination [5, 11, 12]. The temperature should be >36 °C and the blood pressure should be >100 mmHg and mean arterial pressure >75 mmHg, or age-appropriate in a pediatric patient [5]. In a patient treated with targeted temperature management, the evaluation should not be performed until at least 24 h after rewarming to at least 36 °C, and an ancillary blood flow study should be considered in addition to the clinical evaluation and apnea test if there is any concern that a confounding condition that cannot be corrected may be delaying recovery of function [5]. Severe metabolic, acid–base, or endocrine derangements should be corrected, and new guidance was provided for this in the 2023 US guideline update. Only 8% of national BD/DNC standards provide finite guidance on electrolyte levels and 5% on acid–base derangements. A survey of neurointensivists demonstrated that they are most concerned about sodium, arterial pH, and glucose [5, 11]. Residual effects of medications that depress the central nervous system should be excluded by measuring drug levels or allowing five half-lives to pass prior to initiation of the evaluation (or longer in the setting of hepatic or renal dysfunction, obesity, age-related metabolism or hypothermia) [5]. Pharmacologic paralysis should be excluded using a train-of-four electrical stimulation or demonstration of the presence of deep tendon reflexes [5].

The clinical evaluation for BD/DNC includes assessment for coma and brainstem areflexia (loss of the pupillary reflex, corneal reflex, oculocephalic reflex, oculovestibular reflex, gag reflex, and cough reflex) [5]. To be consistent with BD/DNC, the evaluation should demonstrate no evidence of arousal or awareness in response to noxious visual, auditory, and tactile stimulation and no movement of the face or extremities (other than spinally-mediated reflexes) upon application of deep pressure at the temporomandibular joints, supraorbital notches, the sternal notch, and both proximally and distally on all extremities [5]. The pupillary reflex is absent if the pupils remain fixed in a midsize or dilated position when a bright light is shined into both eyes [5]. The corneal reflex is absent if there is no eyelid movement when the cornea is touched with a cotton tipped applicator adjacent to the iris [5]. The oculocephalic reflex is absent if there is no eye movement when the head is briskly rotated horizontally to both sides [5]. The oculovestibular reflex is absent if, after demonstrating patency of the auditory canal, there is no eye movement when ice water is injected into each ear for 1 min (with 5 min between ears) while the head of bed is elevated to 30° [5]. The gag reflex is absent if there is no gag in response to stimulation of the posterior pharyngeal wall bilaterally [5]. The cough reflex is absent if there is no cough in response to stimulation of the tracheobronchial wall via in-line suctioning down the endotracheal tube [5]. The evaluation for BD/DNC in an infant also includes assessment for the sucking and rooting reflexes [5].

If all prerequisites are met and a patient is found to be comatose with brainstem areflexia, the next step in the BD/DNC evaluation is apnea testing [5]. After adjusting the ventilator settings to achieve normocarbia, the patient should be disconnected from the ventilator and oxygenated via placement of an insufflation catheter down the endotracheal tube or application of continuous positive airway pressure via a resuscitation bag with a positive end-expiratory valve or the ventilator [5]. The test is consistent with BD/DNC if the patient does not take any spontaneous breaths and the $PaCO_2$ rises to at least 60 mmHg (and ≥ 20 mmHg above a known elevated baseline in patients with preexisting hypercapnia due to chronic retention) [5]. The WBDP and 2023 US guidelines update also require ensuring the pH is <7.3 before concluding the test is consistent with BD/DNC, as acidosis is felt to be the necessary stimulation for the medullary chemoreceptors [5]. If the patient breathes during the apnea test, they are not dead [5]. If the test needs to be aborted due to respiratory/hemodynamic instability (hypoxia, hypotension, unstable arrhythmia), the test should be repeated when the patient is stable, or ancillary testing is needed [5].

For patients on extracorporeal membrane oxygenation (ECMO), the fundamental principles of apnea testing are unchanged, but the ECMO circuit can be used to raise the $PaCO_2$ and provide apneic oxygenation [5]. The patient must still be disconnected from mechanical ventilation and observed for spontaneous respiratory effort. Given the potential for lack of pulsatile flow, the minimum blood pressure for patients on veno-arterial ECMO is a mean arterial pressure of 75 mmHg (or age-appropriate in children), and again the pH <7.30. To ensure the $PaCO_2$ in the cerebral circulation has exceeded the threshold for BD/DNC determination, blood gases should be sampled from both the distal arterial line and post-oxygenator ECMO circuit, and both values must be greater than the threshold, in conjunction with apnea, to be consistent with BD/DNC. To facilitate hypercarbia, the sweep gas flow can be adjusted to 0.5–1 L/min.

If the full clinical examination and apnea test cannot be completed or the interpretation of the examination is confounded, ancillary testing is needed [5]. Some examples of circumstances in which this is warranted are anophthalmia, ophthalmic surgery that precludes pupillary evaluation, corneal trauma, severe facial trauma, severe orbital/scleral edema/chemosis, skull base fracture, high cervical cord injury, or a pre-existing severe neuromuscular disorder [5]. Other situations in which ancillary testing may be performed include isolated brainstem pathology, institutional/regional/national requirement or to assist a family in understanding/accepting BD/DNC. A review of standards around the world found that 28% of countries require ancillary testing for all evaluations for BD/DNC [5, 9]. The guidance on performance and interpretation of ancillary tests in national standards is inconsistent [12]. Although there are descriptions of a myriad of blood flow and electrodiagnostic tests to evaluate for BD/DNC, the WBDP recommends use of digital subtraction angiography, radionuclide studies, or transcranial Doppler (TCD) ultrasonography and suggests electroencephalography (EEG) only be used in the setting of an open skull fracture/fontanelle or decompressive craniectomy or if required institutionally/regionally [5]. Further, the WBDP suggests EEG be used in conjunction with somatosensory or auditory-evoked potentials because of the limitations evaluating the brainstem [5]. The 2023 US guideline update states that EEG should no longer be used as an ancillary test, and CT/CTA and MRI/MRA have not been validated and also should not be used.

The WBDP suggests the time of death is the time the arterial $PaCO_2$ and pH reach the targets during apnea testing, if ancillary testing is not needed, or the time the ancillary test results are documented by the interpreting attending physician, if ancillary testing is performed [5].

Organ support should be discontinued after death is declared, though the WBDP suggests it can be continued for a brief finite period (<48 h) and the AAN encourages members to include provisions for management of requests to continue support after BD/DNC in institutional protocols [5, 7]. If a family/LAR objects to discontinuation of support, institutional administrative and legal guidance is needed, as laws across the United States and around the world vary, and institutional standards often do not provide guidance for this type of situation. While New Jersey and Israel allow continuation of organ support until death by cardiopulmonary criteria if a family/LAR objects to BD/DNC based on their religion, the law is silent about management of these objections in most other US states and countries, and vaguely references provision of "reasonable accommodation" in others, like California and New York) [5, 13]. Organ support may be continued to facilitate organ donation, but it is worth noting that hemodynamic instability and multiorgan dysfunction may develop without attentive critical care [5]. Lastly, if the patient is pregnant and their family/LAR request continuation of support for the sake of the fetus, this can be feasible for days to months, provided a multidisciplinary team is involved and the family/LAR understands the patient could have a cardiopulmonary arrest at any time and that fetal outcome is uncertain [5, 7].

Near Misses

A BD/DNC evaluation can yield a false-positive result (the patient does not truly meet criteria for BD/DNC, but it falsely appears that they do) if the prerequisites are not met, the clinical examination or apnea test are not completed correctly or ancillary testing is improperly performed or interpreted. Confounders to the clinical evaluation include the following: central nervous system depressing medications, hypothermia, hypotension, hypoglycemia, pharmacologic paralysis, and metabolic derangements [5]. Central nervous system depressing medications that can interfere with the evaluation include, but are not limited to: antibiotics (aminoglycosides, tetracycline, and vancomycin); baclofen; benzodiazepines; bupropion; opiates; tricyclic antidepressants; and valproic acid [5]. There have been numerous reports of reversible conditions that mimic BD/DNC, including rabies encephalitis, snake bites, botulism, high cervical cord injury, Guillain-Barré Syndrome, and leptomeningeal carcinomatosis [5]. Lastly, some conditions can confound the assessment of brainstem reflexes including cervical spine injury, skull base fracture, facial trauma, or anophthalmia [5].

Key Radiologic Findings

Neuroimaging can help determine the etiology, severity, and reversibility of brain injury, but BD/DNC is a clinical, not radiographic, diagnosis. Imaging that shows evidence of intracranial hypertension (severe cerebral edema and herniation) can indicate the potential for progression to BD/DNC [5]. However, it is worth noting that it is unclear if the presence or severity of edema/herniation is predictive of progression to BD/DNC. Ray et al. reported that prediction of BD/DNC, the sensitivity and specificity (respectively) of (1) brain herniation was 79% and 24%, (2) diffuse sulcal effacement was 93% and 17%, (3) basal cistern effacement was 91% and 20%, and (4) loss of gray/white differentiation was 46% and 80% [14]. However, imaging was not performed at the time of the BD/DNC evaluation, so interpretation is somewhat limited (the median duration of time between imaging and evaluation was >24 h for patients both with and without herniation). The WBDP advised the need for caution when considering performance of an evaluation for BD/DNC in the absence of herniation on neuroimaging [5].

The neuroimaging-based ancillary studies for BD/DNC accepted by the WBDP include digital subtraction angiography, radionuclide studies, and TCDs, the latter of which are only validated for use in adults) [5]. Digital subtraction angiography (4-vessel) is considered the gold standard ancillary test; findings are consistent with BD/DNC if there is absent filling at the points where the internal carotid arteries and vertebral arteries enter the skull base, but a patent external carotid circulation. Regarding radionuclide studies, the WBDP suggests preferentially using (1) diffusible (lipophilic) radiopharmaceuticals and (2) single-photon emission computed tomography (SPECT) over planar imaging (or if unavailable, perfusion scintigraphy with anterior and lateral planar imaging with appropriate time intervals to demonstrate static filling of the posterior fossa). The absence of intracranial isotope is consistent with BD/DNC. If TCDs are used, the exams need to be performed bilaterally, anteriorly, and posteriorly. To be consistent with BD/DNC, there should be biphasic oscillating flow and systolic spikes with reversal of flow in diastole on two separate studies performed ≥ 30 min apart.

Key Monitoring

To perform an evaluation for BD/DNC, the WBDP suggests there should be neuroimaging evidence of intracranial hypertension, as discussed above, or evidence that intracranial pressure equals or exceeds the mean arterial pressure [5]. Once it is believed a patient is in a permanent coma with brainstem areflexia and inability to breathe spontaneously, (1) temperature and blood pressure should be measured to ensure prerequisite thresholds are met, (2) a basic metabolic panel and arterial blood gas should be checked to exclude severe derangements, (3) a toxicology screen should be sent and drug levels should be measured (as appropriate) to ensure drugs/toxins have been cleared and levels are not supratherapeutic, and (4) a blood alcohol level should be measured if there is concern for intoxication. Throughout the evaluation, particularly during apnea testing, the blood pressure must be monitored closely. Intravenous fluid boluses, vasopressors, and/or inotropes should be administered as needed to maintain blood pressure above the target range. Serial arterial blood gases must be sent prior to and during apnea testing to ensure the initial $PaCO_2$ and pH levels are appropriate and to demonstrate adequate development of hypercarbia and acidemia; an arterial line can help facilitate this testing.

Take Home Message

Although BD/DNC is rare, clinicians who are involved in the evaluation of patients for BD/DNC must be adept at ruling out mimics of BD/DNC, ensuring prerequisites are met; conducting the clinical evaluation and apnea testing, identifying when ancillary testing is indicated and interpreting the results and communicating with families and LARs about BD/DNC. Clinicians should be educated about BD/DNC to ensure the evaluation is performed accurately and consistently, and that there are no false positives [5]. To facilitate this, the Neurocritical Care Society created an interactive electronic didactic course and toolkit [15, 16]. It has been suggested that a regulatory organization, such as the Joint Commission, could audit institutional standards to confirm that they conform with national standards, and that certification is required for any clinicians performing BD/DNC determinations [5, 10].

References

1. Seifi A, Lacci JV, Godoy DA. Incidence of brain death in the United States. Clin Neurol Neurosurg. 2020;195:105885. Epub ahead of print
2. Al-Eyadhy A, Temsah M-H, Hasan GM, et al. Causes, timing, and modes of death in a tertiary pediatric intensive care unit: five years' experience. Saudi Med J. 2021;42:1186–94.
3. Kirschen MP, Francoeur C, Murphy M, et al. Epidemiology of brain death in pediatric intensive care units in the United States. JAMA Pediatr. 2019;173:469–76.
4. Madelaine T, Cour M, Roy P, et al. Prediction of brain death after out-of-hospital cardiac arrest. Chest. 2021; https://doi.org/10.1016/j.chest.2021.01.056.
5. Greer D, Shemie S, Lewis A, et al. Brain death/determination of death by neurologic criteria around the world: the world brain death project. JAMA. 2020;324:1078–97.
6. Lewis A, Adams N, Chopra A, Kirschen M. Organ support after death by neurologic criteria in pediatric patients. Crit Care Med. 2017;45:e916–24.
7. Russell JA, Epstein LG, Greer DM, Kirschen M, Rubin MA, Lewis A. Brain death, the determination of brain death, and member guidance for brain death accommodation requests. Neurology. 2019; https://doi.org/10.1212/WNL.0000000000006750.
8. Lewis A, Kitamura E. The intersection of neurology and religion: a survey of hospital chaplains on death by neurologic criteria. Neurocrit Care. 2021;35:322–34.
9. Lewis A, Bakkar A, Kreiger-Benson E, Kumpfbeck A, Liebman J, Shemie S, Sung G, Torrance S, Greer D. Determination of death by neurologic criteria around the world. Neurology. 2020;95:e299–309.
10. Greer DM, Kirschen MP, Lewis A, Gronseth GS, Rae-Grant A, Ashwal S, Babu MA, Bauer DF, Billinghurst L, Corey A, Partap S, Rubin MA, Shutter L, Takahashi C, Tasker RC, Varelas PN, Wijdicks E, Bennett A, Wessels SR, Halperin JJ. Pediatric and adult brain death/death by neurologic criteria consensus guidline: report of the AAN Guidelines Subcommittee, AAP, CNS and SCCM. Neurology. 2023;101(24):1112–32.
11. Lerner DP, Bassil R, Tadevosyan A, Ramineni A, Burns JD, Russell JA, Varelas PN, Lewis A. Metabolic values precluding clinical death by neurologic criteria/brain death: survey of neurocritical care society physicians. J Clin Neurosci. 2021;88:16–21.
12. Lewis A, Liebman J, Kreiger-Benson E, Kumpfbeck A, Bakkar A, Shemie SD, Sung G, Torrance S, Greer D. Ancillary testing for determination of death by neurologic criteria around the world. Neurocrit Care. 2020; Epub ahead of print
13. Lewis A, Varelas P, Greer D. Prolonging support after brain death: when families ask for more. Neurocrit Care. 2016;24:481–7.
14. Ray A, Manara AR, Mortimer AM, Thomas I. Brain herniation on computed tomography is a poor predictor of whether patients with a devastating brain injury can be confirmed dead using neurological criteria. J Intensive Care Soc. 2021; Epub ahead of print
15. The Neurocritical Care Society Brain Death Determination Course. https://www.neurocriticalcare.org/higherlogic/s/p/cm/ld/fid=1101. Accessed 9 Dec 2019.
16. Rubin MA, Kirschen MP, Lewis A. The neurocritical care brain death determination course: purpose, design, and early findings. Neurocrit Care. 2021;35(3):913–5. Epub ahead of print

Further Reading

Greer D, Shemie S, Lewis A, et al. Brain death/determination of death by neurologic criteria around the world: the world brain death project. JAMA. 2020;324:1078–97.

Brain Death and Management of the Potential Organ Donor

39

Samuel M. Galvagno Jr, Neeraj Badjatia, and Kenneth E. Wood

Contents

Abstract

A structured and standardized approach to the diagnosis of brain death is essential to ensure that patients are appropriately classified. This involves a physical exam to establish coma and exclude reversible causes of coma, a comprehensive evaluation of the cranial nerves, and an apnea test. The inability to perform any of the physical exam elements necessitates the use of confirmatory studies. Management of the potential organ donor commences after the diagnosis of brain death is established. Donation after cardiac death should be considered in patients whose prognosis is futile and in whom care is to be withdrawn. Specific donor management goals have been established and have been associated with greater organ procurement. Hemodynamic management forms the cornerstone of brain-dead donor management. Echocardiography should be performed in all potential donors to evaluate cardiac function. Fluid resuscitation is frequently necessary as potential donors tend to be intravascularly volume depleted. Vasopressors should be used to support acceptable blood pressure and hemodynamic profiles. Donor lung management should utilize a lung protective strategy with ventilatory manipulations undertaken to ensure adequate systemic oxygenation and lung expansion. A coordinated, active donor management approach utilizing intensivists and OPO coordinators has been shown to more effectively manage the donation process, resulting in more organs procured and transplanted.

S. M. Galvagno Jr
Department of Anesthesiology, University of Maryland School of Medicine, Baltimore, MD, USA

N. Badjatia
Department of Neurology, Section of Neurocritical Care, Program in Trauma, University of Maryland School of Medicine, Baltimore, MD, USA

K. E. Wood (✉)
Lifespan System, Warren Alpert Medical School of Brown University, Providence, RI, USA
e-mail: KWood4@lifespan.org

Introduction

Intensive care management of the potential organ donor represents the most immediate and practical solution to the current crisis in organ donation. While rigorous research to improve organ procurement has been limited [1], accumulating evidence suggests that active and continuous involvement by the intensive care team may help maximize the yield and function of retrieved organs [1–3]. The standardization

E. Mahanna Gabrielli et al. (eds.), *Textbook of Neurointensive Care: Volume 1*, https://doi.org/10.1007/978-3-031-62220-5_39

and the elimination of unwarranted variation in the management of the potential organ donor have led to higher rates of procurement, improved quality of organs procured, and improved outcomes in the transplant recipient [4–9]. Ensuring that there is maximal utilization and optimal management of the existing donor pool can significantly increase the number of donors available for procurement and enable transplantation to save the lives of those with end-stage disease and enhance the quality of life for those individuals maintained on dialysis.

Consent

Consent or authorization for donation is an absolute requirement and frequently the rate limiting step in the process. Despite an extensive body of research on the topic, there is limited consensus on the best approach. Recent literature suggests that an effective request is one that includes factors that impact the consent rate and the family satisfaction with their decision and the process [10]. Various legislative and policy initiatives to include required request and routine notification have failed to significantly improve consent rates [11]. The Organ Donation Breakthrough Collaborative sponsored by the Health Resources and Services Administration's Division of Transplantation revealed that when routine notification was combined with Organ Procurement Organization (OPO) collaboration and participation in the request process, significant benefit was realized [12]. It is generally accepted that an empathetic approach, treating the family with respect and dignity, the provision of physical support and accommodations, a non-pressurized and time sensitive approach along with detailed information related to the donation process and disposition of the deceased after donation and funeral arrangements are associated with improved consent rates.

Decoupling refers to separating the discussion of donation from the preceding notification of death in the case of brain death or the consent to withdrawal support in the setting of donation after circulatory death and traditionally has been the standard recommended approach. However, it has been reported that only a weak effect was found related to the impact of timing and that raising the issue before rather than after death pronouncement may be associated with higher consent [13]. Similarly, the traditional practice of providing a detailed discussion of brain death to ensure family comprehension has been questioned as unnecessary and unduly complicating the consent process [11]. It has been reported that only a minority of families could provide a correct definition of brain death after being told and there was no association between the definition and the willingness to donate [13]. Although requirements vary from state to state, historically two independent brain death exams, usually separated by 6–12 h were required although the American Academy of Neurology has recommended a single exam [14]. The time between the exams has been shown to negatively affect organ donation [15]. Siminoff et al. [11] have identified that effective communication during requests requires:

1. Initiating the request in an empathetic manner with appropriate introductions and acknowledgement of the loss of the patient.
2. Soliciting patient and family information using clear, open-ended questions while avoiding interruption.
3. Soliciting the family's perspectives and beliefs about organ donation and the patient's wishes.
4. Developing and maintain a supportive, trust-based relationship with the family that includes addressing concerns and questions with sensitivity and providing information underscoring the benefits of donation.
5. Providing closure by summarizing the family's position regarding donation, outlining the next steps in the process and expressing gratitude for the family's time and consideration of donation.

Although there is considerable international variation regarding who makes the request, the US requires the request to be made by an individual certified as a Designated Requestor that is frequently an OPO specialist coordinator, but may be a member of the health care team. Previous work suggested that the presence of the coordinator was one of three independent variable associated with success and that a collaborative approach between the OPO specialist and the health care team had the highest consent rate [16]. In contrast, the UK Assessment of Collaborative Requesting Trial compared the collaborative approach to the routine request by the patient's physician and found no difference [17].

Donation After Circulatory Determination of Death (Non-heart Beating Donors)

Donation After Cardiac Death

Donation after cardiac death refers to the recovery of organs from patients that are not brain dead but die secondary to cardiopulmonary causes. This was previously known as a non-heartbeating donor. Donation may occur in several circumstances that are either controlled or uncontrolled. The vast majority of donation after cardiac death occurs during controlled situations when care is withdrawn and the patient is pronounced dead from cardiopulmonary arrest. Uncontrolled donation after cardiac death is far less common and occurs in emergent circumstances such as death from an acute trauma. Prior to 1968, there was no legal definition for brain death and donation after cardiac death was the primary method for obtaining organs for transplantation. After the acceptance of brain death, donation from brain-dead donors has significantly exceeded those from donation after cardiac death. The Institute of Medicine (IOM) formally evaluated the donation after cardiac death practice into separate reports [18, 19]. Specifically, the IOM stipulated that the decision to withdraw or withhold care be undertaken based upon the patient's wishes and not influenced by any potential for organ donation. It was further recommended that a separate team provide end-of-life care that was distinct from the transplant team. Donation after cardiac death must adhere to the dead donor rule, which stipulates that donor organs may only be procured from dead patients. When undertaking donation after cardiac death, the withdrawal of care should be indistinguishable from the withdrawal of care in any other critically ill patient. Death is declared when there is cessation of cardiopulmonary function and after a period of time to ensure that there is no spontaneous recrudescence of respiratory function. Although the initial 1997 recommendation from the IOM was a 5-min period between the diagnosis of death and the initiation of organ recovery, it is currently recommended that this period be at least 2 min and no more than 5 min [20].

Donation After Brain Death Determination of Death (Brain Dead Heart-Beating Donors)

Formal declaration of brain death should be done in a regimented, sequential process. Many institutions utilize prescribed checklists for declaration. In efforts to standardize education, the Neurocritical Care Society recently introduced formal certification process. The first prerequisite to determination is establishing a proximate cause for cessation of brain function. This includes reviewing CT scans for demonstration of extensive brain injury. It is important to note that a CT scan can be initially normal if the patient has been imaged very early after cardiopulmonary arrest; however, cerebral edema or marked hypodensities in deep nuclei (thalamus, caudate, and putamen) are seen on a follow-up CT scan in a patient that may meet criteria for brain death testing. Proceeding with brain death testing in a patient with repeated normal CT scans should never occur. Beyond establishing devastating structural injury, potential confounders that may impair the ability to perform clinical testing must be ruled out. Spontaneous hypothermia and hypotension are common after brain herniation, and both conditions can impair testing of cranial nerve reflexes. Therefore, it is important to support the temperature and blood pressure to maintain normothermia ($T \geq 36.0$ °C) and normotension (SBP ≥ 100) throughout the entire brain death declaration process. Pharmacological influences on the neurological examination should not be present. Often this requires analyzing the drug elimination half-life of any sedatives utilized and allowing for 5–7 times that duration to pass prior to performing the clinical exam. The lingering presence of neuromuscular blockade can be assessed by the presence of four twitches with a train of four applying maximal intensity of stimulation to the ulnar nerve. Concomitant hepatic and renal insufficiency and/or administration of therapeutic hypothermia ($T < 36$ °C) is common in this population and therefore, may be additional factors to consider when assessing the time needed for drug clearance prior to proceeding with testing. The absence of illicit substances should be confirmed, and specifically for alcohol content, levels below the legal limit for driving (blood alcohol level of 0.08% [80 mg/dL]) are considered acceptable for proceeding with brain death determination. Finally, the absence of severe electrolyte, or acid–base disturbances, should be documented; however, there are no established thresholds defining "severe" [21].

Once these prerequisites have been established, clinical examination can proceed. It is widely accepted that a single examination is adequate; however, there may still be regulatory differences that still mandate two examinations, usually separated by at least 6 h [22]. The examination begins by establishing unresponsiveness by administration of noxious stimulation both centrally (e.g., tempomandibular joint compression, supraorbital nerve compression) and peripherally in the extremities. It is important to differentiate spinal responses from cortical or brainstem reflex motor responses. Spinal reflexes do not resemble decorticate or extensor reflex movements and may occur with neck flexion and peripheral stimulation but not with central stimulation. Clear communication and detailed documentation is necessary to mitigate the distress to family members or confusion among medical staff that may occur as are result of the presence of these movements. The remainder of the exam focuses on careful assessment of the pupillary reactivity, corneal response, gag reflex/cough, and oculovestibular and oculocephalic reflex. Subsequently, ventilator adjustments are made to normalize $PaCO_2$ levels (range: 35–45 mmHg by arterial blood gas) to proceed with apnea testing. For this procedure, patients are disconnected from the ventilator, with continued oxygen support (from 4 to 6 L/min O_2 via a cannula inserted in the endotracheal tube) for approximately 10 minutes to assess for the presence of any respiratory effort. During this time period, careful attention to monitor for cardiac arrhythmias, maintain normal blood pressure (SBP ≥ 100 mmHg), and avoid hypoxia. The use of carbogen, exogenous CO_2 with a mixture of 3% CO_2 and 97% O_2 delivered through a ventilator, is an alternative method that provides more cardiopulmonary stability and is the preferred method of testing in patients undergoing V-V or V-A ECMO [23]. The absence of respirations along with a rise in $PaCO_2$ by 20 mmHg above baseline or absolute level >60 mmHg[1] confirms the absence of the medullary respiratory reflex. All reflexes must be tested to complete the assessment of brain death. The presence of any of these reflexes precludes the diagnosis of brain death.

There are instances whereby the clinical examination cannot be completed. Most commonly, it is due to cardiopulmonary instability precluding apnea testing. However, there may be facial disfiguration (e.g., traumatic enucleation, hemotympanum) that precludes full completion of the clinical examination. In these instances, secondary, or ancillary, tests are required in order to complete brain death assessment. Accepted ancillary tests include cerebral angiography, radionuclide angiography, electroencephalogram, and transcranial doppler [24]. It is important to note that each ancillary test has limitations and prespecifications that must be followed for the test to be an accurate assessment for presence of brain death. More recently, reports of using CT angiography or MR angiography [25] have emerged as a means by which to obtain noninvasive assessments of cerebral blood flow; however, these neuroimaging methods have not been well studied in the assessment of brain death [26]. It is important to recognize that all of these tests have considerable inaccuracy and should not replace, in any way, a clinical assessment. Furthermore, none of these tests by themselves establish the diagnosis of brain death. Nor are these tests considered confirmatory, and they should not be performed if the clinical examination and apnea testing have already been completed.

Pathophysiology of Brain Death

In a landmark manuscript published in 1901, Harvey Cushing described the physiology of intracranial hypertension and its effect on systemic hemodynamics [27]. Cushing's observations were described as a triad: irregular respirations, decreased heart rate, and increased blood pressure. In contrast to animal models used by Cushing and others where the experimentation was undertaken in a controlled setting, the physiology of human brain death remains challenging for multiple reasons: the time of actual brain death may be significantly different from the certification time with significant physiologic changes occurring in the interval, treatment of the patient in the period antecedent to brain death and in the immediate post-brain death period may result in abnormalities independent of brain death, and, last, there will never be a human model of brain death [28]. As a consequence, an understanding of brain death physiology is derived from animal models and data inferred from human case series.

Management of the potential organ donor requires not only an implicit understanding of the pathophysiology of brain death but an appreciation of the traumatic or physiologic events that contributed to or precipitated brain death and which may act synergistically with brain death physiology to impair organ function during the management period. Following a declaration of brain death, a series of pathophysiological events ensue with attendant organ-specific dysfunction. Hence, transplanted organ dysfunction is not only related to peri-transplant ischemic time and reperfusion injury but also pretransplant systemic inflammation, blood brain disruption, dysautonomia, hormonal failure, and activation of the coagulation cascade, among many other pathophysiological events [3].

This is best exemplified in the cardiovascular system where it is recognized that hemodynamic instability in the potential organ donor is likely reflective of a series of events conspiring to produce coincident cardiac dysfunction and vasodilatation. It has long been recognized that brain injury may lead to cardiac dysfunction, which is reflected in EKG abnormalities and cardiac enzymatic elevations [29].

Pre-brain death endocrine dysfunction may be precipitated by direct injury to the hypothalamic–pituitary axis, neuroendocrine effects from catecholamines and cytokines, disruption of the vascular supply, or from systemic infection or inflammation. In a review of endocrine failure after traumatic brain injury in adults, the estimated incidence of hormonal reduction was adrenal 15%, thyroid 5–15%, growth hormone 18%, vasopressin 3–37%, and gonadal 25–80%. Hyperprolactinemia was present in more than 50% of patients. The authors concluded that severe traumatic brain injury when accompanied by basilar skull fracture, hypothalamic edema, prolonged unresponsiveness, hyponatremia, and/or hypotension was associated with a high incidence of endocrinopathy [30, 31]. As with antecedent cardiac dysfunction, it would seem reasonable that pre-brain death endocrine dysfunction, in conjunction with the brain death process, may contribute to instability during the donor management period.

In concert with the previously described pre-brain death physiology associated with severe brain injury, the brain death process precipitates significant pathophysiologic changes in all organ systems with the most pronounced effect upon the cardiovascular system. The rostral–caudal progression of ischemia is known as coning. Ischemia at the cerebral level produces vagal activation associated with a decreased heart rate, decreased cardiac output, and decreased blood pressure. Although underappreciated, the first signs of

[1] A rough rule for calculation of apnea time is as follows: The $PaCO_2$ normally increases 3 mmHg per minute with apnea. Thus, if the starting $PaCO_2$ is 35 mmHg and we want to achieve a $PaCO_2$ of 60 mmHg or greater: 60–35 = 25 mmHg/3 = ~8–9 min of apnea to achieve the $PaCO_2$ value of at least 60 mmHg. We usually add on 2–3 min to the calculated value. As long as SpO_2 is acceptable and there is no hemodynamic instability, this works well.

incipient herniation may simply be bradycardia in a severely brain-injured patient. Ischemia at the pons level produces the mixed vagal and sympathetic stimulation known as the Cushing's response characterized by bradycardia and hypertension associated with irregular breathing. Further progression of the coning process to involve ischemia of the medulla oblongata is associated with a sympathetic stimulation termed the autonomic storm. During this period, dramatic increases in catecholamines are reported with significant tachycardia and elevations in blood pressure. This represents the severely brain-injured patient's attempt to maintain cerebral perfusion pressure gradients in the face of elevated increased intracranial pressure (ICP) and evolving herniation. During this period, there is ischemic destruction of the hypothalamic–pituitary axis resulting in thermoregulatory impairment and purported endocrine dysfunction. Further progression of ischemia results in spinal cord destruction with herniation and sympathetic deactivation characterized by bradycardia, vasodilatation, and a low cardiac output state. Somatic death after clinical brain death will inevitably occur in the absence of aggressive support. In an era when brain death was not accepted, prolonged survivorship, with a mean duration of 23 days, was noted in a study that aggressively maintained brain-dead patients [32]. Autopsy studies of patients that were declared brain dead revealed histopathologic evidence of necrosis and liquefaction [33].

The catecholamine surge or autonomic storm produces multiple EKG and hemodynamic abnormalities along with biochemical and histologic changes in the cardiac system. In a series of sentinel observations and experiments, Novitzky initially defined the cardiovascular pathophysiology associated with brain death [34–37]. Catecholamines induce a sudden increase in cytosolic calcium which jeopardizes ATP production and activates lipases, proteases, and endonucleases. Xanthine oxidase activation reportedly produces free radicals which further impair organ function. Histopathologic changes reported in experimental animals reveal various degrees of focal myocyte necrosis located predominantly in the subendocardial area consisting of contraction bands and myocytolysis with mononuclear cell infiltrates precipitating edema proximate to the necrotic areas. Contraction bands were observed in the smooth muscle of coronary arteries and electron microscopy revealed a hypercontractile state of the sarcomere visualizing mitochondrial deposition of electron dense material and secondary lysosome containing injured mitochondria. The loss of ATP production jeopardizes myocardial energy stores and mediates the transition from the aerobic to anaerobic metabolism compromising myocardial function.

Animal data and observations from human series have defined multiple abnormalities related to the catecholamine surge and brain death including impaired coronary endothelial dysfunction [38], selective expression of inflammatory molecules [39], downregulation of myocardial contractility [40], abnormalities in loading conditions and impaired coronary perfusion [40], abnormalities of left ventricular myocardial gene expression [41], and changes in myocardial beta-adrenergic receptor function and high-energy phosphates along with beta-adrenergic receptor deregulation [42, 43]. From animal models, it appears that a sudden rise in ICP is more provocative of the hyperdynamic–hemodynamic response with significantly higher catecholamine levels and is associated with greater histopathologic damage. A more gradual intracranial pressure increase resulting in brain death is associated with a milder hyperdynamic response, less catecholamine release, and milder ischemic changes in the myocardium [44]. Clinically, this has been correlated with the development of cardiac allograft vasculopathy in the recipient. The coronary artery vasoconstriction, subendocardial ischemia, and focal myocardial necrosis associated with the autonomic storm have been reported to be associated with a high incidence of intimal thickening of the transplanted heart coronary arteries, myocardial infarction, and the need for subsequent revascularization surgery [45].

The hemodynamic abnormalities and their impact are illustrated in a recent study that compared post-brain death cardiac function in a group of potential organ donors whose autonomic storm was attenuated compared to donors whose autonomic system storm was untreated. Using a definition of autonomic storm characterized by a systolic blood pressure greater than or equal to 200 mmHg and tachycardia with heart rates exceeding 140 beats per minute, the authors treated this hemodynamic response, which was observed in 63% of donors for a mean duration of 1.2 h, with beta-blockers. Treatment resulted in a significantly higher post-brain death left ventricular ejection fraction (63.9% vs 49%), a higher rate of cardiac transplantation (91.7% vs 41.2%), and better heart recipient survival at 2 months (100% vs 43%). The authors concluded that treatment of the autonomic storm enabled better cardiac function post-brain death, higher rates of cardiac transplantation, and better recipient outcomes [46]. The study illustrates the significant impact of brain death upon cardiac function. However, recommendations regarding the treatment of the autonomic surge should be viewed with caution as this physiologic compensatory mechanism represents the patient's attempt to maintain cerebral perfusion in the face of herniation. Abolition of this response constitutes active intervention, and donor management in patients who have not been declared brain dead raises significant ethical concerns.

Globally, the intense systemic vasoconstriction of the autonomic storm compromises blood flow in various organs during this period. Subsequently, with herniation/brain death and associated denervation with vasodilatation, there is reperfusion which forms the basis of the global ischemia–

reperfusion (IR) injury which is thought to contribute significantly to organ dysfunction in the donor and facilitates the development of an immunologic continuum between the donor and recipient. In addition to the IR injury that occurs with the brain death process, IR may occur antecedent to the brain death event during resuscitation from the initial trauma or may follow brain death during the periods of cold storage and transplantation. Ischemia precipitates the loss of aerobic oxidative metabolism which is associated with cellular energy loss along with changed ion gradients promoting calcium influx. With reperfusion of oxygen-rich blood, there is generation of oxygen radicals, lipid peroxidation, and further membrane permeability to calcium. IR activates the vascular endothelium and donor leukocytes with resultant cytokine expression. This precipitates local inflammation, which is thought to contribute to graft immunogenicity by producing major histocompatibility antigens and adhesion molecules.

In concert with this, there are substantial animal and some human data to support that hypothalamic–pituitary destruction produces an endocrinopathy of brain death which is additive to the issues noted previously. Dominated by the thyroid and adrenal deficiencies, it is proposed that the absence of these key hormones contributes to cellular dysfunction, metabolic abnormalities, and hemodynamic deterioration. Deficiency of thyroid hormone is proposed to impair mitochondrial function and consequently diminish energy substrate with the resultant transition from aerobic to anaerobic metabolism. Proponents of HRT propose that diminished cardiac contractility consequent to low thyroid hormone levels can be reversed with exogenous hormone supplementation. However, significant disparities exist related to hypothalamic–pituitary axis dysfunction when comparing animal and human studies. An abundance of animal data suggest that low circulating thyroid hormone levels are responsible for abnormal energy sources, impaired cardiac function, and hemodynamic instability [36, 37, 47]. Animal studies and some human reports suggest that there is a dramatic reversal of the anaerobic metabolism, improvement in cardiovascular stability, and normalization of lab parameters and EKG changes as well as improved organ suitability for transplantation when the exogenous hormonal therapy is employed [36, 37].

However, it is important to recognize that several studies have failed to define the presence of endocrine dysfunction [29, 48, 49], show improvement with the addition of exogenous hormones [50, 51], or correlate hemodynamic instability with hormone levels [48, 49]. Consequently, the use of hormone replacement therapy remains controversial and will be further discussed under cardiovascular management.

The impact of brain death upon graft function and transplanted organs was first recognized in the early 1980s by Cooper and coworkers in a landmark series of experiments and observations related to the pathophysiologic effects of brain death on transplanted organs. During this period, the authors observed that hearts procured from healthy anesthetized baboons, stored for 48 h, when subsequently transplanted, functioned immediately with no evidence of cardiac dysfunction. However, hearts procured from brain-dead donors and stored in a similar fashion required several hours to achieve adequate function. The authors recognized that the only difference between the two groups was brain death and determined that the brain death process was a risk factor for poor outcomes after transplantation [47]. These observations began to establish that the brain death process is not static and that the graft is not biologically inert. Tilney and colleagues have proposed the existence of an immunologic continuum between donors and the recipients as a mechanism to understand the influence of brain death on recipient organ function [52]. Utilizing this model, they hypothesize that IR events associated with brain death and pre–/post-brain death events precipitate immunologic and non-immunologic injuries that impact upon short- and long-term graft function. A major component of the immunologic continuum is the IR injury that is proposed to initiate a significant inflammatory response, which triggers and amplifies the acute post-immunologic activity impacting upon multiple organs and contributing to their dysfunction in the short and long term.

Recently, it has been reported that increased plasma interleukin-6 levels in donors have been associated with lower recipient hospital-free survival after cadaveric organ transplantation [53]. Similarly, elevated plasma interleukin-6 levels in donors were associated with greater degrees of preload responsiveness that correlated with fewer organs transplanted [54]. In a study of cardiac donors, serum and myocardial levels of tumor necrosis factor alpha and interleukin-6 were elevated in all donors but were more markedly elevated in the dysfunctional unused donor hearts [55]. An intense inflammatory environment defined by elevated levels of interleukin-1, interleukin-6, tumor necrosis factor alpha, C-reactive protein, and procalcitonin has been reported in potential heart and lung donors. In this study, elevated procalcitonin levels were related to worse cardiac function and potentially thought to attenuate any improvement in cardiac function gained by donor management [56]. Similar elevations of inflammatory markers have been reported in liver transplantation. In a comparison study of hepatic tissue from brain-dead donors and living donors, the authors reported significant elevations in inflammatory cytokines in brain-dead donors compared to living donors. Cellular infiltrates were appreciably increased in parallel to the cytokine levels. This correlated with elevated liver enzymes and bilirubin levels and increased rates of rejection and primary graft nonfunction [57]. Attenuation of the increased inflammatory response with methylprednisolone was shown to significantly decrease soluble interleukins and the inflammatory response, significantly ameliorating IR injury in the post-transplant course, which was accompanied by a decreased incidence of acute rejection [58]. In summary, there is appreciable evidence that brain death and the associated inflammatory response has a substantial impact upon the transplanted organs. Future strategies will likely seek to not simply preserve organs but attenuate the inflammatory response in the donor.

Specific Organ Support

Hemodynamic and cardiovascular management form the cornerstone of potential organ donor management. A standardized and structured approach to hemodynamic management ensures that the donor somatically survives for procurement and maintains the remainder of potential organs in the best possible condition. Similar to the care of any critical patient, a collaborative approach utilizing the skills of physicians, nurses, respiratory therapists, and the OPO coordinator is pivotal for optimum management. Although the traditional management of the potential organ donor has been taken by the OPO transplant coordinator, there has been an evolution towards a collaborative approach between the intensivist/critical care community and the OPO. Standardization of donor management from the referral process through consent, followed by management and recovery, has been shown to significantly increase the number of organs recovered and organs transplanted [4–9, 59, 60]. Up to 20% of organs may be lost due to challenges with organ support of the post-brain dead donor [5, 61, 62]; institution of bedside checklists and intensivist-led management of potential organ donors has been associated with an increase in the number of transplanted organs and a decrease in post-brain death donation losses due to cardiac arrest [4–9, 59, 60, 62, 63]. Suggested donor management goals, based on US and international expert consensus guideline committees [62, 64–68], are listed in Table 39.1.

Table 39.1 Donor management goals

Variable	Target value
Mean arterial blood pressure, mmHg	>65
Central venous pressure, mmHg (range)	6–8
Ejection fracture, % (range)	45–55%
Number of vasopressors required	<1
pH (range)	7.3–7.5
PaO_2/FiO_2 ratio	>300
Sodium, mEq/L	135–155
Urine output, mL/kg/h	>0.5
Glucose, mg/dL	<150
Hemoglobin, mg/dL	>7
Platelets, $\times 10^9$/L	10
Tidal volume, mL/predicted body weight (range)	6–8

Although no clear current consensus exists, the traditional approach to organ donor management was to minimize the time between brain death and procurement because of the perception that prolonged management was detrimental to the donor organs and bed utilization in busy intensive care units necessitated admission for salvageable patients. This concept has been challenged as evolving literature reports that a longer period of donor management may be beneficial. In a retrospective study with a mean time from brain death to procurement of 35 h, it was reported that there was no decrease in the procurement to consented ratio with increasing time after brain death. When individual organs were analyzed separately, heart and pancreas procurement improved with an increased management period after brain death and some organs were successfully procured greater than 60 h after brain death [69]. Similarly, in a study of 100 consecutive organ donors whose mean donor management time was 23 h, it was reported that donors managed in excess of 20 h resulted in significantly more heart and lung procurements, more organs procured per donor (4.2 vs 3.2) and more organs transplanted per donor (3.7 vs 2.6). Interestingly, there was no significant difference noted in the obtainment of donor management goals [70].

Cardiovascular and Hemodynamic Management

Hemodynamic instability is reported to occur in a vast majority of potential organ donors and can be sustained in 20% of donors, despite ongoing vasoactive support [71]. Initial assessments of stability should be undertaken in all potential donors and include echocardiography, mean arterial blood pressure, vasoactive requirements, urine output, measurement of the left ventricular ejection fraction, and assessment of other dynamic indices. Figure 39.1 represents an algorithmic approach to the cardiovascular and hemodynamic management of the potential organ donor.

Potential organ donors achieving the thresholds identified in Fig. 39.1 should be continuously monitored and formally evaluated for cardiac donation. Traditionally, cardiac catheterization has been required for potential organ donors over 40 years of age. Given the significant myocardial stress associated with brain death, echocardiography should not be performed immediately after brain death declaration as this may provide misleading information related to cardiac function [72]. Initial attempts at stabilization should include normalizing blood pressure, metabolic abnormalities, and electrolyte disturbances. Transthoracic echocardiography (TTE) should be performed in all patients to evaluate structural abnormalities that may preclude cardiac donation and evaluate the left ventricular ejection fraction [73]. Echocardiographic abnormalities are reported to be responsible for 26% of non-used hearts with an odds ratio of 1.48 per 5% decrease in ejection fraction [74]. Although instrumental in the evaluation of cardiac function in the potential

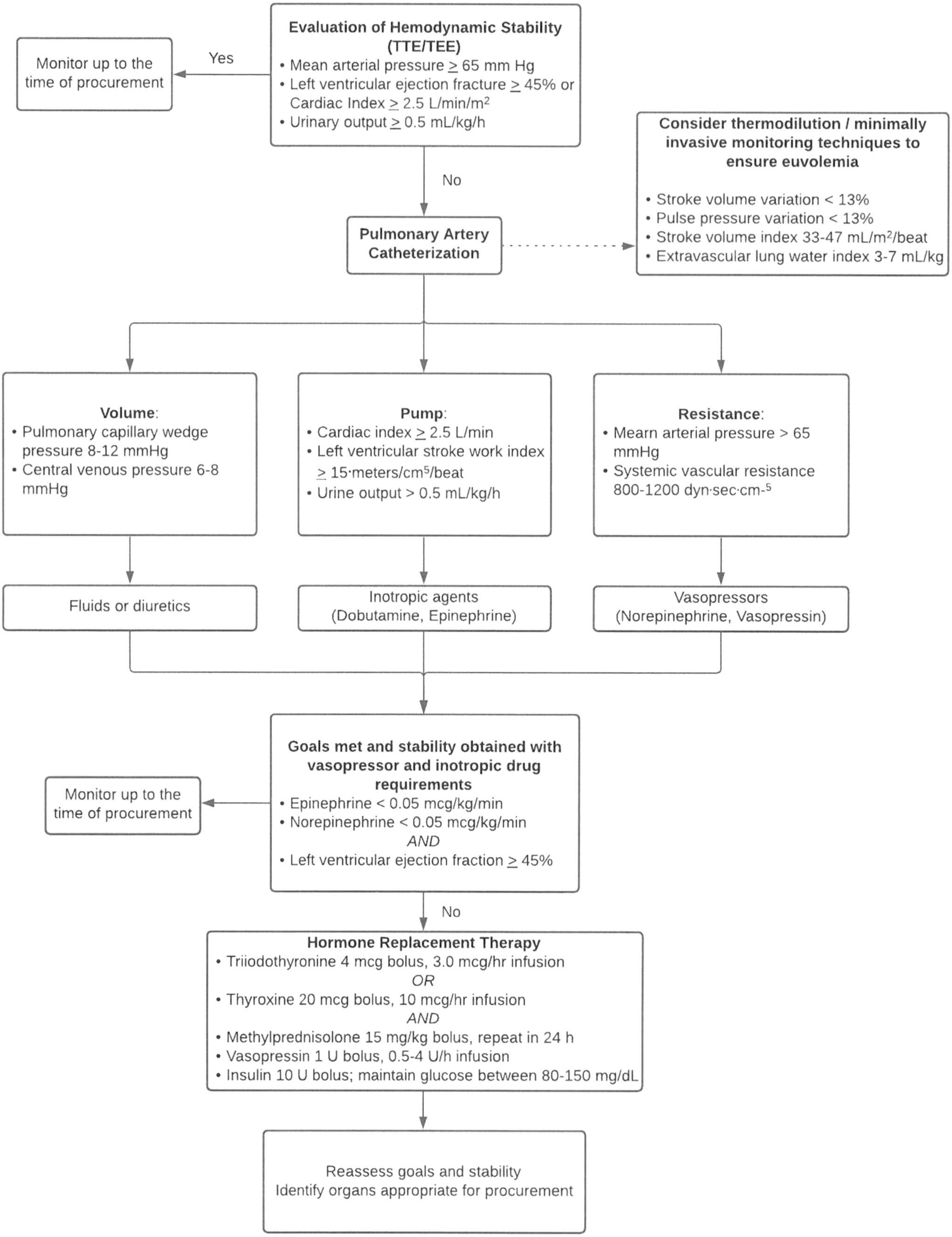

Fig. 39.1 Hemodynamic management algorithm and goals for the brain dead donor with a beating heart

organ donor, several issues warrant consideration regarding echocardiographic evaluation. These include the difficulty in securing the test, technical challenges with imaging in critically ill patients, and the accuracy and impact of the echocardiographic interpretation. When adequate images cannot be obtained with TTE, transesophageal echocardiography (TEE) should be performed as this modality has the additional benefit of detecting valvular lesions that could be underdiagnosed with TTE [75]. Serial echocardiographic examinations with either TTE or TEE are often indicated in patients with severe neurological injury for the identification of potentially reversible cardiac conditions [76].

Brain death predisposes potential donors to cardiac dysfunction with regional wall motion abnormalities that may be reversible. Similarly, it is important to appreciate that left ventricular ejection fraction is a load-dependent measure of contractility with variance noted when there are changes in preload and afterload [73]. It is also important to recognize that temporal changes occur in left ventricular systolic function. In a study that evaluated sequential echocardiograms in potential organ donors, with ejection fractions less than 50% or regional wall motion abnormalities on the initial cardiogram, 12 of 13 patients improved after donor management. Utilizing a strategy that employed high-dose corticosteroids and dopamine without the use of thyroid hormone, the 12 donor hearts were transplanted with a survival rate of 92% over a mean follow-up of 16 months [77]. In work by Madan et al., similar results were observed as hearts with transient left ventricular systolic dysfunction were resuscitated and successfully transplanted [78]. The literature suggests that more than 50% of the hearts with initial abnormal function may attain hemodynamic transplantation criteria with aggressive donor management. In a prospective study of 66 potential organ donors, an initial normal left ventricular ejection fraction independently predicted end-assessment hemodynamic suitability for transplantation. An initial abnormal left ventricular systolic function was identified in almost half of donor hearts, of which 58% achieved hemodynamic stability criteria for procurement [72]. Although there are limited data from small case series, low-dose dobutamine stress tests may be able to detect myocardium that appears dysfunctional in the donor and may be capable of recrudescing function in the recipient [79].

When echocardiography (i.e., TTE or TEE) cannot be reliably obtained, a pulmonary artery catheter (PAC) may be used. Most major guidelines recommend use of hemodynamic monitoring tools such as the PAC or other noninvasive monitors [1, 65, 80]. In one of the largest protocol-guided studies that randomized 556 brain-dead donors to protocolized therapy (i.e., an algorithm targeting cardiac index, mean arterial blood pressure and pulse pressure variation), the study was stopped early as the number of organs transplanted per donor was not found to be statistically significantly improved [81]. Moreover, while most current donor management guidelines endorse central venous pressure, this monitoring modality is fraught with inaccuracy in critically ill patients [82]. Other hemodynamic monitoring tools, such as noninvasive arterial waveform monitors or thermodilution techniques that monitor dynamic changes in systolic pressure, pulse pressure, and stroke volume have been found to have high sensitivity and specificity for predicting volume responsiveness in patients undergoing mechanical ventilation [83]. Regardless of the modality, hemodynamic monitoring tools—including use of more than one modality—aid in the assessment of volume status and response to therapy. Either PAC or noninvasive monitoring techniques should be considered, as described in Fig. 39.1.

In patients failing to achieve stability and defined endpoints listed in Fig. 39.1, vasopressors are frequently necessary to maintain perfusion pressures. Firm recommendations regarding the choice of vasopressors remain limited by an absence of controlled trials and perceived negative effects of catecholamines from studies that did not reliably measure the adequacy of intravascular volume. When vasopressors are utilized, the endpoints of therapy should be clearly defined and vasopressor use titrated to specific physiologic abnormalities. Once intravascular volume resuscitation has been adequately attained, the choice of vasoactive support depends upon the predominant physiologic abnormalities. In organ donors with predominant myocardial dysfunction and inadequate flow despite adequate volume resuscitation, dobutamine should be used for inotropic support. In potential organ donors whose hemodynamic instability is dominated by vasodilatation, vasopressors should be used to maintain mean arterial pressure and ensure adequacy of perfusion pressure gradients. Most current recommendations support the use of vasopressin as a first-line agent to maintain vascular tone [76, 84] those others have endorsed norepinephrine given its additional beta-1 receptor actions [85]. Although not well appreciated, catecholamines have immunomodulatory properties. A large retrospective study conducted by Schnuelle reported that the donor use of dopamine and/or norepinephrine was associated with beneficial results related to acute rejection that were attributed to the immunomodulatory ability of catecholamines. This benefit was dominantly confined to renal graft survivorship, although a potential negative impact of norepinephrine was noted on heart transplantation [86, 87]. Additional literature suggests that the use of low-dose dopamine (4 mcg/kg/min) independent of hemodynamic instability was associated with a decrease in the need for dialysis after kidney transplantation [88]. In another study, use of dopamine in donors was associated with an improved survival after 3 years (87% vs 67.8%). The authors concluded that fewer recipients of a pretreated graft required hemofiltration after transplantation (21.7% vs 40.4%) and that treatment of potential brain-dead donors with dopamine of 4 mcg/kg/min did not harm cardiac allographs and improved the clinical course of the recipient [42].

Hormonal Replacement Therapy (HRT)

The use of hormonal replacement therapy (HRT) in organ donors is predicated upon the assumption that the ischemic damage to the hypothalamic–pituitary axis occurring with brain death creates an endocrinopathy dominated by the absence of thyroid and adrenal hormones that contribute to donor instability. The anterior pituitary and posterior pituitary have distinct differences in blood supply, innervation, and hormonal production. There is no specific direct arterial blood supply to the anterior pituitary, which receives its blood supply via drainage from the hypothalamus. Blood emerging from the hypothalamus empties into a portal system that bathes the anterior pituitary. Blood supply for the posterior pituitary is via the inferior hypophyseal artery and the connection to the hypothalamus is predominantly neuronal. HRT infers that there is significant damage to the blood supply to the hypothalamic and pituitary areas that precipitate an endocrinopathy with the attendant physiologic sequelae of a low thyroid hormone state and adrenal insufficiency.

There are substantial animal data and some human data to support a state of profound thyroid/adrenal depletion with exogenous supplementation reported to dramatically improve hemodynamic instability and suitability for transplantation [36]. In the original work utilizing HRT, which consisted of thyroid hormone, corticosteroids, and insulin, dramatic improvements in organ donor stability were achieved resulting in significant improvements in transplant suitability, diminutions in the requirements for vasoactive support, and dramatic improvements in cardiac function [37]. Large retrospective reviews of brain-dead donors reported significant benefit through the use of steroids and vasopressin and utilization of either triiodothyronine or thyroxine. In the group of potential organ donors that received HRT, the number of organs procured was significantly higher than the donors that did not receive HRT. This resulted in a 23% increase in the number of organs procured with dramatic improvements in the likelihood of an organ being transplanted [60]. However, more recent reviews of thyroid hormone administration during adult donor care concluded that no publications support the routine administration of thyroid hormone for all donors [85]. Rescue replacement for cardiac inotropic support was supported by some studies, although the methodologic designs were not detailed enough to support a recommendation for routine use [89]. In one of the few prospective randomized double-blind trials, 80 potential cardiac donors were allocated to receive triiodothyronine (0.8 mg/kg/bolus followed by a 0.113 mg/kg/h infusion), methylprednisolone 1000 mg bolus, both drugs, or placebo following an initial hemodynamic assessment. Independent of the use of HRT, an explicit donor management algorithm with optimization variables was initiated that used vasopressin as the primary vasoactive agent. During the 6-h management period, cardiac index was noted to significantly increase in virtually all donors. However, the administration of thyroid hormone and methylprednisolone, either alone or in combination, did not affect the hemodynamics nor has any impact upon heart retrieval. Importantly, 35% of the hearts initially deemed marginal or dysfunctional were suitable for transplantation at the end of the assessment. The authors concluded that donor circulatory status can be improved by active management with the potential to increase transplantable hearts when organ acceptance is deferred until a period of resuscitation and assessment is completed. Hemodynamic management utilizing a PAC was felt to be the cornerstone of donor management and the introduction of hormonal therapy was not a substitute for a detailed hemodynamic assessment and management optimization approaches [90]. Consequently, the use of HRT in potential organ donor management remains controversial and of uncertain benefit. Some experts recommend broad use of HRT [37, 91] while others reserve HRT for use only in hemodynamically unstable patients [65, 92]. Pragmatically, it would appear that HRT should be utilized in hemodynamically unstable donors with ongoing instability, despite aggressive optimization management [65, 93]. Both T3 and T4 are acceptable for HRT. Dosing regimens are described in Fig. 39.1.

Vasopressin deficiency is a frequent complication of brain death resulting from brainstem infarction. Up to 80% of patients with brain death develop central diabetes insipidus [94]. The absence of vasopressin can contribute to multiple donor management issues, including hyperosmolarity, electrolyte disturbances, and intravascular volume depletion. It is important to differentiate diabetes insipidus from mannitol-induced osmotic diuresis. Diabetes insipidus is generally associated with polyuria (> 3–4 L/d), normal or increased serum osmolality, inappropriately dilute urine (specific gravity <1.005, urine osmolality <200 mOsm/kg H_2O), and hypernatremia (sodium concentration > 145 mMol/L) [65, 67]. Diabetes insipidus should be treated with hypotonic solutions, and frequently, 5% dextrose in water is used to match urine output mL for mL. For diabetes insipidus with significant hypernatremia without hypotension, desmopressin acetate (DDAVP) or arginine vasopressin may be utilized. Desmopressin may be given intravenously as 1–4 mcg with additional doses titrated to urine output, urine osmolality, and serum sodium [65]. A typical dose of 2 mcg every 6 h is required, although higher doses may be needed. Vasopressin exerts its effect on three receptors: V1 receptors on the smooth muscle and is responsible for vasopressor effects, V2 receptors located in the kidney which promote the antidiuretic effect, and V3 receptors in the pituitary which regulate corticotropin-releasing hormone. Arginine vasopressin has antidiuretic and vasopressor effects, whereas DDAVP has greater affinity for the V2 receptor and consequently a predominant antidiuretic effect. Subsequent dosing is dependent upon the response. In the setting of hypotension, arginine vasopressin is preferred at a dose between 0.01 and 0.04 U/min with or without an initial bolus dose of 1 U [65, 95].

The hormonal alterations following brain death result in additional endocrine disorders to include hyperglycemia. Although the effects of hyperglycemia are understudied in the organ donor population [67, 96], hyperglycemia is believed to impair organ function. Hyperglycemia is thought to lead to metabolic exhaustion of pancreatic islet cells with potential detrimental effects on pancreatic donor function [65]. Consequently, hyperglycemic donors should be managed similarly to other critically ill patients using an empiric concentration of 150 mg/dL as a threshold for initiation of therapy while avoiding IV fluids containing dextrose [3, 65, 67].

Following brain death, a massive inflammatory response supervenes, characterized by elevations in cytokines [96]. Steroids are recommended to counteract the inflammatory cascade and to reduce concentrations of cytokines such as intetrleukin-6 and tumor necrosis factor [56]. While varying rates of relative adrenal insufficiency have been reported in brain dead donors [67], steroids may also be of benefit for this indication [97]. Despite conflicting data on the beneficial effects of steroids on graft function [98], most clinical pathways and donor management guidelines recommend methylprednisolone 15 mg/kg, followed by an infusion of 100 mg/h or 15 mg/kg every 24 h to help reduce the deleterious effects of the inflammatory cascade [1, 3, 58, 65]. Some authors have advocated for lower doses of steroids (i.e., hydrocortisone 300 mg IV followed by 100 mg every eight h) [99].

Pulmonary and Respiratory Care Management

Multiple competing pathophysiological factors conspire to jeopardize pulmonary function in the potential organ donor. Neurogenic pulmonary edema is frequently associated with brain death [100]. Consequent to the catecholamine surge, there are significant elevations in systemic vascular resistance which result in elevations in left arterial pressure. This represents a transient massive hydrostatic pressure gradient generating fluid flux into the lung that is coupled with structural damage to the capillary endothelium. Against this background of capillary permeability, ongoing fluid resuscitation is purported to increase extravascular lung water, which is associated with changes in the chest x-ray appearance and diminution in lung function which have precluded procurement. Initial work in animal models revealed a dramatic distribution of blood to the right atrium and right ventricle consequent to venoconstriction and augmentation of venous return. Dramatic increases in pulmonary artery pressure were reported that resulted in 72% of the effective circulating volume being contained in the lungs for several minutes during the brain death event [37]. Subsequent to this hydrostatic and capillary burst injury pattern associated with brain death, Fisher recognized the presence of an inflammatory response associated with brain death. In a study that compared inflammatory signals in brain-dead patients compared to controls, dramatic increases in neutrophil concentration and lavage concentrations of interleukin-8 were reported [101]. The interleukin-8 signal in the donor was found to be correlative with the degree of impairment in graft oxygenation, the development of severe early graft dysfunction, and the early recipient mortality [102].

Management of the potential organ donor invokes the same principles of ventilator management used in patients with acute respiratory distress syndrome [67, 103, 104]. Whereas a lung protective strategy has been established as the standard of care for patient with acute lung injury, traditional donor management has utilized relatively high tidal volumes in an effort to minimize de-recruitment and improve gas exchange. In the Protective Ventilatory Strategy in Potential Lung Donors Study, donors were randomized to a protective ventilator strategy using tidal volumes of 6–8 mL/kg predicted body weight and positive end-expiratory pressures (PEEP) of 8–10 cm H_2O vs. tidal volumes of 10–12 mL/kg predicted body weight and lower levels of PEEP (3–5 cm H_2O) [103]. Donors ventilated with lower tidal volumes and higher PEEP were significantly more likely to be eligible for lung donation and had lower concentrations of inflammatory mediators [103]. These results suggest that hyperinflation has an adverse effect on lung function and compromises the eligibility of lung donors. Several studies have shown dramatic increases in the rate of lung procurement when an aggressive strategy focused upon ventilator management and respiratory care was employed [101, 103, 105, 106].

Suggested goals for the management of respiratory function in potential organ donors are listed in Table 39.2.

Alternative ventilatory modes, such as airways pressure release ventilation (APRV), have been inadequately studied in the brain dead donor population though in one exploratory study of 45 donors randomized to either APRV or a conventional lung protective strategy, an association with more lung procurements was observed in the APRV group [107]. Prone ventilation may be considered for donors with basilar or posterior opacities on chest imaging. In a prospective study of 40 lung-eligible donors with hypoxemia, prone ventilation improved oxygenation, decreased atelectasis, and increased the number of lungs transplanted from 24% to 45% ($P = 0.03$) [108]. As has been shown for the management of acute respiratory distress syndrome, restrictive fluid

Table 39.2 Ventilator and respiratory management goals for the potential organ donor

Parameter	Goal
Tidal volume	6–8 mL/kg using predicted bodyweight
Positive end expiratory pressure	8–10 cm of water, titrated higher as needed to maintain oxygenation
Arterial pH	7.35–7.45
Plateau pressure	<30 cm of water
PaO_2	>100 mmHg
Fraction of inspired oxygen	<0.40
Goals of bronchoscopy	Anatomical evaluation Foreign body assessment/removal Assessment of aspiration Secretion clearance
Goals of fluid management	Cautious diuresis Extravascular lung water < 10 mL/kg Pulmonary capillary wedge pressure < 6–10 mmHg Central venous pressure 6–8 mmHg
Use of antimicrobial agents	Used on the basis of results of culture and Gram's staining of aspirated secretions
Preventative care	Head of bed elevation >30°

strategies have been associated with greater numbers of functional organs in brain dead donors, including kidney donors [109]. Although widely used in critical care units, regular use of nebulized albuterol has not been associated with improved lung oxygenation or lung utilization and is not routinely recommended [110]. Measures to prevent ventilator-associated pneumonia are recommended, including elevation of the head of the bed to 30°, as well as other standardized recommendations for the prevention of hospital acquired infections [111].

Renal, Fluids, and Electrolyte Management

Avoidance of hypovolemia and prevention of electrolyte derangements are essential goals for the critical care management of the potential organ donor. Volume depletion may be precipitated by hyperglycemia-induced osmotic diuresis, diabetes insipidus, or a cold diuresis in a hypothermic patient. Vasodilatation is a consistent feature in the potential organ donor predominantly related to herniation-mediated denervation and the loss of vasomotor control and autoregulation. Whenever possible, fluid resuscitation in the potential organ donor should be guided by objective measurements and defined endpoints (Fig. 39.1). Inadequacy of initial volume resuscitation has been shown to precipitate a significant increase in inflammatory mediators with fewer organs procured and transplanted [54]. Prompt correction of hypovolemia may be accomplished with the use of either crystalloids (0.9% saline, PlasmaLyte, Normosol, or lactated Ringers) or colloids, though the use of hydroxyethyl starch should be avoided owing to its association with coagulopathy and renal dysfunction [65, 96].

Hypernatremia has been described as one of the most deleterious electrolyte derangements in regard to hepatic outcomes after transplantation. Diabetes insipidus and hypovolemia can lead to hypernatremia, with concentrations greater than 155 mMol/L being associated a higher incidence of graft loss and metabolic abnormalities in liver transplant recipients [112]. Therefore, cautious attention to correcting the serum sodium and appropriately transitioning from normal saline to a hypotonic solution is appropriate once intravascular volume has been repleted and there is evidence of adequate perfusion. Similarly, it is important to recognize that the infusion of significant amounts of hypotonic solutions containing dextrose, which are frequently used to treat diabetes insipidus, may precipitate hyperglycemia, osmotic diuresis, and hyperglycemia-mediated immune dysfunction.

There are often antagonistic and competing strategies related to fluid resuscitation in the potential organ donor. Several studies have sought to clarify the approach to an appropriate fluid balance which will ensure the optimum procurement of both lungs and kidneys. In a study that compared the relationship between HRT and CVP on increasing organs for transplantation, the authors reported that when HRT was infused for greater than 15 h and a CVP was maintained at less than 10 mmHg, there was a dramatic increase in the number of hearts and lungs procured. When a final CVP was less than 10 mmHg, 44% more hearts, 95% more lungs, and 13% more kidneys were transplanted [113]. A similar retrospective study sought to evaluate the impact of a restrictive fluid balance that focused upon increasing lung procurement and evaluating renal function after kidney transplantation. The authors reported that a negative or equal fluid balance with a CVP less than or equal to 6 mmHg had no effect on kidney recipient graft function or the development of delayed graft function. A positive fluid balance between the brain death event and organ procurement did not reduce the risk of graft survivorship of delayed graft function. In summary, fluid resuscitation should be guided by objective measurements and defined endpoints similar to that used in the management of other critically ill patients. Previous strategies that focused upon aggressive overhydration to enhance renal perfusion have been shown to jeopardize pulmonary function and preclude procurement. A moderate or restrictive fluid resuscitative strategy is appropriate for both lung procurement and maintenance of renal function similar to the management approach for other critically ill patients.

Additional Supportive Care

Notwithstanding limited data, there is speculation that hepatic glycogen stores may be depleted in the brain death period and that support with enteral nutrition may play an important role in modulating organ function after transplantation [114]. In the absence of contraindications, many posit that it is appropriate to continue enteral nutrition following for any evidence of hyperglycemia [65]. Others have advocated for the cessation of enteral nutrition due to the loss of vagal tone that accompanies brain death, resulting in loss of intestinal transit and malabsorption of nutrients [85, 115]. Coagulation abnormalities are frequently encountered in potential organ donors, and ongoing assessment of coagulopathy and hemoglobin is necessary during the course of donor management. Although there are no outcome data for potential organ donors, the approach advocated is similar to that of other critically ill patients utilizing a transfusion threshold for hemoglobin of 7 mg/dL and normalization of coagulation parameters [65, 92]. Deceased organ donors are at increased risk for venous thromboembolism; prophylaxis with enoxaparin (40 mg every 12 h) is recommended in patients with normal renal function and unfractionated heparin is used for patient with renal dysfunction. Pituitary injury predisposes to thermoregulatory impairment and it is imperative that the donor receive warmed fluids and body temperature be monitored routinely, as hypothermia can further impair coagulation and predispose to cardiac rhythm disturbances. Alternatively, the role of mild therapeutic hypothermia (34–35 °C) remains uncertain, although promising results have been reported when used in donors, with improved 1-year graft survival and reductions in delayed graft function [116, 117].

References

1. Frenette AJ, Williamson D, Weiss MJ, et al. Worldwide management of donors after neurological death: a systematic review and narrative synthesis of guidelines. Can J Anaesth. 2020;67(12):1839–57. https://doi.org/10.1007/s12630-020-01815-0.
2. Dhanani S, Shemie SD. Advancing the science of organ donor management. Crit Care. 2014;18(6):612. https://doi.org/10.1186/s13054-014-0612-z.
3. Maciel CB, Greer DM. ICU management of the potential organ donor: state of the art. Curr Neurol Neurosci Rep. 2016;16(9):86. https://doi.org/10.1007/s11910-016-0682-1.
4. Kothari R, Tolles J, Adelmann D, Lewis RJ, Malinoski DJ, Niemann CU. Organ donor management goals and delayed graft function in adult kidney transplant recipients. Clin Transpl. 2022;36(2):e14528. https://doi.org/10.1111/ctr.14528.
5. Patel MS, De La Cruz S, Sally MB, Groat T, Malinoski DJ. Active donor management during the hospital phase of care is associated with more organs transplanted per donor. J Am Coll Surg. 2017;225(4):525–31. https://doi.org/10.1016/j.jamcollsurg.2017.06.014.
6. Rosendale JD, Chabalewski FL, McBride MA, et al. Increased transplanted organs from the use of a standardized donor management protocol. Am J Transplant. 2002;2(8):761–8. https://doi.org/10.1034/j.1600-6143.2002.20810.x.
7. Salim A, Velmahos GC, Brown C, Belzberg H, Demetriades D. Aggressive organ donor management significantly increases the number of organs available for transplantation. J Trauma. 2005;58(5):991–4. https://doi.org/10.1097/01.ta.0000168708.78049.32.
8. Wheeldon DR, Potter CD, Oduro A, Wallwork J, Large SR. Transforming the "unacceptable" donor: outcomes from the adoption of a standardized donor management technique. J Heart Lung Transplant. 1995;14(4):734–42. (https://www.ncbi.nlm.nih.gov/pubmed/7578183)
9. Venkateswaran RV, Patchell VB, Wilson IC, et al. Early donor management increases the retrieval rate of lungs for transplantation. Ann Thorac Surg. 2008;85(1):278–86.; discussion 286. https://doi.org/10.1016/j.athoracsur.2007.07.092.
10. Chandler JA, Connors M, Holland G, Shemie SD. "Effective" requesting: a scoping review of the literature on asking families to consent to organ and tissue donation. Transplantation. 2017;101(5S Suppl. 1):S1–S16. https://doi.org/10.1097/TP.0000000000001695.
11. Siminoff LA, Agyemang AA, Traino HM. Consent to organ donation: a review. Prog Transplant. 2013;23(1):99–104. https://doi.org/10.7182/pit2013801.
12. Howard DH, Siminoff LA, McBride V, Lin M. Does quality improvement work? Evaluation of the organ donation breakthrough collaborative. Health Serv Res. 2007;42(6 Pt 1):2160–73.; discussion 2294–323. https://doi.org/10.1111/j.1475-6773.2007.00732.x.
13. Siminoff LA, Lawrence RH, Zhang A. Decoupling: what is it and does it really help increase consent to organ donation? Prog Transplant. 2002;12(1):52–60. https://doi.org/10.7182/prtr.12.1.t2ph6gtg70351460.
14. Wijdicks EF, Varelas PN, Gronseth GS, Greer DM, Academy A, of N. Evidence-based guideline update: determining brain death in adults: report of the Quality Standards Subcommittee of the American Academy of Neurology. Neurology. 2010;74(23):1911–8. https://doi.org/10.1212/WNL.0b013e3181e242a8.
15. Lustbader D, O'Hara D, Wijdicks EF, et al. Second brain death examination may negatively affect organ donation. Neurology. 2011;76(2):119–24. https://doi.org/10.1212/WNL.0b013e3182061b0c.
16. Gortmaker SL, Beasley CL, Sheehy E, et al. Improving the request process to increase family consent for organ donation. J Transpl Coord. 1998;8(4):210–7. https://doi.org/10.7182/prtr.1.8.4.2g64j1x161620765.
17. Collaborators AT. Effect of "collaborative requesting" on consent rate for organ donation: randomised controlled trial (ACRE trial). BMJ. 2009;339:b3911. https://doi.org/10.1136/bmj.b3911.
18. Potts JT Jr, Herdman R. Non-heart-beating organ transplantation: medical and ethical issues in procurement. Washington (DC): National Academies Press (US); 1997.
19. Division of Health Care Services, Committee on Non-Heart-Beating Transplantation II, The Scientific, Ethical Basis for Practice, Protocols. Non-heart-beating organ transplantation: practice and protocols. Washington (DC): National Academies Press (US); 2000.
20. Ethics Committee ACoCCM, Society of Critical Care M. Recommendations for nonheartbeating organ donation. A position paper by the Ethics Committee, American College of Critical Care Medicine, Society of Critical Care Medicine. Crit Care Med. 2001;29(9):1826–31. https://doi.org/10.1097/00003246-200109000-00029.
21. Greer DM. Determination of Brain Death. N Engl J Med. 2021;385(27):2554–61. https://doi.org/10.1056/NEJMcp2025326.
22. Varelas PN, Rehman M, Mehta C, et al. Comparison of 1 vs 2 brain death examinations on time to death pronouncement and organ donation: a 12-year single center experience. Neurology. 2021;96(10):e1453–61. https://doi.org/10.1212/WNL.0000000000011554.

23. Madden M, Andrews P, Rector R, Menaker J, Habashi N. Carbogen for apnea testing during the brain death declaration process in subjects on extracorporeal membrane oxygenation. Respir Care. 2020;65(1):75–81. https://doi.org/10.4187/respcare.06378.
24. Rizvi T, Batchala P, Mukherjee S. Brain death: diagnosis and imaging techniques. Semin Ultrasound CT MR. 2018;39(5):515–29. https://doi.org/10.1053/j.sult.2018.01.006.
25. Gastala J, Fattal D, Kirby PA, Capizzano AA, Sato Y, Moritani T. Brain death: radiologic signs of a non-radiologic diagnosis. Clin Neurol Neurosurg. 2019;185:105465. https://doi.org/10.1016/j.clineuro.2019.105465.
26. Bohatyrewicz R, Pastuszka J, Walas W, et al. Implementation of computed tomography angiography (CTA) and computed tomography perfusion (CTP) in polish guidelines for determination of cerebral circulatory arrest (CCA) during brain death/death by neurological criteria (BD/DNC) diagnosis procedure. J Clin Med. 2021;10(18) https://doi.org/10.3390/jcm10184237.
27. Cushing H. Some experimental and clinical observations concerning states of increased intracranial tension. Am J Med Sci. 1901;124:375.
28. Power BM, Van Heerden PV. The physiological changes associated with brain death--current concepts and implications for treatment of the brain dead organ donor. Anaesth Intensive Care. 1995;23(1):26–36. https://doi.org/10.1177/0310057X9502300107.
29. Gramm HJ, Meinhold H, Bickel U, et al. Acute endocrine failure after brain death? Transplantation. 1992;54(5):851–7. https://doi.org/10.1097/00007890-199211000-00016.
30. Powner DJ, Boccalandro C, Alp MS, Vollmer DG. Endocrine failure after traumatic brain injury in adults. Neurocrit Care. 2006;5(1):61–70. https://doi.org/10.1385/ncc:5:1:61.
31. Schneider HJ, Kreitschmann-Andermahr I, Ghigo E, Stalla GK, Agha A. Hypothalamopituitary dysfunction following traumatic brain injury and aneurysmal subarachnoid hemorrhage: a systematic review. JAMA. 2007;298(12):1429–38. https://doi.org/10.1001/jama.298.12.1429.
32. Yoshioka T, Sugimoto H, Uenishi M, et al. Prolonged hemodynamic maintenance by the combined administration of vasopressin and epinephrine in brain death: a clinical study. Neurosurgery. 1986;18(5):565–7. https://doi.org/10.1227/00006123-198605000-00009.
33. Black PM. Brain death (first of two parts). N Engl J Med. 1978;299(7):338–44. https://doi.org/10.1056/NEJM197808172990705.
34. Novitzky D. Donor management: state of the art. Transplant Proc. 1997;29(8):3773–5. https://doi.org/10.1016/s0041-1345(97)01150-0.
35. Novitzky D, Cooper DK, Chaffin JS, Greer AE, DeBault LE, Zuhdi N. Improved cardiac allograft function following triiodothyronine therapy to both donor and recipient. Transplantation. 1990;49(2):311–6. https://doi.org/10.1097/00007890-199002000-00017.
36. Novitzky D, Cooper DK, Morrell D, Isaacs S. Change from aerobic to anaerobic metabolism after brain death, and reversal following triiodothyronine therapy. Transplantation. 1988;45(1):32–6. https://doi.org/10.1097/00007890-198801000-00008.
37. Novitzky D, Cooper DK, Reichart B. Hemodynamic and metabolic responses to hormonal therapy in brain-dead potential organ donors. Transplantation. 1987;43(6):852–4. (https://www.ncbi.nlm.nih.gov/pubmed/3296351)
38. Szabo G, Buhmann V, Bahrle S, Vahl CF, Hagl S. Brain death impairs coronary endothelial function. Transplantation. 2002;73(11):1846–8. https://doi.org/10.1097/00007890-200206150-00027.
39. Segel LD, vonHaag DW, Zhang J, Follette DM. Selective overexpression of inflammatory molecules in hearts from brain-dead rats. J Heart Lung Transplant. 2002;21(7):804–11. https://doi.org/10.1016/s1053-2498(02)00382-0.
40. Szabo G, Hackert T, Buhmann V, Sebening C, Vahl CF, Hagl S. Myocardial performance after brain death: studies in isolated hearts. Ann Transplant. 2000;5(4):45–50. (https://www.ncbi.nlm.nih.gov/pubmed/11499360)
41. Yeh T Jr, Wechsler AS, Graham LJ, et al. Acute brain death alters left ventricular myocardial gene expression. J Thorac Cardiovasc Surg. 1999;117(2):365–74. https://doi.org/10.1016/S0022-5223(99)70435-6.
42. Benck U, Hoeger S, Brinkkoetter PT, et al. Effects of donor pre-treatment with dopamine on survival after heart transplantation: a cohort study of heart transplant recipients nested in a randomized controlled multicenter trial. J Am Coll Cardiol. 2011;58(17):1768–77. https://doi.org/10.1016/j.jacc.2011.05.060.
43. D'Amico TA, Meyers CH, Koutlas TC, et al. Desensitization of myocardial beta-adrenergic receptors and deterioration of left ventricular function after brain death. J Thorac Cardiovasc Surg. 1995;110(3):746–51. https://doi.org/10.1016/s0022-5223(95)70107-9.
44. Shivalkar B, Van Loon J, Wieland W, et al. Variable effects of explosive or gradual increase of intracranial pressure on myocardial structure and function. Circulation. 1993;87(1):230–9. https://doi.org/10.1161/01.cir.87.1.230.
45. Mehra MR, Uber PA, Ventura HO, Scott RL, Park MH. The impact of mode of donor brain death on cardiac allograft vasculopathy: an intravascular ultrasound study. J Am Coll Cardiol. 2004;43(5):806–10. https://doi.org/10.1016/j.jacc.2003.08.059.
46. Audibert G, Charpentier C, Seguin-Devaux C, et al. Improvement of donor myocardial function after treatment of autonomic storm during brain death. Transplantation. 2006;82(8):1031–6. https://doi.org/10.1097/01.tp.0000235825.97538.d5.
47. Cooper DK, Novitzky D, Wicomb WN. The pathophysiological effects of brain death on potential donor organs, with particular reference to the heart. Ann R Coll Surg Engl. 1989;71(4):261–6. (https://www.ncbi.nlm.nih.gov/pubmed/2774455)
48. Howlett TA, Keogh AM, Perry L, Touzel R, Rees LH. Anterior and posterior pituitary function in brain-stem-dead donors. A possible role for hormonal replacement therapy. Transplantation. 1989;47(5):828–34. https://doi.org/10.1097/00007890-198905000-00016.
49. Powner DJ, Hendrich A, Lagler RG, Ng RH, Madden RL. Hormonal changes in brain dead patients. Crit Care Med. 1990;18(7):702–8. https://doi.org/10.1097/00003246-199007000-00004.
50. Goarin JP, Cohen S, Riou B, et al. The effects of triiodothyronine on hemodynamic status and cardiac function in potential heart donors. Anesth Analg. 1996;83(1):41–7. https://doi.org/10.1097/00000539-199607000-00008.
51. Randell TT, Hockerstedt KA. Triiodothyronine treatment in brain-dead multiorgan donors—a controlled study. Transplantation. 1992;54(4):736–8. https://doi.org/10.1097/00007890-199210000-00034.
52. Pratschke J, Wilhelm MJ, Kusaka M, et al. Brain death and its influence on donor organ quality and outcome after transplantation. Transplantation. 1999;67(3):343–8. https://doi.org/10.1097/00007890-199902150-00001.
53. Murugan R, Venkataraman R, Wahed AS, et al. Increased plasma interleukin-6 in donors is associated with lower recipient hospital-free survival after cadaveric organ transplantation. Crit Care Med. 2008;36(6):1810–6. https://doi.org/10.1097/CCM.0b013e318174d89f.
54. Murugan R, Venkataraman R, Wahed AS, et al. Preload responsiveness is associated with increased interleukin-6 and lower organ yield from brain-dead donors. Crit Care Med. 2009;37(8):2387–93. https://doi.org/10.1097/CCM.0b013e3181a960d6.

55. Birks EJ, Burton PB, Owen V, et al. Elevated tumor necrosis factor-alpha and interleukin-6 in myocardium and serum of malfunctioning donor hearts. Circulation. 2000;102(19 Suppl 3):III352–8. https://doi.org/10.1161/01.cir.102.suppl_3.iii-352.
56. Venkateswaran RV, Dronavalli V, Lambert PA, et al. The proinflammatory environment in potential heart and lung donors: prevalence and impact of donor management and hormonal therapy. Transplantation. 2009;88(4):582–8. https://doi.org/10.1097/TP.0b013e3181b11e5d.
57. Weiss S, Kotsch K, Francuski M, et al. Brain death activates donor organs and is associated with a worse I/R injury after liver transplantation. Am J Transplant. 2007;7(6):1584–93. https://doi.org/10.1111/j.1600-6143.2007.01799.x.
58. Kotsch K, Ulrich F, Reutzel-Selke A, et al. Methylprednisolone therapy in deceased donors reduces inflammation in the donor liver and improves outcome after liver transplantation: a prospective randomized controlled trial. Ann Surg. 2008;248(6):1042–50. https://doi.org/10.1097/SLA.0b013e318190e70c.
59. Malinoski DJ, Daly MC, Patel MS, Oley-Graybill C, Foster CE 3rd, Salim A. Achieving donor management goals before deceased donor procurement is associated with more organs transplanted per donor. J Trauma. 2011;71(4):990–5.; discussion 996. https://doi.org/10.1097/TA.0b013e31822779e5.
60. Rosendale JD, Kauffman HM, McBride MA, et al. Aggressive pharmacologic donor management results in more transplanted organs. Transplantation. 2003;75(4):482–7. https://doi.org/10.1097/01.TP.0000045683.85282.93.
61. Patel MS, Zatarain J, De La Cruz S, et al. The impact of meeting donor management goals on the number of organs transplanted per expanded criteria donor: a prospective study from the UNOS Region 5 Donor Management Goals Workgroup. JAMA Surg. 2014;149(9):969–75. https://doi.org/10.1001/jamasurg.2014.967.
62. Martin-Loeches I, Sandiumenge A, Charpentier J, et al. Management of donation after brain death (DBD) in the ICU: the potential donor is identified, what's next? Intensive Care Med. 2019;45(3):322–30. https://doi.org/10.1007/s00134-019-05574-5.
63. Hoste P, Ferdinande P, Vogelaers D, et al. Adherence to guidelines for the management of donors after brain death. J Crit Care. 2019;49:56–63. https://doi.org/10.1016/j.jcrc.2018.10.016.
64. Ball IM, Hornby L, Rochwerg B, et al. Management of the neurologically deceased organ donor: a Canadian clinical practice guideline. CMAJ. 2020;192(14):E361–9. https://doi.org/10.1503/cmaj.190631.
65. Kotloff RM, Blosser S, Fulda GJ, et al. Management of the potential organ donor in the ICU: society of critical care medicine/American college of chest physicians/association of organ procurement organizations consensus statement. Crit Care Med. 2015;43(6):1291–325. https://doi.org/10.1097/CCM.0000000000000958.
66. Souter MJ, Blissitt PA, Blosser S, et al. Recommendations for the critical care management of devastating brain injury: prognostication, psychosocial, and ethical management : a position statement for healthcare professionals from the neurocritical care society. Neurocrit Care. 2015;23(1):4–13. https://doi.org/10.1007/s12028-015-0137-6.
67. Patel MS, Abt PL. Current practices in deceased organ donor management. Curr Opin Organ Transplant. 2019;24(3):343–50. https://doi.org/10.1097/MOT.0000000000000638.
68. Becker F, Roberts KJ, Nadal M, et al. Optimizing organ donation: expert opinion from Austria, Germany, Spain and the UK. Ann Transplant. 2020;25:e921727. https://doi.org/10.12659/AOT.921727.
69. Inaba K, Branco BC, Lam L, et al. Organ donation and time to procurement: late is not too late. J Trauma. 2010;68(6):1362–6. https://doi.org/10.1097/TA.0b013e3181db30d3.
70. Christmas AB, Bogart TA, Etson KE, et al. The reward is worth the wait: a prospective analysis of 100 consecutive organ donors. Am Surg. 2012;78(3):296–9. (https://www.ncbi.nlm.nih.gov/pubmed/22524766)
71. Whelchel J, Diethelm A, Phillips M. The effect of high dose dopamine in cadaveric donor management in delayed graft function and graft survival following renal transplant. Transplant Proc. 1986;18:523–7.
72. Venkateswaran RV, Townend JN, Wilson IC, Mascaro JG, Bonser RS, Steeds RP. Echocardiography in the potential heart donor. Transplantation. 2010;89(7):894–901. https://doi.org/10.1097/TP.0b013e3181cfe8e9.
73. Zaroff J. Echocardiographic evaluation of the potential cardiac donor. J Heart Lung Transplant. 2004;23(9 Suppl):S250–2. https://doi.org/10.1016/j.healun.2004.03.015.
74. Zaroff JG, Babcock WD, Shiboski SC. The impact of left ventricular dysfunction on cardiac donor transplant rates. J Heart Lung Transplant. 2003;22(3):334–7. https://doi.org/10.1016/s1053-2498(02)00554-5.
75. Stoddard MF, Longaker RA. The role of transesophageal echocardiography in cardiac donor screening. Am Heart J. 1993;125(6):1676–81. https://doi.org/10.1016/0002-8703(93)90758-2.
76. Lazzeri C, Bonizzoli M, Guetti C, Fulceri GE, Peris A. Hemodynamic management in brain dead donors. World J Transplant. 2021;11(10):410–20. https://doi.org/10.5500/wjt.v11.i10.410.
77. Zaroff JG, Babcock WD, Shiboski SC, Solinger LL, Rosengard BR. Temporal changes in left ventricular systolic function in heart donors: results of serial echocardiography. J Heart Lung Transplant. 2003;22(4):383–8. https://doi.org/10.1016/s1053-2498(02)00561-2.
78. Madan S, Saeed O, Vlismas P, et al. Outcomes after transplantation of donor hearts with improving left ventricular systolic dysfunction. J Am Coll Cardiol. 2017;70(10):1248–58. https://doi.org/10.1016/j.jacc.2017.07.728.
79. Kono T, Nishina T, Morita H, Hirota Y, Kawamura K, Fujiwara A. Usefulness of low-dose dobutamine stress echocardiography for evaluating reversibility of brain death-induced myocardial dysfunction. Am J Cardiol. 1999;84(5):578–82. https://doi.org/10.1016/s0002-9149(99)00382-3.
80. Yoshikawa MH, Rabelo NN, Welling LC, Telles JPM, Figueiredo EG. Brain death and management of the potential donor. Neurol Sci. 2021;42(9):3541–52. https://doi.org/10.1007/s10072-021-05360-6.
81. Al-Khafaji A, Elder M, Lebovitz DJ, et al. Protocolized fluid therapy in brain-dead donors: the multicenter randomized MOnIToR trial. Intensive Care Med. 2015;41(3):418–26. https://doi.org/10.1007/s00134-014-3621-0.
82. Marik PE, Baram M, Vahid B. Does central venous pressure predict fluid responsiveness? A systematic review of the literature and the tale of seven mares. Chest. 2008;134(1):172–8. https://doi.org/10.1378/chest.07-2331.
83. Marik PE, Cavallazzi R, Vasu T, Hirani A. Dynamic changes in arterial waveform derived variables and fluid responsiveness in mechanically ventilated patients: a systematic review of the literature. Crit Care Med. 2009;37(9):2642–7. https://doi.org/10.1097/CCM.0b013e3181a590da.
84. Swanson EA, Patel MS, Groat T, et al. Vasopressor selection during critical care management of brain dead organ donors and the effects on kidney graft function. J Trauma Acute Care Surg. 2020;88(6):783–8. https://doi.org/10.1097/TA.0000000000002688.
85. Chamorro-Jambrina C, Munoz-Ramirez MR, Martinez-Melgar JL, Perez-Cornejo MS. Organ donor management: eight common rec-

ommendations and actions that deserve reflection. Med Intensiva. 2017;41(9):559–68. https://doi.org/10.1016/j.medin.2017.01.012.
86. Schnuelle P, Berger S, de Boer J, Persijn G, van der Woude FJ. Effects of catecholamine application to brain-dead donors on graft survival in solid organ transplantation. Transplantation. 2001;72(3):455–63. https://doi.org/10.1097/00007890-200108150-00017.
87. Schnuelle P, Lorenz D, Mueller A, Trede M, Van Der Woude FJ. Donor catecholamine use reduces acute allograft rejection and improves graft survival after cadaveric renal transplantation. Kidney Int. 1999;56(2):738–46. https://doi.org/10.1046/j.1523-1755.1999.00567.x.
88. Schnuelle P, Gottmann U, Hoeger S, et al. Effects of donor pretreatment with dopamine on graft function after kidney transplantation: a randomized controlled trial. JAMA. 2009;302(10):1067–75. https://doi.org/10.1001/jama.2009.1310.
89. Powner DJ, Hernandez M. A review of thyroid hormone administration during adult donor care. Prog Transplant. 2005;15(3):202–7. https://www.ncbi.nlm.nih.gov/pubmed/16252625
90. Venkateswaran RV, Steeds RP, Quinn DW, et al. The haemodynamic effects of adjunctive hormone therapy in potential heart donors: a prospective randomized double-blind factorially designed controlled trial. Eur Heart J. 2009;30(14):1771–80. https://doi.org/10.1093/eurheartj/ehp086.
91. Rosengard BR, Feng S, Alfrey EJ, et al. Report of the Crystal City meeting to maximize the use of organs recovered from the cadaver donor. Am J Transplant. 2002;2(8):701–11. https://doi.org/10.1034/j.1600-6143.2002.20804.x.
92. Hoste P, Hoste E, Ferdinande P, et al. Development of key interventions and quality indicators for the management of an adult potential donor after brain death: a RAND modified Delphi approach. BMC Health Serv Res. 2018;18(1):580. https://doi.org/10.1186/s12913-018-3386-1.
93. Wood KE, Becker BN, McCartney JG, D'Alessandro AM, Coursin DB. Care of the potential organ donor. N Engl J Med. 2004;351(26):2730–9. https://doi.org/10.1056/NEJMra013103.
94. Smith M. Physiologic changes during brain stem death—lessons for management of the organ donor. J Heart Lung Transplant. 2004;23:S217–22.
95. Copeland H, Hayanga JWA, Neyrinck A, et al. Donor heart and lung procurement: a consensus statement. J Heart Lung Transplant. 2020;39(6):501–17. https://doi.org/10.1016/j.healun.2020.03.020.
96. Sally M, Malinoski D. Current research on organ donor management. Anesthesiol Clin. 2013;31(4):737–48. https://doi.org/10.1016/j.anclin.2013.08.004.
97. Pinsard M, Ragot S, Mertes PM, et al. Interest of low-dose hydrocortisone therapy during brain-dead organ donor resuscitation: the CORTICOME study. Crit Care. 2014;18(4):R158. https://doi.org/10.1186/cc13997.
98. van Erp AC, van Dullemen LFA, Ploeg RJ, Leuvenink HGD. Systematic review on the treatment of deceased organ donors. Transplant Rev (Orlando). 2018;32(4):194–206. https://doi.org/10.1016/j.trre.2018.06.001.
99. Dhar R, Cotton C, Coleman J, et al. Comparison of high- and low-dose corticosteroid regimens for organ donor management. J Crit Care. 2013;28(1):111. e1–7. https://doi.org/10.1016/j.jcrc.2012.04.015.
100. Kopelnik A, Zaroff JG. Neurocardiogenic injury in neurovascular disorders. Crit Care Clin. 2006;22(4):733–52.; abstract ix-x. https://doi.org/10.1016/j.ccc.2006.06.002.
101. Fisher AJ, Donnelly SC, Hirani N, et al. Enhanced pulmonary inflammation in organ donors following fatal non-traumatic brain injury. Lancet. 1999;353(9162):1412–3. https://doi.org/10.1016/S0140-6736(99)00494-8.
102. Fisher AJ, Donnelly SC, Hirani N, et al. Elevated levels of interleukin-8 in donor lungs is associated with early graft failure after lung transplantation. Am J Respir Crit Care Med. 2001;163(1):259–65. https://doi.org/10.1164/ajrccm.163.1.2005093.
103. Mascia L, Pasero D, Slutsky AS, et al. Effect of a lung protective strategy for organ donors on eligibility and availability of lungs for transplantation: a randomized controlled trial. JAMA. 2010;304(23):2620–7. https://doi.org/10.1001/jama.2010.1796.
104. Swanson EA, Patel MS, Hutchens MP, et al. Critical care and ventilatory management of deceased organ donors impact lung use and recipient graft survival. Am J Transplant. 2021;21(12):4003–11. https://doi.org/10.1111/ajt.16719.
105. Gabbay E, Williams TJ, Griffiths AP, et al. Maximizing the utilization of donor organs offered for lung transplantation. Am J Respir Crit Care Med. 1999;160(1):265–71. https://doi.org/10.1164/ajrccm.160.1.9811017.
106. Angel LF, Levine DJ, Restrepo MI, et al. Impact of a lung transplantation donor-management protocol on lung donation and recipient outcomes. Am J Respir Crit Care Med. 2006;174(6):710–6. https://doi.org/10.1164/rccm.200603-432OC.
107. Hanna K, Seder CW, Weinberger JB, Sills PA, Hagan M, Janczyk RJ. Airway pressure release ventilation and successful lung donation. Arch Surg. 2011;146(3):325–8. https://doi.org/10.1001/archsurg.2011.35.
108. Marklin GF, O'Sullivan C, Dhar R. Ventilation in the prone position improves oxygenation and results in more lungs being transplanted from organ donors with hypoxemia and atelectasis. J Heart Lung Transplant. 2021;40(2):120–7. https://doi.org/10.1016/j.healun.2020.11.014.
109. Minambres E, Rodrigo E, Ballesteros MA, et al. Impact of restrictive fluid balance focused to increase lung procurement on renal function after kidney transplantation. Nephrol Dial Transplant. 2010;25(7):2352–6. https://doi.org/10.1093/ndt/gfq054.
110. Ware LB, Landeck M, Koyama T, et al. A randomized trial of the effects of nebulized albuterol on pulmonary edema in brain-dead organ donors. Am J Transplant. 2014;14(3):621–8. https://doi.org/10.1111/ajt.12564.
111. Mazzeffi M, Galvagno S, Rock C. Prevention of healthcare-associated infections in intensive care unit patients. Anesthesiology. 2021;135(6):1122–31. https://doi.org/10.1097/ALN.0000000000004017.
112. Totsuka E, Dodson F, Urakami A, et al. Influence of high donor serum sodium levels on early postoperative graft function in human liver transplantation: effect of correction of donor hypernatremia. Liver Transpl Surg. 1999;5(5):421–8. https://doi.org/10.1002/lt.500050510.
113. Abdelnour T, Rieke S. Relationship of hormonal resuscitation therapy and central venous pressure on increasing organs for transplant. J Heart Lung Transplant. 2009;28(5):480–5. https://doi.org/10.1016/j.healun.2009.01.018.
114. Singer P, Cohen J, Cynober L. Effect of nutritional state of brain-dead organ donor on transplantation. Nutrition. 2001;17(11–12):948–52. https://doi.org/10.1016/s0899-9007(01)00671-2.
115. Hergenroeder GW, Ward NH, Yu X, et al. Randomized trial to evaluate nutritional status and absorption of enteral feeding after brain death. Prog Transplant. 2013;23(4):374–82. https://doi.org/10.7182/pit2013996.
116. Malinoski D, Patel MS, Axelrod DA, et al. Therapeutic hypothermia in organ donors: follow-up and safety analysis. Transplantation. 2019;103(11):e365–8. https://doi.org/10.1097/TP.0000000000002890.
117. Niemann CU, Feiner J, Swain S, et al. Therapeutic hypothermia in deceased organ donors and kidney-graft function. N Engl J Med. 2015;373(5):405–14. https://doi.org/10.1056/NEJMoa1501969.

Index

E. Mahanna Gabrielli et al. (eds.), *Textbook of Neurointensive Care: Volume 1*, https://doi.org/10.1007/978-3-031-62220-5

D

E

MIX
Papier aus verantwortungsvollen Quellen
Paper from responsible sources
FSC® C105338

If you have any concerns about our products,
you can contact us on
ProductSafety@springernature.com

In case Publisher is established outside the EU,
the EU authorized representative is:
Springer Nature Customer Service Center GmbH
Europaplatz 3, 69115 Heidelberg, Germany

Printed by Libri Plureos GmbH
in Hamburg, Germany